# HYPERBARIC MEDICINE PRACTICE

## 3RD EDITION

# HYPERBARIC MEDICINE PRACTICE

## 3RD EDITION

*ERIC P. KINDWALL, M.D.*

*HARRY T. WHELAN, M.D.*

*EDITORS*

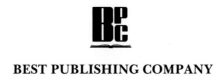

**BEST PUBLISHING COMPANY**

Cover Design: William Owen
Text Layout and Design: William Owen, Travis Moore
Editorial: Jim Joiner

First Edition 1994
Second Edition 1999
Second Edition-Revised 2002
Second Edition-Revised 2004
Third Edition 2008

Copyright © 2008 by Best Publishing Company

International Standard Book Number: 9781930536494
Library of Congress catalog card number: 2008923157

For more information contact:
Best Publishing Company
2355 North Steves Blvd.
Post Office Box 30100
Flagstaff, AZ 86003-0100, USA
Telephone: 928.527.1055
Fax: 928.526.0370
E-mail: divebooks@bestpub.com
Website: www.bestpub.com

# CONTENTS

## *SECTION II*
## DISORDERS APPROVED FOR HYPERBARIC TREATMENT

## SECTION III
## HYPERBARIC OXYGEN USED IN OFF-LABEL DISORDERS AND INVESTIGATIONAL AREAS

# PREFACE

## 3ᴿᴰ EDITION

It has been nine years since the Second Edition of this text was published in 1999. Many changes and advancements have been made in the interim. The number of active hyperbaric facilities has increased immensely. Whereas in 1999 there were about 300 hyperbaric units, at this writing there are now over 800. Continuing the previous trend, almost all of the new chambers are situated in wound care centers.

The management of compromised wounds now can be considered a *de facto* new subspecialty. As the obesity rates rise and the average age of the population increases, with a surge from the baby boomers, diabetic ulcers, radionecrosis, and other manifestations of age attendant to unhealthy diets and smoking will vastly increase the number of compromised wounds, some of which may benefit from HBO.

The treatment of carbon monoxide with HBO has become the standard of care with the publication in 2002 of "Hyperbaric Oxygen for the Treatment of Acute Carbon Monoxide Poisoning" in the New England Journal. This was a double blind controlled study by Lin Weaver showing that neurologic function and cognitive functioning at 6 months and one year post treatment were significantly better for patients treated with HBO. No hyperbaric patients had sequelae.

The American College of Hyperbaric Medicine was a new society, started some years ago by a group of physicians who felt the Undersea and Hyperbaric Medical Society (UHMS) guidelines were too restrictive. They created a fairly long list of conditions they felt were treatable with HBO. A majority of physicians in the hyperbaric community felt that hyperbaric treatment of a number of the diseases on their list was unproven. Some flew in the face of research that proved HBO didn't work and today would be considered quackery. As a result, the American College gained a tainted reputation. Gradually, however, many UHMS members infiltrated the College and their "approved" list was drastically reduced to comply with the UHMS guidelines. As time went on, incorporation of the College lapsed and further activity was scant.

The American College of Hyperbaric Medicine was reincorporated in Wisconsin in 2005 by Robert Bartlett and Jeffrey Niezgoda. I serve as Executive Director. Only physicians are eligible for membership and the College is designed specifically to serve their needs. The College conducts seminars on the intricacies of producing documents to enable reimbursement by Medicare and other insurers as well as approved courses in clinical hyperbaric medicine. It also sponsors clinical research. A registry of radionecrosis patients looking at outcomes following HBO treatment is ongoing. To date we have amassed data on over 1,000 patients. The trends are highly encouraging.

A critical factor impeding the establishment of more hyperbaric units has been the lack of trained hyperbaric physicians. There are several centers that offer courses in clinical hyperbaric medicine but there is a definite need for more. Before I "retired" in 2008 and stopped seeing patients, I could almost define myself as an itinerant teacher. I conducted 5-day courses in clinical HBO in nearly 70 hospitals in the United States as well as several in Europe. Unfortunately no one is offering such "portable" courses at present. There are distinct advantages in having the teacher go to the students instead of visa-versa. Only one airfare is required instead of one for each student. The doctors don't leave town so they remain close to their practices and are available for emergencies. Generally I scheduled classes over the weekends so the doctors were away from their offices or O.R.s for only three days instead of five. The only requirement was that the hospital have a functioning hyperbaric chamber for the "hands-on" part of the course.

The book retains its original three-part format; Part one: General Considerations, Part two: Disorders Approved for Hyperbaric Treatment and Part three: Investigational Areas. There is a brand new chapter on wound healing by Jeffrey Niezgoda. There have been major advances in that field in the last nine years.

This Third Edition has been three years of hard work. For health reasons I did not have time to actively work on editing for a large part of 2007. Harry Whelan, my co-editor and his hard working secretary, Debbie Dye, stepped up to the plate and kept the editing process on the rails. Fortunately the health problems are now in the past, and I am back to full-time functioning. Additionally, our thanks to Mary Verhage for her support in the editing.

Hyperbaric quackery continues to be a problem, as desperate parents seek cures for cerebral palsy and autism. Stroke victims also turn to the hyperbaric chamber weeks or months after the event when treatment will be of no avail. Unfortunately there are a number of practitioners who will treat anything that walks in the door and have no qualms about relieving the victim of his or her money.

The only way we have of minimizing quackery is to train more physicians in approved courses. As always more controlled studies need to be published to educate doctors as well as to protect the public.

Our hope is that this book will remain an up-to-date reference text in this and in future editions and that clinicians as well as researchers may find it useful.

Eric P. Kindwall M.D.
Milwaukee, Wisconsin
February, 2008

# Eric P. Kindwall, M.D.

Dr. Kindwall began diving in 1950 and later developed an interest in diving physiology while majoring in zoology at the University of Wisconsin. He is a 1960 graduate of Yale University School of Medicine, where his M.D. thesis was entitled "Some Observations on Decompression Sickness". After leaving Yale, he did postgraduate research at the Laboratory of Aviation and Naval Medicine, Department of Physiology, Karolinska Institute in Stockholm. On returning to the United States, he entered a rotating internship at the University of Virginia and completed a residency at Harvard.

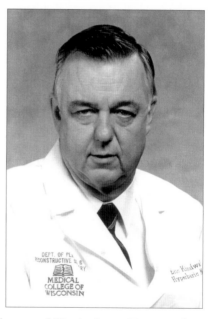

During the Vietnam War, Dr. Kindwall served in nuclear submarines and became Assistant Director of the U.S. Navy School of Submarine Medicine, where he was Senior Officer in Charge of the Diving Medicine Program. After leaving the Navy in 1969, Dr. Kindwall was chief of the Department of Hyperbaric Medicine at St. Luke's Medical Center in Milwaukee for twenty years. In 1989 he accepted a full-time combined appointment on the faculty of the Medical College of Wisconsin in the Department of Plastic and Reconstructive Surgery and the Department of Pharmacology and Toxicology. He served as Director of Hyperbaric Medicine for the medical school until being granted Emeritus status in 1998, to devote his time to teaching and consulting.

Currently, Dr. Kindwall is the Medical Director of Hyperbaric Wound Care Associates and the Executive Director of The American College of Hyperbaric Medicine.

A past president of the Undersea and Hyperbaric Medical Society (UHMS), Dr. Kindwall founded *Pressure*, the UHMS newsletter, and was founding chairman of the UHMS Committee on Hyperbaric Oxygen Therapy. He is former chairman of the Commission on Underwater Physiology and Medicine for the International Union of Physiological Sciences. He retired as a commander from the U.S. Navy Reserve in 1995. Over 90 publications and book chapters in the fields of diving, clinical hyperbaric medicine, and compressed air construction work are attributed to him. In addition, he has consulted internationally for commercial diving companies, tunnel construction companies, foreign navies, and hospitals acquiring clinical hyperbaric facilities.

# Harry T. Whelan, M.D.

Dr. Whelan, a Milwaukee native, is Professor of Neurology, Pediatrics, and Hyperbaric Medicine at the Medical College of Wisconsin, is a Captain and a Diving Medical Officer (DMO) in the U.S. Navy, and a consultant to the Navy Experimental Diving Unit (NEDU). and currently serves as Undersea Medical Officer for "Deep Submarine Unit," which is the navy's submarine rescue team and it's deep sea research component.

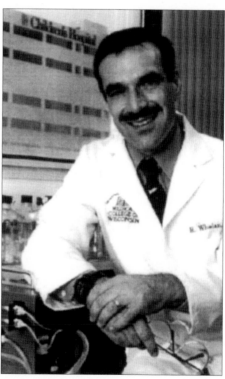

He began diving in 1968, and developed his interest in cellular metabolism during a National Science Foundation Summer Research Program in biochemistry at Wesleyan University in Connecticut. Later, after graduating cum laude in chemistry (biochemistry option) from the University of Wisconsin – Milwaukee, he attended the University of Wisconsin Medical School in Madison, where he received his M.D. degree. He completed pediatrics internship and residency training at the University of Florida in Gainesville, and a neurology fellowship at the University of Minnesota in Minneapolis.

Dr. Whelan then joined the faculty of Vanderbilt University in Nashville, TN. While there he developed a laboratory research project involving new types of treatment for brain tumors. For this he received the American Cancer Society's Clinical Oncology Career Development Award.

Moving back to Milwaukee, he became Professor of Neurology and Pediatrics at the Medical College of Wisconsin. There he joined the U.S. Naval Reserve. He formed research ties with the Hyperbaric Medicine Unit at the Medical College of Wisconsin, and the U.S. Navy Experimental Diving Unit in Panama City, FL. There the navy trained him at its dive school to become a Diving Medical Officer. When he was promoted to full Commander, his fellow officer pinned his new rank onto his uniform in an underwater ceremony, 190 feet below sea level. He has since been promoted to Captain in the U.S. Navy.

Dr. Whelan continued his research with funding and collaboration from NASA Marshall Space Flight Center. Using space based light-emitting diode (LED) technologies developed for growing plants on the Space Shuttle, he now has over fifteen years experience conducting studies on the use of near-infrared light for photodynamic therapy of cancer, and in combination with hyperbaric oxygen, for stimulation of human tissue growth and wound healing, during space flight and for patients here on earth. In the year 2000, Dr Whelan was inducted into the NASA space technology Hall of Fame. More recently, he has done extensive research on Combat Casualty Care for DARPA as a principle investigator and is currently conducting research on the use of hyperbaric medicine for stroke patients.

Dr. Whelan assumed Directorship of the Medical College of Wisconsin's Hyperbaric Unit in 1998. He has over 80 publications including cancer, laser, LED and diving/hyperbaric studies.

# CONTRIBUTORS

**Dirk Jan Bakker, MD, PhD**
Academic Medical Center
University of Amsterdam
Meibergdreef 9
1105 AZ Amsterdam-Zuidoost, The Netherlands
Phone: +31 294 291429
       +31 20 5663468
Fax:   +31 294 291199
Email: *D.J.Bakker01@amc.uva.nl*
       *D.JBakker01@freeler.nl*

**Ronald P. Bangasser, MD (Deceased)**

**Diane M. Barratt, MD, MPH**
Staff Neurologist
Neuroscience Division
Baptist Hospital
Miami, FL  33176

**Bob Bartlett, MD, FACEP, FAPWCA, FACHM**
Associate Professor of Surgery
Ohio State University
President, American College of Hyperbaric Medicine
Senior Clinical Advisor, National Healing
149 Rudder Court
Lexington, SC 29072
Phone: 866.280.9718
Email: *bobbartlettmd@msn.com*

**Richard C. Baynosa, MD**
Division of Plastic Surgery
Microsurgery & Hyperbaric Laboratory
University of Nevada School of Medicine
2040 West Charleston Blvd STE 302
Las Vegas, NV 89102
Phone: 702.671.2273
Fax:   702.671.2245
Email: *rbaynosa@medicine.nevada.edu*

**Valerie J. Bonne, MD**
> Assistant Professor of Medicine
> Medical College of Wisconsin
> 9200 W. Wisconsin Ave., Suite 5200
> Milwaukee, WI 53226
> Phone: 262.928.2391
> Fax: 262.928.2718
> Email: *vbonne@mcw.edu*

**Robert C. Borer, Jr., MD**

**Paul E. Cianci, MD, FACP**
> Emeritus Professor of Medicine
> University of California, Davis
> Medical Director/Hyperbaric Medicine
> Doctors Medical Center
> 2000 Vale Road
> San Pablo, CA 94806
> Phone: 510.235.3483
> Fax: 510.970.5770
> Email: *pcianci@aol.com*

**James M. Clark, MD, PhD**
> 943 West Woodlawn Avenue
> San Antonio, TX 78201-5726

**Richard 'Dick' Clarke, CHT**
> National Baromedical Services
> 5 Richland Medical Park
> Columbia, SC 29203-8002
> Phone: 803.434.7101
> Fax: 803.434.4354
> Email: *dick.clarke@palmettohealth.org*

**Tomas Dvorak, MD**

**Myrvin H. Ellestad, MD, FACC**
> Heart Institute
> Long Beach Memorial Medical Center
> 2801 Atlantic Ave., P.O. Box 1428
> Long Beach, CA 90801-1428
> Phone: 213.426.3333
> Fax: 213.595.2110
> Email: *mellestad@memorialcare.org*

## David H. Elliot, OBE, DPhil, FRCP, FFOM

The Civilian Consultant in Diving Medicine to the Royal Navy
Retired Shell Professor Research Fellow
University of Surrey
United Kingdom
Rockdale, 40 Petworth Road
Haslemere, Surrey, GU27 2HX, United Kingdom
Fax:     011.44.1428.658678
Email:  *Davidelliot001@aol.com*

## LT Charles C. Falzon, MC, USN

Undersea Medical Officer
USS Tranquility Medical Clinic 1007
3420 Illinois Street
Great Lakes, IL  60088
Phone: 847.688.6755 x 6235
Fax:     847.688.2721
Email:  *Charles.Falzon@med.navy.mil*

## Joseph C. Farmer, MD

P.O. Box 3805
Duke University Medical Center
Durham, NC  27710

## Guenter Frey, MD

Federal Armed Forces Hospital
Oberer Eselberg 40
D-89081 Ulm, Germany
Phone: +49.731.1710.2040
Fax:     +49.731.1710.2028
Email:  *GuenterFrey@bundeswehr.org*

## Lisardo García-Covarrubias, MD

Cardiothoracic Surgery Fellow
Division of Cardiothoracic Surgery
University of Miami Miller School of Medicine
Jackson Memorial Hospital
Miami, FL 33136-1096

## Michael L. Gimbel, MD

Assistant Professor of Surgery
Division of Plastic Surgery & Reconstructive Surgery
University of Pittsburgh Medical Center
5750 Centre Avenue No 180
Pittsburgh, PA 15206
Phone: 412.661.5380
Fax:     412.661.5381
Email:  *gimbelml@upmc.edu*

**Christer E. Hammarlund, MD**

Helsingborg Hospital
Department of Anesthesia & Intensive Care
S-251 87 Helsingborg, Sweden
Phone: +011.46.42.102140
Fax:    +011.46.42.260454

**George B. Hart, MD**

Thoracic Surgeon
Long Beach Memorial Medical Center
University of California, Irvine
4162 Pierson Drive
Huntington Beach, CA  92649-3000
Phone: 714.840.4911
Cell:   714.745.4911
Fax:    562.533.6060
Email: *gbabehart@hotmail.com*

**Richard D. Heimbach, MD**

San Antonio Wound Care & Hyperbaric Medicine Center
4499 Medical Dr., SLZ
San Antonio, TX  78229

**Ann K. Helms, MD, MS**

Assistant Professor
Department of Neurology
Medical College of Wisconsin
9200 W. Wisconsin Avenue
Milwaukee, WI  53226
Phone: 414.805.5223
Fax:    414.805.5252
Email: *ahelms@mcw.edu*

**Thomas K. Hunt, MD, FACS, FRCS, DMMC**

Professor Emeritus
Department of Surgery
University of California, San Francisco,
513 Parnassus Avenue, Room S-320
San Francisco, CA  94143-0104
Phone: 415.476.3049
       415.476.1236 (Kate Hanlin)
Email: *huntt@surgery.ucsf.edu*
       *hanlink@surgery.ucsf.edu* (secretary)

**Thomas M. Kidder, MD**

Professor, Department of Otolaryngology & Communications Sciences
Medical College of Wisconsin
9200 W. Wisconsin Avenue
Milwaukee, WI  53226
Phone: 414.805.5584
       414.805.7890
Email: *tkidder@mcw.edu*

## Eric P. Kindwall, MD

Associate Professor Emeritus
Medical College of Wisconsin
Executive Director
American College of Hyperbaric Medicine
260 Bunker Hill Drive
Brookfield, WI 53005
Phone: 262.751.4520
       262.641.0393
Fax:    262.641.0394
Email: *EricK@aya.yale.edu*
      *Ekindwall@sbcglobal.net*

## Diane L. Krasner, PhD, RN, CWCN, CWS, BCLNC, FAAN

## Lorenz A. Lampl, MD

Professor of Anesthesiology
Federal Armed Forces Hospital
Oberer Eselsberg 40
D-89081 Ulm, Germany
Phone: +49.731.1710.2000
Fax:    +49.731.1710.2028
Email: *LorenzLampl@bundeswehr.org*

## Frank J. Martorano, MD

## Robert E. Marx, DDS

6000 Chapman Field Drive
Miami, FL 33156
Phone: 305.256.5270
Fax:    305.661.1808
Email: *rmarx@med.miami.edu*

## Luis A. Matos, MD

## Yehuda Melamed, MD

Director, Hyperbaric Medical Center
Rambam & Elisha Hospitals
Haifa, Israel
Email: *hbomed@netvision.net.il*

## Valerie J. Messina, RN, BSN

Long Beach Memorial Medical Center
2801 Atlantic Avenue
Long Beach, CA 90806
18321 Oxboro Lane
Huntington Beach, CA 92648
Phone: 562.933.6960
Fax:    562.933.8964
Email: vmessina@memorialcare.org

**Stuart S. Miller, MD, FAAEM**

Education Director, Department of Hyperbaric Medicine
Attending, Department of Emergency Medicine
Long Beach Memorial Medical Center
2801 Atlantic Avenue
Long Beach, CA 90806
Phone: 562.933.6950
Fax:    562.933.6060
Email: *smiller1@memorialcare.org*

**Roy A. M. Myers, MD**

M.I.E.M.S.S
20 South Greene Street
Baltimore, MD 21201-1595

**Joseph Myslinski, MD**

**Paul M. Nemiroff, MS, PhD, MD, FACS ICA**

Vanderbilt University
420 Lowell Drive SE-STE 300
Huntsville, AL 35801-3762

**Jeffrey A. Niezgoda, MD**

Center for Comprehensive Wound Care &
        Hyperbaric Oxygen Therapy
Aurora Health Care
2901 W KK Pkwy, Suite 311
Milwaukee, WI 53215
Phone: 414.649.6577
Pager: 414.222.1235
Email: *niezgoda@execpc.com*

**Diane M. Norkool, RN, MN (Deceased)**

**Matthew K. Park, MD**

10 Center Drive
Niaid Blvd, 10, RM11N228
Bethesda, MD 20892-1888

**Max F. Riddick, MD (Retired)**

1553 Winter Springs Blvd.
Winter Springs, FL 32708
Phone: 407.359.4999
Fax:    321.238.2006
Email: *mfriddick@cfl.rr.com*

### Daniel N. Reis, Professor, F.R.C.S.E.

Horev Medical Centre,
15 Horev St. Haifa, Israel
Phone: 04 8349011; mobile 0525407218
Fax:      04 8349022
Email:  daniel30@012.net.il

### Gaylan L. Rockswold, MD, PhD

Hennepin County Medical Center
701 Park Avenue
Minneapolis, MN  55415
Phone: 612.873.2810
Fax:      612.904.4297
Email:  *gaylan.rockswold@hcmed.org*

### Sarah B. Rockswold, MD

Hennepin County Medical Center
701 Park Avenue #P5
Minneapolis, MN  55415
Phone: 612.873.8700
Fax:      612.904.4297
Email:  *sarah.rockswold@hcmed.org*

### R. Gary Sibbald, BSc, MD, FACS, AAOS, ABPM/UHM, FRCPC (Med)(Derm), ABIM, DABD, MEd

### Michael B. Strauss, MD, FACS, AAOS, ABPM/UHM

Medical Director, Hyperbaric Medicine
Long Beach Memorial Hospital
Clinical Professor, Orthopedic Surgery
University of Irvine School of Medicine
Attending Physician PACT (Prevention-Amputation, Care Treatment)
2801 Atlantic Avenue
Long Beach, CA 90806
Phone: 562.933.6950
Fax:      562.933.6060
Email:  *MStrauss@memorialcare.org*

### Hideyo Takahashi, MD, PhD

Clinical Associate Professor
Medical Director
University of Nagoya School of Medicine
Showa-ku, Nagoya 466, Japan

### Stephen R. Thom, MD, PhD

## Paul A. Thombs, MD

Presbyterian/ St. Luke's Medical Center
1719 E. 19th Avenue
Denver, CO 80218
Phone: 303.839.6900
Fax:    303.839.6157
Email: *pthombs@msn.com*

## Lindell K. Weaver, MD

804 Terrace Hills Drive
Salt Lake City, UT 84103-4021
Phone: 801.408.3623
Fax:    801.321.1668
Email: *Lindell.Weaver@intermountainmail.org*

## Harry T. Whelan, MD

Bleser Professor of Neurology & Hyperbarics
Medical College of Wisconsin
8701 W. Watertown Plank Rd.
Milwaukee, WI 53226

## James A. Williams, Jr., MD

University of South Carolina
School of Medicine
6311 Garners Ferry Rd.
Columbia, SC 29208

## David A. Youngblood, MD, MPH, TM

P.O. Box 699
Haleiwa, HI 96712-0699
Phone: 808.216.0166
Fax:    808.638.0834
Email: *nradoc@yahoo.com*

## William A. Zamboni, MD, FACS

Professor & Chairman, Department of Surgery Chief
Division of Plastic Surgery
University of Nevada School of Medicine
2040 West Charleston Boulevard, Suite 301
Las Vegas, NV 89102
Phone: 702.671.2278
Fax:    702.671.2245
Email: *wzamboni@medicine.nevada.edu*

# SECTION I
# HYPERBARIC OXYGENATION-
# GENERAL CONSIDERATIONS

CHAPTER 1

# A HISTORY OF HYPERBARIC MEDICINE

## CHAPTER ONE OVERVIEW

# A History of Hyperbaric Medicine

*Eric P. Kindwall*

## COMPRESSED AIR THERAPY

The concept of putting patients in a recompression chamber and raising the ambient pressure around them for therapeutic purposes was, at first, without scientific basis. Perhaps intuitively, it "seemed like a good idea" to a British clergyman, Henshaw. In 1662, he built a sealed chamber he called a "Domicilium" (15). Chamber pressure was controlled by valved organ bellows which could either raise or lower pressure depending on adjustment of the valves. Henshaw felt that acute disease of all kinds would respond to increased ambient pressure, whereas chronic diseases were better treated with more rarefied air. Therefore if the disease became chronic, he reversed the valving on the bellows to produce a slight vacuum. Considering the apparatus and the pressure changes possible, any effect on the patients he treated had to be purely psychological.

In the 19th century, others followed his early example by creating pneumatic institutes on the European continent. These large chambers able to sustain pressures of two or more atmospheres, could often accommodate up to 10 people, and rivaled the popularity of the mineral water spas of the era (2). They produced no scientifically valid results. See Figure 1.

In 1879, a French surgeon named J. A. Fontaine built a mobile operating room on wheels that could be pressurized (12). See Figure 2. Over 20 surgical procedures were performed in this unit using nitrous oxide as the anesthetic. Deep surgical anesthesia was possible because its increased effective percentage, accompanied by a higher oxygen partial pressure, rendered it safer. Compressed air at two atmospheres gives an effective level of 42% inhaled oxygen. Hernias were seen to reduce more easily and the patients were not their normal cyanotic color when coming out of anesthesia. Fontaine's experiments with hyperbaric surgery were the only semi-scientific efforts made during the entire compressed-air era, which ended in 1930.

In 1891, J. L. Corning, the first physician to administer a spinal anesthetic, introduced compressed air therapy to the United States and was the first to operate his compressor with electric power (7).

Orville J. Cunningham, a professor of anesthesia at the University of Kansas in Kansas City, was the last of the great compressed-air enthusiasts (8). He started out legitimately enough, noting that people with heart disease and

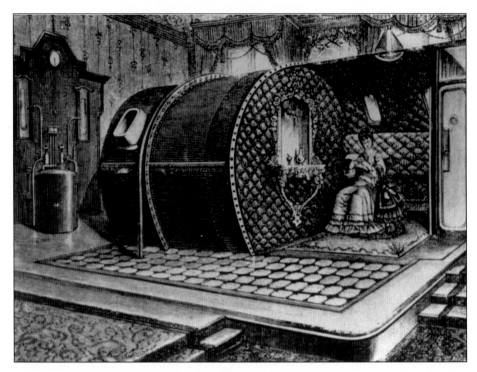

*Figure 1. This chamber, built for Forlanini (1875), the pioneer of artificial pneumothorax therapy, shows the luxurious appointments which were often found in pneumatic institutes or "spas." (Reprinted with permission of the New York Academy of Sciences).*

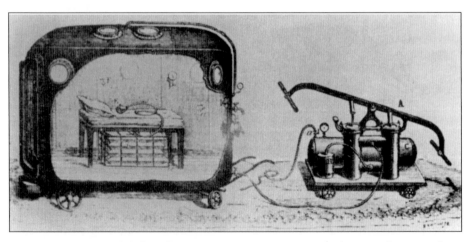

*Figure 2. Fontaine's mobile hyperbaric operating room (1879). Note the manually operated two cylinder compressor, the anesthesia gas container under the operating table and the mask. (Reprinted with permission of the New York Academy of Sciences).*

certain other circulatory disorders did poorly when living at altitude, but improved on return to sea level. Taking this concept one step further, he felt that increased atmospheric pressure would be still more beneficial. During the flu epidemic of 1918, he placed a moribund young resident physician in a chamber which had been used for animal studies and, by compressing him to two atmospheres, was able to successfully oxygenate him during his hypoxic crisis. Having thus proved to himself that his concept was sound, he constructed an 88-foot long chamber, (Figure 3) 10 feet in diameter, in Kansas City, and began to treat a multitude of diseases, most of them without scientific rationale (16).

A Mr. Timkin of the Timkin Roller Bearing Company apparently had a spontaneous recovery from a uremia while in Dr. Cunningham's chamber. In gratitude, Timkin built Dr. Cunningham the largest hyperbaric chamber ever constructed. See Figure 4. It was a steel sphere, six stories high, and 64 feet in diameter. This "steel ball hospital," located in Cleveland, Ohio, accommodated a smoking room on the top floor, plush carpeting, dining rooms with white tablecloths, and individual rooms. It could reach three atmospheres pressure (14).

Cunningham believed that some anaerobic organism, "which could not be cultured," was responsible for a host of diseases, including hypertension, uremia, diabetes, and cancer, and that compressed air therapy helped inhibit this organism. The AMA and the Cleveland Medical Society, failing to receive any scientific evidence for his rationale, finally forced him to close in 1930 (1). Unfortunately, the steel ball hospital was broken up for scrap during World War II. It would have made a magnificent museum.

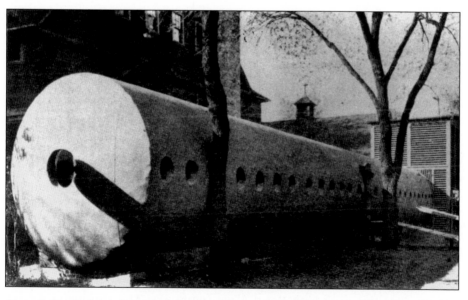

Figure 3. Cunningham's first clinical chamber in Kansas City (1921). It measured 10 feet in diameter by 88 feet in length. (Reprinted with permission of the New York Academy of Sciences).

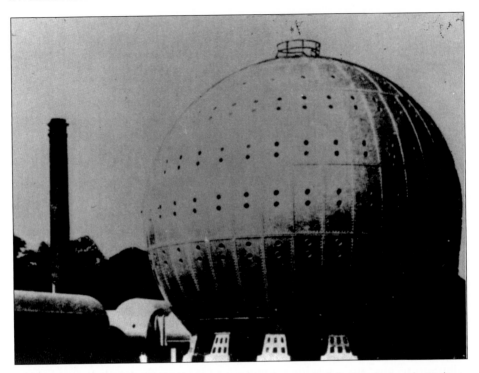

*Figure 4. The "Steel Ball Hospital." This hyperbaric chamber was built for Cunningham by Timkin in 1928. It is six stories high, has 72 rooms with 12 bedrooms per floor, a grand piano and other amenities. (Reprinted with permission of the New York Academy of Sciences.)*

## MILITARY CONTRIBUTIONS

As early as 1878, Paul Bert demonstrated the toxic properties of oxygen, showing that it produced grand mal seizures when breathed at elevated pressure for only moderate periods of time (3). In 1899, J. Lorrain-Smith showed that oxygen produced pulmonary damage when breathed at lesser pressures for longer exposures (18).

These findings became clinically important during WW II when underwater demolition teams, combat swimmers, and two-man torpedo operators, known as "charioteers," had to breathe pure oxygen from closed-circuit diving gear. Closed, pure oxygen apparatus left no tell tale bubbles rising to the surface. The open circuit Aqualung using air as the breathing gas was not invented until 1943 when Gagnon and Cousteau built the first one in occupied France. The critical time depth envelope for oxygen breathing with which clandestine operations could be safely carried out needed to be defined (10).

K. W. Donald of Edinburgh University, Edinburgh, Scotland, carried out much of this work with Royal Navy volunteers. They formed a special unit in which men swam at various depths under different levels of exercise and cold, until convulsions occurred (11). The U.S. Navy sponsored similar studies. Were it not for these hard-won data, safe exposure times for civilian hyperbaric oxygen (HBO) treated patients could not be quantified.

It has frequently been said that the history of "hyperbaric oxygenation" goes back "over 300 years," probably referring to the work of Henshaw. This is incorrect, as oxygen was not even discovered until 1775 by Priestley. All the early chambers were pressurized with compressed air, and oxygen was not a consideration. Clinical hyperbaric oxygenation goes back only about 45 years, beginning with the work of Churchill-Davidson and Boerema.

## THE ADVENT OF HYPERBARIC OXYGEN

Modern scientific use of the hyperbaric chamber in clinical medicine began in 1955 with the work of I. Churchill-Davidson (6). He was the first to attempt using high oxygen environments to potentiate the effects of radiation therapy in cancer patients. That same year, Ite Boerema, Professor of Surgery of the University of Amsterdam in Holland, proposed using hyperbaric oxygen in cardiac surgery to prolong a patient's tolerance to circulatory arrest.

## HBO AND SURGERY

Boerema had conceived the idea of "drenching" the tissues with oxygen, but realized that this would require increasing the ambient pressure surrounding the patient. He contacted the Royal Dutch Navy at Den Helder, Netherlands, and secured its cooperation in letting him use one of its chambers. The ensuing animal experiments, done with the cooperation of Dr. N.G. Meijne, were so promising that he had a large operating-room chamber built at the Wilhelmina Gasthuis, the academic hospital of the University of Amsterdam. There he conducted surgical operations under pressure for a variety of conditions, including surgical correction of transposition of the great vessels, tetralogy of Fallot, and pulmonic stenosis. His first publication appeared in 1956 (4).

Meanwhile, W.H. Brummelkamp of the University of Amsterdam found that hyperbaric oxygen could also inhibit anaerobic infections. This was particularly useful in Clostridial gas gangrene, and his group published their first paper in 1961 (5). The following year, George Smith and G.R. Sharp were the first to report treatment of carbon monoxide poisoning in humans at the Western Infirmary in Glasgow, Scotland (19). Because of early favorable studies regarding hyperbaric oxygenation, a clinical chamber was built at Duke University in 1960, although it was too small to support surgical operations. That same year in New York, Mt. Sinai Hospital acquired a large, 12-feet in diameter, surgical hyperbaric chamber that was operated under the aegis of Julius Jacobson, a cardiovascular surgeon.

Similar surgical chambers were built at Presbyterian Hospital in Chicago, Illinois, Hennepin County Hospital in Minnesota, Lutheran General Hospital in Park Ridge, Illinois, Good Samaritan Hospital in Los Angeles, California, St. Barnabus Hospital in New Jersey, and Harvard University installed a chamber at Children's Hospital in Boston, Massachusetts. Large, non-surgical chambers were also installed at Edgewater Hospital in Chicago, Illinois, and St. Luke's Hospital in Milwaukee, Wisconsin.

## INTERNATIONAL MEETINGS

Because of the striking results produced in cardiovascular surgery, gas gangrene and carbon monoxide poisoning, it seemed only fitting that there should be an International Congress on Hyperbaric Oxygenation, where information could be freely exchanged among those doing research in the area. The first such congress took place in 1963, under the auspices of the Department of Surgery at the University of Amsterdam. Its president was Dr. Boerema. In quick succession, international meetings were held in Glasgow in 1964, and at Duke University in 1965. At that point, because progress in research seemed to be flagging (perhaps because many researchers were leaving the field), the next international meeting was deferred until 1969, when it was held in Sapporo, Japan. Subsequently, these congresses were held every four years in Vancouver, Canada; Aberdeen, Scotland; Moscow, U.S.S.R.; and then on a tri-annual basis in Long Beach, California; Sydney, Australia; and, in 1990, once again in Amsterdam, Holland. Meetings continued in 1993 in Fuzhow, the People's Republic of China and in Milan, Italy, in 1996. Subsequent meetings were in Kobe, Japan in 1999, San Francisco in 2002 and Barcelona in 2005.

These hyperbaric congresses were initially organized informally and there was no international organization to schedule them. The leaders in the field simply met at the conclusion of each congress and voted among themselves where the next congress would convene. The lack of an organized body to oversee the regulation of hyperbaric therapy eventually would prove to be a major drawback.

In 1990, largely through the efforts of Dirk Bakker and Fred Cramer, a permanent office was established in Amsterdam to oversee these congresses.

## INVOLVEMENT OF THE NATIONAL ACADEMY OF SCIENCES

In 1966, the whole field of hyperbaric oxygenation was drawn to the attention of the U.S. National Academy of Sciences/National Research Council by Christian J. Lambertsen, and a committee on hyperbaric oxygenation was formed in the Division of Medical Sciences. This committee was chaired by Captain George Bond of the U.S. Navy Submarine Service and included representatives from Duke University (Ivan Brown), the University of Maryland (R. Adams Cowley), the U.S. Navy Medical Research Institute (Leon J. Greenbaum, Jr.), the State University of New York at Buffalo (Edward Lanphier), the University of California (John Severinghaus), the U.S. Navy Experimental Diving Unit (R. D. Workman), and the University of Pennsylvania (Dr. Christian Lambertsen). They produced an extremely useful basic text, Fundamentals of Hyperbaric Medicine, which described in detail the physical and physiological effects of oxygen under pressure, anesthesia and related drug effects, and the engineering requirements for hyperbaric chambers with their ancillary equipment (13). This volume, however, did not discuss any of the clinical conditions being treated currently with hyperbaric oxygen.

## DECLINE OF THE FIELD

With hyperbaric oxygen producing seemingly dramatic results in cardiac surgery, carbon monoxide poisoning and gas gangrene, researchers were eagerly seeking other uses for the chamber. Patients with a variety of other chronic conditions were treated in chambers, often without much scientific rationale. Patients suffering from emphysema, stroke, senility, arthritis, and other debilitating conditions which had not responded to conventional therapy, were treated in the hope that some change might be noted. Unfortunately, many of these experiments were poorly controlled, and "good results" were usually reported anecdotally.

Meanwhile, the development of improved cardiopulmonary bypass equipment had progressed and, with the advent of better heart-lung machines and deep hypothermia, the need for doing surgery under hyperbaric conditions decreased dramatically. By the early 1970s, many large chambers were closing or gathering dust. Most of the surgeons whose primary interest had been in cardiovascular work left the field, and the early enthusiasm and good quality research precipitously declined. About the only headlines made in the hyperbaric field during this period were made by HBO zealots or dedicated fanatics who were treating a multitude of disorders with little concern for science. By 1977, there were only 37 hyperbaric chambers operating in hospitals in the United States.

Just as important as the lack of scientific progress in the research fields, were problems in the regulatory area. Furthermore, insurance companies had few guidelines to follow with regard to reimbursement for hyperbaric treatment.

By 1975, it was clear that the field had to be more formalized. Except for a treatment manual, **Hyperbaric Medicine Procedures**, written by the author at St. Luke's Hospital in Milwaukee, there was no general textbook available. This manual, which has been in print since 1970 with periodic revisions, simply listed disorders that had been treated in the hyperbaric chamber, along with the protocols that had been used. The references were few and no distinction was made between those conditions for which good evidence of the efficacy of hyperbaric oxygen existed, and those for which such evidence was sparse. The most recent edition, published in 2006 is a practical chamber-side guide to carrying out treatment, and only clinically established disorders are covered. Experimental indications and diseases that have been treated with no apparent scientific basis are listed in separate chapters at the end. To help establish such guidelines, in 1972, Medicare convened a panel of Undersea Medical Society members in the clinical hyperbaric field, chaired by Capt. George B. Hart of the U.S. Navy. However, that panel met informally only once, for a few hours, and issued some broad recommendations which were only slowly implemented over the ensuing years. The Medicare list was still sadly out of date.

## A TEXT BOOK AND NEW BEGINNINGS

The late Jefferson C. Davis of the United States Air Force was particularly active in the clinical hyperbaric field and established a vigorous clinical program at the School of Aerospace Medicine at Brooks Air Force Base in Texas. Davis felt that a general textbook was needed in the field and convinced the Undersea Medical Society (UMS) to convene a workshop that met in San Francisco, in the summer of 1975. At that workshop, experts from the international hyperbaric community assembled to outline what the contents of such a textbook should be. From that outline ensued an excellent text, **Hyperbaric Oxygen Therapy**, edited by Davis and Thomas K. Hunt, Professor of Surgery at the University of California-San Francisco (9). Funds for the publication of the book were provided in part by the National Library of Medicine and the United States Air Force. This multi-authored volume first appeared in 1977 and represented a real milestone.

By 1976, a number of hyperbaric clinicians in the Undersea Medical Society had become appalled by the indiscriminate use of hyperbaric oxygen. No organization had yet taken responsibility for the field, and insurers were still working largely without guidelines that identified when the use of hyperbaric oxygenation was valid as a treatment modality.

## THE UNDERSEA MEDICAL SOCIETY ENTERS THE FIELD

For many years, there had been debate among the members of the executive committee of the UMS whether the society should become involved in clinical hyperbarics.

The UMS had been founded in 1967 by six U.S. Navy Diving and Submarine medical officers and, originally, had been conceived as an organization dedicated to diving and undersea medicine. Over the years it has grown to a society of about 2,800 members internationally.

After much soul searching, an ad hoc Committee on Hyperbaric Oxygenation was authorized at the executive committee meeting held in Bethesda, Maryland, on November 5, 1976. The author was made its chairman and appointed 18 members from around the United States, mostly from academia and the military, to help in reviewing the field.

## THE REPORT OF THE COMMITTEE ON HYPERBARIC OXYGENATION

The committee consulted with the Social Security Administration, which handled Medicare, and with the Blue Cross/Blue Shield Association in Chicago, the largest private medical insurer in the United States. These organizations were asked what their requirements were and what issues they would wish to see addressed in a report concerning hyperbaric oxygenation.

By May of 1977, a report had been formalized and approved by the Executive Committee of the UMS (17). This report divided hyperbaric disorders into four categories. Category One encompassed those diseases for which there was no question of the efficacy of hyperbaric oxygen, and for which the data were indisputable. Category Two listed those diseases which had a physiologically sound basis for treatment, but for which fewer data were available. The evidence adduced for the efficacy of HBO in Category Two disorders had to be at least as good as the evidence for those treatments routinely reimbursed by medical insurers. It was recommended that treatment of Categories One and Two be reimbursed by third-party payers. Category Three were those diseases which were considered to be investigational and might have promise, while to Category Four were allocated those disorders which were considered to have no scientific basis, and in which treatment was based simply on wishful thinking.

Copies of the report were sent to the Health Care Finances Administration (which had taken over Medicare from Social Security) and to the National Blue Cross/Blue Shield Association. After review by the medical advisory board of Blue Cross/Blue Shield, the report was accepted in toto as their source document on September 14, 1977.

Since that time, the report has been updated periodically and the committee has changed from an ad hoc committee to a standing committee of the UMS. The report was greatly expanded and improved under the successive chairmanships of Richard D. Heimbach, Jefferson C. Davis, Roy A. M. Myers, Jon T. Mader, Enrico Camporesi, and Neil B. Hampson and most recently by John J. Feldmeier. With the revision of the report chaired by Dr. Davis, the original four categories were abolished and only two categories were recognized: diseases approved for treatment and those considered investigative. Disorders considered to be without specific scientific basis were dropped from the report. As of 2008, only 13 disorders were approved for hyperbaric treatment.

## SPECIALTY JOURNALS

The UMS had published its own journal, Undersea Biomedical Research, since 1974, which chiefly contained diving medicine papers. Only occasional articles appeared dealing with clinical hyperbarics.

Dr. Charles W. Shilling, who had become the mainstay of the UMS as its Executive Secretary in 1973, was the moving force in developing a journal devoted to HBO. He launched *Hyperbaric Oxygen Review* in 1980, a quarterly abstract journal of which the author became editor. This journal contained a collection of the latest abstracts from the literature, and at least one substantial review article with exhaustive references in each issue. It was the first journal to deal exclusively with clinical hyperbarics. By 1986, however, the executive committee of the UMS felt that a full-fledged journal containing original papers was warranted. Thus, in January 1986, *Hyperbaric Oxygen Review* was supplanted by the new quarterly, *Journal of Hyperbaric Medicine*, with Enrico Camporesi as its editor. In January of 1993, *Undersea Biomedical Research* and the *Journal of Hyperbaric Medicine* were combined as *Undersea and Hyperbaric Medicine* in order to obtain listing by the National Library of Medicine for reference retrieval.

## CERTIFICATION FOR HYPERBARIC PHYSICIANS AND NURSES

In 1983, attempts were made to devise pathways for certification in hyperbaric medicine for physicians, nurses, respiratory therapists, and hyperbaric technicians. Little progress was made in this area, however, until quite recently. The Baromedical Nurses Association, created in 1985, took the initial lead in establishing a basis for eventual certification of hyperbaric nurses through the American Nursing Association (ANA). As of this writing (2006), they have created a nationally recognized certifying examination and criteria for certification.

The UMS wished to keep hyperbaric oxygenation within the mainstream of medicine and, therefore, had no desire to create an "American Board of Hyperbaric Medicine" that would not be a member of the American Board of Medical Specialties. The American Board of Preventative Medicine was approached and, largely through the efforts of Jefferson Davis, agreed to administer an examination for the award of a certificate of special competence in the hyperbaric field. An examination was created, but it dealt exclusively with diving medicine. Only a few people boarded in occupational medicine bothered to take the examination.

There was an ongoing problem. Members of many different specialties run hyperbaric facilities, and there was difficulty in getting agreement among the various boards. A single exam, oriented to both clinical hyperbaric and diving medicine, and a unified set of criteria for eligibility to take the exam were created by the American Board of Preventative Medicine, largely through the efforts of Jefferson C. Davis. This enabled all board certified specialists to be given a certificate of added qualification through a standard examination. The first examination was given, under the auspices of the American Board of Preventive Medicine in November of 1999. In addition to being board certified in one of the 28 specialties recognized by the American Board of Medical Specialties and passing the exam, candidates for certification had to have had a 40 hour introductory course in HBO approved by the UHMS and two years of clinical practice in the field. This allowed experienced hyperbaric physicians to be "grandfathered" for certification. By 2001, the board examination was also recognized by the American Board of Emergency Medicine. However, in 2005 the "grandfathering" provision had run out and now candidates for board certification must have completed a formal one-year fellowship in the field to sit for the exam and be board certified.

It was anticipated that very few mid-career physicians with extensive hyperbaric experience would be able to take a year off from their practices to complete one of the few hyperbaric fellowships approved by the UHMS. Thus there was no way for their hyperbaric expertise to be formally recognized by hospital credentialing committees. To fill this gap, a newly reconstituted American College of Hyperbaric Medicine with Robert Bartlett as its President, developed a stringent examination comparable to the one given by the American Board of Preventative Medicine. Additionally, candidates for the exam must have essentially the same qualifications recognized by the American Boards of Preventative Medicine and Emergency Medicine during the "grandfathering" period. The American College does not award a "board certification" to candidates who pass the exam, but a certificate of competence in the field that can be recognized by hospital credentialing committees.

In 1991, the National Association of Diving Medical Technicians (NADMT), through the efforts of its president, Dick Clarke, announced the creation of a certifying body for hyperbaric technicians who operate the hyperbaric chambers. The new organization, called the National Board of Diving and Hyperbaric Medicine Technology (NBDHMT), gave its first certification examination at the annual UHMS Scientific Meeting held in 1991, in San Diego, California. It was a thorough examination and resulted in nationally recognized accreditation for those who passed it. Initially, hyperbaric technicians, respiratory therapists, and nurses who had at least 2,000 hours of HBO treatment experience could be "grandfathered" to qualify to take the exam. The "grandfather clause" expired in 1996. After that, candidates for the examination had to be graduates of a UHMS or NBDHMT-approved training course. As of 1999, a 40-hour course for technicians must be specifically approved by the NBDHMT, and those passing the examination must have 480 hours of hyperbaric chamber experience to be certified.

## COOPERATION WITH THE JOINT COMMISSION

In 1977, the author compiled a list of suggested guidelines for the Joint Commission on Accreditation of Hospitals (JCAH) for use in inspecting hyperbaric facilities. Because of the shortage of facilities in operation at that time, the guidelines were not incorporated in the JCAH manual. By 1989, however, these guidelines were being observed by some inspecting teams visiting hospitals with hyperbaric chambers. Revised guidelines, along with a suggested quality assurance program, have now been developed and published as an appendix to the UHMS Hyperbaric Oxygen Committee Report. In 2004, the UHMS embarked on a program of formally credentialing individual hyperbaric units that met high standards of care. To accomplish this, units volunteering to be credentialed are visited by a UHMS hyperbaric team consisting of one physician, a certified nurse or technician and the accreditation leader where all aspects of safety, record keeping and treatment standards are reviewed over a two-day period. On completion of the review, the team meets with the hyperbaric unit personnel and again with the hospital administrators to point out any discrepancies and how they are to be remedied. When any deficiencies are corrected, the unit receives official approval of the UHMS.

## CLINICAL HYPERBARICS JOINS THE UNDERSEA MEDICAL SOCIETY

In 1972, when the author founded *Pressure*, the newsletter of the Undersea Medical Society, the opening editorial remarks stated that the name Pressure was chosen to embrace both the diving and clinical hyperbaric fields. At that time some of us already had the hope that the society could represent both groups.

This did not happen immediately, and clinical hyperbaric papers were not well represented at the annual UMS scientific meeting. To provide a forum for hyperbaric clinicians, George Hart initiated an annual clinical hyperbaric oxygen conference, hosted by Long Beach Memorial Hospital. These extremely valuable and well-attended conferences ran annually from 1976 through 1986, after which they were melded into the UHMS Annual Meeting. In 1986, the members at the UMS annual scientific meeting held in Kobe, Japan, voted to change the name of the Undersea Medical Society to the Undersea and Hyperbaric Medical Society (UHMS).

## EUROPEAN GROWTH OF HYPERBARIC MEDICINE

Starting from its birth in Amsterdam, hyperbaric treatment centers soon developed in other parts of Europe. In the United Kingdom, Slack, Perrins, Smith, Sharp, Skene, Ledingham, Cameron, and Thurston began active research in surgical uses of the chamber, carbon monoxide poisoning, and myocardial infarction. This research abated, however, as the heart-lung machine came into use. On the continent, work continued in France and Italy, with contributions by Wattel, Mathieu, Ohresser, Oriani, and many others. In the Soviet Union, Academician Petrovsky became interested in HBO and spent time as a fellow with Julius Jacobson at Mt. Sinai in New York. Subsequently, he popularized HBO in his homeland when he became Commissar of Public Health, and dozens of chambers were installed. One of the largest hyperbaric complexes in the world, consisting of six interconnected chambers, was constructed in Moscow, where it was directed by Sergei Efuni. At this writing there are some 2,000 chambers being operated in Russia. As in the United States, enthusiasm for HBO waxed and waned in Europe. Initially, few chambers were built in Scandinavia or Germany. Beginning in about 1985, however, interest in the field began to increase, and multiple clinical chambers came on line in Germany. Sweden in recent years has produced many scientific papers in the field of HBO by Barr, Lind, Nylander, Granström, and Hammarlund. Today there are active clinical chambers in Stockholm, Gothenburg, and Helsingborg.

In 1992, the first European Consensus Congress was convened in Lille, France, and there it was decided which disorders should be approved for hyperbaric treatment. The list that came out of the congress largely coincided with the UHMS approved list. In 1998, a consensus congress on the parameters necessary for patient selection for HBO treatment of the diabetic foot was convened in London. Meanwhile, HBO had begun a scientific resurgence in the U.K. with the establishment of a Hyperbaric Society made up of the clinical HBO units.

## HYPERBARIC MEDICINE IN ASIA AND THE PACIFIC RIM

In the mid 1960s, Professor Juro Wada in Sapporo, Japan became interested in HBO for cardiac surgery and established a large chamber there. In Nagoya, Professor Kinsaku Sakakibara started a program for cardiac surgery and quickly branched out into treatment of other disorders. A vigorous society for hyperbaric medicine was created, with many chambers being installed throughout Japan. Professor Hideyo Takahashi at the University of Nagoya became a Japanese leader in the field.

In Taiwan, the growth of hyperbarics was due to the influence and interest of the Surgeon General of the Navy, Admiral Tu Tzu Chu, who, in 1976, inaugurated a hyperbaric program. He sent naval officers as fellows to the United States to learn HBO; two of them participated in the author's program for one-year tenures. His efforts were continued by the subsequent Surgeons General, Admiral Kwan, and more recently, Admiral An-Jen Lee. Captain Alan Ko Chi Niu, one of my former fellows, became a leader in the hyperbaric field in Taiwan and has authored the largest comparative study of HBO in burn treatment published to date. Large clinical facilities are in operation in Taipei at the Tri-Service General Hospital and the Veteran's General Hospital. Clinical chambers are also operating in Keelung and at the Tsoying Military Hospital in Kaohsiung. Taiwan University has now entered the hyperbaric field with a chamber in their department of Plastic Surgery, and there are chambers at several private hospitals.

Clinical chambers are also operational in Indonesia, through the influence of the former Naval Surgeon General Soesanto Mangoensajito, now retired. A large clinical chamber is in operation in Surabaya, with a smaller one in Jakarta.

On mainland China, there are 3,800 hyperbaric chambers in operation for clinical work, of which 2,600 are multiplace units. Much research from Chinese investigators has been published. The late Professor Wen-Ren Li was a leader in the field in mainland China.

In Australia, Ian Unsworth pioneered clinical hyperbaric treatment in Sydney. Large multiplace chambers are now active there and in university centers in Hobart, Melbourne, Adelaide, Freemantle, Townsville and Brisbane. Australian researchers have contributed much to the diving literature and are beginning to produce work of equal importance in the clinical hyperbaric field. Des Gorman, an avid researcher in both diving and hyperbaric medicine, is now active in New Zealand, after having been with the faculty in Adelaide.

## DEVELOPMENT OF HBO TRAINING

Prior to 1976 there were no regular hyperbaric training courses for civilian physicians available in the U.S. Dr. Harry Alvis had conducted one ad hoc course in the principles and theory of hyperbaric medicine in the mid-1960s, for interested physicians at the State University of New York at Buffalo, but there was no follow-up. Most doctors, who ran hyperbaric chambers, if they had any formal training, received it in the military. Submarine medical officers were taught about decompression sickness and air embolism, but little else.

United States Air Force flight surgeons were also taught the management of decompression sickness and air embolism. Beginning about 1972, they started hearing about other clinical uses of the chamber in their training, largely through the interest and efforts of Jefferson C. Davis. At that time, he was in charge of the Aerospace Medicine Residency Program, and Director of the Hyperbaric Medicine Division at the School of Aerospace Medicine in San Antonio, Texas. Davis managed to interest the Surgeon General of the Air Force in clinical HBO. This later resulted in the Air Force contributing much information and research in the field. Of the three military services, the Air Force is now designated the lead agency. Large multiplace chambers are located at the Wright Patterson air force base and at Travis air force base.

Captain George Hart of the Naval Regional Medical Center in Long Beach, California, became interested in HBO as early as 1967. He established monoplace chambers at that hospital while he was Chief of Surgery. Although Hart, as well as Davis, was a true pioneer in this field, U.S. Navy involvement with HBO remained isolated to the Long Beach facility and was not officially recognized. Aside from the work of George Hart, who published extensively, the U.S. Navy has added relatively little to clinical hyperbarics.

Although others had previously offered ad hoc courses, the author offered the first regularly scheduled formal course in hyperbaric medicine to civilian physicians in the United States, in the summer of 1976. The first course ran two weeks and his class of one student, Dr. Steven Strong, came to Milwaukee all the way from Maui, Hawaii. This course was offered twice a year at St. Luke's Medical Center, Milwaukee, until 1995. It was reinstituted in 1999.

Other hyperbaric physicians soon initiated training programs in the clinical field. George Hart and Michael Strauss began teaching regularly scheduled courses in 1977, and now offer four to five courses a year to physicians and other health professionals. Since 1984, the Hart-Strauss team has trained over 100 students a year. Carraway Methodist Hospital in

Birmingham, Alabama, began offering courses in 1985, and was instructing about 50 students a year. In 1983, Roy Meyers began teaching HBO courses at the University of Maryland.

Jefferson Davis, who left the Air Force to run the chambers at Methodist Hospital in San Antonio, Texas, in 1983, began teaching multiplace chamber operation to physicians who bought Perry Oceanographics chambers. Later he opened the course to all those interested. His course, originally designed exclusively for multiplace chamber physicians, was two weeks long. Since his tragic and untimely death from cancer in July of 1989, these courses continued under the direction of Dean Heimbach and now Paul Sheffield. Dick Clarke at Richland Memorial Hospital in Columbia, South Carolina, also organizes a variety of clinical HBO courses, teaching over 400 students per year. The author taught two courses per year at the Medical College of Wisconsin in Milwaukee until 1998, and gives on-site courses as new wound-care centers are established. At the present time, there are at least six institutions featuring courses in clinical hyperbaric medicine.

## DIVING MEDICINE COURSES

Since 1970, there have been dozens of courses in diving medicine taught principally at Caribbean resorts. In recent years, most of these courses have also included additional lectures on the non-diving uses of the chamber in clinical medicine. Often, this is the first exposure to clinical HBO for many of these physicians, who represent all the specialties. A number of new hyperbaric units have been started by these doctors following their introduction to the subject through participation in sport-diving medicine courses.

## COURSE CERTIFICATION

Starting in 1972, the Undersea Medical Society began to play an important role in hyperbaric education. Some of the diving-medicine courses being offered in the Caribbean were of poor quality, and really were little more than tax-deductible scuba-diving holidays masquerading as medical education. A number of us in the Undersea Medical Society were disappointed in these inadequate offerings and agreed some kind of quality assurance was necessary.

To provide this, the Medical Education and Standards Committee was formed and the author became its first chairman. The purpose was to review the proposed curriculum and the list of lecturers for scheduled diving medicine courses, and to give official UMS approval to those that met certain standards. Such a system was valuable to the organizers of the courses as they could then advertise an "approved course," and it raised the course standards considerably. Dr. Edward Tucker taught the first UMS-approved diving-medicine course. Dr. Tucker had succeeded the author as Assistant Director of the U.S. Navy School of Submarine Medicine in New London and, after leaving the Navy, adapted the relevant parts of the Navy diving-medicine course for civilian diving physicians. His course final examination was the same as that used at the submarine school, excluding the helium diving and "hard hat" portions.

## ADVENT OF CME CREDITS

At the same time, the American Medical Association (AMA) was beginning its program of certification in Continuing Medical Education (CME) for all physicians. If a physician took 30 hours of CME courses approved in advance by the AMA, he could get a Physician's Recognition Award. Most states in the U.S., which do the licensing of physicians, put teeth into the program by demanding that every physician must take a minimum number of CME credit hours each year to retain his or her license to practice medicine, regardless of specialty or seniority. The author approached the AMA and secured its approval of the Undersea Medical Society, as a certifying agency, to choose the diving-medicine courses for which the AMA would grant official CME credit. As a result, all courses approved by the Education and Standards Committee of the UMS receive automatic AMA recognition.

It was fortunate that this recognition of the UMS was already affirmed when the first formal courses in Clinical Hyperbaric Medicine appeared. The Medical Education and Standards Committee (later simply called the Education Committee) began monitoring and approving clinical HBO courses as well. For a clinical HBO course to receive approval, it had to be taught by competent teachers at a facility that treated only those disorders approved by the Committee on Hyperbaric Oxygen. If the facility treated non-approved disorders, those treatments had to be carried out on a strict research protocol, approved by the hospital's Institutional Review Board. In the United States, the federal government requires an Institutional Review Board for every hospital to pre-approve all research and insure that patients are afforded full protection and are not subjected to unethical research.

Because the responsible hyperbaric community since 1976 has voluntarily restricted itself to treating only a limited number of disorders for which there is a rational basis backed by good scientific evidence, the field has begun to achieve recognition by mainstream medicine. Indiscriminate treatment of large numbers of patients, out of enthusiasm supported only by wishful thinking, inevitably angers both responsible physicians and insurance companies alike, be they governmental or private. Over the years, such occurrences greatly slowed the acceptance of HBO.

## HYPERBARIC FELLOWSHIPS

Fellowships in Clinical Hyperbaric Medicine have been offered by the United States Air Force, and by at least seven civilian institutions. The United States Air Force created the first formal fellowship in clinical hyperbaric medicine in 1978, accommodating two to three fellows, at the School of Aerospace Medicine in San Antonio, Texas. Dr. Hart at Long Beach Memorial Hospital also offered a fellowship program, selecting up to two incumbents per year.

A formal fellowship, approved by the Education Committee of the UHMS was established at St. Luke's Hospital in Milwaukee in 1984. Although not filled every year, four graduates completed year-long fellowships during the author's tenure as director. Dr. Roy Myers offered a fellowship approved through the University of Maryland and graduated five fellows. Other one-year fellowships have been created at the University of Pennsylvania (Dr. Stephen Thom), Tulane University (Dr. Keith Van Meter), the University of Miami

(Dr. Luis Matos), and the University of Texas, Galveston (by the late Dr. Jon Mader). The University of Texas fellowship placed heavy emphasis on infectious disease, with both clinical and animal research.

Physicians who complete fellowships have demonstrated a deep interest in the specialty and are usually destined to become prominent in the field, either as researchers and clinicians or teachers.

## RENEWED NAVAL INTEREST

In March of 1993, while a reservist on active duty at the Trident submarine base at Bangor, Washington, the author broached the subject of teaching clinical hyperbaric medicine to the Undersea Medical Officers with Captain Henry Schwartz, Force Medical Officer for Submarines Pacific. Dr. Schwartz supported the idea and arrangements were made to include it in the training received by Undersea Medical Officers at the Naval Undersea Medical Institute, New London (formerly the School of Submarine Medicine). Since May of 1994, each class of Undersea Medical Officers has received three days of HBO instruction, in addition to their diving-medicine training, as part of their course.

## TEACHING OF MEDICAL STUDENTS

In order to introduce physicians to hyperbaric medicine and have them maintain an interest in it, instruction must begin in medical school. The author accepted medical students for one-month elective rotations during their senior year for over 15 years, and other institutions do likewise. However, this usually meant that only two or three students per year at each institution were exposed to the concepts of HBO. With so much medicine to learn in only four years, curriculum committees were reluctant to add even more new subjects. However, for three years, the author was fortunate to give a two-hour lecture to all second-year pharmacology students at the Medical College of Wisconsin on "Oxygen as a Drug," as part of their required course. HBO is not an esoteric treatment procedure. It is best introduced to medical students as a pharmacologically active element and an important addition to the physician's armamentarium.

## THE FUTURE

In the past, most hyperbaric facilities were run by physicians who practiced hyperbaric medicine part-time. They used it as a useful adjunctive tool, but continued to actively practice their own medical specialty, be it surgery, pulmonary medicine, emergency medicine, critical care, or other specialty. This may not be the case in the future.

In the past few years, it has been demonstrated that chronic non-healing wounds are best and most efficiently managed in wound-care centers, where a team or multi-specialty approach is used. Each patient has a case manager who assures that standardized diagnostic and treatment algorithms are used. Each specialist in internal medicine, vascular, orthopedic, plastic surgery, or dermatology, is consulted in a timely fashion and wounds are cared for meticulously with modern dressings. About 15% of the patients referred to wound-care centers will potentially be benefited by HBO. Today, for this reason, most new chambers are being installed in wound-care centers.

For a physician to be paid a "procedural fee" by governmental insurance for supervision of HBO treatment, he must be present and immediately available for the entire time the patient is in the chamber. Indeed for the hospital to be paid a technical fee for treatment, the physician must be present. This only becomes feasible if the physician is engaged full time in the wound-care clinic where the chamber is located. He is assumed in such case to be attending patients with wounds, and by being present, is immediately available in case of need at chamber-side. We may anticipate that a trend will develop in which generalists and internists sub-specialize in chronic wound care.

As of 1981, the number of clinical chambers in operation had grown to 110, and by 1988 the number was 240. At this writing (2008), there are over 800 chambers operating in the United States. This number will continue to grow.

The single most important need for this specialty continues to be published, controlled studies, done in academic settings and citing outcomes. Such studies are becoming increasingly common. Of great importance today are those studies which compare the total costs of treatment with and without adjunctive HBO. Hyperbaric oxygen is increasingly being seen not only to lower morbidity, but also to save health-care dollars.

## REFERENCES

1. American Medical Association Bureau of Investigation. The Cunningham "Tank treatment". The Alleged Value of Compressed Air in the Treatment of Diabetes Mellitus, Pernicious Anemia and Carcinoma. JAMA. 1928;90: 1494.

2. Arntzenius, AKW. De Pneumatische Therapie. Scheltema and Holkemas Boekhandel, Amsterdam, 1887.

3. Bert, P. Barometric Pressure. 1878, p571. (Translated by M.S. and F.A. Hitchcock) Reprinted by the Undersea Medical Society, Bethesda, 1978.

4. Boerema, I, JA Kroll, NG Meijne, E Lokin, B. Kroon and JW Huiskes. "High atmospheric pressure as an aid to cardiac surgery." Arch. Chir. Neerl. 1956;8:193-211.

5. Brummelkamp, WH, J Hogendijk and I Boerema. "Treatment of anaerobic infections (Clostridial myositis) by drenching the tissues with oxygen under high atmospheric pressure." Surgery. 1961;49:299-302.

6. Churchill-Davidson, I, C Sanger and RH Thomlinson. "High-pressure oxygen and radiotherapy." Lancet. 1955;1:1091-1095.

7. Corning, JL. "The use of compressed air in conjunction with medicinal solutions in the treatment of nervous and mental affections, being a new system of cerebrospinal therapeutics." Med Record. 1891;40:225.

8. Cunningham, OJ. "Oxygen therapy by means of compressed air." Analgesie. 1927, 6:64.

9. Davis, JC and TK Hunt. Hyperbaric Oxygen Therapy. Undersea Medical Society, Bethesda, 1977.

10. Davis, RH. Deep Diving and Submarine Operations, 7th Edition. Siebe, Gorman & Company, Ltd., Chessington, Surrey, 1962;291.

11. Donald, KW. "Oxygen poisoning in man." Brit. Med. J., May 24, 1947;712-717.

12. Fontaine, JA. "Emploi chirurgical de l'air comprimé." Union Med. 1879;28:445.

13. Fundamentals of Hyperbaric Medicine. Publication #1298, National Academy of Sciences, National Research Council, Washington DC, 1966.

14. Funk and Wagnalls "Book of Marvels." 1931;12.

15. Henshaw, In: (Simpson, A.) Compressed Air as a Therapeutic Agent in the Treatment of Consumption, Asthma, Chronic Bronchitis and Other Diseases. Sutherland and Knox, Edinburgh, 1857.

16. Jacobson, JH II, JCH Morsch and L Rendell-Baker. "The historical perspective of hyperbaric therapy." Annals of the New York Academy of Sciences. 1965;117(Art.2):651-670.

17. Kindwall, EP (Chairman) Report of the Committee on Hyperbaric Oxygenation. Undersea Medical Society, Bethesda, 1977.

18. Lorrain-Smith, J. "The pathological effects due to increase of oxygen tension in the air breathed." J. of Physiology. 1898, 24:19-35.

19. Smith, G and GR Sharp. "Treatment of coal gas poisoning with oxygen at two atmospheres pressure." Lancet. 1962;1:816-819.

CHAPTER 2

# THE PHYSICS OF DIVING AND HYPERBARIC PRESSURES

## CHAPTER TWO OVERVIEW

# THE PHYSICS OF DIVING AND HYPERBARIC PRESSURES

*Eric P. Kindwall*

## INTRODUCTION

The physics of diving and hyperbaric pressure are very straight forward and are defined by well-known and accepted laws. Gas under pressure can store enormous energy, the amounts of which are often surprising. Also, small changes in the percentages of the various gases used are greatly magnified by changes in ambient pressure. The resultant physiologic effects differ widely depending on the pressure. Thus, diving or operating a hyperbaric facility requires gaining complete knowledge of the laws involved to ensure safety.

## UNITS OF MEASURE

This is often a confusing area to anyone new to hyperbaric medicine as both American and International Standard of Units (SI) are used. In addition to meters, centimeters, kilos, pounds, and feet, some pressures are given in atmospheres absolute and millimeters of mercury. Table 1 gives the exact conversion factors between SI and American units.

## TABLE 1. PRESSURE CONVERSION TABLE

| Multiply given unit by the factor in the appropriate column below | | | | |
|---|---|---|---|---|
| **GIVEN UNIT** | **BAR** | **ATMOSPHERES** | **PSIG** | **Kg/cm$^2$** |
| **1 Bar** | 1 | 0.98692 | 14.504 | 1.01944 |
| **1 Standard Physical Atmosphere** | 1.0133 | 1 | 14.696 | 1.03322 |
| **1 PSIG** (gauge pressure) | 0.06895 | 0.68046 | 1 | 0.07031 |
| **1 Kg/cm$^2$** | 1.01944 | 0.98692 | 14.504 | 1 |
| **1 Kilopascal** | 0.01 | 0.009869 | 0.14504 | 0.010194 |
| **1 Torracelli** (torr) | 0.001332 | 0.001316 | 0.01934 | 0.0013046 |
| **1 Cubic foot** = 28.316 liters | | | | |
| **33 feet of sea water** = 10.0584 meters | | | | |
| **Pressure equivalent of 33 feet of seawater** = 1.0256 Kg/cm2 = 14.685 psig | | | | |

The table above gives exact equivalents, but for the diver or clinical hyperbaric specialist, such precision is not required and the figures given below are more than adequate for practical use.

## The American System

I use the term "American System" because even though the units of measurement were originally English, the United Kingdom has now officially gone over to the metric system. The United States is the only country which still uses the original English units.

The pressure of one atmosphere is equal to 14.7 pounds per square inch. This is considered to be the ambient pressure at sea level. By convention, when the term "atmospheres" is used, it always refers to atmospheres absolute. This means that if one is referring to elevated atmospheric pressure in atmospheres, one always includes the ambient air pressure on the surface at sea level, plus the added pressure. Therefore, if one descends 33 feet in sea water, one is at an absolute pressure of two atmospheres. Thirty-three feet is equal to 14.7 pounds per square inch as read on the gauge. This is abbreviated psig. Descending another 33 feet to 66 feet produces an absolute pressure of 3 **atmospheres absolute**, abbreviated ATA. When physicians prescribe treatment pressures, they customarily refer to those pressures in atmospheres absolute. This is an extremely **important point to understand** since taking a patient to a pressure of 99 feet or four atmospheres absolute would quickly produce oxygen toxicity in a patient if the order were understood to mean three atmospheres as measured on the gauge. Gauge pressures do not show the ambient pressure from which one begins pressurization.

The American system is cumbersome. Pressure changes cannot be treated decimally and one must multiply by a conversion factor every time one wants to achieve an equivalency between pounds and feet, or between pounds and atmospheres. The conversion factor for converting feet of sea water (fsw) to pounds per square inch gauge (psig) is 0.445. Thirty-three feet multiplied by 0.445 equals 14.7 pounds per square inch, when rounded to nearest tenth of a pound. Thus, a depth of 100 feet of sea water would equal 44.5 pounds per square inch gauge (psig). **Pounds** and **feet** always denote gauge pressure unless they are specifically labeled absolute. The conversion factor of 0.445 should be memorized by anyone using the American system.

## The Metric System

The metric system vastly simplifies pressure and depth calculations for diving and hyperbaric work. As a practical matter, 14.7 psig is taken to be the equivalent of 1 kilogram per square centimeter.

In Europe the term "bar" is often used, being equivalent to one atmosphere. However, **bar** is always a **gauge pressure** as opposed to atmospheres which are always absolute. For practical purposes, the pressure at sea level is considered to be one kilogram per square centimeter absolute. Thus, one atmosphere is equal to one kilogram per square centimeter. Going to a depth of 10 meters in sea water, "very close to 33 feet," produces a pressure of two atmospheres. Thus for every 10 meters one descends in the sea, one adds an additional atmosphere of pressure. In the metric system,

**atmospheres** are always given as **absolute**, just as in the American system, and **meters** and **kilograms per square centimeter** are always expressed as **gauge pressures.**

As an aside, it should be pointed out that it is only fortuitous that 10 meters equals one atmosphere and that one kilogram per square centimeter equals atmospheric pressure. The framers of the metric system originally defined the meter as being one ten-millionth of the distance between the North Pole and the Equator.

In the American system it is useful to memorize the number of feet to a given number of atmospheres and to count by 33s (i.e., 33 feet, 66 feet, 99 feet, 132 feet, and 165 feet, corresponding to 2, 3, 4, 5, and 6 atmospheres respectively). In the course of clinical hospital practice, one rarely if ever exceeds a pressure of 165 feet, and going to that pressure would only be in the treatment of decompression illness.

In the metric system, ten-meter increments are usually calculated as additional atmospheres are applied. Thus, it is easy to equate 50 meters with 6 atmospheres absolute (ATA), whereas in the American system one has to memorize that the pressure at six atmospheres is 73.4 pounds per square inch gauge (psig) or 165 feet.

## Kilopascals

There is a growing trend to express pressures in terms of SI units or kilopascals. One hundred kilopascals equals 1 atmosphere or 1 kilogram per square centimeter. Rigid convention specifies that kilopascals are always an expression of absolute pressure. Thus, 250 kilopascals equals 2.5 atmospheres, or 1.5 kilograms per square centimeter gauge. The reader should be cautioned, however, that not all authors use kilopascals as absolute pressures and occasionally one may find them expressed as gauge pressures. Thus, be careful to double check the author's frame of reference when reading manuscripts in which pressures are expressed as kilopascals.

## Millimeters of Mercury

An older unit of measure typically used to express pressures of one atmosphere or less is the millimeter of mercury sometimes called the Torr. Normal atmospheric pressure at sea level is accepted as being equal to 760 millimeters of mercury. This is abbreviated mmHg. Partial pressures of gases dissolved within the body are often expressed in mmHg. For practical purposes, the ambient pressure of oxygen in air at normal sea level pressure is 160 mmHg. The partial pressure of nitrogen is taken to be 600 mmHg. The trace gases, helium, neon, argon, krypton, and xenon are usually ignored, even though argon represents nearly one percent of the inert gas moiety.

## BOYLE'S LAW

In the 1670s, Robert Boyle observed that for a body of ideal gas at constant temperature, the volume is inversely proportional to the pressure. Thus, if the temperature does not change, compressing a given volume of gas to twice its original absolute pressure will halve its volume. Tripling the pressure reduces the volume to one-third. It is easily observed that there is proportionately less change in volume as each additional atmosphere of pressure is added. This has practical significance in treating patients. At the beginning of pressurization, volume changes affecting the middle ear are maximal, whereas the deeper one goes, possibilities of barotrauma become less and less. Doubling the pressure from the surface to 2 atmospheres halves the volume, whereas going from three atmospheres to 4 ATA changes the volume only from one-third to one-fourth of its original surface equivalent. For this reason, to minimize the chance of barotrauma, pressurization should begin slowly and then accelerate only as the patient is exposed to greater and greater pressure.

## CHARLES' LAW

Charles, a French physicist, observed that for a body of ideal gas at constant pressure, the volume is directly proportional to the absolute temperature. From a practical standpoint, we are interested in the inverse of this statement: Compressing a gas will make it hotter. This is the principle on which the diesel engine works; as air is greatly compressed in the engine cylinder, it becomes hot enough to ignite the diesel oil when it is injected into the cylinder at the top of the power stroke. Fortunately, temperatures do not reach such heights in hyperbaric chambers, but, with fast compression, the chamber can become uncomfortably warm. Boyle's Law and Charles' Law are combined in the general gas equation:

$$\frac{P1\ V1}{T1} = \frac{P2\ V2}{T2}$$

Where P = pressure of the gas, V = volume of the gas, and T = the absolute temperature. P1, V1, and T1 indicate the original pressure, volume, and temperature; P2, V2, T2 indicate the changed pressure, volume, and temperature. It must be noted, however, that temperature is expressed in terms of absolute temperatures, "denoted as temperatures Kelvin." Absolute zero on the Celsius scale is –273°C. Thus a room temperature of 20°C equals 293 Kelvin. It can be seen from the above equation that if temperature is kept constant and pressure is doubled, volume will be halved. It will also be seen that if pressure is doubled and volume is kept constant (i.e., V2 has the same number of molecules occupying the space as V1); the absolute temperature will be doubled to 586 Kelvin. Subtracting 273K from 586K gives us 313K, which is what a standard thermometer would read. However, in reality cold air is constantly being forced into the chamber to increase the pressure so the rise in temperature is, by contrast, minimal. The above equation assumes instant compression. In practice, compression rates in hyperbaric chambers are so slow that an appreciable warming will be noted, but is easily tolerated. The excess heat is radiated quickly. The converse is true on decompression as the chamber will become cold and fog often will form as the temperature drops below the dew point. The formation of fog has nothing to do directly with pressure change, but is due solely to a drop in temperature.

## DALTON'S LAW

John Dalton was an English chemist and physicist who formulated the law which states that in a mixture of gases, the sum of the partial pressures of the gases in the mixture equals the total pressure. Thus with regard to air, the oxygen pressure is 160 mmHg and the nitrogen pressure is 600 mmHg at sea level. Combining these two pressures equals 760 mmHg which is atmospheric pressure. If this law is kept in mind, it will remove a great deal of confusion in calculating the effects of pressure changes we shall see below.

## HENRY'S LAW

Henry's law states that the partial pressure of a gas dissolved in a liquid is equal to the partial pressure of that gas exerted on the surface of the liquid at equilibrium. For this reason, a cup of water sitting on a table at sea level will contain a partial pressure of oxygen equaling 160 mmHg and a partial pressure of nitrogen equaling 600 mmHg. It does not matter what kind of liquid one is dealing with since the partial pressure would be the same in a cup of oil or a cup of water. It will also be seen that the partial pressure of nitrogen in sea water will be 600 mmHg one centimeter below the surface, as well as at 36,000 feet (11,000 meters) at the bottom of the Marianas Trench. Henry did not specify the depth of the container and one can assume equilibrium in the case of air or sea water.

## EFFECTIVE PERCENTAGES

If one enters a hyperbaric chamber, closes the door, and pressurizes it with compressed air to a depth of 33 feet (10 meters), one doubles the atmospheric pressure and also the density of the oxygen one is breathing. The partial pressure of oxygen in the inspired compressed air rises from 160 mmHg to 320 mmHg. Thus, for every lung-full of air, one is receiving twice as many molecules of oxygen impinging on the alveolar membrane. This is equivalent to breathing 42% oxygen at a pressure of one atmosphere. Thus, we say that the individual is breathing an **effective** percentage of 42%. At 4 atmospheres pressure, the effective percentage breathing compressed air would be 84%. It can be seen that scuba divers (who breathe compressed air not oxygen, for reasons of oxygen toxicity) are extremely well oxygenated at a depth of 99 feet (30 meters), or 4 atmospheres absolute (ATA).

## USING DALTON'S LAW

I often ask my students if they would be willing to enter a hyperbaric chamber, have the door closed and then be pressurized to 7 atmospheres (60 meters, or 198 feet) admitting only pure helium to the chamber. I usually get no takers because people realize that the oxygen in the chamber would be diluted to 3% by the time one arrived at depth.

Here Dalton's Law comes to our rescue. Everyone agrees that upon closing the chamber door, the oxygen partial pressure would be 160 mmHg, assuming the chamber was air filled. Likewise, the partial pressure of nitrogen would be 600 mmHg. If one then added 6 additional atmospheres of pure helium (4,560 mmHg), the total pressure in the chamber would be 5,320 mmHg upon reaching 7 atmospheres. Everyone can agree that an oxygen partial pressure of 160 mmHg is quite satisfactory for preserving life. When one arrives at 7 atmospheres pressure, although the inert partial pressures are enormous, one still is breathing oxygen at a partial pressure of 160 mmHg. Thus, if we were satisfied with 160 mmHg at sea level, why can we not be satisfied with it at 7 atmospheres absolute? Indeed, one will survive very nicely and this is how commercial divers earn their living when they carry out saturation dives in the oil fields.

In those situations, the chamber is initially pressurized with compressed air to raise the partial pressure of oxygen to an effective percentage somewhere between 30 and 60% (0.30-0.60 ATA), then pressurization is continued using pure helium until the desired depth is reached, which can range anywhere from 300 to 1,000 feet. They then remain at pressure for periods up to two weeks, living in a deck decompression chamber at the desired storage pressure, and commuting to work using a personnel-transfer capsule also pressurized to the storage pressure.

The personnel transfer capsule "PTC" is a diving bell which is mated on to the deck-decompression chamber, allowing the divers to enter it under the storage pressure. The hatches are then shut and the diving bell detached from the deck-decompression chamber (DDC), and the divers lowered to the working depth. There, the pressure within the bell is equalized with the pressure outside and the hatch is opened at the bottom, allowing the divers to exit and go about their work tethered to the diving bell by an umbilical cord which supplies their breathing gas, hot water to heat their wet suits, and the telephone cable. Working at such extreme depths is called saturation diving since, within about 36 hours of continuous exposure, no more inert gas will go into solution in the diver's tissues. For this reason, decompression time is the same whether the divers stay for two days or two weeks. Saturation diving avoids daily decompressions which would be prohibitive in length at those very deep depths. Subsequent decompression is at the rate of about 100 feet (30 meters) per 24 hours when their task is completed.

## NORMOXIC MIXES

Normoxic mixes equal 0.21 atmospheres of oxygen under all circumstances, no matter what the pressure. This would equate to an oxygen partial pressure of 160 mmHg. Thus, we see that the diver pressurized with pure helium to 198 feet (60 meters) is breathing a normoxic mix, even though the actual percentage of gas he is inspiring is only 3% of all the gases in the chamber. It can also be seen that the diver pressurized to 33 feet with compressed air, even though 21% of the gases he is breathing is oxygen, is not breathing a normoxic mix, but breathing an effective percentage of 42%. Our lungs are "molecule counters" and are interested only in the number of molecules striking the alveolar membrane at any given time; they are not interested in what percentage of oxygen is in the mix. Oxygen monitors are also "molecule counters." We can adjust a portable oxygen monitor to read 21% oxygen at sea level, but when we take it into a hyperbaric chamber and compress to 2 atmospheres, it will read 42% because of the doubled density of the oxygen molecules. Likewise, if we take the same monitor adjusted to read 21% at sea level and take it into the chamber pressurized with pure helium to a depth of 198 feet (60 meters), it will continue to read 21%, even though the actual percentage in the mix is only 3%. The effective percentage is found by multiplying the actual percentage times the number of atmospheres of pressure it is under.

## DECOMPRESSING WHILE BREATHING A NORMOXIC MIX

We have discovered that one can breathe 3% oxygen quite safely at a pressure of 7 atmospheres. Now let us examine what will happen when we begin to decompress. As the pressure is lowered, the helium is vented from the chamber, as well as the nitrogen and the oxygen; thus, if we were to decompress directly to the surface, on arrival at the surface, we would be breathing a true 3% oxygen mix equal to only 23 mmHg. Obviously, this is insufficient to support life. For this reason, when decompressing after one has been using a normoxic mix at depth, oxygen must be continually injected into the chamber to maintain a suitable inspired partial pressure of oxygen.

## BUNSEN'S SOLUBILITY COEFFICIENT

Bunsen's solubility coefficient determines the amount of gas in solution in a liquid. From Henry's Law we learned that at equilibrium, the partial pressure of nitrogen in a cup of water or a cup of oil equals 600 mmHg at sea level, if it has been equilibrated with air. However, if we were to count the number of nitrogen molecules present in the cup of oil, we would discover that there are 5 times as many nitrogen molecules in the oil as there are in the water, despite their partial pressures being identical. This is because nitrogen is five times more soluble in oil than it is in water. Bunsen's solubility coefficient has been determined for all combinations of gases and liquids. Multiplying the partial pressure by the coefficient will indicate the amount of gas actually dissolved. Therefore, it is important to remember that the partial pressure is not indicative of the amount of gas actually in solution.

## PHYSICS OF WHOLE BODY SQUEEZE

The classic deep-sea diving rig consisting of a rigid copper helmet and breast plate connected to a flexible rubberized canvas dress was in use by the navies of the world, as well as commercial divers for 150 years. It was a very safe suit as if offered the diver good protection from cold as well as from pollutants in busy harbors. One potentially fatal accident could occur with this suit if the diver suddenly fell more than a few feet under water or if air pressure was lost in the helmet. The disparity between the water pressure outside the suit and the lesser pressure within the suit would compress the flexible portion of the dress and tend to force the diver up into the helmet. The pressure disparity could produce catastrophic results because of the large flexible area of the dress. Assume that a diver has a total body surface area of two square meters. This translates to an area of 3,100 square inches. If 25% of the area were taken up by the rigid helmet and breast plate, which leaves 2,325 square inches of flexible (and thus compressible) dress. The water pressure at 30 feet (9 meters) is 13.35 pounds per square inch. Multiplying 2,325 sq. in. by 13.35 pounds gives us 31,039 pounds or 15.5 tons. This would be the force driving the body up into the helmet. In the days before helmets were equipped with non-return valves which checked backward flow out of the helmet, a diver in New York's East River was killed when his air supply was inadvertently opened to atmospheric pressure at the surface. At the time he was working on a sunken oil barge in only 30 feet of water. The softer parts of his body were found twelve feet up the air hose.

## PHYSICS OF SHALLOW WATER BLACKOUT

There are actually two types of shallow water blackout, one purely physiological and the other dependent on physics.

In type one, the individual attempts to swim under water as far as he can while breath-holding. Typically, he takes many deep breaths to blow off his $CO_2$ and then with a maximal inspiration, begins his swim just below the surface. Because of his muscular exercise, his arterial $PO_2$ drops below levels capable of sustaining consciousness before his $CO_2$ levels have risen high enough to cause him to breathe and he becomes unconscious. This type is purely physiological in origin.

In type two, the individual is again breath-holding, but with a full inspiration dives to a much greater depth which would be typical of a spear fisherman. Let us assume that the partial pressure of oxygen in the man's alveolae is 160 mmHg at the surface, ignoring water vapor and $CO_2$. If he instantly were to arrive at 33 feet, the compression of his lungs in accordance with Boyle's law would halve their volume. Also in accordance with Boyle's law, the oxygen partial pressure would be doubled to 320 mmHg. This represents a surfeit of oxygen, and he could very happily function until the oxygen was metabolized down, let us say, a partial pressure of 76 mmHg. On return to the surface, the partial pressure would precipitously drop to 38 mmHg, which would most likely render him unconscious shortly before his arrival. This type of shallow water blackout is dependent on the physics of Boyle's law.

## CHARACTERISTICS OF INERT GASES

### Nitrogen

Most diving is carried out using compressed air. Under pressure, the nitrogen in the air goes into solution in the tissues where it remains completely inert; it does not enter into any chemical bond or reaction. If one remains long enough at a depth deeper than 33 feet (10 meters) nitrogen will accumulate to the point where subsequent decompression, if carried out precipitously, will cause the evolution of gas bubbles within the tissue and the syndrome of decompression illness. Actually, bubbles form during every decompression from depth, but they only become large enough to cause symptoms when the depth is greater than 33 feet. The other effect of nitrogen at depth is nitrogen narcosis. Symptoms of nitrogen narcosis begin to appear at depths deeper than 100 feet (30 meters) and become essentially incapacitating at depths greater than 300 feet (90 meters). Nitrogen narcosis was discovered by Behnke in the mid 1930s when he found that nitrogen behaved like an aliphatic anesthetic. The anesthetic potency of any aliphatic anesthetic can be predicted by its oil/water solubility ratio as described by the Meyer-Overton hypothesis. Meyer and Overton, at the turn of the century, discovered that any aliphatic anesthetic exerts its potency in direct proportion to its solubility in oil or lipids. Using the Meyer-Overton hypothesis, nitrogen's anesthetic potency appears exactly where it would be predicted. Heavier gases such as argon, krypton, and xenon have even higher lipid solubility's and are, therefore, extremely narcotic under pressure. Neon is less potent than nitrogen and helium exerts little narcotic effect since it is not very soluble in lipid.

The exact mechanism whereby an inert gas that is soluble in lipid exerts its anesthetic effect remained a mystery for many years, until Peter Bennett discovered that it causes edema of the neuron cell membrane and disrupts the protein channels that regulate the egress and entrance of sodium and potassium into the cell during firing and repolarization. In nitrogen narcosis, the neuron cell membrane becomes much more permeable to ion transport. Because little could be done to counteract this effect, it was long thought that diving would have to be limited to depths of less than 300 feet (90 meters).

## Helium

Helium diving was suggested by the physiologist Elihu Thompson as early as 1919 because it had only a fraction of the density of air and would therefore be easier to breathe. Nitrogen narcosis was not understood at that time. The Royal Navy and the U.S. Navy experimented with helium, but found that severe decompression sickness could result, even with extra long decompressions. Helium diving was put "very much on the back burner" by 1924, Admiral Momsen recalled. After nitrogen narcosis was discovered by Albert Behnke, Edgar End, a 26-year-old intern at the Milwaukee County General Hospital, thought it would be useful to try helium for diving. Since helium defuses rapidly, he reckoned that it would come out of solution rapidly, and that deeper decompression stops would be required, much deeper than those used for air diving. Accordingly, he constructed a decompression table which he tested upon himself in the recompression chamber located in the basement of the county emergency hospital. He suffered no ill effects and was able to interest Max Nohl, a Milwaukee diver, in trying this gas.

Nohl had constructed a self-contained diving rig eminently suited to using precious, donated helium in a closed circuit. Using only two large "H" cylinders of helium, they completed work-up dives; then with the remaining helium, Nohl descended 420 feet into Lake Michigan in December of 1937 to break the previous world depth record of 306 feet. Helium diving was taken up by the U.S. Navy, after End proved it was feasible, and soon put it to use when the submarine *USS Squalus* sank in 240 feet of water on sea trials in 1939. Thirty-six survivors were successfully rescued after a helium diver replaced the broken down-haul cable for the rescue bell. A previous diver, breathing air, became so disoriented he was unable to carry out this task.

For the next 15 years, only the U.S. Navy had helium-diving capabilities. In 1956, the Royal Navy set another world record of 600 feet in the open sea using helium, but discovered a brand new phenomenon. Symptoms consisted of uncontrollable tremors, nausea, "periods of micro-sleep," akin to petit mal seizures, and loss of the alpha waves on the EEG. Initially labeled "the helium shakes," it was later termed high pressure nervous syndrome, "HPNS." This new phenomenon was encountered when depths of 600 feet were reached. This barrier seemed impenetrable until Peter Bennett, working at the Royal Naval Physiological Research Laboratory in Alverstoke, England, took two divers to a simulated depth of 1,500 feet of sea water in a dry chamber. He did this by using an extremely slow compression that took six days. The French soon eclipsed this record by going to 1,700 feet; then 1972, to a depth record of 2,001 feet. However, despite slow compressions, the French divers were nearly incapacitated by HPNS at maximum depth.

Bennett later moved to Duke University where he continued his experimentation with ultra-deep diving. There it was postulated that helium had the opposite effect of nitrogen and actually compressed the neuron cell membrane, slowing the transport of ions across the membrane during firing and repolarization. He noted that helium seemed to block the effects of normal gas anesthetics, or the "helium reversal effect". For example it was impossible to anesthetize someone with halothane when breathing helium at 700 feet. Bennett found that adding back 10% nitrogen to the inert moiety of the breathing gas blocked the effects of HPNS. Using this discovery, he was able to pressurize dogs to a depth of 1,000 feet in one-half hour with no apparent ill effects. Soon, his divers at Duke set a new world depth record of 2,250 feet in the chamber. With these extreme pressures, however, even the relatively light gas helium was quite dense when compressed, and it was found that the work of breathing consumed half of all the calories expended as work. Another factor that became important was that helium under pressure is an excellent conductor of heat, and unless the breathing gas was pre-warmed while diving in cold water to great depths, the diver could die of hypothermia secondary to respiratory heat loss within a matter of minutes.

## THE USE OF HYDROGEN GAS

During World War II, a few German submarines sank off the Swedish coast in very deep water, and the Swedes were interested in recovering code books and the electric torpedoes in these boats. However, the depths called for the use of helium. Possessing no helium within Sweden, Arne Zetterstrom experimented, using a mixture of hydrogen and oxygen for the breathing gas. He found that when mixed with 3% oxygen or less, the hydrogen-oxygen mixture was not explosive. To use this gas, he descended to 60 meters breathing air, and then thoroughly flushed his suit and the supply hoses with a mixture of 97% nitrogen and 3% oxygen. Following this he shifted to 97% hydrogen and 3% oxygen. Successful dives were made in the Baltic Sea in the summer of 1945 to a maximum depth of 526 feet.

Unfortunately, Zetterstrom was killed in a winch accident which had nothing to do with his breathing gas and further experimentation with hydrogen in Sweden was terminated. Hydrogen was reinvestigated by Peter Edel in New Orleans under an Office of Naval Research contract in the 1970s and also by William Fife at Texas A and M University. Hydrogen-oxygen mixtures or hydrox apparently caused no ill effects on dogs and human volunteers. Soon it was discovered that even though hydrogen was the lightest of the gases, being half the weight of helium, it possessed a narcotic effect, based on its oil/water solubility ratio of about 25% of that of nitrogen. This fortuitous finding was capitalized on by the French who mixed helium and hydrogen with small amounts of oxygen to dive to very extreme depths. The hydrogen supplanted nitrogen as the antagonist of HPNS. Using a mixture of 45% hydrogen, 54% helium, and 1% oxygen, or "hydreliox", Comex, a diving company, was able to make a record-breaking 1,700-foot, open sea dive. That French company now holds the world record for a dry chamber dive using hydreliox, of 2,300 feet, set in May, 1985.

## CHAMBER SAFETY CONSIDERATIONS

It seems appropriate to include in this chapter on diving and hyperbaric physics something of chamber construction and the various codes which apply.

### The American Society of Mechanical Engineers Code

Should a chamber rupture or a door carry away, the results would be catastrophic due to the cumulative effect of large areas exposed to pressure. For example, a door measuring 36 inches by 72 inches (91 cm x 182 cm) exposed to 3 atmospheres would have a total force exerted on it of 38 tons. For this reason, chambers built in the United States are constructed in accordance with the American Society of Mechanical Engineers (ASME) Code, Section 8, Division 2, for unfired, pressure vessels. This code calls for a safety factor of 4 to 1 between burst pressure and operating pressure. In Europe, similar codes are enforced by Lloyds and by Det Norske Veritas. The reason for the 4 to 1 safety factor (or more recently 3 to 1 in Europe) is to prevent weakening of the chamber through cycle fatigue. Whenever a chamber is pressurized, it is actually "inflated" due to stretching of the steel or aluminum. It was found that by having a 4 to 1 safety factor, the stretching effect on pressurization would not be enough to engender cycle fatigue. Both aluminum and steel chambers are built to a 4 to 1 safety factor in the United States. The chambers which are fashioned from plastic cylinders are required to have a 20 to 1 safety factor since plastic is inherently more elastic and the safety factor has to be greater to prevent stretching and subsequent cycle fatigue. Following manufacture, chambers are given a hydrostatic test to 1.5 times their normal working pressure to test their integrity. After the initial hydrostatic tests, there is no requirement for repeated hydrostatic testing.

Gas cylinders normally pressurized to 2,250 psig (approximately 150 kg/cm$^2$) must be hydrostatically tested every 5 years. This is because they are subjected to more repeated trauma, rough handling and possible corrosion. During hydrostatic testing of cylinders, their volume is monitored and it must return to within 10% of the original volume within 3 minutes following depressurization, or the cylinder is condemned.

Following a hydrostatic test of the chamber, no welding, cutting, or boring of holes in the chamber hull is permitted without voiding the hydrostatic test. Welding may cause nitrogen embrittlement at the edge of the weld, weakening the chamber, and the new hole, termed a "nozzle" by chamber manufacturers, will present a new stress point. More recently, ASME has added a new code for pressure vessels for human occupancy (PVHO). The PVHO code gives specifications for windows, which now must be plastic, as well as many other specifics of chambers designed for this purpose.

### The National Fire Protection Association Code

The National Fire Protection Association (NFPA) also has a code for hyperbaric chambers which undergoes periodic updating. It specifies characteristics of fire protection systems, electrical wiring, and other hazardous items involved in chamber operation. When the NFPA code was first written for clinical hyperbaric chambers in 1970, surgery was being performed and flammable anesthetics were a possibility. For this reason the

NFPA classified the chamber atmosphere as potentially explosive. With that in mind, the regulations for wiring and electrical equipment that could be used in the chamber were restrictive in the extreme. Recently, this code has been revised and the chamber atmosphere has been classified as hazardous, not explosive, because of the absence of any explosive or flammable gases. It is hazardous because of the increased oxygen pressure. The multi-place chamber wiring code under NFPA has been undergoing drastic revision to reflect this and now it is much more practical.

Fire marshals vigorously enforce the NFPA code and it is only prudent to be sure that the entire chamber facility is in strict compliance with the NFPA code. Of particular importance is that oxygen levels within the multiplace chamber must be monitored continuously to prevent their rising over 23%. Even at atmospheric pressure, a rise in the oxygen level from 21 to 28% will double the burning rate. At hyperbaric pressures with oxygen over 30%, it may be impossible to extinguish a fire. It is especially important that the deluge system required by NFPA within the chamber be tested at monthly intervals, and the results of the tests logged. To avoid flooding the chamber with each test, suitable bypass systems should be incorporated in the design. Hard experience has shown that with inactivity, the valves for fire suppression systems can corrode and stick shut when actuation is attempted.

## WINDOWS

The design life of plastic windows for PVHO chambers has been defined by ASME to be ten years or ten thousand cycles. The original interpretation of this rule by ASME was that the windows had to be changed at the end of design life. However, recent experience has shown that there is little, if any, deterioration in plastic windows that are properly maintained, have not been subjected to trauma, or exposed to ultraviolet light. For this reason, it is left up to the user to determine the service life of the window, which may far exceed the design life. Now, the user determines whether windows need replacing, depending on the type of service, the condition of the window, and environmental factors. Unlike glass windows, when a plastic window is beginning to fail it develops "crazing" or the appearance of fine cracks within the plastic before exploding. Should crazing be seen in the plastic shell of a monoplace chamber (where incidentally, it is classified as a "window" in the ASME code), it must be immediately taken out of service.

## SUGGESTED FURTHER READING

- Bove, AA and Davis JC (Eds.) Diving Medicine, 3rd Edition 1997 WB Saunders Company, Philadelphia, Best Publishing Company, Flagstaff

- Bennett, PB and Elliott, DH (Eds.) The Physiology and Medicine of Diving 4th Edition 1993 WB Saunders Company, Philadelphia, Best Publishing Company, Flagstaff

- ASME PVHO-1 Published by the American Society of Mechanical Engineers, United Engineering Center, 345 East 47th Street, New York, NY 10017

- NFPA 99, Chapter 19 Published by the National Fire Protection Association, 1 Battery March Park, P.O. Box 9101, Quincy, MA 02269-9904

- UHMS Report—Monoplace Hyperbaric Chamber Safety Guidelines

- UHMS Report—Guidelines For Clinical Multiplace Hyperbaric Facilities

The UMHS Reports above are published by the Undersea and Hyperbaric Medical Society, 21 West Colony Place, Suite 280, Durham, NC 27705

## NOTES

CHAPTER 3

# THE PHYSIOLOGIC EFFECTS OF HYPERBARIC OXYGENATION

## CHAPTER THREE OVERVIEW

# THE PHYSIOLOGIC EFFECTS OF HYPERBARIC OXYGENATION

*Christer E. Hammarlund*

## INTRODUCTION

There are only two basic effects of hyperbaric oxygenation on the human body: the mechanical effect which is useful in reducing bubble size (following diving accidents or the iatrogenic introduction of intravascular air), and the effects of an increased partial pressure of oxygen (which is multifaceted depending on physiologic or pathophysiologic conditions in organs and tissues).

Pressures much higher than normal invest oxygen with properties not observed at atmospheric pressure. Under these circumstances oxygen typically behaves as a drug with specific indications and side effects.

## MECHANICAL EFFECTS OF PRESSURE

### Effects on Bubble Size

Bubbles and gas-containing cavities within the body are subject to the mechanical effects of changing pressure. These effects follow Boyle's law, which states that volume is inversely proportional to the absolute pressure. Volume is changed in a geometric progression related to the pressure change; large reductions take place near the surface, with subsequent reductions becoming smaller at high pressure. The mechanical effects of pressure are also the source of unwanted barotrauma in the form of middle-ear distress, sinus squeeze, lung squeeze during compression (any significant pressure differences will cause blood vessels in the area of lower pressure to distend to equalize pressures, causing middle-ear bleeding, sinus bleeding, or pulmonary bleeding associated with squeeze), and burst lung if the person holds his/her breath during decompression. If a patient is suffering from gaseous distension of the bowel, compression in the chamber will ease his discomfort while the inhalation of oxygen will establish a high gradient for the removal of nitrogen from the distended gut. Gas trapped in the bowel decreases by approximately 50% when a patient breathes oxygen over a six-hour period at two atmospheres absolute (15, 16).

In gas gangrene, if gas bubbles produce tissue distension, compression in the chamber will reduce bubble size as well as tissue pressure, permitting better perfusion. Pain is also reduced when this occurs.

In decompression sickness and air embolism, essentially all of the bubbles are intravascular. Both nitrogen and helium diffuse very rapidly through the cytoplasm of the cell to the nearest capillary. It is there that the problem arises in terms of gas transport. The capillary blood can only carry a limited amount of inert gas subject to the constraints of Bunsen's solubility coefficient at 37 degrees C. If more gas is presented to the vasculature from the tissues than the blood can carry in solution, it must inevitably bubble. When bubbles form, vastly greater amounts of gas can be carried, up to the point where the bubbles become too large and begin to significantly activate platelets and impinge on vessel walls. When a gas bubble is compressed to six atmospheres (6 ATA), its volume decreases to 16% of what it was at the surface. A spherical bubble, however, decreases its diameter by only approximately one half at 6 ATA. This fact may initially seem discouraging to anyone treating decompression sickness since, with each increasing atmosphere beyond 6 ATA, the reduction in bubble diameter becomes even more meager (68). It must be remembered, however, that the only kind of bubble that does not mechanically injure the bends victim is spherical. As long as a bubble remains spherical, we can infer that it is not touching any surface. The spherical bubble becomes a pure carrier of inert gas in the blood stream and thus can become beneficial. It does, however, retain its ability to cause platelet aggregation and distort plasma proteins.

The only bubbles that are mechanically detrimental are those that are cylindrical in shape, tending to block blood vessels. On recompression to three atmospheres, these bubbles are reduced in length by two thirds; at six atmospheres, bubbles are reduced to one-sixth of their original length. This represents a significant change in bubble architecture and may cause the bubble to assume a spherical form and move on. The vessels become continually larger returning to the lung, where the bubble is then trapped and eliminated by gas diffusion through its wall. The ultimate mechanism for bubble removal occurs when spherical bubbles become microscopically small. Surface-tension forces, which cause bubble collapse, reach many thousands of dynes per square centimeter. At that point, the bubble either collapses and disappears or shrinks to a nucleus.

## Effects of Oxygen Solubility in Plasma

Placing the patient in a hyperbaric chamber raises oxygen tensions 10 to 13 times above their normal level when the patient is breathing 2.8 ATA oxygen; six volumes percent (6 ml per 100 ml of plasma) of oxygen are dissolved in the plasma - the mean extraction rate of oxygen in the body. This is a simple physical event. The plasma is thus capable of carrying enough oxygen to meet the needs of the body's tissues. The overall effect is that the hemoglobin is still fully saturated on the venous side.

Depending, however, on the physiologic or pathophysiologic status of the patient, the effects of high oxygen pressure on the functions of various organs, structures, and biochemical reactions, can be myriad. These include suppression of alpha-toxin production in gas gangrene, enhancement of leucocyte-killing activity, decrease in white cell adherence to capillary walls, vasoconstriction in normal vessels, restoration of fibroblast growth and collagen production, stimulation of superoxide dismutase production, preservation of adenosine triphosphate in cell membranes with secondary reduction in tissue edema, suppression of selected immune responses (experimental allergic encephalomyelitis in the guinea pig), enhancement of osteoclast activity, increased capillary proliferation, decreased flexibility of the ocular lens (visual changes), suppression of surfactant production in the lung, termination of lipid peroxidation in CO poisoning, hastening removal of CO from hemoglobin, etc.

These physiologic events which assume varying degrees of importance during treatment, depending on the disease process being managed, will be discussed in more detail below, and in other chapters.

## Effects of $CO_2$ Retention

During hyperbaric oxygen breathing, the hemoglobin is still fully saturated on the venous side, effectively blocking $CO_2$ transport by hemoglobin. This rarely causes any problems because carbon dioxide is 50 times more soluble than oxygen and is buffered by bicarbonate, or is physically dissolved and transported in the blood plasma. It causes the pH to shift only slightly to the acid side.

## EFFECTS OF ELEVATED PARTIAL PRESSURES OF OXYGEN

The clinical use of hyperbaric oxygenation is limited to a maximal partial pressure of 3 ATA oxygen. Exceeding this pressure gives no advantage and increases the toxic effect of oxygen. Oxygen behaves like any other drug: too little is not enough and too much will cause harm.

## Reduction of Blood Flow in Hyperoxic Tissues

Bird (8) found a 20% flow reduction in limb circulation in man during oxygen breathing, but suggested that this vasoconstriction is well compensated due to the increased amount of oxygen dissolved in the plasma. Lindblom et al. (68), studied the influence of oxygen on perfused capillary density and capillary red cell velocity in rabbit skeletal muscle. They showed that closure of normal capillaries is probably related to the level of oxygen, but they were unable to say whether or not injured capillaries react in a similar way.

Ohta et al. (80) measured cerebral blood flow (CBF) during HBO in healthy volunteers. They found that up to 2 ATA, CBF gradually decreased in accordance with the elevation of the arterial $pO_2$. Above this pressure, the CBF showed a tendency to increase, but normalized when HBO was terminated. They stated that too much oxygen disturbs the oxygen regulatory response of CBF.

Hordnes et al. (46) studied the effect of high ambient pressure and oxygen tension on organ blood flow in conscious, trained rats. They found decreases in blood flow to the myocardium, kidney, brain, the ocular globe, and splanchnic areas.

HBO changes hemodynamics in man, as shown by Villanuci et al. (111). Cardiac output decreases (24 – 35%) as well as the left ventricular index (11–30%), whereas afterload increases by 30 to 60%. These results are in agreement with earlier studies.

The documented vasoconstrictive effect in various organs rendered hyperoxic, and the changed hemodynamics due to HBO might change the traditional view of optimal oxygen pressures for treatment of decompression sickness. Anderson et al. (2) found that hyperoxia induced vasoconstriction and reduced tissue perfusion, resulting in a slowed $N_2$ washout -8.9% and -16.9% for 2.0 and 2.5 ATA $O_2$ respectively, compared to controls at 0.2 ATA. Hypoxia (0.12 ATA $O_2$) resulted in a significant increase in $N_2$ washout (9.4%) compared to controls. This is in contrast to the elimination of helium during the decompression phase. Helium washout seems to be more insensitive to the oxygen induced vasoconstriction (57).

In a rather unique study looking at cure rates for different treatment tables, it seems as if early HBO combined with high pressure is important when treating Type II decompression sickness (DCS). In that study by Lee et al. (66) on 374 very severe cases of Type II DCS, 75% of them delayed more than 48 hours, the cure rate using table 6A, which incorporates an initial excursion to 6 atmospheres was 51% (n=98). Previous cases treated with oxygen at a maximum pressure of 2.8 atmospheres produced a cure rate of only 8.3% Adding three more stops to Table 6A (120 ft for 1 minute, 80 ft for 8 minutes and 70 ft for 15 minutes) gave a cure rate of 59.9% (n=177). The extended table was named 6A1. Using a table allowing early HBO using 40% oxygen at 6 atmospheres (Table 6A1M) had a cure rate of 70.7% (n=99). They used nitrogen as the inert gas, but now helium is preferred to avoid an increase in nitrogen load.  Gorman and co-workers (29) are carrying out controlled studies in the treatment of decompression illness, comparing the relative efficacy of oxygen breathing at 2.0 versus 2.8 atmospheres using nitrox and heliox mixtures.

## No Reduction of Blood Flow in Hypoxic Tissues

One of the major objections to possible effects of HBO treatment in clinical practice has been the generalized vasoconstriction caused by oxygen breathing, as there had been no studies to show that hypoxic areas were not affected in the same way.

Hammarlund et al. (35) using laser Doppler flowmetry, studied the effects of oxygen breathing on the dermal microcirculation in healthy volunteers. They found a dose-dependent vasoconstriction in the skin in response to oxygen breathing. In a separate experiment, a patient with a chronic venous leg ulcer was tested. He responded to oxygen breathing with the expected vasoconstriction in the fingertip, while the blood flow in the diseased skin near the ulcer remained unchanged. Following successful treatment, the dermal vascular response to hyperoxia was normalized in the lower limb. The authors suggested that the dermal flow reduction observed in healthy volunteers is not a general reaction, but rather a physiologic response to hyperoxia. Presence of the reaction might thus indicate that the inhaled oxygen has reached the tissues and caused hyperoxia.

In another human study, Dooley and Mehm (19) found that HBO at 2.0 and 3.0 ATA results in an increase in peripheral tissue-oxygen delivery, despite vasoconstrictive reductions in peripheral (calf) blood flow.

HBO treatment improves distal microvascular perfusion as measured by laser Doppler flowmetry in ischemic skin flaps in the rat. This effect is observed for HBO treatment given either during or following eight hours of global ischemia (117).

Sirsjö and Lewis (89) evaluated the effect of HBO in post-ischemic skeletal muscle in the rat. They found no difference in blood flow between the ischemic groups after 1 hour of reperfusion (40% and 30% respectively of the control group), but after 4.5 hours reperfusion, the blood flow was significantly increased in the HBO group compared with the untreated group (66% and 40% respectively of the control group). These results are in agreement with Zamboni et al. (118). Zamboni and co-workers used an intravital microscopy preparation with a transilluminated rat gracilis muscle as a model. The control group showed no significant changes in arteriolar diameter as did the no-ischemia HBO group. In the four-hour ischemia group, the initial vasodilatation following ischemia was followed at one hour by a severe vasoconstriction. The HBO-treated, four-hour ischemia group, however, maintained the initial vasodilatation for the three-hour reperfusion period.

Blood supply to an acute dermal wound is not only maintained, but actually increased during hyperoxemia, as shown by Hammarlund et al. (38). The vasoconstrictive response in intact skin to oxygen breathing with a concomitant increase in systemic blood pressure results in a redistribution of blood flow to the wound where tone is already released through local mechanisms (the Robin Hood effect). The redistribution of blood flow to hypoxic areas during oxygen breathing has been confirmed in a clinical setting by the use of a Laser Doppler imaging device (39). See Figures 1 thru 3.

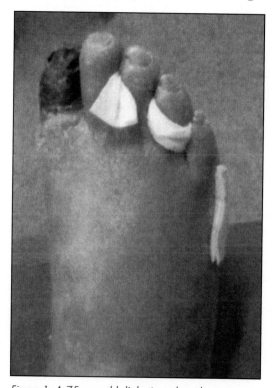

*Figure 1. A 75-year-old diabetic male with uremia.*

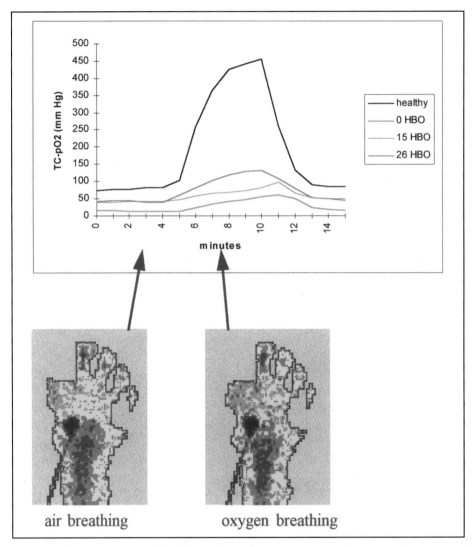

Figure 2. The male in Figure 1 breathing 1 ATA oxygen during minute 4 to 10 (wash-in phase of oxygen). From minute 10, the wash-out phase of oxygen.

## Increase in Healing of Hypoxic Wounds

Lactate synthesized by macrophages is the most fundamental trigger stimulating fibroblasts to make collagen (48). Fibroblasts cannot synthesize collagen without a reasonable amount of oxygen, which is required for the post-translational processing of collagen necessary for its crosslinking. There is a delicate balance of vessel growth and collagen deposition that is easily upset when host circulatory and nutritional support fails. Because macrophages release lactate, even while well oxygenated, some stimulus to collagen synthesis remains, even during hyperoxygenation.

Tensile strength of wounds, collagen deposition, and the rate at which they close a dead space are affected by the amount of available oxygen. The decrement due to hypoxia is significant, and so is the improvement in ischemic

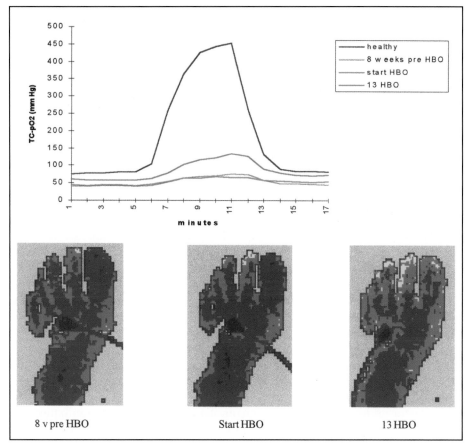

*Figure 3. A 50-year-old female diabetic. Small necrosis on lateral side of dig 2, left foot. 1 ATA oxygen breathing during minute 5 to 11 (wash-in phase of oxygen). From minute 11, the wash-out phase of oxygen. Treatment shows increased microcirculation from 13 HBO sessions.*

wounds with clinically obtainable hyperoxia. The increment relates to faster rather than excessive healing. This may seem a paradox unless one accepts that hypoxic macrophages drive repair. When hypoxia is no longer a feature of the central dead space, healing stops and thus is not allowed to become excessive. Because angiogenesis is accelerated in ischemic wounds when extra oxygen is supplied by the circulation, the time to healing is shortened (48).

Poor perfusion and decreased oxygen tension increases infectability, as illustrated by a series of experiments on skin flaps in dogs (54). One myocutaneous flap (with excellent blood flow and tissue oxygenation) and the other a random pattern flap (with progressively poorer perfusion and oxygenation from base to tip), were elevated simultaneously. Bacteria injected into the flaps survived, multiplied, and caused visible lesions in inverse relation to both blood flow and oxygen supply. The myocutaneous flap, which was perfused as well as normal skin, resisted infection equally well. On the other hand, the distal portion of random-pattern flaps, where perfusion was low and tissue $pO_2$ had fallen below 30 mmHg, was literally destroyed by infection. Necrosis was worst where blood flow and oxygenation were least.

"Contrary to years of belief, there is a physiology of wound healing, not just a biochemistry," as noted by Hunt (48).

Live bacteria, including *S. aureus* and *E. coli*, were injected into the dermis of guinea pig backs (61). Heat-killed bacteria in the same concentration were injected as a control in order to determine the influence of bacterial protein on the lesion size. Half of the animals were injected with ampicillin 6 mg intraperitoneally. The inoculated animals were then caged in controlled environments and breathed 45%, 21%, or 12% oxygen. The guinea pigs were examined at 24 and 48 hours, and the dimensions of the infectious necroses that developed at each inoculation site were measured. The results revealed that the effect of raising oxygen tension was marginally superior to that of giving antibiotics. The most important finding was that hyperoxia and antibiotics were additive, so that only rarely was there evidence of infection seen in animals treated with both hyperoxia and antibiotics, while every injection site became infected in hypoxic animals that had not received any antibiotics.

HBO exposure could have important consequences for cellular activities essential for effective wound healing, such as migration of cells into the wound, and control of cell function, as shown by Roberts and Harding (86). They found an increased synthesis of hyaluronic acid and proteoglycans by fibroblasts from wounds and normal skin exposed to HBO.

Increase in endothelial cell proliferation is seen after 15 minutes of HBO, while fibroblasts require 120 minutes to produce a response (lasting for 72 hours after exposure) as shown by Tompach et al. (106). They exposed cultured endothelial cells and fibroblasts to HBO. A second exposure on the same day or an increase in pressure from 2.4 to 4.0 ATA did not enhance the proliferative response. Hehenberger (45B) and coworkers have shown *in vitro* effects of HBO on proliferation of human fibroblasts from normal skin and from chronic foor ulcers in non-insulin-dependent diabetics. A 1-hour exposure to HBO increased the proliferation in both groups. They also found a dose-dependent stimulatory effect, with a peak increase in normal fibroblasts at 250 kPa, and at 200 kPa in diabetic fibroblasts. They speculated that HBO additionally might activate mitogenic growth factors.

Ischemia intensifies the impairment of healing seen in old age, but can be reversed by HBO, as shown by Quirinia and Viidik (84). They studied the healing of normal incisional wounds and ischemic flap wounds in young and old rats, together with the effect of HBO treatment on day 0–3 after wound making. Treatment of ischemia with hyperbaric oxygenation was much more effective in old animals, despite the fact that it also had a pronounced effect in young animals. In a similar study by Uhl et al. (109), HBO accelerated normal wound healing by 2 days and ischemic wound healing by 4.4 days. Laser Doppler data showed no difference in tissue blood flow between treated and untreated animals. They concluded that the beneficial effect was not associated with changes in microvascular perfusion and, therefore, probably was due to high arteriolar oxygen content and oxygen diffusion.

The addition of growth factors to HBO treatment produced a synergistic total reversal of the wound-healing deficit produced by ischemia in a study by Zhao et al. (122). They studied the influence of HBO, platelet-derived growth factor-BB (PDGF-BB), and transforming growth factor-beta 1

(TGF-beta 1) on the healing rate of ischemic wounds. They used a noncontractile, dermal-ulcer, standardized model in the rabbit ear and showed that HBO alone increased the production of new granulation tissue by approximately 100% at 7 days, without significantly affecting new epithelial growth. In contrast, PDGF-BB and TGF-beta 1 each increased the new granulation tissue volume by greater than 200% in 7 days and also had a significant effect on new epithelial growth. However, the combination of HBO with either of the growth factors has a synergistic effect.

Thirty HBO sessions in 6 weeks caused significant reduction of the wounds at week 4, and at week 6, in a randomized double-blind study of chronic, nondiabetic leg ulcers by Hammarlund and Sundberg (37). They concluded that HBO may be used as a valuable adjunct to conventional therapies when nondiabetic wounds do not heal.

HBO significantly reduced diabetic wound size in a small, non-randomized prospective study by Zamboni et al. (121). The result was in coherence with an earlier open study by Baroni et al. (5). These results should serve as a basis for prospective, randomized, double-blind, controlled studies to definitively evaluate the effect of HBO on the healing of diabetic foot wounds.

In humans, HBO is a well-known therapy for radiation-induced damage to bone and soft tissues (30-32, 44, 53, 71, 74, 112), causing new capillary growth.

## Inhibition of *Clostridium perfringens*

HBO inhibits the production of clostridial alpha-toxin, a lecithinase, which destroys cell membranes and increases capillary permeability (110).

HBO also acts directly on *Clostridium perfringens* (CP) and has an indirect effect through polymorphonuclear leucocyte (PMN) killing. Oxygen is only bacteriostatic at 150 mmHg. Adams et al. (1) concluded in their study that increased oxygen tensions may only have a small direct role in the killing of CP. A more important role was the indirect effect of increasing oxygen tension on the PMN killing of CP.

## Reduction of Carbon Monoxide (CO) Toxicity

Assessing the efficacy of HBO in CO poisoning is difficult. Understanding of how much tissue hypoxia is necessary to increase morbidity in CO poisoning is limited. Ultraviolet absorption spectra show progression of lipid peroxidation over a 24-hour period subsequent to CO poisoning, but Thom (101, 102) showed that HBO, only when administered at a pressure greater than 2 ATA, prevents brain lipid peroxidation in a CO-poisoned rat model. Cho and Yun (13) found that the fetuses of CO-poisoned rats treated with HBO did not show any significant growth retardation, compared to controls who sustained significant damage during pregnancy. They exposed primiparous Sprague-Dawley rats for 1 hour to a CO level of 1,800 ppm or 2 hours to a CO level of 1,400 ppm, resulting in COHgb levels of 68-72% on day 11 of gestation.

Brown and Piantadosi (12) exposed anesthetized rats to CO, produced 70% COHgb levels and caused profound reductions in blood pressure and the brain redox state. After CO exposure had stopped, blood pressure recovered, but COHgb fell more rapidly at 2.5 ATA O$_2$ than at 1.0 ATA, but the two groups were similar physiologically at 45 and 90 minutes. Cytochrome redox state, however, recovered to only 75–80% of control after 90 minutes at 1 ATA, while it recovered 95% at 2.5 ATA after 90 minutes. The [PCr], [ATP], and pH continued to decline for 45 minutes in animals treated at 1 ATA, but returned towards normal at 45 minutes in animals treated at 2.5 ATA. By 90 minutes, the energy metabolite concentrations still had not recovered fully in the animals treated at 1 ATA. These data indicate that HBO can restore cytochrome redox state, pH and energy metabolites after acute CO poisoning, while O$_2$ at 1 ATA may lead to cerebral energy failure and cellular acidosis despite the elimination of CO from the blood.

HBO, but not NBO, prevented the severe increase in the CSFp and was thus life saving after CO exposure in a study by Jiang and Tyssebotn (52) on conscious rats with an occluded left carotid artery. They investigated the influence of cerebral edema after acute carbon monoxide poisoning on cerebrospinal fluid pressure (CSFp). After the CO exposure, all non-edema control rats (without carotid artery ligation) recovered. All untreated and NBO- treated rats developed a severely increased CSFp (> 50 mmHg) with neurologic motor dysfunction, and died of a severely increased CSFp (> 100 mmHg) with considerable cerebellar herniation. Except in one rat, the CSFp did not reach a dangerous level (> 25 mmHg) after the HBO session (3 atmospheres O$_2$ for 1 hour, beginning at 20 minutes post CO. Compared to the normoxic treatments, HBO significantly reduced the mortality and the neurologic morbidity in a similar study by the same authors (51). The results support the value of HBO in improving short-term outcome of acute CO poisoning.

In a prospective, randomized study in humans, HBO treatment decreased the incidence of delayed neurologic sequelae (DNS) after CO poisoning (104). The patients in the study presented within 6 hours with mild to moderate CO poisoning. The incidence of DNS was compared between groups treated with NBO or HBO. In 7 of 30 patients, DNS developed after treatment with NBO, whereas no sequelae developed in 30 patients after HBO treatment (P < 0.05). DNS occurred 6 ±1 (mean ±SE) days after poisoning and persisted 41 ±8 days.

What is the mechanism of DNS? It is known that the oligodendroglial precursor cells are exquisitely sensitive to reactive oxygen species (49). Foncin and LeBeau described an unusual clinical case where a cerebral biopsy was obtained 3 days post poisoning in a patient who later died (23). The specimen, consisting of right frontal cortex and white matter, was fixed immediately and studied with electron microscopy. It showed that the white matter was selectively attacked, with destruction of the myelin coverings of the axons. Most striking, however, was the selective damage to the oligodendrocytes, which showed pyknotic or absent nuclei and homogenization of the cytoplasm with empty mitochondria. The blood vessel endothelial cells had occasional areas of tumefaction, but had normal nuclei and in other respects were normal. The neuronal axons were unchanged with normal synapses. Kindwall suggests (59) that a plausible explanation for DNS is the selective destruction of the nuclei of the oligodendroglia. The oligodendrocytes (ODC) produce the myelin that insulates the axons in the

CNS, but unlike the Schwan cells in the peripheral nervous system, the oligodendrocytes produce myelin for a number of axons. If the ODC die there is no reparative mechanism for myelin. This will cause loss of function in the demyelinated axons and typically, after two to three weeks, delayed neurologic sequelae develop.

## Improvement of Bone Repair

In his review of the treatment of chronic osteomyelitis with a combination of HBO, surgery, and antibiotics, Strauss (98) commented that once union was achieved, a 33% stress-fracture rate occurred. He claimed that the profound stimulation of the osteoclast activity by HBO explained the phenomenon, but mechanisms by which bone-resorbing osteoclasts form and are activated by hormones are poorly understood.

The generation of oxygen-derived free radicals in cultured bone is associated with the formation of new osteoclasts and enhanced bone resorption, identical to the effects seen when bones are treated with hormones, such as parathyroid hormone (PTH) and interleukin (IL-1). When free oxygen radicals are generated adjacent to bone surfaces *in vivo*, osteoclasts are also formed. PTH and IL-1-stimulated bone resorption is inhibited by both natural and recombinant superoxide dismutase, an enzyme that depletes tissues of superoxide anions. Garret et al. (25) suggest that oxygen-derived free radicals, and particularly the superoxide anion, are intermediaries in the formation of osteoclasts.

The rebound effect noted in the work done by Persson (82) on growth in the length of bones secondary to changes in oxygen and carbon dioxide tensions might be explained to some extent by increased osteoclast activity, but this is conjectural.

The effect of HBO on the healing of standardized metaphyseal defects in the cortices of rat femurs was studied by Barth et al. (6). Once-a-day treatment appeared to accelerate bone repair and vessel ingrowth compared to controls, while twice-a-day treatment seemed to retard these processes.

Ueng et al. (108) investigated the effect of HBO on bone healing by studying surgical tibial lengthening in rabbits. A bone mineral density (BMD) study was performed for all of the animals at 1 day before operation and at 3, 4, 5, and 6 weeks after operation. Using the preoperative BMD as an internal control, they found that the BMD of the HBO group was increased significantly compared with the non-HBO group during the whole study. Using the contralateral nonoperated tibia as an internal control, they found that torsional strength of lengthened tibia of the HBO group was increased significantly compared with the non-HBO group.

Wang et al. (112) studied the protective effect of HBO and basic fibroblast growth factor (bFGF) on bone growth after irradiation. Control C3H mice received hind leg irradiation at 0, 10, 20, or 30 Gy. HBO-treated mice received radiation 1, 5, or 9 weeks before beginning HBO. Radiation effects on bone growth was reduced by HBO after 10 or 20 Gy, but not after 30 Gy. At 30 Gy, bFGF still reduced the degree of bone shortening, but HBO provided no added benefit to bFGF therapy.

In a prospective randomized study by Lindström et al. (69), 20 consecutive patients, with closed and simple tibial shaft fractures treated with reamed intramedullary nailing, were assigned randomly to HBO or control groups. HBO therapy was given postoperatively at 2.5 ATA for 90 minutes daily for a total of five treatments. The first HBO therapy was given 1 hour after the operation. There was a significant improvement in tibialis posterior arterial peak signal (TPA) in the nailed legs in the HBO group after the first postoperative day, and these values remained at a significantly higher level until the end of the study when compared to the nailed legs in the control group. Further, there was a significant improvement in $PtcO_2$ values in the nailed legs in the HBO group after the third HBO treatment. The improvement in TPA and $PtcO_2$ values may result from the vasoconstrictive and edema reductive effect of HBO.

## Suppression of Autoimmune Responses

Suppression of selected immune responses may occur. Warren et al. (113) reported that development of allergic encephalomyelitis in guinea pigs and rats was delayed up to 34 days after injection of antigen when animals immediately began treatment with HBO at 2 ATA. However, to achieve these results it was necessary to expose the animals for 6 hours per day.

Eiguchi et al. (20) claimed that their results studying the immuno-regulatory effects in rats showed that there was an immunosuppressive action of HBO both in the immunohumoral response and in the immunocellular response. On the other hand, Feldmeier et al. (21) investigated the effects of a standard HBO treatment protocol (2.4 ATA for 90 min QD) on normal human volunteers, who received 20 HBO treatments over a four-week period. No change was seen in the complete blood count (CBC); the differential immune globulins, IgG, IgM, and IgA; complement CH50, C3, C4, or the total lymphocyte count, the lymphocyte subpopulation, and the helper-to-suppressor ratio. Delayed skin hypersensitivity tests were done at week one and at week eight. Measurements were carried out to week twelve.

The effect of HBO (2.8 ATA for 4 hours daily over 3-7 days) on the immune system of normal (BALB/c and MRL- +/+) and autoimmune (MRL-lpr/lpr) mice showed a remarkable decrease in the cell population of the spleen and thymus in normal mice, in a study done by Xu et al. (114). The sensitivity to HBO varied among subpopulations of lymphocytes. Despite the decrease in total cell number in the spleen, the proliferative response of T cells from the spleen to Con A was not impaired. Exposure of autoimmune mice to HBO caused a marked reduction of weight and cell population of the otherwise enlarged spleen and lymph nodes (amongst others B220+Thy-1+ double positive abnormal cells). The conclusion was that HBO therapy may be applicable for the treatment of some autoimmune diseases.

TNF-alpha seems to have a role in mediating HBO effects on different tissues and their immune responses as shown by Lahat et al. (64). They exposed rats for 90 minutes to either 100% oxygen or air at 2.8 ATA, and then mononuclear cells were isolated from blood, spleen, and lungs and cultured for 18 hours. The secretion of TNF-alpha from the cultured monocytes/macrophages was determined with and without stimulation with lipopolysaccharide (LPS). Exposure to hyperbaric oxygen induced a significant increase in the spontaneous *ex vivo* secretion of TNF-alpha (without LPS) by mononuclear cells from the blood, spleen, and lung.

Stimulation with LPS induced a marked increase in secretion of TNF-alpha from blood monocytes after exposure to air, but not after exposure to HBO.

HBO might be effective in treating cluster headache, but the mechanism of the action is not clear. A marked decrease in the content of immunoreactivity for substance P was found in patients exposed to HBO compared to placebo in a study by Di Sabato et al. (18).

## Effect on Blood Cells

HBO may cause a reduction in the hematocrit, and it reduces platelet aggregation. It also increases the deformability of the red blood cells and thus improves the ability of the red blood cells to pass through narrowed capillaries (22, 47, 57, 62).

Neutrophils require molecular oxygen as a substrate for microbial killing. The oxidative burst seen in neutrophils after phagocytosis of bacteria involves a 10 to 15-fold increase in oxygen consumption. This oxidative killing depends on oxygen captured by the leucocytes, then converted to high-energy radicals such as hydroxyl radical, peroxides, and superoxide. The rate at which leucocytes produce these toxic radicals is directly proportional to the amount of oxygen available (4).

Neutrophil activation and the generation of oxygen-derived free radicals may adversely affect capillary integrity during reperfusion. Zamboni et al. (118) hypothesized that systemic HBO may block the action of neutrophils by altering leukocyte adherence properties and activation efficiency. Perhaps HBO is downregulating intercellular adhesion molecule (ICAM 1) expression.

They used an intravital microscopy preparation with a transilluminated rat gracilis muscle to investigate this hypothesis. The most striking effect of HBO was the sharp reduction in adherent leucocytes in the venules as compared to the ischemic no-treatment group. The authors believe leucocytes play a major role in the ultimate production of the no-reflow phenomenon and that HBO may be beneficial in blocking leucocyte action. Previous investigations in their laboratory of muscle microcirculation after ischemia showed increased neutrophil adherence during reperfusion. On the other hand, Sirsjö and Lewis (89) studied changes in post-ischemic skeletal muscle in the rat. They found no significant increase of PMNs in the post-ischemic muscle of untreated rats compared to controls, but with HBO treatment, there was a significant accumulation of PMNs. They concluded that HBO treatment improves the bloodflow in post-ischemic skeletal muscle after 4 hours ischemia without affecting edema formation and despite the accumulation of PMNs.

Poston et al. (83) studied the impact of increased donor cardiac intercellular adhesion molecule (ICAM-1) expression on both reperfusion injury and chronic graft vascular disease after transplantation. They concluded that the induction donor inflammatory state before harvest, leading to increased cardiac ICAM-1 expression, promotes reperfusion injury and chronic graft vascular disease after transplantation in their rodent heterotopic heart model. A study by Toursarkissian et al. (107) showed that arterial thrombosis, but not surgical injury, induces pronounced early and sustained upregulation of ICAM expression in smooth muscle-containing regions of the arterial media. Upregulation of ICAM is likely to promote recruitment of inflammatory cells or mediate vascular remodeling after luminal thrombosis. In a study by Formigli et al. (24), it was shown that vitamin E administration was able to prevent the accumulation of neutrophils within the ischemic and reperfused muscle in humans. This beneficial effect of Vitamin E was due to its ability to hinder the expression of E-selectin and ICAM-1, molecules known to increase the adhesiveness of endothelium to circulating neutrophils. After treatment with Vitamin E, a marked attenuation of the repercussion injury was also evident. In conclusion, Vitamin E treatment may be considered a valuable tool for protection against the ischemia-reperfusion damage of human skeletal muscle.

## Decrease in Lipid Peroxidation

Lipid peroxidation (LP) is believed to be one of the main causes of tissue injury occasioned by a transient ischemic-hypoxic insult, as well as that caused by pharmacologic and noxious substances. LP is absolutely oxygen dependent but, paradoxically, HBO can decrease injury in conditions where oxidative injury is involved, e.g. muscle reperfusion injury (69), and bowel reperfusion syndrome (9).

Lipid peroxidation occurs as an early event during oxidant exposure (nitrogen dioxide) in the lungs of healthy volunteers; but, vitamins C and E diminish lipid peroxidation and preserve the elastase inhibitory capacity of the alveolar lining fluid during oxidant stress (73).

Thom (101) used a rat model of CO poisoning to identify brain lipid peroxidation. This peroxidation, measured as conjugated dienes, was increased by 89% over controls only when the rats were "soaked" with CO at 1,000 ppm prior to experiencing an interval of unconsciousness caused by brief exposure to 3,000 ppm CO. His results suggested that the consequent brain injury might be a form of "ischemia-reperfusion" injury; unconsciousness is always associated with a transient hypotension, and lipid peroxidation occurs only after the rats breathed air for 90 minutes subsequent to CO exposure. He concluded that HBO over 2 ATA, but not 1 ATA $O_2$ exposure, prevented lipid peroxidation.

## Improvement of Tissue Salvage in Burns

During the first 24 hours, a progression of the burn wound in histological depth or extension is often noted. This can only be prevented partially by the routinely used protocols of fluid resuscitation and burn wound dressing.

In a rat burn model (5% TBSA), HBO and piracetam were evaluated for their ability to further prevent this early deepening of the burn wound in a study by Germonpré et al. (26). It was found that both HBO and piracetam had significant effects on the preservation of epidermal basal membrane. HBO, but not piracetam, had further significant effects on the destruction of skin appendages and on the degree of subepidermal inflammation, as measured by leucocyte infiltration. Furthermore, the HBO group showed significantly less leucocyte infiltration than the piracetam group. It was concluded that the effect on subepidermal leucocyte infiltration was striking and warrants further investigation of the anti-inflammatory effects of HBO and possibly piracetam.

Stewart et al. (94) studied tissue ATP levels in a rat burn model. Their results indicated a significant rise in tissue ATP levels in all HBO groups versus burned controls. At 36 hours post injury, with 2 HBO treatments, there was more than a tenfold increase in tissue ATP compared to the 36-hour control group.

Among the useful effects of HBO therapy in burn injuries is a decreased fluid requirement during the first few days after thermal injury. Clinical trials report less edema formation and extravasation of fluids from the wounds (14, 34, 45). Another benefit of HBO treatment is the diminished number of surgical procedures needed, which reduces the length of hospital stay (10).

This clinical picture was confirmed in a series of experiments. Nylander et al. (76) showed a significant reduction in the generalized post-burn edema remote from the burn site (the contralateral ear), by using HBO treatment in a rabbit ear model. The edema formation in the burned ear was not affected by HBO. Burn wound levels of hydroxyproline increase as a measure of collagen turnover (116).

A human study was performed by Hammarlund et al. (37) on healthy male volunteers, who were wounded by skin blistering, excision of the blister roof and ultraviolet irradiation of the dermal wound bed. They concluded that HBO had beneficial effects on this superficial dermal lesion. Edema and exudation decreased, as did the peripheral hyperemia, but the rate of epitheliazation was not significantly accelerated. A similar and blind study by Niezgoda et al. (75) further supports that hyperbaric oxygenation is beneficial in a superficial dermal wound.

## Improvement of Viability in Tissue Flaps

Superoxide dismutase is an essential antioxidative defense mechanism and blocks the generation of superoxide radicals from xanthine oxidase. A substantial increase in xanthine oxidase activity, a major source of oxygen free radicals, has been observed in flap tissues during prolonged periods of preservation. The degree of increase in xanthine oxidase activity correlates well with the fate of free flaps. Inhibition of the xanthine oxidase system may be one of the mechanisms of improved success of skin flap transplantation. A single dose of allopurinol or SOD prior to flap elevation significantly improves the area of flap viability as shown by Im et al. (50). Similar results were obtained when either of these agents was administered 60 minutes after flap elevation. These findings suggest that oxygen-derived free radicals play an important role in the development of tissue necrosis in the critical transition zone between the proximal viable portion and the distal nonviable margin of large skin flaps.

The effects of HBO on flap survival during tissue preservation have been investigated in free flaps in rats, by Tai et al. (99). Groin skin flaps were harvested, stored in either room air or HBO (2.9 ATA at 23 degrees C for 18 hours), and transplanted to the contralateral groin. Free flaps exhibited a high incidence of complete necrosis in the room air control. The survival of free flaps stored under HBO increased significantly (from 10% to 60%) after 18 hours of preservation. Skin flaps exhibited an increase in tissue hypoxanthine by 3.6-fold normal after 18 hours of storage in room air. HBO preservation prevented the accumulation of hypoxanthine and inhibited xanthine oxidase.

Stewart et al. (95) has shown in similar experiments that moderate doses of radical scavengers or antioxidants coupled with HBO can result in the increased survival of random-pattern skin flaps in an animal model with male Sprague-Dawley rats.

In oxygen-tolerance studies, an increase in SOD activity has been demonstrated in the lungs of oxygen-adapted rats (43). The observed changes in activity were moderated by intermittent air breathing periods. Systemic administration of exogenous SOD increases tissue SOD activity and improves the transplantation success rate of skin flaps. HBO increases SOD activity significantly. The beneficial effect of HBO on flap survival may be partially explained by increased SOD activity induced by intermittent exposure to HBO (55).

In a study designed to evaluate the effect of HBO on flap survival when exposed to critical combinations of primary ischemia, reperfusion, and secondary ischemia times, Stevens et al. (93) showed that HBO (90 minutes BID for 7 days) enhances the tolerance of normothermic, microvascular flaps to prolonged secondary ischemia. A similar effect was not noted in the 100% oxygen group.

HBO treatment improved distal microvascular perfusion as measured by laser Doppler flowmetry in ischemic skin flaps in the rat. This effect was observed for HBO treatment given either during or following eight hours of global ischemia (117).

The cutaneous area in a prefabricated myocutaneous flap surviving after elevation is dependent on the rate and amount of vascular ingrowth that occurs from the underlying muscle. Bayati et al. (7) used basic fibroblast growth factor and HBO separately and together in a prefabricated myocutaneous-flap animal model to improve flap survival. There was a significant increase in flap survival area when either basic fibroblast growth factor or HBO was used alone. Further improvement was noted with combination therapy. Histology confirmed improved vascularity in the basic fibroblast growth factor and HBO-treated flaps. The use of either basic fibroblast growth factor or HBO caused a significant increase in the area of prefabricated myocutaneous flap survival. There was a further complementary effect when these two modalities are combined, leading to near complete flap survival through improved vascularity.

## Improvement of Tissue Salvage in Ischemia-Reperfusion Injury

In traumatic injury to the extremities, causing circulatory insufficiency, the resultant ischemia leads to decreasing levels of the energy-rich compounds adenosine triphosphate (ATP) and phosphocreatine (PCr) and increasing levels of lactate in muscle. In the skeletal muscle of man, anaerobic metabolism starts after 10–15 minutes of ischemia and tissue $PO_2$ reaches low values after 20–25 minutes. Tissue glucose levels decrease because of an increased rate of glycolysis and glycogenolysis which, due to the anaerobic situation, leads to production and accumulation of lactate (55). The effect of ischemia on phosphocreatine (PCr) levels of skeletal musculature is an early and rapid decrease. The changes in tissue ATP of skeletal muscle are comparatively small; a significant decrease is not present until after some hours of ischemia. A continuous resynthesis of ATP is necessary for the transport of ions and molecules across the cell membrane, and for maintaining the cell membrane. Most energy in the form of ATP is produced by oxidative phosphorylation (Krebs cycle), a process that is oxygen dependent. HBO reduces the fall in ATP and PCr following ischemia and reduces the increase in lactate during the ischemic period (78, 88, 94).

Phosphorylase activity, a sensitive marker for muscle-cell damage, is to a great extent prevented by HBO treatment in the post-ischemic phase, but repeated HBO treatments are necessary to maintain this effect (78). Thus, repeated HBO treatments in the post-ischemic phase stimulate aerobic metabolism.

In an experimentally-produced, compartment syndrome in dogs, HBO significantly reduced muscle necrosis (50%) after the hind limb had been held at 100 mmHg for 8 hours. This was demonstrated both by histologic examination and radioactive pyrophosphate uptake. The study suggests that HBO may be helpful in treating patients with compartment syndrome, but should be considered an adjunct to standard treatment (96). The investigators continued to follow up the effects of delayed HBO treatment, and found that there was also a significant reduction of edema and muscle necrosis in animals treated by HBO (97).

Nylander et al. (77) studied post-ischemic muscle in rats and were able to show a significant increase in water content after restoration of circulation. With HBO treatments, the post-ischemic edema was significantly reduced.

Zamboni and co-workers (118) used an intravital-microscopy preparation with a transilluminated rat gracilis muscle as a model. The control group showed no significant changes in arteriolar diameter, nor did the no-ischemia HBO group. In the four-hour ischemia group, the initial vasodilatation following ischemia was followed at one hour by a severe vasoconstriction. The HBO treated, four-hour ischemia group, however, maintained the initial vasodilatation for the three-hour reperfusion period. In a similar study, Sirsjö et al. (90) found that after 1-1.5 hours of reperfusion following 4 hours of total ischemia, postischemic blood flow was severely depressed in both the HBO and control groups (HBO and control). However, after 4.5-5 hours of reperfusion, blood flow rates in the post-ischemic muscle in the HBO-treated animals did not differ significantly from those in non-ischemic muscle, compared to a persistent, significant decrease in blood flow in the untreated animals. After 5 hours of reperfusion, capillary density was significantly improved in HBO-treated animals compared to untreated animals. These results suggest that HBO treatment enhances the recovery of blood flow and functional capillary density in post-ischemic muscle tissue, indicating attenuation of the microvascular dysfunction, or damage in the post-ischemic period.

Haapaniemi et al. (41) studied (in a rat hind limb model) the effect of HBO on skeletal muscle submitted to 3 or 4 hours of ischemia after 48 hours of reperfusion. The injury to skeletal muscle was quantified from the uptake of 99m technetium-pyrophosphate in anterior tibial muscle harvested 3 hours later. The uptake was significantly lower in HBO-treated rats than in untreated rats. After 4 hours of ischemia, the changes in levels of the intracellular muscle compounds–adenosine triphosphate, phosphocreatine, and lactate–were less in the hyperbaric oxygen-treated rats than in the untreated ones. In a similar study (40), they found that HBO treatment lessens the metabolic, ischemic derangements, and improves recovery in post-ischemic muscle after 3 hours of ischemia followed by reperfusion.

Sterling et al. (92) studied the effect of HBO in modifying necrosis in an open-chest rabbit model of myocardial ischemia and reperfusion. A branch of the left coronary artery was occluded for 30 minutes, followed by 3 hours of reperfusion. Untreated rabbits were ventilated with 100% oxygen at 1 ATA (control hearts). Treatment animals were exposed to HBO at 2.5 ATA. The control hearts developed 41.5 +/- 4.6% infarction of the ischemic zone. Animals exposed to HBO during ischemia only, reperfusion only, or ischemia and reperfusion, all had significantly smaller infarcts compared to control animals (16.2 ±2.9%, 14.5 ±3.7%, and 9.8 ±2.7%, respectively), indicating that they had been protected by the procedure. When HBO was begun 30 minutes after the onset of reperfusion, no protection was seen (35.8 ±3.8%). They concluded that HBO limits infarct size in the reperfused rabbit heart, when HBO is begun at reperfusion.

Kolski et al. (62) studied the effect of HBO on testicular ischemia-reperfusion injury in a rat model. They found that HBO administered during ischemia (4 hours), or at reperfusion, significantly reduced injury to the testicle. They concluded that the results suggest a potential benefit of HBO treatment in clinical situations of testicular torsion.

Yamada et al. (115) found that HBO was able to ameliorate ischemia-reperfusion injury in the rat small intestine.

In a human study by Bouachour et al. (10), 36 patients with crush injuries were assigned in a blinded, randomized fashion, within 24 hours after surgery, to treatment with HBO (100% $O_2$ at 2.5 ATA for 90 minutes, twice daily, over 6 days) or placebo (21% $O_2$ at 1.1 ATA for 90 minutes, twice daily, over 6 days). All the patients received the same standard therapies (anticoagulant, antibiotics, wound dressings). The two groups (HBO group, n=18; placebo group, n=18) were similar in terms of age; risk factors; number, type or location of vascular injuries, neurologic injuries, or fractures; and type, location, or timing of surgical procedures. Complete healing was obtained for 17 patients in the HBO group vs. 10 patients in the placebo group (p < 0.01). New surgical procedures (such as skin flaps and grafts, vascular surgery, or even amputation) were performed on one patient in the HBO group vs. six patients in the placebo group (p < 0.05). Analysis of groups of patients, matched for age and severity of injury, showed that in the subgroup of patients older than 40 with Gustilo-Anderson grade III soft-tissue injury, wound healing was obtained for seven patients (87.5%) in the HBO group vs. three patients (30%) in the placebo group (p < 0.05).

How can HBO improve outcome of reperfusion injuries? Animal studies have suggested that this improvement may be due to an inhibition of leukocyte adherence to injured endothelium (10, 97). This suggestion is supported by a study, using human neutrophils (13, 97), showing that HBO, at 2.8 or 3.0 ATA for 45 minutes, inhibited the function of human neutrophil beta2-integrins by a process linked to impaired synthesis of cGMP.

Using the rat gracilis-muscle microcirculation model, Zamboni et al. (120) showed that the increase in pedicle arterial leukocyte and neutrophil concentrations following ischemia-reperfusion injury was significantly reduced to control levels by HBO treatment. The observed reduction was not attributable to HBO-induced pulmonary sequestration, which did not significantly change with HBO administration. In conclusion, Vitamin E treatment (24), as well as HBO (10, 41, 87, 106, 107, 115, 118, 120), may be considered valuable tools for protection against ischemia-repercussion damage to human skeletal muscle.

## Improvement of Nerve Cell Regeneration

HBO, performed in the early post-ischemic period, accelerated neurologic recovery and improved the survival rate in dogs after 15 minutes of complete global cerebral ischemia in a study by Takahashi et al. (100) in a canine model. Complete global ischemia was induced in 19 dogs by occlusion of the ascending aorta and the caval veins. Nine dogs were randomized to treatment with HBO at 3 ATA for 1 hour at 3, 24, and 29 hours after ischemia under spontaneous respiration; the other ten dogs served as the control group without HBO. The survival rates were 3/10 (30%) in the control group vs. 7/9 (78%) in the HBO group (p < 0.05). Over the 14-day post-ischemic period, the best EEG scores of each dog were significantly better in the HBO group, and the best neurologic recovery scores of each dog were significantly higher. The number of dogs which attained a neurologic recovery assessed as a slight disability were 1/10 in the control group, and 6/9 in the HBO group.

The preventive effect of HBO against delayed neuronal death was investigated in the gerbil following transient forebrain ischemia, by Konda et al. (63). Delayed neuronal death in the gerbil was produced by clips on both the common carotid arteries (10 minutes). More neurons in the hippocampal CA1 were better preserved in the gerbils treated with HBO than in the gerbils with no HBO. Moreover, more neurons were preserved in the CA1 treated with HBO within 6 hours of the ischemia, than when the HBO was started 24 hours after the ischemia. No oxygen toxicity to the neurons was detected, up to at least 2 ATA.

Radiation-induced necrosis (RIN) of the brain is a complication due to the use of aggressive focal treatments such as radioactive implants and stereotactic radiosurgery. In a a small study by Chuba et al. (13B), ten patients with central nervous system (CNS) RIN received 20–30 HBO sessions at 2.0 to 2.4 ATA for 90 minutes to two hours. All patients had presented with new or increasing neurologic deficits associated with imaging changes, and had clinically failed steroid therapy prior to the initiation of HBO. Initial improvement of stabilization of symptoms and/or imaging findings were documented in all patients. During follow up, four patients died due to tumor progression (6–10 months) later. Four of six surviving patients were still improved by clinical and imaging criteria at last follow up (3-36 months). The authors concluded that in a group with few treatment options available, HBO was well tolerated and most patients improved, although a large number of patients are needed to prove whether HBO is an adjunct to surgery and steroid therapy for CNS RIN.

Kihara et al. (56) evaluated whether HBO rescues peripheral nerve, rendered ischemic by microembolization, from ischemic fiber degeneration.

The arteries supplying rat sciatic nerve were embolized with microspheres of 14 microns diameter at high and moderate doses. Rats were randomized to receive HBO (2.5 ATA 100% oxygen for 2 hours/day for 7 days, beginning within 30 minutes of ischemia), or room air. Nerve blood flow and nerve-action potential were uniformly absent, and more than 90% of fibers had degenerated in both the control and treatment groups receiving high doses. Control and treatment groups receiving moderate doses were significantly different by behavior score, nerve action potential and histology. On single teased-fiber evaluation, the predominant abnormality was E (axonal degeneration). They concluded that hyperbaric oxygenation will effectively rescue fibers from ischemic fiber degeneration, providing the ischemia is not extreme.

The effect of HBO on peripheral-nerve recovery following transection, devascularization, and repair was studied by Zamboni et al. (119), using the rat sciatic-nerve model. The right sciatic nerve was mobilized, stripped of the extrinsic blood supply, transected, and repaired in an epineurial fashion, using microsurgical technique. Following repair, animals were randomized into: control – no HBO (n = 20), or HBO at 2.5 ATA twice daily for one week (n = 16). Nerve recovery was assessed weekly (total of 10 weeks) by walking-track analysis, from which the sciatic function index (SFI) was calculated for each animal. Mean SFI scores were improved in the HBO-treatment group over controls, becoming significant at weeks 7 through 10. These results suggest that functional recovery in transected, devascularized, peripheral nerves may be improved by one week of HBO treatment following microsurgical repair.

Bradshaw et al. (11) studied the regenerative effects of HBO on crushed sciatic nerves in 30 adult male rabbits. Treatments were initiated 4 days post injury. The morphology of crushed nerves after 7 weeks of treatment with HBO resembled normal uncrushed nerves, with nerve fibers uniformly distributed throughout the section. Myelination in the animals resembled undamaged nerves. The control groups received 2 ATA compressed air, 100% normobaric oxygen, or ambient air. The nerves in these animals were edematous and contained disarrayed nerve fibers. Collagen and blood vessels were more evident in the control groups. These differences in morphology suggest that HBO can accelerate a peripheral nerve's recovery from a crush injury.

In a similar study Haapaniemi et al. (42), concluded that the regeneration distances at all time points were significantly longer in animals exposed to HBO (45-minute exposures to 100% $O_2$ at 3.3 ATA at 0, 4, and 8 hours postoperatively, and then every 8 hours for up to 5 days). No more treatments after 25 hours, appeared as effective as when treatments were being given every 8 hours until evaluation. They concluded that HBO treatment stimulates axonal outgrowth following a nerve crush lesion.

## The Role of Free Radicals and Their Formation in the HBO Environment

Raskin et al. (85) suggested in their study, based on findings in the mouse lung, that HBO oxidizes ascorbic acid and ferrous iron, resulting in quantities of ascorbic acid and ferrous iron insufficient to permit lipid peroxidation *in vitro* or *in vivo*. When they added additional ascorbic acid and ferrous iron, *in vitro* peroxidation occurred.

In 1982, Dirks & Faiman (17) showed in an *in vitro* rat brain that, as the oxygen pressure is increased and more oxygen is made available to the brain, free radical formation is increased. No increase in malondialdehyd, a breakdown product of polyunsaturated fatty acids, was seen until 2 ATA of oxygen had been reached, and then only as a slight increase up to 8 ATA. According to their study, exposure at 2.5 ATA of oxygen would not cause any significant increase in radical formation, compared to untreated controls.

Harabin et al. (43) exposed rats and guinea pigs to $O_2$ at 2.8 ATA, delivered either continuously or intermittently (repeated cycles of 10 minutes of 100% $O_2$ followed by 2.5 minutes of air). The $O_2$ time required to produce convulsions and death was increased significantly in both species by intermittent exposure to oxygen. HBO increased lung superoxide dismutase, and decreased catalase and glutathione peroxidase activity in brain and lung. Intermittency benefited both species by postponing gross symptoms of toxicity, but changes in enzyme activity and other variables were more pronounced in guinea pigs, suggesting additional mechanisms for tolerance.

Thom et al. (103) carried out a series of studies to investigate the effects of $O_2$ on lipid peroxidation *in vitro*. Increasing the concentration of $O_2$ from 160 mmHg to between 494 and 988 mmHg $O_2$, slows the rate of linoleic acid peroxidation in a xanthine oxidase/hypoxanthine system. This effect depends on the presence of monounsaturated fatty acids. The mechanism for this effect involves the occurrence of a new termination reaction between hydroperoxyl ($HO_2$) radicals stabilized by pi bond-charge transfer complexes, and monounsaturated fatty acids.

In smoke-inhalation injuries (eight adult intubated patients), 90 minutes of HBO treatment did not lead to oxidative stress that could be measured by elevation of plasma malondialdehyd and expired breath hydrogen peroxide. This suggests that oxidative stress may play a lesser role in the development of inhalational lung injury (33).

HBO, as used therapeutically, has been shown to induce DNA damage in the alkaline comet assay with leukocytes from test subjects. Using formamidopyrimidine-DNA glycosylase, a DNA repair enzyme which specifically nicks DNA at sites of 8-oxoguanines and formamidopyrimidines, Speit et al. (91) have detected enhanced DNA migration, indicating significant oxidative base damage, after HBO treatment. Increased DNA damage was seen immediately at the end of treatment, while 24 hours later no effect was found. They showed that HBO-induced DNA strand breaks and oxidative base modifications are rapidly repaired, leading to a reduction in induced DNA effects of > 50% during the first hour. A similar decrease was found in blood taken immediately after exposure and post-incubated for 2 hours at 37 degrees C *in vitro*, and in blood taken and analysed 2 hours after exposure, suggesting similar repair activities *in vitro* and *in vivo*. When the same blood samples showing increased DNA damage after HBO in the comet assay were analysed in the micronucleus test, no indications of induced chromosomal breakage in cultivated leukocytes could be obtained. The results suggest that the HBO-induced DNA effects observed with the comet assay are efficiently repaired and are not manifested as detectable chromosome damage.

### Decrease in Surfactant Production

Oxygen inhibits enzymes involved in the synthesis of surfactant and may also inhibit the transport of surfactant to the alveoli, as shown by Gilder and McCherry (27, 28).

### Production of Visual Disturbances (Myopia, Cataracts)

Myopia is the most common side effect of HBO (3, 60, 81), causing a blurred distant vision or a sudden ability to read without glasses. It is presumed to be due to changes in the lens, either a change in the shape, or a change in the refraction. Changes have not been found in the curvature of the cornea, but the development of an average of 1.6 diopters of myopia in a group of patients undergoing repeated HBO therapy at 2.5 ATA has been reported (3, 87). Myopia resolved within 3 months following the last treatment, in most cases. Increasing myopia is also a prodromal sign of cataract in the older patient (3, 81). Development of cataracts have been reported in patients receiving more than 150 treatments (81).

### CONCLUSION

The effects of oxygen under pressure on the organs and tissues of the body are multifaceted. Oxygen under these conditions behaves as a drug. The mechanical effects are sometimes important, but of most interest are those aspects of metabolism where oxygen is no longer seen as a simple oxidizer.

## REFERENCES

1. Adams KR., Roberts RM. & Mader JT. "*In vitro* killing of *Clostridium perfringens* by oxygen with and without polymorphonuculear leucocytes." Undersea Biomed Res. 1990;17(Suppl):123. (Abstract only)

2. Anderson D, Nagasawa G, Norfleet W, Olszowka A. and Lundgren C. "$O_2$ pressures between 0.12 and 2.5 atm abs. Circulatory function, and $N_2$ elimination." Undersea Biomed Res. 1991;18(4):279-292.

3. Anderson, B. "Hyperoxic myopia." Trans. Am Ophthalmol Soc. 1978;7:116-124.

4. Badwey JA & Karnovsky ML. "Active oxygen species and the functions of phagocytic leucocytes." Ann Rev Biochem. 1980;49:695 726.

5. Baroni, G., Porro, T., Faglia, E., Pizzi, G., Mastropasqua, A., Oriani, G., Pedesini, G., and Favales, F. Hyperbaric oxygen in diabetic gangrene treatment. Diabetes Care 1987;10:81-86.

6. Barth, E., Sullivan, T and Berg, E. "An animal model for evaluating bone repair with and without adjunctive hyperbaric oxygen therapy (HBO): Comparing dose schedules." J. Invest. Surg. 1990;3:387-392.

7. Bayati, S., Russell, R.C., and Roth, A.C. Stimulation of angiogenesis to improve the viability of prefabricated flaps. Plast.Reconstr.Surg.1998; 101:1290-1295.

8. Bird, AD. and Telfer, ABM. "Effect of hyperbaric oxygen on limb circulation." Lancet. 1965;Feb.13(1):355-356.

9. Bitterman, H., et al. "Effects of hyperbaric oxygen in circulatory shock induced by splanchnic artery occlusion and reperfusion in rats. Can J. Physiol. Pharmacol. 1989;67:1033-1037.

10. Bouachour, G., Cronier, P., Gouello, J.P., Toulemonde, J.L., Talha, A., and Alquier, P. Hyperbaric oxygen therapy in the management of crush injuries: a randomized double-blind placebo-controlled clinical trial. J.Trauma. 1996;41:333-339.

11. Bradshaw, P.O., Nelson, A.G., Fanton, J.W., Yates, T., and Kagan-Hallet, K.S. Effect of hyperbaric oxygenation on peripheral nerve regeneration in adult male rabbits. Undersea.Hyperb.Med.1996;23:107-113.

12. Brown, SD. and Piantadosi, CA. "Recovery of energy metabolism in rat brain after carbon monoxide (CO) poisoning." J Clin Invest 1992 Feb;89(2):666-672.

13. Cho, S. and Yun, DR "Effects of acute carbon monoxide intoxication during pregnancy on fetal growth in rat." Undersea Biomed. Res. 1989;16 (Suppl):45. (Abstract only)

13b. Chuba PJ; Aronin P; Bhambhani K; Eichemhorn M, Zamarano L; Cianci P; Muhlbauer M; Porter AT; Fontanesi J. "Hyperbaric oxygen therapy for radiation-induced brain injury in children." Cancer 1997 Nov 15;80(10):2005-12

14. Cianci, P, Lueders H, Shapiro, R, Sexton, J and B Green, "Current status of adjunctive hyperbaric oxygen in the treatment of thermal wounds." Proceedings of the Second Swiss Symposium on Hyperbaric Medicine. 1988;163-172 (D J Bakker & J. Schmutz Eds.) Foundation for Hyperbaric Medicine, Basel.

15. Cross, FS. "Effects of increased atmospheric pressures and the inhalation of 95% oxygen and helium oxygen mixtures on the viability of the bowel wall and the absorption of gas in closed loop obstructions." Surgery. 1954;36:1001-1026.

16. Cross, FS and Wangensteen OH. "Effect of increased atmospheric pressures on the viability of the bowel wall and the absorption of gas in closed loop obstructions." Surg. Forum. 1952;3:111-116.

17. Dirks, RC and Faiman MD. "Free radical formation and lipid peroxidation in rat and mouse cerebral cortex slices exposed to high oxygen pressure." Brain Res. 1982;248:355-360.

18. Di Sabato, F., Giacovazzo, M., Cristalli, G., Rocco, M., and Fusco, B.M. Effect of hyperbaric oxygen on the immunoreactivity to substance P in the nasal mucosa of cluster headache patients. Headache. 36:221-223, 1996.

19. Dooley JW and Mehm, WJ, "Noninvasive Assessment of the Vasconstrictive Effects of Hyperoxygenation." J. Hyperbaric Medicine. 1990;4(4):177-187.

20. Eiguchi K., Bertholds M., Grana D. Malateste, E. Mareso, E. Gomez, and Falasca, CA, "Immunoregulatory effect of HBO on rats." J. Hyperbaric Medicine. 1990;5(3):187-191.

21. Feldmeier JJ., Boswell RN, Brown M. and Shaffer P. "The effects of hyperbaric oxygen on the immunologic status of healthy human subjects." Proceedings of the Eighth Internat. Cong. on Hyperbaric Med. (E. Kindwall, Ed.) Best Publishing Company, Flagstaff, Arizona. 1987;41-46.

22. Fischer B. and Jain KK. "Blood lactate and ammonia levels during exercise under hyperbaric oxygen." Proceedings of the XIIIth Annual Meeting of the European Undersea Biomedical Society. (Marroni G., Oriani G. Eds.) Palermo, Italy, Sept. 8-12, 1987.

23. Foncin, J.F. and LeBeau J. (French) Myélinopathie par intoxication oxycarboné: Neuropathologie ultrastructurale, Acta Neuropathol. (Berlin) 43:153, 1978

24. Formigli, L., Ibba Manneschi, L., Tani, A., Gandini, E., Adembri, C., Pratesi, C., Novelli, G.P., and Zecchi Orlandini, S. Vitamin E prevents neutrophil accumulation and attenuates tissue damage in ischemic-reperfused human skeletal muscle. Histol.Histopathol.1997.Jul. 12:663-669

25. Garret IR., Boyce BF, Oreffo RO, Bonewald L., Poser J and Mundy GR, "Oxygen-derived free radicals stimulate osteoclastic bone resorption in rodent bone *in vitro* and *in vivo*." J. Clin. Invest. 1990;85(3):632-639.

26. Germonpre, P., Reper, P., and Vanderkelen, A. Hyperbaric oxygen therapy and piracetam decrease the early extension of deep partial-thickness burns. Burns.1996;22:468-473.

27. Gilder H. and McCherry CK, "Mechanism of oxygen inhibition of pulmonary surfactant synthesis." Surgery. 1974;76:72-79.

28. Gilder H and McCherry CK "Phosphatidylcholine synthesis and pulmonary oxygen toxicity. Biochem. Biophys. Acta. 1976;441:48-56.

29. Gorman, D. 1992, 1998; Personal Communication to the Editor

30. Granström, G., Jacobsson, M., and Tjellström, A. Titanium implants in irradiated tissue: benefits from hyperbaric oxygen. Int.J.Oral Maxillofac. Implants.1992;7:15-25.

31. Granström, G., Tjellström, A., Brånemark, P.I., and Fornander, J. Bone-anchored reconstruction of the irradiated head and neck cancer patient. Otolaryngol.Head.Neck Surg. 1993;108:334-343.

32. Granström, G. Hyperbaric oxygen therapy decreases the rejection rate of osseointegrated implants after radiotherapy. Strahlenther.Onkol.1996;172 Suppl 2:20-21.

33. Grim PS., Nahum A., Gottlieb L., Wilbert C., Hawe E, and Sznajder J. "Lack of measurable oxidative stress during HBO therapy in burn patients." Undersea Biomed. Res. 1989;16(Suppl):22. (Abstract only)

34. Grossman, AR, "Hyperbaric oxygen in the treatment of burns." Ann. Plast. Surg. 1978;1:163-171.

35. Hammarlund C., Castenfors J., and Svedman P. "Dermal vascular response to hyperoxia in healthy volunteers." Proceedings of the Second Swiss Symposium on Hyberbaric Medicine. DJ Bakker & J Schmutz (Eds.) Foundation for Hyperbaric Medicine. Basel. 1988;55-59.

36. Hammarlund C., Svedman C., and Svedman P "Hyperbaric oxygen treatment of healthy volunteers with u.v.-irradiated blister wounds." Burns. 1991;17(4):296-301.

37. Hammarlund, C. and Sundberg, T. Hyperbaric oxygen reduced size of chronic leg ulcers: a randomized double-blind study. Plast.Reconstr.Surg.1994;93(4):829-33; discussion 834.

38. Hammarlund C, Kutlu N, Gustafson P,Thorsen C, and Svedman P. Effects of Oxygen Breathing on Blister Wound Microcirculation in Man. In Hyperbaric Oxygenation and Wound Repair. Effects on the Dermal Microcirculation. Doctoral Dissertation. Lund University, Sweden 1995.

39. Hammarlund, C. Increase of Blood Flow in Hypoxic Tissue During Oxygen Breathing. A Laser Doppler Imaging Study. In manuscript.

40. Haapaniemi, T., Sirsjö, A., Nylander, G., and Larsson, J. Hyperbaric oxygen treatment attenuates glutathione depletion and improves metabolic restitution in postischemic skeletal muscle. Free Radic.Res.1995;23(2):91-101.

41. Haapaniemi, T., Nylander, G., Sirsjö, A., and Larsson, J. Hyperbaric oxygen reduces ischemia-induced skeletal muscle injury. Plast.Reconstr.Surg.1996;97(3):602-7; discussion 608-9.

42. Haapaniemi, T., Nylander, G., Kanje, M., and Dahlin, L. Hyperbaric oxygen treatment enhances regeneration of the rat sciatic nerve. Exp.Neurol.1998;149:433-438.

43. Harabin AL, Braisted JC and Flynn ET "Response of antioxidant enzymes to intermittent and continuous hyperbaric oxygen." J. Appl. Physiol. 1990;69(1):328-335.

44. Hart GB and Mainous EG. "The treatment of radiation necrosis with hyperbaric oxygen." Cancer. 1976;37:2580.

45. Hart GB, O'Reilly RR, Broussard ND, Cave RH, Goodman DB and Yanda RL. "Treatment of burns with hyperbaric oxygen." Surg. Gynacol. Obstet. 1974;139:693-696.

45b. Hehenberger K., Brismar K., Lind F. and Kratz G. "Dose-dependent hyperbaric oxygen stimulation of human fibroblast proliferation." Wound Rep Reg. 1997;5:147-50.

46. Hordnes C. and Tyssebotn I. "Effect of high ambient pressure and oxygen tension on organ blood flow in conscious trained rats." Undersea Biomed Res. 1985;12:115-118.

47. Hsu P., Zan-Shun W., and Yong-Xing M. "The effect of HBO on platelet aggregation, blood rheology, $PaO_2$ and cognitive function in the elderly." Proceedings of the Eighth Internat. Cong. on Hyperbaric Med. E. Kindwall (Ed.) Best Publishing Company, Flagstaff, Arizona. 1984;19

48. Hunt, TK. "The Physiology of Wound Healing." Ann of Emerg. Med. 1988;17:1265-1273.

49. Husain J and Juurlink BH. Oligodendroglial precursor cell susceptibility to hypoxia is related to poor ability to cope with reactive oxygen species. Brain Res. 1995:6;698 (1-2): 86-94

50. Im MI. Manson PN, Bulkley, GB and Hoopes, JE. "Effects of superoxide dismutase and allopurinol on the survival of acute island skin flaps." Ann Surg. 1985;201:357-359

51. Jiang, J. and Tyssebotn, I. Normobaric and hyperbaric oxygen treatment of acute carbon monoxide poisoning in rats. Undersea.Hyperb.Med.1997.Jun. 24:107-116.

52. Jiang, J. and Tyssebotn, I. Cerebrospinal fluid pressure changes after acute carbon monoxide poisoning and therapeutic effects of normobaric and hyperbaric oxygen in conscious rats. Undersea.Hyperb.Med.1997;24:245-254.

53. Johnsson, K., Hansson, A., Granström, G., Jacobsson, M., and Turesson, I. The effects of hyperbaric oxygenation on bone-titanium implant interface strength with and without preceding irradiation. Int.J.Oral Maxillofac.Implants.1993;8:415-419.

54. Jönsson K, Hunt TK, Mathes SJ, "Oxygen as an Isolated Variable Influences Resistance to Infection." Ann Surg. 1988;208(6):783-787.

55. Kaelin CM, Im MJ, Myers RA, Manson PN & Hoopes, JE. "The effects of hyperbaric oxygen on free flaps in rats." Arch. Surg. 1990;125(5):607-609.

56. Kihara, M., McManis, P.G., Schmelzer, J.D., Kihara, Y., and Low, P.A. Experimental ischemic neuropathy: salvage with hyperbaric oxygenation. Ann.Neurol. 1995;37(1):89-94.

57. Kindwall E. "Measurement of helium elimination from man during decompression breathing air or oxygen." Undersea Biomed. Res. 1975;2(4): 277-284.

58. Kindwall E. and Johnson JP. "Outcome of hyperbaric treatment in 32 cases of air embolism." Undersea Biomed. Res. 1990;17(Suppl):90. (Abstract only)

59. Kindwall, EP Delayed sequelae in Carbon Monoxide Poisoning and Their Possible Mechanisms In: Carbon Monoxide (DG Penney, Ed) pp 248-250 New York. CRC Press 1996

60. Kindwall E. Personal Communication 1998.

61. Knighton DR., Halliday B and Hunt TH "Oxygen as an antibiotic: A comparison of inspired oxygen concentration and antibiotic administration on *in vivo* bacterial clearance." Arch. Surg. 1986;121:191-195.

62. Kolski, J.M., Mazolewski, P.J., Stephenson, L.L., Texter, J., Grigoriev, V.E., and Zamboni, W.A. Effect of hyperbaric oxygen therapy on testicular ischemia-reperfusion injury. J.Urol.1998;160:601-604.

63. Konda, A., Baba, S., Iwaki, T., Harai, H., Koga, H., Kimura, T., and Takamatsu, J. Hyperbaric oxygenation prevents delayed neuronal death following transient ischaemia in the gerbil hippocampus. Neuropathol.Appl.Neurobiol.1996;22:350-360.

64. Lahat, N., Bitterman, H., Yaniv, N., Kinarty, A., and Bitterman, N. Exposure to hyperbaric oxygen induces tumour necrosis factor-alpha (TNF-alpha) secretion from rat macrophages. Clin.Exp.Immunol.1995;102(3):655-659.

65. Larsson, J. and Hultman, E. "The effect of long-term arterial occlusion on energy metabolism of the human quadriceps muscle." Scand J. Clin Lab Invest. 1979;39:257-264.

66. Lee C.H., Niu K.C., Chen L.P., Chang K.L., Tsai J.D. and Chen L.S. îTherapeutic Effects of Different Tables on Type II Decompression Sickness.î J Hyperbaric Med 1991;6:11-17.

67. Li, W. and Li X. "The hemo-rheologic changes in patients treated with hyperbaric oxygenation at 3 ATA." Undersea Biomed Res. 1990;17(Suppl):61. (Abstract only)

68. Lindblom L., Tuma RF and Årfors KE. "Influence of oxygen on perfused capillary density and capillary red cell velocity in rabbit skeletal muscle." Microvasc. Res. 1980;19:197-208.

69. Lindström, T., Gullichsen, E., Lertola, K., and Niinikoski, J. Effects of hyperbaric oxygen therapy on perfusion parameters and transcutaneous oxygen measurements in patients with intramedullary nailed tibial shaft fractures. Undersea.Hyperb.Med.1998;25:87-91.

70. Lyne AJ. "Ocular effects of hyperbaric oxygen." Trans Opthalmol. Soc UK 1978;98:66-68.

71. Marx RE "A new concept in the treatment of osteoradionecrosis." J. Oral Maxillofac. Surg. 1983;41(6):351-357.

72. Mathieu D. Coget J. Vinckier L, et al. "Red blood cell deformity and hyperbaric oxygenation." Proceedings of the Eighth Internat. Cong. on Hyperbaric Med. E. Kindwall (Ed.) Best Publishing Company, Flagstaff, AZ. 1987;27-28

73. Mohsenin, V. "Lipid peroxidation and antielastase activity in the lungs under oxygen stress: role of antioxidant defenses." J. Appl. Physiol. 1991;70(4):1456-1462.

74. Neovius, E.B., Lind, M.G., and Lind, F.G. Hyperbaric oxygen therapy for wound complications after surgery in the irradiated head and neck: a review of the literature and a report of 15 consecutive patients. Head.Neck 1997;19:315-322.

75. Niezgoda, J.A., Cianci, P., Folden, B.W., Ortega, R.L., Slade, J.B., and Storrow, A.B. The effect of hyperbaric oxygen therapy on a burn wound model in human volunteers. Plast.Reconstr.Surg.1997.May. 99:1620-1625,

76. Nylander G. Nordström H, and Eriksson E. "Effects of hyperbaric oxygen on edema formation after a scald burn." Burns. 1984;10(3):193-196.

77. Nylander G., Lewis DH, Nordström H, and Larsson J., "Reduction of post-ischemic edema with hyperbaric oxygen." Plast. Reconstr. Surg. 1985;76:596-601.

78. Nylander G., Nordström H., Lewis DH and Larsson J., "Metabolic effects of hyperbaric oxygen in post-ischemic muscle." Plast. Reconstr. Surg. 1987;79(1):91-97.

79. Nylander G., et al. "Effects of hyperbaric oxygen treatment in post-ischemic muscle. A quantitative morphological study." Scand. J. Plast. Reconstr. Surg. 1988;22(1):31-39.

80. Ohta H., Yasui N., Suzuki E., and Yasui N., et al. "Measurement of cerebral blood flow under hyperbaric oxygenation in man - relationship between $PaO_2$ and cerebral blood flow." Proceedings of the Eighth Internat. Cong. on Hyperbaric Med. E. Kindwall (Ed.) Best Publishing Company, Flagstaff, AZ. 1987;62-67

81. Palmquist BM., Philipsson B., and Barr PO. "Nuclear cataract and myopia during hyperbaric oxygen therapy." Br. J. Opthalmol. 1984;68(2):113-117.

82. Persson, BM. Doctoral Dissertation. Acta Orthop. Scand. (Suppl) 1968;117:1-99.

83. Poston, R.S.,Jr., Billingham, M.E., Pollard, J., Hoyt, E.G., and Robbins, R.C. Effects of increased ICAM-1 on reperfusion injury and chronic graft vascular disease. Ann.Thorac.Surg.1997.Oct. 64:1004-1012

84. Quirinia, A. and Viidik, A. The impact of ischemia on wound healing is increased in old age but can be countered by hyperbaric oxygen therapy. Mech.Ageing Dev.1996;91:131-144.

85. Raskin P., Lipman RL, and Oloff CM. "Effect of hyperbaric oxygen on lipid peroxidation in the lung." Aerosp. Med. 1971;42:28-30.

86. Roberts, G.P. and Harding, K.G. Stimulation of glycosaminoglycan synthesis in cultured fibroblasts by hyperbaric oxygen. Br.J.Dermatol.1994;131(5):630-633.

87. Ross, M.E., Yolton, D.P., Yolton, R.L., and Hyde, K.D. Myopia associated with hyperbaric oxygen therapy. Optom.Vis.Sci.1996;73:487-494.

88. Sirsjö A., Larsson J., Haapaniemi T., Lewis D. and Nylander G. "Reduction of necrosis and increased levels of adenosine triphosphate (ATP) and phosphocreatine (PCr) in post-ischemic skeletal muscle after hyperbaric oxygen treatment." Int. J. Microcirc: Clin Exp. (Suppl) 1990;1:24.

89. Sirsjö A., and Lewis D. "Improved bloodflow in post-ischemic skeletal muscle after hyperbaric oxygen treatment." Int. J. Microcirc.: Clin Exp. (Suppl) 1990;1:156.

90. Sirsjö, A., Lehr, H.A., Nolte, D., Haapaniemi, T., Lewis, D.H., Nylander, G., and Messmer, K. Hyperbaric oxygen treatment enhances the recovery of blood flow and functional capillary density in postischemic striated muscle. Circ.Shock 1993;40:9-13.

91. Speit, G., Dennog, C., and Lampl, L. Biological significance of DNA damage induced by hyperbaric oxygen. Mutagenesis 1998;13:85-87.

92. Sterling, D.L., Thornton, J.D., Swafford, A., Gottlieb, S.F., Bishop, S.P., Stanley, A.W., and Downey, J.M. Hyperbaric oxygen limits infarct size in ischemic rabbit myocardium *in vivo*. Circulation1993;88:1931-1936.

93. Stevens, D.M., Weiss, D.D., Koller, W.A., and Bianchi, D.A. Survival of normothermic microvascular flaps after prolonged secondary ischemia: effects of hyperbaric oxygen. Otolaryngol.Head.Neck Surg. 1996;15:360-364.

94. Stewart RJ, Yamaguchi KT, Mason SW, Roshdieh BB, Dabassi NI, and Ness VT. "Tissue ATP levels in burn injured skin treated with hyperbaric oxygen." Undersea Biomed. Res. (Suppl) 1989;16:53.

95. Stewart, R.J., Moore, T., Bennett, B., Easton, M., Newton, G.W., and Yamaguchi, K.T. Effect of free-radical scavengers and hyperbaric oxygen on random-pattern skin flaps. Arch.Surg.1994;129(9):982-7; discussion 987-8.

96. Strauss MB, Hargens AR, and Gershuni DG, et al. "Reduction of skeletal muscle necrosis using intermittent hyperbaric oxygen in a model compartment syndrome." J. Bone Joint Surg. 1983;65A(5):656-662.

97. Strauss MB, Hargens AR., Gershuni DH, et al. "Delayed use of hyperbaric oxygen for treatment of a model anterior compartment syndrome." J. Orthop. Res. 1986;4(1):108-111.

98. Strauss MB., "Refractory osteomyelitis." J. Hyperbaric Med. 1987;2:3:147-159.

99. Tai, Y.J., Birely, B.C., Im, M.J., Hoopes, J.E., and Manson, P.N. The use of hyperbaric oxygen for preservation of free flaps. Ann.Plast.Surg.1992;28:284-287.

100. Takahashi, M., Iwatsuki, N., Ono, K., Tajima, T., Akama, M., and Koga, Y. Hyperbaric oxygen therapy accelerates neurologic recovery after 15-minute complete global cerebral ischemia in dogs. Crit.Care Med. 1992;20:1588-1594.

101. Thom SR., "CO poisoning in a rat model: Physiological correlation with clinical events and the effects of HBO." Undersea Biomed Res. (Suppl) 1989;16:51-52. (Abstract only)

102. Thom SR., et al. "Carbon monoxide mediated brain lipid peroxidation in the rat." J. Appl. Physiol. 1990;68(3):997-1003.

103. Thom SR., "Molecular mechanism for the antagonism of lipid peroxidation by hyperbaric oxygen." Undersea Biom. Res. (Suppl) 1990;17:53-54.

104. Thom, S.R., Taber, R.L., Mendiguren, I.I., Clark, J.M., Hardy, K.R., and Fisher, A.B. Delayed neuropsychologic sequelae after carbon monoxide poisoning: prevention by treatment with hyperbaric oxygen :see comments: Ann.Emerg.Med.1995;25(4):474-480.

105. Thom, S.R., Mendiguren, I., Hardy, K., Bolotin, T., Fisher, D., Nebolon, M., and Kilpatrick, L. Inhibition of human neutrophil beta2-integrin-dependent adherence by hyperbaric $O_2$. Am.J.Physiol.1997;272:C770-7.

106. Tompach, P.C., Lew, D., and Stoll, J.L. Cell response to hyperbaric oxygen treatment. Int.J.Oral Maxillofac.Surg.1997;26:82-86.

107. Toursarkissian, B., Schwartz, D., Eisenberg, P.R., and Rubin, B.G. Arterial thrombosis induces early upregulation of intercellular adhesion molecule in the media. J.Vasc.Surg.1997.Oct. 26:663-669

108. Ueng, S.W., Lee, S.S., Lin, S.S., Wang, C.R., Liu, S.J., Yang, H.F., Tai, C.L., and Shih, C.H. Bone healing of tibial lengthening is enhanced by hyperbaric oxygen therapy: a study of bone mineral density and torsional strength on rabbits. J.Trauma.1998;44:676-681.

109. Uhl, E., Sirsjö, A., Haapaniemi, T., Nilsson, G., and Nylander, G. Hyperbaric oxygen improves wound healing in normal and ischemic skin tissue. Plast.Reconstr.Surg.1994;93:835-841.

110. Van Unnik AJM. "Inhibition of toxin production in Clostridium perfringens *in vitro* by hyperbaric oxygen." Antonie von Leeuwenhoek. 1965;31:181-186.

111. Villanucci S., Di Marzio GE., Scholl M., Pivorine C., d'Adamo C., and Settimi F. "Cardiovascular changes induced by hyperbaric oxygen therapy." Undersea Biomed. Res. (Suppl) 1990;17:117.

112. Wang, X., Ding, I., Xie, H., Wu, T., Wersto, N., Huang, K., and Okunieff, P. Hyperbaric oxygen and basic fibroblast growth factor promote growth of irradiated bone. Int.J.Radiat.Oncol.Biol.Phys.1998.Jan.1. 40:189-196

113. Warren J., Sacksteder MR., and Thuning CA. "Oxygen immunosuppression: modification of experimental allergic encephalomyelitis in rodents." J. Immunol. 1978;121:315-320.

114. Xu, X., Yi, H., Kato, M., Suzuki, H., Kobayashi, S., Takahashi, H., and Nakashima, I. Differential sensitivities to hyperbaric oxygen of lymphocyte subpopulations of normal and autoimmune mice. Immunol.Lett. 1997;59:79-84.

115. Yamada, T., Taguchi, T., Hirata, Y., Suita, S., and Yagi, H. The protective effect of hyperbaric oxygenation on the small intestine in ischemia-reperfusion injury. J.Pediatr.Surg.1995;30(6):786-790.

116. Yamaguchi KT, Hoffman C., Stewart RJ, Cianci PA, Vierra M, and Naito M. "Effect of oxygen on burn wound tissue levels of ATP and collagen." Undersea Biomed. Res. (Suppl) 1990;17:65. (Abstract only)

117. Zamboni, W.A., Roth, A.C., Russell, R.C., and Smoot, E.C. The effect of hyperbaric oxygen on reperfusion of ischemic axial skin flaps: a laser Doppler analysis. Ann.Plast.Surg.1992;28:339-341.

118. Zamboni, W.A., Roth, A.C., Russell, R.C., Graham, B., Suchy, H., and Kucan, J.O. Morphologic analysis of the microcirculation during reperfusion of ischemic skeletal muscle and the effect of hyperbaric oxygen. Plast.Reconstr.Surg.1993;91:1110-1123.

119. Zamboni, W.A., Brown, R.E., Roth, A.C., Mathur, A., and Stephenson, L.L. Functional evaluation of peripheral-nerve repair and the effect of hyperbaric oxygen. J.Reconstr.Microsurg. 1995;11(1):27-9; discussion 29-30.

120. Zamboni, W.A., Wong, H.P., and Stephenson, L.L. Effect of hyperbaric oxygen on neutrophil concentration and pulmonary sequestration in reperfusion injury. Arch.Surg.1996;131:756-760.

121. Zamboni, W.A., Wong, H.P., Stephenson, L.L., and Pfeifer, M.A. Evaluation of hyperbaric oxygen for diabetic wounds: a prospective study. Undersea.Hyperb.Med.1997;24:175-179.

122. Zhao, L.L., Davidson, J.D., Wee, S.C., Roth, S.I., and Mustoe, T.A. Effect of hyperbaric oxygen and growth factors on rabbit ear ischemic ulcers. Arch.Surg. 1994:129:1043-1049.

CHAPTER 4

# OXYGEN TOXICITY

## CHAPTER FOUR OVERVIEW

# OXYGEN TOXICITY

*James M. Clark, Valerie J. Bonne, Charles C. Falzon, Harry T. Whelan*

## RECOGNITION AND PREVENTION OF OXYGEN POISONING IN HYPERBARIC OXYGEN THERAPY

Although any therapeutic application of hyperbaric oxygen (HBO) is intrinsically associated with the potential for producing mild to severe toxic effects (12, 17, 37, F), the appropriate use of hyperoxia is one of the safest therapeutic procedures available to the modern medical practitioner. A wide margin of safety for oxygen use is provided by potent antioxidant defense mechanisms (29) that slow the development of oxygen poisoning and hasten recovery from its subclinical manifestations. In conditions of prolonged oxygen exposure, however, antioxidant defenses are overwhelmed and toxic manifestations eventually occur. Susceptibility to oxygen toxicity may be influenced by the clinical state of the patient, or by the effects of concurrent drug therapy. Both the awareness of such influences and the ability to recognize early manifestations of oxygen poisoning can further enhance the safety and efficacy of HBO therapy.

## BIOCHEMICAL MECHANISMS OF OXYGEN POISONING

There is now general agreement that the formation of reactive oxygen species is an intermediate event in the production of oxidant damage to cell membranes and their constituents. The degree of damage appears to be determined by the stoichiometric relationship between the rate of formation of reactive oxygen species and their rate of elimination by antioxidants. Evidence for and against this current concept has recently been the subject of extensive discussion by several authors (35, B, D, S).

Reduction of molecular oxygen by the sequential addition of electrons results in the formation of superoxide, hydrogen peroxide, hydroxyl radical, and, finally, water. There are indications that superoxide radicals generated in mitochondria are rapidly dismutated to hydrogen peroxide, and that these products interact further in the presence of catalytic amounts of iron to potentially generate both highly reactive hydroxyl radicals and singlet oxygen. Initiation of lipid peroxidation by either of these highly reactive radicals could greatly increase oxidant damage by propagating a series of reactions, resulting in possible oxidation of proteins and lipids, inactivation of critical enzymes, and, ultimately, cellular membrane damage. Protein cross-linking, fatty acid oxidation, and oxidation of amino acids are all potential results of free radical production in hyperoxic environments (3, 4, 11, 13, 35).

There are several antioxidant enzymes that oppose the formation of reactive oxygen species, including superoxide dismutase, catalase, glutathione peroxidase, glutathione reductase, and the enzymes of the Hexose Monophosphate (HMP) Shunt. Other compounds that appear to have important antioxidant activity include glutathione, selenium, vitamin E, and vitamin C. The nature and degree of oxidant damage during hyperoxia exposure is determined by the net results of the radical-producing and radical-quenching actions. The oxidant damage is determined by the interaction of antioxidant defenses and tissue repair mechanisms (B, D, F).

Potential insights into mechanisms that cause oxygen convulsions are provided by studies of pharmacologic agents that delay the onset of seizures in animals exposed to toxic oxygen pressures. These agents include diethyldithiocarbamic acid, 1-aminobenzotriazole, 21-aminosteroid compounds (lazeroids) (31, 33, 44), propranolol (45, 46), and low dose caffeine (9, X).

Diethyldithiocarbamic acid and 1-aminobenzotriazole are two examples of anti-oxidants that effectively inhibit the cytochrome P-450 mono-oxygenases, a class of enzymes that are known to form reactive oxygen species. These anti-oxidant compounds are selectively distributed and at their highest concentrations in neuronal tissue, or non-glial cells, where they are most effective (25). A potential physiological role for cytochrome P-450 dependent enzymes is explained by the fact that neurons contain biochemical machinery for the synthesis of neurotransmitters, neurohormones, and other physiologically active endogenous substances. Inhibiting these enzymes limits the extent of oxidative injury that can occur by decreasing the rate of formation of reactive oxygen species.

Free radical-induced peroxidation of neuronal, glial, vascular cell membranes, and myelin within the central nervous system is catalyzed by release of free iron from injured cells. This suggests a possible role for iron-chelating drugs, such as the 21-amino steroids, in the prevention of lipid peroxidation (10, B, D, F).

The protective effects of propranolol against neurological manifestations of oxygen toxicity have been attributed to its adrenergic blocking properties (45, 46). However, propranolol also decreases cerebral blood flow and cerebral oxidative metabolism. These additional actions could contribute to the delayed onset of oxygen convulsions by pre-exposure administration of propranolol (45, 46.)

Low dose caffeine produces cerebral vasoconstriction by acting as an adenosine receptor agonist, and as an anti-oxidant, which may have antiepileptic properties, delaying the onset of oxygen convulsions (9, X).

## MANIFESTATIONS OF OXYGEN POISONING

### Central Nervous System Effects

Grand mal convulsions caused by central nervous system (CNS) oxygen toxicity can occur in patients breathing oxygen at pressures of 2.0 ATA or greater (K, L, M, O). Convulsions may occur abruptly, or may be preceded by other signs of central nervous system irritability (Table 1).

## TABLE 1. SIGNS AND SYMPTOMS OF CNS OXYGEN POISONING IN NORMAL MEN (ADAPTED FROM DONALD)

| | |
|---|---|
| Facial pallor | Inspiratory predominance |
| Sweating | Diaphragmatic spasms |
| Bradycardia | Nausea |
| Palpitations | Spasmodic vomiting |
| Depression | Fibrillation of lips |
| Apprehension | Lip twitching |
| Visual field constriction | Twitching of cheek, nose, eyelids |
| Tinnitus | Syncope |
| Auditory hallucinations | Convulsions |
| Vertigo | |

Detection of one or more of the premonitory symptoms of CNS oxygen poisoning should be treated by switching the patient's source of breathing gas from oxygen to chamber air. Reversal of the symptoms while breathing chamber air is consistent with recovery from oxygen poisoning. Once the patient has recovered by showing no evidence of persistent CNS toxicity, treatment with oxygen may be resumed after the patient's treatment protocol is modified to prevent recurrence of toxic symptoms by either inserting additional "chamber air" intervals, or by ascending to the depth where the patient was previously asymptomatic (W). As long as mechanical trauma is avoided while the patient is actively seizing, there should be no residual effects to the oxygen convulsions.

## Pulmonary Effects

Prolonged exposure to oxygen pressures greater than 0.5 ATA is associated with the development of intra-tracheal and bronchial irritation, such as substernal burning, chest tightness, cough, and dyspnea (13, 17, 18, G, H, Q, U, V). With continued oxygen exposure, the patient develops progressive impairment of pulmonary function, and, eventually, acute respiratory distress syndrome (ARDS). Initially, there are indications of capillary endothelial damage, followed by pulmonary edema, protein exudation, and progressive respiratory failure. These changes are seen over the course of days to weeks at lower oxygen pressures, and occur more rapidly as the oxygen pressure is increased. The early changes of pulmonary oxygen toxicity generally reverse upon cessation of oxygen therapy. No residual (irreversible) pulmonary effects have been observed after a single administration of any of the therapy protocols listed in Table 2. When oxygen therapy is provided in accordance with the standard HBO treatment protocols outlined in this text, there is little or no danger that patients will experience pulmonary oxygen toxicity.

## TABLE 2. CUMULATIVE PULMONARY OXYGEN TOXICITY INDICES FOR COMMONLY USED OXYGEN THERAPY TABLES

| THERAPY TABLE | UPTD* |
|---|---|
| Refractory osteomyelitis/radionecrosis | |
| 120 min oxygen at 33 fsw | 300 |
| 90 min oxygen at 45 fsw | 270 |
| Anaerobic infection | 401 |
| 45 min oxygen/15 min air/45 min oxygen at 60 fsw | |
| 45 min oxygen at 60 - 0 fsw with 8 min at 20 fsw and 27 min at 10 fsw | |
| CO intoxication | 361 |
| 30 min oxygen at 60 fsw | |
| 4 min oxygen at 60 - 33 fsw | |
| 90 min oxygen at 33 fsw | |
| 10 min oxygen at 33 - 0 fsw | |
| USN 5** | 33 |
| USN 6 | 645 |
| USN 6 extended | |
| 20 min oxygen/5 min air at 30 fsw | 718 |
| 15 min air/60 min oxygen at 30 fsw | 787 |
| 20 min oxygen/5 min air at 60 fsw and 15 min air/60 min oxygen at 30 fsw | 860 |
| USN 6A | 690 |
| USN 6A extended | |
| 20 min oxygen/5 min air at 60 fsw | 763 |
| 15 min air/60 min oxygen at 30 fsw | 833 |
| 20 min oxygen/5 min air at 60 fsw and 15 min air/60 min oxygen at 30 fsw | 906 |
| IFEM 7A*** (air and oxygen) | 1813 |
| IFEM 7A alternating 50/50 Nitrox with | |

*UTPD value indicates duration (minutes) of oxygen breathing at 1.0 ATA that would cause equivalent degree of pulmonary intoxication (measured as decrease in vital capacity). From the Institute for Environmental Medicine. Revision of UPTD concept with addition of new data (16, 20) is ongoing.
**USN (United States Navy)
***IFEM (Institute for Environmental Medicine, University of Pennsylvania)

When patients show signs of pulmonary oxygen toxicity, they must be provided with sufficient time to fully recover before being treated with another course of HBO or receiving supplemental oxygen between treatments. Otherwise, thee patients are risk of developing harmful side effects, as a result of their cumulative oxygen dose. The progression of intoxication is best monitored by serial pulmonary-function studies; however, direct measurement in this fashion may be difficult or unduly expensive (11, 18, 22, 41). Consequently, attempts have been made to quantify the degree of pulmonary intoxication from a single hyperoxic exposure (12, 13, 17) for two purposes: 1) to compare the degree of toxicity expected from exposure to different oxygen pressures for different lengths of time, and 2) to calculate the cumulative toxicity from repeated hyperoxic exposures. These attempts have led to development of the concept of the unit pulmonary toxic dose (UPTD) (6, 47) a standard value that allows physicians to compare the potential pulmonary effects from the various treatment tables. The UPTD is designed to express any pulmonary toxic dose in terms of an equivalent exposure to oxygen at 1.0 ATA. The calculations are based on vital capacity measurements that describe the rate of development of pulmonary intoxication at oxygen pressures above 0.5 ATA.

The UPTD values shown in Table 2 are derived from averaged data obtained during single, continuous-oxygen exposures in healthy male subjects. They should be regarded only as general guidelines for assessing degrees of pulmonary oxygen poisoning in any individual patient. The cumulative effects of pulmonary oxygen toxicity with repeated exposures can be estimated by multiplying the UPTD of the treatment by the number of treatments. In the absence of adequate information about the time course for reversal of pulmonary oxygen poisoning, this value does not provide an estimate of the amount of recovery that can be expected to occur between treatments.

For example, this method would predict that 10 oxygen treatments at 2.4 ATA, or 45 feet of sea water (fsw), for 90 minutes each would give a patient a UPTD of 2,700, and should produce significant pulmonary symptoms, and a 20% reduction in vital capacity (47). However, it is common clinical experience that patients are able to tolerate this daily regimen, 6 days a week, for up to 6 to 8 weeks without reporting any side effects (23). Pulmonary symptoms, such as inspiratory burning or chest tightness, are occasionally experienced by sensitive individuals during administration of a USN Table 6 or 6A, especially when these tables are extended or repeated for treating severe gas lesion diseases, such as decompression sickness or an arterial gas embolism. In the event that saturation with intermittent hyperoxygenation at increased ambient pressure (Institute for Environmental Medicine, University of Pennsylvania 7A or equivalent) is required for gas-lesion diseases that are refractory to standard HBO treatment protocols, the timing and duration of intermittent oxygen periods may be determined partially by the severity of pulmonary symptoms.

## Ocular Effects

Progressive myopia has been reported by some patients who receive daily 90- to 120-minute oxygen treatments at 2.0 to 2.4 ATA for various chronic disease states (3, 4, 39, 42). The overall incidence is approximately 20 to 40%, with some indications of an increased incidence in diabetics and elderly patients. Complete recovery usually occurs within 6 weeks of terminating HBO therapy, but can also be irreversible in exceptional cases (39, 42). Although the observed myopia appears to be lenticular in origin (4, T), the exact mechanism remains obscure. Direct exposure of the eye to 100% $O_2$ in a hood or monoplace chamber is likely, though not yet demonstrated, to produce a higher lens $PO_2$ than when oxygen is delivered via facemask at depth.

The growth of preexisting nuclear cataracts may be stimulated by prolonged series of hyperbaric oxygen therapies, and new cataracts were found in 7 of 15 patients exposed to 150-850 daily therapies at 2.0-2.5 ATA (42). The nuclear cataracts were not reversible after cessation of these extremely prolonged therapy series. Published reports, (3, 4, 39, 42) as well as extensive clinical experience in major HBO centers, indicate that new cataracts do not develop within the series of 20-50 therapies that are used to treat most chronic disease states.

Other reversible effects of hyperoxia on visual function in humans include contraction of peripheral visual fields (8, 38) and reduction in the electrical response of retinal glial cells to a light flash (15, 21). These effects have been observed only with continuous or intermittent, experimental oxygen exposures that greatly exceed the limits of all standard HBO regimens. Visual effects of hyperoxia that have occurred in uniquely susceptible individuals include the development of retrolental fibroplasia in premature infants after exposure to relatively low levels of hyperoxia (43), and a reversible, unilateral loss of vision during a 6-hour oxygen exposure at 2.0 ATA in an individual who had a previous history of retrobulbar neuritis (40).

## MODIFICATION OF OXYGEN TOLERANCE

Susceptibility to developing overt manifestations of pulmonary or CNS oxygen toxicity varies widely among different individuals and animal species (12, 17). Specific chemical manifestations may prove to be less variable. The development rate can also be modified extensively by a variety of conditions, procedures, and drugs. Although most of the factors found to modify oxygen tolerance in laboratory animals have not been evaluated in clinical trials, it is assumed that agents with prominent effects on oxygen tolerance in animals should produce similar effects in human subjects.

### Factors that Decrease Oxygen Tolerance

Examples of factors that either hasten the onset or increase the severity of overt manifestations of oxygen toxicity are shown on the left side of Table 3. While none of these factors should be considered an absolute contraindication to hyperbaric oxygen therapy for a patient who would benefit from treatment, the presence of one or more of the listed influences should be regarded as an indication for caution. Consideration should be given either to reducing the inspired oxygen pressure, or to decreasing the total duration of oxygen exposure.

## TABLE 3. FACTORS THAT MODIFY RATE OF DEVELOPMENT OF OXYGEN POISONING

| HASTEN ONSET OR INCREASE SEVERITY | DELAY ONSET OR DECREASE SEVERITY |
|---|---|
| Adrenocortical hormones | Acclimatization to hypoxia |
| $CO_2$ inhalation | Adrenergic blocking drugs |
| Dextroamphetamine | Antioxidants |
| Epinephrine | Caffeine (low-dose) |
| Hyperthermia | Chlorpromazine |
| Insulin | Gamma-aminobutryic acid |
| Norepinephrine | Ganglionic blocking drugs |
| Paraquat | Glutathione |
| Hyperthyroidism | Hypothyroidism |
| Vitamin E deficiency | Propranolol |
| | Reserpine |
| | Starvation |
| | Succinate |
| | Trisaminomethane |
| | Intermittent exposure* |
| | Disulfiram* |
| | Hypothermia* |
| | Vitamin E* |

*Potentially useful as protective agents (Adapted from Clark and Lambertsen) (10).*

## Factors that Increase Oxygen Tolerance

Other factors, listed on the right side of Table 3, have been found to delay the onset or decrease the severity of overt toxic manifestations. Some factors (indicated by *) are potentially useful as protective agents under appropriate conditions of oxygen exposure. For example, physicians should be cautious when administering Disulfiram (Antabuse) as a neuroprotective agent. While Disulfiram does provide the benefit of delaying the onset of convulsions in animals exposed to oxygen at 4.0 ATA (27, 28), it also enhances the progression of pulmonary intoxication in oxygen at 1.0 ATA (24) or 2.0 ATA (30).

At present, the most rational and practical means for extension of oxygen tolerance in man is the systematic alternation of oxygen-exposure periods with relatively brief intervals of normoxia. Early studies at the University of Pennsylvania (32, 36, W) established the effectiveness of providing these "air breaks" to animal subjects, which led to subsequent validation in humans (34). Additional studies (14, 15, 19) extending these observations have been completed, and open literature documentation is in progress.

## MANAGEMENT OF OXYGEN-INDUCED SEIZURES

Convulsions are hazardous in all patients, but particularly so in those with fractures, osseous nonunion, head injury, cardiac abnormality, or recent surgery. In addition to ensuring standard safety measures that prevent the patient from injuring themselves or aspirating during a seizure, the attending physician must remember that it is extremely important to avoid decompression during the tonic phase of the convulsion, since expanding pulmonary gas could then rupture the lung and produce a possibly fatal arterial-gas embolism. Once there is evidence of tonic-clonic movements and resumes a normal breathing pattern, the patient may undergo decompression.

One chamber requirement that is critical to preventing CNS toxicity is selecting an oxygen-delivery apparatus that limits the amount of carbon dioxide that patients can re-breath while at depth. The simultaneous intake of carbon dioxide with oxygen markedly accelerates the onset of oxygen convulsions, even at pressures as low as 2.0 ATA. Elevation of arterial $PCO_2$ causes cerebral vasodilation with an associated increase in brain oxygen tension. Increased tensions of arterial carbon dioxide partial pressures can also be caused by ventilatory depression following administration of narcotic analgesic drugs such as morphine or meperidine hydrochloride.

Epileptic patients may undergo HBO treatment, but they should be considered much more susceptible to oxygen-induced seizures than patients without a history of seizure disorders. It is prudent to ensure that the patient's anticonvulsant medication regimen has been administered and that they are at therapeutic blood levels prior to starting treatment with HBO.

Oxygen-induced seizures are usually self limited and do not require pharmacologic agents to terminate the seizure activity. The occurrence of an oxygen-induced seizure is not a contraindication to further HBO therapy. Additional seizures can be prevented by shortening the duration of oxygen exposure (inserting more air breaks) and/or by decreasing the oxygen pressure. Although administration of diazepam (Valium) before each treatment can also be used to suppress seizures, instituting an anticonvulsant therapy regimen after the completion of an HBO treatment protocol is not indicated for patients without a pre-existing seizure history.

# REFERENCES

1. Alderman J, Culver BW, Shellenberger MK. "An examination of the role of gamma-aminobutyric acid (GABA) in hyperbaric oxygen-induced convulsions in the rat. I. Effects of increased gamma-aminobutyric acid and protective agents." J Pharmacol Exp Ther 1974; 190:334-40.

2. Allen JE, Goodman DB, Besarab A, Rasmussen H. "Studies on the biochemical basis of oxygen toxicity." Biochem Biophys Acta 1973; 320:708-28.

3. Anderson B Jr., Farmer JC Jr. "Hyperoxic myopia." Trans Am Opthalmol Soc. 1978;76:116-124.

4. Anderson B Jr., Shelton DL. "Axial length in hyperoxic myopia." Bove AA, Bachrach AJ, Greenbaum LJ, eds. Underwater and Hyperbaric Physiology IX. Proceedings of the Ninth International Symposium on Underwater and Hyperbaric Physiology. Bethesda, MD: Undersea and Hyperbaric Medical Society. 1987;607-611.

5. Balentine JD. "Pathology of oxygen toxicity." New York: Academic Press. 1982.

6. Bardin H, Lambertsen CJ. "A quantitative method for calculating pulmonary toxicity. Use of the "Unit pulmonary toxicity dose" (UPTD)." Institute for Environmental Medicine Report. Philadelphia, University of Pennsylvania, 1970.

7. Becker NH, Galvin JF. "Effect of oxygen-rich atmospheres on cerebral lipid peroxides." Aerosp Med 1962; 33:985-7.

8. Behnke AR, Forbes HS, Motley EP. "Circulatory and visual effects of oxygen at 3 atmospheres pressure." Am J Physiol. 1936;114:436-442.

9. Bitterman N, Schaal S. "Caffeine attenuates CNS oxygen toxicity in rats." Brain Research. 1995; 696(1-2):250-3.

10. Braughler JM, Burton PS, Chase RL, et al. "Novel membrane localized iron chelators as inhibitors of iron-dependent lipid peroxidation." Biochem Pharmacol 1988; 37:3853-60.

11. Caldwell PRB, Lee WL Jr, Schildkraut HS, Archibald ER. "Changes in lung volume, diffusing capacity, and blood gases in men breathing oxygen." J Appl Physiol. 1966;21:1477-1483.

12. Clark JM. "Oxygen toxicity." Bennett PB, Elliott DH (Eds.) The Physiology and Medicine of Diving, 3rd Ed. London: Bailliere, Tindall and Cox. 1982;200-238.

13. Clark JM. "Pulmonary limits of oxygen tolerance in man." Experimental Lung Research. 1988;14:897-910.

14. Clark JM, Gelfand R, Stevens WC, Lambertsen CJ. "Extension of pulmonary oxygen tolerance in man at 2.0 ATA by intermittent exposure on 60:15 oxygen:normoxic pattern in Predictive Studies VI." Undersea Biomed Res. (Suppl) 1990;17:25.

15. Clark JM, Gelfand R, Stevens WC, Lambertsen CJ. "Comparison of human visual and pulmonary responses to continuous and intermittent oxygen exposure at 2.0 ATA in Predictive Studies V and VI." Undersea Biomed Res. (Suppl) 1991;18:86.

16. Clark JM, Jackson RM, Lambertsen CJ, Gelfand R, Hiller WDB, Unger M. "Pulmonary function in men after oxygen breathing at 3.0 ATA for 3.5 h." J Appl Physiol. 1991;71:878-885.

17. Clark JM, Lambertsen CJ. "Pulmonary oxygen toxicity: A review." Pharmacol Rev. 1971;23:37-133.

18. Clark JM, Lambertsen CJ. "Rate of development of pulmonary oxygen toxicity in man during oxygen breathing at 2.0 ATA." J Appl Physiol. 1971;30:739-752.

19. Clark JM, Lambertsen CJ. "Principles of oxygen tolerance extension defined in the rat by intermittent oxygen exposure at 2.0 and 4.0 ATA." Undersea Biomed Res. 16 (Suppl) 1989;99.

20. Clark JM, Lambertsen CJ, Gelfand R, Flores ND, Pisarello JB, Rossman MD, Elias JA. "Effects of prolonged oxygen exposure at 1.5, 2.0, or 2.5 ATA on pulmonary function in men (Predictive Studies V)." J Appl Physiol. 1999;86(1): In press.

21. Clark JM, Lambertsen CJ, Montabana DJ, Gelfand R, Cobbs WH. "Comparison of visual function effects in man during continuous oxygen exposures at 3.0 and 2.0 ATA for 3.4 and 9.0 hours." Undersea Biomed Res. 15(Suppl) 1988;32.

22. Comroe JH Jr, Dripps RD, Dumke PR, Deming M. "Oxygen toxicity. The effect of inhalation of high concentrations of oxygen for twenty-four hours on normal men at sea level and at a simulated altitude of 18,000 feet." JAMA. 1945;128:710-717.

23. Davis JC, Dunn JM, Heimbach RD. "Hyperbaric medicine: Patient selection, treatment procedures, and side effects." Davis JC, Hunt TK, (Eds.) Problem Wounds: The Role of Oxygen. New York: Elsevier. 1988;225-235.

24. Deneke SM, Bernstein SP, Fanburg BL. "Enhancement by disulfiram (Antabuse) of toxic effects of 95 to 97% oxygen on the rat lung." J Pharmacol Exp Ther. 1979;208:377-380.

25. Dhawan A, Parmar P, Seth D, Seth PK. "Cytochrome P-450 dependent monooxygenases in neuronal and glial cells: inducibility and specificity." Bio Chem Biophys Research Comm 1990; 170(2):441-7.

26. Donald KW. "Oxygen poisoning in man. I and II." Br Med. J. 1947;1:667-672, 712-717.

27. Faiman MD, Mehl RG, Oehme FW. "Protection with disulfiram from central and pulmonary oxygen toxicity." Biochem Pharmacol. 1971;20:3059-3067.

28. Faiman MD, Nolan RJ, Oehme FW. "Effect of disulfiram on oxygen toxicity in beagle dogs." Aerospace Med. 1974;45:29-32.

29. Forman HJ, Fisher AB. "Antioxidant defenses." Gilbert DL (Ed.) Oxygen and Living Processes. New York: Springer-Verlag. 1981;235-249.

30. Forman HJ, York JL, Fisher AB. "Mechanism for the potentiation of oxygen toxicity by disulfiram." J. Pharmacol Exp Ther. 1980;212:452-455.

31. Frank L, McLaughlin GE. "Protection against acute and chronic hyperoxic inhibition of neonatal rat lung development with the 21-aminosteroid U-74389F." Pediatr Res 1993; 33:632-8.

32. Hall DA. "The influence of the systematic fluctuation of $PO_2$ upon the nature and rate of development of oxygen toxicity in guinea-pigs." Master's Thesis, University of Pennsylvania, 1967.

33. Haynes J, Seibert A, Bass JB, Taylor AE. "U74500A inhibition of oxidant-mediated lung injury." Am J Physiol 1990; 259:H144-H148.

34. Hendricks PL, Hall DA, Hunter WL Jr, Haley PJ. "Extension of pulmonary oxygen tolerance in man at 2 ATA by intermittent oxygen exposure." J Appl Physiol. 1977;42:593-599.

35. Jamieson D. "Oxygen toxicity and reactive oxygen metabolites in mammals." Free Radical Biology and Medicine. 1989;7:87-108.

36. Lambertsen CJ. "Respiratory and circulatory actions of high oxygen pressure." Goff LG (Ed.) Proceedings of the Underwater Physiology Symposium. Washington, DC, National Academy of Sciences-National Research Council, Pub 377, 1955;25-38.

37. Lambertsen CJ. "Effects of hyperoxia on organs and their tissues." Robin E (Ed.) Extrapulmonary Manifestations of Respiratory Disease. New York: Marcel Dekker. 1978;239-303.

38. Lambertsen CJ, Clark JM, Gelfand R, Pisarello J, Cobbs WH, Bevilacqua JE, Schwartz DM, Montabana DJ, Leach CS, Johnson PC, Fletcher DE. "Definition of tolerance to continuous hyperoxia in man. An abstract report of Predictive Studies V." Bove AA, Bachrach AJ, Greenbaum LJ (Eds.) Underwater and Hyperbaric Physiology IX. Proceedings of the Ninth International Symposium on Underwater and Hyperbaric Physiology. Bethesda, MD: Undersea and Hyperbaric Medical Society. 1987;717-735.

39. Lyne AJ. "Ocular effects of hyperbaric oxygen." Trans Opthalmol Soc. 1978;98:66-68.

40. Nichols CW, Lambertsen CJ, Clark JM. "Transient unilateral loss of vision associated with oxygen at high pressure." Arch Opthalmol. 1969;81:548-552.

41. Ohlsson WTL. "A study on oxygen toxicity at atmospheric pressure." Acta Med Scand.(Suppl) 1947;190.

42. Palmquist BM, Philipson B, Barr PO. "Nuclear cataract and myopia during hyperbaric oxygen therapy." Br J Opthalmol. 1984;68:113-117.

43. Patz, A. "Effect of oxygen on immature retinal vessels." Invest Opthalmol. 1965;4:988-999.

44. Richards IM, Griffin RL, Fidler SF, Jacobsen EJ. "Effect of the 21-aminosteroid U-74389F on hyperoxic lung injury in rats." Agents Actions 1993; 39:C136-8.

45. Torbati D. "Effect of propranolol on brain electrical activity during hyperbaric oxygenation in the rat." Undersea Bio Res 1985; 12:423-9.

46. Whelan HT, Bajic DM, Karlovits SM, Houle JM, Kindwall EP. "Use of Cytochrome-P450 Mono-Oxygenase 2 E1 Isozyme Inhibitors to Delay Seizures Caused by Central Nervous System Oxygen Toxicity." Aviation, Space, and Environmental Medicine 1998; 69(5):480-5.

47. Wright WB. "Use of the University of Pennsylvania Institute for Environmental Medicine procedure for calculation of cumulative pulmonary oxygen toxicity." US Navy Experimental Diving Unit. 1972;Report 2-72.

A. Balestra C, Germonpre P, Poortmans JR, Marroni A. Serum erythropoietin levels in healthy humans after a short period of normobaric and hyperbaric oxygen breathing: The "normobaric oxygen paradox". J Appl Physiol. 2006 Feb;100(2):512-8.

B. Ahmad S, White CW, Chang LY, Schneider BK, Allen CB. Glutamine protects mitochondrial structure and function in oxygen toxicity. American Journal of Physiology - Lung Cellular & Molecular Physiology. 2001 Apr;280(4):779-91.

C. Liang LP, Ho YS, Patel M. Mitochondrial superoxide production in kainate-induced hippocampal damage. Neuroscience. 2000;101(3):563-70.

D. Liang LP, Patel M. Mitochondrial oxidative stress and increased seizure susceptibility in Sod2(-/+) mice. Free Radic Biol Med. 2004 Mar 1;36(5):542-54.

E.  Sheffield PJ. How the davis 2.36 ATA wound healing enhancement treatment table was established. Undersea & Hyperbaric Medicine. 2004;31(2):193-4.

F.  Shinkai M, Shinomiya N, Kanoh S, Motoyoshi K, Kobayashi H. Oxygen stress effects on proliferation rates and heat shock proteins in lymphocytes. Aviation Space & Environmental Medicine. 2004 Feb;75(2):109-13.

G.  Suttner DM, Sridhar K, Lee CS, Tomura T, Hansen TN, Dennery PA. Protective effects of transient HO-1 overexpression on susceptibility to oxygen toxicity in lung cells. Am J Physiol. 1999 Mar;276(3 Pt 1):443-51.

H.  Topal T, Oter S, Korkmaz A, Sadir S, Metinyurt G, Korkmazhan ET, Serdar MA, Bilgic H, Reiter RJ. Exogenously administered and endogenously produced melatonin reduce hyperbaric oxygen-induced oxidative stress in rat lung. Life Sci. 2004 Jun 11;75(4):461-7.

I.  van Hulst RA, Haitsma JJ, Lameris TW, Klein J, Lachmann B. Hyperventilation impairs brain function in acute cerebral air embolism in pigs.[see comment]. Intensive Care Med. 2004 May;30(5):944-50.

J.  Vann RD. Lambertsen and $O_2$: Beginnings of operational physiology. Undersea & Hyperbaric Medicine. 2004;31(1):21-31.

K.  Bitterman N. CNS oxygen toxicity. Undersea & Hyperbaric Medicine. 2004;31(1):63-72.

L.  Chavko M, Xing G, Keyser DO. Increased sensitivity to seizures in repeated exposures to hyperbaric oxygen: Role of NOS activation. Brain Res. 2001 May 11;900(2):227-33.

M.  Hampson N, Atik D. Central nervous system oxygen toxicity during routine hyperbaric oxygen therapy.[see comment]. Undersea & Hyperbaric Medicine. 2003;30(2):147-53.

N.  Helms AK, Whelan HT, Torbey MT. Hyperbaric oxygen therapy of cerebral ischemia. Cerebrovascular Diseases. 2005;20(6):417-26.

O.  Yildiz S, Aktas S, Cimsit M, Ay H, Togrol E. Seizure incidence in 80,000 patient treatments with hyperbaric oxygen.[see comment]. Aviation Space & Environmental Medicine. 2004 Nov;75(11):992-4.

P.  Plafki C, Peters P, Almeling M, Welslau W, Busch R. Complications and side effects of hyperbaric oxygen therapy.[see comment]. Aviation Space & Environmental Medicine. 2000 Feb;71(2):119-24.

Q.  Weaver LK, Churchill S. Pulmonary edema associated with hyperbaric oxygen therapy. Chest. 2001 Oct;120(4):1407-9.

R.  Huang TY, Tsai PS, Wang TY, Huang CL, Huang CJ. Hyperbaric oxygen attenuation of lipopolysaccharide-induced acute lung injury involves heme oxygenase-1. Acta Anaesthesiol Scand. 2005 Oct;49(9):1293-301.

S.  Smerz RW. Incidence of oxygen toxicity during the treatment of dysbarism. Undersea & Hyperbaric Medicine. 2004;31(2):199-202.

T.  Bantseev V, Oriowo OM, Giblin FJ, Leverenz VR, Trevithick JR, Sivak JG. Effect of hyperbaric oxygen on guinea pig lens optical quality and on the refractive state of the eye. Exp Eye Res. 2004 May;78(5):925-31.

U.  Buhrke T, Lenz O, Krauss N, Friedrich B. Oxygen tolerance of the $H_2$-sensing [NiFe] hydrogenase from ralstonia eutropha H16 is based on limited access of oxygen to the active site. J Biol Chem. 2005 Jun 24;280(25):23791-6.

V. Capellier G, Beuret P, Clement G, Depardieu F, Ract C, Regnard J, Robert D, Barale F. Oxygen tolerance in patients with acute respiratory failure. Intensive Care Med. 1998 May;24(5):422-8.

W. Clark JM. Extension of oxygen tolerance by interrupted exposure.[comment]. Undersea & Hyperbaric Medicine. 2004;31(2):195-8.

X. Stephens M, Frey M, Mohler S, Khamis H, Penne R, Bishop J, Bowden A. Effect of caffeine consumption on tissue oxygen levels during hyperbaric oxygen treatment. Undersea & Hyperbaric Medicine. 1999;26(2):93-7.

## APPENDIX - MEASURING PULMONARY OXYGEN TOXICITY

### The Unit Pulmonary Toxicity Dose Concept (Original Definition)*

Using the standard treatment protocols as outlined in this manual, there is little or no danger that patients will experience pulmonary oxygen toxicity. If, however, patients must be carried on supplemental $O_2$ between treatments, pulmonary oxygen toxicity can become a real problem. The UPTD method allows one to predict how soon someone will become toxic when continuously exposed to high partial pressures of oxygen.

The following section is adapted from Rutkowski and Wells' outline of this method for "bookkeeping" the pulmonary effects of oxygen exposure as presented in the UHMS/NOAA diving medicine course for physicians. This method was originally developed at the University of Pennsylvania (1, 4).

The "Unit Pulmonary Toxicity Dose" (UPTD) concept of Wright (1972) allows one to estimate the degree of pulmonary toxicity incurred by breathing oxygen at partial pressures in excess of 0.5 ATA. Oxygen exposures should be planned so as not to exceed the following limits. During decompression and for treatment of mild decompression sickness, the total oxygen exposure should be limited to that which yields a UPTD of 615 or less. In the use of oxygen for medical therapy or treatment of serious decompression sickness which is responding poorly, an extreme limit of oxygen exposure which yields a UPTD of 1425 or less should be planned. A dose of 1425 will produce a predicted 10% decrease in vital capacity. U. S. Navy Table 6 (2, 3) gives a UPTD of 645. Occasionally these limits are knowingly exceeded when medically required (a Table 6 with multiple extensions, for example).

Having derived a formula for calculating a UPTD, Wright developed a simplified arithmetic method and constructed a table which may be used to calculate oxygen exposure from 0.6 to 5.0 atmospheres. The following arithmetic method enables the calculation of the total UPTD for a given oxygen exposure or sequences of exposures. This method, however, makes no provision for interrupted exposures to elevated oxygen partial pressures. Such interruptions are known to increase oxygen tolerance, but the expected improvement in tolerance has not yet been fully quantitated for humans. Doses of 600 UPTD given in two treatment sessions have been administered on a daily basis with no evidence of cumulative toxicity.

*UPTD concept is under revision with addition of new data.

## ARITHMETIC METHOD

1. Convert the partial pressure of oxygen breathed at each depth to $PO_2$ in atmospheres ($PO_2$ = fraction of inspired $O_2$ x total pressure in atmospheres).

2. Select the corresponding Kp from Table 1 (below).

3. Multiply the time of exposure (in minutes) at that $PO_2$ by the corresponding Kp to get the UPTD for that depth.

4. Add the UPTD's for each $PO_2$ in the complete exposure together to get the total UPTD for the exposure (1).

## TABLE 1. KP FACTORS FOR CALCULATING UPTD

| $PO_2$ | Kp | $PO_2$ | Kp | $PO_2$ | Kp | $PO_2$ | Kp |
|------|------|------|------|------|------|------|------|
| 0.50 | 0.00 | 1.70 | 2.07 | 2.90 | 3.70 | 4.10 | 5.18 |
| 0.60 | 0.26 | 1.80 | 2.22 | 3.00 | 3.82 | 4.20 | 5.30 |
| 0.70 | 0.47 | 1.90 | 2.36 | 3.10 | 3.95 | 4.30 | 5.42 |
| 0.80 | 0.65 | 2.00 | 2.50 | 3.20 | 4.08 | 4.40 | 5.54 |
| 0.90 | 0.83 | 2.10 | 2.64 | 3.30 | 4.20 | 4.50 | 5.66 |
| 1.00 | 1.00 | 2.20 | 2.77 | 3.40 | 4.33 | 4.60 | 5.77 |
| 1.10 | 1.16 | 2.30 | 2.91 | 3.50 | 4.45 | 4.70 | 5.89 |
| 1.20 | 1.32 | 2.40 | 3.04 | 3.60 | 4.57 | 4.80 | 6.01 |
| 1.30 | 1.48 | 2.50 | 3.17 | 3.70 | 4.70 | 4.90 | 6.12 |
| 1.40 | 1.63 | 2.60 | 3.31 | 3.80 | 4.82 | 5.00 | 6.24 |
| 1.50 | 1.78 | 2.70 | 3.44 | 3.90 | 4.94 | | |
| 1.60 | 1.93 | 2.80 | 3.57 | 4.00 | 5.06 | | |

**REFERENCES FOR APPENDIX**

1. Bardin H, Lambertsen CJ. "A quantitative method for calculating pulmonary toxicity. Use of the "Unit Pulmonary Toxicity Dose" (UPTD)." Institute for Environmental Medicine Report. Philadelphia: University of Pennsylvania, 1970.

2. NOAA Diving Manual, GPO #003-017-00468-6, Best Publishing Company.

3. U. S. Navy Diving Manual, NAVSEA 0994-LP-001-9010, Best Publishing Company.

4. Wright WB: "Use of the University of Pennsylvania Institute for Environmental Medicine procedure for calculation of cumulative pulmonary oxygen toxicity." U. S. Navy Experimental Diving Unit Report 2-72, 1972.

**References 0806**

Biochemical Mechanisms of Oxygen Poisoning

(1-10)

Manifestations Of Oxygen Poisoning
Central Nervous System Effects

(9, 11-16)

Pulmonary Effects

(7, 16-19)

Ocular effects

(20)

Modifications of Oxygen Tolerance

(7, 21-23)

Management of Oxygen-Induced Seizures

(11, 13, 15, 24)

CHAPTER 5

# THE MONOPLACE CHAMBER

## CHAPTER FIVE OVERVIEW

# THE MONOPLACE CHAMBER

*George B. Hart*

## INTRODUCTION

Our interest in the monoplace chamber began upon starting an investigation using hyperbaric oxygen (HBO) to treat acute thermal burns. (9) The device solved two problems with HBO that confronted that research in the late 1960s. A mask to deliver oxygen was unnecessary in a monoplace chamber compressed with oxygen. Specifically, patients with thermal burns or other conditions (osteomyelitis or radiation burns) about the head and neck may not tolerate a mask or hood delivery system available in the multiplace chamber. Also, the patient's mattress would be easily adapted into the existing hospital environment of the time. The latter was considered the most important because of the ease of operation, maintenance, and low cost of operation. A recent evaluation (23) notes this equitable operation cost. It further notes the equity of having oxygen recycling in areas where liquid oxygen (LOX) is not either available or nor equitable.

The history of the monoplace chamber, however, spans greater than 175 years. It is briefly touched on in the following notes.

## HISTORY OF THE MONOPLACE CHAMBER

### First Report

Junod (12) first described the clinical use of a monoplace hyperbaric chamber in 1834. The chamber was a hollow sphere of copper measuring 1.4 meters (approximately five feet) in diameter. Remarkably, the first patients were treated at hypobaric pressures with the internal working pressures lowered to 500 mmHg air absolute. He discarded this technique when the patients consistently became short of breath and cyanotic. He then used pressures of two to four atmospheres absolute (ATA) air with more observed success.

### Recent Developments

Following Junod, monoplace chambers were relegated to the treatment of decompression illness until Churchill-Davidson (5) reported HBO as a radiation sensitizer for malignancies. He used it concurrently with radiation therapy in 1955. It's noteworthy that "a modified naval diving recompression chamber" was used in this report, assisted by the "surgeons and diving officers of *H.M.S. Vernon* and *H.M.S. Reclaim*." This was a unique human trial, as it was the first clinical trial using anesthetized patients in a monoplace chamber. Each patient was monitored with an electrocardiograph and electromyograph. The middle ear was protected against barotrauma by elective myringotomy prior to pressurization. The spontaneously breathing patients' respirations were monitored by a thermistor mounted on an outlet of the carbon-dioxide absorbing canister.

The majority of monoplace chambers, at that time, were cylindrical in shape and made mostly of metal with small, tempered-glass view ports. These chambers usually measured 26 to 36 inches in diameter and were seven to eight feet in length. A patient tray is required in this type, usually of similar length to gain entrance and exit, and requiring a clearance of an additional six feet or more in room length for patient insertion.

The Vickers hyperbaric oxygen bed was designed to operate in a smaller space (approximately seven feet) than the preceding cylindrical chambers. This is accomplished by placing the patient in a seated position using a bivalve top hinged at the foot end of the chamber. The top is opened by elevating the top from the bottom. The first prototype of the "clam-shell" device (1) was installed in the Westminster Hospital (England) in 1964. The English have since stopped production of this model, but its configuration found favor in Russia, and there it was mass produced in a similar model. See Figure 1 which displays a Russian copy of the Vickers "clam-shell' operating in Cuba.

An important contribution during this period of development was making the monoplace hull out of clear plastic, allowing improved visual contact with the patient and greatly reducing claustrophobia. Emery et al. (6) inspired the development of this design when setting out the following goals:

1. Production of a mobile chamber, able to withstand at least one atmosphere above ambient, which would allow continuous visual and auditory contact with the patient.
2. Elimination of any features which make the conscious patient unwilling to undergo this form of treatment.

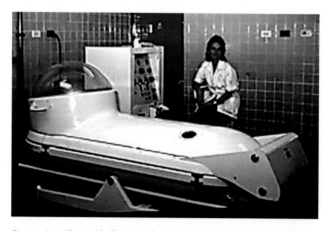

Figure 1. "Clam" Shell Monoplace Chamber a Russian copy of an English design with recycling of oxygen through a $CO_2$ absorber in geographic locations that liquid $O_2$ is not available or in short supply.

3. Elimination of the risk of explosive decompression, which may endanger bystanders and adversely affect the patient because of a sudden drop in pressure.
4. Development of a system of pressurization to minimize ear and sinus pain or damage (otic/sinus barotrauma). These syndromes are caused by differences of pressure between the environment, the sinus, and middle-ear cavities.
5. Provision of adequate ventilation, giving full oxygenation and to prevent retention of water vapor, and carbon dioxide inside the chamber.

Ambulances were reportedly equipped with these plastic chambers in the early 1960s to treat carbon monoxide intoxication (15) and myocardial infarction (19). The portability of monoplace chambers has made it suitable for close support of military diving activities from World War II to the present. It has been successfully used in treating commercial (2) and sports divers (16, 17). Uniquely, it's been used as a transfer device, transporting the chamber by helicopter to a stricken diver, and then returning the patient back, under pressure, to a larger treatment facility.

## ADVERSE OCCURRENCES
Historically, eight significant chamber accidents have occurred with monoplace chambers (some times and locations are approximate).

1. 1968 in the USA, a plastic curved window exploded at the bolt holes fastening it to a metal hull, causing severe lacerations to a nearby radiotherapist. The patient died some time later from the malignancy for which he was being treated at the time of the accident. This accident was the sole stimulus for the development of the double-hulled, acrylic chamber for use in the USA so as to prevent injury to personnel in the immediate area, if there is sudden material fatigue. Note: the enlarged monoplace chambers of the 1990s and now into the 20th millennium have returned to a single shell design.
2. 1969 in Mexico, a telescopically-collapsible, metal chamber exploded at an unknown operating pressure with the occupant reportedly dying from the event. This type has been discontinued by the manufacturer.
3. 1960s in the USA, a patient suffered a runaway pacemaker after reaching 2.5 ATA pressure. The patient was decompressed emergently due to the shock-like state from a heart rate of 240 per minute. Fortunately, the attending Naval Medical Officer (thoracic surgeon) rapidly excised the malfunctioning internal pacemaker and replaced it temporarily with an external model. The manufacturers were notified of this occurrence and now produce implantable models that are pressure resistant (14). The pacing electrical stimulus is insufficient to create an ignition point within the myocardium. Please note: temporary external cardiac pacemakers are unsafe within an oxygen environment under pressure, but may

be safely used when placed external to the chamber and the leads glanded through the bulkhead of the system.

4. In the 1970s in the USA, a fiberglass patient tray burst into flames outside the chamber due to a break in the electrical grounding wire running through the matrix of the material. The patient and attendants in the room were not injured. The flaming tray was thrown from the room to the exterior of the building through a glass window. The fiberglass trays were rapidly replaced by the manufacturer with conductive metal (ferrous material) trays.

5. In the 1970s in Japan, a patient was burned to death in a prototype monoplace chamber. An ignition device was allowed in with the patient. No further development of this particular model has occurred to date.

6. In the 1980s in Italy, a four-year-old child was incinerated in a monoplace chamber when a rolling toy which produced sparks as it moved was allowed inside, where it became an ignition source. The use of monoplace chamber was summarily banned by the Italian government. A pertinent reminder is that electrical devices introduced into an oxygen environment *must be tested and shown to be intrinsically safe for the rated pressures conforming to Underwriter's Laboratories Code 913.*

7. In the 1980s in Japan, two patients were fatally burned in monoplace chambers when butane fueled hand warmers were allowed in with the patients.

8. In 1996 in Japan, another patient was killed when he was placed in an acrylic chamber with a chemical hand warmer on his chest hidden under two plastic fiber blankets. On transfer from another hospital, he was not stripped and dressed in all cotton clothing. The enormous fuel load provided by the synthetic blankets caused the chamber to rupture, the ends blowing off, failing as designed, before the plastic shell ruptured. The patient's wife was outside and fatally injured when struck by the chamber door which went on to exit the room through a wall.

## MONOPLACE CHAMBER PROBLEMS SOLVED IN THE 1970s

Explosive decompression from "O" ring door seal failure was resolved by developing the flanged "O" ring. We observed explosive decompressions from time to time with the available monoplace equipment until 1974. The patient was instantaneously decompressed and the observers were uniformly startled by a loud report similar to a shotgun being fired in very close proximity. In the three or four instances in which this has occurred, the only patient morbidity noted that by this author was moderate barotrauma to the ears and sinuses, and resulted in a perforated eardrum in one patient.

A ventilator was developed for monoplace chamber use. Respirator-dependent patients may now be supported on ventilators during treatment. The driving mechanism is external to the chamber environment. The chamber operator may externally adjust the tidal volume and rate to meet the demands of the patient. Close attendance of a trained and experienced operator is required for this application. It is recommended that technicians maintain their skills with these devices by repetitive training on artificial lungs. Rarely, when the availability of pediatric ventilators is exceeded due to several children exposed to smoke inhalation/carbon monoxide, a physician/respiratory technician qualified in such ventilation may assist the moribund patient. See Figure 2.

Further, this author does not recommend placement of water in the humidifier, as it will lead to a very wet airway requiring frequent suctioning. Note: the time of exposure to dry oxygen in the usual treatment protocols has not been reported as causing any long term effects on the airway mucosa.

Externally operated displacement pumps were developed so that required intravenous fluids and medications may be administered while the patient is under pressure. This particular application requires close observation to prevent the accidental injection of gas.

Patients requiring temporary cardiac pacing may be successfully paced with a device external to the chamber. The pacer wires are glanded through the bulkhead to the patient. Coordination of chamber personnel to effect the change for chamber entry and exit is essential for patient safety.

Discomfort from heating of the chamber atmosphere during pressurization and cooling during decompression may be ameliorated by passing the oxygen through a heat exchanger. The heat exchanger is a type of radiator where the gas is piped through a water jacket. The gas is then warmed or cooled by the circulating water to maintain the desired temperature for patient treatment.

The back bleeding, which could occur from an accidental disconnection of an intravascular line, is now prevented by a check valve in the tubing, before the pass-through port in the door or bulkhead. However, the blood loss in the past from these disruptions was insufficient to cause alterations in the patients' vital signs. It does prevent soiling of the equipment and reduces anxiety during an accident made obvious by the spilled red cells.

Ways were developed to continue chest tube drainage under pressure by using a Heimlich valve with a non-return valve in sequence with a drainage bag. Please note it is not advisable to place a patient with brisk bleeding from

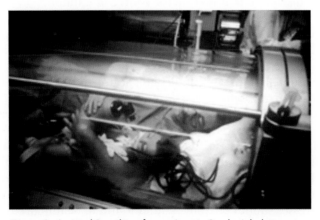

*Figure 2. Assisted Breathing for an Apneic Smoke Inhalation.*

the thoracic cavity (>200 cc per hour) into a monoplace chamber with the Heimlich valve system being the only means to evacuate the blood loss.

A suction system can be created within a monoplace chamber by connecting a vacuum regulator valve exterior to the chamber. This gives the chamber operator the ability to aspirate fluids or gas, as in the preceding case of chest drainage, or it can make possible blood sampling from intravenous or arterial lines. The check valves in the tubing of these lines must be removed in order to make this system work.

Blood analysis at pressure may also be accomplished by the preceding action. Tissue-gas determinations are possible at pressure using continuous micro sampling Teflon-tipped cannulae placed in the selected tissue. The gases are measured by mass spectrometry in a device external to the chamber environment.

An adjustable flow rate of oxygen solves the occasional problem of hypothermia in susceptible children. Decreasing the flow decreases the evaporative heat loss. In reverse fashion, the flow rate may be increased, thereby accelerating the evaporative heat loss and cooling the patient.

## MONOPLACE CHAMBER PROBLEMS SOLVED IN THE 1980s

A non-invasive, automated blood-pressure device became available. This device uses Doppler technology to detect systolic and diastolic pressures.

A non-invasive, laser capillary-flow meter was introduced. The device uses a fiber-optic cable that is passed through the bulkhead at a suitable point, and topical blood flow may be measured by an externally located flow meter.

Radiometer developed a transcutaneous, oxygen-partial-pressure monitor that could be used in the monoplace chamber. Transcutaneous tissue partial pressures of oxygen and carbon dioxide can now be safely measured via an intrinsically safe electrode placed directly on the patient's skin. The electrode cable is glanded through the bulkhead from the patient to an external digital display on the transcutaneous oxygen meter.

## ITEMS PROHIBITED IN THE MONOPLACE CHAMBER

1. Clothing, pillows, and coverings made from plastic fibers may collect a static discharge that may be the source of ignition.
2. Air-activated chemical warming devices. these products in a hyperbaric oxygen environment greatly increases the supply of oxidant and thus increases the rate of reaction and maximum temperature to unacceptable levels.
3. Combustible liquids such as alcohol, acetone, or ether to remove adhesive from skin.
4. Vaseline or oil on open wounds. Vaseline gauze dressings are acceptable, if covered. Remove spilled oil from the black conductive rubber flash covers, as the oils may build up on the conductive mattress reducing its conductivity. Also, oils may accumulate within the filters, presenting a potential for ignition. Routine cleaning of the filters is recommended. Routine tests of the conductivity of the mattresses should be done, and, if found to be impaired, they should be replaced.

5. External pacemakers represent a source of ignition and may not be pressure resistant. Do not allow them in the chamber.
6. Prostheses such as artificial limbs should be removed, particularly if hinged with metallic joints, because of the possibility of scratching the acrylic-chamber surface.
7. Removable dentures, retainers, and/or bridges should be removed to avoid possible airway blockage if the patient sustains an oxygen seizure.
8. Hard contact lenses may become tightly adhered to the cornea, requiring the services of an ophthalmologist to remove.
9. Hearing aids are not pressure resistant. Conceivably, it could be a problem if the fit is occlusive; as pressure rises, the aid could be forced into the external auditory canal. In the absence of the aid, the internal speaker volume of the chamber may be increased to meet the needs of the patient.
10. Wigs, cosmetics, hair sprays are excluded. Patients are advised to bathe and shampoo using soaps without oils.

## ITEMS PERMITTED IN THE MONOPLACE CHAMBER

1. A cotton sheet to cover the conductive mattress and the patient is to be used, as well as a cotton pillow case for the patient's pillow. Cotton blankets are used for warmth. Please note: cotton herein refers to pure cotton, and not a mixture of plastic fiber with cotton fiber. These items must be specially acquired. Although cotton is nonconductive, the moisture derived from sweating skin effectively grounds the patient through the sheets to the underlying conductive mattress cover.
2. Patients wear a pure cotton smock (preferred by author) or jump suit without pockets.
3. Cervical traction tray with radiolucent underside may be used if the patient is separately grounded to the underlying grounding strip.
4. External skeletal fixation devices may be used, as the bolts that pass into and/or through the underlying bone ground them. Any sharp edges on the external device must be padded with cotton pads to prevent scratching of the acrylic hull.
5. Fiberglass casts may be used for local extremity skeletal support, if proper patient grounding is insured. It is noteworthy that the binding matrix of fiberglass becomes with time a very combustible substance. Please note: the patient tray of the Vickers CH3 monoplace chamber was made of fiberglass and one ignited following its removal. Apparently, this was due to a spark from a broken grounding wire running through the matrix of the patient tray.

## MONOPLACE CHAMBER TYPES

**Modifications:** The officers, nurses, and corpsmen of the United States Navy at the Naval Hospital, Long Beach, California, (1967 through 1975) were especially responsible directly or indirectly for many of the modifications of the monoplace chamber presently available to treat critically ill patients. To those enlightened young people this author is particularly grateful. A composite of the optimal system as envisioned in 1971 is displayed in Figure 3.

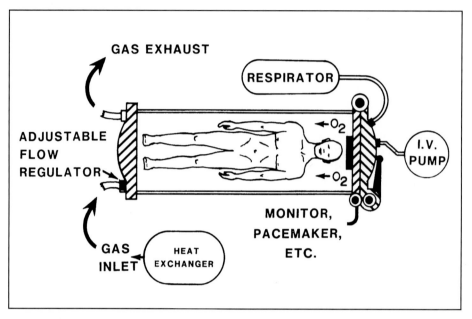

GAS EXHAUST

RESPIRATOR

ADJUSTABLE FLOW REGULATOR

I.V. PUMP

MONITOR, PACEMAKER, ETC.

GAS INLET    HEAT EXCHANGER

*Figure 3. The optimal monoplace chamber system.*

## Geometric Shapes of the Chamber

The chamber hull may be with or without bilges (wet or dry) which are fabricated as specified by the ANSI/ASME PVHO Code. A bilge is the space beneath the tray supporting the patient. Most are maintained as a dry bilge, but a wet bilge conceivably may be of benefit, as it may add to the moisture content within the chamber.

**Sphere, spheroid, or cylinder-on-end:** The patient is treated in a seated position. Patient access is usually through a clamshell, hinged, or sliding door hatch. It is usually reserved for chronically ill patients who can tolerate the seated position.

**Horizontal cylinder:** The patient is treated in a supine or prone position. Patient access is usually through an opened, hinged end plate. This model has been the most popular geometric form, as it may be used not only for the acutely ill, but may also service the chronically ill. Several models are available in this class. See Figure 4 for composite and portable types. See Figures 5, 6, 7, and 8. Please note in Figure 8, this model is equipped so that an attendant may be seated inside at the head of the patient. Any of the presently available models require a longitudinal space of at least 16 feet for ease of insertion and extraction of the patient.

**Sphere and cylinder combination:** The patient is treated in a partially seated or Fowler's laying position. Patient access is through a cantilevered, horizontal clamshell opening. This is popular in areas where there is limited space for withdrawal of a patient tray. See Figure 1.

## CHAMBER MATERIALS

The material composition of the pressure hull must be of sufficient strength to contain the designated treatment pressures. Importantly, if it is used to contain oxygen at pressure, it must be fire resistant and compatible with oxygen. See Figure 4.

**Rigid and non-collapsible:** These are designed to be durable and may be heavy enough to require reinforcement of the underlying floor. Importantly, if one is concerned about weight distribution (weight over 1000 pounds in a four-point distribution) in a proposed area, then inquiry must be made of a hospital architect. These heavy models may be designed to withstand exceptional pressures, such as 165 feet of sea water (6 ATA) or greater. Most models designed for hospitals have a maximum operating pressure of 3 ATA. The 3 ATA pressure was elected for hospital applications to preclude their inadvertent use at higher pressures, thus avoiding accidental oxygen toxicity.

**Note:** *Fiberglass construction is not recommended for hyperbaric chambers or for parts of chambers, as the epoxy bonding materials deteriorate with time into highly combustible compounds.*

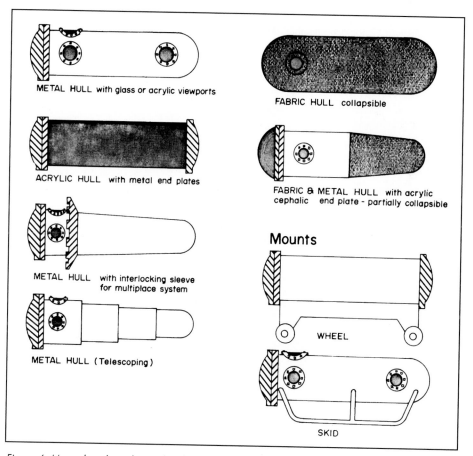

Figure 4. Monoplace hyperbaric chamber systems.

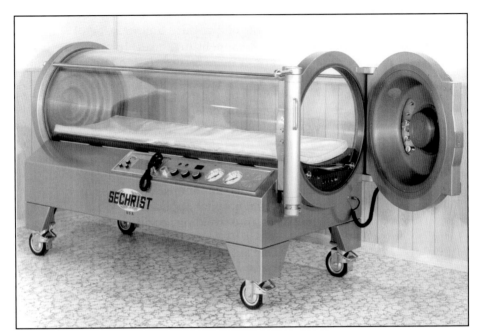

Figure 5. Sechrist Monoplace Chamber - Model 2500B.

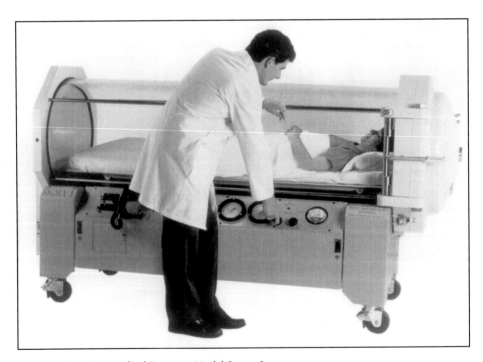

Figure 6. Perry Baromedical Services - Model Sigma 1.

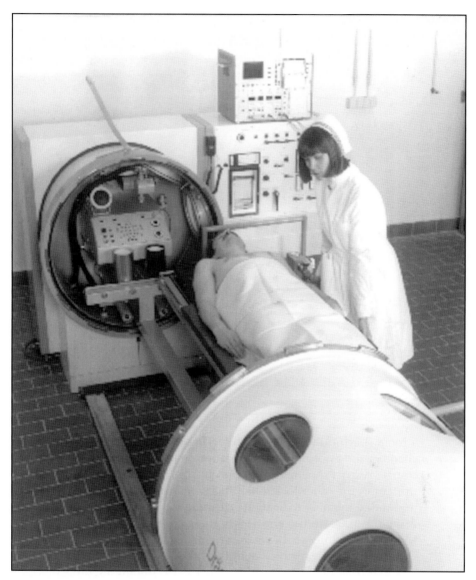

*Figure 7. Dräger Monoplace Chamber - Model 1200.*

A. Chambers with a metal hull, metal end plates, and portholes of glass or acrylic are preferred by organizations requiring portability. The metal hull is more durable and the replacement of damaged portholes is less expensive than replacing an acrylic chamber hull. Usually, skid mounts are preferred for improved portability, as they are more easily attached to a truck bed or aircraft floor. These are usually of single-hull design and are lighter than the following type.

B. A chamber with an acrylic hull and metal end plates is preferred where viewing of the entire patient is important. To insure durability, the acrylic hull must be protected against scraping, ultraviolet irradiation and falling objects. They are usually placed in

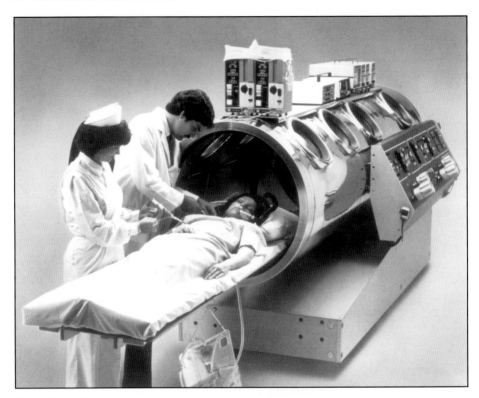

*Figure 8. The Reneau Unit.*

a room specifically altered for hyperbaric oxygen operation, i.e., the chamber does not move from location to location. This does not, of course, restrict such motion if the appropriate safeguards are present in the other locations. This type is usually fitted with wheels for limited mobility to facilitate cleaning underneath the chamber. From the 1960s to the mid 1990s, these chambers were designed with an inner hull which retains the pressure, and an outer hull which acts as a protective shield (6) – a tube within a tube concept. The external hull is designed specifically to contain the force of a sudden fatigue rupture of the internal hull, thus protecting personnel from any missiles that may develop if the event is explosive. The overall weight is more than the preceding metal hull design due to the double hull configuration. The enlarged chambers presently available have a single acrylic hull, and, aside from weight considerations, may present a placement problem in the facility, i.e. space allocation. In order to reach pressure efficiently, these larger chambers require specific piping and gas flow volumes.

**Collapsible:** The collapsible design was adopted as a space-saving advantage aboard military ships or aircraft. Primarily, they are used for close support of military diving activities, or to transport patients to a treatment facility. They are lightweight in construction and can usually be moved, with a patient under pressure, by four men. A separate cradle is useful to support this chamber and it may be adapted to a wheeled or skid base for transport. Insertion of the patient is usually through the rigidly-constructed door and frame at one end of the chamber. These chambers are easily adapted for combat situations with compressed-air diving cylinders, as the gas source for compression and ventilation.

A. The metal, telescopically-collapsing hull with a porthole in the door. This is a collapsing "tea cup" design, wherein interlocking cylinders extend for operation. The larger cylinder was at the door end, with a progression to the smallest at the foot. It was popularized for close naval support, as it was conveniently small for storage on small vessels where space was at a premium. It is no longer commercially available in the USA.

B. A nonmetallic, non-rigid, reinforced plastic chamber, with small acrylic or glass portholes at the head end and with pressure maintained using metallic "O" clamps. A model is available for entry through a zipper along the longitudinal axis. This was only available for close support of military activities.

C. A combination of the two preceding types of metal and nonmetallic non-rigid reinforced plastics. These are designed so that the head and torso are resting in the rigid portion of the chamber, while the lower limbs extend into the collapsible portion.

## Mobility Configuration

**Fixed:** This is the favored configuration of those models that require additional structural support due to the intrinsic weight of the chamber or supporting equipment. It prevents wear and tear on the chamber, while protecting the institution from an ill-advised movement to an area where the floor supports may be inadequate to support the weight of the device.

**Movable**: Mobility is often desirable for hospital use. Should the chamber only be used occasionally, it may be stored out of the way. This is also an advantage if it is to be retired or replaced with more advanced equipment. The hospital bed is a prime example of this trend toward increasing mobility as bed design shows constant improvement.

A. Wheel mounted: This is the favored model for hospital use and facilitates cleaning of the local area. These are easily moved by two adults. Most models, presently available for use within a hospital, weigh 1000 pounds or less unoccupied, on a four point distribution. Importantly, the aforementioned weight distribution conforms to weight support tolerances for hospital building codes throughout the USA.

B. Skid mounted: This is a favored model for hand transportable models usable in unpredictable terrain. It is used on site to support activities such as diving, excursion into toxic environments, or close medical support for the military. The skid lends itself to being securely attached to vehicles, boats, or aircraft using clamps or lines.

### Design of the Patient Seat or Tray

The patient-resting surface may be fixed or adjustable in a reclining and/or sitting position. The patient should be electrically grounded during each treatment while resting on the seat or tray. This is usually accomplished using mattresses or padded seats covered with a conductive material. The pad or mattress is then so placed as to be in contact with conductors that are in turn connected to an external ground. If the preceding is not possible, then a grounding strap must be applied to the patient and attached to the grounding system. The latter maneuver is particularly appropriate for the cervical traction device, as the tray is made of nonconductive material.

### Design of the Gas Supply

The gas is piped directly from the source to the treatment area via insulated piping. In-line heat exchangers are recommended to heat or cool the gases entering the chamber for patient comfort, and to avoid hypothermia or hyperthermia in the unconscious patient. A heat exchanger is recommended to maintain the ambient chamber temperature between 68 to 72 degrees Fahrenheit (20-22°C) for comfort. A simple radiator design using hot and/or cold water with a thermistor to actuate water flow is recommended, warming below 66°F and cooling above 72°F. However, these may not be the desired settings; in the case of children with acute thermal burns, a somewhat warmer environment is appropriate to prevent hypothermia.

The gas may require humidification in extremely dry areas to insure patient grounding and to suppress static discharges. The humidity within a monoplace chamber is usually maintained, to some degree, by insensible water loss from the occupant. See Figure 9. A simple solution to increasing humidification if desired is to place a wet towel over the oxygen inlet within the chamber. The moisture may be replenished by pumping water into the towel from an external positive-displacement pump. A free flow of the pressurizing gas through a permanently installed humidifier may be more appropriate in those areas where excessive dryness is a constant problem.

### Gas Storage Designs

This deals with the types of bulk storage available for the gases used in compression and treatment.

**Compressed gas:** Stored in high-pressure cylinders. This is the preferred method to use with the transportable chamber due to weight, space, and economic considerations. However, compressed gases are more expensive in hospital settings in the United States and are four to six times as expensive as cryogenic gas such as LOX. The costs are further increased in a seismically sensitive area due to the additional security that must be afforded to a large number of the high-pressure cylinders. However, the author prefers compressed gas (oxygen) cylinders as an emergency supply. The emergency system reacts to a loss of line pressure in the cryogenic system by automatically switching to the compressed gas. The gas derived from high-pressure reservoirs should be warmed prior to use with the monoplace chamber; otherwise the adiabatic cooling may be significant.

**Cryogenic gas:** This is the preferred oxygen supply source within the USA, but it may be unrealistic for use in those countries where liquid oxygen

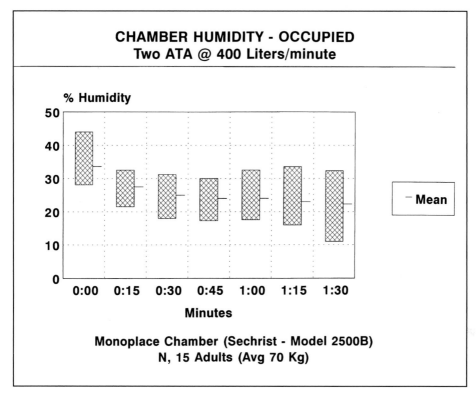

Figure 9. Percentage of humidity vs. time in monoplace chamber.

is not generally available to the medical community. Importantly, the gas should be warmed to the temperature that it is to be used, and further protected from warming or cooling by passage through insulated pipes to the treatment area. The cryogenic source is essentially a large "thermos" bottle, and as such is usually placed a distance from the hospital. It is recommended that a separate piping system be established directly to the hyperbaric department. This is necessary so that life-support-ventilating equipment may not be placed in jeopardy of failure if there is a sudden drop in line pressure and flow due to the actuation of the hyperbaric chamber(s).

 **Mixed sources:** It is common to use a compressed gas such as air as a compressing agent, and/or alternating with oxygen from a cryogenic source. The air is compressed, filtered, and stored at the site. We elect to use compressed oxygen as an alternate source, with a cascade configuration for emergency use in a seismically sensitive area. Great care must be taken to avoid contamination of each gas supply if two or more use a common valve system into the chamber. There are several methods to prevent the contamination of one gas or the other secondary to "back-bleeding" into the line with less pressure. However, we recommend routine inspections of the equipment by experienced engineering personnel and chamber operators to preclude this occurring. We prefer oxygen sensors with in-line alarms to note contamination.

## Operating Gases

These are the individual gases to be used in pressurization and/or treatment of patients.

**Single gas:** In the hospital setting this is usually oxygen, USP, where the patient is compressed in and breathes the gas. In the USA, it's from a cryogenic supply ideally, and evaporated to 70°F, and delivered to the chamber area at a line pressure of 60 to 80 pounds per square inch gauge (psig). Portable chambers used in the field to support diving activities frequently use air as the compressing and treating gas. Some navies adapt portable chambers to use available diving cylinders for transport of the pressurized diver to a more suitable treatment site.

**Multiple gases:** This configuration is favored, with oxygen as the primary treatment gas and air available for oxygen air breaks and personnel training. Many combinations are available when using a closed ventilation circuit such as an endotracheal tube, regulator, mask, or hood:

A. Compressed in one and breathing another – such as compressed in air, and breathing oxygen.
B. A change of gases or mixtures during a specified treatment protocol – such as the delivery of Trimix, or the use of "air breaks" to avoid oxygen toxicity.

## Ventilation Rates

The purge rate of most monoplace systems is set at a minimum flow rate of 200 liters per minute (L/min), as delivered from the factory. Some models have no mechanism by which the flow can be increased or decreased. Certain manufacturers will, upon request, modify designated chambers so that the flow rates may be significantly reduced and/or increased to avoid certain therapeutic misadventures. Examples: 1. A child with a large burn placed in a chamber with the treating gas at 70° F flowing at 200 L/min may have an unacceptable evaporative heat loss – becoming severely hypothermic. 2. A high flow rate of 400 L/min is required in certain models to improve comfort for adults of 70 kilograms or greater by increasing the evaporative heat loss. 3. A low flow will allow the increase of water vapor within the chamber when desired.

Recycled gas with subtraction and/or addition is a favored approach in areas where the cost of the treatment gases is of concern. Available models have some degree of purging where about 50% is exhausted from the system and recycling is incomplete. Chemical absorbents must be used in this type to remove the carbon dioxide and odors from the recycled portion. However, with chemical absorbents, filtration scrubbers, and molecular sieves, a system theoretically could be produced to rid the circuit of unwanted gases.

Non-recycled gas is favored in the USA, as the costs of LOX, liquid nitrogen, or filtered compressed air are below that of maintaining and operating a recycling unit.

## Exhaust Gas

All exhausted gases must be vented to the exterior of the building and clear of all neighboring hazards to prevent reentry into the building. The exhaust port at the exterior of the building must be protected by a grille and/or fence to prevent the intrusion, accidentally or purposefully of a hazardous substance. Hazardous substances are defined as those which may be ignited or which are ignition sources such as cigarette butts. The exhaust port to the exterior must be so placed so as not to contaminate the intake system that compresses air for use within the facility.

## Filtration of Supplied Gases

**Chamber filters:** The filters supplied within the chamber by the manufacturer must be periodically cleaned to prevent buildup of any deposits. In chambers presently available, there are both ingress filters and egress filters. The egress filter, located in the exhaust line, is usually referred to as a "lint trap," as the debris most commonly found within the filter are fibers from bedding or garments. Placing a filter in the exhaust line is desirable to prevent an accumulation of lint in relief valves or exhaust conduits.

**Institutional filters:** Filters must be placed at convenient locations in the piping to the hyperbaric chambers. These filters must be capable of removing particulate material. If there is concern over the possible introduction of any noxious contaminant, such as a hydrocarbon gas or vapor, into a hyperbaric chamber, then appropriate monitors must be installed. If aqueous lubricants are used in Teflon compressors, one-micron filters must be placed in the piping in order to prevent the clogging of the monoplace control mechanisms with calcite crystals. Periodic gas analysis must be performed on the gases supplied for chamber use to detect any contamination. Furthermore, in those areas where it is possible for the gas intake for medical grade air to be contaminated by the exhaust from an internal-combustion engine, a continuous carbon monoxide monitor with alarm must be fitted to the chamber supply piping. The exhaust pipe from the institution to the exterior of the building, if convenient to passersby, should be covered with a grating to avoid intentional insertion of combustible materials.

## Design of the Two-Way Communication System

Intercommunication is mandatory for the safe operation of a monoplace chamber, and the system used must be intrinsically safe. The components within the chamber must be positioned so as to minimize contamination or patient manipulation. Ideally, the system should be designed so that chamber operators cannot squelch the output for their convenience. A modular design facilitates rapid replacement of the components such as the chamber operator's hand microphone. This component gets the most "wear and tear" of the monoplace equipment.

## Lighting

The illuminating device must not be a source of heat within the chamber. The lighting for monoplace chambers must be mounted outside the chamber and conducted into the chamber by glass or acrylic ports, or by fiber-optic cable. Illumination striking acrylic should not have high levels of ultraviolet irradiation, as it will weaken the acrylic with time. With repetitive exposures, ionizing irradiation will similarly weaken the structure of the acrylic. We recommend that fluorescent lights, which may shine directly into the patient's eyes, be turned off during normal treatments and only used for emergency purposes. This step is intended to reduce the possibility of photically-stimulated seizures (strobe effect of fluorescent light) through the concave surfaces of the chamber. (13) Alternatively, animal research (3, 20) would indicate that ambient light does not enhance oxygen seizures. However, this was using the rat model, a nocturnal mammal. Thus, until this controversy is resolved, we continue to use indirect lighting in the chamber area.

## Grounding

The chamber shall be installed in such a way that it may be safely grounded during its operation. These grounds must be checked routinely to insure proper function. Check with the hospital engineer to assure you have a safe and secure ground.

## EQUIPMENT ADAPTATIONS

Adapting equipment for use with or within a hyperbaric chamber depends on the patient's needs. The adaptation should be designed or approved by a competent biomedical engineer, if one is available. The engineer must fully appreciate the demands of the hyperbaric oxygen environment as it applies to the design of the device, and the applicability of the relevant NFPA or ASME codes. This will normally require on-site visits during the development phase to assist in the fine-tuning.

### Monitors

Electrically-driven monitors and recorders shall be placed external to the monoplace chamber for control by the chamber operator, but most importantly as a safety consideration. These electrical devices must be designed so as not to allow an electrical surge of a magnitude to create an ignition source within the chamber. An ignition source is defined as that place in an electrical system where there is sufficient energy to cause combustion. The electrical glands (pass-through or plug) built into the chambers must be routinely checked for malfunction.

### Adaptations to Modify Therapy

**Gas delivery:** A patient's ventilating gases may be altered from the gas in which they are compressed by scuba regulator, mask, closed-circuit ventilation device (when intubated), or a hood. This allows the use of "air breaks" or the delivery of blended gases, wherein the clinician may use Navy Treatment Table 6 (USN TT 6). Minor modifications to existing equipment may be necessary to accomplish these changes in gas delivery (27).

**Pharmacologic agents:** Certain drugs may be delivered at the time of treatment by a positive-displacement pump external to the chamber, when the target cells and/or organisms are sensitized by the abundance of oxygen. Caution should be taken when treating those patients with an implanted medication pump (i.e. insulin pumps). These implanted pumps deliver measured amounts of a medication for patients that are dependent upon that drug. It is recommended that this device be rendered inoperative and the medicament withdrawn from the reservoir prior to treatment with hyperbaric oxygen. This avoids overmedicating the patient should there be any gaseous interface within the reservoir.

**Radiotherapy:** Radiation sources may be positioned externally to ports or translucent hulls to irradiate tumors after they have become radiosensitive by the hyperbaric oxygen (4, 22)

## PATIENT CHAIR OR TRAY

These are engineered to be electrically safe within the environment they are placed. Comfort is an important factor for the awake patient, but it must not compromise the safety of the treatment process.

**Fixed:** These remain within the chamber at all times. The supporting frame is fabricated from conductive materials; the seat pads or mattresses are covered with a conductive material.

A. Chair: The chair may be adjusted to recline or it may be in a fixed, upright position. This adaptation is appealing in treating patients where there are space limitations for chamber operation. The chamber may be constructed with less required operational length than a cylindrical chamber with end loading capabilities.

B. Tray: The patient must be placed on this tray at the chamber site, as it is not detachable in the usual sense for use as a transport device. The device may be capable of raising or lowering the head of the patient.

**Mobile (i.e., easily detached from the chamber and may be used to transport the patient from one point in the health care facility to another):** These are engineered to become electrically safe by contact points placed in such a position that the tray is grounded when positioned for treatment within the chamber. An alternative is separate grounding of the patient by a grounding lead or probe when the tray or chair cannot be grounded.

A. Wheelchair: The chair may be adjustable to a reclining position or in a fixed upright mode.

B. Mobile tray: The tray is usually transported on top of a wheeled lower portion, using the combined arrangement as a hospital gurney. The tray easily detaches and slides from the wheeled transport frame into the chamber. Special trays may be acquired for cervical traction, x-rays, or magnetic-resonance studies. A special traction tray, upon which the patient lies, is described by Sukoff (21) wherein cervical traction is maintained during transport and care. This device is versatile and, as it is radiolucent, may be used in CT scans, as it will fit through the machine aperture. It does require attention to properly ground the patient; this is accomplished with appropriate grounding straps. Thus, with the availability of this device or one of equal capabilities, a quadriplegic patient may safely be treated with HBO. Patients fitted with a "Halo" skull fixation device (Gardner-Wells traction) may also be safely treated in a HBO chamber.

## COMFORT ITEMS

No item whose purpose is to provide for patient comfort shall be inserted into the chamber if it is not intrinsically safe for the rated gases and pressure of the chamber.

**Mattresses or chair cushions:** These are covered with conductive material that lies upon a conductive surface, thereby insuring electrical grounding of the patient within the chamber. If the mattresses/cushions are not covered, or if they are not provided with conductive contacts, then the patient shall be grounded separately.

**Entertainment:** A television may be placed externally within the patient's field of vision and the accompanying sound piped into the interior of the chamber to entertain the patient during the treatment. Music and biofeedback sounds may also be broadcast into the chamber to comfort and to allay anxiety.

**Expanded visual field:** Wide-angle mirrors should be placed so that the chamber operator may have continual visual contact with the patient. This has been found to be a comfort to the patient.

## EMERGENCY OPERATION

Please note: these preparations are important to sustain operation of the chambers for emergencies in seismically and/or climatically-sensitive geographical locations.

### An Alternate Gas Supply Shall be Available

This is solved by a storage manifold of oxygen cylinders arranged in a cascade to continue necessary treatment. The alternate supply is turned on when there is a drop of the main supply pressure below a designated level. Periodic checks of these supplies are important to maintain a state of readiness.

### An Alternate Electrical Supply Shall be Available

This is a requirement of all health care facilities; if the chamber is used for therapeutic purposes, it must be in compliance. This includes emergency lighting for the chamber area. Monitors and life-support equipment shall be connected to this system at all times. It is recommended that the communication system with the patient be supported by a direct-current system, with a battery backup, or be continuously connected to the emergency electrical supply.

## EMERGENCY EXTRACTION OF THE PATIENT

In chambers that are designed with a maximum operating pressure of 3 ATA, the design should permit patient removal from the chamber within 90 seconds or less, if compressed in oxygen and breathing oxygen. This may also be used in those patients where air breaks of 5 minutes are being used to reduce the complication of CNS oxygen toxicity. It is most important to be able to evacuate the patient quickly in the event of either internal or external calamity. It should be carefully explained to each patient that this capability exists should an emergency arise. Referring physicians and other medical professionals within the community should be kept apprised that these safety requirements exist.

Importantly, monoplace chambers that exceed 3 ATA operating pressures using inert gas mixtures must adhere to other well-established safety constraints in emergency decompression, as outlined for multiplace chambers. These must conform to those schedules that require decompression stops when the situation will allow.

## FIRE SUPPRESSION DEVICES

A redundancy of fire suppression devices is recommended for the immediate vicinity of the monoplace chambers. The chamber operators must be disciplined in the use of the available equipment. The following are recommended:

A. Sprinkler system.
B. $CO_2$ extinguisher.
C. Chemical extinguisher.
D. High-pressure water hose.

## GAS SUPPLY VALVES

There shall be gas supply valves within and immediately outside of the chamber area that may be used to stop the inflow of the gases. Having alternate methods to shut off the oxygen supply is important to reduce the intensity of a fire that may be supported by oxygen entering the chamber area. It is further recommended that the monoplace chamber used in hospitals be designed to decompress to ambient pressure should there be a loss of pressure of all supplied gases.

## CONDUCT OF TREATMENT IN THE MONOPLACE CHAMBER

The patient must be carefully informed about all facets of the treatment, unless unconscious. Each facet should be covered such as adiabatic heating during compression, sinus squeeze, maneuvers to relieve pressure within the middle ear, length of stay in the chamber, etc. Punctual delivery of treatments by courteous, skilled, and informative operators is the hallmark of a successful HBO unit.

The following are some frequently asked questions:

**When does a treatment commence?** The treatment time is considered to commence at pressurization and lasts until the depressurization is complete. The reasoning for this practice is as follows: 1. Oxygen saturation/desaturation of the tissues is not immediate and requires greater than 30 minutes in the human (10). 2. The patient is at risk from the start of pressurization through depressurization. The risks are barotrauma, gas embolism, confinement anxiety, and oxygen toxicity.

**How fast do you compress the unconscious patient?** The unconscious patient is routinely compressed at one pound per square inch per minute. Thus, it requires approximately 10 to 15 minutes in reaching the pressure of 2 ATA. If myringotomies have been performed, one may pressurize more rapidly.

**When do you use the emergency decompression routine?** The following types of decompression are presently being practiced:

A. Emergency decompression: The exhaust valves are opened as wide as possible after turning off the operating gases. Some monoplace systems are equipped with emergency decompression valves or "red button" interrupters and the time of decompression varies between 30 and 60 seconds. We have reserved this particular type of exit for situations such as cardiac arrest, fire in the vicinity, or natural disasters, such as earthquakes. This use for oxygen seizures is not advocated as there is the possibility of decompressing the patient with a closed glottis that would possibly give rise to a pneumothorax.

B. Urgent decompression: The source gas is turned off or changed to air, and the chamber is allowed to decompress in approximately two to three minutes depending on whether the glottis is opened or closed. This is the recommended rate for oxygen seizures.

C. Standard decompression: The chamber is decompressed over a ten-minute period. This is recommended for most treatment protocols.

**What is an appropriate purge rate for the monoplace chamber?** A purge rate of 200 liters per minute or greater is recommended for the adult, and may be increased in some chambers to 500 liters per minute when an increase in evaporative heat loss may be comforting to the patient.

## NUMBER OF MONOPLACE CHAMBERS IN USE

Personal communications with manufacturers of monoplace chambers would indicate that approximately 35,500 are in service around the world at this time. The former USSR has a significant number of this type.

## REFERENCES

1. Ashfield R., and Drew CE. "Clinical use of the hyperbaric oxygen bed." Postgrad Med J. 1969;45.643-647.

2. Bennett PB. "The treatment offshore of decompression sickness. A European undersea biomedical workshop," London. UMS Report. No. 4-9-76. 1976.

3. Bitterman N, Melamed Y and Perlman I. "CNS oxygen toxicity in the rat: Role of ambient illumination." Undersea Biomed Res. 1986; 13:19-25.

4. Churchill-Davidson I, Sanger C and Thomlinson RH. "Oxygenation in radiotherapy. II. Clinical applications." Brit J. Radiol. 1957;30:406-422.

5. Churchill-Davidson I, Sanger G and Thomlinson RH. "High pressure oxygen and radiotherapy." Lancet. 1955;1:1091-1095.

6. Emery EW, Lucas BGB and Williams KG. "Technique of irradiation of conscious patients under increased oxygen pressure." Lancet. 1960;1:248-250.

7. Foust G and Golden EB. "Alternative instructions for the Sechrist Model 500A Hyperbaric Ventilator." J Hyperbaric Med. 1989;4(3):143-145.

8. Hart GB, Meyer GW, Strauss MB and Messina VJ. "Transcutaneous partial pressure of oxygen measured in a monoplace hyperbaric chamber at 1,1.5, and 2 atm abs oxygen." J Hyperbaric Med. 1990;5(4):223-229.

9. Hart GB, O'Reilly RR, Broussard ND, Cave RH, Goodman DB and Yanda RL. "Treatment of burns with hyperbaric oxygen." SGO. 1974;139:693-696.

10. Hart GB, Wells CH, Guest MM, Goodpasture JE and Sanders W. "Inert gas diffusion and hyperoxia." Proceedings of the Sixth International Congress on Hyperbaric Medicine. Smith, G., (Ed.) Aberdeen University Press, Publ. 1979;130-139.

11. Johnson JK and King WL. "Materials design requirements for implantable pacemakers." Biomater Med Devices Artif Organs. 1974;2(4):353-356.

12. Junod VH. "Recherches physiologiques et therapeutiques sur les effets de la compression et de la raréfaction de l'air, tant sur le corps que sur les membres isolés." Rev Med Franc Étrange. 1834;3:350.

13. Kasteleijn-Nolst Trenité_ DGA. "Photosensitivity in epilepsy. Electrophysiological and clinical correlates." Acta Neurol Scan. (Suppl) 1989;80(125):3-149.

14. Kratz JM, Blackburn JG, Leman RB and Crawford FA. "Cardiac pacing under hyperbaric conditions." Ann Thor Surg. 1983;36:66-68.

15. Li RC.The monoplace hyperbaric chamber and management of decompression illness.Hong Kong Med J. 2001 Dec;7(4):435-8.

16. Maudsley RH, Hopkinson WI and Williams KG. "Vascular injury treated with high pressure oxygen in a mobile chamber." J Bone Joint Surg. 1963;45B:346-350.

17. Melamed Y and Ohry A. "The treatment and neurological aspects of diving accidents in Israel." Paraplegia. 1980;18:127-128.

18. Melamed Y, Sherman D, Wiler-Ravell D and Kerem D. "The transportable recompression rescue chamber as alternative to delayed treatment in serious diving accidents." Aviat Space Environ Med. 1981;52:480-484.

19. Meyer GW, Hart GB and Strauss MB. "Noninvasive blood pressure monitoring in the monoplace chamber: A new technique." J Hyperbaric Med. 1989;4(4):211-216.

20. Moon AJ, Williams KG and Hopkinson WI. "A patient with coronary thrombosis treated with hyperbaric oxygen." Lancet. 1964;1:18-20.

21. Ngai SH, Levy A, Finck AD, Yang JC and Spector S. "Central nervous system toxicity of hyperbaric oxygen - effects of light, norepinephrine depletion and beta-adrenergic blockade." Neuropharmacology. 1977;16:675-679.

22. Raleigh G, Rivard R, Fabus S. Air-activated chemical warming devices: effects of oxygen and pressure. Undersea Hyperb Med. 2005 Nov-Dec;32(6):445-9.

23. Sukoff MH. "Use of hyperbaric oxygenation for spinal cord injury." Modern Neurosurgery. M Brock (Ed.) Springer-Verlag, Berlin. 1982;272-283.

24. Sutherland WH. "Instrumental and technical notes. A new method of beam direction, with particular application in hyperbaric oxygen therapy." Br J Radiol. 1966;41:633-636.

25. Treweek S, James PB.A cost analysis of monoplace hyperbaric oxygen therapy with and without recirculation. J Wound Care. 2006 Jun;15(6):235-8.

26. UL 913. Northbrook IL; Underwriter's Laboratory Inc, 1979.

27. Weaver LK, Greenway L and Elliott CG. "Performance of the Sechrist 500A hyperbaric ventilator in a monoplace hyperbaric chamber." J Hyperbaric Med. 1988; 3(4):215-225.

28. Weaver LK. "A functional suction apparatus within the monoplace chamber." J Hyperbaric Med. 1988;3(3):165-171.

29. Weaver LK. "Air breaks with the Sechrist 500A monoplace hyperbaric ventilator." J Hyperbaric Med. 1988;3(3):179-186.

30. Weaver LK: Monoplace hyperbaric chamber use of U.S. Navy Table 6: a 20-year experience. Undersea Hyperb Med. 2006 Mar-Apr;3392):85-8.

CHAPTER 6

# MANAGEMENT OF CRITICALLY ILL PATIENTS IN THE MONOPLACE HYPERBARIC CHAMBER

## CHAPTER SIX OVERVIEW

# MANAGEMENT OF CRITICALLY ILL PATIENTS IN THE MONOPLACE HYPERBARIC CHAMBER

*Lindell K. Weaver*

## AUTHOR'S NOTE

*The most important element of treating critically ill patients with hyperbaric oxygen in the monoplace chamber is the experience of the staff. At our facility, the monoplace chamber is an extension of the critical-care environment: in proximity, in equipment, and in personnel. Having extensive experience in critical care is vital to managing critically ill patients. This is especially true when performing interventions that affect significant cardiovascular changes, such as hyperbaric therapy. This chapter is an overview of the manner in which we treat critically ill patients with hyperbaric oxygen at our institution. To apply some of the techniques that are presented in this chapter to any monoplace unit would be clearly inappropriate. For example, I state that we often intubate, sedate, and paralyze critically ill or comatose patients to carry out hyperbaric treatment. These are skills that are performed on a daily basis in the critical care units. We feel competent with the procedures, drugs, and expected patient responses. However, hyperbaric staff without this background may not feel as comfortable with these aspects of care. Certainly, a brief book chapter cannot train people in critical care. This requires years of experience in the appropriate environment. It is the goal of this chapter to focus on the treatment of critically ill patients in the monoplace hyperbaric chamber. What I hope to do, is demonstrate our hyperbaric unit as part of a critical care system, which may be of value to others caring for patients in the monoplace hyperbaric chamber.*

## INTRODUCTION

In the past several years, there has been rapid growth in the number of clinical hyperbaric facilities; this is due, in part, to the availability of the monoplace, or single-person hyperbaric chamber. These chambers are relatively inexpensive, require less personnel, and require less space to operate and maintain than multiplace (walk-in) chambers. These are some of the reasons that most clinical hyperbaric facilities operate monoplace chambers (24). Another advantage of the monoplace over the multiplace chamber is that attendants need not enter the hyperbaric chamber with the patient. However, some hyperbaric physicians express concerns about treating unstable or critically ill patients in the monoplace chamber, because of the lack of "hands-on" care during hyperbaric exposure, the lack of suitable equipment for optimal patient care, and the limitations of treatment pressures to 3 atmospheres absolute pressure (ATA). We have found that with a well-trained staff and the availability of appropriate equipment, critically ill patients can be treated safely in the monoplace chamber. We and others have presented monoplace chamber use in critically ill patients (3, 15, 19, 20, 26, 36, 37, 43). Anyone who anticipates treating critically ill patients in a monoplace chamber should be familiar with this work.

## APPROACH TO THE CRITICALLY ILL PATIENT

The team concept is an important element of the optimal management of patients in the intensive care unit (ICU). Successful patient management depends upon the integration of physicians, nurses, respiratory therapists, social workers, ethicists, and others. For the ICU-patient requiring hyperbaric oxygen therapy (HBO), it is imperative that the hyperbaric unit be staffed and configured as an extension of the ICU; otherwise, there is risk that the level of care may be lower than in the ICU, which is potentially dangerous to the patient. Therefore, the HBO unit should be staffed with nurses, therapists, and physicians knowledgeable in the management of the critically ill patient, as well as possessing a thorough understanding of hyperbaric physiology and the medical techniques unique to HBO.

Furthermore, since the patient must be transported to and from the ICU to the chamber, perhaps several times per day, the patient may be exposed to additional risks (2). The risk/benefit ratio of HBO and the risk of transport must be carefully evaluated in critically ill patients. A hypothetical example would be a patient with respiratory distress syndrome with multiple chest tubes requiring intravenous pressors, high partial pressures of oxygen ($O_2$), and high airway pressures, who develops clostridial gas gangrene. Most hyperbaric physicians would agree that gas gangrene should be treated with HBO, but to move such a patient to the chamber, much less to treat him/her in the chamber (monoplace or multiplace) may present more risk than not using HBO at all. Experience and careful weighing of the risk versus the benefit in these situations is important.

There are many details of the ICU patient that require attention prior to the transport of the patient to the chamber for hyperbaric treatment. These include informed consent, recording of the ventilator settings and blood gases, filling the endotracheal tube cuff with sterile saline, capping off unnecessary intravenous catheters and drains, placing chest tubes to Heimlich one-way valves, changing arterial pressure and electrocardiograph (ECG) monitors to the appropriate portable units, and adequately sedating the patient if clinically indicated. In addition, the patient will need to be able to equalize middle-ear pressure during compression and decompression. These items will be discussed in more detail below.

## THE HYPERBARIC UNIT

If the hyperbaric unit anticipates treating critically ill patients, appropriate emergency medical equipment and supplies need to be readily available. This includes equipment for maintenance of an artificial airway, ventilators, hemodynamic monitors, a defibrillator, suction apparatus, oximeters, intravenous (IV) catheters, IV sets, tubing, infusion pumps, chest tube insertion trays, and the drugs employed in the management of critically ill patients.

Ample space in the chamber area is requisite. There may be several medical personnel attending to the critically ill patient prior to the HBO treatment, so it is important to have enough room for access to both sides of the patient. See Figure 1.

Special equipment is necessary to deal with the ICU patient in the monoplace chamber. This includes electrical pass-throughs for monitoring of the ECG and pressures from invasive catheters, IV pass-throughs, and a gas pass-through for the ventilator. We have designed or modified other equipment that permits:

1) Suctioning of tubes and drains [Appendix I, (33)].
2) Use of air-breaks with mechanical ventilation during HBO [Appendix II, (34)].
3) Noninvasive blood pressure (BP) monitoring [Appendix III, (39)].
4) Monitoring of pulmonary artery hemodynamics, measurement of thermodilution of cardiac output, and mixed venous blood oximetry (35).
5) Simultaneous use of up to four IV lines through a single monoplace chamber hatch penetrator.

Subsequent sections will discuss these modifications and techniques.

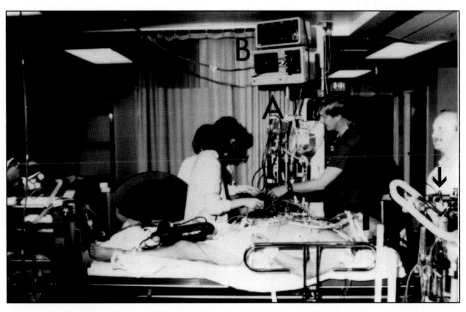

Figure 1. Preparing to place a critically ill patient with necrotizing fascitis and septic shock in the monoplace chamber. A liquid oxygen powered transport ventilator (arrow) ventilated the patient during transport. The patient receivied intravenous total parenteral nutrition, blood transfusion, continuous infusions of dobutamine and midazolam (A). The physiologic monitor and end-tidal $CO_2$ Monitor (B) is located in a position that is easily observed by the chamber operator. Ample room is important.

## DEFIBRILLATION

I have defibrillated one patient and cardioverted another patient who were rapidly removed from the monoplace chamber for dysrhythmias, both successfully. Some hyperbaric practioners have recommended that patients exiting the oxygen-filled chamber be moved some distance away from the chamber prior to defibrillation, because of concerns about the risk of combustion. The patient's tissues (including the brain and heart) presumably will have high concentrations of $O_2$, so taking a few extra seconds to move the patient to an area with a lower ambient concentration of $O_2$ should be acceptable. In the two cases commented upon above, a few seconds elapsed following extraction of the patients from the chamber before defibrillation. Both patients were defibrillated/cardioverted while on the gurney attached to the monoplace chamber. There was no evidence of sparks or fire. Provision for cardiac monitoring, defibrillation, bag-valve-mask ventilation, and intubation must be readily available if the hyperbaric unit anticipates treating critically ill patients.

> **Editor's Note:** *We have measured oxygen levels in the room after emergency decompressing and opening a monoplace chamber. The cold oxygen falls to the floor and dissipates in about 30 seconds. It does not measurably remain elevated at the level of the patient or rise in other parts of the room.*

## INTRA-HOSPITAL TRANSPORT OF CRITICALLY ILL PATIENTS

Paramount in the safe transport of critically ill patients is a knowledgeable and experienced staff. Critically ill patients can be safely transported to the HBO chamber, but it is important to recognize that ICU-care must continue without major disruptions during the transport to minimize adverse consequences to the patient. If the patient requires mechanical ventilation and positive-end expiratory pressure (PEEP), ventilation with a portable transport ventilator (see Figure 1), or a manually operated bag-valve incorporating a PEEP attachment are suggested. If PEEP is removed for patient transport, the patient's pulmonary efficiency may decrease, which may reduce the ability of the patient to oxygenate into the hyperbaric range during HBO. If there is concern about the adequacy of ventilation, arterial blood gases (ABG) may be necessary to inspect the pH and arterial carbon dioxide tension ($PaCO_2$). Monitoring of the end-tidal $CO_2$ ($EtCO_2$) and pulse oximetry during transport can serve as an aid in determining the adequacy of pulmonary gas exchange and alert the transport team to potential ventilation and/or oxygenation problems.

The ECG rhythm and BP should be monitored if the patient is at risk for hemodynamic instability, or if the patient is receiving continuous infusions of cardiovascular-active drugs such as dopamine or nitroprusside. Several portable transport monitors are available that are compact and battery operated. A transport defibrillator may be necessary if the patient has dysrhythmias.

Critically ill patients commonly have continuous IV infusions of maintenance fluids, cardiovascular drugs, total parenteral nutrition (TPN), insulin, antibiotics, analgesics, and sedatives. See Figure 1. Some of these can be withheld for the transport, but some must be continued. Utilizing volumetric infusion pumps facilitates the administration of IV agents during transport. The team needs to take emergency drugs (e.g. lidocaine, epinephrine, etc.) along with the patient.

A transport cart that attaches to the patient's gurney is useful to carry multiple IV pumps, monitors, $O_2$ cylinders, a portable suction device, and containers with clearly labeled emergency drugs.

## PREPARING THE CRITICALLY ILL PATIENT FOR MONOPLACE HBO

The cardiac rhythm and BP (if an arterial catheter is present) should be monitored during the time that preparations are underway for placing the patient in the chamber. The patient's endotracheal tube can be connected to the hyperbaric ventilator circuit and appropriate adjustments can be made in the minute ventilation (VE). The Sechrist 500A hyperbaric ventilator (Sechrist Industries, Inc., Anaheim, California) entrains ambient gas (air if the chamber hatch is open) to deliver an appropriate tidal volume (VT). If the patient requires high fractional inspired concentrations of $O_2$ (FiO$_2$), (s)he may develop arterial hypoxemia, unless supplemental $O_2$ is provided to the entraining valve area. One suggestion to minimize patient hypoxemia prior to chamber compression would be to connect the patient to the Sechrist 500A ventilator just prior to HBO. Pulse oximetry can be useful to warn care givers of patient hypoxemia. The patient needs to be clothed in a gown made of antistatic materials (100% antistatic cotton or non-static flame-proof material) (43). Comatose patients should be physically restrained to prevent them from inappropriately pulling on lines and tubes, and to position their arms in a safe position. We restrain patients by placing soft restraints on wrists, pulling one of the restraints under their ipsilateral buttock and up through their groin, then tying the restraint from the contralateral wrist to the other. If the elbows splay out too far, or if the IV catheters are kinked by binding of the arms at the elbow, we wrap Kerlex gauze around the elbows, and tie the ends together, pulling the elbows inward. Care must be taken to ensure that the gauze does not cause too much local pressure. Combative or anxious patients should be sedated, and, if intubated, sedated and possibly paralyzed. Surgical drains may be capped off. If the drain requires suction during HBO, it can be performed in the monoplace chamber (Appendix I) (33). Chest tubes need to have the drainage system removed and a Heimlich valve inserted. The drainage tubing can then be placed to suction or left open to ambient pressure.

Most monoplace chambers are limited in the number of IV pass-through ports. This requires careful consideration of which drugs and IV solutions are necessary during HBO. For example, if the patient is receiving separate infusions of TPN and insulin, those two infusions could be joined together before infusing the solution through the chamber. If the patient is receiving drugs such as dopamine, nitroprusside, midazolam, or potent analgesics by continuous infusion, then anticipate not using that particular IV line for anything else during the course of HBO, since "pushing" another drug in that IV line would result in a bolus of a potent cardiovascular agent to the patient, with concomitant potential adverse consequences. A knowledge of which drugs are compatible with one another is important when combining IV agents in the same IV line.

Some critically ill patients require more IV lines than are available in some monoplace chambers. Our solution to this limitation was to develop special pass-through penetrators that allow up to four IV lines to pass through one chamber hatch orifice. See Figures 2-5. This 4-in-1 split bolt is not presently available commercially, but if one were so inclined, a machine shop should be able to configure it (Machining details of the split-bolts are available in the Appendix of reference #35). Similarly, another special chamber hatch penetrator permits passage of the Sechrist 500A ventilator gas supply, provides pass-through ports for the suction device (33) and for monitoring EtCO$_2$ during HBO (7, 14). See Figure 6. A port for supplying either O$_2$ or air to an anesthesia bag fixed about the Sechrist 500A ventilator entraining venturi, a modification that permits air breaks to be given to mechanically ventilated patients undergoing HBO (34). This specially manufactured pass-through conserves the other chamber hatch orifices, permitting them to be available for IV use, an important factor in treating critically ill patients in the monoplace chamber.

Preferably, intubated patients should have an endotracheal (ET) tube that is a low pressure, high volume design (to reduce the risk of tracheal necrosis). Prior to HBO, air is evacuated from the ET tube cuff and the cuff is filled with sterile saline to achieve an appropriate seal with as minimal pressure as possible. After HBO, the saline is removed and the cuff is filled with

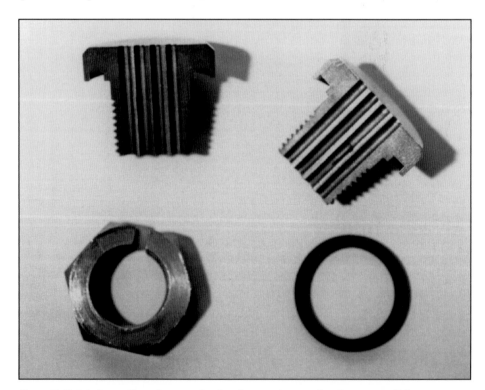

Figure 2. Split bolt pass-through, nut and o-ring that permits up to four intravenous (IV) pressure lines to pass through a single Sechrist chamber hatch pass-through orifice.

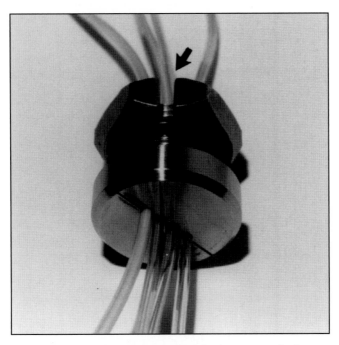

Figure 3. Assembled split bolt pass-through. The nut is notched (arrow) to fit over IV lines.

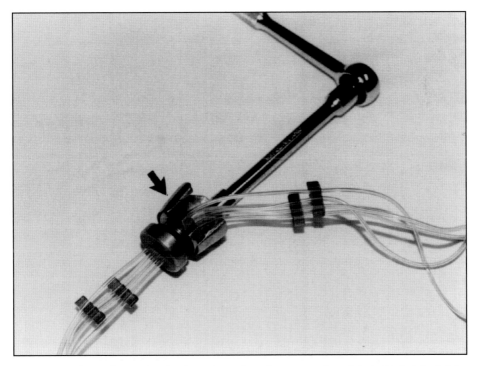

Figure 4. Ratchet and special socket (arrow) to tighten the nut onto the split bolt. The bolt is slightly tapered so as the nut is tightened, the bolt halves are drawn tightly together.

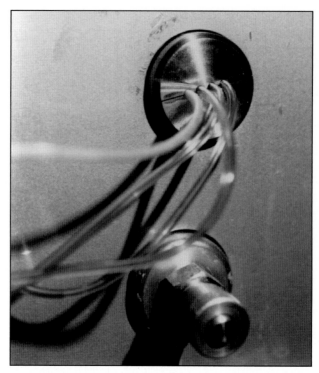

Figure 5. Split bolt pass-through and four IV lines installed in the door of the Sechrist chamber. One-way back-check valves are located between the IV tubing connections and the catheters inside the chamber (not shown).

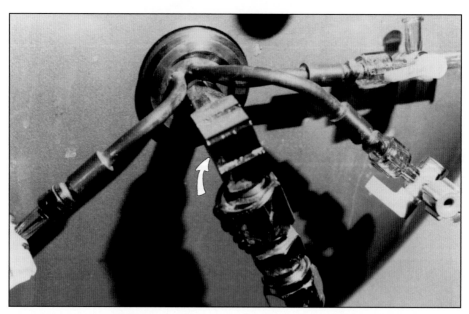

Figure 6. Four-in-one modified pass-through. This pass-through permits passage of a 1/8-inch NPT for the ventilator gas supply (arrow) and three additional ports (e.g., suction $EtCO_2$ monitoring and operation of the Doppler noninvasive blood pressure device).

air, with documentation of an acceptable cuff pressure. The ET tube needs to be securely tied in the appropriate position. Restraining the patient, to prevent the patient from self-extubation or from pulling IV catheters, should be considered.

Some hyperbaric physicians recommend that myringotomies be performed on all intubated patients to prevent middle and inner ear barotrauma (10). However, other hyperbaric practitioners, including myself, do not routinely perform prophylactic myringotomies in intubated patients. If myringotomies are not performed, our practice style has been to sedate, and occasionally paralyze the intubated patient to facilitate passive inflation of the middle ear space during hyperbaric compression. Presently, there is no controlled clinical information indicating that myringotomies are absolutely required in intubated patients treated with HBO.

If the individual hyperbaric physician deems that the patient requires myringotomies, the procedure is performed as follows:

The patient is sedated to facilitate the procedure. Cerumen is removed from the auditory canals to visualize the tympanic membrane (TM). Using an otolaryngologic operating microscope (or an otoscope and magnifying lens) to visualize the TM, the auditory canal is filled with 2% lidocaine with epinephrine. This drug is used primarily to induce TM vasoconstriction to reduce bleeding after the myringotomy, but also will lessen the momentary pain of the procedure. The patient's head is positioned for a few minutes so the lidocaine does not flow out of the ear canal. Rotating the patient's head in the opposite direction allows the lidocaine to flow out of the dependent ear canal. A neonatal suction catheter or auditory suction catheter is useful to remove additional lidocaine. After the TM has been anesthetized, a 21-gauge spinal needle or myringotomy knife is used to perforate the TM in the anterior-inferior quadrant (4 o'clock position in the patient's right ear, 8 o'clock position in the left) under direct vision. Using an otoscope with a sliding or rotating magnifying lens is necessary. The lens is positioned so that the physician can see the TM and simultaneously can insert the needle through the otoscope. (An operating otolaryngologic microscope is optimal for visualizing the TM and performing the myringotomy. This scope makes removing cerumen and performing the myringotomy safer and easier.) The perforation should have no blood clot present. If there is minimal TM hemorrhage, the perforation remains patent for generally 1 to 5 days. Bilateral tympanotomies should be considered if chronic HBO of intubated patients is anticipated. Obtaining special training in myringotomy procedures from otolaryngologic colleagues is helpful and highly recommended.

## PATIENT MONITORING IN THE MONOPLACE CHAMBER

The majority of patients (non-critically ill) treated in monoplace chambers can be safely monitored by direct observation alone. The respiratory rate is evident, as well as manifestations of anxiety, which can be a warning sign of central nervous system (CNS) $O_2$ toxicity (6). Critically ill patients require additional monitoring, which is determined clinically.

The cardiac rhythm is easily monitored during HBO by placing electrocardiographic leads on the patient who pass out of the chamber via an

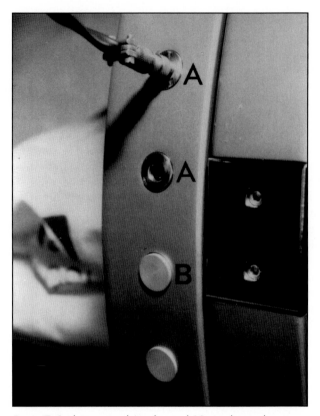

*Figure 7. Sechrist monoplace electrical 19-pin electrical pass-throughs (A) and blank plugs (B).*

electrical pass-through (The Sechrist 2500B monoplace chamber incorporates a 19-pin electrical pass-through) (see Figure 7), and are, in turn, connected to a physiologic monitor. The monitoring system should permit graphing, and the delayed inspection of adverse or suspected dysrhythmic events.

In critically ill patients, BP is generally measured by an indwelling arterial catheter connected to a pressure transducer through which an electrical signal is passed out of the chamber to a physiologic monitor. See Figure 8. The catheter and transducer (Transpac IV, Disposable Transducer, #42589-05, Abbott Critical Care Systems, Abbott Laboratories/Hospital Products Division, North Chicago, IL 60064 ) are continually flushed with sterile saline at 3 ml per hour by a continuous flush device (Intraflo-III, #42013-02, Abbott Critical Care Systems) (13). The flush solution is heparinized saline, or saline without heparin (our facility does not use heparin in catheter flush devices having found it unnecessary), to prevent catheter occlusion or dampening of the arterial waveform. The continuous flush device is connected to a bag of saline maintained at 300 mmHg pressure by a Surgi-press pressure infuser made for HBO applications (Ethox Corp., 251 Seneca St., Buffalo, NY 14204). A formerly available pressure infuser (Tycos) had a petroleum-based grease as a bearing lubricant, which should not be used in the hyperbaric $O_2$ environment because of the risk of fire (32). Prior to chamber compression, the pressure transducer should be zeroed to the appropriate

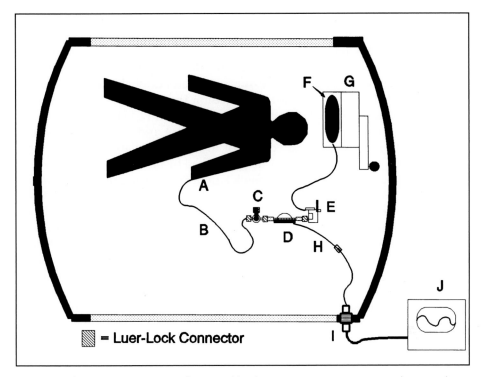

**= Luer-Lock Connector**

*Figure 8. Schematic representation of invasive blood pressure monitoring system in the monoplace chamber. The arterial catheter (A) is connected to four foot neonatal Cobe pressure tubing (B). A stopcock (C) is placed proximal to the pressure transducer (D). An intraflow (E) flushes the transducer and catheter continuously at 3 ml/hr. Saline (F) is pressurized (300 mmHg) by a Tycos Infuser (G) to provide the intraflow with adequate pressure to maintain system patency. The transduce signal is passed out of the chamber by its electrical leads (H) connected to the Sechrist 19-pin electrical pass-through (I) and displayed by a physiologic monitor (J).*

reference level. Also, the arterial pressure waveform should be inspected to ensure that adequate dynamic response is present in the system for interpretation (8, 9). If the BP monitoring system has inadequate dynamic response, the pressure will not be an accurate representation of the patient's true BP; this is a significant implication considering the potent drugs we often use to raise or lower the BP. Gardner's review and recommendations are strongly encouraged for anyone practicing invasive monitoring (12).

Non-invasive BP monitoring can be accomplished in the monoplace chamber. We developed a system for noninvasive BP monitoring, incorporating a Doppler flow detector to determine the systolic BP (39). A complete description of this non-invasive BP monitoring system is described in Appendix III of this chapter so will not be reiterated here (39). We found a good correlation between this Doppler system and concurrent arterial pressure measurements (39).

An automated BP system (Oscillomate 1630, CAS Medical Systems, Inc., Branford, CT) is commercially available (23). This BP monitoring device inflates the cuff automatically from outside the chamber, at a pre-set interval. The instrument also displays the mean arterial pressure and the heart rate, and has adjustable alarms.

Mechanically ventilated patients should have several respiratory variables monitored during HBO. These include: ventilatory rate (VR), expired VT, PEEP, peak airway pressure, ventilator $O_2$ supply pressure, and presence of spontaneous breathing by the patient. Airway pressure, respiratory rate, and alarms for pressures and rates can be measured with the Tau Pressure Monitor (Core-M, Inc., Precision Instruments, Allston, MA; it is also available from Perry Baromedical, Rivera Beach, FL) (17).

The $EtCO_2$ can be followed during HBO and may provide useful information regarding the adequacy of alveolar ventilation (7, 14). Side-stream $EtCO_2$ measurements may be performed by placing the sampling port at the proximal airway adjacent to the ET tube and passing this sampling line out of the chamber. Gas is analyzed by a $CO_2$ detector. We use a POET $EtCO_2$ analyzer (Criticare Systems, Inc., Milwaukee, WI). The expected $CO_2$ would be the predicted value x Atmospheric pressure/Chamber pressure (in absolute units). For example: assume the $EtCO_2$ is 40 torr at our altitude (0.85 ATA). At a chamber pressure of 3.0 ATA the displayed $EtCO_2$ ideally would be 11.3 torr (40 x 0.85/3.0). We have found that the POET monitor measures about 7 torr higher than predicted (16 torr in this example) at 2.9 ATA and 6 torr higher at 2 ATA in normal subjects when compared to simultaneously measured $PaCO_2$. See Table 1 (14). (There are errors in the table shown in reference 19 (Corrections are displayed in Table 1.)

Measuring $EtCO_2$ is helpful in adjusting the mechanical ventilator, and provides a continuous display for respiratory rate. $EtCO_2$ can also be monitored in non-intubated spontaneously breathing patients who are wearing a nasal cannulae as a sampling catheter, that is passed out of the chamber and analyzed by the POET monitor. As expected, there is more

## TABLE 1. SIMULTANEOUSLY MEASURED END-TIDAL $CO_2$ ($EtCO_2$) AND ARTERIAL CARBON DIOXIDE TENSION ($PaCO_2$)

| PCH (ATM) | PREDICTED $PaCO_2$ | $EtCO_2$* | $EtCO_2$ | PREDICTED $EtCO_2$* |
|---|---|---|---|---|
| 0.85 | 33.8+2.5 | 33.8+2.5 | 31.2+1.7 | -2.6+2.3 |
| 2.9 | 31.6+2.6 | 9.3+0.8 | 16.4+1.1 | 7.1+0.9 |
| 2.5 | 31.3+2.2 | 10.7+0.8 | 17.6+1.3 | 6.9+0.8 |
| 2.0 | 30.8+2.9 | 13.1+1.3 | 19.0+1.5 | 5.9+0.7 |
| 1.2 | 30.9+1.7 | 21.9+1.3 | 26.8+2.4 | 4.8+1.4 |
| 0.85 | 33.0+2.9 | 33.2+2.9 | 30.9+2.5 | -2.4+3.3 |

* mean (mmHg) + 1 S.D.

*Measurements in normal subjects breathing through a mouthpiece while wearing a nose clip. Expired gas was sampled continuously in a side-stream fashion, passed out of the chamber and analyzed in a POET $EtCO_2$ analyzer. Predicted $EtCO_2$ = $PaCO_2$ atmospheric pressure / chamber pressure. As can be appreciated, the POET analyzer over estimates the predicted $EtCO_2$ of subjects compressed in the chamber.*

variability in the measurement, but it can be useful to follow trends in the individual patient, particularly if the patient is given sedatives or analgesics.

Arterial blood gases (ABGs) of patients treated with HBO can be monitored. This technique requires a set-up permitting aspiration of arterial blood out of the pressurized chamber. See Figure 9. It is important to use Luer lock connections and hard-pressure tubing. The continuous flush device (i.e., Intraflo) is not necessary with this system since the arterial catheter can be flushed from outside the chamber. However, the continuous flush device can be used by placing a 4-way stopcock between the arterial pressure transducer and the Intraflo, which permits connecting the arterial blood sampling line. The handle of the 4-way stopcock should be positioned so that the continuous flush device, the sampling line, and the transducer are all in direct communication. Incorporating the continuous flush device in this system prevents the arterial catheter from clotting. We have demonstrated that the ABL 330 blood gas laboratory (Radiometer, Copenhagen, Denmark) can accurately measure $O_2$ tension of saline and blood in tonometry experiments (Appendix IV) (42). Further studies have verified that the ABL 330 can also measure the arterial $O_2$ tension ($PaO_2$), pH, and arterial carbon dioxide tension ($PaCO_2$) of subjects (40) and patients exposed to HBO. See Table 2

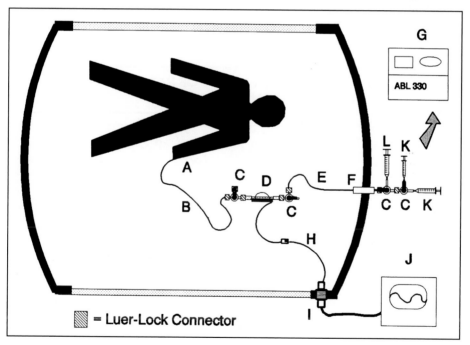

Figure 9. Schematic representation of the system we use to aspirate arterial blood out of the compressed monoplace chamber. The pressure monitoring system is analogous to Figure 8. Arterial blood can be withdrawn by connecting a stopcock (C) to the distal side of the pressure transducer (D). A four or six foot neonatal Cobe pressure line (E) connects to a Cobe hyperbaric sterile, disposable pass-through (F) (See blow-up of pass-through in Figure 10). A 10 ml Luer lock syringe (L) collects the dead-space volume during sampling and a 3 ml blood gas syringe (K) is used to collect the arterial sample in a midstream fashion. The sample is anyalyzed immediately in the Radiometer ABL 330 (G) (See Appendix IV and text).

(41). The arterial sample needs to be obtained anaerobically with careful attention to prevent dilutional errors in the sample during aspiration. Prior to analysis, the arterial sample needs to be maintained under pressure by sealing the hub end closed with a stopcock, and holding firm pressure on the syringe plunger. This pressure prevents $O_2$ from coming out of solution from the supersaturated blood sample. After obtaining the arterial blood sample, the arterial sampling line is flushed with sterile saline until the line is clear of blood. The blood sample needs to be analyzed quickly (< 2 minutes), or the $PaO_2$ value may not represent the actual value accurately (a complete discussion of the technique is available) (42).

We often measure ABGs to determine the adequacy of mechanical ventilation (pH and $PaCO_2$) during HBO. Personnel who perform ABG measurements of patients in the monoplace chamber need to be aware of several potential risks. Retrograde arterial gas embolism can occur if any gas is introduced into the arterial catheter (4). Inadvertent rapid loss of blood could ensue if a catheter or connector becomes accidentally disconnected. Embolic phenomena may occur if clots or thrombi are infused into the arterial catheter. Iatrogenic blood loss is possible, since one should ideally withdraw 3 times the system dead space prior to obtaining the arterial blood sample. Typically this is approximately 10cc. If heparinized and aspirated using sterile technique, this blood could be given back to the patient in a venous line.

Patients who have pulmonary dysfunction, requiring supplemental $O_2$ at atmospheric pressure to have adequate arterial $O_2$ saturation, would

## TABLE 2. ARTERIAL OXYGEN TENSION OF PATIENTS WITH ABNORMAL PULMONARY FUNCTION

| Pch (ATM) | N | $P_AO_2$* | $P_AO_2$ meas | $(P_aO_2)$ Corr | $P_aO_2/P_AO_2$ (a/A2 ratio) | $P_aO_2$ pred (from pre HBO a/A) |
|---|---|---|---|---|---|---|
| 0.85** | 22 | 564±10 | 269±81 | 269±81 | 0.487±0.14 | 0 |
| 2 | 6 | 1433±10 | 1083±232 | 1162±232 | 0.76±0.16 | 278±138 |
| 2.4 | 15 | 1740±8 | 1168±293 | 1272±293 | 0.67±0.17 | 394±242 |
| 2.9 | 32 | 2113±11 | 1282±230 | 1416±230 | 0.61±11 | 396±266 |
| 3 | 19 | 2195±7 | 1420±185 | 1561±185 | 0.61±0.17 | 531±306 |
| 0.85*** | 9 | 562±7 | 254±144 | 254±144 | 0.45±0.25 | 0 |
| 0.85**** | 18 | 219±75 | 95±49 | 95±49 | 0.48±0.25 | 0 |

\* Alveolar $PO_2$–$O_2$ values expressed as mean ± 1 S.D.
\*\* a/A ratio from 0.85 ATA pre $HBO_2$ data
\*\*\* 100% $O_2$
\*\*\*\* < 100% $O_2$

Blood gases were analyzed by a Radiometer ABL 330 operated at atmospheric pressure. Hyperbaric tonometry experiments (30) provided a correction factor for chamber pressures >1.0 atm abs, converting measured $PaO_2$ values ($PaO_2$ meas) to corrected $PaO_2$ values ($PaO_2$ corr):

$$PaO_2 \ corr = [PAO_2 *0.919 + 37.3] + PaO_2$$

The predicted $PaO_2$ ($PaO_2$ pred) derives from using the atmosphere's pressure a/A ratio to predict the hyperbaric $PaO_2$.

require higher treatment pressures to have similar hyperbaric $PaO_2$ than would patients with normal lungs at lower chamber pressures (41). See Table 2. Therefore, it may be reasonable to treat patients with abnormal lungs (i.e., an increased right-to-left intrapulmonary shunt fraction) with chamber treatment pressures higher than for patients with normal lungs.

Accurate measurement of $PaO_2$ during treatment may be important to titrate the treatment pressure. This observation also has implications for patients who are mechanically ventilated with the Sechrist 500A ventilator, because its performance is marginal at chamber pressures > 2.0 ATA (38). The optimal $PaO_2$ of patients requiring HBO is unknown. Tissue $PO_2$ is the measurement that is likely to aid in titrating the dose of HBO. Unfortunately, tissue $O_2$ tension measurements are not performed and are certainly not yet practical as a useful tool to titrate the HBO dose.

We generally do not offer HBO to patients requiring > 50% $FiO_2$ for adequate arterial saturation at atmospheric pressure unless the risk/benefit ratio clearly favors treating with HBO. If we do treat such patients with HBO, ABG measurements are performed during HBO. Even at 3 ATA, some of these patients have such severe pulmonary dysfunction that they are unable to achieve $PaO_2$ values > 1,000 torr, and frequently considerably lower. Furthermore, these patients generally require PEEP and high VE so adequate ventilation becomes a significant problem with the Sechrist 500A ventilator. The HBO $PaO_2$ cannot be predicted in patients with abnormal pulmonary function (arterial/alveolar ratio < 0.75) from measurements made at atmospheric pressure (41). In patients with considerable pulmonary dysfunction who require high $FiO_2$s, we generally withhold HBO until the patient's pulmonary function improves.

The data available from a flow-directed, pulmonary artery oximetric (Swan-Ganz) catheter can be obtained from patients treated in the monoplace chamber. We have simultaneously measured the right arterial pressure, pulmonary artery pressure, pulmonary capillary occlusion (wedge) pressure, thermodilution cardiac output, continuous core body temperature, mixed pulmonary venous blood oxyhemoglobin saturation by continuous oximetry, and the arterial-venous blood $O_2$-content difference in patients treated with HBO (35, 43). The techniques are time-consuming, require special hatch penetrators not commercially available, and possibly should be performed only if the data are absolutely required or if part of a defined and approved research protocol. The details of this technique are beyond the scope of this chapter.

It is possible to monitor the intracranial pressure (ICP) during HBO in the monoplace chamber with a transducer system analogous to the invasive BP monitoring system (29). Similarly, the electroencephalogram (EEG) signal can be passed out of the chamber via the 19-pin electrical pass-throughs.

Transcutaneous oxygen ($TcPO_2$) measurements are commonly employed by multiplace chambers (28). $TcPO_2$ measurements can also be performed in the monoplace chamber (16). Radiometer (Copenhagen, Denmark) has developed a transcutaneous $O_2$ monitor that is intrinsically, electrically-safe passing Underwriter's Laboratories criteria for use in a 100% $O_2$ environment (27). Special cables to pass the probe into the Sechrist chamber are available from Sechrist Industries. The $TcPO_2$ data may be useful in predicting the response to HBO in problem wounds (9, 22, 30, 31).

To summarize, with innovation and a few modifications to equipment, patients can be extensively monitored in the monoplace hyperbaric chamber. The degree of monitoring required for the individual patient should depend upon the clinical scenario, and the physician and hyperbaric staff's experience with critical care in the monoplace chamber. Most patients can be sufficiently monitored with the ECG and BP, whether noninvasive or invasive. Only rarely, if ever, are data from a Swan-Ganz catheter necessary to treat patients in the monoplace chamber. If clinically indicated, other monitoring modalities such as EEG, ICP, and $TcPO_2$ measurements are relatively straightforward to accomplish.

## PATIENT MANAGEMENT DURING HBO

A staff that has experience treating critically ill patients is the most important element of delivering HBO to critically ill patients. Of course, the hyperbaric staff needs to be familiar with hyperbaric physiology, but it is also mandatory that they are skilled in dealing with critical care. If the HBO unit only sees critically ill patients rarely (e.g., a septic patient with gas gangrene once per year), that level of experience may be inadequate to maintain proper skills. Training evolutions can be constructed to attempt to maintain practice skills of treating critically ill patients. Also, rotating the HBO staff through the ICU is a method of maintaining their critical care medicine skills. The HBO unit must have physicians trained in critical care and hyperbaric medicine immediately available if the unit is treating critically ill patients.

If the patient is not alert, it may be prudent to intubate the patient for airway protection. Assuming the staff has adequate expertise, it is probably safer to pharmacologically control combative or semi-comatose patients that require HBO. Patients who are at risk of vomiting and aspiration, or of awakening abruptly inside the chamber in an anxious or combative state, may pull out lines and possibly harm themselves before sedatives can be provided. It is mandatory that paralytic agents such as vecuronium not be used unless the patient is adequately sedated. For adults, 5 mg IV diazepam may be used, titrated in frequent doses to an adequate response. Patients often may require 20 to 30 mg of diazepam to be adequately sedated for a 2-hour treatment. Occasionally, a continuous IV infusion of midazolam is used, titrating the infusion rate to provide adequate sedation. Boluses of midazolam are not favored for patients treated with HBO, due to its short half-life. Bolus injections of midazolam seem to wear off abruptly in compressed patients and they can become quite agitated. Propofol is also attractive as an agent for continuous sedation if only intermittent sedation (e.g., during HBO therapy) is desired. If pain is a prominent feature, we titrate morphine IV (or fentanyl), generally 5-10 mg morphine every 30 to 60 minutes, sometimes with intermittent IV diazepam. Since analgesics and sedatives blunt the ventilatory drive, careful attention must be paid to the patient's adequacy of ventilation (with ABGs) and with airway patency. As mentioned, our threshold to intubate these patients is low, so they may be appropriately sedated and mechanically ventilated. By the same line of reasoning, we may delay extubation in patients with necrotizing fasciitis to permit the continuance of HBO twice per day until the patient is well on the way to recovery, as well as to adequately control pain during dressing changes and whirlpool therapy.

Neuromuscular blocking agents are used to paralyze patients. The author favors vecuronium (0.1 mg per kg) because it has essentially no cardiovascular side-effects, has a rapid onset, and has relatively short half-life. The patient must be adequately sedated prior to use, since this drug has no sedative or amnestic properties. Obviously, if patients are paralyzed, or even sedated, they will not demonstrate with compression the typical expected clinical responses from a pneumothorax, seizure, or auditory or sinus pain. It is critical that chamber personnel pay close attention to returned VT, airway pressures, and evidence of auto-PEEP. Air breaks [Appendix II (34)] may be provided to intubated patients to reduce the risk of CNS $O_2$ toxicity, especially in patients who are paralyzed and who cannot demonstrate the typical manifestations of $O_2$ toxicity.

## INTRAVENOUS THERAPY

Intravenous infusions are provided to compressed patients in the monoplace chamber by passing the IV tubing through the chamber bulkhead via a special sterile IV pass-through. See Figures 10, 11.

The IV line passes from inside the chamber hatch to outside. It is unnecessary to completely disassemble the IV pass-through device. By loosening the knurled pass-through fitting, the sterile, disposable pass-through can be inserted. Once inserted, the knurled fitting is tightened down to achieve a seal. The hyperbaric IV pass-through and back-check valve (Argon, Maxxim Medical Corp., Athens, TX; formerly Cobe, Lakewood, CO) is favored (Figure 11) because of its versatility, ease of use, and low internal dead-space volume. The IV line must be flushed with IV solution. For maintenance lines, this can be Lactated Ringers, normal saline, or 5% dextrose in water. For continuous infusions of drugs or TPN, the line is flushed with the appropriate solution.

High pressure IV pumps permit the controlled delivery of IV fluids. Presently there are two pumps available that can generate sufficient pressures to infuse IV solutions into patients compressed to 3 ATA. See Figures 12, 13. They are the IVAC 530 (IVAC Corp., San Diego, CA; available from Sechrist, Inc.; Hyperbaric Clearinghouse, Inc., Springfield, VA; and American IV Products; Inc., Hanover, MD) (see Figure 12) and the Abbot Shaw Hyperbaric Pump (Abbott Laboratories, North Chicago, IL). See Figure 13. The Flowguard #6201 volumetric pump (Baxter, Deerfield, IL) can deliver up to 1,999 ml per hour of IV crystalloid to a patient compressed to 19 psig (2.1 ATA at our altitude of 1,500 m). During compression the occlusion alarm is activated, but once 2 ATA pressure is reached, the alarm can be reset and the pump operates satisfactorily. The Flowguard pump will not infuse IV fluids above approximately 2 ATA, unless the occlusion alarm sensitivity is altered or defeated, an alteration that is not endorsed by the manufacturer.

The IVAC and Abbott pumps both have inaccuracies at very low and high infusion rates, especially at high chamber pressures (> 2.0 ATA) (8, 44). For delivery of potent drugs such as dopamine or nitroprusside, calibration of the particular pump, under the treatment pressures is important (8). The

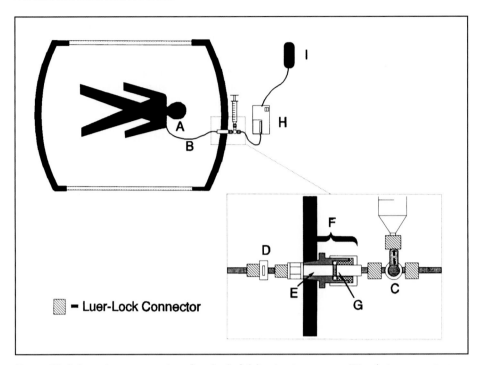

Figure 10. Schematic representation of method of delivering intravenous (IV) solutions to patients compressed in the monoplace chamber. The IV catheter (A) is Luer lock connected to pressure tubing (B). The pressure tubing is connected to a one-way back-check valve (D) located inside the chamber. This valve permits unidirectional flow of fluids towards the patient. Shown is a Cobe hyperbaric pass-through (E). The pass-through is passed out of the chamber by a Swage-lock metal fitting (F). A pressure seal is accomplished by an o-ring (G). A stopcock (C) is located just outside the chamber. Medications are pushed at this point. IV solutions (I) are pumped into the patient by a high pressure pump (H).

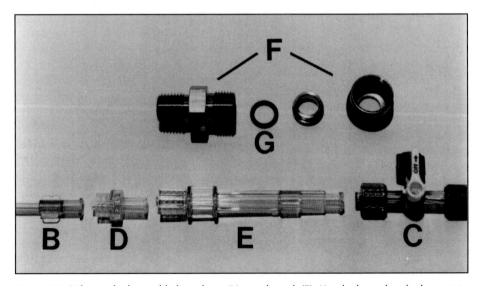

Figure 11. Cobe sterile disposable hyperbaric IV pass-through (E). Use the legend and schematic in Figure 10. The Swage-lock fitting (F) is shown disassembled.

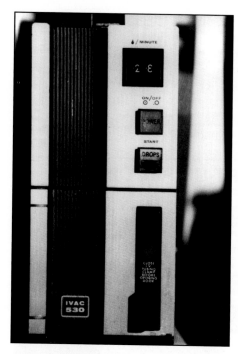

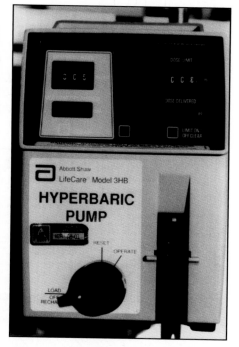

Figure 12. IVAC 530 pump - peristaltic pump that is suitable for infusing IV fluids into patients compressed in the monoplace chamber.

Figure 13. Abbott Shaw Hyperbaric Pump - a volumetric infusion pump suitable for monoplace hyperbaric applications.

IVAC pump is a peristaltic pump, so infused volume is a function of the pump rate and the drip chamber type. See Figure 14. The Abbott pump is a volumetric pump, but a conversion chart needs to be used to provide the desired rate, which is a function of chamber pressure. See Figure 15. Information regarding the accuracy of the Baxter pump used in hyperbaric applications is unavailable.

It is important to have a one-way or back-check valve in-line in the IV tubing. See Figures 10, 11. The back-check valve prevents retrograde blood return in case of an IV line disconnect outside the chamber. The Amron back-check valve can be located inside the chamber anywhere along the IV line. Luer-lock pressure tubing should be used inside the chamber to prevent inadvertent IV-tubing disconnections, or kinking of the IV tubing. Several different manufacturers have hyperbaric tubing sets available. At the present time, these include Sechrist, Amron, and Abbott. The Sechrist tubing, is a larger bore (i.e., dead-space volume, or volume of fluid necessary to fill the tubing is larger), but is useful if delivering highly viscous solutions at rapid rates (e.g., blood or plasma). The Amron tubing is highly versatile since the back-check valve, pass-through and IV tubing are connected with Luer locks permitting tubes of differing lengths and internal diameters to be used. This feature is particularly useful if one desires to sample blood from a compressed patient (e.g., monitoring the ABG or inspecting blood glucose). Also, the Amron IV tubing is available in a neonatal variety, which has a smaller internal diameter, hence less internal dead-space. This is important in treating infants for whom the volume of infused IV fluid needs to be carefully titrated, or when withdrawing blood from a compressed patient. The Abbott tubing is designed to be used with the Abbott Hyperbaric pump. The Sechrist and Amron tubing sets are designed to be used with the IVAC 530 pumps. The Baxter pump requires a specially designed, IV infusion set, as well.

Intravenous medications are given as controlled infusions or as bolus injections. To give a bolus injection, the drug is drawn up in a 3 ml Luer lock syringe. The needle is removed and the syringe Luer lock tightly connected to

# INFUSION PUMP START-UP PROCEDURE

FOR DETAILED INSTRUCTIONS, REFER TO USER INFORMATION

1. START I.V. ACCORDING TO STANDARD PROCEDURE.
2. PROPERLY POSITION DROP SENSOR ON DRIP CHAMBER.
3. SET PRESCRIBED RATE OF INFUSION ON DROPS PER MINUTE SELECTOR.
4. OPEN PUMP DOOR, PLACE I.V. TUBING BETWEEN GUIDES. MAKE SURE THAT DIRECTION OF FLOW IS FROM TOP TO BOTTOM AS INDICATED BY ARROW.
5. CLOSE DOOR AND OPEN CLAMP ON I.V. TUBING.
6. TURN INSTRUMENT "ON" BY DEPRESSING ON/OFF BUTTON.
7. PRESS START BUTTON TO START INFUSION.

CAUTION: · CLOSE I.V. SET CLAMP BEFORE OPENING PUMP DOOR.
· MAXIMUM RECOMMENDED RATE: 200 ml PER HR.

NOTE: FOR NORMAL OPERATION, INSTRUMENT MUST BE CONNECTED TO 3-WIRE GROUNDED OUTLET. BUILT-IN BATTERY WILL OPERATE INSTRUMENT FOR A LIMITED TIME ONLY.     125718A

## INFUSION PUMP FLOW RATE CONVERSION CHART
### SETTINGS IN DROPS PER MINUTE

| ml PER HOUR | IVAC | TRAVENOL | McGAW | ABBOTT | CUTTER | PEDS SET | IVAC | TRAVENOL | McGAW | ABBOTT | CUTTER | PEDS SET | IVAC | TRAVENOL | McGAW | ABBOTT | CUTTER | PEDS SET |
|---|---|---|---|---|---|---|---|---|---|---|---|---|---|---|---|---|---|---|
| 5 | 2 | 1 | 1 | 2 | 2 | 5 | 2 | 1 | 2 | 1 | 2 | 5 | 2 | 1 | 2 | 2 | 2 | 6 |
| 10 | 3 | 2 | 3 | 3 | 4 | 10 | 3 | 2 | 3 | 2 | 4 | 10 | 4 | 2 | 3 | 4 | 5 | 12 |
| 15 | 5 | 3 | 4 | 4 | 6 | 15 | 5 | 3 | 4 | 4 | 7 | 15 | 6 | 4 | 5 | 6 | 6 | 17 |
| 20 | 6 | 4 | 6 | 6 | 8 | 20 | 7 | 4 | 6 | 6 | 9 | 21 | 7 | 5 | 7 | 7 | 10 | 25 |
| 25 | 8 | 5 | 7 | 7 | 10 | 25 | 8 | 5 | 7 | 7 | 11 | 26 | 10 | 6 | 9 | 9 | 12 | 31 |
| 30 | 9 | 6 | 9 | 9 | 12 | 30 | 10 | 6 | 9 | 9 | 13 | 31 | 12 | 7 | 10 | 10 | 15 | 37 |
| 35 | 11 | 7 | 10 | 10 | 13 | 35 | 12 | 7 | 11 | 10 | 15 | 36 | 13 | 9 | 12 | 13 | 17 | 39 |
| 40 | 12 | 8 | 12 | 11 | 15 | 40 | 13 | 8 | 12 | 11 | 17 | 42 | 15 | 10 | 13 | 14 | 20 | 50 |
| 45 | 14 | 9 | 13 | 13 | 17 | 45 | 15 | 9 | 14 | 12 | 19 | 47 | 18 | 11 | 15 | 16 | 22 | 56 |
| 50 | 15 | 10 | 14 | 14 | 19 | 50 | 17 | 10 | 15 | 15 | 21 | 52 | 20 | 12 | 17 | 18 | 25 | 63 |
| 55 | 17 | 11 | 16 | 16 | 21 | 55 | 18 | 11 | 17 | 17 | 23 | 57 | 21 | 13 | 19 | 20 | 27 | 69 |
| 60 | 19 | 12 | 17 | 17 | 23 | 60 | 20 | 12 | 18 | 18 | 25 | 62 | 23 | 15 | 20 | 21 | 30 | 75 |
| 65 | 21 | 13 | 19 | 18 | 25 | 65 | 22 | 14 | 20 | 20 | 27 | 67 | 25 | 17 | 22 | 23 | 32 | 81 |
| 70 | 23 | 14 | 20 | 20 | 27 | 70 | 24 | 15 | 21 | 22 | 30 | 72 | 27 | 18 | 24 | 24 | 34 | 88 |
| 75 | 24 | 15 | 22 | 21 | 29 | 75 | 25 | 16 | 23 | 23 | 32 | 78 | 29 | 19 | 25 | 26 | 37 | 94 |
| 80 | 26 | 16 | 23 | 22 | 30 | 80 | 27 | 17 | 24 | 25 | 35 | 82 | 31 | 20 | 27 | 28 | 39 | 99 |
| 85 | 27 | 17 | 25 | 23 | 33 | 85 | 29 | 18 | 26 | 26 | 37 | 88 | 32 | 21 | 29 | 30 | 42 | |
| 90 | 29 | 18 | 26 | 25 | 35 | 90 | 31 | 19 | 27 | 28 | 39 | 93 | 34 | 22 | 31 | 31 | 44 | |
| 95 | 30 | 19 | 27 | 27 | 36 | 95 | 32 | 20 | 28 | 29 | 41 | 98 | 36 | 24 | 32 | 33 | 46 | |
| 100 | 32 | 20 | 28 | 28 | 39 | 99 | 34 | 21 | 30 | 31 | 43 | | 37 | 25 | 34 | 35 | 49 | |
| 105 | 33 | 21 | 29 | 29 | 40 | | 35 | 22 | 31 | 32 | 44 | | 38 | 26 | 35 | 36 | 51 | |
| 110 | 34 | 22 | 30 | 31 | 43 | | 37 | 23 | 33 | 33 | 46 | | 40 | 27 | 37 | 37 | 54 | |
| 115 | 36 | 23 | 32 | 32 | 45 | | 39 | 24 | 34 | 34 | 48 | | 41 | 29 | 39 | 39 | 56 | |
| 120 | 37 | 24 | 34 | 33 | 46 | | 40 | 25 | 36 | 36 | 50 | | 43 | 30 | 41 | 41 | 59 | |
| 125 | 39 | 25 | 35 | 35 | 48 | | 42 | 27 | 38 | 37 | 52 | | 45 | 31 | 42 | 42 | 61 | |
| 130 | 41 | 26 | 37 | 36 | 50 | | 43 | 28 | 40 | 39 | 54 | | 47 | 33 | 44 | 44 | 64 | |
| 135 | 42 | 27 | 38 | 38 | 52 | | 45 | 29 | 42 | 41 | 56 | | 50 | 34 | 46 | 46 | 65 | |
| 140 | 43 | 28 | 39 | 39 | 54 | | 47 | 30 | 44 | 42 | 58 | | 52 | 35 | 48 | 47 | 67 | |
| 145 | 44 | 29 | 41 | 40 | 55 | | 48 | 31 | 45 | 44 | 60 | | 54 | 36 | 49 | 49 | 68 | |
| 150 | 46 | 30 | 43 | 42 | 58 | | 50 | 32 | 47 | 46 | 62 | | 56 | 37 | 52 | 51 | 69 | |
| 155 | 48 | 31 | 44 | 43 | 59 | | 51 | 33 | 48 | 47 | 64 | | 59 | 39 | 55 | 52 | 72 | |
| 160 | 49 | 32 | 46 | 44 | 60 | | 53 | 34 | 49 | 48 | 66 | | 61 | 40 | 56 | 54 | 74 | |
| 165 | 51 | 33 | 47 | 46 | 62 | | 54 | 35 | 51 | 50 | 68 | | 62 | 41 | 58 | 56 | 77 | |
| 170 | 53 | 34 | 48 | 47 | 64 | | 56 | 36 | 53 | 52 | 70 | | 64 | 42 | 61 | 57 | 78 | |
| 175 | 54 | 35 | 49 | 48 | 65 | | 57 | 37 | 54 | 53 | 72 | | 66 | 44 | 62 | 59 | 80 | |
| 180 | 55 | 36 | 51 | 50 | 66 | | 59 | 38 | 56 | 55 | 73 | | 68 | 45 | 63 | 61 | 81 | |
| 185 | 57 | 37 | 52 | 51 | 67 | | 60 | 39 | 57 | 57 | 75 | | 69 | 46 | 65 | 62 | 82 | |
| 190 | 58 | 38 | 53 | 53 | 69 | | 62 | 40 | 59 | 59 | 77 | | 71 | 47 | 66 | 64 | 83 | |
| 195 | 59 | 39 | 55 | 54 | 70 | | 63 | 41 | 60 | 60 | 79 | | 73 | 49 | 68 | 66 | 84 | |
| 200 | 61 | 40 | 56 | 56 | 71 | | 64 | 42 | 61 | 61 | 81 | | 75 | 50 | 69 | 67 | 85 | |

**APPROXIMATE SET RATING:**

IVAC — 20 DROPS PER ml

TRAVENOL — 10 DROPS PER ml

McGAW — 15 DROPS PER ml

ABBOTT — 15 DROPS PER ml

CUTTER — 15 DROPS PER ml

PEDS (ALL) — 60 DROPS PER ml

| GROUP I SOLUTIONS ELECTROLYTE 5%-10% DEXTROSE | GROUP II SOLUTIONS HYPERALIMENTATION 20%-25% DEXTROSE | GROUP III SOLUTIONS ALCOHOL |
|---|---|---|

Figure 14. IVAC 530 infusion pump conversion chart. Infused volumes are a function of pump set flow rate and the type of IV tubing and drip chamber.

a 3-way stopcock located just outside the chamber bulkhead hatch. See Figures 10, 11, 16.

The drug is injected into the IV line. The drug must be flushed through the IV tubing dead-space to arrive at the patient. This is easily accomplished by drawing up approximately 10 ml of compatible IV solution

# HYPERBARIC PUMP

**CAUTION:** Delivery Rate and Dose Limit Settings and Volume/Dose Delivered are Valid at 2 ATA only. For Settings and Dose/Rate Values at Different Hyperbaric Chamber Pressure Settings (ATA). See Conversion Chart Below.
**Pump Not To Be Used Inside Hyperbaric Chamber**

Delivery Rate and Dose Limit Settings vs Actual Delivery Rates/Dose Limits for Different Hyperbaric Chamber Pressure Settings (ATA)

| Desired Rate (mL/hr) or Dose (mL) | 1 ATA | 1.5 ATA | 2.0 ATA | 2.5 ATA | 3.0 ATA |
|---|---|---|---|---|---|
| | Set Thumbwheel Selector at Value Below | | | | |
| 10 | 8 | 9 | 10 | 11 | 12 |
| 15 | 13 | 14 | 15 | 16 | 18 |
| 20 | 17 | 18 | 20 | 22 | 24 |
| 25 | 21 | 23 | 25 | 27 | 30 |
| 30 | 25 | 28 | 30 | 33 | 37 |
| 35 | 30 | 32 | 35 | 38 | 43 |
| 40 | 34 | 37 | 40 | 44 | 49 |
| 45 | 38 | 41 | 45 | 49 | 55 |
| 50 | 42 | 46 | 50 | 55 | 61 |
| 55 | 47 | 50 | 55 | 60 | 67 |
| 60 | 51 | 55 | 60 | 66 | 73 |
| 65 | 55 | 60 | 65 | 71 | 79 |
| 70 | 59 | 64 | 70 | 77 | 85 |
| 75 | 64 | 69 | 75 | 82 | 91 |
| 80 | 68 | 73 | 80 | 88 | 98 |
| 85 | 72 | 78 | 85 | 93 | 104 |
| 90 | 76 | 83 | 90 | 99 | 110 |
| 95 | 80 | 87 | 95 | 104 | 116 |
| 100 | 85 | 92 | 100 | 110 | 122 |
| 150 | 127 | 138 | 150 | 165 | 183 |
| 200 | 169 | 183 | 200 | 220 | 244 |
| 250 | 212 | 229 | 250 | 275 | 305 |
| 300 | 254 | 275 | 300 | 330 | 366 |
| 350 | 296 | 321 | 350 | 385 | 427 |
| 400 | 339 | 367 | 400 | 440 | 488 |
| 450 | 381 | 413 | 450 | 495 | 549 |
| 500 | 424 | 459 | 500 | 550 | 610 |
| 550 | 466 | 504 | 550 | 604 | 671 |
| 600 | 508 | 550 | 600 | 659 | 732 |
| 650 | 551 | 596 | 650 | 714 | 793 |
| 700 | 593 | 642 | 700 | 769 | 854 |
| 750 | 635 | 688 | 750 | 824 | 915 |
| 800 | 678 | 734 | 800 | 879 | 976 |
| 850 | 720 | 780 | 850 | 934 | – |
| 900 | 762 | 825 | 900 | 989 | – |
| 950 | 805 | 871 | 950 | – | – |

*Figure 15. Abbott pump conversion chart demonstrating that the delivered IV volume is a function of the set pump rate and chamber pressure.*

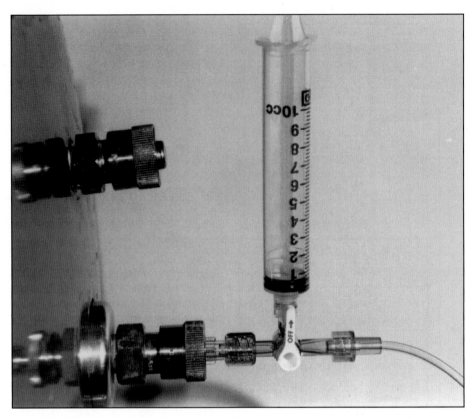

*Figure 16. Medications are pushed into the IV line by a syringe Luer lock connected to a 3-way stopcock located at the chamber pass-through. Adequate volumes of IV fluid must be pushed behind the medication to push it through the tubing dead-space (generally 6-15 ml) in order for the medication to reach the patient.*

and injecting it behind the medication. The smaller the syringe plunger diameter, the easier it is to push the fluid into the IV line (Force = Pressure x Area). The amount of flush solution is determined by the volume of tubing dead-space. With adult 6-foot Amron tubing the system dead-space is 6 ml. With 6-foot Amron neonatal tubing the dead-space is 2.5 ml. The Sechrist tubing dead-space volume is 15 ml. To initiate a potent pressor, such as dopamine, a hypotensive compressed patient requires either that dopamine has been primed in a dedicated IV line in anticipation, or must be started once the patient has been compressed. To begin dopamine in the latter circumstance requires the clinical team to know precisely when the dopamine has been flushed through the tubing dead-space and when it reaches the patient, to avoid giving the patient a dopamine bolus that could be potentially lethal. One method of initiating dopamine in a compressed patient is to inject a few mls of methylene blue into the IV tubing just proximal to the dopamine infusion. The dopamine is quickly injected into the IV system while observing the methylene blue. When the methylene blue reaches the patient, the infusion may be controlled at the desired rate. This line may not subsequently be used for providing drugs in a bolus fashion, since to do so would result in the patient receiving a bolus of dopamine.

Total parenteral nutrition and insulin infusions are sometimes discontinued during HBO (25). We generally do not discontinue TPN or insulin during HBO. Generally, we favor continuing TPN during HBO because discontinuing the TPN predisposes to hypoglycemia, reduces the net caloric balance per day, and potentiates swings in the patient's nutritional balance. Total parenteral nutrition requires a dedicated IV line. Also, enteral feeding can be continued during HBO. By passing the enteral feeding tube into the chamber via a Amron disposable IV pass-through, continuous enteral feeds can be continued during HBO by infusing the feeding solution with the IVAC 530 peristaltic pump.

The patient's response should be monitored after infusing medications. Sedatives may contribute to hypercarbia, a risk factor for CNS $O_2$ toxicity (6). Analgesics can cause hypotension, so BP monitoring of patients who are receiving these agents may be necessary. A flow sheet can be helpful in documenting physiologic responses to medications. Also, communication and documentation in the patient's in-patient record of the type, dose, route, and time of medications is important.

Some monoplace hyperbaric chambers have limited numbers of IV pass-through ports. The Sechrist 2500B monoplace chamber only has 5 pass-through orifices in the chamber hatch, each of 13/16-inch diameter. See Figure 17. The hatch may not be altered, according to American Society of Mechanical Engineers - Pressure Vessel for Human Occupancy (ASME-PVHO) guidelines (American Society of Mechanical Engineers, United Engineering Center, New York, NY). It is difficult, and potentially dangerous for the physician to treat critically ill patients with HBO if there are inadequate numbers of IV pass-throughs. For the HBO session, certain IV infusions can be discontinued or run piggy-back. However, some critically ill patients may still require more than 5 IV lines (fewer than 5 are available if mechanically ventilating the patient, or if inspecting ABGs during HBO). Our solution to the limited number of pass-throughs in the 2500B chamber was to design a pass-through permitting several IV lines to pass through a single chamber hatch orifice.

As previously discussed, a "split-bolt" IV tubing pass-through was designed (See Figure 2-4) that permits 4 IV tubes to enter the chamber through one hatch orifice. See Figures 5, 17. These pass-throughs are not available commercially, but anyone with sufficient interest could have similar pass-throughs machined (35).

Septic patients requiring pressors frequently drop their BP during chamber compression and decompression. Intravascular volume expansion and/or increasing the dose of their pressor is often required to treat the hypotension. The BP reduction during chamber compression may be due to a reduction in the dose of pressor delivered to the patient by the IVAC 530 (personal observation). This BP drop is generally transient, lasting only a few minutes. Once treatment pressure is reached, the BP usually increases, but may require a higher IVAC pump drip rate of pressor. The BP reduction when exiting the chamber may be due to a relaxation of vascular tone with a reduction in hyperbaric induced vasoconstriction. If clinically required, we try to time transfusions of blood or plasma until the end of a chamber treatment to volume in order to expand these patients prior to the anticipated

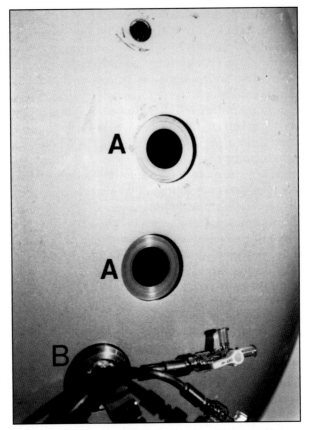

Figure 17. Sechrist 2500B monoplace chamber hatch. Depicted are two open orifices which measure 13/16-inch diameter (A). It is possible to pass more that one line or tube through these orifices (See Figures 4 and 5). Notice the four-in-one pass-through (B) (See Figure 6).

hypotension. Otherwise, increased doses of pressors and infusion of crystalloid solutions generally treat the hypotension adequately.

## VENTILATION

Patients with gas gangrene, necrotizing fasciitis, carbon monoxide poisoning or arterial gas embolism may be intubated and require mechanical ventilation. Mechanical ventilation can be performed in the monoplace chamber. Some aspects of mechanical ventilation that are particularly important are described here.

The endotracheal tube (ET) needs to have an adequate internal diameter. Gas density is greater in the compressed chamber, so VE and the ability of the patient to exhale will be limited if the ET tube lumen is too small. This is a problem if the VE is high (>10 liters/minute) and if the lungs are stiff, requiring high airway pressures and PEEP>5 cm $H_2O$.

If the maintenance of an adequate airway is questionable, the patient should be intubated prior to HBO. Likewise, if the patient is combative, requiring IV sedation, it may be prudent to intubate such a patient to prevent possible aspiration and hypercarbia, a risk factor for CNS $O_2$ toxicity during HBO (6).

There are two ventilators commercially available for use in the monoplace chamber in the U.S.A., the Sechrist 500A hyperbaric ventilator (Sechrist) and the Omni-Vent (Allied Healthcare Products Inc., St. Louis, MO; also available from Perry Baromedical, Rivera Beach, FL). The 500A ventilator circuit is located inside the chamber hatch (See Figure 18) and the ventilator controls are located outside the chamber. See Figure 19. The Omni-vent is generally located outside the chamber, with the airway circuit passing through the chamber hatch. The Omni-vent can be used inside the monoplace chamber with the ventilator controls operated from outside the chamber (5, 21).

A single $O_2$ hose leads from the controls, through a ventilator pass-through in the chamber hatch, and connects to the inlet hose of the ventilator block. See Figure 18. The 500A is a pneumatic, time-cycled ventilator that permits adjustments for flow, inspiratory time and expiratory time. See Figure 19. When the ventilator cycles, $O_2$ moves through the ventilator control unit into the ventilator block supply hose and into the ventilator block, simultaneously closing the exhalation valve to augment VT. Some $O_2$ is routed through a water-filled nebulizer to provide humidity to the inspiratory circuit. VT is measured with a spirometer located inside the

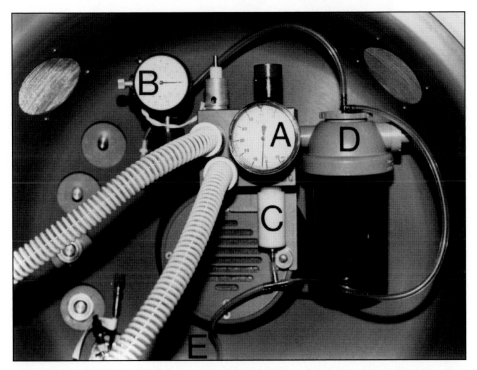

Figure 18. Sechrist 500A hyperbaric ventilator block and circuit are positioned inside the chamber hatch. Airway pressure is measured by a manometer (A). A spirometer (B) located on the exhalation side of the circuit measures exhaled tidal volumes. The entraining venturi (C) augments tidal volume. The nebulizer (D) is also powered from the control module (Figure 19) located outside the chamber.

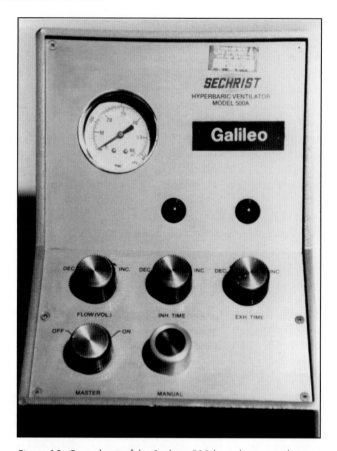

Figure 19. Control unit of the Sechrist 500 hyperbaric ventilator.
Flow, inhalation time, and exhalation time are adjusted by turning
the appropriate knobs.

chamber connected to the expiratory limb of the ventilator circuit. Airway
pressure is measured in the ventilator block, not at the proximal airway. See
Figure 18. PEEP is provided by placing PEEP valves in the expiratory
circuit. See Figure 20.

A peak pressure pop-off valve is located on the 500A ventilator block
and should be adjusted prior to use for each particular patient. A one-way
valve permits the patient to inspire (non-mechanical breath). As originally
designed, the 500A only provides a fractional inspired concentration of 1.00
$O_2$. With modifications, the 500A ventilator can deliver air as well as $O_2$
(Appendix II) (34), which may be important to prevent CNS and pulmonary
$O_2$ toxicity (1, 6, 18).

Because the 500A operates in the control mode only, we generally
sedate the compressed patient (e.g., IV diazepam and morphine or propofol),
and occasionally provide neuromuscular blocking agents (e.g., IV
vecuronium) to sedate and paralyze the intubated, mechanically ventilated
patient in the chamber. We sedate and paralyze the patient to minimize
patient-ventilator asynchrony, which could result in gas-trapping, auto-PEEP;
or, the patient could resist a breath during a controlled mechanical breath,

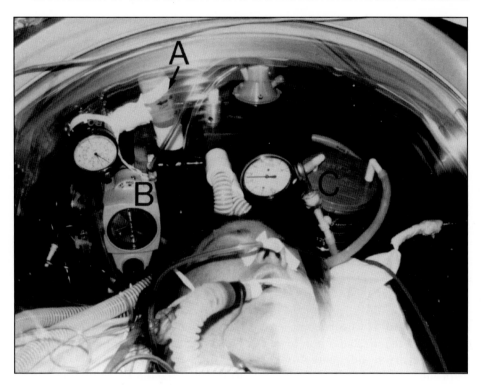

Figure 20. Positive and expiratory pressure (PEEP) is provided to patients in the monoplace chamber by placing PEEP valves (A) at the exhalation port of the 500A ventilator circuit. A vacuum regulator (B) and suction canister (C) are also being used in this patient with necrotizing fasciitis and myonecrosis.

which could result in pulmonary barotrauma, a serious complication in a compressed patient.

The 500A performance is particularly limited with a VE > 15 liters/minute, especially at chamber pressures > 2.0 ATA (Appendix V) (38). For optimal ventilator performance, the ventilator driving pressure must be at least 65 psig, and, preferably up to 85 psig. Most hospitals have wall $O_2$ pressures of only 50 to 55 psig, which is unacceptable to supply the 500A ventilator. The 500A performance was evaluated over a range of inlet supply pressures, test lung compliances, and chamber pressures (Appendix V) (38). The 500A ventilator performance is inadequate to ventilate patients with a compliance < 60 ml/cm $H_2O$ who require > 5 cm $H_2O$ PEEP, with a VE > 15 liters/minute at chamber pressures > 2.0 ATA. Furthermore, the VT and VR change significantly during pressurization and depressurization of the chamber (Appendix V) (38). Careful monitoring of VT, VR and airway pressures is necessary, as the chamber pressure is altered with titration of flow, inspiratory time, and expiratory time to achieve the desired VE. There are no alarms incorporated in the 500A ventilator, so astute attention to detail is mandatory when using it. The Tau Monitor can be used to monitor the VR and airway pressures of both the 500A and the Omni-Vent (17). One needs to weigh carefully the risk-benefit ratio of treating mechanically-ventilated patients in the monoplace chamber, especially if the patient has pulmonary dysfunction requiring higher airway pressures and high VE. The measurement of pH and $PaCO_2$ can help guide the adequacy of mechanical ventilation. Inspecting ABG measurements prior to compression, while the patient is ventilated with the 500A, and during HBO, should be considered.

In order to provide a VE > 10 liters/minute, the 500A ventilator uses an inverted/expiratory ratio (I-time exceeds E-time). An inverted I/E ratio is not necessarily harmful, but operators of this ventilator must be vigilant of auto-PEEP. If the patient is hypotensive, especially with a reduced pulse pressure, it very likely may be due to the ventilator. The treatment is not to increase the dose of dopamine. The treatment consists of adding expiratory time and shortening inspiratory time. Even with the 500A flows set to maximum, small VT are the rule. Some mechanically-ventilated patients must be hypoventilated (increased $PaCO_2$) to prevent auto-PEEP. Presumably, hypoventilation increases the risk of CNS $O_2$ toxicity (6). Use of the 500A ventilator in critically ill patients treated in the monoplace chamber is one of the skills requiring the highest level of expertise and attention.

## CONCLUSION

Critically ill patients can be treated with HBO in the monoplace chamber. Just as with treating critically ill patients in general, treating them with HBO requires attention to detail. The critically ill patient needs to have an adequate airway, adequate numbers of IV lines and care-givers who possess a thorough understanding of the limitations of mechanical ventilation in the monoplace chamber. Suction, $EtCO_2$ monitoring, measurement of hyperbaric $PaO_2$ and increased numbers of IV lines increase the ability of monoplace units to offer HBO to critically ill patients.

A thoroughly knowledgeable staff, skilled in the management of critically ill patients, is the most important element in delivering HBO to these patients. The next most important element is a chamber unit that has the required additional equipment readily available to treat critically ill patients. The close proximity of the HBO unit to the ICU area facilitates the delivery of HBO to critically ill patients. Obviously a sound foundation in HBO physiology, risks, and benefits is central to applying HBO to patients, especially if they are critically ill.

## ACKNOWLEDGMENTS

I wish to thank Steve Howe, M.A., for drawing the schematic figures and his thoughtful review. Appreciation is extended to George Hart, M.D., Eric Kindwall, M.D., and Robert Goldmann, M.D., for building the foundation for treating critically ill patients in the monoplace chamber. Without their prior work and the development of a suitable chamber by Sechrist Industries, Inc., I might not have contributed further to the field.

# REFERENCES

1. Bleiberg B, Kerem D. Central nervous system oxygen toxicity in the resting rat: postponement by intermittent oxygen exposure. Undersea Biomed Res. 1988;15(5): 337-352.

2. Braman SS, Dunn SM, Amico CA, et al. Complications of intra-hospital transport in critically ill patients. Ann Int Med. 1987;107:469-473.

3. Camporesi EM, Moon RE. Management of critically ill patients in the hyperbaric environment (editorial). J Hyperbaric Med. 1987;2(4)195-198.

4. Chang C, Dughi J, Shitabata P, et al. Air embolism and the radial arterial line. Crit Care Med. 1988;16:141.

5. Churchill S, Weaver LK, Haberstock D. Omni-vent: Another option for mechanical ventilation in the monoplace hyperbaric chamber. Undersea Hyperbaric Med 1998; 25(Suppl): 24.

6. Clark JM: Oxygen toxicity: In: Bennett PB, Elliott DH (eds): The Physiology and Medicine of Diving, ed 4. London, WB Saunders Company, Ltd., 1993, pp 121- 169.

7. Eskelson MI, Weaver LK, Greenway LG. End-tidal $CO_2$ monitoring within the monoplace hyperbaric chamber (abstract). Undersea Biomed Res. 1989;16(Supple): 18-19.

8. Evans P, Weaver LK. The use of IVAC 530 infusion pumps in the monoplace hyperbaric chamber. (abstract) Undersea Biomed Res. 1991;18(Supple):91.

9. Faglia E, Favales F, Aldeghi A, et al. Change in major amputation rate in a center dedicated to diabetic foot care during the 1980s: Prognostic determinants for major amputation. J Diabetes Complications 1998; 12(2):96-102.

10. Farmer JC Jr. Ask the expert. In Pressure 1998; 27(5): 12-3.

11. Gardner RM. Direct blood pressure measurement - dynamic response requirements. Anesthesiology. 1981;54:227-236.

12. Gardner RM. Hemodynamic monitoring: from catheter to display. In Weil MH, ed. Acute Care. Basel, Switzerland: S. Karger AG, 1986;12:3-33.

13. Gardner RM, Bond EL, Clark JS. Safety and efficacy of continuous flush systems for arterial and pulmonary artery catheters. Ann Thorac Surg. 1977;23:534-538.

14. Greenway L, Weaver L, Howe S, et al. Comparison of $E_2CO_2$ & $PaCO_2$ in normals at various chamber pressures. (abstract) Undersea Biomed Res. 1991;18(Supplement):23.

15. Hart G. Equipment and procedures - monoplace chambers. In Shilling CW, Carlson CB, Mathias RA, eds. The Physician's Guide to Diving Medicine. New York: Plenum Press, 1984;621-625.

16. Hart GB, Meyer GW, Strauss MB, et al. Transcutaneous partial pressure of oxygen measured in a monoplace hyperbaric chamber at 1, 1.5, and 2 ATA oxygen. J Hyperbaric Med. 1990;5(4):223-229.

17. Hein S, Weaver L, Howe S. Mechanical ventilator monitoring inside the monoplace hyperbaric chamber. (abstract) Undersea Biomed Res 1994; 21(Suppl):34.

18. Hendricks PL, Hall DA, Hunter WH Jr, Haley PJ. Extension of pulmonary oxygen tolerance in man at 2 ATA by intermittent oxygen exposure. J Appl Physiol: Resp Environ Exercise Physiol. 1977;42:593-599.

19. Holcomb JR, Matos-Navarro AY, et al. Critical care in the hyperbaric chamber. In Davis JC, Hunt TK, eds. Problem Wounds. New York: Elsevier, 1988;200-209.

20. Kindwall EP, Goldmann RW: Hyperbaric Medicine Procedures, 7th edition. St. Luke_s Medical Center. Milwaukee, Wisconsin, 1995.

21. Layton W, Weaver L, Haberstock D. Modifications to the Omni-Vent ventilator for use within the monoplace hyperbaric chamber. Undersea Hyperbaric Med 1998; 25(Suppl): 56.

22. Mathieu D, Wattel F, Bouachour G, et al. Post-traumatic limb ischemia: prediction of final outcome by transcutaneous oxygen measurement in hyperbaric oxygen. J Trauma. 1990;30(3): 307-314.

23. Meyer GW, Hart GB, Strauss MB. Noninvasive blood pressure monitoring in the hyperbaric monoplace chamber. J Hyperbaric Med. 1990;4(4):211-216.

24. Myers RA. Functional Hyperbaric Chamber Facilities. Summary of questionnaires compliled by Maryland Institute of Emergency Medical Services (MIEMSS). Baltimore, Maryland: January, 1988.

25. Riseman JA, Zamboni WA, Curtis A, et al. Hyperbaric oxygen therapy for necrotizing fascitis reduces mortality and the need for debridements. Surgery. 1990;108:847-850.

26. Rockswold GL, Ford E, Anderson JR, et al. Patient monitoring in the monoplace chamber. Hyperbaric Oxygen Review. 1985;6(3):161-168.

27. Salomon A. Safety of the Radiometer' transcutaneous monitors when measuring in hyperbaric chambers. TC109 Bulletin, Radiometer'. A/S, Copenhagen, Denmark, 1990;1-10.

28. Sheffield PJ. Tissue oxygen measurements. In Davis JC, Hunt TK, eds. Problem Wounds. New York: Elsevier, 1988;17-51.

29. Sukoff MH, Ragatz RE. Hyperbaric oxygenation for the treatment of acute cerebral edema. Neurosurgery 1982; 10:29-38.

30. Wattel FE, Mathieu DM, Fossati P, et al. Hyperbaric oxygen in the treatment of diabetic foot lesions. J Hyper Med 1991; 6(4): 263-8.

31. Wattel F, Pellerin P, Mathieu D, et al. Hyperbaric oxygen therapy in the treatment of wounds, in plastic and reconstructive surgery. Ann Chir Plast Esthet. 1990;35(2):141-146.

32. Weaver LK. Tycos Pressure Infuser: some precautions before using in the chamber. Pressure. 1987;16(6):15.

33. Weaver LK. A functional suction apparatus within the monoplace hyperbaric chamber. J Hyperbaric Med. 1988;3(3):165-171.

34. Weaver LK. Air breaks with the Sechrist 500A monoplace hyperbaric ventilator. J Hyperbaric Med. 1988;3(3):179-186.

35. Weaver LK. Technique of Swan-Ganz catheter monitoring in patients treated in the monoplace hyperbaric chamber. J Hyperbaric Med. 1992;7(1):1-18.

36. Weaver LK. Clinical applications of hyperbaric oxygen-monoplace chamber use. In Moon RE, Camporesi EM, eds. Problems in Respiratory Care-Clinical Application of Hyperbaric Oxygen. Philadelphia: JB Lippincott, 1991;4(2):189-214.

37. Weaver LK. Operational use and patient monitoring in the monoplace chamber. In Moon R ed. Respiratory Care Clinics of North America. W.B. Saunders Company, In press, 9/98.

38. Weaver LK, Greenway L, Elliott CG. Performance characteristics of the Sechrist 500A hyperbaric ventilator in a monoplace hyperbaric chamber. J Hyperbaric Med. 1988;3(4):215-225.

39. Weaver LK, Howe S. Noninvasive doppler blood pressure monitoring in the monoplace hyperbaric chamber. J Clin Monit 1991;7:304-308.

40. Weaver LK, Howe S. Normobaric measurement of arterial oxygen tension of normal human subjects exposed to hyperbaric oxygen. Chest 1992; 102:1175-1181.

41. Weaver LK, Howe S. Arterial oxygen tension of patients with abnormal pulmonary function during hyperbaric oxygen therapy (abstract). Undersea Biomed Res. 1991;18(Suppl): 107-108.

42. Weaver LK, Howe S, Berlin SL. Normobaric measurement of $O_2$ tension of blood and saline tonometered under hyperbaric $O_2$ conditions. J Hyperbaric Med 1990;5(1):29-38.

43. Weaver LK, Strauss MB (eds): Monoplace Hyperbaric Chamber Safety Guidelines. Bethesda, Maryland, Undersea and Hyperbaric Medical Society, 1997.

44. Ziegler BA, Weaver LK. Intravenous infusion pumps: evaluation for use with the monoplace hyperbaric chamber. (abstract) Undersea Biomed Res. 1991;18(Suppl):91.

## APPENDICES

**Appendix I** - Weaver LK. "A functional suction apparatus within the monoplace hyperbaric chamber." J Hyperbaric Med. 1988;3(3):165-171.

**Appendix II** - Weaver LK. "Air breaks with the Sechrist 500A monoplace hyperbaric ventilator." J Hyperbaric Med. 1988;3(3):179-186.

**Appendix III** - Weaver LK, Howe S. "Noninvasive Doppler blood pressure monitoring in the monoplace hyperbaric chamber." J Clin Monit. 1991;7:304-308.

**Appendix IV** - Weaver LK, Howe S, Berlin SL. "Normobaric measurement of $O_2$ tension of blood and saline tonometered under hyperbaric $O_2$ conditions." J Hyperbaric Med. 1990;5(1):29-38.

**Appendix V** - Weaver LK, Greenway L, Elliott CG. "Performance of the Sechrist 500A hyperbaric ventilator in a monoplace hyperbaric chamber." J Hyperbaric Med. 1988;3(4):215-225.

## APPENDIX I. A FUNCTIONAL SUCTION APPARATUS WITHIN THE MONOPLACE HYPERBARIC CHAMBER

*Lindell K. Weaver*

## Critical Care Medicine, LDS Hospital, Eighth Avenue and C Street, Salt Lake City, UT 84143

## ABSTRACT

Most hyperbaric oxygen (HBO) treatments in the United States are delivered within the monoplace chamber. Patients who require HBO may have nasogastric (NG) tubes, thoracostomy tubes, or wound drains that require suction, which has not been well documented during monoplace HBO therapy. This paper describes a method of providing suction during HBO therapy within a Sechrist monoplace hyperbaric chamber. An Ohio vacuum regulator with a 1.4-liter suction receptacle canister was mounted on a stainless steel bracket that attaches to the hyperbaric chamber hatch in a manner similar to the Sechrist 500A ventilator. The vacuum regulator and canister were configured so that the 500A ventilator could be mounted on the hatch and still allow access to all IV pass-throughs. A vacuum regulator is adjusted to the desired degree before compression. The hose that typically connects the vacuum regulator to the wall outlet is passed out of the chamber via an IV pass-through. It is not necessary to connect the unit to the wall vacuum, because, when chamber pressure exceeds 5 psi, there is an adequate gradient from inside to outside the chamber to drive the vacuum regulator. The vacuum regulator can be turned on or off by turning a 3-way stopcock open or closed. The vacuum regulator should not be turned to "full" as this could expose the suctioned part to an extreme vacuum; rather it should be regulated to the desired level by the variable suction knob. This system has proved satisfactory suction for NG drainage, surgical drains, and oropharyngeal suctioning in a patient who could not swallow.

## INTRODUCTION

The majority of patients treated with hyperbaric oxygen (HBO) therapy receive this therapy in monoplace HBO chambers (1). Patients who are treated with HBO may have nasogastric (NG) tubes, thoracostomy tubes, or wound drains that require suction, either intermittently or continuously. Others who operate monoplace chambers either cap-off surgical drains or NG tubes or place a glove or bag around the tube to collect passive drainage. Chest tubes are used with Heimlich valves that are not applied to suction. Inadequately drained NG tubes may be an increased risk of aspiration of gastric contents, particularly during decompression. Similarly, for surgical drains, it may be important to not interrupt continuous suction during HBO treatment. Chest tube drainage may be inadequate if removed from suction, which could lead to a tension pneumothorax, a serious complication worsened by decompression.

At this time, no medical equipment manufacturer in the United States offers a suction apparatus designed or adapted for use in the monoplace hyperbaric chamber. Drager offers an optional suction unit with its HTK 1200 monoplace hyperbaric chamber (Drägerwerk AG, Lübeck-Travemünde, FRG). Therefore, I sought to develop an adjustable suction apparatus for patients treated within the monoplace hyperbaric chamber. This suction apparatus uses the pressure gradient that exists between the hyperbaric chamber and the ambient environment.

## MATERIALS AND METHODS

An Ohmeda vacuum regulator (#306-1008-880, Ohmeda, Madison, WI) was chosen because of its relative compact size and availability. This vacuum regulator was disassembled to verify that there was no evidence of oxygen-incompatible substances such as grease, thus avoiding any potentially combustible products before placing it into the HBO chamber (2).

The reassembled vacuum regulator was mounted on one end of a stainless steel plate attached to the hatch of the chamber. On the opposite end of the plate, a 1.4-liter suction receptacle canister (#43423-01, Sorensen Research Co., Salt Lake City, UT) was added. See Figure 1. The mounting plate was cut and grooved so it could be held in the chamber hatch as the ventilator block is. The Sechrist 2500B monoplace chamber hatch has two grooved bushings that accept the Sechrist 500A hyperbaric ventilator block. These bushings were extended (see Figure 2) so that both the suction apparatus and ventilator could be mounted in the hatch simultaneously. See

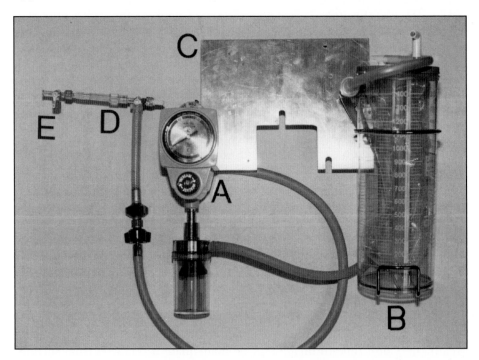

*Figure 1. The Ohio vacuum regulator (A) fand Sorensen suction camister (B) mounted on a bracket (C) configured so that the assembly fits onto the Sechrist 500A ventilator block mounting bushings in the hatch of the Sechrist 2500B hyperbaric chamber. Note the Cobe pass-through (D) connected to the vacuum hose of the Ohio unit. The 3-way stopcock (E) regulates the degree of vacuum once the chamber is pressurized.*

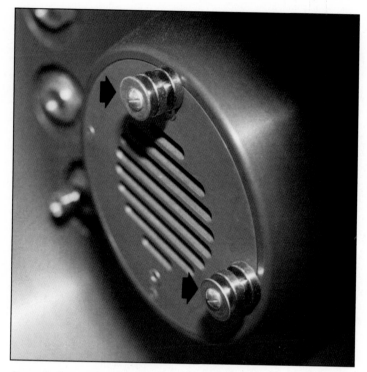

Figure 2. The ventilator block mounting bushings (arrowheads) extended to accept both the suction assembly and the ventilator block simultaneously.

Figure 3. A similar configuration could be applied to any monoplace hyperbaric chamber.

The vacuum hose that normally connects the vacuum regulator to the hospital wall vacuum was cut. To the severed end, a 3-way Luer lock stopcock was attached and secured with Tygon ties. The female Luer lock was then attached to the Luer lock (male) on an IV pass-through (HBO pass-through, #041-600-500, Cobe, Lakewood, CO) to exit the chamber hatch. The Cobe one-way backcheck valve must be removed. Another 3-way stopcock was connected to the Cobe pass-through on the outside of the chamber hatch.

For testing, the latex suction tubing that connects the suction receptacle canister to the item to be suctioned was occluded. The system was mounted in the hatch as specified, and the chamber was pressurized. The vacuum regulator was turned to "full" or to "regulate" before closing the hatch.

## RESULTS

When the chamber was pressurized to approximately 5 psi, there was an adequate gradient to operate the vacuum regulator to full suction (200 to 300 mmHg). The vacuum regulator could be turned on and off merely by opening and closing the outside 3-way stopcock. However, at higher chamber pressures (>10 psig), there was enough suction to collapse the latex suction tubing with the vacuum regulator turned to "on." Therefore, if the vacuum regulator was turned to "regulate" instead of "on," and the degree of vacuum

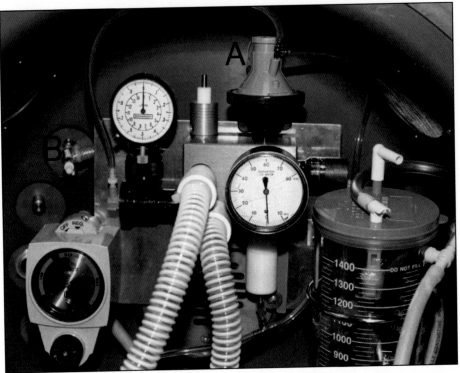

*Figure 3. Configuration of the suction assembly and Sechrist 500A ventilator when used simultaneously. A bird micronebulizer (A) has replaced the standard Bird 500-cc nebulizer. The vacuum hose of the Ohio unit runs behind the assembly and exits the chamber via a Cobe pass-through (B).*

was regulated (by turning the variable adjustment control) before compression, an appropriate degree of suction could be applied. If full vacuum was set with the regulator variable-adjustment control, a suction gradient of 200 to 300 mmHg could be maintained. However, if the vacuum regulator were turned to full, the suctioned item would be exposed to the gradient of pressure from inside to outside the chamber, which is much too high for patient use.

This system has been used at our center to provide continuous or intermittent suction to NG tubes, to suction surgical drains, and to provide oral suction for a cooperative patient who had difficulty swallowing her own secretions. We have not yet had the opportunity to use this suction unit with chest tubes, but we have no reason to believe it would not function adequately.

## DISCUSSION

This system of providing suction to patients treated within a monoplace hyperbaric chamber is appealing because it uses a standard hospital vacuum regulator and easily mounts in the monoplace chamber hatch.

The need to provide suction to patients will increase as HBO therapy is applied to a growing patient population encumbered with NG tubes, chest tubes, and surgical drains.

Several points deserve emphasis. First, it is paramount that the vacuum regulator never be turned to the full position. This can be prevented by placing a screw in the control knob to act as a stop. See Figure 4. In the full position, the vacuum regulator exposes the suctioned item to the maximum "wall" suction which, in the case of a chamber pressurized to 2.0 to 2.8 ATA, is many times the gradient available from the usual hospital wall outlet. Next, the vacuum regulator should be adjusted to the desired level or gradient of vacuum before beginning treatment. This can be accomplished by connecting the outside hatch 3-way stopcock (open position) to the hospital wall vacuum by a vacuum hose made especially for this purpose. Then the vacuum regulator may be adjusted by turning the adjustment knob the appropriate amount. When the chamber is pressurized to the desired treatment level, the vacuum regulator can be turned on and off by turning the 3-way stopcock located outside the chamber hatch, and can be adjusted to any value between on and off by putting the handle of the 3-way stopcock in a position midway between on and off. The degree of vacuum can be read off the dial of the vacuum regulator located in the chamber.

If the patient requires suction continuously (before the chamber is pressurized), the outside hatch stopcock is positioned to the open position and the open lumen is connected to a vacuum regulator powered by the hospital vacuum source. This places two vacuum regulators in a series and works quite well. Once the chamber is pressurized to >5 psi, the wall-vacuum regulator, may be turned off because there is now an adequate gradient available to drive the vacuum regulator located inside the chamber (e.g., a patient has a tube thoracostomy and is receiving positive pressure ventilation, has adult

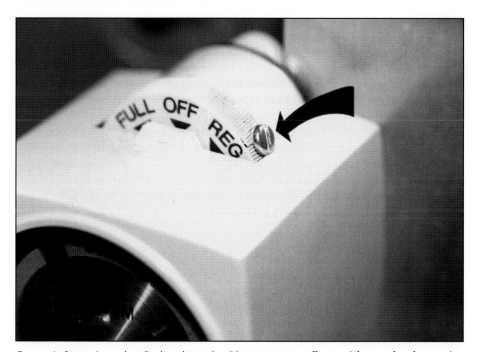

*Figure 4. Screw (arrowhead) placed into the Ohio vacuum on-off control for a safety feature that prevents the regulator from being turned to full on (see Discussion).*

respiratory distress syndrome with a reduced thoracic compliance, and may reaccumulate a pneumothorax unless continuous suction can be provided).

It is expected that $O_2$ will escape through the outside hatch 3-way stopcock when the chamber is pressurized and the stopcock is open. If the resulting sound is distracting, it can be reduced by attaching latex tubing and running it out of the chamber area or, just as simply, by connecting the tubing to the hospital wall-vacuum regulator, and adjusting it to low continuous suction (approximately 80 mmHg). This escaping gas originates from a bypass valve in the vacuum regulator, and does not represent the mass movement of gas from the suctioned item.

This system can be used safely if set up in the manner described, and if the caution about never operating the vacuum regulator in the full on position is adhered to.

Endotracheal (ET) suction can be provided, but at an increased risk. To accomplish this, the suction catheter would have to be inserted into the ET tube and left in that position. A unit similar to the Ballard suction system (Ballard Trach Care Closed Tracheal Suction System, Ballard Medical Products, Midvale, UT) would have to be incorporated. The suction catheter would have to remain inserted through the ET tube lumen for the duration of an HBO treatment (2 to 2.5 hours including compression and decompression time). Increased flow resistance would result, even with large ET tubes, resulting in the potential for auto-PEEP (3). This could have an adverse clinical consequence, including hemodynamic compromise, pulmonary barotrauma, and alveolar hypoventilation (with an increased risk of CNS $O_2$ toxicity if hypercarbia ensues) (4). Furthermore, if the vacuum regulator is inadvertently left on continuously instead of only turned on for brief durations (>15 s), the patient could experience profound hypoxemia (5, 6). For these reasons, the ET tube suction in the monoplace chamber is not recommended.

The Sechrist 500A hyperbaric ventilator will mount on the hatch of the Sechrist 2500B monoplace chamber if configured in the manner described, with one change. The 500-cc Bird nebulizer must be removed from the side of the ventilator block, because there is inadequate space for it and the suction canister. The one-way entraining valve is then positioned there. A Bird micronebulizer (Bird, Palm Springs, CA) is placed on the top of the block, and the gas line that drove the 500 cc nebulizer plugs into the Bird micronebulizer. See Figure 3. We typically operate the ventilator without filling the nebulizer with sterile water. However, with patients who have mucus or blood in the airways, or who have airflow obstruction, nebulized gas may be advantageous. Relocation of the suction canister and use of the 500-cc Bird nebulizer is then recommended.

## CONCLUSIONS

A method of providing suction to patients treated in the monoplace hyperbaric chamber has been presented. An available hospital vacuum regulator is placed within the chamber and driven by the gradient of pressure provided by the pressurized chamber. Intermittent, continuous, and variable suction can be used. The vacuum regulator should never be turned to full; rather, the regulator should be adjusted to the appropriate degree (the pre-HBO amount) before chamber pressurization. With proper configuration, the vacuum regulator, suction canister, and the Sechrist 500A ventilator can be mounted simultaneously in the chamber hatch. This system has been used to suction NG tubes, surgical drains, and for oral suction in a cooperative patient who could not swallow. I caution against using this system with endotracheal tube suction because of potential risks to the patient, including the effects of auto-PEEP, alveolar hypoventilation, and the potential for severe hypoxemia if the suction were inadvertently left on continuously.

## ACKNOWLEDGMENTS

I thank C. Gregory Elliott, M.D., C. DuWayne Schmidt, M.D., and Terry Clemmer, M.D. for reviewing the manuscript. A special thanks to Keith Green and Pat Petersen for preparing the manuscript.

## APPENDIX I REFERENCES

1. Myers RA. Functional hyperbaric chamber facilities. Summary of questionnaires compiled by Maryland Institute of Emergency Medical Services (MIEMSS), April 1986.

2. Weaver LK. Tycos pressure infuser: some precautions before using in the chamber. Pressure 1987; 16(6):15.

3. Pepe PE, Marini JJ. Occult positive end-expiratory pressure in mechanically ventilated patients with airflow obstruction. Am Rev Respir Dis 1982; 126:166.

4. Clark JM. Oxygen toxicity. In: Bennett PB, Elliott DH, eds. The physiology and medicine of diving, 3rd ed. pp. 229-230. London: Bailli_re Tindall, 1982.

5. Caldwell SL, Sullivan KN. Artificial airways. In: Burton GG, Hodgkin JE, eds. Respiratory care: a guide to clinical practice, 2nd ed. Philidelphia: JB Lippincott, 1977:519.

6. Greenway L, King J, Napoli L, et al. The effect of Ballard Closed Tracheal Suction System (BCTSS) on desaturation and saturation recovery time [Abstract]. Respir Care 1986; 31(10):988.

## APPENDIX II. AIR BREAKS WITH THE SECHRIST 500A MONOPLACE HYPERBARIC VENTILATOR

*Lindell K. Weaver*

### Critical Care Medicine, LDS Hospital, Eighth Avenue & C Street, Salt Lake City, UT 84143

### ABSTRACT

Multiplace hyperbaric chambers routinely provide air breaks for spontaneous breathing, as well as for mechanically-ventilated patients receiving hyperbaric oxygen (HBO) to lessen the risk of $O_2$ toxicity. However, patients who are mechanically ventilated within monoplace chambers currently must receive an inspired concentration of 100% $O_2$ without air breaks, even though critically ill patients have an increased risk of $O_2$ toxicity. This paper describes a method of providing air breaks to mechanically ventilated, intubated patients who receive HBO in monoplace chambers. The modification consists of an anesthesia bag fitted around the entraining venturi valve of the Sechrist 500A ventilator. The bag is filled with gas from a source external to the chamber, which allows the ventilator operator to select either $O_2$ or air as the inspired gas by switching the ventilator and venturi bag to the appropriate gas. Approximately 15 breaths using this technique are required to achieve the new $O_2$ concentration at the proximal airway. The gas concentration is not a function of tidal volume, ventilatory rate, or chamber pressure.

### INTRODUCTION

Increasing numbers of critically ill patients receive hyperbaric oxygen (HBO) in monoplace chambers. Kindwall et al. (1), Raleigh (2), and Weaver (3) have discussed methods of providing air breaks in the monoplace hyperbaric chamber to cooperative, spontaneously breathing patients. Intubated, mechanically ventilated patients who are treated in monoplace chambers in the United States are typically ventilated with the Sechrist 500A monoplace hyperbaric ventilator. This ventilator was intended to deliver 100% oxygen to the patient treated with HBO, without the provision for air breaks. However, critically ill patients have an increased risk of oxygen toxicity due to HBO (4:24, 5, 6). Air breaks extend the period of oxygen tolerance (7). Changing the breathing gas from $O_2$ to air is the preferred treatment of $O_2$ toxicity due to HBO (4:18, 8). This paper describes a method of providing air breaks to patients mechanically ventilated with the Sechrist 500A hyperbaric ventilator, by modifying the Sechrist 500A ventilator so that any $FiO_2$, including air, can be delivered.

### MATERIALS AND METHODS

The Sechrist 2500B monoplace chamber was operated according to the owner's manual (9), and the Sechrist 500A ventilator was mounted in the hatch of the chamber. This ventilator has a one-way gas entraining venturi valve mounted on the lower surface of the ventilator block. See Figure 1. The

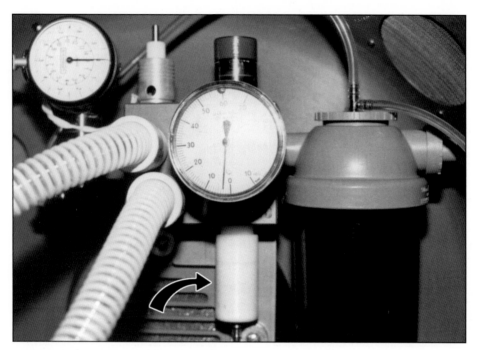

*Figure 1. Sechrist 500A monoplace hyperbaric ventilator one-way entraining venturi valve (arrowhead).*

ventilator control module delivers gas to the venturi valve via the ventilator pass-through in the chamber hatch. This gas flow causes the venturi valve to entrain ambient gas about the valve to provide the desired tidal volume (VT). See Figure 2. Therefore, we placed a gas-tight bag around the entrainment area so that a gas of controlled $O_2$ concentration could be provided from a source external to the chamber. A cut (5-mm long) was made in the lower surface of a 3-liter anesthesia bag (3-liter Breathing Bag, Anesthesia Associates, Inc., San Carlos, CA). The gas tubing that drives the venturi was passed through this cut and fitted to the nipple on the venturi valve. See Figure 3. Next, the open end of the bag was rolled onto the venturi valve and secured.

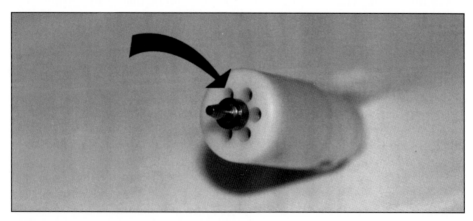

*Figure 2. Entraining orifices (arrowhead) of venturi valve.*

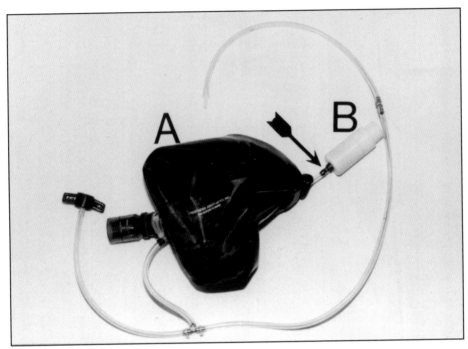

*Figure 3. Three-liter anesthesia bag (A) pulled back off venturi valve (B) to depict tubing placed through the venturi bag and connected to the nipple (arrow) of the venturi valve.*

The opposite end of the anesthesia bag was tucked around this tube and tied with Tygon ties. Similarly, an oxygen tube (Airlife, #001301, American Pharmaseal Co., American Hospital Supply Corp., Valencia, CA) was passed about 10 cm into the bag through another 5-mm cut in the lower surface of the bag and secured with Tygon ties. The other end of the tubing was secured to a female Luer lock tubing connector (Female Tubing Adaptor for 1/8" i.d. tubing, #3081, Becton-Dickinson, Rutherford, NJ). This in turn was attached to an IV pass-through (HBO pass-through, #041-600-500, Cobe, Lakewood, CO) to exit the chamber hatch. See Figure 4. (The one-way IV back check valve needs to be removed.) The anesthesia bag now can be filled with oxygen, air, or a gas of any $FiO_2$ (if one uses an $O_2$ blender, for example.) Our set-up is designed to provide only $O_2$ or air. Oxygen tubing connects the pass-through to an $O_2$ flow meter (Ohio Medical Products, Airco, Inc., Madison, WI) supplied by $O_2$ or air from the hospital wall (at 55 psi). An adaptor allows the $O_2$ flow meter to be supplied with air. All tubing is secured with Tygon ties to prevent disconnections. To prevent the bag from inadvertently becoming overexpanded, with the potential for causing an increased VT and/or positive end expiratory pressure (PEEP), a low-resistance, one-way check valve (#5537, Bird Corp., Palm Springs, CA) was inserted through a larger slit made near the bottom of the bag and secured with Tygon ties. See Figure 4.

The 500A ventilator control module is supplied with either $O_2$ or air from H-cylinders with a driving pressure maintained at generally 75 psi by a 2-stage variable regulator (Harris 2-stage regulator, model 25-100, Harris Calorific Co., Cleveland, OH). Quick connects ($O_2$ diamond adapter, #221-

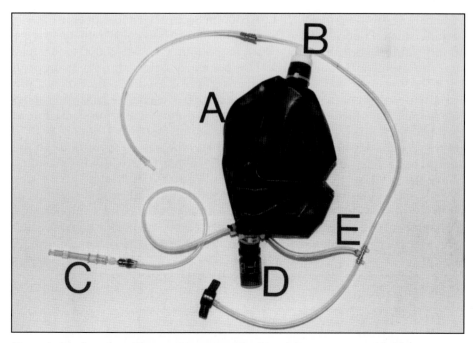

*Figure 4. Anesthesia bag (A) secured to venturi valve (B) with Tygon tie. Bag is filled from a gas source external to the HBO chamber via a Cobe IV pass-through (C). A one-way Bird check valve (D) prevents over-expansion of the bag. Ventilator block gas driving tube (E) goes through the bag and connects to the venturi valve nipple (see Figure 3).*

2683-800, Ohmeda, Madison, WI) with backcheck valves (primary checklist with primary and secondary checks, #221-2694-800, for $O_2$ Ohmeda) enable the gas supply to be switched rapidly from $O_2$ to air.

To validate efficacy of the system, a test lung (Manley Lung Ventilator Performance Analyzer, Medial Developments, Ltd, Chesham, Bucks, England) was connected to the ventilator tubing. The test lung was ventilated over a range of VT and rates over a range of chamber pressures. An oxygen analyzer (Polarographic Oxygen Monitor, model 5570 with model 5580 Sensor, Ventronics, Division of Hudson, Temecula, CA) sampled gas from the proximal airway. The $O_2$ analyzer was calibrated to 100% $O_2$ and air before testing. At atmospheric pressure the $O_2$ sensor was placed in line at the proximal airway. When the chamber was pressurized, gas was provided to the analyzer at a rate of approximately 5 liter/min (atpd) by having a sampling line at the proximal airway, which was passed out of the chamber to the $O_2$ analyzer via a Cobe IV pass-through.

The $FiO_2$ was measured with the $O_2$ analyzer as the ventilator control module gas supply and the venturi bag gas were switched simultaneously from $O_2$ to air and vice versa. The venturi bag gas flow was regulated to keep the bag softly expanded. Generally this required 10 to 15 liter/min (atpd).

## RESULTS

The $FiO_2$ changed rapidly following the switch from $O_2$ to air and vice versa. At atmospheric pressure (0.85 ATA at Salt Lake City, UT), as well as chamber pressures up to 2.9 ATA (maximum Sechrist chamber pressure at our altitude), the $FiO_2$ measured at the proximal airway was equal to that in the gas supply within 15 breaths of the switch in gas source for VT of 500 to 900 ml.

Careful attention to the flow meter gas flow during changes in chamber pressure and after ventilator control module adjustments was important to prevent the venturi bag from being overfilled or collapsing about the venturi. The Bird over-pressure valve prevented gas from being forced through the venturi, which could result in an increase in VT and/or PEEP if the valve were not in place. If the gas flow to the bag were insufficient, the venturi bag collapsed around the venturi valve (See Figure 5), which resulted in a reduced VT.

Since implementing this modification to the Sechrist 500A ventilator we have used it with several patients without evidence of complications. Examples include the treatment of intubated carbon monoxide patients at 2.9 ATA (our chamber limit due to our altitude, instead of the recommended 3.0

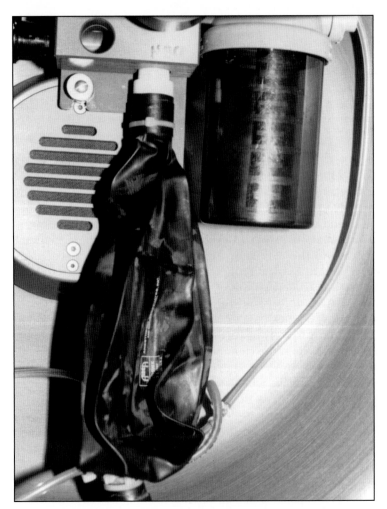

Figure 5. Inadequate venturi bag flow resulting in collapse of the bag with a concomitant reduction in VT.

ATA) and providing the appropriate air breaks according to Kindwall and Goldmann's schedule (10) and routine 10-min air breaks on the 2.4 ATA x 90 min schedules for necrotizing fasciitis and ischemic flaps.

## DISCUSSION

This paper describes a method of modifying Sechrist 500A hyperbaric ventilator so that air breaks can be delivered to intubated, mechanically-ventilated patients treated with HBO in a Sechrist 2500B monoplace hyperbaric chamber.

Concern is often expressed about treating critically ill patients or patients who require air breaks during HBO in the monoplace chamber. However, most HBO facilities operate monoplace chambers, and the majority of patients who receive HBO are treated in monoplace chambers (11). Inasmuch as multiplace chambers probably will not be installed at every HBO center in the United States, it is reasonable to consider how to optimize HBO therapy of patients in the monoplace chamber.

Kindwall et al. (1), Raleigh (2), and Weaver (3) have discussed a technique of providing air breaks in monoplace chambers in cooperative patients. The method described here can be used to provide air breaks to mechanically ventilated patients as well.

Weaver et al. (12) describe the performance characteristics of the Sechrist 500A ventilator, and recommend that the Sechrist 500A ventilator driving (inlet) pressure be adjustable from 65 to 85 psi to optimize ventilator performance to the particular patient. We use gas supplied from H-cylinders and the pressure is adjusted with a variable regulator. Our hospital $O_2$ and air pressure (55 psi) is inadequate to optimally operate the 500A ventilator. The venturi bag could also be filled from the same source as that which drives the ventilator, but the flow to the venturi bag uses considerable volumes of gas, necessitating frequent H-cylinder changes. For that reason we fill the venturi bag from a flow meter that acquires its gas from the hospital wall outlet and only drive the ventilator with gas from H-cylinders. When changing from $O_2$ to air and vice versa, both the ventilator supply and the venturi bag supply must be changed. The flow meter has a one-way valve that prevents retrograde gas flow from the venturi bag, thereby preventing bag collapse during the time it takes to switch gas supply.

The chamber operator should pay close attention to the venturi bag to ensure it is properly filled. This is particularly true during compression, decompression, and with ventilator setting changes. The venturi valve has a flapper valve that offers some resistance to flow. The very low flow resistance of the Bird one-way valve works well to prevent venturi bag over-expansion, although it is recommended that the venturi bag be kept loosely filled by appropriate adjustments to the flow meter. Also, it is useful to adjust the sound volume of the chamber to listen to the ventilator gas flow within the chamber. A change in the sound intensity should prompt the operator to ensure that the bag is properly filled, and that an appropriate VT is being delivered. A further modification to this system could incorporate another bypass valve so that if the venturi bag were to become inadvertently collapsed and the VT reduced, another valve would open, bypassing the venturi bag so that the VT would remain constant.

If intubated patients are spontaneously breathing, or if they are over-breathing the 500A ventilator, they may entrain chamber gas from the one-way valve located on the ventilator block. During air breaks we typically adjust the ventilator so this does not occur. If the patient is sedated and/or paralyzed, this is less likely to occur. The venturi bag could also be configured in a way to provide gas to this valve, but we saw little need to do that given the above discussion.

When treating a patient who has arterial hypoxemia requiring an elevated $FiO_2$ and/or PEEP to maintain an adequate arterial partial pressure of oxygen ($PaO_2$), caution is advised when ventilating these patients with an unmodified Sechrist 500A ventilator before chamber pressurization (for example, during patient set-up just before compression it is reasonable to ventilate the patient with the 500A ventilator while the chamber door is open to room air). However, the unmodified venturi valve entrains ambient gas, which is room air in this situation, therefore diluting the $FiO_2$ to less than 1.00. We have observed one case of arterial hypoxemia due to this mechanism, before utilizing the venturi bag. Presently, we connect the patient to the Sechrist 500A ventilator equipped with the venturi bag, which is filled with oxygen and, if clinically indicated, check adequacy of ventilation and oxygenation with an arterial blood gas before compression (or follow arterial hemoglobin oxygen saturation continuously before compression with a pulse oximeter).

Similarly, in profoundly hypoxemic patients it is possible that hypoxemia could result when the patient's $FiO_2$ is switched to air during hyperbaric therapy, because the alveolar partial pressure of oxygen ($PaO_2$) is reduced by a factor of 5 during the air break. However, this would be relatively uncommon, because at 2.4 ATA the patient breathing air would have the same alveolar concentration of $O_2$ as if he were breathing an $FiO_2$ of approximately 0.5 at sea level. If the patient requires greater than 50 to 60% $O_2$ at sea level to provide an adequate $PaO_2$ arterial hypoxemia may ensue with air breaks during hyperbaric treatment, particularly at chamber pressures that are relatively modest (<2.4 ATA).

We machined another pass-through plug to replace the Sechrist ventilator pass-through plug. This new pass-through plug has another tube (for the venturi bag gas supply) as well as the ventilator 0.25 inch. National Pipe Thread $O_2$ fitting orifice, thus freeing up one of the remaining 4 pass-through ports on the Sechrist chamber hatch in case an additional IV port is needed. Without this change in patients who may have multiple IV infusions, one would have to prioritize the ability to deliver air breaks to the mechanically ventilated patient.

## CONCLUSION

A modification to the Sechrist 500A hyperbaric ventilator allowing mechanically ventilated patients to receive air breaks during HBO treatment in the monoplace chamber is presented. Several patients have received HBO with mechanical ventilation utilizing this modification to the Sechrist 500A ventilator without any untoward effects.

## ACKNOWLEDGMENTS

I thank Dr. C. Gregory Elliott for his critical review of this manuscript, and much appreciation is given to Pat Petersen for preparation of the manuscript.

## APPENDIX II REFERENCES

1. Kindwall EP, Goldmann RW, Thombs PA. Use of the monoplace vs. multiplace chamber in the treatment of diving diseases. J Hyper Med 1988; 3(1):11-14.

2. Raleigh GW. Air breaks in the Sechrist model 2500-B monoplace hyperbaric chamber. J Hyper Med 1988; 3(1):11-14.

3. Weaver LK. Monoplace chamber use of USN Table 6 to treat DCS and AGE. Undersea Biomed Res 1988; 15(suppl):63.

4. Myers RA, Chairman. Hyperbaric oxygen therapy - a committee report. Bethesda, MD: Undersea and Hyperbaric Medical Society, 1986.

5. Kindwall EP, Goldmann RW. Hyperbaric medicine procedures. Milwaukee, WI: St. Luke's Hospital, 1984:55.

6. Darke SG, King AM, Slack WK. Gas gangrene and related infection: classification, clinical features and etiology, management and mortality. A report of 88 cases. Br J Surg 1977;64:104-112.

7. Hendricks PL, Hall DA, Hunter WL Jr, Haley PJ. Extension of pulmonary oxygen tolerance in man at 2 ATA by intermittent oxygen exposure. J Appl Physiol 1977;42:593-599.

8. Flynn ET, Catron PW, Bayne CG. Diving medical officers student guide. Naval Technical Training Command. Washington, DC: Government Printing Office, 1981:10-20,21.

9. Model 2500B monoplace hyperbaric system operational instructions. Anaheim, CA: Sechrist Industries, 1987.

10. Kindwall EP, Goldmann RW. Hyperbaric medicine procedures. Milwaukee, WI: St. Luke's Hospital, 1984:95.

11. Myers RA. Functional hyperbaric chamber facilities. Summary of questionnaires compiled by Maryland Institute of Emergency Medical Services (MIEMSS), January 1988.

12. Weaver LK, Greenway L, Elliott CG. Performance of the Sechrist 500A hyperbaric ventilator in a monoplace hyperbaric chamber. J Hyper Med 1988; 3(4):215-225.

## APPENDIX III. NONINVASIVE DOPPLER BLOOD PRESSURE MONITORING IN THE MONOPLACE HYPERBARIC CHAMBER

*Lindell K. Weaver, Stephen Howe*

## ABSTRACT

We describe a noninvasive method of monitoring blood pressure in the monoplace hyperbaric chamber. A standard blood pressure cuff was placed on the patient's arm. A Doppler probe, linked to an ultrasonic Doppler flow detector outside the chamber, was secured over the patient's radial artery. Cuff inflation tubing and the Doppler probe wires were passed into the chamber by modifying a standard disposable hyperbaric intravenous pass-through. Blood pressure readings were determined by inflating and slowly deflating the cuff from outside the chamber while observing the sphygmomanometer within the chamber, and listening for the first audible flow signal from the Doppler detector, corresponding to the systolic blood pressure. To minimize the risk of fire in the oxygen-filled monoplace hyperbaric chamber, the patient, Doppler detector, and chamber were grounded. Doppler readings obtained from nine normal subjects whose arterial pressures were being measured with indwelling radial arterial catheters (approved as part of another study by the hospital's Investigational Review Board) compare closely with the subject's blood pressures measured with this noninvasive method: 114 + 7.6 mmHg (mean + 1 S.D.) compared to 112 + 8.1 mmHg, respectively (n = 92 measurements in 8 subjects). We conclude that this noninvasive method of monitoring blood pressure within the monoplace hyperbaric chamber is accurate and suitable for monoplace clinical purposes.

## INTRODUCTION

Most hyperbaric oxygen treatments (HBOT) delivered to patients requiring HBOT (1) in the United States are performed in the monoplace hyperbaric chamber (2). Patients who are acutely ill or hemodynamically unstable warrant electrocardiographic and blood pressure (BP) monitoring during HBOT. Electrocardiographic monitoring is straightforward (3) and commonly practiced at monoplace chamber facilities. Invasive BP monitoring in the monoplace chamber has been described (4, 5), but it is cumbersome and exposes the patient to the risks of an indwelling arterial catheter. To our knowledge, there is no product commercially available in the United States for measuring BP noninvasively in the monoplace chamber.

With helicopter medical transport, the problem of measuring noninvasive BP (caused by loud background noise) has been solved by taping an ultrasonic Doppler probe over the radial or brachial artery, and inflating an upper arm BP cuff while observing the sphygmomanometer. The first signal heard from the transducer, corresponding to the systolic BP, is audible above the background noise of the helicopter. The Doppler method of BP measurement has been demonstrated to be accurate in nonhyperbaric applications (6-8). We chose a similar method to measure systolic BP in the monoplace chamber.

## METHODS AND MATERIALS

Systolic BP was measured noninvasively while central arterial BP was being measured invasively in nine patients receiving hyperbaric air and HBOT.

A standard adult or pediatric BP cuff (Tycos, Arden, NC) was fitted to the upper arm of the patient. An ultrasound Doppler probe (Parks Medical Electronics, Inc., Aloha, OR) was taped over the radial or brachial artery, and a water-soluble gel (K-Y Jelly, Johnson & Johnson Products, Inc., New Brunswick, NJ) was placed between the probe and the skin to decrease impedance and improve the signal to noise ratio. The sphygmomanometer (Tycos) pressure relief knob is opened one-eighth to one quarter turn from the closed position to inflate the BP cuff from outside the chamber, yet allow the cuff to deflate through the partially opened valve when the gas flow from outside the chamber was reduced. The knob was taped in this slightly opened position. See Figure 1.

The hatch of the monoplace hyperbaric chamber (Sechrist, Inc., Anaheim, CA) is equipped with several pass-through penetrators that are used to pass intravenous (IV) tubing in and out of the chamber. A disposable IV pass-through (#041-600-500, Cobe, Inc., Lakewood, CO) was modified to pass the Doppler probe electric wires and the BP cuff inflation tubing from inside to outside the chamber. See Figure 2. The Doppler probe wires and the BP cuff inflation tubing were passed through a single Sechrist chamber hatch

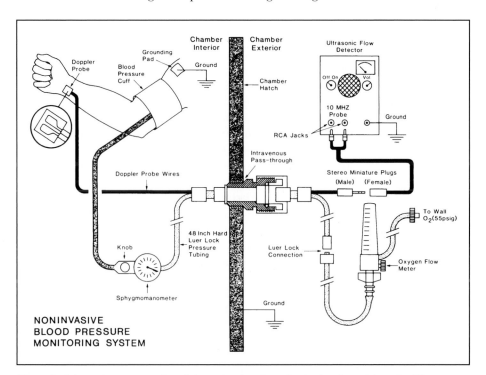

Figure 1. Schematic representation of the monoplace hyperbaric chamber noninvasive BP system. The cuff is inflated from outside the chamber by adjusting oxygen flow to the cuff with the flow meter. The arterial flow sounds corresponding to the systolic BP are detected with the ultrasonic Doppler flow detector. Note that the patient and the detector must be grounded (see text).

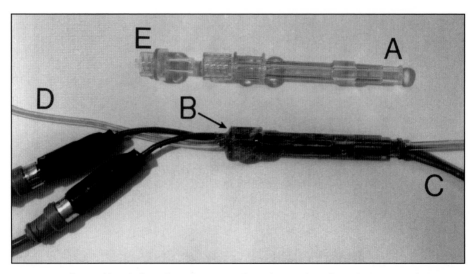

*Figure 2. A disposable adrylic IV hyperbaric pass-through (A) is bored to a larger inner diameter (B) to permit shielded Doppler wires (C) and hard IV pressure tubing (D) to be slipped through the enlarged lumen. The lumen is then sealed with Epoxy glue. The one-way backcheck valve (E) is removed.*

penetrator. The inner lumen of the IV pass-through was bored out to one-quarter inch diameter, allowing standard Cobe IV tubing and the Doppler probe wires to fit through a single Cobe pass-through. Splicing the wires into the standard 19-pin, electric pass-through connector degenerated the quality of the Doppler signal so that the flow signal was inaudible. Cutting the female Luer lock from the IV tubing allowed the tubing to fit through the bored-out IV pass-through. The modified pass-through was installed with the cut end of the tubing outside the chamber. The female end of the Luer lock (tubing side) was drilled to one-eighth-inch diameter, and to a depth of one-quarter inch. The cut IV tubing was secured into the drilled lumen of the female Luer lock with acrylic cement (Free Flow Acrylic Cement, Tap Plastics, Inc., Dublin, CA). After the Doppler probe wires were cut and passed through the pass-through (oriented so that the cut end would be on the outside of the chamber with the modified pass-through installed in the Sechrist IV penetrator), a male stereo miniature plug (#274-286, Radio Shack Tandy, Inc., Houston, TX) was connected to the cut end of the probe wires. See Figures 1, 3. The wire's shielding was maintained to prevent interference to the high frequency Doppler signal. A female stereo miniature plug (#274-274 Radio Shack) was connected to an appropriate length of shielded Doppler probe wire that, in turn, was plugged into the Ultrasonic Flow Dectector (Model 811, Parks Medical Electronics, Inc.) with RCA jacks. Epoxy glue (EE-4198 Resin/HD -3561 Hardener, Hysol Company, City of Industry, CA) was injected into the pass-through to seal the wires and tubing within the drilled lumen. The female Luer lock and the male stereo miniature plug can be inserted through the Sechrist hatch IV penetrator. The male stereo miniature plug and the female Luer lock could not pass through the assembled IV penetrator. We inserted them through the Sechrist hatch IV by following these steps:

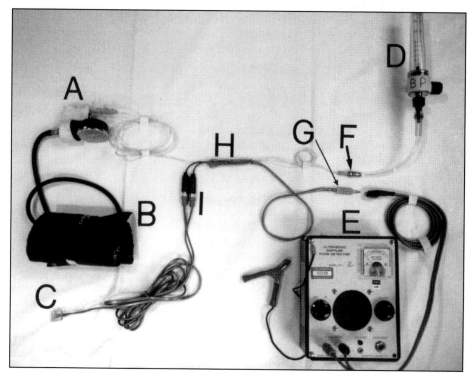

Figure 3. Components of the monoplace hyperbaric BP system. The sphygmomanometer (A) is taped one-eighth of a turn open to provide a leak. The cuff (B) is fitted to the patient's arm and the Doppler probe (C) is taped over the radial artery. The cuff is inflated by controlling the $O_2$ flow meter (D). The ultrasonic flow detector (E) enables the operator to determine BP. The female Luer lock (F) and the miniature stereo plug (G) permit easy insertion and removal of the modified pass-through (H) from the chamber hatch penetrators. RCA plugs (I) allow the probe to be removed for non-hyperbaric use.

1. Removed the IV penetrator cap, O-ring collar and O-ring.
2. Passed the cuff inflation tubing, the male stereo miniature plug, and the attached Doppler probe wires through the IV penetrator from chamber inside to outside direction.
3. Placed the tubing, plug, and wires through the O-ring, O-ring collar and penetrator cap.
4. Repositioned the O-ring, O-ring collar, and penetrator cap on the IV penetrator and secured onto the modified Cobe IV pass-through in the standard fashion.

We reversed the sequence of the above steps to remove the Luer lock and the plug from the hatch. The tubing that is passed out of the chamber is connected to an air flow meter (Ohmeda, Madison, WI) supplied with air from the standard wall source.

As a safety precaution, the patient is grounded to the chamber by placing an electrocardiogram pad on the patient and connecting it to metal within the chamber. The ultrasonic flow detector and the chamber are both grounded to a suitable source in the hospital. While in use, the ultrasonic flow detector must never be charging with the AC adaptor.

By controlling air flow with the flow meter, the cuff was inflated from outside the chamber. Since the sphygmomanometer had been adjusted to leak slightly when gas flow from the flow meter was reduced, the BP cuff pressure fell. Systolic BP was read when the first flow signal from the ultrasonic flow detector was heard.

Central arterial BP was measured simultaneously in all subjects* with an arterial catheter (C.A.P. Intrafuser, 20 gauge; Sorenson Research, Abbott, Chicago, IL). After confirmation of ulnar and radial artery patency by Allen's test, the catheter was inserted percutaneously, maintaining aseptic technique, into the radial artery and advanced to the subclavian artery position. The arterial pressure waveform was observed through a physiologic monitor (Model 7010, Marquette Electronics, Inc., Milwaukee, WI). The BP cuff was fitted to the contralateral upper arm.

Each subject received two hyperbaric exposures: the first with the chamber compressed with air while the subject breathed air, and the second with the chamber filled with 100% oxygen and the subject breathing oxygen. Systolic BP was measured and recorded at atmospheric pressure (0.85), 2.9, 2.5, 2.0 and 1.1 atmospheres absolute (ATA) for each subject. Systolic BP was then measured and recorded again for each subject at atmospheric pressure on each of the two hyperbaric exposures.

A paired t-test was used to compare the systolic BP measured by Doppler to the systolic BP obtained by arterial catheter.

## RESULTS

Noninvasively determined systolic BP correlated well with systolic BP measured by an indwelling arterial catheter (BP, noninvasive = 112 " 8.1 [mean " 1 S.D.]; BP, arterial catheter = 114 " 7.6 mmHg ($p < 0.001$, paired t-test, n = 92 measurements in 8 subjects over a range of chamber pressures 0.85 to 2.9 ATA)]. See Figure 4. Chamber pressurization did not change the correlation of cuff to arterial catheter BP. The Doppler pulse tone depended on positioning of the ultrasonic probe directly over the area that produced the loudest intensity sound. Taping the probe in place and wrapping the wrist in Kerlex gauze kept the probe from shifting position. The cuff and Doppler probe were well tolerated. Most of the subjects complained of pain at the radial artery insertion site, and one individual demonstrated an index digit petechial hemorrhage on the same side as the arterial catheter the evening of his participation in the study. The hemorrhage, likely representing an arterial embolism, resolved spontaneously.

Data for one individual were excluded from the analysis because the patient demonstrated a bilateral, 16 mmHg pressure difference between the cuff and the arterial measurements bilaterally (cuff BP > arterial BP). Auscultory BP measurements with a cuff at atmospheric pressure confirmed the Doppler observations. This finding was incidental.

## DISCUSSION

We have presented a workable, inexpensive method of measuring systolic BP noninvasively during HBOT in a monoplace hyperbaric chamber. The system uses a standard BP cuff, sphygmomanometer, and a Doppler ultrasonic flow detector. The arterial catheter we used measured central

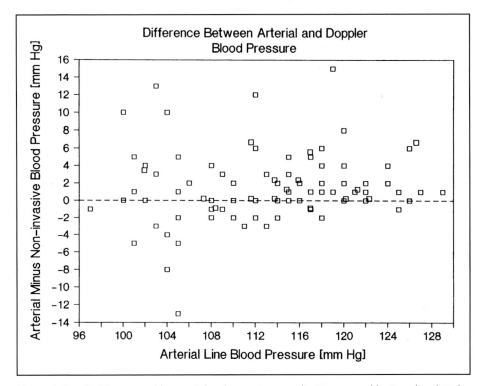

Figure 4. Stytolic BP measured by arterial catheter minus systolic BP measured by Doppler plotted against arterial catheter BP. Ninty-two percent of the BP measurements by Doppler were within 6 mmHg of simultaneously measured arterial catheter pressures.

arterial pressure (subclavian artery position), whereas the cuff measured BP at a more distal contralateral site. These two methodologies are quite different, so any agreement between the measurements may be only coincidental. The results of a paired t-test suggest that the two methods are statistically different, although the magnitude of the difference is small. Ninety-two percent of the Doppler-measured values were within 6 mmHg of the simultaneously measured arterial catheter values. See Figure 4. We believe, therefore, that the Doppler method is clinically acceptable. In most instances in which the clinician is concerned about hypotension, the determination of systolic pressure is adequate. However, we suggest that arterial pressure be measured continuously in hemodynamically unstable patients, or in patients who require potent vasoactive drugs.

We do not use the noninvasive BP system for all patients. Critically ill patients who are treated with HBOT generally have arterial catheters in place. Most routine outpatients do not warrant BP measurements during HBOT. However, we do use it for patients who exhibit hypertension before HBOT, for those that may be receiving sedatives during HBOT, and for children who may be acutely ill, but who do not have an arterial catheter. We also use the system when we do not want to delay HBOT in order to insert an arterial catheter.

It is imperative that the patient, flow detector, and chamber be grounded. The manufacturer believes that, with appropriate grounding, the probe and ultrasonic flow detector should be safe when used in this system, provided the Doppler probe is not cracked and the flow detector is not AC-charged while in use (personal communication, Mr. Parks, Parks Medical Electronics, Inc., February, 1989). The specified epoxy cement used in the pass-through is the same type used by Sechrist, Inc. in the construction of the 19-pin electrical pass-through, and is considered to be acceptable in the monoplace hyperbaric environment (personal communication, Judy Johnson, Sechrist Inc., September, 1990).

As yet, we have not used this system in the monoplace chamber in patients in hemodynamic shock with profound hypotension. The literature supports the accuracy of Doppler measurements of BP during profound hypotension (9), but it has not been demonstrated that this data can be extrapolated to measurements made in the monoplace chamber.

We hope that medical manufacturers will see the need to apply standard noninvasive clinical monitors, such as a noninvasive BP device, to the monoplace HBOT setting; however, until that time, this system, or devices similar to it (Dräger, Drägerwerk AG Lübeck Werk Drückkammertechnik, Auf dem Baggersand 17, Postfach 150 149, D-2400 Lübeck-Travemünde, Germany, uses an electronic stethoscope instead of a Doppler flow detector) will suffice to increase patient safety during monoplace HBOT.

## ACKNOWLEDGMENTS

This study was supported by a grant from the Deseret Foundation of the LDS Hospital, Salt Lake City, Utah. We wish to thank the subjects who volunteered for this investigation, and we appreciate the help of Pam Evans, RRT and the rest of the hyperbaric staff who assisted in the data collection.

**APPENDIX III REFERENCES**

1. Mader JT, Chairman. Hyperbaric oxygen therapy: a committee report. Bethesda, MD: Undersea and Hyperbaric Medical Society, 1989.

2. Myers RA. Functional hyperbaric chamber facilities. Summary of questionnaires compiled by MD, Institute of Emergency Medical Services (MIEMSS). Baltimore, Maryland, January, 1988.

3. Holcomb JR, Matos-Navarro AY, Goldman RW. Critical Care in the hyperbaric chamber. In: Davis JC, Hunt TK, eds. Problem wounds. New York: Elsevier, 1988:206-207.

4. Rockswold GL, Ford E, Anderson JR, Blanchfield E. Patient monitoring in the monoplace hyperbaric chamber. Hyperbaric Oxygen Rev 1985;6(3):161-168.

5. Kindwall EP, Goldman RW. Hyperbaric medicine procedures. 6th Ed. Milwaukee: St. Luke's Medical Center, 1988:115.

6. Ware RW. New approaches to the indirect measurement of human blood pressure. Third Nat Biomed Sci Instr Symp (ISA) 1965, BM-65.

7. Kirby RW, Kemmerer WT, Morgan JL. Transcutaneous Doppler measurement of blood pressure. Anesthesiology 1969;31:86-89.

8. Janis KM, Kemmerer Wt, Hagood CO Jr. Doppler blood pressure measurement in infants and small children. J Pediatr Surg 1971;6(1):70-72.

9. Waltemath CL, Preuss DD. Determination of blood pressure in low-flow states by the Doppler technique. Anesthesiology 1971;34(1):77-79.

## APPENDIX IV. NORMOBARIC MEASUREMENT OF O$_2$ TENSION OF BLOOD AND SALINE TONOMETERED UNDER HYPERBARIC O$_2$ CONDITIONS

*Lindell K.Weaver, Steven L. Berlin, Stephen Howe*

## ABSTRACT

Measuring arterial oxygen tension( PaO$_2$) in patients receiving hyperbaric oxygen therapy (HBOT) may be important to assess adequacy of the HBOT protocol and to limit O$_2$ toxicity. Therefore, we designed a study to assess the ability of the ABL330 to measure the O$_2$ tension of saline and blood tonometered at $37+0.1°C$ under hyperbaric conditions and analyzed immediately at atmospheric pressure. The measured PO$_2$ was compared to the predicted PO$_2$ over a range of chamber pressures (0.85-3.0 ATA). For saline the relationship of measured-to-predicted O$_2$ under hyperbaric conditions is linear: PO$_2$ (meas) = 0.961 x PO$_2$ pred + 78.6, r2 = 0.994; and for blood: PO$_2$ (meas) = 0.919 x PO$_2$ pred + 37.3, r2 = 0.9096. We conclude that the ABL330 operated at atmospheric pressure can accurately measure O$_2$ tension of blood and saline tonometered with O$_2$ at 0.85 to 3.0 ATA when analyzed immediately by an ABL330 operated at atmospheric pressure.

## INTRODUCTION

Measuring arterial oxygen tension (PaO$_2$) and arterial carbon dioxide tension (PaCO$_2$) in patients treated with hyperbaric oxygen therapy (HBOT) may be important to assess the adequacy of the HBOT protocol, to ensure adequacy of ventilation, and to minimize oxygen toxicity. Before this work, blood gas determinations of patients receiving HBOT were either measured in a multiplace chamber (1) or were extrapolated from arterial blood gas (ABG) measurements made at sea level pressure (2). The measurement of ABGs inside multiplace chambers is cumbersome, time consuming, and is performed at only a few institutions. Although the technique of determining the PaO$_2$ at any given hyperbaric pressure by extrapolating the PaO$_2$ measured at normobaric pressure is useful (2), the extrapolation becomes inaccurate for patients with significant lung disease (2) and obviously provides no information about ventilation (PaCO$_2$).

While inspecting the adequacy of ventilation by measuring the PaCO$_2$ in a sample of a patient's arterial blood aspirated out of the chamber through a pass-through (Cobe, Inc., Lakewood, CO) during HBOT from an intubated, mechanically ventilated patient treated in a monoplace hyperbaric chamber (Sechrist, Inc., Anaheim, CA), we incidentally observed a PaO$_2$ approximating the predicted PaO$_2$ (1,400 mmHg). Only one of our three different blood gas analyzers (ABL330, Radiometer, Copenhagen, Denmark) was capable of measuring hyperbaric O$_2$ tensions (> 900 mmHg). Therefore, we designed an *in vitro* study to determine the accuracy of the ABL330 to measure the O$_2$-tension of saline and blood tonometered with 100% O$_2$ under hyperbaric conditions but analyzed at our atmospheric pressure (0.85 ATA - Salt Lake City, Utah is 4,500 ft. above sea level).

## METHODS AND MATERIALS

A blood gas tonometer (Model 237, Instrumentation Laboratories, Lexington, MA) was placed inside a monoplace hyperbaric chamber (model 2500B, Sechrist, Inc., Anaheim, CA). The 110-V power cord was passed through the Sechrist intravenous (IV) penetrator by taking the electrical receptacle off the cord, inserting it through the penetrator, then replacing the receptacle. The penetrator O-ring furnished an appropriate seal. We used a thermodilution pulmonary artery catheter (Sorensen Research, Abbott Laboratories, Salt Lake City, UT) to validate the temperature of the sample being tonometered, and to aspirate the sample from the tonometer bowl out of the chamber. The catheter passed out of the chamber via a specially machined penetrator. Other catheters were initially considered, but we chose this particular one because its deep space volume is low (0.5 ml) and the thermistor was useful to ensure physiologic temperature of the tonometered sample (measured with a 7010 Marquette Bedside Monitor, Marquette Electronics, Milwaukee, WI). The tonometer bath temperature was maintained at 37°C, as verified by an analytical thermometer. Gas supplied to the tonometer was regulated by an $O_2$ flow meter (Ohmeda, Madison, WI) located outside the chamber.

To minimize the risk of fire, the chamber was pressurized with medical grade compressed air. In addition, a plastic bag fitted around the tonometer allowed continuous exposure of the tonometer to a reduced partial pressure of $O_2$ by purging the bag with nitrogen from a source external to the chamber ($O_2$ concentration verified as low or absent). The $O_2$ exiting the tonometer bowl was vented via tubing to the effluent end of the chamber.

A hydraulic switch was developed that allowed us to turn the tonometer agitator on and off from outside the chamber. Samples were aspirated when the agitator was off.

Saline or blood was tonometered with 100% $O_2$ (400 ml x min-1 inside the chamber) over a range of chamber pressures (0.85 to 3.0 ATA). The chamber pressure gauge was verified accurate with a mercury column. For heparinized (20 U/ml) fresh whole blood, carbon dioxide ($CO_2$) was mixed with $O_2$ to provide a physiologic blood pH and $PCO_2$ (7.2 - 7.6, and 15 - 60 mmHg, respectively). The volume of saline or blood introduced into the tonometer bowl was 0.4 ml, which was removed and replenished for each new chamber pressure. One drop of antifoam (Corning Glass Works, Medfield, MA) was added to each aliquot of blood. The sample was aspirated out of the tonometer for assay when it had reached thermal equilibrium, generally about 20 minutes, with the assumption that $PO_2$-equilibrium was expected to occur in approximately the same time as thermal equilibrium.

An ABL330 blood gas analyzer was positioned adjacent to the chamber. Samples were aspirated from the tonometer and immediately analyzed. To minimize preanalytic errors it was important to aspirate the sample in a midstream fashion using the following technique. See Figure 1.

The syringes and catheters were flushed with $O_2$ before obtaining the sample. Saline or blood (0.75ml) was drawn first into the proximal 3-ml syringe. Next, the stopcock handles were positioned allowing saline or blood to flow into the distal 3-ml syringe (0.25 ml). Finally, 0.25 ml of saline or blood was directed into the mid-stream 3-ml blood gas glass syringe (Glaspak 2 1/2

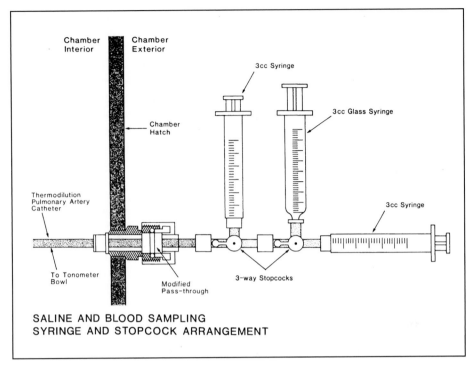

SALINE AND BLOOD SAMPLING
SYRINGE AND STOPCOCK ARRANGEMENT

Figure 1. Schematic representation of pass-through, syringe, and stopcock arrangement used to obtain the saline or blood sample from the tonometer. The sample is directed into the glass syringe in a midstream fashion after clearing the catheter and stopcock dead space with tonometered saline or blood to minimize dilution of the hyperoxic sample (see text).

ml, Beckton-Dickinson, Rutherford, NJ), then pushed into the distal 3-ml syringe. This was repeated two additional times (to rinse the syringe that would be receiving the final sample with oxygenated saline or blood, thereby minimizing the likelihood of dilutional errors). After this, the blood gas sample was obtained by directing 0.75 ml of saline or blood into the mid-3-ml glass syringe, then closing the glass syringe stopcock and the proximal 3-ml syringe stopcock. The 3-ml glass syringe was removed and the sample analyzed. The dead space aliquots were injected back into the tonometer bowl and fresh blood or saline was added to replace the amount withdrawn.

During a measurement, the ABL330 monitors the output of the $PO_2$ electrode 11 times, at 8-sec intervals. It applies response and stability criteria to the individual measurements at several intervals to determine acceptability of the final value (3). Rather than rely only on the ABL330's programmed criteria, we found it was more effective to observe the values at each interval ourselves. The highest degree of accuracy was achieved when the analyzer initially displayed a modest value for $O_2$ tension (e.g., approximately 60% of the predicted $O_2$-tension), with subsequent values each higher than the one before, up to the 8th or 9th value, generally reaching a plateau. On the other hand, highly inaccurate values for $O_2$ tension were obtained if there was considerable scatter in the intermediate $O_2$-tension measurements or if the $O_2$ tension was high initially with subsequent intermediate-measurements decreasing. The only data retained for statistical purposes were obtained from the former situation. After several practice sample collections, the likelihood of appropriate measurements by this criteria was high. All samples were collected by one investigator (LKW).

To provide information about the rate of change of the $O_2$ tension as a function of time, the same sample was analyzed at 3-minute intervals, up to 6 minutes. The syringe stopcock was closed and the syringe plunger held under firm pressure between assays to minimize sample bubble formation.

The ABL330 was 2-point calibrated at the beginning and the end of each day's experiments. Single-point calibrations occurred every 2 hours. All calibrations were within accepted norms.

## RESULTS

The measured $O_2$ tension was compared to the predicted $O_2$ tension [(Predicted $PO_2$ mmHg = (Pchamber ATA) x (760 mmHg) - (47 mmHg, $H_2O$-vapor pressure) - ($PCO_2$ mmHg, if $CO_2$ were added—blood only)]. See Table 1. There is a highly significant correlation of the measured with the predicted $O_2$ tension at all evaluated chamber pressures. The linear regression for saline is: $PO_2$meas = 0.961 x $PO_2$ pred + 78.6, r2 = 0.994 and for blood: $PO_2$meas = 0.919 x $PO_2$pred + 37.3, r2 = 0.9096. See Figure 2. The measured $PO_2$ of blood was approximately 7% lower than the predicted $PO_2$ between 0.85 and 2.8 ATA.

A plot of the difference (measured minus predicted $PO_2$) against the predicted $PO_2$ described by Bland and Altman (4) demonstrates the relationship between the measurement error and the true value. See Figure 3. The measured $PO_2$ of saline was within 70 mmHg of the predicted $PO_2$. This is within the range of measurement error of samples analyzed at atmospheric pressure (100% $O_2$), implying that the ABL330 measures saline tonometered with 100% $O_2$ as accurately at 2.9 ATA as at 0.85 ATA. The measured $PO_2$ of blood was lower than the predicted, with the difference increasing up to a maximum of -200 mmHg for predicted $PO_2$s above 1,400 mmHg.

Preliminary observations suggest that the rate of change of the blood $PO_2$ over time was approximately 3% per min-1 while stored in a sealed glass syringe (up to 6 min at 2.0 and 3.0 ATA). However, this was not always predictable. Often the 3-min measurement was essentially the same as the 0-min value, whereas the subsequent measurements of the same sample were lower.

## DISCUSSION

We have described the accuracy of one commercially available blood gas analyzer (Radiometer ABL330) in measuring $O_2$ tension of saline and blood tonometered inside a hyperbaric chamber, but measured at atmospheric pressure. If the saline sample was obtained carefully and assayed immediately, the ABL330 was able to measure the hyperbaric $PO_2$ accurately. For blood, the measured $PO_2$s were consistently lower than predicted. See Figures 2, 3. The data obtained by Moon, et al. (2) also demonstrated that the measured $PO_2$s were lower than the predicted when the $PO_2$ was > 1,300 mmHg, although only a few data points are demonstrated. Moon's measurements were made with blood gas instruments calibrated and operated within the hyperbaric environment. Our technique for measuring hyperbaric blood $O_2$-tension

## TABLE 1. COMPARISON OF MEASURED TO PREDICTED OXYGEN TENSION (PO$_2$) OF SALINE AND BLOOD

| P$_{Chamber}$ ATA | SALINE, mmHg | | BLOOD, mmHg | |
| --- | --- | --- | --- | --- |
| | PO$_2$-pred | PO$_2$-meas | PO$_2$-pred | PO$_2$-meas |
| 0.85 | 592 | 644 mean (4, 27.4)a | 583 | 547 mean (5, 30.5)a |
| 1.00 | 713 | 753 (4, 8.1) | 709 | 657 (2, 12.0) |
| 1.50 | 1099 | 1150 (5, 24.4) | 1047 | 1012 (10, 24.1) |
| 2.00 | 1473 | 1509 (10, 13.9) | 1438 | 1376 (17, 31.2) |
| 2.10 | 1549 | 1590 (5, 19.0) | | |
| 2.20 | 1625 | 1648 (4, 6.9) | 1584 | 1519 (13, 32.4) |
| 2.30 | 1704 | 1666 (4, 14.8) | | |
| 2.40 | 1777 | 1747 (5, 21.3) | 1747 | 1622 (15, 39.8) |
| 2.50 | 1848 | 1842 (6, 34.4) | | |
| 2.60 | 1929 | 1932 (5, 14.5) | 1899 | 1735 (6, 37.2) |
| 2.70 | 2005 | 2029 (6, 31.5) | | |
| 2.80 | 2081 | 2075 (5, 20.1) | 2048 | 1885 (9, 20.0) |
| 2.90 | 2157 | 2160 (5, 62.1) | 2141 | 2013 (4, 19.1) |
| 3.00 | | | 2188 | 2114 (5, 23.6) |

a (N, SD)

Comparison of measured (meas) to predicted (pred) oxygen tension (PO$_2$) of saline and blood tonometered under HBO conditions, but analyzed at atmospheric pressure by a Radiometer ABL330 blood gas laboratory.

seems to be as accurate as those of investigators making measurements of $PO_2$ under hyperbaric conditions. Of course, the work of Moon, et al. is *in vivo* whereas ours is *in vitro*, so a strict comparison between the two may not be completely reasonable.

There are several reasons why the curves for saline and for blood are different: 1) all blood gas analyzer electrode outputs differ from ideal, linear responses; 2) carryover of gas or fluids from previous rinse cycles; 3) diffusion of gases through the materials of the sample pathway (due to differences in oxygen content and viscosity of sample volumes of gas, saline and blood); 4) the inherent electrode response to a given $PO_2$ in saline is slightly different from the response to the same $PO_2$ in blood; 5) $O_2$-consumption by blood [however, the ABL330 compensates for the expected blood metabolism under normobaric conditions during the measuring period (3)]. To remedy such problems a mathematical correction is determined by comparing the responses of many uncorrected analyzers to a reference method (i.e., tonometry). Radiometer incorporates correction factors into the ABL330 analyzer software to be applied to all $PO_2$ measurements (3). These corrections are determined on blood under normobaric conditions. Radiometer verifies accuracy of the analyzer only within the range $PO_2 = 0 - 800$ mmHg. It is remarkable that the ABL330 measures and reports reasonable values from samples tonometered under

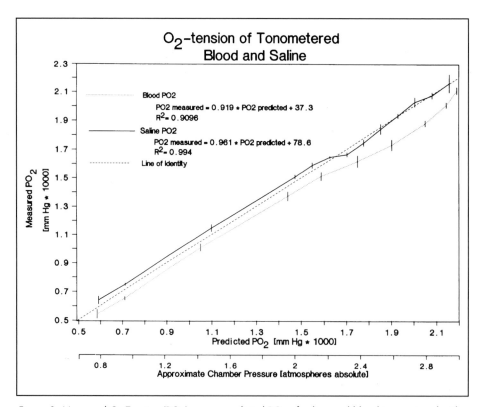

Figure 2. *Measured $O_2$-Tension ($PO_2$) versus predicted $PO_2$ of saline and blood tonometered with 100% $O_2$ over a range of chamber pressures (Chamber pressure is approximate due to the contribution of water vapor and physiologic carbon dioxide pressures being reflected in the predicted $PO_2$). The vertical bars represent +1 S.D.*

hyperbaric conditions. Blood $PO_2$s are as much as 200 mmHg lower than predicted (see Figure 3), but if this difference is expressed as a percentage it represents only approximately 5 to 7% for predicted $PO_2$s > 1,700 mmHg. This is the same percent error we observed at atmospheric pressure, so it might be reasonable to assume that the measured $PO_2$ of blood should be upward corrected by approximately 6% to represent the true value. Although it might be possible to express equations that would bring the measured $PO_2$ value back to baseline, much as Radiometer has done for the ABL330 over the normobaric range (3), this would require extensive testing to be confident of every ABL330's performance in the hyperbaric range.

These observations may be clinically relevant because ABGs from patients treated in monoplace hyperbaric chambers could be analyzed by blood gas laboratories at atmospheric pressure. The HBOT protocol could be chosen to provide the optimal arterial $O_2$ tension, especially for patients with lung disease or a significant right-to-left shunt, as the prediction of their particular $PaO_2$-based atmospheric blood gases is not highly accurate (2).

Withdrawing arterial blood from a patient compressed in the monoplace hyperbaric chamber is not difficult technically, but does expose the patient to some risks. Since the catheter that is used to obtain the sample does not have a backcheck valve, rapid blood loss could occur if there were an inadvertent disconnection of the catheter. This risk can be minimized by using Luer lock connections and being careful when withdrawing blood from a

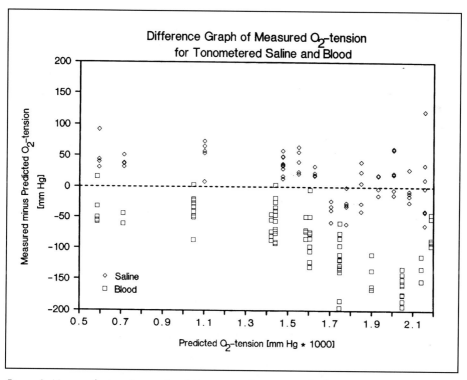

Figure 3. Measured minus the predicted $O_2$-tension of tonometered saline and blood versus predicted $O_2$-tension. $O_2$-tension of saline varied only slightly from the predicted, whereas the blood $O_2$-tension was lower than the predicted.

compressed patient. There is also a risk of retrograde arterial gas embolism if any gas is introduced into the arterial catheter while flushing (5). Emboli can potentially result from flushing an arterial catheter, but that risk should be minimal if only small volumes of heparinized saline are used to flush the catheter.

We have discussed only our ABL330's ability to measure supranormal $PO_2$s *in vitro*. We do not know if other ABL330 analyzers are capable of measuring hyperbaric $O_2$ tension as accurately as ours. We have no reason to assume however that they would not be able to perform this measurement accurately. Our ABL 3 (Radiometer) and the Corning 178 (Corning Glass Works) are not able to measure $PO_2$s into the hyperbaric range (observations made at our institution). It is possible that other blood gas analyzers are capable of measuring supranormal $PO_2$s, but we would advise that tonometry experiments be carried out with the device in question to determine its accuracy before using it clinically.

Eliminating dilutional errors by clearing the aspiration catheter, stopcocks, and collection syringe with hyperbaric oxygenated blood (or saline) just before the actual sample collection was important. In withdrawing arterial blood for gas analysis from patients, 3-4 times the arterial catheter and pass-through tubing (generally 0.8 to 0.10 ml) should be aspirated and discarded, or may be reinfused to the patient via a venous access catheter if heparinized. The blood gas syringe should be filled and cleared with arterial blood 2-3 times just before sampling. Finally, the sample should be sealed and the syringe plunger maintained under firm pressure until analyzed (< 3 min). It should not be disturbed by shaking or rolling.

The rate of change of $O_2$ tension over time was unpredictable, although the trend approximated 3% min-1 decrement of $O_2$ tension • min-1 up to 6 min of blood samples tonometered at 2 and 3 ATA. The falling $O_2$ tension values could be explained by leaking of gas through the syringe or by $O_2$ uptake by leukocytes. Further research could, perhaps, more precisely define the rate of change of $O_2$ tension in blood over time. This information may be important if the blood gas analyzer is not adjacent to the HBOT unit.

We did not expect that an accurate determination of $PO_2$ up to 2,200 mmHg could be performed reproducibly by a blood gas analyzer operating at atmospheric pressure (perhaps made even worse at our altitude). The literature suggests it would be unlikely that this could be done (6, 7). Radiometer did not anticipate this use for the ABL330 and seemed surprised when informed of our results. Obviously, the hyperbaric-tonometered sample is supersaturated with gas when rapidly dropped to atmospheric pressure. This is evident if the sample is tapped or shaken, because numerous small bubbles appear. The ABL330 did not display a "bubble-error" message with the samples that were gently and carefully handled.

In conclusion, we have demonstrated that the $PO_2$ of saline, and blood tonometered to full $O_2$ saturation, under hyperbaric pressures up to 3 ATA, can be accurately measured by a Radiometer ABL330 blood gas laboratory operated at atmospheric pressure, provided the sample is obtained in a manner that minimizes preanalytic errors, and is analyzed immediately. Extrapolation of this data to the clinical situation may or may not be appropriate. Presently, we are investigating the measurement of arterial blood gases at atmospheric pressure in normal human subjects exposed to HBO. Pending conclusion of this *in vivo* study, we would urge caution at applying our *in vitro* results to the clinical setting.

## ACKNOWLEDGMENTS

We thank Terry P. Clemmer, M.D., for his considerate review of this manuscript.

## APPENDIX IV REFERENCES

1. Clark JM, Lambertson CJ. Alveolar-arterial $O_2$ differences in man at 0.2, 1.0, 2.0, and 3.5 ATA inspired $PO_2$. J Appl Physiol 1971;30:753-763.

2. Moon RE, Camporesi M, Shelton DL. Prediction of arterial $PO_2$ during Hyperbaric treatment. In: Bove A, Bachrach AJ, Greenbaum LJ, Jr., eds. Proceedings of the ninth international symposium on underwater and hyperbaric physiology. Bethesda, MD: Undersea and Hyperbaric Medical Society, 1987:1127-1131.

3. Holbek CC. The Radiometer ABL330 blood gas analyzer. J Clin Monit 1989;5:4-16.

4. Bland JM, Altman DG. Statistical method for assessing agreement between two methods of clinical measurements. Lancet 1986;February 8:307-310.

5. Chang C, Dughi J, Shitabata P, et al. Air embolism and the radial arterial line. Crit Care Med 1988;16:141.

6. Lanphier EH. Special requirements of gas administration and physiological measurement in hyperbaric procedures. In: Whipple HE, ed. Hyperbaric oxygenation. Acad Sci, 1965; 117(2):824-827.

7. Litscher G, Friehs G, Maresch H, Pfurtscheller G. Electroencephalographic and evoked potential monitoring in the hyperbaric environment. J Clin Monit 1990;6:10-17.

## APPENDIX V. PERFORMANCE OF THE SECHRIST 500A HYPERBARIC VENTILATOR IN A MONOPLACE HYPERBARIC CHAMBER

*Lindell K. Weaver, Gregory Elliott, Loren Greenway*

### ABSTRACT

In our initial use of the Sechrist 500A hyperbaric ventilator operating within a Sechrist 2500B monoplace chamber, we observed that the patient's tidal volume ($V_T$) decreased as chamber pressure ($P_{CH}$) increased more than -10%, the maximum allowable decrement in $V_T$ from the ambient $V_T$ (500A operators manual). Therefore we decided to quantitate this decrement in $V_T$, and to determine what variables were important for the ventilator to deliver an adequate $V_T$. The 500A ventilator was set up within the chamber in the manner described by the 500A operators manual. First, an adult Boehringer spirometer was calibrated over the range of monoplace $P_{CH}$ (0.85 to 2.9 ATA at our altitude). This was accomplished by collecting a volume of gas at various $P_{CH}$, then measuring the volume of gas at atmospheric pressure and calculating the true $V_T$. Comparing measured $V_T$ to true $V_T$ the percent error discrepancy was: -1.5, +2.4, +2.8, +6.1, +6.0% at $P_{CH}$ = 0.85, 1.5, 2.0, 2.5, 2.9 ATA, respectively (the (+) value means that the spirometer underestimates the actual $V_T$ by that %). Once the spirometer calibration was known, we varied the static compliance ($C_L$ = 15 to 8.7 cc/cm $H_2O$) of a test lung and ventilator control module inlet pressure ($P_{IN}$) from 55 to 85 psig (the allowed range of $P_{IN}$ by Sechrist, Inc.) and measured $V_T$ as the dependent variable. We found that $V_T$ is a function of $C_L$, $P_{CH}$, and $P_{IN}$. Even with a normal $C_L$, $V_T$ decreased more than -10% when $P_{CH}$ exceeded 1.5 to 2.0 ATA. With a $C_L$ = 15 cc/cm $H_2O$, $P_{CH}$ = 2.5 ATA and $P_{IN}$ = 55 psig, $V_T$ was reduced 38% from that at ambient pressure. We recommend monitoring $V_T$ continuously during mechanical ventilation of patients in a monoplace hyperbaric chamber with a hyperbaric-calibrated spirometer, making appropriate ventilator adjustments to maintain an adequate $V_T$.

### INTRODUCTION

Most hyperbaric treatments provided to patients in the United States are delivered within monoplace hyperbaric chambers (1). Many of the conditions approved to receive hyperbaric oxygen (HBO) therapy (2) occur in critically ill, mechanically-ventilated patients. If these patients are to receive HBO in a monoplace chamber, they must be mechanically ventilated with a ventilator either adapted to, or designed for, use within the monoplace hyperbaric environment. The Sechrist 500A hyperbaric ventilator was designed to be used in the monoplace hyperbaric chamber (3). It has been in use since 1979. According to Sechrist, Inc., there are presently 123 500A hyperbaric ventilators in use (personal communication, May, 1987).

It is important to prevent hypercarbia during the hyperbaric treatment. Hypercarbia potentiates CNS oxygen toxicity (4) and acidemia may ensue if the arterial partial pressure of carbon dioxide ($PaCO_2$) increases (5).

Since $CO_2$ production remains nearly constant, minute ventilation is the major determinant of $PaCO_2$. Thus, prevention of hypercarbia requires that tidal volume ($V_T$) and ventilatory rate ($V_R$) remain nearly constant as pressure increases in the monoplace chamber.

The Sechrist 500A ventilator operator's manual states: "As the chamber is pressurized, the control module automatically adjusts the delivery pressure to maintain the preset tidal volume ($V_T$) within $\pm 10\%$. Inhalation and exhalation times remain unaffected" (3). During our initial use of this ventilator with an intubated, mechanically-ventilated patient we observed that the $V_T$ decreased markedly as chamber pressure ($P_{CH}$) increased. This was due, in part to a sticking venturi valve, which we have reported previously (6). However, even with a non-sticking venturi valve, we observed that $V_T$ decreased as $P_{CH}$ increased. Therefore, we decided to study the performance of this ventilator. We addressed the following questions:

1. How accurate are spirometers at measuring $V_T$ in the HBO environment?
2. What is the relationship between $V_T$ and $P_{CH}$?
3. Is the delivered $V_T$ a function of lung compliance ($C_L$)?
4. Is the delivered $V_T$ a function of ventilator control module inlet pressure ($P_{IN}$)? If so, what is (are) the optimal pressure(s)?

## METHODS AND MATERIALS

The Sechrist 500A hyperbaric ventilator was set up within a Sechrist monoplace hyperbaric chamber (Type 2500B) in the manner described(3). Ventilatory rate was set at 15 breaths/min by adjusting expiratory time. The ambient $V_T$ was adjusted to 500-800 cc by adjusting inspiratory time and flow. An adult mechanical spirometer (#8800, Boehringer, Wynnewood, PA) was placed on the expiratory limb of the circuit. A test lung (Manley Lung Ventilator Performance Analyzer, Medical Developments, LTD, Chesham, Bucks, England) for lung $C_L$ = 15 and 32 cc/cm $H_2O$ or two 3-liter anesthesia bags (3-liter Breathing Bag, Anesthesia Associates, Inc., San Marcos, CA 92069) connected in parallel (for lung $C_L$ = 61 and 87 cc/cm $H_2O$) were attached between the inspiratory circuit and the expiratory circuit. Airway resistance was set at zero, and $C_L$ varied. The standard Sechrist breathing circuit was employed (tubing compliance is 2.2 cc/cm $H_2O$).

To validate the accuracy of the Boehringer spirometer (3-min collection time, $V_R$ = 15/min., $V_T$ = 700 to 1,050 cc at 0.85 ATA) a volume of gas was collected at each data point (0.85, 1.5, 2.0, 2.5, 2.9 ATA, respectively) in a Douglas bag (Warren E. Collins, Inc., Braintree, MA), which was connected to the exhalation port of the spirometer via a one-way valve. With inspiration, $O_2$ flowed into the test lung. With exhalation, $O_2$ flowed through the spirometer and was collected in the Douglas bag. At the completion of the $O_2$ collection the chamber was decompressed. The gas volume was then measured (atps) in a 120-liter, chain-compensated Tissot gasometer (Warren E. Collins, Inc.). Through the application of Boyle's Law (pressure x volume = constant) at a fixed temperature the volume of gas at each chamber pressure was calculated. The $V_R$ was known so the $V_T$ could be calculated. This value was compared to the volume measured by the Boehringer spirometer. Each collection of gas was performed 3 times and was reproducible. Once the accuracy of the Boehringer spirometer was known, it was the only spirometer used throughout the remaining data collection.

The hospital's biophysics department validated accuracy of the chamber pressure gauge. A thermistor (Yellow Springs Instrument Co., OH, model 700) was passed through an IV pass-through port (after fashioning an appropriate seal), allowing the measurement of temperature in the distal airway (in the Sechrist 500A ventilator block). Temperature was read off a Marquette Monitor (Marquette, Inc., Milwaukee, WI).

To answer the question, "How does $V_T$ change as $P_{CH}$ varies?" the $V_T$ was calculated by measuring the volume delivered by the ventilator through the circuit used in the spirometer calibration, for 1 min, divided by the $V_R$. We chose to perform this same data collection with test lung settings of varying lung compliance (15, 32, 61, and 87 cc/cm $H_2O$), with zero airway resistance over a range of $P_{INS}$.

To see the effect of varying $P_{IN}$ on ventilator performance, a 2-stage, variable oxygen regulator (Harris Oxygen 2-stage regulator, model 25-100, Harris Calorific Co., Cleveland, OH) was attached to a standard oxygen cylinder ("H" cylinder). The Sechrist 500A ventilator operator's manual states that a pressure of 70 psi gauge $\pm10$ psig should be used. On the back of the ventilator control module it is stamped "use 60 psig $\pm5$ psig." Therefore, we elected to test ventilator performance over a range of pressures from 50 to 85 psig using the same previously tested lung compliances (15, 32, 61, and 87 cc/cm $H_2O$).

Before and after each test we inspected the venturi valve to ensure that it was not sticking.

## RESULTS

The accuracy of the Boehringer spirometer that we used for the entire set of data collection in this study is shown in Table 1 (for $V_T$s between 700 to 950 cc at atmospheric pressure). As chamber pressure increases, the spirometer underestimates $V_T$ up to a maximum of 6.1% at 2.5 ATA.

## TABLE I. CALIBRATION ERROR OF A BOEHRINGER SPIROMETER OVER A RANGE OF HYPERBARIC PRESSURES

| CHAMBER PRESSURE (ATA) | % ERROR |
|---|---|
| 0.85* | - 1.5 |
| 1.5 | + 2.4 |
| 2.0 | + 2.8 |
| 2.5 | + 6.1 |
| 2.9** | + 6.0 |

*The (+) symbol means that the Boehringer spirometer underestimates the actual tidal volume.*
*\* (Salt Lake City, Utah is at an altitude of 1,341 m above sea level)*
*\*\* (This is the chamber pressure limit at 1,341 m)*

The temperature in the ventilator block increased $< 3°C$ with chamber compression to 2.9 ATA. This gives $< 1\%$ change in volume, so this calculation was excluded from the spirometer validation.

Table 2 displays the data. At each $P_{CH}$, $V_T$ is listed for each $P_{IN}$ and $C_L$ tested. Figure 1 shows the percent change in $V_T$ ($\Delta V_T$) plotted against $P_{CH}$ for $C_L = 1.5$ and 87 cc/cm $H_2O$, which represent the extremes of the test. The broken and solid lines, respectively, define the range of $V_T$s over the range of $P_{IN}$ tested. Clearly, $V_T$ is a function of $P_{CH}$, $P_{IN}$ and $C_L$. The greatest $\Delta V_T$ occurred with the lowest $P_{IN}$, the lowest $C_L$ (stiffest lung), and at the highest $P_{CH}$. Increasing $P_{IN}$ at the higher $P_{CH}$ ($> 1.5$ ATA) decreased the $\Delta V_T$.

Figure 2 shows $\Delta V_T$ as a function of $P_{CH}$ and $C_L$, holding $P_{IN}$ constant at 70 psig (the recommended $P_{IN}$). When $P_{CH}$ exceeds approximately 1.5 ATA, the $\Delta V_T$ is greater than -10% for all $C_L$ tested, although the least $\Delta V_T$ is with the highest $C_L$.

We observed that the time required to deliver a preset $V_R$ ($t_V$) depends on $P_{IN}$ as well. See Figure 3. The volume of gas ventilated during 1 min was measured. As we decreased $P_{IN}$ we observed that $V_R$ also decreased (the control module knobs were not adjusted during each change in $P_{IN}$). $V_R$ was set to 15 breaths/min at a $P_{IN}$ equal to 70 psig at 0.85 ATA. The ordinate shows the time required to deliver 15 breaths as $P_{IN}$ was varied. We noted that more time was required to deliver the 15 breaths. As $P_{IN}$ was decreased, by measuring inspiratory and expiratory time (by graphing airway pressure as a function of time) we found the major component of the above change was a change in expiratory time. See Figure 4. $V_R$ was not affected by changing $P_{CH}$ if $P_{IN}$ was constant.

The performance of our ventilator was verified as acceptable by Sechrist, Inc. (letter, 3 September 1987). A second ventilator was also tested in the same manner. It performed identically to the first ventilator with the exception of a $C_L = 16.7$ cc/cm $H_2O$, where the $\Delta V_T$ was even more markedly increased at $P_{CH} > 1.5$ ATA and when $P_{IN} < 75$ psig.

## DISCUSSION

With a normal functioning venturi valve, the ability of the Sechrist 500A hyperbaric ventilator to deliver the preset (atmospheric) $V_T$ is a function of chance $P_{CH}$, $C_L$, and $P_{IN}$. The variability of $V_T$ is significant. For example, assume one is mechanically ventilating a patient with adult respiratory distress syndrome (ARDS) who requires hyperbaric therapy. If we assume $C_L = 15$ cc/cm $H_2O$ and $P_{IN} = 55$ psig, a preset $V_T$ of 1,050 cc would be reduced to a $V_T$ of 650 cc at a chamber pressure of 2.5 ATA. This represents a reduction of 38% in the preset $V_T$. If the $V_R$ is not concomitantly increased (assuming no change in $CO_2$ production and ventilatory deadspace), the alveolar ventilation would also fall 38% allowing the $PaCO_2$ to increase. This could result in two untoward effects: CNS oxygen toxicity (4) and acidemia (5) due to the respiratory acidosis.

This example may be a worst-case scenario, but it is not unreasonable to expect patients with stiff lungs to occasionally require HBO therapy. Many of the approved indications for HBO therapy may be associated with a low $C_L$ (e.g., gas gangrene with ARDS, carbon monoxide poisoning with smoke inhalation injury, acute crush injury with chest or lung contusion or aspiration).

## TABLE 2. TIDAL VOLUMES TABULATED AS FUNCTION OF CHAMBER PRESSURE, CONTROL MODULE PRESSURE, AND COMPLIANCE

| $P_{ch}$ (ATA) | $P_{in}$ (psig) | $V_T$ (cc)[a] | | | |
|---|---|---|---|---|---|
| | | $C_L$ = 87b | $C_L$ = 61 | $C_L$ = 32 | $C_L$ = 15 |
| | 85 | 788 | 919 | 804 | 1070 |
| | 80 | 796 | 945 | 822 | 1067 |
| 0.85 | 75 | 816 | 950 | 833 | 1067 |
| | 70 | 833 | 968 | 843 | 1067 |
| | 65 | 841 | 980 | 849 | 1061 |
| | 60 | 922 | 995 | 858 | 1064 |
| | 55 | 926 | 1022 | 867 | 1063 |
| | 85 | 780 | 880 | 769 | 1019 |
| | 80 | 790 | 903 | 783 | 1022 |
| | 75 | 790 | 911 | 793 | 1034 |
| 1.00 | 70 | 800 | 928 | 802 | 1019 |
| | 65 | 810 | 943 | 811 | 1031 |
| | 60 | 840 | 956 | 819 | 1020 |
| | 55 | 850 | 977 | 827 | 1029 |
| | 85 | 737 | 780 | 710 | 943 |
| | 80 | 727 | 811 | 726 | 947 |
| | 75 | 737 | 828 | 735 | 951 |
| 1.50 | 70 | 763 | 839 | 742 | 953 |
| | 65 | 768 | 852 | 753 | 955 |
| | 60 | 768 | 868 | 761 | 957 |
| | 55 | 788 | 814 | 768 | 955 |
| | 85 | 699 | 719 | 673 | 903 |
| | 80 | 709 | 752 | 691 | 901 |
| | 75 | 709 | 774 | 697 | 904 |
| 2.00 | 70 | 720 | 784 | 709 | 904 |
| | 65 | 730 | 794 | 715 | 903 |
| | 60 | 730 | 801 | 720 | 836 |
| | 55 | 720 | 791 | 706 | 790 |
| | 85 | 711 | 717 | 672 | 903 |
| | 80 | 711 | 748 | 681 | 903 |
| | 75 | 711 | 754 | 684 | 892 |
| 2.50 | 70 | 721 | 761 | 695 | 831 |
| | 65 | 690 | 746 | 671 | 778 |
| | 60 | 690 | 688 | 608 | 711 |
| | 55 | 637 | 625 | 541 | 639 |
| | 85 | 700 | 696 | 720 | 884 |
| | 80 | 689 | 718 | 660 | 845 |
| | 75 | 689 | 714 | 646 | 782 |
| 2.90 | 70 | 678 | 667 | 595 | 727 |
| | 65 | 647 | 613 | 537 | 662 |
| | 60 | 572 | 551 | 473 | 592 |
| | 55 | 498 | 474 | 395 | 513 |

a  All Vt are corrected by the spirometer error (TABLE I); b cc/cm $H_2O$

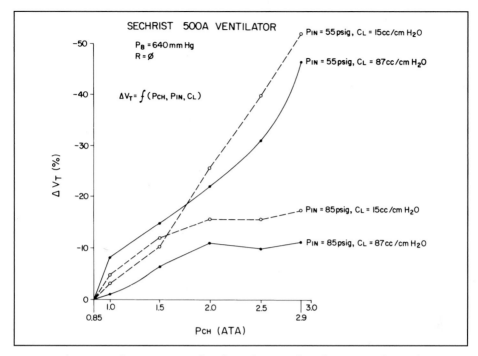

Figure 1. The percent change in $\Delta V_T$ is plotted as a function of $P_{CH}$ for $C_L$ 15 and 87 cc/cm $H_2O$. Broken and solid lines represent 2 families of curves defined by the ventilator $P_{IN}$. Although not depicted, the $\Delta V_T$ for $C_L$ = 32 and 61 cc/cm $H_2O$ fall within the boundaries shown here. Barometric pressure (PB) is as shown. Airway resistance (R) = 0.

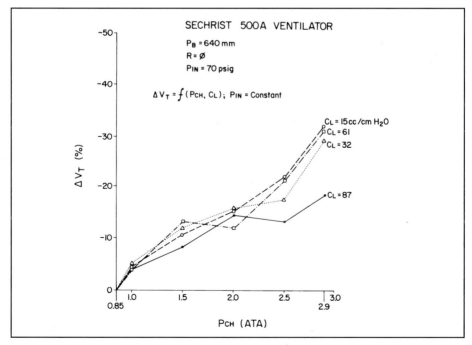

Figure 2. $\Delta V_T$ plotted against $P_{CH}$ with $P_{IN}$ held constant at 70 psig for varying $C_L$. $\Delta V_T$ exceeds - 10% for all lung $C_L$ tested when $P_{CH}$ is > approximately 1.5 ATA.

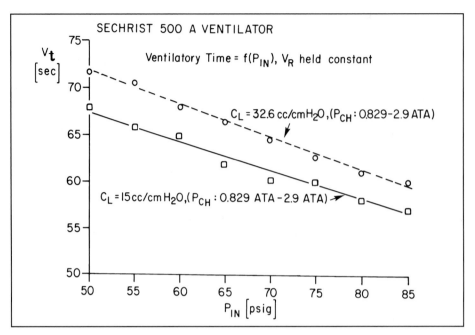

Figure 3. Ventilatory time ($t_V$) as a function of sechrist 500A hyperbaric ventilator control module inlet pressure ($P_{IN}$). Ventilatory rate ($V_R$) was set at 15 breaths per minute with $P_{IN}$ = 70 psig ($C_L$ = 15cc/cm $H_2O$). As $P_{IN}$ was varied, the time required to deliver 15 breaths ($t_V$) also varied. Chamber pressure ($P_{CH}$) changes did not affect the change in $t_V$.

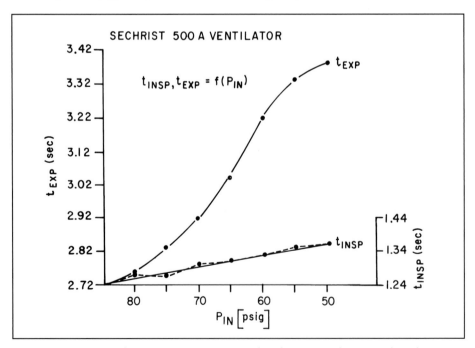

Figure 4. Inspiratory and expiratory times ($t_{exp}$, $t_{insp}$) plotted against Sechrist 500A hyperbaric ventilatory control module inlet pressure ($P_{IN}$). The major determinant of the effect of $P_{IN}$ on ventilatory rate ($V_R$) depicted in Figure 3 is a change in expiratory time, particularly prominent at the lower $P_{IN}$ ($V_T$ = 850 cc @ $P_{CH}$ = 0.85 ATA, $C_L$ + 32 cc/cm $H_2O$).

Even with a normal $C_L$ the $V_T$ decreased greater than 10% when $P_{CH}$ exceeded 1.5 ATA.

With stiff lungs ($C_L$ < 30 cc/cm $H_2O$) and at the higher $P_{CH}$ (> 2.0 ATA), the ability of the Sechrist 500A ventilator to deliver a high minute ventilation (VE) is limited. If one is treating a patient who requires a high VE (for example, 15 liter/min) to maintain an adequate pH with a low $C_L$, the 500A may be unable to deliver that VE even by increasing $P_{IN}$ to 85 psig at a $P_{CH}$ much over 2.0 ATA. Chamber pressures between 2.0 to 2.8 ATA are required for most of the disorders for which HBO is indicated (2).

With the marked reduction in $V_T$ that occurs with low compliance lungs at high $P_{CH}$, the operator of the ventilator may be tempted to increase $V_T$ by increasing inspiratory time. Likewise, the operator may increase VE by increasing $V_R$. Both of these maneuvers should be done cautiously as the patient may "stack breaths" which could result in intrathoracic gas trapping. Major adverse hemodynamic consequences could ensue as well as pulmonary overpressurization and barotrauma if there is inadequate exhalation time (7-8).

Hospital oxygen delivery pressures (at the wall outlet) generally are limited to 50 to 55 psig (9). The 500A ventilator requires a $P_{IN}$ of at least 65 psig and perhaps even up to 85 psig for optimal delivery of a given $V_T$ when $P_{CH}$ exceeds 1.5 ATA. Consideration of operating the 500A ventilator at higher than most hospital oxygen delivery (wall) pressures is reasonable. We operate our 500A ventilator with oxygen supplied from H-cylinders with a variable 2-stage regulator used to control $P_{IN}$ (between 70 and 85 psig). The present data suggest that there is a flow-resistive drop in the supply lines that may be hose-orifice diameter dependent. A future experiment could determine if ventilator performance is improved if the oxygen supply line, control module outlet line, and the pass-through fittings are changed to a larger diameter.

Inspiratory and expiratory time are also dependent upon $P_{IN}$. If $P_{IN}$ remains constant over the operational range of the Sechrist chamber (0.85-2.9 ATA), inspiratory and expiratory time remain constant and the $V_R$ does not change. This observation could be important, however, if $P_{IN}$ dropped for any reason during the course of treating a mechanically ventilated patient. Not only does $V_T$ change if $P_{IN}$ changes, but $V_R$ as well. The VE ($V_T$ x $V_R$) may or may not change, depending upon $P_{CH}$, $C_L$, and the $P_{IN}$. If the VE decreased (which is likely at $P_{CH}$ > 2.0 ATA, if $P_{IN}$ decreased) there could be an abrupt change in $PaCO_2$ and pH.

The present study was performed at an altitude of 1,341 m above sea level (0.85 ATA). The lower ambient pressure accounts for some of the reduction in $V_T$ that we observed. However, even if we assume the $V_T$ measured at 1.0 ATA as our starting $V_T$, $V_T$ still fell below the volume calculated by multiplying the $V_T$ at 1.0 ATA times 90% when $P_{CH}$ exceeded approximately 2.0 ATA, dependent, of course, on $C_L$ and $P_{IN}$. The Sechrist 500A operator's manual does not discuss a possible reduction in $V_T$ with chamber pressurization, which may be enhanced with operation of the ventilator at an elevated altitude. We would expect the reduction of $V_T$ as $P_{CH}$ increased to be even more marked at altitudes higher than 1,341 meters. (The slope of $\Delta V_T$ vs. $P_{CH}$ is fairly steep between 0.85 and 1.0 ATA, see Figures 1, 2).

The Sechrist ventilator tubing has a compliance factor of 2.2 cc/cm $H_2O$. Therefore the tubing losses will be minimal, even with high peak airway pressures. If other circuits are substituted that have a higher tubing compliance factor, it may be difficult to deliver an adequate gas volume from the ventilator block to provide the volume lost in the compliance of the circuit, and to provide an adequate $V_T$ to the patient, particularly with high peak airway pressures and at high $P_{CH}$.

We have presented a method of spirometer calibration within the monoplace hyperbaric environment and have provided the accuracy of our adult Boehringer spirometer. We do not know if other spirometers, or even if another Boehringer spirometer, would have the same percent error discrepancy as ours. Kindwall and Goldman (10) state that a $V_T$ measured with a Wright's spirometer can be corrected by specific factors that are a function of $P_{CH}$ (10). The single Boehringer spirometer we tested exhibited a greater error than what Kindwall and Goldman describe (-3% at $P_{CH}$ = 3.0 ATA, $V_T$ = 1,060 cc), underestimating $V_T$ as $P_{CH}$ increases. It is likely that this error is not solely due to a change in gas density. If it were, we would expect a percent-error curve linearly dependent on $P_{CH}$ in which the $V_T$ (measured by spirometry) would overestimate the actual $V_T$.

This study did not deal with variable airway resistance. Airway resistance was set equal to zero, which clinically is unlikely in intubated patients. Therefore the findings reported here may also apply to patients who exhibit high airway resistance, even if their static lung compliance is relatively normal.

## CONCLUSIONS

1. Continuously measure $V_T$ with a spirometer that has been calibrated to the hyperbaric environment.

2. Continuously monitor $P_{IN}$.

3. Use a $P_{IN}$ that is at least 70 psig which can be adjusted up to 85 psig, allowing the ventilator operator to provide a $V_T$ closest to the preset $V_T$ over the operational range of $P_{CH}$.

4. Ensure that if $P_{IN}$ falls for any reason during HBO treatment the $V_T$ is appropriately adjusted by manipulating flow or inspiratory time, or both. Also ensure that the $V_R$ is adjusted in order to deliver an adequate minute ventilation while also providing adequate exhalation time.

5. Monitor $V_T$ during decompression to maintain an adequate $V_E$ to prevent delivering too large a $V_T$, which could result in pulmonary barotrauma or hemodynamic compromise, or both.

6. Be aware that a patient may stack breaths if an attempt is made to increase $V_T$ by increasing inspiratory time. This may be manifested by an increasing peak or end expiratory pressure, or both.

7. Use a ventilator circuit that has a low tubing compliance factor for patients who have high peak airway pressures and a high $V_E$ (demanding a rather large $V_T$) to minimize volume loss in the circuit.

## ACKNOWLEDGMENTS

We thank Dr. T.P. Clemmer for reviewing the manuscript. Preparation of the manuscript was done by Suzanne Stagg and Pat Petersen, whose help was greatly appreciated. We also thank Judy Johnson, Sechrist, Inc., for her assistance with loaning a ventilator and validating the performance of our ventilator.

## APPENDIX V REFERENCES

1. Myers RA. Functional Hyperbaric chamber facilities. Summary of questionnaires compiled by Maryland Institute of Emergency Medical Services (MIEMSS), January 1988.

2. Myers RAM, chairman. Hyperbaric oxygen therapy - a committee report. Bethesda, MD; Undersea and Hyperbaric Medical Society, 1986.

3. Model 500A hyperbaric ventilator operational instructions. Sechrist Industries, 1986.

4. Clark JM. Oxygen toxicity. In: Bennett PB, Elliott DH, eds. The physiology and medicine of diving, 3rd ed, Flagstaff, AZ: Best Publishing Co., 1982; 229-233.

5. Bracket NC Jr, Coher JJ, Schwartz WB. Carbon dioxide titration curve of normal man: Effect of increasing degrees of acute hypercapnia on acid-base equilibrium. N Engl J Med 1965:272.

6. Greenway L, Weaver L, Elliott G. Performance of the Sechrist 500A hyperbaric ventilator as monoplace chamber pressure increases. Undersea Biomed Res 1987; 14(Suppl):20-21.

7. Egan DF. Fundamentals of respiratory therapy, 2nd ed. St. Louis, Missouri: C.V. Mosby Co., 1973; 352-369.

8. Pepe PE, Marini JJ. Occult positive end-expiratory pressure in mechanically ventilated patients with airflow obstruction. Am Rev Resp Dis. 1982; 126:166.

9. McPherson SP, Spearman CB. Respiratory therapy equipment, 2nd ed. St. Louis, MO: C.V. Mosby Co., 1981; 50.

10. Kindwall EP, Goldmann RW. Hyperbaric medicine procedures, 6th ed. Milwaukee: St. Luke's Hospital, 1984; 39.

# NOTES

CHAPTER 7

# THE MULTIPLACE CHAMBER

## CHAPTER SEVEN OVERVIEW

# THE MULTIPLACE CHAMBER

*Eric P. Kindwall*

## INTRODUCTION

Multiplace, or Class A, chambers, as they are defined by the National Fire Protection Association (NFPA) (4) are capable of accommodating two or more persons. They range in size from a little over a meter (48 in) in diameter to diameters of four meters (12 feet) or more. Most commonly, they are cylinders lying on their side, but a few facilities have very large cylinders with the end bells forming at the top and bottom. About a quarter of all the hyperbaric oxygen (HBO) facilities in operation in the United States have multiplace chambers. Recently, rectangular chambers have been installed chiefly in Australia, built by Eric Fink who pioneered them, one in Stockholm built by Haux in Germany and a Fink chamber to be installed in Milwaukee. All are capable of 6 ATA. There are other rectuangular chambers in place or on order.

Some very old chambers have only one compartment, but most modern hyperbaric chambers have at least two locks, or compartments, and some have three. A second compartment or entry lock permits personnel to lock in and out of the chamber while the patient or patients are maintained at pressure. Additionally, most modern chambers have a small, quick-opening, pass-through lock for introducing drugs or supplies into the chamber while under pressure, or for locking out blood samples or other specimens.

Clinical multiplace chambers are pressurized with compressed air. not oxygen, for reasons of safety. Usually they are supplied by at least two high-volume, relatively low-pressure compressors, for redundancy. Volume tanks are interposed between the compressors and the chamber for storage of reserve air, to allow cooling of the air after compression, and to smooth out pulsation from the compressors.

Compressed air is used for pressurization, as the use of pure oxygen would be too dangerous in a large chamber where people are free to move around, where drawers are opened and closed, and where static electricity might build up due to interaction between patients, attendants, and equipment. Additionally, selected electronic equipment can often be introduced into the chamber with relative safety, which would be impossible in a pure-oxygen environment. Because the chamber is filled with compressed air, patients receive oxygen by tight-fitting oronasal mask, head tent, or endotrachial tube. The head tents are sealed either with a neck-dam seal or are taped tightly to the skin. "Overboard dump" systems are mandatory; through which, exhaled oxygen is conducted out of the chamber in a closed system via vacuum reducers to minimize oxygen build up in the chamber air.

Most multiplace chambers are capable of reaching pressures equivalent to 50 or 60 meters of equivalent sea water depth (165 to 198 fsw), or 6 to 7 atmospheres absolute (ATA), but for the vast majority of treatments, they are operated at pressures in the range of 10 to 20 msw (33 to 66 fsw) or 2 to 3 ATA.

## COMPRESSED AIR SOURCES

Air compressors should be of sufficient capacity that, when combined with the volume tank reserve, they are able to pressurize the chamber to 50 meters within about five minutes. The capacity should be large enough to continuously ventilate the chamber during treatment and prevent oxygen levels from rising over 23%. The maximum pressures created by these compressors are relatively low, usually ranging between 8.5 and 17 kg/cm$^2$ (125 to 250 psig). It is an absolute requirement that the air be free of impurities, especially carbon monoxide and oil vapors. For this reason, the most recent preference is to use high volume, oil-free rotary compressors or alternatively piston compressors with non-lubricated cylinders utilizing Teflon piston rings. Water-lubricated compressors, although more expensive, have also been used.

If compressors with oil-lubricated cylinder walls are used, there must be an effective air clean-up system using appropriate filters to remove impurities and odors. The compressor plant must be chosen carefully after a consultation with an engineer experienced in designing clinical hyperbaric facilities. The use of rotary-air compressors is becoming increasingly popular, as they require little maintenance, can provide large volumes at adequate pressure, and are so designed that oil cannot enter into the discharge air. Thus, oil clean-up systems become unnecessary. Their only potential drawback is that they are quite noisy. However, this is overcome by placing the entire unit in a sound-insulating box.

The use of high pressure (150 kg/cm$^2$ 2200 psig) compressors with large reservoirs of stored air as the primary source for pressurization is to be discouraged. Maintenance costs are much higher, and if the chambers are used continuously for any reason, the compressors will not be able to keep up with the volume requirements.

## CHAMBER CONFIGURATION

At least two compartments, one being an entry lock, are now considered mandatory for clinical facilities. The doors to all compartments must be rectangular to facilitate wheeling hospital stretchers in and out of the chamber, and to allow easy access for patients who have difficulty ambulating. The threshold for these doors obviously must be flush with the floor inside and outside the chamber. Most chambers have their entry lock designed as a separate compartment within the same cylinder.

In those chambers that have a vertical axis for the cylinder, entry locks are usually attached as satellites to the main lock. An advantage to using a vertical axis, with the end bells as the floor and ceiling, is that the curvature of the end bells may more efficiently house ventilation and air conditioning equipment, leaving more space for patients, personnel, and patient-care equipment. Stretchers can be pushed against the wall as the walls do not slope in at the bottom. A limiting factor, however, is the extreme width of these chambers and the subsequent difficulty in transportation from the site of manufacture to the site of installation. Expense is another consideration, as at least two cylinders and four end bells are required for a chamber with a single entry lock. The end bells are also proportionately of a very large diameter and are quite expensive to manufacture. All multiplace chambers in the United States must be manufactured to comply with Section 8 of the ASME Code which requires a 4 to 1 safety factor for pressure in steel or aluminum chambers. All the requirements of the Pressure Vessel for Human Occupancy (PVHO) code of the ASME regulations must also be met.

A recent development is the rectangular steel chamber with wall reinforcement of steel ribs or beams. Fairly large chambers with widths of 10 to 12 feet can be constructed using this design. Such a chamber has been installed at the Royal Adelaide Hospital in Adelaide, Australia. Smaller rectangular locks which can reach 6 ATA have been designed and installed, with the 6 ATA lock serving as the inner chamber attached to a 3 ATA rectangular outer lock. The first of these installations is in Melbourne, Australia. The advantage of the rectangular chamber is that the floor space available utilizes the entire chamber width. The disadvantage is the greater initial cost.

Rectangular concrete chambers are another concept. A prototype was built and successfully tested at the School of Aerospace Medicine at Brooks Air Force Base in San Antonio, Texas. The advantage of reinforced concrete is that it is quite cheap to construct, it provides vertical chamber walls and it can be built quickly. The chamber can be of large volume and there is ample space for cooling and heating coils under the floor or in the overhead. The bilge can be built to any desired depth to contain ancillary equipment. Sliding doors are easily accommodated. Mass production of these chambers awaits code approval from the American Society of Mechanical Engineers (ASME) committee on Pressure Vessels for Human Occupancy (PVHO). At this writing (2008), rectangular, concrete chambers are still only a concept.

## HYBRID CHAMBERS

In the past few years, there have been some very small chambers designed for a single patient and one inside attendant. These technically are multiplace chambers, but are often modular and can be used either as a monoplace chamber, or a second module can be attached to allow the inside tender to reach the patient's head and manage his airway. These chambers are not suitable for the treatment of mass casualties, and claustrophobia remains more of a problem. However, in situations where space limitations are severe and an inside tender is a requirement, the hybrid chamber may be worth considering.

## THE MULTIPLACE CHAMBER ADVANTAGES

If one is treating 10 patients or more per day on a regular basis, the multiplace chamber becomes the better choice economically. Treating several patients at a time permits "batch treatment" and greatly reduces overtime costs. The hyperbaric physician need be present for only one or two chamber runs per day, instead of being in constant attendance as is necessary when multiple patients are treated serially in the monoplace unit. It is a good idea for monoplace facilities that acquire a multiplace chamber to keep at least one monoplace chamber for the occasional patient who cannot come at the scheduled time of the morning or afternoon chamber run. It will also be useful in treating carbon monoxide or smoke inhalation in small children as the child does not have to fight with a mask during treatment.

The most important single consideration is that direct hands-on care that may be given to the patient during treatment in the multiplace chamber, including suctioning. A neurologic examination can be carried out during treatment; this may be quite useful, if one is following the changing neurologic state of a resolving case of decompression sickness. Furthermore, if one is treating an extremely ill patient with multiple IVs, an arterial line, and full monitoring, patients may be taken directly into the chamber with all of their lines and leads still attached. There is no necessity for disconnecting and reconnecting them after placement in the chamber. Claustrophobia is rarely a problem, with only about one in 50 patients exhibiting any confinement anxiety.

In the event of a mass casualty, such as an entire family stricken with carbon monoxide poisoning, more than one patient can be treated at a time, and one is not forced to choose only the most serious to be treated initially.

If cardiac arrest occurs, defibrillation can be carried out in the air-filled multiplace chamber. This is an impossibility in the monoplace chamber where the patient must be decompressed to the surface before resuscitative efforts can begin. However, it is usually best under such circumstances to decompress the patient to the surface and turn a hyperbaric emergency into a normobaric one. Should a patient sustain a pneumothorax while at pressure in the multiplace chamber, a thoracentesis tube may be inserted before the patient is decompressed. This avoids the potential of cardio-pulmonary embarrassment. Should an IV infiltrate, a new one may be started during treatment.

Finally, multiplace chambers usually have a 50 meter (165 foot) depth capability which can be a requirement when treating severe decompression sickness (DCS) and arterial gas embolism (AGE). Depth capability and mixed gas availability can make the difference between success and failure, particularly if one is treating the delayed case, or a diver with DCS following a deep dive. The multiplace chamber is the optimal choice for treating DCS and AGE.

## THE MULTIPLACE CHAMBER DISADVANTAGES

The initial cost of the multiplace chamber is higher, as it must be provided with heavy foundations, a separate room for the compressors and volume tanks, and a more complicated control panel. Environmental control equipment such as heating and cooling coils are often added which carry a high price tag. Once the chamber is in operation, at least two people will be required to run it at all times, the outside chamber operator and the inside attendant. The presence of an inside tender is mandatory for safety reasons. This obviously involves higher personnel costs per chamber dive.

Since the chamber atmosphere is air, every patient must be equipped with an oxygen mask, head tent, or be ventilated via endotrachial tube. Masks and head tents are not a requirement in the monoplace chamber as the atmosphere is 100% oxygen. This can be an advantage when treating small children who may be frightened or uncooperative when required to wear a mask. However, mask leaks are potential problems, and there is a danger that a patient may not receive 100% oxygen if the leak is not detected.

It should be noted that the tightness of the mask fit is critical to delivering a specific, known dosage of oxygen. Unfortunately, in Japan, the Netherlands, and perhaps some other countries, a light plastic mask is often used which does not seal tightly on the face. As a result, actual $O_2$ levels when measured in the hypopharynx is only be 55% to 65%, which would correspond to a lower chamber pressure where a tight mask is used. My own feeling is that the mask should be tight enough that the patient could breathe from it were he lying on his back underwater. Fortunately, very sick patients are frequently intubated which leaves no question as to the $O_2$ delivered.

The reason a tightly-fitting mask or head tent is desirable is that data from one country can then be compared with data from another. With the present state of affairs, anyone comparing patient outcomes would have to know if the patients were intubated or not.

The reason given for using the loose fitting masks are that tight masks are "too uncomfortable," or "that it has been standard practice in the past, and there is no apparent reason to change." Today this reasoning is unacceptable, as tight masks or hoods can be made comfortable. We all must know the exact dosage of the drug, oxygen, we are using in the interests of scientific accuracy and honesty.

Finally, since the inside tender always breathes air in order to avoid any potential oxygen toxicity, he or she is always potentially at risk for decompression sickness. Proper decompression schedules must be observed (see below) to prevent decompression sickness in chamber personnel. This can sometimes pose problems if one wishes to remove a patient from a chamber rapidly. The patient, having breathed oxygen, is at no risk of experiencing decompression sickness and can be decompressed quite rapidly. However, in that case, the inside tender must be in a separate lock if exposed to maximum treatment pressure and time beyond the so called "no decompression" limits. Alternatively, the tender can be decompressed with the patient and then rapidly recompressed in the chamber within 5 minutes and put on a so-called surface decompression schedule.

## CHAMBER HULL PENETRATIONS

From the outset, it is very important that there be sufficient hull penetrations incorporated into the chamber design. New penetrations cannot be drilled or cut into the hull later without violating the hydrostatic acceptance test. Any welding, drilling, or cutting on the pressure hull will require a complete recertification with a repeat hydrostatic test.

Most diving chambers have very few hull penetrations as compared with clinical chambers. Hull penetrations are termed "nozzles" by chamber manufacturers.

Typical hull penetrations for diving chambers:

1. Air supply
2. Air exhaust

3. Telephone port
4. Oxygen system supply port
5 Safety valve
6. View ports
7. Lighting wire port
8. Bilge drain (if not incorporated in safety valve)
9. Pressure gauge

On the other hand, clinical hyperbaric chambers may require some or all of the following additional ports:

1. Mixed-gas supply port
2. Electrical supply port for equipment
3. Speaker-system supply port
4. TV-cable supply port
5. One or more patient-monitoring ports (multi-pin, electrical)
6. Separate ports for the fire hose and deluge systems
7. Defibrillator cable port
8. Chamber atmosphere-monitoring port
9. Remote pressure-gauge line port
10. Patient respiratory gas monitoring port
11. Telephone port

With clinical chambers in teaching hospitals, it is probable that research work will also be carried out. This may involve multiple additional penetrations for special purposes. Therefore, in planning for a clinical hyperbaric chamber, it is best to plan for all of the necessary penetrations, and then double that number to be on the safe side.

A common solution to this problem is the placement of several six or eight-inch (15 to 20 cm) apertures in the chamber hull, each covered by a blanking plate bolted to a flange. It is permissible to drill holes and modify the blanking plates. Since they are bolted to the pressure hull, they are not considered part of the normal hydrostatic test. As modifications are needed over the years, these blanking plates can be exchanged for ones modified to meet specific needs. It is prudent to place some of these blanking plates below the chamber floor, as well as a few high in the overhead.

## FIRE SAFETY IN THE MULTIPLACE CHAMBER

Fires can occur anywhere at normal atmospheric pressure in ambient air containing 21% oxygen. However, with hyperbaric treatment, the air in the multiplace chamber contains more oxygen molecules by volume, while at pressure, causing fires to burn faster.

The basic premise is that fires are to be prevented. Since all fires require fuel, oxygen, and an ignition source, in the absence of anyone of these, a fire cannot occur. When using high partial pressures of oxygen, it is theoretically possible to eliminate only two of three elements, fuel and ignition sources. Sometimes, it is only possible to eliminate one of the elements. This is the most dangerous situation, as only a single critical failure is required to start a fire. If two of the three elements are missing, it would take two simultaneous failures, a much less likely occurrence.

It must be remembered that compressed air at 4.76 atmospheres (equivalent to 37 meters or 124 feet of seawater) contains the same number of oxygen molecules per liter (in the chamber) as a one liter volume of 100% oxygen on the surface. Nevertheless, a fire in air at a pressure of 4.76 atmospheres will not burn with the intensity of a fire in 100% oxygen at sea level due to the quenching effect of the nitrogen present. In compressed-air tunneling operations, torches are routinely used for cutting through steel at air pressures of 30 psig (3 ATA) without any particular increased danger, as long as reasonable precautions are taken. Using the same torch in a 100% oxygen environment would be suicidal.

For this reason, the fire safety requirements for multiplace and monoplace chambers are quite different so long as the oxygen level, measured in the gas exhausted from the chamber, never exceeds 23%. It is possible to defibrillate a patient in the air-filled multiplace chamber, and to use some forms of electronic equipment that are not subject to implosion due to pressure changes. Standard oscilloscopes or cathode ray tubes are not useable in the pressurized chamber because they will implode at higher pressures.

Chamber fire safety is explicitly defined in the National Fire Protection Association (NFPA) code for Class A hyperbaric chambers. (4) Every hospital hyperbaric unit should have an updated copy of this code. The code undergoes frequent revision, so it is important that one has a current edition. At this writing, (2008) the NFPA code for multiplace hyperbaric chambers has undergone substantial revision with the goal of redefining the chamber atmosphere as "hazardous", but not "explosive" as it was defined in 1970, when the code first went into effect. The reason for labeling the atmosphere "explosive" was that surgery was being carried out in some chambers at that time and there was the possibility that a flammable anesthetic (cyclopropane) might be used. Today, surgery is rarely done at pressure in the chamber, but more importantly, flammable anesthetics are not used. Thus, there is no rational reason to label the chamber atmosphere explosive. Changing the definition to "hazardous" immediately permits the use of more electrical equipment (with adequate safeguards), and vastly lowers the cost of placing ancillary equipment in the chamber with fewer adaptations required.

## Fuel

All unnecessary flammable materials should be kept out of the chamber. Flammable liquids such as tinctures should be avoided, as well as solvents which can burn. We allow books and magazines into the air-filled multiplace chamber as a compromise with patient comfort and toleration of treatment. Appreciable quantities of cloth and paper dressings should not be stored in the chamber, but locked-in as needed. All-cotton sheets, pillow cases, and blankets should be treated with a fire-retardant material and color coded so that they can be recognized at the laundry for delivery back to the hyperbaric unit and identified before use. Recently the NFPA has permitted the introduction of 50%-50% cotton/polyester fabrics into the chamber. Chamber personnel should be clothed in snug cotton or cotton/polyester jumpsuits or coveralls, which have been treated with a fire retardant. Cotton is used, as it does not promote static electrical charge build-up. Synthetic materials are avoided in garments and bedclothes. Fiberglass cloth does not burn, but is unacceptable because it produces urticaria. Nomex fiber garments, used by racing car drivers and pilots, are very expensive and appear to be unnecessary. Patients with Vaseline gauze dressings under bulky cotton gauze dressings are routinely treated in both monoplace and multiplace chambers, and these dressings have not caused problems. The new fiberglass or synthetic casts are also safely used in both mono and multiplace chambers.

The walls of the chamber should be painted with a fire-resistant epoxy paint. Avoid a multi-layer buildup of paint. Epoxy paint is available which has a burning index of one, on a zero to 100 scale, where zero is granite and 100 is kiln-dried redwood. The chamber floor should be non-combustible and conductive. It should never be waxed. Aluminum flooring is non-sparking. Wooden furniture and ordinary upholstery are to be avoided. Mattresses and pillows should be of open-cell foam and have conductive rubber flash covers.

## Ignition Sources

Since it is impossible to remove oxygen and all forms of fuel from the chambers (even the human body will support combustion at high oxygen levels) the absolute absence of ignition sources is the most crucial element of fire prevention. Static electricity can be minimized by the measures described above, and also by maintaining at least a 60% relative humidity in the chamber. Obviously, matches, lighters, and smoking materials are excluded. Recent experiments attempting to ignite cotton and other solid materials in 100% oxygen at 3 ATA with static electricity have shown that combustion will not be initiated. However, static electricity under those conditions will ignite flammable liquids.

Often, sources of accidental ignition are electrical. Any switch, if carrying more than a few volts, can arc when opened or closed. Electrical motors containing brush commutators continuously arc. The accidental breakage of an electrical wire or cord can cause an arc. Plugging or unplugging an electrical appliance or piece of equipment can cause a spark.

Transistors or other solid-state devices have almost universally replaced electronic vacuum-amplifier tubes. However, were a tube to rupture in a pressurized chamber it would be an ignition source. Current regulations call for all electrical devices, equipment, and wiring to be "intrinsically safe," implying that if anything or everything goes wrong with it, it will not spark or provide an ignition source; this is in the process of modification for the multiplace chamber as noted above.

Sometimes electronic equipment is required in the chamber. If it is not intrinsically safe, it must in some way be isolated in a pressure-proof casing or rendered inert by purging with an inert gas such as nitrogen. Brushless or induction motors are used. Plugs must be explosion-proof, etc. The NFPA regulations are very specific as to exactly what is permitted.

There have been other sources of ignition implicated in chamber fires. In one case, a diver wished to sleep and hung his tee shirt over a bare light bulb to shield his eyes from the light. It ignited, killing him. In another instance, three divers were in saturation, when a filter for the incoming oxygen in their chamber atmosphere scrubber system ignited from a spark in the scrubber, caused by an electrical fan. The filter, unknown to them, had previously been used to filter JP-4 jet fuel, and contained a kerosene-like residue. All three died.

Sudden compression of high-pressure oxygen can also cause ignition of hydrocarbons. Ball valves or valves that suddenly become fully open with a quarter turn should never be used in oxygen lines where pressures exceed 250 psig. Even if there is only a tiny amount of dirt or combustible material in the line downstream when oxygen is suddenly released through a quick-opening ball valve, it may "diesel" as high oxygen pressure instantly appears. I know of two cases where this has happened; both, fortunately, occurred outside the chamber. In the first case, the individual who opened the valve sustained a 30% total-body surface burn in the resulting explosion. In the second case, no one was injured, but the fire destroyed some equipment. Thus, under certain circumstances, high-pressure oxygen (> 250 psig) can serve as an ignition source all by itself.

A unique accident occurred when a blanket was "pre-warmed" in a microwave oven just before being locked into the chamber. It was immediately placed in the pass-through lock and the pressure equilibrated with chamber pressure (20 psig or 2.4 ATA). When the nurse removed it from the lock, the blanket burst into flame. It was quickly extinguished with the chamber deluge system and no one was hurt. The microwave had heated the center of the folded blanket to near the kindling point. Subsequent sudden pressurization increased the heat to start an actual fire, which was abetted by the higher oxygen level provided by the compressed air.

A tragic fire occurred in Italy where 11 people perished in a multiplace chamber fire. Patients were admitted to the chamber wearing their street clothes. One patient had carried a butane-fueled hand warmer in his pants pocket into the chamber. He subsequently placed an oxygen hood with the gas flowing on his lap. When the oxygen reached the hand warmer it exploded engulfing the entire chamber in fire. The water deluge system was non-functional. All of the occupants, including a nurse, died of asphyxia or burns.

The most common cause of chamber fires is an ignition source brought into the chamber by one of the occupants, either a patient or one of the staff. In another recent chamber fire, which claimed the lives of two divers and a doctor, a cigarette lighter was found in the chamber after the fire. It was the presumed ignition source, as it apparently exploded.

At this writing, (2008) no patient has been involved or injured in a chamber fire in a clinical hyperbaric chamber anywhere in North America. The statement applies to both multiplace and monoplace units. This attests in large part to the diligence of the many chamber crews who operate hyperbaric chambers, as well as good chamber design, and effective enforcement of regulations.

To avoid a repetition of previous accidents, no patient should be treated in his or her street clothes. All garments worn by patients must have the pockets sewn shut or have no pockets. A patient once inadvertently took a cigarette lighter into a monoplace chamber in the pocket of her hospital-supplied jump suit. She discovered it at pressure in 100% oxygen but was safely decompressed. Garments should all be cotton and fireproofed. Some commercial laundries can do fireproofing and the treatment lasts for about 40 washings, typically the life of the garment. Patients who may be suicidal should be carefully checked to see that they are not secreting matches or a cigarette lighter on their person when placed in the chamber. This has happened. A patient once hid a book of matches in the palm of his hand and produced it at pressure in the monoplace chamber announcing that he was going to commit suicide. The chamber operator fortunately was able to engage him in dialog while he was safely decompressed. The deluge system must be regularly checked, usually monthly, to verify its function. A by-pass valve is used to obviate flooding the chamber with each test. The oxygen level in the chamber must be constantly monitored with alarms that sound if the percentage goes over 23%. Keep combustible liquids out of the chamber and hold combustibles in general to a minimum.

The best principle for fire prevention is to continuously assume that "if it can go wrong, it will, and at the worst possible time." Then try to engineer the situation to "fail safe" if possible, so that it can't go wrong.

## PATIENT - RELATED ITEMS PERMITTED IN THE MUTIPLACE CHAMBER

There is often doubt as to what items frequently used in patient care are permitted in the multiplace and monoplace chamber. Below is a partial list:

1. Vaseline gauze dressings. They should be covered with a cloth wrap. (These dressings (covered) can also be used safely in the oxygen filled monoplace chamber.)
2. Implanted pacemakers.
3. Implanted cardiac defibrillators.
4. External metal fracture fixaters.
5. Contact lenses.
6. Hearing Aids. (Only in the air-filled multiplace chamber.)
7. Eye glasses.
8. Books and magazines.
9. Defibrillator paddles (with the switch and electronics external to the chamber). (Only in the air-filled multiplace chamber!)
10. Any of the standard wound care dressings.
11. Petroleum based lotions if used for treatment of pathologic skin conditions.
12. Any electrical or electronic equipment used in the multiplace chamber should be approved by the hospital bioengineering department and by the hyperbaric unit Safety Director.
13. Aortic balloon assist pumps. Only in the multiplace chamber and after testing at pressure and approval by the hospital bioengineering department.
14. Standard battery operated IV pumps.
15. Pleurevac™ or similar continuous thoracic suction devices.
16. The V.A.C.™ vacuum assisted wound closure bags.
17. Tight fitting underwear.

If an item is not on the above list, put it in the chamber only if it is necessary for patient care. Determine that is will not implode with increased pressure or explode during decompression if gas has leaked into it. It should not present any new ignition source or unnecessary fuel source.

# ITEMS PROHIBITED IN THE HYPERBARIC CHAMBER

1. Matches, cigarettes, lighters.
2. Hearing aids in the monoplace chamber.
3. Wrist watches.
4. Hair spray, lipstick, other cosmetics.
5. Chemical hand warmers (actuated by oxygen in ambient air).
6. Volatile fuel burning hand warmers.
7. Thermacare™ self-actuating (with room air) heating packs.
8. Implanted insulin pumps (must be emptied and turned off).
9. No electrical or electronic equipment of any kind in the monoplace chamber except for the intrinsically safe communication system, EKG and EEG leads, arterial line transducer leads and Radiometer™ transcutaneous $pO_2$ electrodes and leads.
10. Walkman™ or similar personal music players and electronics.
11. Cell phones and pocket pagers.

**The above list may not be exhaustive!**

*Note: The ban on cosmetics (lipstick, hairspray, cologne, etc.) may not seem rational as there never has been a lipstick fire nor has static electricity ever ignited hair with spray on it. The real reason for the ban is to continuously drive home to the patient that they are not in a normal environment in the chamber and that they should take no item into the chamber that is not prescribed.*

## SAFE DECOMPRESSION OF INSIDE ATTENDANTS

As the inside tender caring for the patients in the hyperbaric chamber breathes air while the patient breathes oxygen, subsequent decompression must be made in accordance with the decompression requirements of the inside tender. Exposures or dives to pressures of 10 meters (33 feet or 2 ATA) or less are well tolerated, with the tender being able to decompress directly to the surface, even after two-hour exposures. Over a period of years it was found that inside tenders did not experience decompression sickness when making dives to ten meters (33 feet, 2 ATA), even when two such exposures were made per day, separated by a surface interval of as little as one hour. Most naval decompression tables would classify those exposures as within safe limits and not requiring decompression stops on ascent.

The difficulty arises when going to pressures in excess of 10 meters or 2 atmospheres. It must be pointed out, however, that the U.S. Navy limits for "no-decompression" dives in excess of 2 ATA are not safe enough for clinical hyperbaric work. For example, a very common exposure is 2.5 atmospheres for 110 minutes. This corresponds exactly to the U.S. Navy no-decompression dive of 50 feet (15 meters) for 110 minutes. Using the Navy approved decompression schedule calls for a three minute stop breathing air at 10 feet (3 meters). On ascent to the surface, the author has observed vestibular decompression sickness, limb pain in multiple sites, chokes, and spinal cord decompression sickness in inside tenders using that schedule.

When the present U.S. Navy air decompression tables were tested, on acceptance trials, they were found to produce an incidence of decompression sickness of no more than 5%. This incidence is relatively low, and is acceptable for most Naval operations where exposures are infrequent. However, in clinical hyperbaric work where the table is used at its maximum limit for time and depth on every occasion, one would expect to see two cases of decompression sickness per month in inside tenders, if 40 exposures were made during that time. This poses an unacceptable risk of unnecessary pain and possible permanent central nervous system damage to the inside tender, and would invoke an unacceptable expenditure of time and money having to treat a case of bends in one's own personnel every two weeks. For this reason decompression schedules for inside tenders must be liberally padded, far beyond the U.S. Navy requirements.

There is experimental and historical evidence to indicate that the present U.S. Navy decompression stops for the standard air tables are too shallow and that optimal inert gas elimination probably occurs at deeper depths (1-3). An additional stop, at least three meters (10 feet) deeper than the first stop required by the table is probably beneficial. The second measure used to improve the safety of decompression is oxygen breathing. This increases nitrogen elimination by approximately a factor of five and there is experimentally demonstrated evidence that oxygen also decreases blood sludging, and reduces white cell adherence to capillary walls. Using these concepts, the typical decompression profile we use for an exposure at 2.4 atmospheres for 110 minutes is decompression to six meters (20 feet), with two minutes of oxygen breathing accomplished at that stop. This is followed by a stop at three meters (10 feet), where oxygen is breathed for 10 minutes. Using such a decompression schedule, decompression sickness in chamber personnel is an extreme rarity. As stated above, the U.S. Navy schedule indicates that the only decompression required from such an exposure would be three minutes breathing air at three meters (10 feet).

When one is treating a critically ill, gas gangrene patient, for example, the protocol calls for 90 minutes of oxygen breathing at 3 ATA or 66 feet (20 meters). This puts the inside tender on the U.S. Navy 70-foot decompression table for 100 to 110 minutes (considering air breaks and compression time). Even the unsafe U.S. Navy schedule requires 34 to 44 minutes total decompression time. If the patient is critical, it is highly desirable to return him to the ICU and not have him delayed by having to wait out the inside tender's decompression time at 20 and 10 feet. To avoid this kind of delay we use two inside tenders whenever possible. The first tender spends an hour or 70 minutes with the patient at depth and then the second tender locks into relieve him. The first tender takes his required decompression (breathing oxygen) in the outer lock while the patient is finishing the last thirty minutes of his treatment. The second tender having been exposed for only thirty or forty minutes is making a "no-decompression dive" and decompresses directly to the surface with the patient at the conclusion of the treatment.

If an emergency arises where the patient must be emergently decompressed to the surface with the inside tender who has a decompression obligation, this can be managed safely. When the patient has been locked out, the inside tender is returned to 12 meters (40 feet) with a surface interval of no more than 5 minutes. He is subsequently decompressed on a padded version of the U.S. Navy Surface Decompression Table using oxygen.

It is an excellent policy never to routinely use the same inside tender for more than one chamber run per day at pressures greater than 33 feet. This involves a repetitive dive under the best of circumstances, and invokes costly additional decompression time for the second exposure. Again, for clinical work, the standard repetitive-dive tables are not conservative enough to effectively guarantee freedom from bends. In emergency situations, the same tender has been used on more than one dive per day, but then decompression has been considerably lengthened from what is required in the U.S. Navy repetitive-dive schedules, and has been well padded with an additional deeper stop lengthened times at the stops and with oxygen breathing instead of air.

Normally, the inside tender breathes air continuously while attending patients undergoing treatment for decompression sickness on U.S. Navy Table 5 or 6. Oxygen breathing or extra decompression is not officially required for the inside attendant. However, bends have developed in the inside tender following a standard U.S. Navy Table 6 dive. For this reason, most facilities routinely require the inside tender to breathe oxygen during the last 30 minutes of the table while decompressing from 9 meters (30 feet). If Table 6 is extended for any reason, oxygen breathing by the inside tender is an absolute requirement during the last 30 minutes of the table. If more than one extension is made, oxygen breathing should be used by the inside tender for the last hour of the table.

Historically, under U.S. Navy regulations, all of the occupants of the chamber could not be breathing oxygen at the same time, although this rule has recently been modified. Frequently, however, in civilian clinical practice, this rule was and is ignored. The reasons for this are that extra tenders may not be available and the risk of oxygen seizure, while sitting quietly breathing oxygen, is extremely remote at pressures of nine meters (30 feet) or less. While the inside tender is breathing oxygen, he or she should not be active (such as trying to restrain a combative patient) and should not do any form of physical work.

On decompression from U.S. Navy Table 6A, there is no official requirement for oxygen breathing by the inside tender. However, it is highly recommended that oxygen be breathed by the inside tender for the last 30 minutes, even if Table 6A is not extended.

For other specific chamber exposures, the inside tender should be decompressed using a recognized air decompression table as a guide; but then, a two minute stop, on oxygen, should be taken three meters deeper than required by the schedule, along with extensive padding of the subsequent decompression stops while the tender breathes oxygen instead of air.

The author has found the above guidelines to be satisfactory over the past 20 years. The only caveat is that the chamber pressure gauges be calibrated at least once every six months and that all gauge lines be checked for leaks to be sure that critical pressures are not being exceeded. Gauge line leaks and the resultant false low readings have been implicated in more than one case of decompression sickness in inside tenders.

## REFERENCES

1. Behnke, A.R. and T.L. Willmon "Gaseous Nitrogen and Helium Elimination from the Body During Rest and Exercise." American Journal of Physiology. 1941;131(3):619-626.

2. Hills, B.A. "Limited Super-Saturation versus Phase Equilibration." Predicting the Occurrence of Decompression Sickness. Clin. Sci. 1970;38:251-267.

3. Kindwall, E.P., A. Baz, E. Lanphier, E. Lightfoot and A. Seirig. "Nitrogen elimination in man during decompression." Undersea Biomedical Research. 1975;2(4):285-297.

4. Klein, B.R. (Ed.) Health Care Facilities Handbook, Third Edition, Chapter 19, Hyperbaric Facilities, PP 475-512. NFPA 99, National Fire Protection Asociation. 1990. 1 Battery March Park, P.O. Box 9101, Quincy, MA 02269.

## APPENDIX: U.S. Navy Treatment Table 6

1. Descent rate — 20 ft/min.
2. Ascent rate — Not to exceed 1 ft/min. Do not compensate for slower ascent rates. Compensate for faster rates by halting the ascent.
3. Time on oxygen begins on arrival at 60 feet.
4. If oxygen breathing must be interrupted because of CNS Oxygen Toxicity, allow 15 minutes after the reaction has entirely subsided and resume schedule at point of interruption. *
5. Table 6 can be lengthened up to two additional 25–minute periods at 60 feet (20 minutes on oxygen and five minutes on air), or up to two additional 75–minute periods at 30 feet (15 minutes on air and 60 minutes on oxygen), or both.

6. Tender breathes 100% $O_2$ during the last 30 minutes at 30 fsw and during ascent to the surface for an unmodified table or where there has been only a single extension at 30 or 60 feet. If there has been more than one extension, the $O_2$ breathing at 30 feet is increased to 60 minutes. If the tender has had a hyperbaric exposure within the past 12 hours, an additional 60–minute $O_2$ period is taken at 30 feet.

# Depth/Time Profile

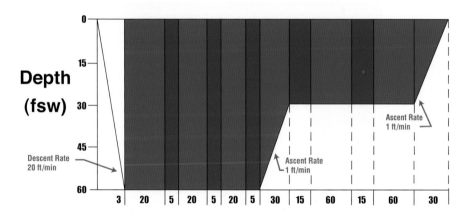

**Depth (fsw)**

Descent Rate 20 ft/min

Ascent Rate 1 ft/min

Ascent Rate 1 ft/min

| 3 | 20 | 5 | 20 | 5 | 20 | 5 | 30 | 15 | 60 | 15 | 60 | 30 |

## Time at Depth (minutes)

**Total Elapsed Time: 285 Minutes (Not Including Descent Time)**

**Breathing Media**

= Oxygen    = Air

*Procedures In the Event of Oxygen Toxicity.* At the first sign of CNS oxygen toxicity, the patient should be removed from oxygen and allowed to breathe chamber air. Oxygen breathing may be restarted 15 minutes after all symptoms have subsided. If symptoms of CNS oxygen toxicity develop again, interrupt oxygen breathing for another 15 minutes. If CNS oxygen toxicity develops a third time, contact a Diving Medical Doctor as soon as possible to modify oxygen breathing periods to meet requirements.

# APPENDIX: U.S. Navy Treatment Table 6A

1. Descent rate — 20 ft/min.
2. Ascent rate — 165 fsw to 60 fsw, not to exceed 3 ft/min, 60 fsw and shallower, not to exceed 1 ft/min. Do not compensate for slower ascent rates. Compensate for faster rates by halting the ascent.
3. Time at treatment depth does not include compression time.
4. Table begins with initial compression to depth of 60 fsw. If initial treatment was at 60 feet, up to 20 minutes may be spent at 60 feet before compression to 165 fsw. Contact a Diving Medical Doctor.
5. If a chamber is equipped with a high-$O_2$ treatment gas, it may be administered at 165 fsw and shallower, not to exceed 2.8 ata O2. Treatment gas is administered for 25 minutes interrupted by five minutes of air. Treatment gas is breathed during ascent from the treatment depth to 60 fsw.
6. Deeper than 60 feet, if treatment gas must be interrupted because of CNS oxygen toxicity, allow 15 minutes after the reaction has entirely subsided and resume schedule at point of interruption. *
7. Table 6A can be lengthened up to two additional 25-minute periods at 60 feet (20 minutes on oxygen and five minutes on air), or up to two additional 75-minute periods at 30 feet (60 minutes on oxygen and 15 minutes on air), or both.
8. Tender breathes 100% oxygen during the last 60 minutes at 30 fsw and during ascent to the surface for an unmodified table or where there has been only a single extension at 30 or 60 fsw. If there has been more than one extension, the $O_2$ breathing at 30 fsw is increased to 90 minutes. If the tender had a hyperbaric exposure within the past 12 hours, an additional 60 minute $O_2$ breathing period is taken at 30 fsw.
9. If significant improvement is not obtained within 30 minutes at 165 feet, consult with a Diving Medical Doctor before switching to Treatment Table 4.

# Depth/Time Profile

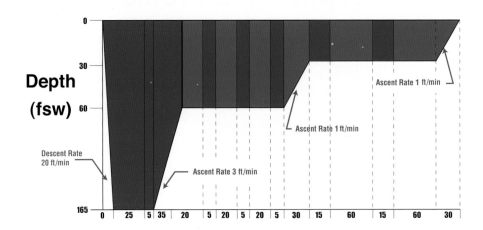

## Time at Depth (minutes)

**Breathing Media**

■ = Oxygen    ■ = Air

**Total Elapsed Time: 350 Minutes (Not Including Descent Time)**

*Procedures In the Event of Oxygen Toxicity. At the first sign of CNS oxygen toxicity, the patient should be removed from oxygen and allowed to breathe chamber air. Oxygen breathing may be restarted 15 minutes after all symptoms have subsided. If symptoms of CNS oxygen toxicity develop again, interrupt oxygen breathing for another 15 minutes. If CNS oxygen toxicity develops a third time, contact a Diving Medical Doctor as soon as possible to modify oxygen breathing periods to meet requirements.

CHAPTER **8**

# ECONOMICS OF HYPERBARIC MEDICINE

## CHAPTER EIGHT OVERVIEW

# ECONOMICS OF HYPERBARIC MEDICINE

*Dick Clarke*

## INTRODUCTION

As with any assessment of the potential for a new medical service, business development personnel will carefully consider each key program success driver. With few expectations they are the determination of market potential and market share; 'buy-in' costs (capital equipment outlay, facility renovations and operating expenses); integration impact on existing service lines; alignment with the provider's mission and philosophy; revenue expectations, and anticipated net margin.

In all likelihood, most diagnostic or therapeutic procedures under review will have already had their role in medical practice defined. Physicians in a position to refer patients will no doubt appreciate the relative benefits of these procedures and recognize those patients within their practice suitable for referral. Positron emission tomography (PET) is a diagnostic service example. PET is developing a unique niche through its ability to detect areas of molecular biology detail prior to any anatomic changes. It is being utilized in clinical oncology and certain diffuse brain diseases. Those who practice within these disciplines, and are in a position to refer, understand PET's role, advantages and limitations. Stereotactic radiosurgery is a therapeutic niche service example. Neurologists and oncologists will likewise appreciate its particular indications within their patient populations.

Because these two examples have a largely established role in medical practice and represent emerging standards of care, business development plans do not usually place great emphasis on the need to educate the regional medical community. Rather, planners are likely to focus more on available market share and anticipated net revenue. Medical science has invariably addressed the educational aspects through journal publications and other dissemination of supportive basic and transitional research.

Unfortunately this is not the case with hyperbaric oxygen (HBO) therapy. Despite over a century of practice, it remains on the periphery of mainstream medical practice. Few medical schools teach hyperbaric physiology and how this translates into the mechanistic basis of HBO therapy. Few residents and fellows are exposed to the practice of hyperbaric medicine during their training. Further complicating any analysis of hyperbaric medicine as a new service is the polarization of opinion as to its clinical efficacy and cost effectiveness. Some in influential positions have decried the lack of sufficient evidence to support the contention that hyperbaric oxygen therapy has a clinically valuable and cost-effective role to play. Their opinions influence elements of the medical community and, equally importantly, those who purchase health care. There is, therefore, increasing pressure on the discipline of hyperbaric medicine to improve clinical evidence levels for its common uses. As a result of these issues, any analysis of the clinical and economical potential of hyperbaric medicine must include a determination of regional physician knowledge, acceptance and bias.

The prompting of an evaluation of hyperbaric medicine's potential may come from several sources. Common among them is an administrative decision to consider its niche market potential or to compete with a regional presence. Physicians may seek its availability for selected patients, particularly those who deal with the various anatomic sites damaged as a consequence of therapeutic radiation. Likewise, an otherwise comprehensive wound-healing center may seek to 'round out' is therapeutic armamentarium.

Whatever the motivation, several issues will be important regarding the planning, successful introduction and effective operation of a hyperbaric medicine service. First and foremost, a sufficient number of referable patients must exist within the hospital's catchment area. This area tends to expand beyond traditional boundaries due to the esoteric nature and oft-limited availability of hyperbaric medicine. In some instances, a traditional service area has more than doubled. Next, physicians must be willing to refer their patients. As a referral service, this component is critical. Given a general lack of exposure to hyperbaric medicine, many physicians are unlikely to appreciate the mechanistic basis of hyperbaric medicine and its treatable indications. This should not be too surprising. Physicians have enough new material to digest in order to keep abreast of advances within their primary specialty to expect them to likewise follow advances in hyperbaric medicine. Again, a broad-based physician education initiative would become vital should the decision be made to introduce hyperbaric medicine. Much of the necessary educational material will be found elsewhere within this textbook. Of course, hospitals and the consulting hyperbaric physician team must be appropriately reimbursed for their respective investments of capital, time and expertise. Finally, one needs an administrative infrastructure robust enough to ensure practice compliance that is consistent with various oversight organizations.

The following sections represent a summary of the key steps considered necessary to critically analyze both clinical and business potential.

## INDICATIONS FOR HYPERBARIC MEDICINE

The question of what represents hyperbaric medicine's common uses has two answers. There is first a scientific position and then there is the reimbursement position.

As the peer scientific body representing the practice of hyperbaric medicine, the Undersea and Hyperbaric Medical Society (UHMS) has long assumed responsibility for the scientific position. Its standing committee on HBO therapy has developed an 'Approved Use' listing of conditions for which the UHMS considers hyperbaric oxygen therapy to be clinically indicated. (Table 1.) This committee's published report, which is revised every three to four years in order to account for emerging evidence regarding existing and

## TABLE 1. UNDERSEA AND HYPERBARIC MEDICAL SOCIETY APPROVED USES (9)

1.  Air or gas embolism.
2.  Carbon monoxide poisoning (Part A).
    Carbon monoxide poisoning complicated by cyanide poisoning (Part B).
3.  Clostridial myositis and myonecrosis (gas gangrene).
4.  Crush injury, compartment syndrome, and other acute ischemias.
5.  Decompression sickness.
6.  Enhancement of healing in selected problem wounds.
7.  Exceptional anemia.
8.  Intracranial abscess.
9.  Necrotizing soft tissue infections.
10. Osteomyelitis (refractory).
11. Delayed radiation injury (soft tissue and bony necrosis).
12. Skin grafts and flaps.
13. Thermal burns.

potential new uses, forms the North and South American foundation for best practice standards.

Those who purchase health care on behalf of their insured beneficiaries have used as their basis for medically necessary payment decisions the recommendations of the UHMS. However, few health care insurers subscribe to the UHMS position in its entirety. Minor variances are common, mostly by not agreeing with some of the UHMS recommendations and in some cases actually including conditions that do not appear on the UHMS listing.

The US government's Center for Medicare and Medicare Services (CMS) is particularly important within this decision-making process because it is the single largest purchaser of HBO therapy in the US. What Medicare will pay for and how much it will pay is a key driver in the evaluation of medical services in general and hyperbaric medicine in particular. Medicare's position on 'Medically Necessary' HBO therapy is listed in Table 2. One will note that missing from the Medicare list, when compared to the recommendations of the UHMS, are chronic wounds not involving an irradiated or diabetic etiology, acute exceptional blood loss anemia, intracranial abscess, mandibular osteoradionecrosis, prophylaxis of planned dental extraction and acute thermal burns. Medicare will, however, reimburse for the provision of HBO therapy in the management of actinomycosis infections, a condition not representing the position of the UHMS.

Private health insurance companies also base their payment decisions on the recommendations of the UHMS, and can be expected to add or delete conditions, as their independent analyses of the available evidence dictates. Two private health insurer examples are Aetna and Anthem Blue Cross Blue Shield.

## TABLE 2. CENTERS FOR MEDICARE AND MEDICAL SERVICES COVERED CONDITIONS FOR HYPERBARIC OXYGEN THERAPY (10)

1. Acute carbon monoxide intoxication.
2. Decompression illness.
3. Gas embolism.
4. Gas gangrene.
5. Acute traumatic peripheral ischemia. HBO therapy is a valuable adjunctive treatment to be used in combination with accepted standard therapeutic measures when loss of function, limb, or life is threatened.
6. Crush injuries and suturing of several limbs. As in the previous conditions, HBO therapy would be an adjunctive treatment when loss of function, limb, or life is threatened.
7. Progressive necrotizing infections (necrotizing fasciitis).
8. Acute peripheral arterial insufficiency.
9. Preparation and preservation of compromised skin grafts (not for primary management of wounds).
10. Chronic refractory osteomyelitis unresponsive to conventional medical and surgical management.
11. Osteoradionecrosis as an adjunct to conventional treatment.
12. Soft tissue radionecrosis as an adjunct to conventional treatment.
13. Cyanide poisoning.
14. Actinomycosis, only as an adjunct to conventional therapy when the disease process is refractory to antibiotics and surgical treatment.
15. Diabetic wounds of the lower extremities in patients who meet the following three criteria:
    a. Patient has Type I or Type II diabetes and has a lower extremity wound that is due to diabetes;
    b. Patient has a wound classified as Wagner grade III or higher; and
    c. Patient has failed an adequate course of standard wound therapy.

Aetna deems hyperbaric treatment medically necessary for acute cerebral edema, idiopathic sudden hearing deafness, acute acoustic trauma and pneumatosis cystoides intestinalis. (Table 3.) Anthem BCBS has specifically listed cerebral edema and perioperative HBO therapy as medically necessary for osteoradionecrosis prophylaxis during dental extractions from the previously irradiated mandible. (Table 4.) While the UHMS feels that latter condition is sufficiently supported by available science, Anthem is the first major health insurer to formally publish an agreed upon payment position.

It is important, therefore, that business development decisions take into account the specific reimbursement position of key national and regional health insurance companies.

## TABLE 3. AETNA POLICY BULLETIN: HYPERBARIC OXYGEN THERAPY (11)

**Aetna considers systemic hyperbaric oxygen therapy (HBOT) medically necessary for any of the following conditions:**

- Non-healing infected deep ulcerations (reaching tendons or bone) of the lower extremity in diabetic adults unresponsive to at least 1 month of meticulous wound care (including aggressive debridement, maximal antibiotic therapy, tight glycemic control, and appropriate treatment of arterial insufficiency, including grevascularization if necessary). HBOT is not considered medically necessary for superficial lesions.
- Acute carbon monoxide poisoning.
- Decompression illness ("the bends").
- Acute air or gas embolism.
- Gas gangrene (Clostridial myositis and myonecrosis).
- Cyanide poisoning (with co-existing carbon monoxide poisoning).
- Acute traumatic peripheral ischemia (including crush injuries and suturing of severed limbs) when loss of function, limb, or life is threatened and HBOT is used in combination with standard therapy.
- Acute peripheral arterial insufficiency (i.e., compartment syndrome).
- Progressive necrotizing soft tissue infections, including mixed aerobic and anaerobic infections (necrotizing fasciitis, Meleney's ulcer.
- Chronic refractory osteomyelitis, unresponsive to conventional medical and surgical management.
- Compromised skin grafts and flaps.
- Radiation necrosis (osteoradionecrosis, myoradionecrosis, brain radionecrosis, and other soft tissue radiation necrosis) as an adjunct to conventional treatment.
- Exceptional blood loss anemia only when there is overwhelming blood loss and transfusion is impossible because there is no suitable blood available, or religion does not permit transfusions.
- Pneumatosis cystoids intestinalis.
- Prophylactic pre-and post-treatment for members undergoing dental surgery of a radiated jaw.
- Acute cerebral edema.
- Idiopathic sudden deafness, acoustic trauma or noise-induced hearing loss, when HBOT is initiated within 3 months after onset.

## DETERMINATION OF PATIENT VOLUME

Several methods have been suggested as useful in determining the number of patients who might be referable for HBO therapy. In 1984, the United States Air Force sought to predict both the number of patients and their respective number of treatments that could be referred to its three clinical

## TABLE 4. ANTHEM BLUE CROSS BLUE SHIELD INDICATIONS FOR HYPERBARIC OXYGEN THERAPY (12)

**Medically Necessary:**

1. Systemic hyperbaric oxygen pressurization is considered medically necessary as a primary therapy in the treatment of any of the following conditions:
   - Carbon monoxide poisoning.
   - Cerebral edema.
   - Cyanide poisoning.
   - Decompression sickness.
   - Gas embolism.
   - Profound anemia with exceptional blood loss: when transfusion is impossible or delayed.
   - Prophylactic pre and post treatment for patients undergoing dental surgery of a radiated jaw.

2. Systemic hyperbaric oxygen pressurization is considered medically necessary when used as adjuvant therapy in conjunction with standard medical and/or surgical treatment for any of the following conditions:
   - Acute or chronic refractory osteomyelitis (refractory osteomyelitis).
   - Acute peripheral arterial insufficiency (compartment syndrome).
   - Acute thermal burns: deep second-degree or third degree in nature.
   - Acute traumatic ischemia.
   - Chronic non-healing wounds.
   - Compromised skin grafts or flaps (enhancement of healing in selected wounds).
   - Crush injuries.
   - Gas gangrene (i.e., clostridial myositis and myonecrosis).

hyperbaric facilities. The resulting School of Aerospace Medicine report considered active duty personnel, their dependents, and military retirees (1). Based upon a retrospective review of Air Force "inpatient only" discharge diagnosis codes, a formula was generated. This formula considered: (1) the actual prevalence of conditions which the report's authors thought appropriate for hyperbaric referral; (2) the percentage of patients within this category of conditions who would be expected to benefit; (3) the acuity of such patients, for multi-place chamber configuration purposes (ambulatory vs. stretcher borne); and (4) the total number of anticipated treatments per condition. The formula was subsequently modified to consider potential outpatient utilization.

This report predicted very high potential volumes that were not borne out in actual practice. There are several reasons as to why this may have been the case. The listing of conditions included some disease states for which HBO therapy was experimental, at best. A continued lack of clinical validation during the intervening period has served to largely eliminate these conditions from further consideration. Importantly, civilian health insurers did not then, and do not now, extend benefits for these conditions to be treated hyperbarically. The USAF report also assumed that a very high number of patients within each condition would be referred. Finally, it used "treatment-per-condition" numbers that exceed modern practice patterns. Today's clinical approach to the wound healing deficient patient, for example, is to employ HBO therapy in order to create a critical mass of angiogenesis which is sufficient to normalize the wound repair process. Once this has been achieved most wounds will then be able to move along their anticipated healing time lines with standard wound care alone. This is in contrast to its earlier use until complete healing had been achieved, now considered clinically unnecessary and cost-ineffective.

While the USAF process was a valiant attempt to identify potential volume, its use has frequently resulted in utilization estimates that are higher than those attainable. Several civilian hyperbaric programs were subsequently over developed, in terms of capacity, with resultant higher capitalization and operational requirements and a failure to meet income expectations. Such programs also failed to consider the potential for subsequent regional competition.

The "one-year data review" principle noted above, and an alternative strategy, which follows, involved several conflicting issues. Together, they served to complicate long-term projections. For instance, it would be expected that a backlog of some of the more chronic indications exists, late radiation tissue injury being one example.

Depending upon the anatomic site, these patients may have been conservatively or otherwise palliatively managed. Immediately upon introduction of a hyperbaric medicine service, referrals would then be disproportionally higher than those which could be sustained on an annual 'steady state' basis. Conversely, the medical education/marketing plan may take time to become fully implemented and uniformly effective. Consequently, referrals would be expected to increase over time, as local and regional physician communities become more knowledgeable, and develop greater confidence in the hyperbaric team. Further, these same physicians would be likely to follow their respective patient outcomes. The more discriminating the patient selection process, the more likely clinical and cost outcomes would be optimized. Failure to employ both suitable screening and an algorithmic approach to hyperbaric dosing, for instance, may have increased patient volume (number of treatments per patient) in the short term, but could raise questions regarding its economic value.

Persels discussed an alternative approach to patient census, one based upon a demographic analysis (2). Volume estimates were based on a population within a 50-mile radius of a proposed facility, a distance the author considered to be the maximum that a patient would be expected to commute daily during a several-week course of therapy. Using retrospective survey information from several newly-introduced programs, Persels proposed that "a reasonable daily treatment volume for the first year of operation can be estimated by applying a factor of 1:100,000 population" within a hospital's service area. Again, it was assumed that physicians would be prepared to refer the identified patient-volumes. Critical to both assumptions would be a carefully thought out medical education program, one based upon the scientific merit and economic value of HBO therapy.

Another method of determining clinical potential is by detailed review of medical records for selected inpatient and outpatient discharge diagnosis codes (3). Such a review will provide a more accurate institutional assessment of those patients with conditions considered appropriate for referral. An advantage of this approach is that it will determine whether a given institution's hyperbaric medicine service can remain viable in the face of local or regional competition. The previous two methods had assumed that all identified patients would be treated at the institution in question. Chart reviews serve to more accurately reflect patient suitability on a case-by-case basis. Contraindications can be identified at this time, as can lesion chronicity and those cases refractory to other interventions. This is particularly useful in that hyperbaric medicine is frequently not the first treatment option. Finally, and equally importantly, such reviews identify the insurance status of each patient. This makes revenue generation estimations much more reliable.

There are disadvantages to this latter approach, of course. The reviewer(s) must be experienced in the art and science of hyperbaric medicine. The review process is time consuming, and it only considers the hospital's potential census. It will also reflect only the study period activity, referred to by some as a less than optimal "snapshot" of a more complete 'longitudinal' picture. One can enhance this snapshot by increasing the number of years under review. Several years versus a single year would certainly provide a greater margin comfort in any final decision.

## BUSINESS MODEL

Fundamental to any determination of the potential for hyperbaric medicine as a new service will be its intended operating model. Over the past decade several alternatives to the traditional 'full-service' (i.e. all patients states) hospital-based 24/7 program have evolved. They are:

1. A hospital- based service but lacking the intent and capability to support critically-ill and ventilator-dependent patients.
2. Hospital-based but 'medical office building' located, available during normal working hours only and commonly instituted in support of a comprehensive wound healing center.
3. Non-hospital-based and non-hospital-owned freestanding private facility practicing UHMS approved uses.
4. Non-hospital-owned freestanding private facility, practicing as a largely 'off-label' service.

Obviously, the costs associated with the provision and support of a hospital-based 24/7 service are inherently greater than one which limits its practice, particularly to outpatient only care. Revenue generation is also an issue. In the majority of US hospitals, compensation is based upon the admitting diagnosis. This usually takes the form of a fixed payment for the illness or disease in question, regardless of the number of diagnostic tests or therapies rendered. The addition of twice-daily inpatient HBO therapy for a necrotizing soft tissue infection, for example, generates no additional revenue yet consumes considerable costs and resources.

If one limits HBO therapy access to outpatients, one can anticipate "treatment by treatment" reimbursement for essentially every patient. Enhanced revenue over expenses will result, particularly as one would not have to staff and compensate for 24/7 on-call coverage.

At first blush then, and when considering net revenue alone, the outpatient hospital-based model is clearly superior (Medicare reimbursement rules prohibit 'technical component' payments to non-hospital affiliated hyperbaric facilities). This model would limit costs and maximize revenue. However, there is another aspect to this equation, one readily apparent to patient advocates. Outpatient only access will eliminate from consideration patients who are likely to benefit most from the provision of HBO therapy. In cases of inatrogenic cerebral arterial gas embolism, for example, prompt provision of HBO therapy can be life saving. For those severely poisoned with carbon monoxide, it has proven central nervous system sparing. In cases of myonecrosis and necrotizing fasciitis, HBO therapy has limited tissue loss, improved mortality and enhanced the soft tissue reconstruction process. Also enhanced is limb salvage in acute foot/extremity infections in the diabetic patient.

So, the human side of the decision-making process needs to be considered despite the fact that these latter patients are, for the most part, not a revenue generating proposition. It does have to be all or nothing, however. The 'wound healing' hyperbaric service can be complimented with a single monoplace hyperbaric chamber located in the hospital, perhaps adjacent to the emergency department or one of the critical care areas, where ready access to physician support is likely.

## DELIVERY SYSTEM

Two hyperbaric delivery systems exist, each involving distinctly different cost, space, and operating characteristics.

One is the traditional 'multiplace' hyperbaric chamber. Its design is based upon the 'caisson lock'. Beginning in the late 19th century, these locks served as decompression chambers for men exiting the compressed air environments of tunnels and caissons, which supported bridge construction and underground mass transit projects. The multiplace chamber, as its name implies, accommodates several patients. It can range in size from those capable of treating two to as many as 20 patients at one time. A staff member usually accompanies multiplace chamber patients. The chamber's main compartment has attached to it a smaller 'entry lock'. This allows the transfer of personnel into and from the chamber while the main compartment remains pressurized.

Supplies can be sent into the chamber through the entry lock or via one or more 'medical locks' attached directly to the main compartment. A cylindrical shape has dominated multiplace chamber design over the past century. Recently, a rectangular design has made better use of the internal space and is gaining popularity. Patients are usually seated but stretcher patients can be accommodated. The chamber is compressed with air, with patients receiving oxygen via an individualized delivery system.

Purchase, delivery, build-out and installation of multiplace hyperbaric delivery systems acquired during 2006 ranged in price from US$1.2 to 7 million. Associated space requirements of 1,800 to 6,000 square feet were necessary to accommodate these relatively large systems.

The alternative hyperbaric delivery system, one that has been responsible for much of the growth of hyperbaric medicine in the US over the past two decades, is the 'monoplace' chamber. This chamber type enjoys a 50-year history and as the name implies is designed to accommodate a single patient. Monoplace chambers are compressed with oxygen, preferably using the hospital's bulk liquid oxygen system. Patients, therefore, breathe oxygen directly from the chamber atmosphere. An individualized air breathing system is incorporated into the monoplace chamber, however, in order to both minimize the risk of developing central nervous system oxygen toxicity and limit its clinical consequences, should premonitory signs and symptoms occur. Ancillary equipment advances now allow the most critically-ill patient to be effectively treated in this chamber type.

Purchase, delivery, build-out and installation of a two-chamber monoplace hyperbaric delivery system can be expected to range from US$400,000 to US$700,000 the major variable being the renovation and medical gas costs. One thousand square feet of space will accommodate up to three chambers, an office, patient examination room and handicap-accessible bathroom and a changing area.

For those who elect to incorporate this system type, starting out with two chambers will help ensure the necessary physician attendance and supervision from an income generating perspective. A single monoplace chamber in a non-wound healing center setting will be unlikely to generate the necessary professional income to support the compliance requirement of an on-site physician.

## CLINICAL TEAM REQUIREMENTS

The make-up of the clinical team will reflect, in large part, both the type of hyperbaric delivery system and its intended business model.

Medicare compliance requirements dictate that a physician credentialed in hyperbaric medicine by the hospital be immediately available to undertake patient supervision and related case management responsibilities. Physicians who bill Medicare for non-hospital based hyperbaric medicine attendance and supervision must likewise be 'immediately available.' What constitutes 'immediately available' is open to some interpretation. One is best advised to review the local coverage determination (LCD) for the position of the Medicare fiscal intermediary responsible for the region in question. 'Immediately available' definitions will be found to range from being on-site in the facility and closely observing the patient throughout their entire hyperbaric treatment, to working within a wound care center which is contiguous to hyperbaric medicine, and finally to a response time for that which a physician feels is appropriate for the state of the patient and their condition. Presently, there are no specific attendance and supervision requirements dictated by non-governmental health insurance companies.

Essentially every clinical specialty has been represented within the make-up of the consulting hyperbaric physician team. Those comfortable caring for acutely-ill patients are more likely to be found in support of the full-service and 24/7 program. Hyperbaric programs integrated into the comprehensive wound healing service will have represented a cross-section of physicians and surgeons who specialize in the management of wound healing deficiencies.

The educational foundation for most physicians intending to practice hyperbaric medicine is a week long (40 hours) introductory course. Ideally, such a course would be formally approved by the UHMS. This will ensure that course content and faculty knowledge meet specified minimum standards.

Board certification in undersea and hyperbaric medicine has been available since 1999. Two pathways are available. The first is practice-based. This permits physicians presently practicing hyperbaric medicine and who have accumulated sufficient clinical experience to challenge the certification examination. This pathway closes in 2010. Completion of a one year undersea and hyperbaric fellowship represents the second pathway. The Board Certification process is administered by the American Board of Preventive Medicine for all specialties, with the exception of Emergency Medicine. In this latter case, the American Board of Emergency Medicine assumes administrative oversight. The actual examination is common to both organizations.

Consistent with the policy of the Joint Commission on Accreditation of Hospitals Organization (JCAHO) a registered nurse must undertake a patient evaluation prior to a therapeutic intervention. This is also a common hospital policy. Given this requirement, at least one registered nurse should be a component of the hyperbaric clinical team. In the monoplace chamber setting, this nurse may or may not be required to operate the chamber. Alternatively, the chamber operations role may be assigned to other licensed health care professionals such as respiratory therapists, other technologists and occasionally to pre-hospital emergency medical personnel.

Nurse training for those who will operate the monoplace chamber is, with few exceptions, through attendance at a one week (40 hours) course. Ideally, this course will be recognized and approved by the Baromedical Nurses Association (BNA) (4). An exception to immediate formal education would be on-the-job training. In many cases, this latter process is subsequently complemented by formal didactic training. The BNA provides certification in hyperbaric nursing. Those who successfully challenge the BNA examination become Certified Hyperbaric Registered Nurses. Eligibility for testing includes formal training and a period of clinical practice preceptorship. The BNA has also established hyperbaric nursing standards.

Those non-RNs who operate the monoplace hyperbaric delivery system will likewise be expected to undergo formal training. Again, this will most likely be a one week introductory course. Professional advancement for technical personnel and nurses is available through the National Board of Diving and Hyperbaric Medical Technology (5). 'Certification in Hyperbaric Technology' is awarded to those who undergo formal training approved by the NBDHMT, acquire the necessary preceptorship experience and successfully challenge the CHT examination.

For multiplace operations, the nurse's role is to accompany patients during their pressurized treatments. Some nurses may also assist in the operation of the multiplace hyperbaric delivery system in conjunction with their in-chamber patient care activities.

Given the nature and complexity of multiplace chamber operations, it is common to find a retired military diver or ex-commercial diver engaged as the technical and safety director. The safety director is a formal title and position mandated by the National Fire Prevention Association (NFPA) (6). Every hospital-based hyperbaric medicine program is required to have a designated hyperbaric safety director. In the monoplace chamber setting, the hyperbaric nurse manager usually assumes this position.

## ADMINSTRATIVE INFRASTRUCTURE

It is common practice for the hyperbaric medicine program to operate as a division of a larger hospital department. Early programs were frequently aligned with Respiratory Therapy, both from staffing and hyperbaric physician (pulmonary-critical care) perspectives. Emergency Medicine was another common alignment, and had the benefit of 24/7 physician coverage. In this latter setting, the designated hyperbaric physician would likely be simultaneously attending in the emergency room and 'available' to hyperbaric medicine as patient needs dictated. Medicare reimbursement compliance requirements have essentially eliminated this approach. By the mid-1990s, and with the introduction of physician-staffed comprehensive wound management centers, hyperbaric medicine has frequently been integrated into wound center operations and administrative oversight.

Regardless of the setting in which hyperbaric medicine operates, its administrative and operational support structure must be clearly defined and consistent with every other hospital service. There has been a tendency to find that hyperbaric medicine has 'fallen through the cracks' to some degree administratively. Examples include lack of a hyperbaric physician credentialing policy, failure to integrate the service into the hospital's infection control policy, and continuity of care lapses as patients are transferred to hyperbaric medicine from critical care areas and left without appropriate nursing coverage.

The hyperbaric medicine program must be supported by policies, procedures and compliance oversight that is broad enough to ensure safe and effective application of hyperbaric medicine. Resources to assist in the development of this process include the NFPA (patient safety), the UHMS (facility operational guidelines), the BNA (nursing standards and nursing certification), and the NBDHMT (technical and safety).

## FACILITY ACCREDITATION

In 2003, the UHMS introduced hyperbaric facility accreditation. Its goal is to enhance all key aspects of hyperbaric medicine operations and related delivery of care. At the present time this is a voluntary process. Consistent with the accrediting of other diagnostic and therapeutic services, however, it can be expected to eventually evolve into a mandatory requirement, perhaps first prompted by health insurance organizations that purchase HBO therapy.

The present JCAHO hospital accreditation process fails to adequately evaluate hyperbaric medicine. There are no hyperbaric-specific inspection probes and surveyors are unlikely to have any hyperbaric-specific knowledge. Consequently, JCAHO visits to a hyperbaric medicine facility are likely to be cursory and do little to determine whether best practice standards and appropriate patient safety measures are in place and being adhered to.

As with the JCAHO process, UHMS hyperbaric accreditation takes place on a three-year cycle. Its survey team consists of a physician, a nurse and a technician, all of whom are experienced in hyperbaric medicine and formally trained as hyperbaric surveyors.

The UHMS has been advised by the JCAHO that once 100 hyperbaric facilities are accredited, consideration will be given to designating the UHMS as a complimentary accreditation body. The effect of this designation would be that the JCAHO no longer incorporates hyperbaric medicine into its hospital survey process, should a given program be accredited through the UHMS. At the time of this writing (July, 2007), the UHMS has accredited 70 hyperbaric medicine programs, 27 of which have been reaccredited.

## PROGRAM SUCCESS DRIVERS

As noted above, hyperbaric medicine is a physician referral service. The regional medical community, therefore, should have an appreciation of the mechanistic basis of hyperbaric medicine, and how this translates into referable indications. One hopes that those in a position to refer would also be generally aware of the supportive science and where hyperbaric medicine sits in the clinical 'evidence' hierarchy. In most cases, this is going to require a thoughtful, comprehensive and ongoing medical education initiative.

The regional medical community must also develop confidence in the hyperbaric physician team. Such is the history of hyperbaric medicine that some will have formed opinions based upon criticisms of available science that is now decades old. Keys to overcoming this bias, and generating referring physician 'buy-in', are several fold. First, the practice of hyperbaric medicine should be evidence-based to the greatest extent possible for a given condition. There is a growing weight of supportive data that favorably compares hyperbaric oxygen therapy with other therapies for a given condition. While hyperbaric medicine lacks high level evidence for several of its 'approved uses', so, too, do many of its therapeutic alternatives. Where no high level evidence exists for any intervention for a given condition, the evidence-based medicine process dictates that one moves down the evidence hierarchy until 'best evidence' is reached (7). It is during this process that hyperbaric medicine may become identified as 'best evidence.'

To further augment referring physician confidence, hyperbaric medicine should be algorithmically applied wherever possible. In many cases, there exist sufficient criteria to permit selection and treatment based upon patient-specific basis. Transcutaneous oximetry is a case in point. An algorithmic screening process, introduced in 1992 (8), permits the selection of would healing deficient patients whose lesions involve reversal local hypoxia. This allows treatment decisions to be based upon evidence rather that simply a failure of other more conventional therapies. Transcutaneous oximetry testing is also likely to identify hyperbaric 'responders' early in the treatment process, thereby avoiding an unnecessary, somewhat risky, and expensive continued courses of HBO therapy. Equally valuable is the ability of transcutaneous oxygen testing to help identify a therapeutic endpoint. The modern application of HBO therapy for problem wounds, the most common hyperbaric referral, is to employ it until the patient has achieved a critical mass of angiogenesis sufficient to normalize the wound repair process. This is in contrast to the early application of HBO therapy when it was applied until complete healing was achieved. Follow-up tissue oximetry testing will identify this endpoint. The net effect of this algorithmic treatment process is to: (1) Select patients who demonstrate the physiologic capacity to respond locally to systemically delivered hyperbaric oxygen, (2) identify early responders, and undertake additional etiologic testing in those who are not responding, and (3) deliver more financially sound dosing in that HBO is halted once local host competency has been achieved.

How effectively one organizes and implements a regional medical education initiative will have a direct bearing on initial and sustainable patient volumes.

A second success driver is the choice of business model. Several options exist, and center around selection of hyperbaric delivery system and the setting in which it will operate. The choice of a delivery system will, in part, be a function of anticipated patient volumes, local and regional competition (present and potential), space availability and hyperbaric physician team preference. The business setting in which it operates will be dictated largely by those who are encouraging its development and availability.

As previously noted, the introduction of hyperbaric medicine involves both clinical and financial positions. Limiting access to outpatients is certainly attractive from a revenue generation perspective. Hopefully, however, the needs of the patient, across the range of referable indications for hyperbaric medicine, will also be represented during the decision-making process. It would not be too challenging a process, either medically or financially, to accommodate a deserving inpatient or the occasional emergent 'call-back' referral.

Those who intend to introduce a multiplace delivery system will have likely planned for 'full service' clinical operations. The chamber will almost certainly be located within a main hospital building and include in its outfitting the necessary ancillary equipment infrastructure to support the full range of anticipated patient states.

Common within today's monoplace hyperbaric program is its incorporation into the comprehensive wound healing center setting. This setting is invariably on a hospital campus but more likely in an office building rather than within the hospital itself. If the program is office building based, then a single monoplace chamber could be located in the hospital.. Available ancillary technologies incorporated into this chamber will likewise provide for the full range of anticipated patient states. A hospital credentialed hyperbaric physician would need to be available on call, as would a hyperbaric nurse or technologist. Some institutions may elect to provide physician on-call compensation.

Others may expect non-compensated physician call based upon a lack of practice expenses incurred by the physician in a setting provided (expensed) by the hospital, and in contrast to a physician medical office-based practice and its related financial overhead.

Adherence to best practice standards and algorithmic case management, close coordination of HBO therapy with other necessary therapies and regular communication with each referring physician will do much to promote acceptance of the service within the regional medical community. All of this sounds intuitive, but it has not been and is not always the case. Treatment protocols may not always be updated to reflect latest evidence. The hyperbaric physician may not be sufficiently available and engaged, with resultant lack of peer-to-peer communication. The problem wound referral may not receive adequate follow-up and standard wound care if the hyperbaric physician is not sufficiently knowledgeable. Equipment inspection and servicing infrastructure may lack necessary compliance with national oversight organizations and even the hospital's policy expectations.

## CONCLUSION

In summary, the planning and introduction of a hyperbaric medicine service requires a great deal more planning beyond that which forms the basis for other diagnostic and therapeutic technologies. Consideration of the elements noted above in conjunction with a dedicated clinical team will do much to ensure that a hospital's regional community is served by a uniquely valuable resource, one that is life-saving, CNS sparing, infection fighting, tissue salving and advanced wound healing.

# REFERENCES

1. Workman WT, Robinette MD, Laird TD, et al.: Medical planning criteria for implementation of clinical hyperbaric facilities. Brooks Air Force Base, Texas: USAF School of Aerospace Medicine Report 1984.

2. Persels JB: Developing the hyperbaric medicine service. Journal of Hyperbaric Medicine 1987; 2(2):97-105.

3. Clarke D: Economics of Hyperbaric Medicine. Hyperbaric Medicine Practice, Second Edition 1999:143-167, Eds. EP Kindwall & HT Whelan, Best Publishing Co., Flagstaff, AZ.

4. *www.hyperbaricnurses.org* (accessed June 28, 2007).

5. *www.nbdhmt.org* (accessed June 28, 2007).

6. *www.nfpa.org* (accessed June 28, 2007).

7. Sackett DL, Rosenberg WMC, Gray JAM, et al.: Evidence-Based Medicine: What It Is and What It Isn't. BMJ 1996; 312:71-72.

8. Clarke D: An Evidence-Based Approach to Hyperbaric Wound Healing. Blood Gas News 1998; 7(2):14-20.

9. Undersea and Hyperbaric Medical Society Hyperbaric Oxygen Committee Report, 2003. ISBN-0-930406-23-0.

10. Centers for Medicare and Medical Services: National Coverage Determination for Hyperbaric Oxygen Therapy (20.29). Published number 100-3; Manual section number 3 20.29; version 3. 6/19/2006.

11. Aetna Clinical Policy Bulletin: Hyperbaric Oxygen Therapy (HBOT); Number 0172 1/16/2007.

12. Anthem Blue Cross Blue Shield; Medical Policy on Hyperbaric Oxygen Therapy; Number MED.00005 8/01/2006.

CHAPTER 9

# HYPERBARIC NURSING

## CHAPTER NINE OVERVIEW

# HYPERBARIC NURSING

*Valerie J. Messina, Diane M. Norkool*

## INTRODUCTION

The specialty of hyperbaric nursing has evolved since the 1950s along with the practice of hyperbaric medicine. Nurses, qualified by education, experience, and professional licensure, provide care for patients in the altered environment of the hyperbaric chamber. The art and science of nursing are uniquely combined in this setting as nurses not only deal with the technology of the hyperbaric chamber, the physiological monitoring and life support equipment, but also with the art of psychologically adapting the patient, and providing emotional support and patient and family education.

The administrative aspects of setting up a hyperbaric medicine department and training and developing staff also fall into the realm of nursing. This chapter discusses these aspects as well as the practical aspects of hyperbaric nursing.

## HISTORICAL PERSPECTIVES

Clinical hyperbaric oxygen therapy as we know it today evolved from the research and clinical experience of physicians in Europe, primarily in Holland, England and Scotland. Most noted of these was Dr. Ite Boerema in Amsterdam. Prior to 1959, experimental work was conducted in the hyperbaric chambers of the Dutch Royal Navy in Den Helder. At that time, there was one male operating-room nurse who accompanied Dr. Boerema and his colleagues in the hyperbaric chambers while doing experiments. All other members of the hyperbaric team were Dutch Navy divers/technicians who worked both inside and outside the chambers.

In 1959, a large multiplace hyperbaric chamber facility was installed at the Wilhelmina Gasthuis in Amsterdam, and was used primarily for open-heart surgery. Thus, the first hyperbaric nurses were selected from qualified operating-room nurses who volunteered to participate in this unique work environment. At that time, there were beliefs that females might have a higher risk of intraperitoneal infections with hyperbaric exposures; this is now known to be untrue, but for that reason hyperbaric work for nurses was strictly voluntary (4, 12).

When victims of carbon monoxide poisoning, gas gangrene, and other anaerobic necrotizing infections began being treated with hyperbaric oxygen at the Wilhelmina Gasthuis, patient care inside the chambers was provided primarily by anesthesiologists, resident physicians, and young surgeons, since the hyperbaric chamber was so closely integrated into the surgery department. Occasionally, nurses accompanied patients inside the chambers.

Initially, these pioneer hyperbaric nurses received on-the-job training. Later, formal training in hyperbaric therapy was provided by the Dutch Royal Navy in Den Helder, and by the hyperbaric medicine department at the Wilhelmina Gasthuis. When specialization in intensive care and coronary care nursing evolved in the 1960s, this training and experience also became a prerequisite (4).

The multiplace clinical hyperbaric facility at Western Infirmary in Glasgow, Scotland, began in much the same way as the facility in Amsterdam. However, their focus was more on the treatment of various nonhealing wounds, as well as acute carbon monoxide poisoning and anaerobic infections. As one author stated, "Up to the present, medical students and all interested members of the medical staff of the hospital have been rendering valuable and enthusiastic aid. It may well be, however, in the future, when this form of treatment becomes established, that specially trained nursing staff will be integrated as members of the team treating these patients. Such nurses would have to take sole charge of a patient in the chamber on occasions" (20).

The introduction of the Vickers one-man pressure chamber occurred in England; nurses were trained to operate these chambers and to provide care prior to, during, and after hyperbaric treatment. Later nursing auxiliaries were trained as hyperbaric nurse technicians to assist with these treatments (25). In 1964, a Vickers chamber was obtained for a hyperbaric program in Stockholm, Sweden (7) and use of these monoplace chambers spread throughout the world in the later 1960s. A variety of personnel, from nurses to technicians and respiratory therapists, were trained to operate these chambers. See Figure 1.

In the late 1950s in the United States, clinical hyperbaric research was also underway. For example, surgeons from Harvard used an old U.S. Navy decompression chamber to evaluate surgical procedures for correcting heart

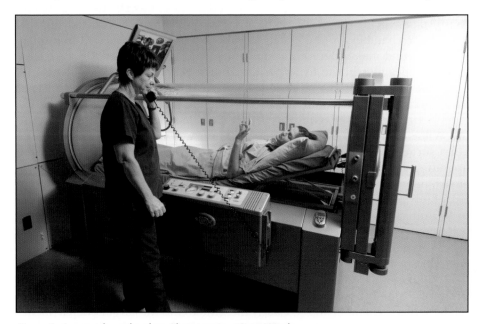

*Figure 1. A monoplace chamber. Photo courtesy Scott Windus.*

abnormalities under pressure. This led to the installation of a huge multiplace hyperbaric facility in the early 1960s at Children's Hospital Medical Center in Boston which was used primarily for cardiovascular surgery (2).

In 1960, Lutheran General Hospital in Park Ridge, Illinois, installed a multiplace hyperbaric facility. Other multiplace facilities at Duke University in North Carolina, Mount Sinai in New York, St. Barnabas Medical Center in New Jersey, Millard Fillmore Hospital in Buffalo, New York and the University of Maryland Hospital, to name a few, soon followed (1, 36). The Royal Victoria Hospital in Montreal established the first Canadian medical hyperbaric facility in 1963. Toronto General Hospital opened its unit in 1964, and Vancouver General Hospital opened its facility in 1965 (45). Vickers monoplace chambers were also being installed in some hospitals. Most noted of these was the unit at the United States Naval Hospital in Long Beach, California (15).

As in Europe, some of the first American hyperbaric nurses were operating-room nurses. HBO was being used to treat many other conditions, so nurses with experience primarily in critical care, as well as emergency room nursing and medical-surgical nursing, were being trained in the specialty of hyperbaric oxygen therapy. An interest in research was also a prerequisite. Some hyperbaric units like the one at Lutheran General used registered nurses exclusively for patient care during hyperbaric treatment (18, 35).

Nursing had the opportunity to be involved in the planning and development of some of these early hyperbaric programs. The most publicized of these was at Mount Sinai Hospital in New York. Venger and Jacobson described this program's development as an ideal project for showing the value of cooperation between the nurse, the clinician, and the administrator (41). Nursing needs were identified and divided into two areas: selection of personnel and staffing; training and staff development. Patient care needs focused around emotional support, patient teaching, medical therapy, surgical procedures, and experimental research. Venger described the potential of hyperbaric nursing as being founded on the medical program, and on the findings relative to research (42). Further, she challenged that nurses had an innate responsibility to keep pace as their role broadened and expanded (40). It is noteworthy that the chamber at Mount Sinai was organizationally under the department of nursing.

During the 1960s and early 1970s, the subject of hyperbaric oxygen therapy received considerable attention in nursing journals around the world. Although physicians contributed some of these articles, the majority of these were published by nurses working in hyperbaric therapy (9, 13, 16, 19, 21, 28, 30, 31, 32, 38, 39). While these articles addressed nurses in general, one publication in a nursing textbook provided an in-depth analysis of the nurse's role in hyperbaric therapy. This information, written over four decades ago, remains current to this day (26).

Communication between nurses working in hyperbaric oxygen therapy occurred on an informal basis for many years. It wasn't until the Fifth International Hyperbaric Congress in Vancouver, B.C., Canada, in 1973, that a small group of nurses and respiratory therapists met for half a day and presented papers, as well as shared experiences. Another formal meeting of this kind did not occur again until 1982 in Norfolk, Virginia, when the

Undersea Medical Society (UMS) Associates sponsored a half-day program of presentations by technicians, nurses, and respiratory therapists. This was the first time that the UMS Associates had conducted their own program in conjunction with the UMS Annual Scientific Meeting. From that time on, the Associates continued to grow into an active organization with a rapid increase in membership, including nurses, and representation on the UMS Executive Committee.

The annual conferences on the clinical application of hyperbaric oxygen therapy sponsored by the Baromedical Department at Memorial Medical Center in Long Beach, California, attracted many hyperbaric nurses as well as physicians, respiratory therapists and technicians. In 1978 this conference began including workshops specifically for nurses.

## HYPERBARIC NURSING AS A SPECIALITY

The specialty of hyperbaric nursing was formally recognized with the founding and incorporation of the Baromedical Nurses Association (BNA) in 1985. The BNA was established with 35 founding RN members at the joint meeting of the UMS Annual Scientific Meeting, and the Long Beach clinical hyperbaric conference. The BNA, which is international in scope, maintains a membership of 200 registered nurses from approximately ten countries. Functions of the BNA include promoting professional activities that enhance the effectiveness of hyperbaric nursing in the health care system, and promoting educational opportunities for nurses practicing in the specialty. The BNA develops and maintains standards of practice in hyperbaric nursing and supports nursing research efforts (5). Hyperbaric nurses may now achieve specialty certification as a certified, or advanced-certified hyperbaric nurse, or as a hyperbaric nurse clinician. Since its inception, the face of the BNA has aged, but its mission to serve nurses practicing in the field of clinical hyperbaric nursing is essentially unchanged. Information and an application for membership can be obtained from the Baromedical Nurses Association through internet access at www.hyperbaricnurses.org.

In hyperbaric medicine, a collegial role between the nurse and the physician exists, roles both independent and interdependent (17). This collegial role has been described throughout the evolution of hyperbaric nursing, and it continues as the BNA joins the Undersea and Hyperbaric Medical Society (UHMS) for their annual scientific meetings, providing a forum for sharing scientific knowledge between the members of the hyperbaric health care team. The BNA is also represented on the UHMS Executive Committee by the BNA President.

## QUALIFICATIONS FOR HYPERBARIC NURSES

The patient population treated at hospital-based hyperbaric departments is quite diverse in age, diagnosis and degree of acuteness. Because of this diversity, the hyperbaric nurse should be experienced and competent in medical-surgical nursing of ill adults and children. One year of critical care experience is highly recommended and is required at most hyperbaric facilities as well as Advanced Cardiac Life Support (ACLS) and Pediatric Advanced Life Support (PALS) certifications. Good communication skills are essential both for patient care and for working with other departments and other hospitals involved in the care of the patient receiving HBO therapy. Good leadership skills are needed to coordinate and provide continuity of care to patients and to direct patient care provided by non-nursing staff. A high degree of technical skill and expertise is also beneficial in the hyperbaric setting, as the hyperbaric chambers and ancillary equipment are technically state-of-the-art. Hyperbaric staff must also be available for on-call emergency coverage (44). Nursing staff must be licensed in the state in which they practice and must function within the guidelines of the Nurse Practice Act of that state.

Nurses who are applying for work inside a multiplace hyperbaric chamber must also meet specific physical requirements (24). These must be rigid in the area of pulmonary, ear, and sinus function. There must be no history of seizure disorder, insulin-dependent diabetes, or claustrophobia which could render the inside attendant unconscious or incapacitated. Pre-existing conditions, such as certain orthopedic injuries, may increase the risk of developing decompression sickness, and would be a disqualifying factor, as would conditions involving chronic pain, even if intermittent, that could be confused with symptoms of decompression sickness.

Pregnancy is an absolute contraindication to working in a high-pressure environment, and all female inside-chamber attendants must be warned of potential danger to the fetus. Any female attendant trying to become pregnant must avoid hyperbaric exposure. While these physical requirements are very specific, hyperbaric inside-attendant staff do not need to meet the physical requirements of recreational divers, such as stamina and the ability to swim. Applicants for hyperbaric inside-attendant positions need to be evaluated by a physician knowledgeable in diving and hyperbaric medicine (10, 37).

Staffing for a hyperbaric department is dictated by the state laws in which the facility operates. Joint Commission on Accreditation of Healthcare Organizations (JCAHO) guidelines influence the staffing and the practice of nursing in hyperbaric units (22). Accountability to these legislative and organizational guidelines is paramount to a department's success.

## HYPERBARIC OXYGEN THERAPY TRAINING

All hyperbaric personnel involved in patient care and chamber operations must be trained in hyperbaric medicine theory and clinical practice, including technical procedures. Effective patient management and safety procedures cannot be learned in the classroom alone. Hands-on training and precepted on-the-job experience are essential to develop a level of expertise necessary for providing safe, comprehensive, quality patient care.

Hyperbaric departments utilizing multiplace chambers usually have a facilities manager with knowledge and expertise in chamber systems operation and maintenance, as well as expertise in the use of diving tables. See Figure 2. Personnel for these positions usually come from the military or from a commercial diving setting. Patient care planning and delivery of patient care, however, is in the domain of nursing. It is important that an RN be in charge of this activity for both multiplace and monoplace chamber facilities. JCAHO guidelines require that nursing services be directed by a nurse executive who is a registered nurse qualified by advanced education and management experience (22).

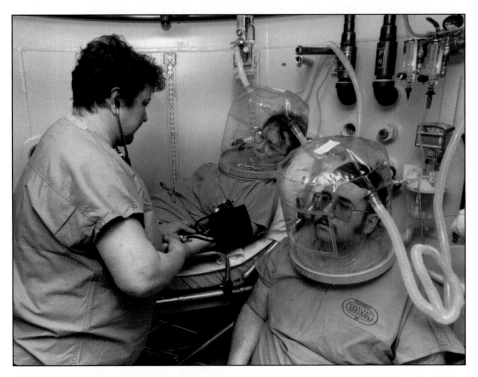

Figure 2. The multiplace chamber's oxygen hoods in use.

The most efficient use of staff in a multiplace hyperbaric facility is obtained through cross-training. Registered nurses should be trained to operate the chamber, and technical staff should have Emergency Medical Technician or Diver Medical Technician training and certification to work inside the chamber during patient treatments. The use of on-call staff in addition to full-time staff provides for better treatment coverage and reduces the risk of staff burn-out, and the risk of developing decompression sickness. The use of on-call staff has a favorable impact on the budget; it decreases overtime pay, nonproductive paid time, and the indirect costs from fringe benefits.

There are several medical centers that sponsor hyperbaric training programs for physicians, nurses, and technicians in either monoplace or multiplace chamber settings. These training programs are ideal for staff starting out in a newly established hyperbaric program. Information on hyperbaric courses can be obtained through the Undersea and Hyperbaric Medical Society, Bethesda, MD. Some hyperbaric chamber manufacturers also provide training in the operation of their equipment. Established hyperbaric departments often provide their own training program for new staff. Businesses that start up hyperbaric medicine departments in clinics and hospitals also provide training for the hyperbaric staff.

Course content for nurses includes didactic sessions and clinical practicum on the following topics: introduction and history of hyperbaric medicine; mechanisms of HBO; gas laws and HBO physiology; standards for the clinical use of HBO; complications of HBO, contraindications, and safety precautions; pharmacology of HBO; application of HBO in medical, diving, orthopedic, neurological, compromised wound healing, infectious disease conditions; the role of the hyperbaric nurse; care of the critically ill patient in the hyperbaric chamber; and reimbursement issues.

Nurses also participate in relevant continuing-education programs to remain prepared for their responsibilities in the hyperbaric specialty unit. In order to practice in this setting, the hyperbaric nurse must be knowledgeable of the complex patient environment found in hyperbaric nursing. Basic and critical care nursing skills, as well as hyperbaric skills such as transcutaneous oxygen monitoring are reviewed and validated yearly per state and JCAHO standards (22).

## THE ROLE OF THE HYPERBARIC NURSE

Hyperbaric nursing was defined by the BNA as "the diagnosis and treatment of human responses to actual or potential health problems in the altered environment of the hyperbaric chamber" (6). This further expands the American Nurses Association's definition of nursing which is "the protection, promotion, and optimization of health and abilities, prevention of illness and injury, alleviation of suffering through the diagnosis and treatment of human response, and advocacy in the care of individuals, families, communities and populations (3). Hyperbaric nursing was further defined in the publication *Hyperbaric Nursing*, a text of essential and practical information devoted to the specialty of hyperbaric nursing (24).

The hyperbaric nurse has a multifunctional role—that of clinician, educator, and researcher. The administrative role may also be an integral function in managing the department and supervising patient care. The goal of hyperbaric nursing is to provide safe, cost-effective, quality patient care, according to established standards (11).

### The Hyperbaric Nurse Clinician

Hyperbaric nurse clinicians utilize the nursing process to provide direct patient care. Hyperbaric patients are first assessed using the nursing theoretical framework of the institution in which the hyperbaric facility is located. Nurses assess for risks related to hyperbaric medicine, and the psychological and physiological status of the patient. The assessment is then used as a database to develop a care plan for the hyperbaric patient. HBO treatment is administered according to hyperbaric protocol, physician orders, and clinical practice guidelines. Patients are continually assessed during treatment and nursing actions are provided as necessary to prevent or manage any complications, and to continue medical and nursing interventions. After treatment, evaluation is done to assess the response to treatment and the presence of complications. The nursing process is documented in the health team record. An example of a treatment documentation format is demonstrated in Table 1. Electronic medical records are being implemented in hyperbaric units for documenting the treatment, nursing process, and outcomes.

Part of nursing practice involves activities within the medical domain. Administering    medications,    performing    treatments,    and    monitoring

## TABLE 1. HYPERBARIC OXYGEN TREATMENT RECORD

| | |
|---|---|
| DATE | _____ |
| TREATMENT NO. | _____ |
| TIME IN/TIME OUT | _____ |
| ATA/TOTAL TIME | _____ |
| OXYGEN/AIR BREAKS | _____ |
| PRE-HBO ASSESSMENT | _____ |
| POST-HBO EVALUATION | _____ |
| HBO TREATMENT ADMINISTERED | _____ |
| PHYSIOLOGICAL MONITOR/ LIFE SUPPORT EQUIPMENT | _____ |
| NURSING DIAGNOSIS: POTENTIAL FOR INJURY RT HBO TREATMENT | _____ |
| PROTOCOL IMPLEMENTED | _____ |
| MULTIDISCIPLINARY TEAM ROUNDS | _____ |
| SIGNIFICANT FINDINGS | _____ |
| | _____ |

physiological changes are delegated medical functions. The domain of nursing practice, however, deals with activities that address human responses to actual or potential problems related to an altered health status (physiological, psychological, sociological, and cognitive). It is the nurse who helps patients and their families manage illness and medical treatment as it impacts on their ability to cope and their activities of daily living (8).

Patient care standards reflect the application of the nursing process for specific patient care situations. They establish nursing diagnosis of patient and family problems associated with illness and medical treatment, they identify patient and family-focused desired outcomes of nursing care, and they develop nursing interventions that will assist the patient and family in preventing, relieving, or coping with identified problems in daily living (34).

Standards help to operationalize the nursing process and to provide baseline criteria for evaluating the quality of nursing care delivered to patients. They provide the basis for continuity of care delivered to one patient by many caregivers, or for continuity within groups of patients with common problems and needs (34).

Within the following patient care standards, there are nursing diagnostic statements related to common human responses, either actual or potential, associated with a medical condition or treatment. The desired outcomes are derived from the nursing diagnosis, and the interventions are specific statements of nursing actions that address the nursing diagnosis. While these interventions are specific in nature, they still allow for flexibility to include the unique variability of individuals. The patient care standards in Table 2 represent examples which are generic to all patients receiving HBO (33).

## The Nurse as Educator

Facilitating the educational process of patients and families is an accountability of the hyperbaric nurse. Patient education helps maximize the

---

## TABLE 2. CARE OF THE PATIENT RECEIVING HYPERBARIC OXYGEN THERAPY

---

I.  A.  NURSING DIAGNOSIS/PROBLEMS
       Potential complications: barotrauma to ears, sinuses, and lungs related to changes in atmospheric pressure inside the HBO chamber, or cerebral gas embolism associated with gas expansion during decompression.

    B.  DESIRED OUTCOMES
        1.  Barotrauma and gas embolism will be prevented.
        2.  Signs and symptoms of barotrauma or gas embolism will be recognized and promptly treated if present.

    C.  NURSING INTERVENTIONS
        1.  Prior to HBO treatment instruct patient in ear equalization techniques such as swallowing, chewing, yawning, tilting head back, and modified Valsalva maneuver.
        2.  Prior to HBO treatment, administer decongestants and assist patient, if necessary, with decongestant nasal spray per physician orders.
        3.  Monitor patients during HBO therapy for signs and symptoms of barotrauma including:
            a. signs and symptoms of middle ear barotraumas,
            b. increased rate or decrease in depth of respirations,
            c. signs and symptoms of pneumothorax
            d. observed swallowing of gas.
        4.  Stop chamber pressurization to allow additional time for pressure equalization if patient is not successful in doing so. Notify physician if patient is unable to clear his/her ears.
        5.  Remind patient to breath normally during pressure changes.
        6.  Document instruction, observations, and patient's ability to follow instructions.

II  A.  NURSING DIAGNOSIS/PROBLEMS
       Potential anxiety and fear related to feelings of claustrophobia associated with confinement in HBO chamber.

---

**TABLE 2.** *(Continued)*

---

B.   DESIRED OUTCOMES
Patient will be able to tolerate being in the HBO chamber for duration of treatment.

C.   NURSING INTERVENTIONS
1.   Monitor and document patient's behavior for symptoms of claustrophobia including:
   a. restlessness,
   b. inability to tolerate face mask or head hood
   c. statements of feeling confined or trapped
2.   Talk to patient with a soft voice.
3.   Ask patient to make eye contact with nurse.
4.   Reassure patient that he/she is safe.
5.   Engage patient in problem-solving his/her feelings of claustrophobia such as visualization, distraction, listening to music, etc.
6.   Notify physician if patient is having problems with claustrophobia.
7.   Administer anti-anxiety medications per physician's orders.
8.   Monitor and document patient response to anti-anxiety medication and other interventions.

III.   A   NURSING DIAGNOSIS/PROBLEMS
Potential complication: oxygen toxicity related to administration of 100% oxygen at increased atmospheric pressure.

B.   DESIRED OUTCOMES
1.   Signs and symptoms of oxygen toxicity will be promptly recognized, reported, and treated.
2.   Oxygen toxicity seizure will be avoided.

C.   NURSING INTERVENTIONS
1.   Instruct patient how to recognize signs and symptoms of oxygen toxicity.
   a. Central nervous system (CNS) oxygen toxicity: numbness and tingling, ringing in ears, vertigo, blurred vision, nausea, restlessness, difficulty breathing, and/or palpitations.
   b. Pulmonary oxygen toxicity: tightness in chest, dry hacking cough, and/or difficulty inhaling a full breath.
2.   Monitor for oxygen toxicity risk factors.
3.   Monitor for signs and symptoms of CNS and pulmonary oxygen toxicity. Notify physician. Document.
4.   Immediately switch breathing gas from oxygen to air if patient has symptoms of CNS oxygen toxicity.
5.   Initiate emergency protocol if patient has a CNS oxygen toxicity seizure. Notify physician. Document.

benefit of hyperbaric therapy's integration into the total health care delivery system, and helps improve cost effectiveness, and maintain patient safety and facilitate care. The principles of teaching/learning are utilized as the nurse assesses for readiness to learn, and adapts the teaching process to the individual patient and family. A thorough orientation to HBO, including the concepts and patient objectives in Table 3 is facilitated with the use of audiovisual aids such as videos and pamphlets.

Participation in educational programs for the community and for the health care team enhances the advancement of the specialty and the effectiveness of hyperbaric medicine in the health care system. As examples of the educator role, nurses facilitate patient care conferences, inservices, and other formal classes on hyperbaric medicine for their medical centers, and

---

## TABLE 3. PATIENT ORIENTATION TO HYPERBARIC OXYGEN THERAPY

---

CONCEPT:     Effects of hyperbaric oxygen therapy.
OBJECTIVES:  Verbalizes purpose and indication for treatment.

CONCEPT:     Psychological adaptation to the hyperbaric chamber.
OBJECTIVES:  Verbalizes self-control for exiting chamber prn.
             Identifies/refines own relaxation techniques.
             Demonstrates technique for calling for nurse.
             Discusses when/how to request sedative for relaxation prn.

CONCEPT:     Signs & Symptoms of possible complications.
OBJECTIVES:  Verbalizes/recognizes S & S of middle ear & sinus barotrauma.
             Identifies/verbalizes S & S of visual acuity changes.
             Identifies/verbalizes S & S of oxygen toxicity.

CONCEPT:     Safety protocols for hyperbaric oxygen treatments.
OBJECTIVES:  Demonstrates knowledge of safety protocols - patient gown on,
                 toiletries removed, jewelry off.
             Recognizes importance of limiting vitamin C & aspirin.
             Verbalizes/recognizes need to empty bladder before treatment.

CONCEPT:     Middle ear equalization.
OBJECTIVES:  Demonstrates technique for "clearing ears."
             Discusses ability to request decongestants for congestion.

CONCEPT:     Smoking cessation.
OBJECTIVES:  Verbalizes importance of cessation: effect on tissue oxygenation.
             Verbalizes resources/mechanisms to assist with cessation.

participate in multidisciplinary rounds on hyperbaric patients. Nurses also contribute to web sites for health care institutions and professional organizations that provide hyperbaric medicine education.

## The Nurse as Researcher

Nurses are frequently involved in the arena of medical research, in cooperation with the hyperbaric physician, administering HBO treatments according to investigational protocols, developing research protocols and their implementation, and reporting and publishing the results. The testing of new technology in the hyperbaric field is often delegated to nurses who will be utilizing the equipment.

Nurses working in hyperbaric departments centered at academic institutions will find opportunities to be involved in research projects at the basic laboratory stage. Working in these types of settings requires the professional nurse to draw upon her scientific background and training. These nurses perform experiments, collect and analyze data, and document results. The nurse becomes integral to the research team when the project advances from the laboratory stage to human studies. Nurses involved in research being conducted in the area of wound healing are helping to define and document the benefit of new technology (43). The unique perspective that nursing provides, aids in the design of functional, effective, and patient-friendly equipment that will be used as an adjunct to hyperbaric oxygen treatments to serve the population of patients with problem wounds.

As healthcare resources diminish, hyperbaric nurses are also challenged to conduct nursing research to define and validate their role, and to describe the client's response to actual or potential health problems in the altered environment (17). Nursing research has been presented at recent BNA and UHMS meetings, but wider publication of these results should be encouraged in order to better disseminate the acquired knowledge.

## The Nurse as Manager

Responsibility for management of resources in the hyperbaric department often is in the realm of the hyperbaric nurse who functions in a management position. Accountabilities may include management of resources—staffing, supplies and services, and supervision of patient care. Responsibilities may include coordination of clinical and educational activities and research within the department. In the multiplace setting, this may be a shared responsibility with a facilities manager. The nurse manager is accountable for directing and monitoring the department's adherence to state laws, JCAHO standards, and NFPA standards. These monitors include fire drills, disaster preparedness, and environment of care reviews (22, 29).

## ADVANCED PRACTICE NURSING IN HYPERBARIC MEDICINE

Advanced practice nurses (APN), nurse practitioners (NP), and/or clinical nurse specialists (CNS) are nurses with a Master's degree in nursing and advanced clinical education. Many states have granted APNs independent prescriptive authority and insurance companies, Medicare and Medicaid, reimburse for care provided by APNs.

Proper utilization of the APN in the hyperbaric medicine unit will increase the opportunity for research and coverage of increased patient populations in the units. The APN may be responsible for pre-treatment history and physicals, as well as care and intervention needed during HBO therapy. APNs maintain quality health care, and add to the research potential of HBO therapy.

## PEDIATRICS

Use of HBO in the pediatric population requires skill and knowledge in the care and treatment of children's physical, as well as emotional conditions. Children present a particular challenge based on age and cognition. Fears of confinement anxiety and separation need to be addressed. Hyperbaric nurses need to show evidence of age-specific training and skills which are reviewed and validated annually. Some facilities require Pediatric Advanced Life Support (PALS) certification for hyperbaric nurses treating children in the hyperbaric chamber.

Parents can and should be present to talk and interact with their child. Reading stories or watching a favorite movie are helpful distractions. In cases in which a child becomes fearful or anxious before entering the chamber, the use of guided imagery is beneficial. Asking the child to name his/her special place, such as a castle, rocket ship, etc., and helping to make up a story about it can keep him/her occupied. Writing the story down or recording it can be used for future treatments. Cognition and age-appropriate guided imagery and movies can be used for distraction in the chambers. Multiplace hyperbaric facilities allow closer contact with children and can alleviate anxiety due to separation.

## TRENDS

Demand for hyperbaric nurses is growing as the number of hyperbaric facilities and the number of patients receiving hyperbaric treatment has grown (14). The focus of most hyperbaric facilities currently centers on the management of problem wounds (23, 27). Some hyperbaric departments have changed their names to reflect the emphasis on wound management. Many hyperbaric nurses have become experts in wound care; some also serve as wound-care consultants to non-hyperbaric patients within their medical centers. Just as the practice of hyperbaric medicine is dynamic, so is the process of defining the role of nurses practicing within this unique specialty. Hyperbaric nursing continues to be responsive to the changing health care needs of our patients and the health care environment. Maintaining patient safety and quality of care while ensuring adequate reimbursement challenges the hyperbaric nurse as we begin the 21st century.

# REFERENCES

1. Abbott C. "The use of the hyperbaric chamber as an auxiliary curing aid." AORN Journal. 1969;9 (5):80-84.

2. Adams J. "Hyperbaric oxygen therapy." American Journal of Nursing. 1964;64 (6):76-79.

3. American Nurses Association. Nursing's Social Policy Statement, 2nd Ed. Silver Spring, Missouri, 2003, American Nurses Association, p.6.

4. Bakker D. Letter of personal communication, April 8, 1991.

5. Baromedical Nurses Association. Rules, Article 1, Section 1, 1985.

6. Baromedical Nurses Association. "Position statement of the BNA." BNA Update. July, 1987.

7. Barr P. Telephone communication, May 2, 1991.

8. Carnevali D, Mitchell P, Woods N, Tanner C. Diagnostic Reasoning in Nursing. Philadelphia: J. B. Lippincott Co., 1984.

9. Cockerill G, O'Conner R. "Hyperbaric oxygenation - a new field opened for nurses." Nursing Times. 1967;63:216-218.

10. Davis J. Medical Examination of Sport Scuba Divers. San Antonio, 1986, Medical Seminars, Inc.

11. De Jesus-Greenberg D, Messina V, Mones C, Chase P. "Hyperbaric oxygen therapy in critical care." In Zschoche D, editor: Comprehensive Review of Critical Care, (3rd Ed.). St. Louis, 1986, The C. V. Mosby Co., pp.301-310.

12. Fegan F. "Hyperbaric oxygen therapy centers." Nursing Forum. 1964; III: (2):90-101.

13. Fegan F. "What is hyperbaric oxygen therapy?" American Association of Industrial Nurses Journal. 1964;12 (2):11-13.

14. Gaskill, M. "Deep Impact." NurseWeek. 2003; 8(1-3).

15. Gaul A, Thompson R, Hart G. "Hyperbaric Oxygen Therapy." American Journal of Nursing. 1972;72 (5):892-896.

16. Gaul A, Hart G. "Baromedical nursing combines critical, acute, chronic care." AORN Journal. 1975;21 (6):1038-1047.

17. Gaul A. Keynote address to First Annual Baromedical Nurses Association Meeting, Key Biscayne, FL, April, 1986.

18. Gaynor, M. Editorial. "Nursing under pressure." Nursing Outlook. 1964;12 (5):29.

19. Greenberg D, Messina V, Reichow W, MacLean C. "Hyperbaric oxygen: Exciting new clinical results." RN. 1979;42 (9):52-57.

20. Griffiths J. "Oxygen therapy in a high pressure environment: recent advance in treatment." Nursing Mirror. 1962;115:171-173.

21. Hanson G. "Hyperbaric oxygenation." Nursing Times. 1967;63:213-216.

22. Joint Commission on Accreditation of Healthcare Organizations. Comprehensive Accreditation Manual for Hospitals: The Official Handbook. Oak Brook, IL, 2007, Joint Commission on Accreditation of Healthcare Organizations.

23. Kob DG, Gesell LB, Spadafora MP, Liu T. "Utilization and staffing of monoplace hyperbaric facilities in the United States." Undersea & Hyperbaric Medicine. 1998;25 (Supplement):25.

24. Larson-Lohr, V. Norvell, H (Ed.) Hyperbaric Nursing. Flagstaff, AZ, Best Publishing Company, 2002.

25. Maudsley R, Mandow G, Lustig E, Daly B. "Experience with a hyperbaric oxygen unit." Nursing Mirror. 1966;9:x-xii.

26. Molbo D. "The nurse's role in hyperbaric therapy." In: (Bergersen BS, [et al.] Eds.) Current Concepts in Clinical Nursing. St. Louis: The C.V. Mosby Co., 1967:57-75.

27. Moon, RE. "Use of hyperbaric oxygen in the management of selected wounds." Advances in Wound Care. 1998;11(7):332-334.

28. Nash M. "Hyperbaric Medicine." The Australian Nurse's Journal. 1974;3(8):24-26.

29. National Fire Protection Association, NFPA-99: Standard for Health Care Facilities. Quincy, MA, 2005, National Fire Protection Association.

30. Neelon V, McIntosh H. "Hyperbaric oxygenation. Part I: therapeutic benefits." Cardiovascular Nursing. 1971;7(3):69-72.

31. Neelon V, McIntosh H. "Hyperbaric oxygenation. Part II: hazards and implications." Cardiovascular Nursing. 1971;7(4):73-76.

32. Norkool D. "Current concepts of hyperbaric oxygenation and its application in critical care." Heart & Lung. 1979;8(4):728-735.

33. Norkool D. "Care of the patient receiving hyperbaric oxygen therapy (HBO)." In: Reiner A, (Ed.) Manual of Patent Care Standards. Gaithersburg, MD, Aspen Publications, 1992.

34. Reiner A (Ed). Manual of Patient Care Standards. Gaithersburg, MD, 1991, Aspen Publications.

35. Robinson A. "Hyperbaric oxygen unit." Nursing Outlook. 1964;12:40-41.

36. Shaw B. "Whatever happened to hyperbaric medicine?" RN. 1969;32(11):50-55.

37. Sheffield P, Davis J, Bell G, Gallagher T. "Hyperbaric chamber clinical support multiplace." In (Davis J, Hunt T, Eds.) Hyperbaric Oxygen Therapy. Bethesda, MD, Undersea Medical Society, 1977;25-39.

38. Thompson M. "Treating a patient in the pressure chamber." Nursing Times. 1964;60:174.

39. Vaughan P. "Success of hyperbarics in modern medicine." The Nursing Journal of India. 1966;57(9):264.

40. Venger M, Jacobson J. "Nursing plans for a hyperbaric unit." American Journal of Nursing. 1964;64(10):79-81.

41. Venger M, Jacobson J. "Hyperbaric oxygenation: a nursing challenge." International Nursing Review. 1965;12(1):17-19.

42. Venger M. "Hyperbaric oxygenation: nursing responsibility in planning for a new clinical service." Nursing Clinics of North America. 1966;1(1):131-142.

43. Whelan HT, Houle JM, Donohoe DL, Bajie DM, Schmidt MH, Reichert KW, Weyenberg GT, Lasron DL, Meyer GA, Caviness JA. "Medical Applications of Space Light-Emitting Diode Technology - Space Station and Beyond." Space Technology & Application International Forum. 1999;458(1):3-15.

44. Wills-Long S, Long C, Laybourne M. "Hyperbaric oxygen therapy - nursing opportunity." Dimensions of Critical Care Nursing. 1989;8(3):176-182.

45. Zilm G. "Hyperbaric oxygen units - high pressure nursing." The Canadian Nurse. 1969;65(2):37-40.

# NOTES

CHAPTER 10

# THE USE OF DRUGS UNDER PRESSURE

## CHAPTER TEN OVERVIEW

# THE USE OF DRUGS UNDER PRESSURE

*Eric P. Kindwall*

## OXYGEN AS A DRUG

Oxygen, under pressure, behaves like a drug. Therefore, one would naturally be concerned that there might be multiple drug interactions of which to be cognizant. Fortunately, however, most drugs do not have any detrimental combined effect with increased oxygen partial pressures. Indeed, there are a number of beneficial synergisms. Although important exceptions exist, it is usually safe to assume that unless there are specific contraindications or precautions regarding the use of a particular substance or drug under pressure, it is safe to administer it. Significant known exceptions are covered in this chapter.

## PRACTICAL CONSIDERATIONS

The mechanical effects of pressure on the drug container are our first concern. It is important that the drugs, which are stocked in the multiplace chamber and which are subjected to continual compressions and decompressions, retain their absolute seal at the maximum pressure anticipated. In our experience, glass vials easily resist pressures ranging up to six atmospheres. When opening small two or three milliliter vials under pressure, we have not experienced any particular problems with implosion. However, caution should be used when opening large 10 ml glass vials at pressures of three atmospheres or greater. The vials should be wrapped in gauze to avoid flying glass generated by implosion. Alternatively, the vial can be opened outside the chamber and the contents locked in (in a syringe). If a rubber-stoppered vial is used into which a needle is introduced to withdraw the contents, the vial should not be pressurized again. Even if only a single dose is used in the multiple-dose vial, the vial should be discarded at the conclusion of decompression because of possible contamination and the fact that air can enter the vial during subsequent compressions and force out the contents during decompression, especially if the vial is lying on its side. One large hyperbaric unit has reported an apparent decrease in potency in certain drugs when subjected to continuous compression-decompression cycles (13).

IV solutions are now generally stocked in plastic bags, which do not present any problem when used in the multiplace chamber. However, certain drugs, such as low molecular weight Dextran, still come in glass bottles. Glass bottles are usable in the chamber so long as a vent tube is provided that reaches to the bottom of the bottle. During compression, a vent tube is not required; increasing pressure causes air to bubble freely through the contents of the IV bottles and gather at the top. During decompression, however, an air vent tube is mandatory, or the expanding air in the IV bottle above the liquid will forcefully drive the entire contents of the bottle into the patient's circulation all at once. This will be followed by a bolus of air, which may vary in amount from a few milliliters to over a liter. If a glass bottle is used with no vent tube extending through the contents to the bottom, the bottle may be turned over so that the vent needle is on top. This will allow any air in the bottle to escape during decompression without emptying the bottle of its contents. In such case, the IV will necessarily be halted during decompression.

Flexible plastic bags holding infusion mixtures or blood require no special vent tubes. Flexible containers actually are ideal for infusion mixtures stored in the chamber for protracted periods. We experienced one case where a sealed, unopened 500 ml glass bottle of normal saline apparently had some air forced into it after being cycled through a number of compressions, and exploded in a storage cabinet during decompression from six atmospheres. It is recommended that all IV fluids used in chambers be stored in bags.

Infusion pumps may be used in the multiplace chamber if battery powered. If supplied from line voltage, the plug must be of the explosion-proof type, which positively locks and the current must be supplied through an isolation transformer. It should be noted that at this writing (2008), the NFPA code has been revised and the chamber atmosphere is no longer classified as explosive, but is now classified as hazardous. This will means that some electrical equipment that was banned in the past is now permitted.

## Routes of Drug Administration

Hyperbaric oxygen causes a vasoconstriction in normal tissues resulting in up to a 20% reduction in blood flow. It was thought that this same vasoconstriction would also severely impede the normal absorption of drugs injected intramuscularly and subcutaneously. However, Emerson et al., in Fremantle, Australia, compared blood levels of midazolam administered in the chamber to the levels attained at atmospheric pressure (7). Twenty normal volunteers were injected with midazolam (Versed®) on the surface breathing air. Later their blood levels were correlated with the levels reached when the drug was injected at 2.8 ATA while the subjects breathed oxygen. In 65% of the subjects peak levels occurred earlier while at 2.8 ATA. Peak levels occurred significantly later at 2.8 ATA in only 15%. The mean time to peak level at 2.8 ATA was 33 minutes, and 41 minutes at 1 ATA. The oral route is not affected, nor is administration of drugs by inhalation degraded. However, the intravenous route is probably the best choice for delivering drugs in the chamber.

## DRUGS INCOMPATIBLE WITH HYPERBARIC OXYGEN

### Cis-Platinum

Cis-Platinum, a chemotherapeutic agent used in testicular, ovarian, head and neck, and other cancers, interferes with DNA synthesis which affects fibroblast production and collagen synthesis. Using mice, Nemiroff studied the use of HBO to determine whether or not HBO might help mitigate those effects. Wound breaking strength was found to be adversely affected by HBO in these animals when compared to controls (25). HBO may increase the cytotoxic effect of the drug in the tissues, thereby impeding wound healing. Any patient who has a wound healing problem (such as radionecrosis) should not be treated concomitantly with hyperbaric oxygen and Cis-Platinum. However, in a life-threatening situation such as CO poisoning, gas gangrene, or necrotizing fasciitis, wound-healing concerns are overridden by the emergency indication and are not an issue.

## Doxorubicin (Adriamycin®)

Animal studies were carried out by Upton, et al., to determine if tissue damage caused by extravasation of doxorubicin could be counteracted by hyperbaric oxygen (35). Other agents such as beta-carotene, sodium bicarbonate, butylated hydroxytoluene (BHT), hydrocortisone, and ice were also tried. All the other ingredients made no difference or produced only a slight improvement in healing. However, those animals exposed to HBO experienced an 87% mortality when concomitantly receiving doxorubicin. The mortality remained equally high using once a day or b.i.d. HBO regimens. Thus, HBO and doxorubicin should never be combined. At least three days should elapse between the last doxorubicin dose and the initiation of a course of HBO.

## Mafenide Acetate (Sulfamylon®)

Pruitt and his group at Brook Army Burn Center popularized this antibacterial agent, which was first developed by the Germans. It has been shown to suppress bacterial growth in burn patients significantly reducing mortality secondary to burn sepsis. However, Sulfamylon® is a carbonic anhydrase inhibitor, which will tend to cause a build up of $CO_2$, which in turn promotes a vasodilatation. Bornside and Nance demonstrated that peripheral vasodilatation in burned animals, coupled with a central vasoconstriction induced by hyperbaric oxygen, produces results which are worse than when using either agent alone (4). For this reason, if a burn patient is referred for hyperbaric therapy, Sulfamylon® must be carefully removed by showering before the patient is put in the chamber. Silver sulfadiazine (Silvadene®) may be substituted effectively and safely.

## DRUGS COMMONLY USED WITH HYPERBARIC OXYGEN OR THAT MAY HAVE SPECIAL CONSIDERATION

## Bleomycin

**Ble·o·my·cin** (ble"o-mi'sin) *any of a mixture of glycopeptide antibiotics produced by a strain of Streptomyces verticillus, designated $A_1$ to $A_6$, $A_2$', and $B_1$ to B6, that bind to DNA causing chain scission and removal of purine and pyrimidine bases, resulting in inhibition of DNA synthesis and, to a lesser extent, RNA and protein synthesis and also accumulation of cells in the $G_2$ phase of the cell cycle. The drug used clinically is a mixture consisting primarily of bleomycins $A_2$ and $B_2$.*

**b. sulfate** [USP] *a mixture of the sulfate salts of the components of bleomycin, especially that of bleomycin A₂, used alone or in conjunction with other chemotherapeutic agents as an antineoplastic, particularly to treat testicular carcinoma, lymphomas, and various squamous cell carcinomas; administered intravenously, intramuscularly, intra-arterially, or subcutaneously.*

With regard to bleomycin, the First Edition of this text (1994) did not even mention it, as there had been no reports of bleomycin lung in HBO patients. In the Second Edition (1999), it was listed as a relative contraindication to HBO because the predominant literature and papers at the time indicated that patients with even a remote history of bleomycin treatment might experience a recurrence of bleomycin lung when given oxygen. Then gradually more papers appeared implicating faulty fluid management and other factors during and after surgery as causing symptoms of bleomycin lung, but that bleomycin was not causative. This more modern point of view is now shared by most experienced anesthesiologists. This Edition reflects these changes and bleomycin is no longer listed as an absolute contraindication.

Only about 4% of cancer patients experience bleomycin lung at the time of their initial treatment. It is possible that this small sub-set of patients might be susceptible to a later recurrence if given an oxygen stimulus, but there is no credible evidence that this is true or not true. Human trials, of course, cannot be carried out. Pulmonary problems are the limiting factor to bleomycin dosage. To be on the side of caution, that small sub-set of patients should be given complete PFTs when considering oxygen in any concentration and must clearly not have any vestiges of pulmonary fibrosis.

Dr. Richard Moon of the Department of Hyperbaric Medicine at Duke University has treated 11 bleomycin patients with impunity while they breathed 100% oxygen at 2.0 to 2.5 atmospheres for 90 minutes to two hours. The time between the last dose of bleomycin and the administration of HBO ranged from a few months to many years. There were no sequelae.

It is felt that as long as the patient has no signs of pulmonary compromise from fibrosis and it has been over three or four months since he or she was treated with bleomycin; his or her exposure to bleomycin should not be a health factor.

In January 2008, an Air Force pilot was seen at Duke Medical Center who had been grounded because of previous bleomycin therapy, his PFTs and CAT scan showed no signs of pulmonary impairment or fibrosis. He was then given an oxygen challenge of 100% oxygen at 2.8 atmospheres absolute for one hour and then the studies were repeated. They remain completely normal.

A previous case, a female F-16 pilot was grounded when it came to her flight surgeon's attention that she had received bleomycin for cancer some 7 years previously. There was a paucity of published reports concerning the lack of data to support bleomycin lung secondary to remote administration of bleomycin, but there had been a great deal of clinical experience. She did an exhaustive search of what literature there was and contacted me and knowledgeable physicians, at Sloan Kettering, the University of Indiana, M.D. Anderson, Roswell Park, the University of Pennsylvania as well as elsewhere.

They unanimously supported her in her quest to return to flight status, and indeed she succeeded in having her flight status restored. She has since reported no problems or complications.

In light of the foregoing, there is no credible evidence that exposure to oxygen, or even hyperbaric oxygen would be harmful.

## Steroids

It is well known that the administration of adrenal corticosteroids can potentiate oxygen toxicity. There seems to be an increase in epinephrine and adrenocortical hormones in response to the stress of hyperbaric oxygen. Normally, the elaboration of these substances in response to stress serves as a protective mechanism. The reverse seems to be true in oxygen toxicity. Steroids and adrenaline seem to further sensitize the organism (3).

In clinical practice, hyperbaricists are often called upon to treat people who are receiving steroids. It is a good idea to carefully watch the patient who is receiving high dose steroids and to give anticonvulsant drugs, prophylactically, if necessary. Frequent air breaks are often used. It has been our experience that patients on steroids may develop premonitory signs of oxygen toxicity more quickly than normal. Steroid mediated seizures have not been seen in patients exposed to U.S. Navy Tables 5 and 6, probably because of the short exposures to oxygen between air breaks.

We treated one patient with Addison's disease who was receiving maintenance steroids. Since in this patient the addition of the hyperbaric oxygen stress caused no further elaboration of adrenocortical hormones, the patient was not at any greater risk for oxygen toxicity, despite the fact that she was receiving exogenous steroid hormones.

## Alcohol

The post-alcoholic state appears to predispose to decompression sickness in divers, probably secondary to dehydration. Fortunately, acute alcoholic intoxication does not seem to seriously predispose to oxygen toxicity or seizures. This has been attested by the numerous CO and trauma patients who may have had significant blood-alcohol levels when they were treated in the chamber. They have not been unduly prone to seizure. As an aside, hyperbaric oxygen does not lower blood-alcohol levels significantly faster or have a sobering effect, as measured by performance testing (14).

## Analgesics, Non-Narcotic

Non-narcotic pain medications, and non-steroidal anti-inflammatory drugs such as aspirin, acetaminophen, Motrin®, Darvon®, and phenacetin, when given in the usual therapeutic dosage, are not known to have any potentiating effects on oxygen toxicity. Their efficiency under increased partial pressure of oxygen appears to be unimpaired. Although some workers feel that aspirin may potentiate oxygen toxicity, there is little clinical evidence to support this, and we have had no problems with it over the past 30 years.

## Analgesics, Narcotic

Be especially alert for oxygen toxicity in patients receiving morphine, meperidine (Demerol®) or one of the other narcotic analgesics. Narcotic drugs depress respiration by reducing the reactivity of the medulla to $CO_2$ (18, 19, 21). When the respiration is decreased, a rise occurs in the alveolar and arterial $pCO_2$. In addition, oxygen can have a depressant effect on respiration as well as a stimulatory effect. Oxygen leads to a further depression of ventilation in the presence of narcotic drugs. This exaggerated depression of ventilation leads to a still greater rise in arterial $pCO_2$ above normal (20). The blood vessels of the brain dilate as a result of this increased $pCO_2$ and, because of the increased blood flow thus afforded, the amount of dissolved oxygen rises in brain tissue. The increased amount of oxygen in brain tissue speeds the development of oxygen convulsions. One should be particularly watchful if the patient has received one of these agents. Because intramuscular and subcutaneous absorption of morphine varies widely (although recent research shows the intramuscular absorption of drugs to be uninfluenced by HBO), the intravenous route is preferred for all hyperbaric patients. If the patient's respirations are noted to be slowed, the patient, if cooperative, should be instructed to take a number of deep breaths to blow down the $CO_2$ levels.

## Anesthetics

Total coverage of this very complex area would require a chapter by itself. The basics concerning the administration of anesthetic drugs have been well covered elsewhere by Severinghaus (32). When volatile or gaseous anesthetics are used, the concentration or percentage must be reduced in proportion to the number of atmospheres of pressure at which it is used. That is to say, the effective percentage is the actual percentage multiplied by the number of atmospheres of pressure at which it is administered. Strict attention must be paid to containing the gas so that it does not contaminate the chamber atmosphere, and adequate chamber ventilation must be assured. Needless to say, flammable anesthetics cannot be used.

Since 1966 when Severinghaus' article appeared, the dissociative drugs such as Ketamine have been put on the market. This type of anesthesia has many potential advantages for use under hyperbaric conditions, in that one does not have to be concerned about the changing effective percentages of anesthetic gas. Ketamine is administered intravenously. Despite its known clinical drawbacks, it deserves investigation under hyperbaric conditions. Its use involves risks similar to all general anesthetics and must be administered by physicians specifically trained in its use. Local anesthetics and regional blocks work well under hyperbaric conditions and require no modification in technique.

Generally, the employment of a general anesthetic in a hyperbaric chamber, regardless of the route of administration, requires all of the safeguards and equipment of a modern operating room. The special conditions imposed by increased barometric pressure are additive to the routine considerations of general anesthesia. Today, surgery requiring general anesthesia in the chamber is a rarity. However, as surgeons acquire more knowledge of the effects of HBO on reperfusion injury and the inhibition of membrane guanylate cyclase as it triggers the leucocyte adhesion molecule, we may well see more surgery carried out in the chamber. Its uses will be in crush injury, acute trauma surgery and replantation of severed limbs and digits.

## Anticonvulsants

The use of anticonvulsants, in connection with hyperbaric therapy, may be either prophylactic or for the treatment of seizures which do not stop when oxygen inhalation is terminated (status epilepticus).

If anticonvulsants are used prophylactically to suppress convulsions, it is **CRITICALLY IMPORTANT THAT THE USUAL OXYGEN PRESSURE/TIME LIMITS BE STRICTLY OBSERVED.** Suppression of convulsions, if exposure is carried beyond the normal latent period for oxygen toxicity, can occasion permanent oxygen-induced damage to the central nervous system (CNS). This has been well demonstrated by Gutsche, et al. (10). In dogs exposed to 5 ATA of oxygen for four hours, convulsive seizures were suppressed by anesthetics. Post-decompression, the surviving animals had permanent paralysis and severe neurologic damage. In clinical exposures of no more than 90 minutes limited to 3 ATA, permanent damage has not been reported in the human. Even though there is still disagreement among some hyperbaricists regarding seizure prophylaxis, we feel it is safe using prophylaxis in selected cases, so long as these limits are not exceeded. It is probable that the commonly used anticonvulsants have no direct effect on oxygen seizures themselves. They seem to prevent seizures only in people with idiopathically-low seizure thresholds. Over 35 years experience in using anti-seizure drugs in the chamber has revealed no complications when the time-depth limits given above have been observed.

In the patient who is febrile, toxic from gas gangrene, taking steroids, or has an idiopathic-low seizure threshold, prophylactic administration of a suitable anticonvulsant is indicated.

## Barbiturates

Phenobarbital has long been known to control grand mal seizures. Its disadvantage is that it tends to produce respiratory depression. Phenobarbital is better than some of the other barbituric acid derivatives in that it seems to possess more seizure suppressant activity relative to its respiratory depressant activity. If the drug's respiratory depressant and hypnotic tendencies do not present a problem, Phenobarbital is probably the most efficacious agent in preventing oxygen **CONVULSIONS**. It does not prevent poisoning of the tissues themselves, however. Dosage is 130 mg to 250 mg intravenously, based on the clinical indication and patient response. Sodium Amytal by intravenous injections is very effective and safe for use in sedation or for status seizures. Dosages of 100 mg given in100 mg increments have been successfully used to arrest refractory status epilepticus. If excessive dosage is administered too quickly, problems with hypotension and respiratory depression may be manifest.

## Diazepam (Valium®)

Diazepam has been recommended for use as an adjunct in the convulsive disorders, and it is used prophylactically in patients who are thought to be at high risk for oxygen convulsions. Diazepam has been proven to be useful in terminating seizures in convulsive disorders of nonhyperbaric origin (29). When given intravenously, the drug should never be injected faster than 5 mg (1 ml) per minute. As with phenytoin (Dilantin®), it should not be added to IV fluids. The usual dose is 5 mg to 10 mg intravenously. Frequently, patients under hyperbaric therapy will require larger doses than would normally be expected. The reason for this is unclear, but Courtiere, et al. have shown a 29% decrease in cortical benzodiazepine receptors under hyperbaric hyperoxia (6). There does not seem to be any evidence of rebound sedation following cessation of therapy when larger than usual dosages of diazepam (15 to 50 mg) have been used. Although the mechanism preventing oxygen seizures in humans has not been defined, we have not yet seen a seizure in any patient premedicated with Valium® at our facility.

## Disulfiram (Antabuse®)

The use of disulfiram in blocking oxygen toxicity was tested by Faiman. He showed that mice could be exposed to six atmospheres of oxygen, exercising for one hour, without convulsing, when pretreated with intraperitoneal disulfiram. Subsequent necropsy failed to demonstrate any CNS or pulmonary oxygen damage. This work was also repeated in beagle dogs at pressures of four atmospheres with little or no evidence of oxygen toxicity (9). Hart (unpublished data) reported its use in one patient treated hyperbarically who had an extremely low seizure threshold. Hart's conclusion was that the effect is dose related. Dosage in the human has ranged between 500 mg and 300 mg per day. Obviously, anyone receiving disulfiram must not be using alcohol or have a recent history of ingesting alcohol. Alcohol swabs, mouthwash, and other sources of alcohol must be vigorously excluded from contact with the patient.

This medication is available for humans only in oral form and its efficacy in blocking seizures has not been demonstrated in a controlled trial with humans. Disulfiram probably acts in competition with enzymes containing SH bonds for the free radical oxygen and thereby exerts a protective effect.

The theoretical problem with using disulfiram in the chamber is that it also blocks the production of superoxide dismutase (SOD) which is the body's major protection against oxygen toxicity (12). Based on the animal data, it was thought that disulfiram might pose a risk if taken in concert with HBO therapy.

It must be borne in mind, however, that the dosages of disulfiram given in the animal experiments were extremely high, corresponding to 14 grams of the drug given intraperitoneally in humans and there have been no reports of a human having a problem with HBO while taking disulfiram. Therefore, it is no longer considered a contraindication. See Disulfiram in the chapter by Kindwall entitled "Contraindications and Side Effects to Hyperbaric Oxygen Treatment," for more detail.

## Lorazepam (Ativan®)

This drug is similar to diazepam in many respects, but is given in one fifth the dosage. It will produce clinical sedation, relief of anxiety, and lack of recall within 15 to 20 minutes of being given IV. The intended effects last 6 to 8 hours. It does not enhance the respiratory depressant effect of meperidine. It is an excellent choice of management of status epilepticus, although the PDR does not list it under that indication at the present time.

## Phenytoin (Dilantin®)

Phenytoin has been widely used in epilepsy since 1937, but its efficacy in preventing oxygen convulsions was not demonstrated. Marks, in early animal experiments, did not find phenytoin to be effective in delaying or preventing oxygen convulsions (23). It is probable that, in animals with a normal seizure threshold, no effect could be observed. The usual anticonvulsants probably do not have an effect on the oxygen seizure mechanism, but are only useful in raising a pathologically-low seizure threshold to normal. Clinical experience, however, indicates that, in very high IV dosage (15 mg/kg), its effect in stopping oxygen seizures can be substantial in the acute situation. It is probable that the mechanism is an indirect one as outlined above (37). Particular care should be taken to insure that this drug does not extravasate around the vein as it is highly alkaline. The drug should be given no faster than 50 mg a minute, and it should not be included in IV bottles because of possible precipitation. In the event that full phenytoin dosage is required, a dosage of 15 to 18 mg/kg is administered at a maximum rate of 50 mg per minute with careful blood pressure monitoring. Oral phenytoin should not be relied on if given just prior to hyperbaric therapy, since up to 48 hours may be required for therapeutic blood levels to be established by this route. The usual or oral maintenance dosage is 100 mg three times a day.

## Vitamin E (Alpha Tocopherol)

Research by Kann, et al., and Okamoto and co-workers showed that alpha Tocopherol deficient mice had a higher mortality in HBO (16, 26). Vitamin E also appears to protect against pulmonary oxygen toxicity. Pauland, Bollinger, et al., have shown that Vitamin E prolonged life in mice an average of 1.6 days compared to Vitamin E deficient mice (4.9 vs. 3.3 days) when exposed to 100% oxygen (27). The seizure threshold also appears to be raised by supplemental Vitamin E. Hart recommends a dosage of 400 units p.o. per 90 minute treatment, given at any time preceding treatment, allowing time for absorption (Personal Communication).

## Lidocaine

When Lidocaine is utilized as an anti-arrhythmic, no specific differences in its use are encountered. In addition, Lidocaine may be helpful, when added to a potassium containing solution, in patients who have large potassium requirements. It prevents pain and irritation at the infusion site. Lidocaine used as a local anesthetic is no different when used in the hyperbaric chamber. Experimentally it has been used with good result in anti-arrhythmic doses to protect the brain after air embolism (8). It was shown to significantly enhance neural recovery in the cat after embolism. An initial bolus of 100 mg administered over 3 minutes would be followed by a continuous infusion in saline of 2 mg/min for 50 minutes. The dosage used in the cat experiments consisted of 1.5 mg/kg for the remaining hour. This method of delivery was described by Salzer (27).

## Digitalis/Digoxin

Hyperbaric oxygenation has not been reported to decrease the effectiveness of the cardiac glycosides. In cases of overdose with digitalis glycosides, there is evidence that hyperbaric oxygenation can afford some protection to the organism.

In experiments with guinea pigs, Bachand and Somani found that the dose of Ouabain needed to produce ventricular tachycardia and ventricular fibrillation was significantly increased when guinea pigs were equilibrated with 100% oxygen at pressures of 2 and 3 atmospheres absolute (1). When pressure alone (3 ATA) with 7% oxygen was used, there was no difference in effect. The dose necessary to initiate ventricular tachycardia was raised from 171 micrograms per kilogram in air to 272 micrograms per kilogram with hyperbaric oxygen at 3 ATA (p<0.001). The authors felt that the decreased toxicity of the digitalis glycosides appeared to be due to an increased amount of dissolved oxygen in the blood under hyperbaric conditions, but were not able to describe the mechanism. It should not be concluded from this that hyperbaric oxygen increases the tolerance to digitalis under clinical conditions. The effectiveness of hyperbaric oxygen in the treatment of digitalis toxicity has not been studied in humans.

Our experience with one elderly patient who was taking a digitalis preparation showed his cardiac sinus rate to gradually DECREASE during a course of twenty hyperbaric treatments. His digitalis dosage was not changed. When his sinus rate reached 40, digitalis was discontinued and then later reinstituted at a much lower dosage. It was inferred that hyperbaric treatment, for some reason, decreased the patient's need, at least temporarily, for digitalis. Elderly people taking digitalis should be monitored closely with the EKG.

## Heparin

Although hyperbaric oxygen does not alter the effects of heparin, it has been used experimentally in disorders treated with HBO.

Cockett, et al., pretreated dogs with heparin prior to rapid decompression from depth, which produced severe decompression sickness. The unheparinized control dogs all died, whereas the heparinized animals survived (5). Philp has shown that it ameliorates DCS and has a lipemia clearing effect in congenitally obese rats (28).

On the other hand, Reeves and Workman found it to have no effect in dogs suffering mild to moderate decompression sickness (30). There are no human studies to determine its effect in bends, but the author has given it empirically in severe cases of bends shock (5,000 IU).

Its use has been suggested in air embolism, as it would appear that the no-reflow phenomenon is mitigated in situations where heparinization is in effect before embolization (cardiovascular pump bypass patients and animal studies). There are no controlled studies in humans where it has been given post-embolization. Farmer discourages its use in vestibular decompression sickness patients (personal communication, 1985), as he has observed hemorrhage into inner ear structures following decompression. In Waite's dog studies of air embolism, one of the dogs developed an intracranial bleed following embolization which was documented photographically (36). In the author's experience, at least one case of air embolism has been observed in a diver where an intracranial hemorrhage was seen on C-T.

Nevertheless, Hart routinely used heparin in the treatment of 30 air embolism cases and 14 decompression sickness patients with no apparent deleterious effect (9).

## Insulin

HBO effects on insulin secretion or its metabolism are not completely understood. However, in insulin-dependent diabetic patients who are undergoing HBO therapy, blood glucose levels have consistently been shown to fall dramatically (15, 22, 33, 34). Average drops in blood glucose levels during a single hyperbaric oxygen treatment ranging between 31 and 51 milligrams per deciliter have been reported in different series. Plasma glucagon levels have also been shown to decrease in diabetics receiving HBO, and this may be the chief mechanism (34). These changes may also be secondary to alteration in insulin receptor activity or other factors. Martindale and Dixon have also shown that mouse diaphragms take up glucose more rapidly during HBO (24). If this is true, increased glucose metabolism may play a role in the falling glucose levels. It should be borne in mind, though, that non-diabetics do not suffer a corresponding drop in glucose levels when exposed to HBO. Insulin levels are not increased by HBO (34). Insulin requirements in diabetics may change rapidly, precipitating unexpected insulin reactions. HBO patients should be constantly monitored for glucose levels and placed on sliding scale dosage. Additionally, the fact that the patient's toxic infectious status may be improving during HBO therapy may be responsible for further reduction in insulin requirements. It is a good idea to have on hand in the hyperbaric unit, orange juice and 50% glucose for injection to manage incipient or frank insulin reactions. All diabetic patients must have their blood glucose levels recorded immediately prior to treatment and after decompression. Supplemental glucose must be given prior to treatment if the level is less than 110 mg per deciliter.

## FACTORS THAT AFFECT OXYGEN TOXICITY

### Hypothermia

Low body temperature (absent shivering) has long been recognized as a deterrent to oxygen toxicity, whereas an elevation of temperature has the opposite effect. The reason for this is believed to be largely due to the attendant changes in metabolism. Thus, the use of hypothermia in clinical procedures in HBO should diminish the possibility of oxygen poisoning, as well as reducing oxygen consumption. This is true only if shivering is suppressed.

### Central Vasodilator (Acetazolamide)

Acetazolamide (Diamox®) is a carbonic anhydrase inhibitor which prevents oxygen-induced vasoconstriction. This is probably not a blocking mechanism, but an indirect, $CO_2$-related effect. Kong (17) who provided photographic evidence of this effect in the retinal vessels first demonstrated this. Its use has been described in the experimental hyperbaric treatment of sickle cell anemia.

The possible disadvantage is that by preventing systemic vasoconstriction, it also permits greater cerebral blood flow during HBO treatment. This may predispose to CNS oxygen toxicity with seizures. The drug should probably not be used at chamber pressures greater than 2 ATA, and it might well be wise to consider prophylactic diazepam, if the drug must be used at higher pressures.

Its usefulness in the management of other hyperbarically treated conditions has not been studied or documented.

If a patient is already taking acetazolamide when referred for treatment, there may be a higher risk of oxygen seizure at pressures greater than 2 ATA.

## Thyroid (Synthroid®)

Iatrogenic production of hyperthyroidism with the administration of thyroid extract or thyroxin in experimental animals results in very pronounced enhancement of $O_2$ toxicity at atmospheric pressure and at increased ambient pressure. A thyroidectomy has the opposite effect. This has been demonstrated in animal studies, and one may reasonably assume that these factors would also be operative in human subjects selected for clinical exposure to hyperbaric oxygen. Presumably, this is due to the increased metabolic rate and its propensity to cause toxicity during exercise. Hypophysectomy also counters oxygen seizures. Active Graves's disease predisposes to seizures as the patient is hyperthyroid. There is no danger of oxygen toxicity in a patient taking thyroxin or Synthroid® to maintain a euthyroid state.

## Phenothiazines

Of the phenothiazines, only chlorpromazine (Thorazine®, Largactil®), has been investigated with regard to its effect on oxygen toxicity. Bean et al. have demonstrated that chlorpromazine has a considerable protective action in the CNS against the seizure-producing propensity of oxygen under high pressure (2). Again, it must be borne in mind that the absence of seizures does not necessarily mean absence of toxicity or the possibility of permanent damage if pressure/time limits are exceeded. This is interesting, as chlorpromazine, if given in large initial dose by itself, can produce convulsions. This is quite apart from its ability to produce a Parkinson-like syndrome. However, Bean felt that the protective action of the drug is due in large measure to the removal or blocking of neurogenic causal factors by a suppressant action on sympathetics at the hypothalamic and medullary levels, as well as an anti-epinephrine effect. He demonstrates in the paper referenced that this protection is not due to chlorpromazine's hypotensive effect and a presumptive consequential decrease in cerebral blood flow and oxygen supply to the CNS. For this reason one would expect other phenothiazines which do not effect vasomotor tone as much as chlorpromazine (such as the piperazine side-chain drugs) to have a similar effect. Suitable research in this regard is lacking, however. Chlorpromazine can safely be given in a dose of 50 mg intramuscularly initially and then 100 mg. three times a day orally.

Of interest is that we have seen two patients who developed moderate to severe extra-pyramidal symptoms on minute or very moderate therapeutic doses of phenothiazines when associated with carbon monoxide poisoning. One patient taking Mellaril® 400 mg q.d. developed extra-pyramidal symptoms and signs during hyperbaric treatment and the other went into oculogyric crisis when given a tiny dose of phenothiazine (Stelazine® 2mg) several days after apparent recovery from severe CO poisoning. This is presumed to be secondary to the damaging effects of CO on the basal ganglia. Both responded to IV diphenhydramine (Benadryl®).

## CONCLUSION

What is known about drug interactions with HBO has been presented above. Most drugs retain their usual effects under hyperbaric conditions and do not interact with oxygen under pressure. Whenever the physician uses a new drug, however, he should at least consider the pharmacology of the drug and think of any theoretical adverse effects before employing it.

## REFERENCES

1. Bachand RT Jr and Somani P. "Digitalis Intoxication: Protection with Hyperbaric Oxygen." Life Sciences. 1967;6:739-742.

2. Bean JW and Wagemacker H. "Brain blood flow, Chlorpromazine (Thorazine and protective action against the toxicity of O2 at high pressure." Am J of Physiol. 1960;198:(2)341-345.

3. Bean JW. "Factors influencing clinical oxygen toxicity." Ann of the NY Acad of Sci. 1966;117:645-755.

4. Bornside GH and Nance FC. "High pressure oxygen combined with antibiotics in the therapy of experimental burn wounds." In: (GL Hobby, Ed.) Proc of the 8th Interscience Conf on Antimicrob Agents and Chemother, Am Soc for Microb, Wash, D.C. 1968:497-500.

5. Cockett ATK. Presentation, Journees Int. d'Hyperbarie et Physiol. Subaquat. Marseille, France, June, 1970.

6. Courtiere A, Reybaud J, Camilla C, Lobert P, Drouet J and Jadot G. Oxygen-induced modifications of benzodiazepine receptors and D2 dopamine receptors in the rat under hyperoxia. Free Rad. Res. Comms. 15(1):29-34, 1991.

7. Emerson, G, and Hackett P, Hyperbaric Oxygen Does Not Delay the Absorption of Intramuscular Midazolam, SPUMS J. 1998;28(3):122-125.

8. Evans DB, McDermott JJ, Kobrine AI, Flynn ET. "Effects of Intravenous Lidocaine in experimental cerebral air embolism." Undersea Biom Res. 1988;15:(Suppl)17. (Abstract only)

9. Faiman MD, Mehl RG, Oehme FW. "Protection with Disulfiram from central and pulmonary oxygen toxicity." Biochem Pharma. 1971;20:3059-3067. Pergamon Press, Great Britain.

10. Gutsche BB, Harp JR, Stephen CR. "Influence of anesthetic drugs on dogs subjected to oxygen at 5 atmospheres." Proc of Third Intl Conf on Hyperbaric Med. Natl Acad Sciences, Natl Research Council, 1966:300-306.

11. Hart GB. "Treatment of Decompression illness and air embolism with hyperbaric oxygen." Aerospace Med. 1974;45(10):1190-1193.

12. Heikkila RE, Cabbat FS, Cohen G. "In Vivo inhibition of superoxide dismutase in mice by Diethyldithiocarbamate." J Biol Chem. 1976;251:2182.

13. Hyperbaric Unit Staff, Mount Sinai Hospital, New York, (1968) Personal Communication. (Deterioration of opened drugs stored in chamber.)

14. Jacobson GR, Kindwall EP. "Effects of hyperbaric oxygenation on acute alcohol intoxication." J of Hyperbaric Med. 1991;6(2):119-131.

15. Kakhnovskii IM, Efuni SN, Khodas MY, Bolshakova TD and Gitel EP The mechanism of hypoglycemic effect of hyperbaric oxygenation in diabetes mellitus patients. Klin Med (Mosk) 59(9):83-88; Sept. 1981 HBO Rev 1983 July;4(3):143.

16. Kann HE Jr., et al. "Oxygen Toxicity and Vitamin E." J of Aerosp Med. 1964;35:840-844.

17. Kong Y, Lunzer S, Heyman A, et al. "Effects of Acetazolamide on cerebral blood flow of dogs during hyperbaric oxygenation." Am Heart J. 1969;78:229-237.

18. Lambertsen CJ. "Drugs and respiration." Ann Rev Pharmacol. 1966;6:327-378.

19. Lambertsen CJ, Kough RH, Cooper DY, Emmel GL, Loeschske HH. "Oxygen toxicity. Effects in man of oxygen inhalation at 1 and 3.5 atmospheres upon blood gas transport, cerebral circulation and cerebral metabolism." J of App Physiol. 1953;5:471-486.

20. Lambertsen CJ. Personal communication. 1971.

21. Lambertsen CJ, Hall P, Wollman H, Goodman MW. "Quantitative interactions of increased pO2 upon respiration in man." Ann of the NY Acad Sci. 1963;109:731-741.

22. Longoni C, Camporesi EM, Buizza M, et al. "Reduction in insulin requirements during HBO therapy." UBR. 1988;15(Suppl):16-17.

23. Marks HP. "Interim report on oxygen intoxication in animals and the effect of drugs on sensitivity to oxygen intoxication." Med Res Counc, R.N. Personnel Res Comm Report. 1944;44/001.

24. Martindale VE and Dixon PA, Fresh dissected mouse diaphragms take up glucose more rapidly during hyperbaric oxygenation. Undersea and Hyperbar Med. 20 (Suppl):33. Jul 1993.

25. Nemiroff PM. "Effects of Cis-Platinum and hyperbaric oxygen on wound healing in mice." Undersea Biomed Res. 1988;15:(Suppl):40. (Abstract only)

26. Okamoto H and Isa P. "Protective effects of alpha-tocopherol nicotinate against oxygen effects in mouse and rat." Jap J of Anesth. 1975;24:468-471. (English abstract)

27. Pauland RL, Bollinger RO, Bozynski ME, Karna P, Perrin EVD. "Effect of Vitamin E deficiency on pulmonary oxygen toxicity." Ped Res. 1977;11(4):577.

28. Philp RB. "The ameliorative effects of heparin and depolymerized hyaluronate on decompression sickness in rats." Can J Physiol and Pharma. 1964;42:819-829.

29. Physician's Desk Reference. 46th Ed. Medical Econ. Data Inc., Oradell, NJ. 1992:1937.

30. Reeves E and Workman RD. "Use of heparin for the therapeutic/prophylactic treatment of decompression sickness." Aerosp Med... 1971;42(1):20-23.

31. Salzer LB, et al. "The comparison of methods of Lidocaine administration in patients." Clin Pharmcol Therapy. 1981;29:617-624.

32. Severinghaus JW. "Anesthesia and related drug effects." Fundamentals of Hyperbaric Medicine., Natl Acad of Sci, Wash., D.C. 1966;9:115-127. (Reprinted by the Undersea and Hyperbaric Medical Society).

33. Springer R. "The importance of glucometer testing of diabetic patients pre and post-dive." UBR. 1991;18(Suppl):20. (Abstract only)

34. Takahashi H, Kobayshi S, Sakakibara K. "Effect of HBO on the endocrine system and metabolism of diabetic patients." Undersea Biom Res. 1990;17(Suppl):52. (Abstract only)

35. Upton PG, Yamaguchi KT, Myers S, Kidwell TD, Anderson RJ. "Effects of antioxidants and hyperbaric oxygen in ameliorating experimental doxorubicin skin toxicity in the rat." Cancer Treatment Reports. 1986;70(4):503-507.

36. Waite CL, Mazzone WF, Greenwood ME. "Cerebral air embolism 1. Basic studies." U.S. Naval Submarine Med Ctr Report #493, Bureau Med and Surg. 1967, Navy Dept., Wash., D.C.

37. Weaver, LK. "Phenytoin sodium in oxygen toxicity-induced seizures." Ann Emerg Med. 1983;12:(1)81-84.

# NOTES

# MYRINGOTOMY

## CHAPTER ELEVEN OVERVIEW

# MYRINGOTOMY

*Thomas M. Kidder*

## INTRODUCTION

Air containing spaces within the skull and facial skeleton include the middle ear cleft (tympanum) and the paranasal sinuses. Air pressure within these spaces must equilibrate with ambient pressure in order for a person undergoing pressurization or depressurization to remain asymptomatic. The most common problem encountered in patients undergoing hyperbaric treatment is ear squeeze, i.e., inability to equalize pressure in the middle ear clefts during compression. Less commonly inability to equalize air pressure in one or more of the paranasal sinuses can occur, resulting in facial or head pain. Acute barotitis (ear) or barosinusitis (paranasal sinuses) are terms used to describe pain, transudation of fluid and/or hemorrhage resulting from failure of this equilibration process. This chapter will deal primarily with acute barotitis and its management.

## PATHOPHYSIOLOGY OF BAROTITIS

A diagnosis of barotis can be inferred if the patient complains of deep ear pain, either unilateral or bilateral, during hyperbaric pressurization. Examination of the ear using an otoscope may show retraction, engorgement or hypervascularity of the tympanic membrane, blood within the middle ear cleft (hemotympanum), or even perforation of the tympanic membrane with or without hemorrhagic otorrhea. Because for whatever reason the auditory (Eustachian) tube is unable to equilibrate middle ear space air pressure with ambient pressure, a relative vacuum develops within the middle ear cleft. Depending on how rapidly this negative pressure develops and how great the pressure differential between the middle ear cleft and the ambient environment, the patient will experience one or more of the signs or symptoms mentioned above. Sometimes patients may be able to equilibrate if the pressurization is done very gradually, but they are unable to do so if the compression is rapid. Although the auditory tube serves other important functions (e.g., protection of the middle ear from pharyngeal secretions), the focus in this chapter is on the auditory tube as a conduit for pressure equalization.

The auditory tube (see Figure 1), the only natural communication between the middle ear cleft and the ambient air, is normally closed in the resting state. It opens briefly with swallowing, yawning, or during a modified Valsalva maneuver. Air can passively exit the middle ear cleft through the

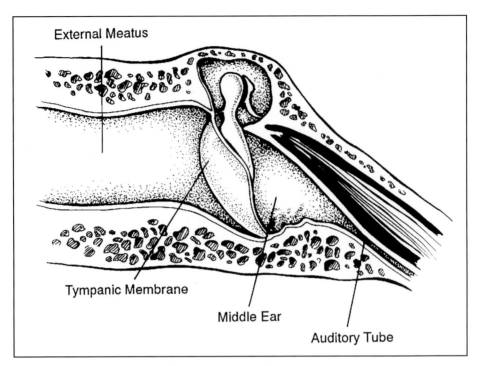

*Figure 1. Cutaway coronal view of external canal, middle-ear, auditory tube, and tympanic membrane.*

auditory tube, since the lateral tympanic portion of the tube is bony and rigid. However, entrance of air into the middle ear cleft depends on active contraction of the palatine and pharyngeal musculature, especially the tensor veli palatini, to open the collapsible cartilaginous medial portion of the auditory tube. Functional integrity of the auditory tube may also be impaired by edema or hypersecretion of the tubal mucosa; failure of the mucociliary blanket within the tube; altered function of the tubal opening muscles, as in patients with cleft palate; or, obstruction of the tube by inspissated mucus or exudates. Mucosal edema and dysfunction of the mucociliary blanket may be due to factors such as infection, allergy, tobacco smoking, dry air and exposure to noxious chemicals.

    The distinction between a Valsalva maneuver and a modified Valsalva maneuver should be understood. A Valsalva maneuver, which has no effect on opening the auditory tube, is performed by closing the glottis and increasing intrathoracic pressure. Examples of the Valsalva maneuver include straining during heavy lifting, defecation or childbirth. The modified Valsalva maneuver is performed by maintaining an open glottis, closing the mouth, occluding the nose (e.g., pinching the nostrils closed), and then increasing intrathoracic pressure). In effect, this latter maneuver should force air up through the auditory tube into the middle ear. The modified Valsalva maneuver is not recommended as a way to equalize middle ear pressure because it can raise intracranial pressure to dangerously high levels and, in susceptible individuals, retrogradely force cerebrospinal fluid through the cochlear aqueduct into the inner ear. A much safer and equally effective method of inflating the middle ear is the Toynbee maneuver. The patient simply pinches the nostrils closed and swallows. This facilitates opening the auditory tube without rising intracranial and cerebrospinal fluid (CSF) pressure.

"Locking" of the auditory tube, such that no amount of swallowing, yawning or modified Valsalva maneuver is able to open the medial pharyngeal end of the tube, occurs when the pressure differential between the ambient air and the middle ear cleft reaches or exceeds about 125 torr. This differential is about one atmosphere of pressure change. When this occurs, the patient must be returned to sea level pressure and compression restarted and progressed very slowly.

## DECONGESTANTS

Spraying the nose liberally with a topical sympathomimetic like oxymetazoline (Afrin®), xylometazoline (Otrivin®), or phenylephrine (Neo Synephrine®) may help to decongest the auditory tube and facilitate tubal opening. The use of oral decongestants or decongestant/antihistamine preparations is less predictable. In general, oral decongestants have no preferential effect on the vascularity of the auditory tube, so in order to obtain meaningful vasoconstriction in the nose and auditory tube doses high enough to also potentially cause cardiac dysrhythmias and hypertension would need to be used.

A fairly effective aid for individuals who chronically have difficulty clearing their ears during flight in an aircraft is Ear Planes®. These proprietary ear plugs, which must be inserted properly in the ear canals before the aircraft begins its descent, contain a small ceramic filter which permits slow and gradual pressurization within the external auditory canal. They are reportedly effective for two uses and can be purchased at nominal cost in most pharmacies. The author is not aware of any controlled trials of these devices for hyperbaric therapy, but they might be worth considering in patients who would otherwise require myringotomy.

## MYRINGOTOMY: INDICATIONS

Myringotomy (a small incision or perforation of the tympanic membrane) is indicated when acute otalgia, secondary to middle ear barotrauma, develops during pressurization and cannot be relieved by nonsurgical measures.

Performing a myringotomy in an unconscious patient (e.g., carbon monoxide poisoning) who is not experiencing pain is not advisable or necessary. If the tympanic membrane does rupture spontaneously or if the middle ear fills with blood or transudate, these occurrences will almost always heal or resolve spontaneously. The risk of inner ear damage resulting from middle ear barotrauma in an unconscious patient is extremely unlikely and does not justify routine performance of myringotomy.

## MYRINGOTOMY: TECHNIQUE

As with any surgical procedure, exposure of the operative site is paramount. In the ear this means a nonobstructed external auditory canal, coaxial bright light, and the largest speculum the ear canal will comfortably

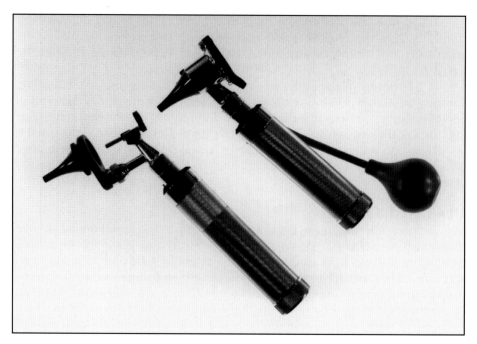

*Figure 2. Two electric otoscopes. Left, open "operating" head. Right, closed "diagnostic" head; pneumatic otoscopy bulb attached.*

accommodate. The light source may be an electric otoscope (Figure 2) with an operating head that allows instrumentation of the ear canal and eardrum, a head mirror, an electric headlight, or a binocular operating microscope. Retracting the pinna upward and backward straightens the cartilaginous ear canal and provides an optimal view of the eardrum, assuming there is no cerumen or desquamated skin debris obstructing the canal.

Cerumen and desquamated skin debris should be removed from the external auditory canal if it interferes with adequate visualization of the tympanic membrane landmarks. Removal of debris must be done gently and carefully, since the skin of the external ear canal, and especially the medial bony portion of the canal, is delicate and easily traumatized. While cerumen removal may be safely performed by an experienced clinician using a wax removal loop, a safer method for removing wax under less than ideal conditions is to irrigate the wax using warm water close to or at body temperature. At body temperature the irrigation will be comfortable and will not elicit vertigo or nausea. While many cerumen irrigation devices are commercially obtainable, an easy method using readily-available supplies is the following: (see Figure 3) a large plastic syringe (preferably 30 to 50 ml) with Luer-Lock tip is attached to a 14- or 16-gauge, 3 to 5 cm long flexible plastic intravenous catheter (e.g., Angiocath®). This apparatus produces a fine hard stream of water which will dislodge and flush out most ear canal debris with little chance of abrading the delicate skin of the external auditory canal. It is important to use a Luer-Lock syringe and to be certain the catheter is securely attached so that it does not become a missile and perforate the tympanic membrane during irrigation.

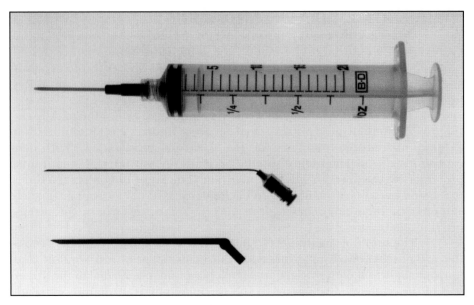

Figure 3. Top, large plastic syringe with flexible short catheter attached; note Luer-Lock tip. Middle, 22 gauge spinal needle, angled near hub. Bottom, disposable Beaver® myringotomy knife blade.

The question of whether it is safe to irrigate an ear canal filled with cerumen before one has determined that there is no perforation is not really a problem. If, during pressurization in the chamber, the patient experiences otalgia, it is virtually certain that the tympanic membrane is intact, since a perforation allows automatic equalization of pressure through the perforation and the patient would experience no pain.

It is best to position the patient supine with the contralateral side of the head resting firmly on the mattress or pillow to minimize movement. Children may need to be restrained and immobilized using a papoose board or similar method to minimize movement and make the procedure safer.

The basic instruments (see Figures 2 and 3) needed for a myringotomy are: an otoscope with an operating head (i.e., one which permits adequate visualization of the tympanic membrane during myringotomy); an ear speculum of adequate size; and, a myringotomy knife, preferably a sharp disposable knife whose blade can be angled to permit an accurately placed incision. Lacking a myringotomy knife, a simple, inexpensive, readily-available substitute is a 25- or 22-gauge disposable spinal needle which may be angled as needed. Alternative ways of visualizing the tympanic membrane are with a head mirror or headlight which provide illumination coaxial to the line of vision, or, with a binocular operating microscope.

Anesthetizing the tympanic membrane is usually not necessary for a myringotomy done as an emergency procedure to relieve acute barotitis. The brief momentary pain of the myringotomy is usually overshadowed by the discomfort the patient is already experiencing and is followed by immediate relief. Actually the application of an anesthetic, either topical or infiltration, is likely to produce as much or more discomfort than the myringotomy itself, assuming the procedure is performed carefully and skillfully.

## TYMPANIC MEMBRANE LANDMARKS

Otologists divide the tympanic membrane into four quadrants (Figure 4). A vertical line through the umbo divides the eardrum into anterior and posterior halves; a horizontal line through the umbo divides it into superior and inferior halves. The intersection of these two imaginary lines produces four quadrants.

Because of the location of structures contained within the middle ear (Figure 5) and their susceptibility to penetrating injuries it is imperative that a blind or random puncture of the eardrum be avoided. With few exceptions the myringotomy should be made in the inferior quadrants, preferably in the anterior-inferior quadrant. The latter option is sometimes precluded by an obstructing bulge in the bony external ear canal. In such cases the myringotomy is made either directly inferiorly or in the posterior-inferior quadrant.

The superior quadrants (Figures 4 and 5) should be avoided because the malleus handle, long process of the incus, stapes, oval window and horizontal portion of the facial nerve (Fallopian) canal lie medial to the upper half of the tympanic membrane. If the myringotomy is made too cephalad, even in the posterior-inferior quadrant, the aforementioned structures could potentially be injured. It is therefore safest to incise either inferiorly or anterior-inferiorly.

The myringotomy need not be a long incision if a ventilation tube is not to be inserted. A simple full-thickness puncture of the tympanic membrane will suffice. Admittedly the perforation usually heals in a day or two, but such an opening will provide immediate pain relief from acute barotitis. The clinician must remember that the tympanic membrane is usually retracted medially and is often, at least in its central portion, in contact with the bony bulge (promontory of the medial wall of the tympanum. Therefore it is advisable to keep the myringotomy entrance site

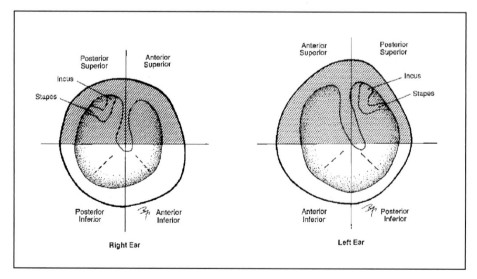

Figure 4. View of tympanic membrane, showing division into quadrants; incise inferior quadrants; avoid incising posterier-superior quadrant.

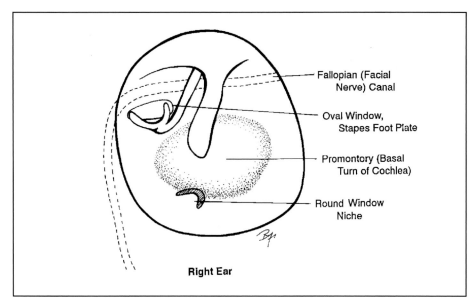

*Figure 5. Drawing of medial wall of tympanum with tympanic membrane removed to show middle-ear structures.*

peripheral, a few millimeters from the tympanic membrane annulus, to minimize the chance of impinging the tip of the knife or needle on the bony wall of the middle ear cleft.

As a result of previous middle ear inflammatory disease some tympanic membranes may contain hard plaques of myringosclerosis, a hyalinization of the submucosal layer of the eardrum. These usually appear as white chalky patches in the tympanic membrane. It is best to avoid incising one of these plaques, since they are often difficult to penetrate.

## PRESSURE EQUALIZATION TUBES

For the patient who is unable to equalize middle ear pressure readily and will require a series of hyperbaric treatments (e.g., for osteomyelitis, flap survival or radionecrosis), otolaryngologic consultation for placement of middle ear vent tubes is recommended. For patients in whom generalized edema is expected to occur as a result of the injury or disease (e.g., burn victims) it is advisable to consider myringotomy and insertion of vent tubes at the time of the first hyperbaric treatment. This can be done, usually at the bedside, using topical or infiltration local anesthesia. Hyperbaric treatments can be commenced immediately after placement of the vent tubes, and the tubes will migrate out of the tympanic membrane spontaneously after several months leaving a healed, intact tympanic membrane. Patients with middle ear vent tubes are usually advised to keep water out of the ear canals until the tubes have extruded from the eardrums. This is easily accomplished by using small soft earplugs during bathing, shampooing, showering and swimming, although diving underwater should be avoided as long as the tubes are functional.

## REFERENCES

1. Cummings C., et al. Otolaryngology - Head and Neck Surgery, Vol. 4. St. Louis, MO: Mosby; 1986.

2. English G. (Ed.). Otolaryngology, Vol 1. New York, NY: Lippincott; 1991.

3. Naumann HH. (Ed.) Head and Neck Surgery: Ear, Vol. 3. Philadelphia, PA Saunders; 1982.

4. Paparella M., et al. Otolaryngology (3rd Edition), Vol. 2. Philadelphia, PA: Saunders; 1990.

5. Shambaugh G. Surgery of the Ear (2nd Edition). Philadelphia, PA: Saunders; 1967.

CHAPTER 12

# CONTRAINDICTIONS AND SIDE EFFECTS TO HYPERBARIC OXYGEN TREATMENT

## CHAPTER TWELVE OVERVIEW

# CONTRAINDICTIONS AND SIDE EFFECTS TO HYPERBARIC OXYGEN TREATMENT

*Eric P. Kindwall*

Of all the medical treatments carried out in hospitals, hyperbaric oxygen therapy is one of the most benign when it comes to side effects. The contraindications are relatively few. Nevertheless, some preexisting conditions or concurrent therapies can present absolute or relative contraindications to HBO.

## ABSOLUTE CONTRAINDICATIONS

### Doxorubicin (Adriamycin®)

Upton and co-workers (30), while investigating the possible use of hyperbaric oxygen among other non-surgical "antidotes" for tissue damage caused by extravasation of doxorubicin, found that this chemotherapeutic drug produced an 87% mortality in rats when combined with HBO. Presumably this was due to cardiac toxicity. The animals were on a b.i.d. treatment schedule, but even when shifted to a once-a-day regimen, there was no significant decrease in mortality. Doxorubicin is probably inactivated and cleared from the tissues in about 24 hours. However, to be prudent, it would be wise to wait at least two to three days after the last dose of doxorubicin before initiating hyperbaric oxygen treatment. HBO has been used safely to aid in healing tissue necrosis secondary to doxorubicin extravasation, but chamber treatment was given after treatment with the drug had been halted.

### Mafenide Acetate (Sulfamylon®)

This antibacterial drug was first synthesized in Germany, but later developed into a useful topical agent by Pruitt and his colleagues at the Brook Army Burn Center in San Antonio, Texas. It was found to be effective in suppressing bacterial infection in burn wounds and superseded silver nitrate therapy.

Mafenide, however, is a carbonic anhydrase inhibitor which tends to promote a $CO_2$ buildup, causing a peripheral vasodilatation. When this is coupled with the central vasoconstriction caused by HBO, the results are worse than when using either agent alone. If a burn patient is referred for hyperbaric therapy, all the mafenide cream must be carefully removed by showering or tubbing before putting the patient in the chamber. Silver sulfadiazine (Silvadene®) may be substituted quite effectively and it is safe for concomitant use with HBO.

## Untreated Pneumothorax

Untreated pneumothorax is considered an absolute contraindication to hyperbaric treatment, as there is always concern that if it becomes a tension pneumothorax while the patient is in the chamber, it will render decompression hazardous or potentially life threatening. Since there is no guaranteeing that a pneumothorax will not continue to enlarge at pressure or be transformed into a tension pneumothorax, a chest tube should always be inserted for control, before the patient is placed in the chamber. It is highly advisable to obtain a chest roentgenogram after placement, or attempted placement, of a subclavian line, before the patient is submitted to HBO.

If the patient does not develop a pneumothorax at pressure, any preexisting pneumothorax will be made smaller when the patient breathes oxygen at treatment depth. The pneumothorax diminishes in size as the nitrogen present is rapidly eliminated secondary to oxygen breathing. Under such circumstances, the pneumothorax will be smaller when the patient is removed from the chamber. A one-liter pneumothorax, present just before decompression, however, will assume a 2.5 liter volume on reaching the surface from 2.5 atmospheres absolute.

## RELATIVE CONTRAINDICATIONS

Listed below are conditions in which caution must sometimes be observed, but which are not necessarily a contraindication to hyperbaric oxygen therapy.

## Cis-Platinum

Cis-Platinum is an agent which is useful in a number of different cancers in that it interferes with DNA synthesis, which in turn delays fibroblast production and collagen synthesis. Nemiroff (22) hoped that HBO might help mitigate these effects, but found that wound breaking strength in mice was adversely affected by HBO. When compared with controls, it appears that HBO may increase the cytotoxic effect of the drug in tissue, ultimately impeding wound healing. Any patient having a nonhealing wound who is receiving Cis-platinum will not be helped, and may be worsened by HBO. If one is forced to treat a patient receiving Cis-platinum emergently (necrotizing fasciitis or CO poisoning, for example) the breaking strength of a wound is not an issue, and one would be governed by the emergency indication for recommending treatment with HBO.

## Seizure Disorders

Patients who have a lower than normal seizure threshold may be more prone to develop seizures due to oxygen toxicity. If HBO treatment is a requirement, additional anticonvulsants can be added to these patients' regimens. We frequently use one of the benzodiazepines.

## Emphysema with $CO_2$ Retention

In some patients with severe emphysema and COPD, the only stimulus to breathe is hypoxemia, as they have lost their sensitivity to normal levels of $CO_2$. These patients may dramatically slow their respiratory rate if placed in the hyperbaric chamber. If treatment is absolutely necessary, they can be intubated and ventilated, but clinical judgment should be used to determine whether this is indicated for treatment of a slow healing ulcer, or some other minor problem.

## High Fevers

Uncontrolled high fever can predispose to oxygen seizures. In such cases, drugs can be given to lower the fever, and a hypothermia blanket can also be used. If absolutely necessary, the patient can be gavaged and the stomach irrigated with iced saline. In situations where the patient must be treated acutely, such as gas gangrene, such measures are sometimes indicated. Also, anti-convulsant medication can be given prophylactically.

## History of Spontaneous Pneumothorax

Although history of spontaneous pneumothorax is an absolute contraindication to scuba diving, it does not really present a problem in clinical hyperbaric treatment. The physician, however, should be aware of the history and be prepared to manage pneumothorax in the chamber, should it subsequently occur. Do not make the mistake of thinking that pneumothorax occurs most commonly when the person is physically active, reaching over his head or stretching. This condition often occurs spontaneously during sleep; therefore, it can easily occur in the chamber, when the patient is at rest.

## Upper Respiratory Infections and Chronic Sinusitis

Upper respiratory infections make it difficult for the patient to clear his or her ears, and the same is true for chronic sinusitis. These patients can often be compressed if decongestants are used, or if myringotomy is performed bilaterally. On the other hand, if a patient is receiving a series of hyperbaric treatments for radionecrosis or osteomyelitis, it is often wise to interrupt treatment for three or four days to allow the respiratory infection to clear.

## History of Otosclerosis Surgery

In recent years, stapes mobilization has been supplanted by replacement of the middle ear ossicular conduction chain with a plastic or wire strut. In these patients, failure to equalize pressure in the middle ear might cause bending or displacement of the strut, with severe degradation of hearing. If a patient has had such an operation, I refer the patient to his ENT specialist for placement of a pressure equalization tube in the affected ear(s). Perforation of the eardrum, previous mastoid surgery or other forms of ear surgery, usually pose no problem.

## Viral Infections

Some authorities feel that acute viral infections are a contraindication to hyperbaric oxygen therapy, in that they may be severely exacerbated. We have not had any negative experience in this regard, although some animal work has indicated that pulmonary viral infections may be worsened by adjunctive HBO. Presumably, this is secondary to the irritation of oxygen being synergistic with the viral process in the lung. Other viral infections have not worsened with HBO treatment. Notably, herpes zoster and herpes simplex types 1 and 2 have not been exacerbated or exhibited flare-ups during hyperbaric treatment. Hyperbaric oxygen appears not to influence the immune system in any negative way (7). HIV positive and AIDS patients have not been deleteriously affected by HBO.

## Congenital Spherocytosis

In this condition, the red cells are quite fragile and increased oxygen levels have been shown on occasion to produce severe hemolysis. If there is an absolute requirement to treat such a patient (i.e., gas gangrene) one should not be deterred by the presence of spherocytosis, however, one should be prepared to manage the complications. Such patients have been successfully treated in the chamber.

## History of Optic Neuritis

There have been anecdotal reports of blindness associated with hyperbaric treatment in some patients with a history of optic neuritis, even if not active at the time of treatment. However, these have been extremely rare. One such case was monocular and reverted to normal spontaneously when treatment ceased. However, the author knows of one case where a woman with a history of optic neuritis was being treated for multiple sclerosis. She went completely blind during the course of HBO treatment and remained so. One should immediately halt any further hyperbaric treatment at the slightest suggestion of any visual changes related to the retina. Visual changes can incorrectly be easily dismissed if the patient complains of decreased vision, as temporary changes in the lens which worsen myopia are well known. However, presbyopia should temporarily improve. If the patient complains of impaired vision, determine if it is for distant vision only. If reading ability is also compromised, urgent ophthalmologic consult should be obtained, and further HBO treatment halted.

Some hyperbaric units defensively insist on an ophthalmologist's evaluation of all patients prior to submitting them to multiple treatments. Our universal concern about patients with a history of optic neuritis is probably somewhat overblown; many patients with multiple sclerosis have such a history, with optic neuritis being the harbinger of their disease. However, hundreds of patients have been treated with HBO for MS (albeit ineffectually over the long term) (15) without any additional reported ophthalmologic complications.

## CONDITIONS FORMERLY THOUGHT TO BE ABSOLUTE CONTRAINDICATIONS BUT NOT CONSIDERED SO AT PRESENT

### Bleomycin

When this drug was first introduced as a potent chemotherapeutic agent against certain tumors, interstital pneumonitis was recognized to be the dose-limiting factor. Over the years it had also been reported that even modest elevations of the $FIO_2$ intraoperatively can endanger severe or fatal pneumonitis in patients previously treated with Bleomycin. This was thought to occur even if Bleomycin therapy had ceased months or years before. With this in mind, a history of Bleomycin therapy was normally considered a contraindication to HBO. However, it now appears that this caveat was overblown. A number of patients with a history of Bleomycin have been successfully treated with HBO, with appropriate screening, with no ensuing pulmonary problems.

## Disulfiram (Antabuse®)

Initially, disulfiram was found to block both pulmonary and central nervous system oxygen toxicity when tested by Faiman et al. (6). They showed that mice could be exposed to six atmospheres of oxygen for one hour without convulsing, when pretreated with disulfiram injected intraperitoneally. Necropsy later failed to demonstrate any trace of pulmonary or CNS damage. The work was also repeated with beagle dogs at pressures of four atmospheres absolute with little or no evidence of toxicity. The drug probably acts in competition with enzymes containing SH bonds for free radical oxygen molecules and thereby exerts a protective influence.

However, Heikkila et al. (12) subsequently discovered that disulfiram also blocks the production of superoxide dismutase (SOD) which is the body's major protection against oxygen toxicity. Thus, a single exposure to HBO (such as might occur in carbon monoxide poisoning) would be perfectly safe, and the patient would be in very little danger of convulsing. However, subsequent exposures would be made without the protection of SOD, with unknown effects. For this reason, its use was felt to be contraindicated in those patients receiving multiple HBO treatments. That, however, could be due to the relative rarity of disulfiram treatment, to say nothing of its combination with HBO. Additionally, the dosage given to the rats would equate to about 14 grams of disulfiram given intraperitoneally to humans. Disulfiram dosage to deter alcohol ingestion usually is only 250 mg daily, taken orally. It should be noted that there has been no report of deleterious effects in humans from the combination of disulfiram and HBO.

## Known Malignancies

For many years it was feared that occult metastases, which had outgrown their blood supply, might be stimulated by exposure to hyperbaric oxygen and subsequently not remain occult. Any improvement with HBO in the ischemia associated with a malignancy was felt to be potentially detrimental. However, when hyperbaric units began treating greater numbers of patients with radionecrosis, who had presumably had their cancer eradicated, some patients with residual tumor were inadvertently treated. In these patients, it was frequently noted that most of the radionecrotic areas improved dramatically, except for the area which was subsequently found to contain tumor. In that sense, it was almost a diagnostic test. Failure to heal a small, circumscribed area with HBO is an indication for biopsy. These patients did not seem to exhibit a more aggressive growth of the tumor, however. Subsequent animal experiments have shown that HBO does not speed the growth of tumors (11, 19, 21). Most recently, Sklizovic et al. implanted two different cell lines of human squamous cell carcinoma in nude mice, a species which does not reject living foreign cells. Half the animals were treated with HBO at 2 ATA while the other half were controls. At six weeks there was no difference in tumor size or invasiveness seen in the two groups (28).

## Pregnancy

Because the fetus is by definition premature, and since high concentrations of oxygen have been known since the 1950s to produce retrolental fibroplasia or retinopathy of the newborn, it was felt that hyperbaric oxygen should be contraindicated. Additionally, since stimulus for closure of the patent ductus arteriosus is an increased arterial $PO_2$, potentially fatal intrauterine closure of the ductus was also feared.

However, research published in Russia between 1979 and 1983 (1, 20, 26, 27, 29, 32) concerning over 700 pregnant women treated, during all stages of gestation, with hyperbaric oxygen for hypoxemia-secondary to congenital heart defects, toxemia, mitral insufficiency, habitual abortion, anemia and diabetes-failed to demonstrate any maternal or fetal complications or mortality. Some of these children were even delivered in the chamber. Apparently, the short exposure times used in hyperbaric oxygen treatment do not result in retinopathy of the newborn, and it is also known that it takes 12 continuous hours of exposure to elevated $PO_2$ to initiate closure of the patent ductus. Thus, there appears to be no contraindication to emergency treatment of the pregnant patient (31). While it possibly would be dangerous to treat premature infants, HBO treatment of full-term babies has been shown to be safe.

In pregnancy, it is important to make a distinction between hyperbaric oxygenation and scuba diving. When the patient is placed in the clinical hyperbaric chamber, she breathes only oxygen at pressure. Oxygen is a metabolic gas which is used up rapidly, and does not form bubbles during decompression. However, when scuba diving, she breathes air which contains 79% nitrogen. On decompression, nitrogen forms bubbles as it reverts to gas phase, even during normal "safe" decompressions, and, presumably, this bubbling also occurs in the fetus. Limited research suggests that there is a greater incidence of birth defects in infants whose mothers have engaged in scuba diving while pregnant.

## Implanted Pacemakers

Early pacemakers (in the 1960s) had voids in them and did not tolerate pressurization safely. One of them went out of control and generated a rate of 240 pulses/minute. (See the chapter by Hart entitled "The Monoplace Chamber.") Modern pacemakers apparently tolerate pressurization safely. S. Simmons (Virginia Mason Hospital) reviewed manufacturers testing of the newer models and summarized the results as follows (by manufacturer).

### CPI: 1(800) 227-3422

CPI pulse generators and automatic implanted cardiac defibrillators (AICDs) are tested to 2.36 ATA. Anecdotally, patients have been to higher pressures with no report of problems, according to the manufacturer.

*Intermedics: 1(800) 231-2330*

Each device was tested from 0 to 85 psig. The devices were left at 85 psig for 24 hours, and then tested. No adverse effects were noted.

Devices tested:    Quantum (254-20      Nova II (281-05))
                   Comos (282-04)       Relay (294-03)

*Medtronic: 1(800) 328-2518*

Several pacemakers were tested. All performed normally up to a pressure equivalent of 60 feet of seawater (fsw). Rate responsive pacing began to diminish at pressures in excess of 60 fsw, causing the devices to pace at the lower rate limit. No loss or degradation of output was seen. At pressures of 132 fsw, deformation of the titanium shield was noted. Maximum pressure testing was to 165 fsw. Following the hyperbaric chamber tests, all devices were analyzed. Each performed within specifications.

Devices tested:    Legend TM            Legend II TM
                   Synergist II TM      Elite TM
                   Thera I              Prodigy
                   Elite II

*Pacesetter: 1(800) 722-3774*

All Pacesetter current design cardiac pacemaker models have been tested to 100 psig pressure while maintaining normal function.

## Thoracic Surgery, History

This is not really a contraindication, but it is something of which the physician should be cognizant. It rarely presents a problem. The concern here was that surgical scarring may have produced air-trapping lesions. This is a very real concern in scuba diving, where ambient pressure changes may be halved in as little as five seconds. (This could occur if a diver fully inflated his life jacket at a depth of 10 meters, which is equivalent to 2 ATA.) In the clinical treatment of patients, decompression from the equivalent of 10 or 15 meters (2 or 2.5 atmospheres) takes up to 10 minutes. This is very much akin to the gentle depressurizations experienced by passengers on commercial aircraft. Despite the very poor state of the lungs of many commercial airline passengers, there have been only one report of lung barotrauma and that patient had a giant congenital cyst. Airline passengers, by regulation, may be taken only to a maximum altitude of 8,000 feet in a pressurized cabin; this corresponds to a sea water pressure change of approximately 2 meters (6.5 feet). Burst lung can occur at a transpulmonic pressure of 80 mmHg, which corresponds to a little over a meter of seawater.

The author has successfully given multiple hyperbaric treatments to a patient who had a thoracoplasty. Patients who are post-pneumonectomy can also be successfully treated in the chamber. If there has been a recent pneumonectomy, and there is an air filled space formerly occupied by the lung, a chest tube can be inserted to avoid distortion of the thorax during compression. On the other hand, the space previously occupied by the surgically removed lung fills with fluid very quickly, and then later consolidates. At this stage, when the air is no longer present, pneumonectomy presents no problem.

## Asthma

Anyone with active asthma or asthma precipitated by inhaling cold air or experiencing asthma with exercise should not dive. In any form of diving where compressed air is breathed, unplanned rapid ascents can occur at any time. If the lungs cannot be rapidly deflated as the diver moves upward, gas embolism is the result. With a rapidly inflated buoyancy compensator vest, a diver leaving 50 feet (15 meters) will be on the surface in 7 seconds. The situation is quite different in the hyperbaric chamber. Here, decompressions take 10 minutes or more from the common treatment pressures and the lungs apparently can exhaust gas slowly but safely. We have treated asthmatics with smoke inhalation and with respiratory distress without ensuing gas embolism. Aminophylline and other bronchodilators can be given improve gas exchange.

## COMPLICATIONS AND SIDE EFFECTS

### Barotrauma of the Ear

Barotrauma or ear squeeze is the most common complication of hyperbaric therapy. It is inherently more difficult to inflate the middle ear because the inner ends of the Eustachian tubes, located in the fossae of Rosenmueller in the naso-pharynx, have slit-like openings. These openings tend to close tighter if they are not opened actively. If the patient has descended more than about one meter without clearing the ears, it will be impossible to voluntarily open the tubes through swallowing, yawning, or doing the Valsalva maneuver. This is referred to as a "locked ear". Then the chamber will have to be brought up slightly to facilitate ear clearing. A classification system for the degree of ear squeeze, based on the appearance of the drum, was devised by Wallace Teed, a United States Navy Submarine Medical officer during World War II.

His four point scale is illustrated below.

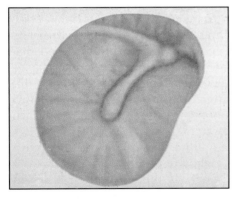 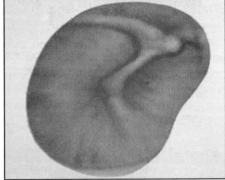

*Figure 1. Teed I - Erythema or injection around the handle of the malleus.*

*Figure 2. Teed II - Erythema or injection of the entire drum.*

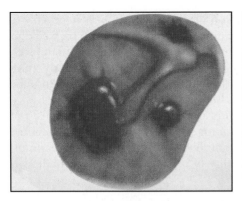 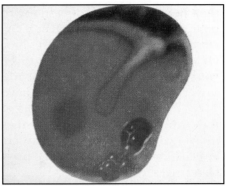

*Figure 3. Teed III - Hemorrhage into the substance of the tympanic membrane itself. These hemorrhages appear as bright red patches on the drum.*

*Figure 4. Teed IV - Deep blue/black appearance of the drum indicating blood filling the middle ear. The eardrum may or may not be ruptured.*

## Round Window Blowout

This extremely rare complication is caused by the vigorous performance of the Valsalva maneuver. When intrathoracic pressure increases maximally, the intracranial pressure also rises, transmitting pressure to the perilymph and endolymph. Increased pressure in the perilymph and endolymph tends to blow out the round and oval windows into the relative vacuum of the middle ear, and if the Valsalva is vigorous enough (as carried out by a highly motivated patient) the round or oval window may rupture. Normally, in an unconscious patient, the tympanic membrane ruptures before the round window gives way. It is only when the Valsalva is applied vigorously that the round or oval window is in jeopardy. Round or oval window blowout usually produces immediate deafness, tinnitus and can produce vestibular symptoms and signs such as nystagmus and vertigo. This syndrome has usually been reported in divers; the author does not know of any occurrence in a clinical hyperbaric patient. Patients should be instructed in the safer Frenzel maneuver in which the intra-pharyngeal pressure is built up using only the muscles of the floor of the mouth and tongue while the nose is pinched shut.

## Sinus Squeeze

Sinus squeeze is caused if any of the openings to the various sinuses to the head are blocked by an overgrowth of tissue, edema, or mucus. Maxillary sinus squeeze may easily be confused with a tooth squeeze of a maxillary tooth. Frontal sinus squeeze usually provokes extremely severe pain, which is rarely tolerable if not relieved by decongestants or very slow compression. The pain of sphenoid sinus squeeze is projected to the occiput or the vertex of the skull.

## Visual Refractive Changes

During the course of multiple hyperbaric treatments (20 treatments or more), some patients may complain of a temporary difficulty in focusing sharply on distant objects, as myopia becomes worse. On the other hand, it tends to improve presbyopia. When patients come to the unit proclaiming their delight at not needing to use reading glasses anymore, it is necessary to point out that the improvement is only temporary, and that within six weeks of cessation of HBO therapy their vision should return to its pretreatment level. Older people (over 50) tend to be affected much more frequently than younger people. It is recommended that new glasses for myopia not be prescribed until at least 8 weeks have passed post HBO treatment.

These changes result from an alteration in the shape of the lens, not the cornea. But the reasons for these changes are not known, and in some individuals refractive error may not completely revert to its pretreatment level, although this is rare. The probability of uric acid buildup in the lens is being investigated.

There has been concern that patients with preexisting cataracts might experience more rapid maturation of the cataracts following hyperbaric treatment. However, Lyne, who studied 26 patients undergoing hyperbaric therapy for more than 30 days, found that no patient who started with a clear lens developed cataracts. In those patients with cataracts present at the start of therapy, the opacities became no more extensive during therapy, and no further changes were found during follow-ups, which ranged from six months to two years (17).

In a Swedish series where patients were treated on a daily basis between 150 and 850 times at pressures ranging from 2 to 2.5 atmospheres, seven of 15 patients with clear lenses before treatment developed well defined nuclear cataracts. The earliest lenticular change was noted at 150 treatments over a four-month period. Three developed nuclear turbidity at 150 to 200 treatments and, 11 developed these changes between 200 and 850 treatments over eight to 19 months. One of the 15 patients showed no lenticular changes (25).

In the United States, the usual maximum number of treatments given ranges between 60 and 75. For this reason the author has not seen cataracts arising *de novo*.

The above data suggest that with a total of fewer than 150 hyperbaric treatments, all lenticular changes should be reversible. Patients with a history of diabetes mellitus, a history of radiation therapy of the head and neck, or a history of systemic steroid therapy are at greater risk for developing cataracts under any circumstances.

In the literature, there have been a number of reports of permanent ocular damage and visual cell death occurring after hyperbaric exposure. However, all of these studies have involved exposures at pressures and durations far greater than would ever be used in clinical therapy (16, 18, 23, 24).

## Numb Fingers

Some patients will complain of numbness and tingling in the ulnar distribution of their fingers after receiving more than 20 hyperbaric oxygen treatments. The mechanism for this is unknown. Treatment consists merely of reassurance, as the paresthesias disappear four to six weeks after HBO therapy ceases. These paresthesias have also been reported as an occupational side effect in Dutch divers who breathe high oxygen mixtures to hasten decompression. There are no known permanent residua.

## Dental Problems, Tooth Squeeze

Rarely, patients will suffer tooth pain during compression or decompression. This is typically caused by a dental restoration that has an air space under the filling. Unfilled teeth or teeth with obvious caries do not pose a problem. When a small air bubble is trapped below the filling in a repaired tooth, upon compression the pulp is forced into the air space within the tooth, which causes exquisite pain. The only solution is replacement of the filling. It is sometimes difficult to distinguish maxillary tooth pain from maxillary sinus squeeze.

## Claustrophobia

*(Some facilities refer to this as "confinement anxiety" to be more politically correct.)*

Davis reported that approximately one out of 50 patients exhibits some degree of confinement anxiety in the multiplace chamber. It is rare, however, that this is severe enough to require sedation. On the other hand, the monoplace chamber can be very anxiety provoking for patients. Approximately one patient in 10, using the 25 inch (63.5 cm) chamber, will have claustrophobia severe enough to make treatment difficult or impossible. However, with the newer 32 and 40 inch (81 and 100 cm) chambers now being manufactured, claustrophobia is much less of a problem. Generally, the more seriously ill the patient is, the less of a problem presented by claustrophobia. It is important to assure the patient that he is in full control at all times and that treatment can be terminated at any time if he or she feels anxious. Should the patient indicate a wish to leave the chamber, this must be accommodated immediately to avoid producing a panic reaction. Later, treatment may be attempted again with appropriate pre-sedation with one of the benzodiazepines.

## Seizures

Davis quoted the incidence of oxygen convulsions to be 1.3 per 10,000 patient treatments, at a pressure of 2.4 ATA. In that series, air breaks of 5 minutes were given every 20 minutes (4). These statistics were based on treatments given over a number of years at the hyperbaric laboratory of the United States Air Force School of Aerospace Medicine. In retrospect, it is now believed that a number of these patients who experienced seizures were hypoglycemic at the time and that they were probably seizures due to low blood sugar. If hypoglycemic seizures were excluded, the true incidence would be more like 0.7 seizures per 10,000 patient treatments. Today, clinical chambers my only give one air break in the middle of a 90 minute protocol. Some chambers use a 5-minute air break every 30 minutes.

## Pulmonary Oxygen Toxicity

Oxygen can produce pulmonary toxicity at one atmosphere, but 24 hours of continuous oxygen breathing is usually required before early signs appear, such as substernal chest pain, dry cough, and a decrease in vital capacity. At 2 ATA, these changes appear within six hours of continuous exposure. However, continuous HBO exposures rarely exceed two hours clinically. In the treatment of decompression sickness on Table 6, the patient breathes oxygen for four hours. Exposure time is interrupted for air-breathing periods, during which time recovery from sub clinical toxicity takes place. Using the normal protocols published for HBO treatment, pulmonary oxygen toxicity has never been reported. If, however, the patient is continuously carried on $FIO_2$s greater than 40% between HBO treatments, toxicity of the lung may become a possibility.

## REFERENCES

1. Aksenova, A., I.V. Proshina, L.K. Smirnova, et al. "Methods of Prenatal Diagnosis of Fetal Hypoxia and Control of the Effectiveness of its Treatment with Hyperbaric Oxygen." Akush. Ginekol. (Russian) 1979;11:15-18.

2. Comis. R.L. (Editorial) Detecting Bleomycin Pulmonary Toxicity: A Continued Conundrum. J. Clin. Oncol. 8(5):765-767 May, 1990.

3. Comis, R.L. Bleomycin Pulmonary Toxicity: Current Status and Future Directions. Seminars in Oncology 19:(2) (Suppl 5) 64-70, April 1992.

4. Davis, J.C. "Complications" Davis, J.C. and T.K. Hunt (Eds.) Problem Wounds: The Role of Oxygen, Elsevier Science Publishing Company, New York. 1988;233.

5. Donat, S.M. and Levy, D.A. Bleomycin Associated Pulmonary Toxicity: Is Perioperative Oxygen Restriction a Necessity? J. of Urology 160:1347-1352 Oct. 1998.

6. Faiman, M.D., R.G. Mehl and F.W. Oehme. "Protection with disulfiram from central and pulmonary oxygen toxicity." Biochem. Pharma. Pergamon Press, Great Britain. 1971;20:3059-3067.

7. Feldmeier, J.J., R.N. Roswell, M. Brown, et al. "The effects of hyperbaric oxygen on the immunologic status of healthy human subjects." Kindwall, E.P. (Ed.) Proceedings of the Eighth International Congress on Hyperbaric Medicine. Best Publishing, Flagstaff, Arizona. 1987;41-46.

8. Gilson, A.J., and Sahn, S.A., Reactivation of Bleomycin Lung Toxicity following Oxygen Administration. A second response to corticosteroids. Chest 55(2): 304-306, August 1985.

9. Goldiner, P.L., Carlon, G.C, Cvitkovic, E., Schweizer, O. and Howland, W.S. Factors influencing Postoperative Morbidity and Mortality in Patients Treated with Bleomycin Brit. Med. J. 1:1664-1667, 24 June 1978.

10. Goldiner, P.L.and Schweizer, O. The Hazards of Anesthesia and Surgery in Bleomycin-Treated Patients, Seminars in Oncology 6:(1) 121-124 March 1979.

11. Granström, G., S. Edström, T. Westin, et al. "Hyperbaric oxygenation does not stimulate experimental tumor growth." Undersea Biomedical Research. 17(Suppl) 1990;66 (Abstract only).

12. Heikkila, R.E., F.S. Cabbat & G. Cohen. "*In vivo* Inhibition of superoxide dismutase in mice by diethyldithiocarbamate." J. Bio. Chem. 1976;251:2182.

13. Ichikawa, T., Studies of Bleomycin: Discovery of its clinical effect, combination treatment with bleomycin and radiotherapy, side effects and long term survival. Jpn J. of Cancer Research 19:99-115, 1976.

14. Jules-Elysee, K. and White, D.A. Bleomycin-Induced Pulmonary Toxicity. Clinics in Chest Medicine 11(1):1-20, March 1990.

15. Kindwall, E.P., M.P. McQuillen, B.O. Khatri, H.W. Gruchow and M.L. Kindwall "Treatment of multiple sclerosis with hyperbaric oxygen." Arch of Neurol. 1991;48:195-199.

16. Kobayashi, T., S. Murakami. "Blindness of an adult caused by oxygen." JAMA. 1972;219:741.

17. Lyne A.J. "Ocular effects of hyperbaric oxygen." Transactions of the Ophthalmologic Society of the UK. 1978;98:66-68.

18. Margolis, G. "Hyperbaric oxygenation: The eye as a limiting factor. " Science. 1966;151:466-468.

19. Marx, R.E. and R.P. Johnson. "Relationship of hyperbaric oxygen to oral cancer." JC Davis and TK Hunt (Eds.) Problem Wounds: the Role of Oxygen. Elsevier Science Publishing Company, New York. 1988;107-110.

20. Molzhaninov, E.V., V.K. Chaika, A.I. Domanova, et al. "Experience and prospects of using hyperbaric oxygenation in obstetrics." Proceedings of the Seventh International Congress on Hyperbaric Medicine, Moscow 1981. Nauka, Moscow. (Russian) 1983;1:139-141.

21. Nemiroff, P.R., R.G. Martin, S.H. Mahafee and N.J. Cassissi. "The effects of hyperbaric oxygen and cyclophosphamide on Lewis Lund tumors in mice." Undersea Biomedical Research. 15(Suppl) 1988;22 (Abstract only).

22. Nemiroff, P.R."Effects of Cis-Platinum and hyperbaric oxygen on wound healing in mice." Undersea Biomedical Research. (Suppl):40 1988;15 (Abstract only).

23. Noell, W.K. "Metabolic injuries of the visual cell." American Journal of Ophthalmology. 1955;40:60-68.

24. Noell, W.K. "Differentiation, metabolic organization and viability of the visual cell." Archives of Ophthalmology. 1958;60:702-733.

25. Palmquist, B.M., B. Phillipson & P.O. Barr. "Nuclear cataract and myopia during hyperbaric oxygen therapy." British Journal of Ophthalmology 1984;68:113-117.

26. Pobedinsky, N.M., I.V. Proshina, N.D. Fanchenko, et al. "Hyperbaric oxygen in the treatment of reproductive function of women." Proceedings of the Seventh International Congress on Hyperbaric Medicine, Moscow 1981. Nauka, Moscow (Russian). 1983;1:133-136.

27. Proshina, I.V., N.V. Kuzmina, S.S. Borisenko. "Hyperbaric oxygenation in the prevention and treatment of toxemia of pregnancy and placental insufficiency." Akush. Ginekol. (Russian) 1983;6:20-23.

28. Sklizovic, D., J.R. Sanger, E.P. Kindwall, J. Fink, B. Grunert, B.H. Campbell "Hyperbaric oxygen therapy and squamous cell carcinoma growth." Head and Neck. 1993;15(3):236-240.

29. Stepanyants, N.A., E.L. Grinshpun, V.A. Popov, et al. "Hyperbaric oxygenation in the complex treatment of late toxicosis of pregnancy." Proceedings of the Seventh International Congress on Hyperbaric Medicine. Moscow 1981. Nauka, Moscow (Russian). 1983;1:137-138.

30. Upton, P.G., K.T. Yamaguchi, S. Myers, T.P. Kidwell and R.J. Anderson "Effects of antioxidants and hyperbaric oxygen in ameliorating experimental doxorubicin skin toxicity in the rat." Cancer Treatment Reports. 1986;70(4):503-507.

31. VanHoesen, K.B., E.M. Camporesi, R.E. Moon, et al. "Should hyperbaric oxygen be used to treat the pregnant patient for acute carbon monoxide poisoning?" JAMA. 1989;261(7):1039-1043.

32. Vanina, L.V., S.N. Efuni, A.L. Beilin, et al. "Obstetrics aid in hyperbaric conditions." Proceedings of the Seventh International Congress on Hyperbaric Medicine. Moscow 1981. Nauka, Moscow (Russian) 1983;1:26-28.

33. Youngblood, D.A., Scuba Diving Following Bleomycin Therapy: Is it Safe? Triage (Newsletter of the Nat. Bd. Of Diving and Hyperbaric Technicians) Vol.4 #1 p. 3, Fall 1991.

CHAPTER 13

# MANAGEMENT OF COMPLICATIONS IN HYPERBARIC TREATMENT

## CHAPTER THIRTEEN OVERVIEW

# MANAGEMENT OF COMPLICATIONS IN HYPERBARIC TREATMENT

*Eric P. Kindwall*

## INTRODUCTION

As has been seen in earlier chapters, hyperbaric oxygen therapy is remarkably free of major side effects, and complications are rare. The most common difficulty is barotrauma, typically of the middle ear, but this usually is more of an annoyance than a major problem.

Although serious problems are not often encountered, it is imperative that the physician be fully capable of managing them should they occur.

## COMPLICATIONS

### Barotrauma

Any gas-containing cavity within the body which has unyielding walls is subject to barotrauma if its communication with ambient pressure is blocked. Those areas which typically cause problems are the middle ear, the cranial sinuses, and, occasionally, a tooth.

In non-emergent situations, if a patient is suffering from an upper respiratory infection with nasopharyngeal congestion, it is often wise to postpone initiation of hyperbaric treatment for a few days. This is often done with patients who have had chronic radionecrosis or osteomyelitis for months or years. If a patient develops an upper respiratory infection during the course of a series of hyperbaric treatments for radionecrosis or osteomyelitis, therapy is often halted for a few days, until the acute phase has passed. Avoidance of the problem is probably better than trying to force gas into the middle ear of a patient who has marginal Eustachian patency. On the other hand, in the acute situation, one will have to proceed regardless of the status of the Eustachian tubes.

It is always easier to clear the ears while sitting up than while lying down. This is well known to divers who may have difficulty descending headfirst but whose ears clear easily if they descend feet first. In the multiplace chamber, a sitting position is possible for ear clearing if the patient is able to sit up. In the older 25-inch (64-cm) monoplace chambers, this is not usually possible. If there are no contraindications, patients are frequently given a vasoconstricting nasal spray, although a controlled study showed it reduces ear clearing difficulty marginally, if at all (2). If used, sufficient time must be allotted for vasoconstriction to take place. Difficulties with the Eustachian tubes can usually be anticipated in those patients who have nasogastric tubes, in those recovering from recent head and neck surgery, and in burn patients.

The patient is instructed in how to clear his/her ears using the Frenzel maneuver, or the Valsalva, if necessary, and by swallowing or yawning. The Frenzel maneuver is performed by pinching the nostrils shut, closing the glottis, and then raising the pressure in the oropharynx by elevating the floor of the mouth and tongue. The Frenzel maneuver is quite effective; in that, the muscle movement involved, per se, tends to open the Eustachian tubes more than the Valsalva, and it does not carry with it the dangers of round-window blowout seen with the Valsalva maneuver. In the monoplace chamber, each patient is usually provided a small squeeze bottle of water from which he/she may take sips during compression. Stretching the neck away from the affected side while performing the Frenzel or Valsalva maneuver is often helpful. It is important to remember that if the patient descends more than about four feet (2 psig, one meter, 10 Kg/Pa) without equalizing middle ear pressure, the slit-like openings of the Eustachian tubes in the nasopharynx will be squeezed shut, rendering further equalization impossible. This is referred to as a "locked ear". For this reason, it is necessary that the patient continually keep up with pressure changes. Should the ears become locked, it will be necessary to decrease pressure by 2 or 3 psig (one to two meters) so that equalization can again occur.

Extremely slow compressions may be used, taking as long as 30 to 40 minutes to reach two atmospheres pressure, if one is committed to continue treatment that day. However, if multiple treatments are to be given, pressure-equalization tubes must be placed in the tympanic membranes before treatment is tried again. In the multiplace chamber, helium/oxygen breathing has sometimes been used to help move gas into the tight Eustachian orifices. If it is absolutely imperative that pressure be reached quickly, and none of the other methods have been adequate to achieve equalization, a myringotomy can be done. See the chapter by Kidder entitled "Myringotomy." In the multiplace chamber, this is typically done at pressure in the chamber. In the monoplace chamber, the patient must be decompressed, removed from the chamber and the myringotomy performed. In the patient who is to be treated chronically, and with whom there is no urgency, it may be wise to decompress the patient, and send him/her to an ENT specialist for pressure equalization tubes before attempting re-treatment. In patients with marginally patent tubes, the administration of an oral decongestant given one to two hours before treatment may be a good solution, but the results may be uncertain. In the unconscious patient, where no myringotomy has been done, if the ears do not clear spontaneously, the eardrums may rupture, which immediately solves the equalization problem. The drums will heal spontaneously, as they do following myringotomy, within 10 to 14 days. In the timid, frightened patient, it is extremely important to pay particular attention to the ears and to minimize the effects of barotrauma.

However, in small children I have found it is often wiser to forego myringotomy. Much cerumen is often present, blocking visualization of the drum at the end of a tiny canal. Lengthy and painful attempts to remove the cerumen and carry out the myringotomy in a squirming, crying patient can be more upsetting to both child and parent than a simple rupture of the tympanic membrane during a quick compression. The tympanic membrane usually heals remarkably quickly if chronic infection is not present. It should be remembered that the eardrum ruptures before the round or oval window, unless the patient is actively doing the Valsalva maneuver.

## Sinus Blockage

This is much more difficult to treat as there is no surgical remedy such as myringotomy, which is readily available. Fortunately, it is not as common as blocked ears. The only practical solutions available are the use of oral decongestant tablets and vasoconstrictive nasal sprays. The frontal sinus is extremely sensitive to barotrauma and the pain from a blocked frontal sinus is nearly unbearable. Pain from the sphenoid sinus will radiate to the occiput or vertex of the skull. If a blocked sinus cannot be cleared, and the patient requires multiple treatments, consultation should be sought with an ENT specialist.

## Round or Oval Window Rupture

If pressure is built up on the tympanic membrane without compensatory inflation of the middle ear, it will usually rupture somewhere between 4 and 7 psig (3 to 5 meters of seawater equivalent). It takes a greater trauma to rupture the round or oval window membranes, which retain the endolymph and perilymph in the inner ear.

Rupture of these structures can occur if the Valsalva maneuver is too vigorously performed. A highly motivated patient may hold his/her nose and vigorously compress the thorax in an effort to equalize the ears. The intrathoracic pressure stops venous return, causing intracranial pressure to rise precipitously. This pressure, in turn, is reflected in the perilymph and endolymph, which causes the round and oval window membranes to bulge out into the relative vacuum of the middle ear. Too much pressure can cause rupture with resultant fluid leakage. Symptoms may be vertigo, tinnitus, and abrupt deafness in the affected ear.

An ENT specialist familiar with round window rupture, cochlear hemorrhage, or tears in Reissner's membrane, should carefully work up deafness, vertigo, and tinnitus following a hyperbaric treatment. The patient should be confined to bed with the head elevated, and any coughing or straining at stool must be suppressed. If symptoms do not clear within 72 hours, surgical exploration is mandatory.

## Painful Teeth

Rarely, there may be a gas pocket under a filling in a restored tooth. If this continues to be a problem, the only remedy is to have a dentist remove the filling and replace it, being careful to completely fill the entire void.

## Gas Embolism

Gas embolism is an exceedingly rare occurrence in clinical hyperbaric oxygen therapy. Its incidence must be minutely small, as the author has never seen it occur in over 35 years of practice. Gas embolism following "burst lung" occurs much more commonly in divers where very rapid changes in the ambient pressure are possible. Ascent from 33 feet (10 meters, 2 ATA) to the surface, with an inflated life vest or buoyancy compensator, can take place in as little as five seconds. Lung gas volume doubles in that time, and unless there is free egress of air from the lungs, lung rupture will result. In the clinical hyperbaric chamber, decompressions typically take 10 minutes or more; in multiplace chamber practice, a decompression stop is often included. Under those circumstances, lung rupture almost becomes a practical impossibility. Should a gas embolism occur in a monoplace chamber, it will always be an oxygen embolism. Since oxygen is a metabolic gas, any bubbles will eventually be metabolized, and, theoretically, the prognosis should be better. Nevertheless, a no-reflow phenomenon may result, even from an oxygen embolism because of bubble-induced damage to the capillary endothelium and blockage by the formed elements of the blood. In the multiplace chamber, if the patient is not wearing an oxygen mask at the time the embolism occurs, it will be an air embolism in which 79% of the bubble volume will be composed of nitrogen. If embolism occurs following a normal hyperbaric treatment, the gradient of nitrogen out of the bubble into the surrounding tissues will be larger than normal, as there will be little nitrogen in the tissues. Therefore, in theory, the nitrogen embolism should clear more rapidly.

The only reasonable mechanism whereby burst lung and a gas embolism could occur in a clinical hyperbaric chamber would be a rapid, emergency decompression with a blocked glottis. This might occur in the event of explosive decompression following rupture of a chamber viewport or catastrophic failure of the chamber itself. Alternately, rapid decompression of a patient during the tonic phase of a seizure (while the patient is breath holding) might also precipitate rupture of the lung. On at least two occasions blockage of outflow from a bronchopulmonary segment has cause burst lung and embolism. In one case it was due to a carcinoma and the other was secondary to a tubercular broncholith that acted as a ball and check valve. Proper treatment of an embolism will only follow proper diagnosis and the availability of recompression. If there has been an equipment casualty, and there is no other chamber available in the vicinity, immediate recompression may be impossible. Diagnosis should be made from the usual criteria of sudden unconsciousness or cerebral signs, a hemiplegia, an enlarged pupil, changes in voice quality, and eventual subcutaneous emphysema in the neck. Subcutaneous emphysema is seen in one-third of the cases embolizing in the open sea where there is a delay before treatment, but is never seen in submarine escape-training casualties, as they are typically recompressed within seconds of symptom onset.  A hallmark of arterial gas embolism usually is sudden onset of the condition, typically as the door of the chamber is opened. If immediate recompression is impossible, or while trying to establish a definite diagnosis in a questionable case, the patient should be placed in steep Trendelenburg position (30 to 60 degrees) for no more than five or six minutes, if other factors permit this (1). Prolonging the head down position for more than a few minutes is harmful and will cause cerebral edema (3). If definite embolism is diagnosed, and it is impossible to retreat at one's own facility due to an equipment casualty, the patient must be transferred to another chamber no matter how far away it is. The patient, minimally, should be recompressed to 60 feet (2.8 ATA), and treated with oxygen. If the treating chamber facility permits, recompression to 6 ATA is recommended. (See treatment protocols in other chapters.) If the patient needs ventilatory support, this should be provided via endotracheal tube and a ventilator. Ancillary problems such as sedation, seizure prevention, maintenance of the airway, etc., must be dealt with. The patient may need to be paralyzed and other critical care provided. Treatment should be as for air embolism occurring in any other setting.

## Decompression Sickness

Patients treated with hyperbaric oxygen are not at risk for decompression sickness as they are being denitrogenated during the entire treatment. In a multiplace chamber, in the event that air has inadvertently been administered by mask as opposed to oxygen, decompression sickness becomes a theoretical possibility. With a clinical protocol such as oxygen breathing for 2 hours at 2 ATA, decompression sickness would not cause a problem, even if the treatment gas had been switched in error. At 2.4 atmospheres it could pose a problem. It is extremely important that there be fail-safe mechanisms to always assure oxygen delivery to the patient. Accidents have occurred in the past secondary to improper breathing gas connections.

Attendants taking care of patients inside the chamber routinely breathe air, and decompression sickness is not unknown in hyperbaric chamber crews. If the decompression recommendations listed in the chapter describing the multiplace chamber are carried out, decompression sickness should be a rarity indeed. Nevertheless, should it occur, treatment is on US Navy treatment tables, as for any other case of decompression sickness. Hyperbaric crews should be well aware of how to contact the hyperbaric physician on call should decompression sickness occur, and provision should be made for immediate treatment of inside tenders, particularly on holidays and weekends when a full staff or the regular hyperbaric physician may not be available. Inside attendants must not engage in scuba diving in the 24 hours prior to working in the hyperbaric chamber, nor should they fly for a period of 24 hours following the last exposure in the chamber. They should be well schooled in the symptoms of decompression sickness and taught not to ignore early signs. There is evidence to suggest that even "pain only" decompression sickness may carry with it possible brain damage, especially if not treated immediately (4).

Inside attendants should be particularly aware of the symptoms of vestibular DCS. They must be taught, as part of their training, the absolute necessity of recompression treatment _within 45 minutes_ of the onset of symptoms of vestibular DCS, if significant immediate relief is to be achieved.

## Respiratory Arrest

Patients with chronic obstructive lung disease may be relatively insensitive to $CO_2$ and when given high concentrations of inspired oxygen under hyperbaric conditions, they theoretically could lose their respiratory drive completely. Patients who could fall into this category should be watched closely, especially during their first treatment, to determine that they are not relying on hypoxic drive alone to maintain their respirations. Should respiratory arrest occur, or should the respirations be noted to become extremely infrequent or shallow, the conscious patient may be instructed to take several deep breaths, and can be coached to maintain a reasonable respiratory rate for the remainder of the treatment. If respirations cease and the patient becomes unconscious, the patient should be mechanically ventilated with an Ambu or Laerdal bag in the multiplace chamber, or promptly decompressed in the monoplace chamber. The arterial $pO_2$ will generally be high and there is little danger of brain damage.

## Seizure

Based on data from the United States Air Force hyperbaric unit in San Antonio, Texas, oxygen seizures occur only about 1.3 times in 10,000 exposures, when 5 minute air breaks are given every 20 minutes at 2.4 ATA. The actual incidence, if hypoglycemic seizures are excluded, may be half of that. Convulsions are usually seen in people with previous brain injury or idiopathically low seizure thresholds. Signs of oxygen toxicity begin with sweating, followed by one or more of the following: Nausea and vomiting, apprehension, shortness of breath, tunnel vision, tinnitus, and muscle twitching, especially around the eyes, or twitching of the diaphragm. I have seen two patients with transient deafness. These may be premonitory to a grand mal seizure. In my experience, however, none of these factors, other than sweating, have preceded the actual seizure, which has always come without warning. Sweating as an early sign of oxygen toxicity is so common (almost universal) that it has no predictive value.

In the multiplace chamber, treatment consists simply of removing the mask. The patient will usually cease seizing within one or two minutes. In the event that the seizure does not stop following mask removal and breathing chamber air, diazepam (10 mg), or lorazepam (2 mg) may be given intravenously. Alternatively, intravenous phenobarbital (250 mg) may be given or intravenous phenytoin in the dosage of 15 to 18 mg/kg at the rate of 50 mg per minute. Blood pressure should be monitored.

In the monoplace chamber, if the patient has an IV running, diazepam or lorazepam can be administered while decreasing the $FIO_2$. The only practical way of lowering the inhaled oxygen pressure in the monoplace chamber is to decompress the patient. Initially, the seizure will consist of a tonic phase where the patient may well be holding his/her breath. Decompression *should never be attempted during the tonic phase*. When the patient ceases being tonic, and begins jerking clonic movement, there will usually be some stertorous, uneven, irregular breathing. During this time, the patient should be emergently decompressed *by pushing the emergency decompression button IN SHORT BURSTS*, allowing equilibration of pressure every two to three pounds. This is to avoid lung rupture. When the patient is removed from the chamber, should the seizure not stop, medication can be administered as described above. In diabetics, the seizure may well be due to hypoglycemia, as blood sugar is seen to fall during hyperbaric treatment. A quick glucometer test can determine the patient's blood sugar level. If indicated, 50% glucose can then be delivered IV.

## Pneumothorax

Pneumothorax occurring in the chamber is a serious, potentially life-threatening event. When the patient is subsequently decompressed, the pneumothorax expands as a function of the number of atmospheres pressure at which it occurred. Correct diagnosis is the key to its management.

The usual signs of pneumothorax are shortness of breath, chest pain, tracheal deviation to the side of the collapsed lung, and absence of breath sounds on the affected side. In the chamber, cyanosis will not be seen. In the multiplace chamber, there often is a good deal of background noise from ventilating fans, incoming air, and the rumble of exhaust air. Under those circumstances, it may be difficult to hear differences in breath sounds between the two sides of the chest. It is advantageous to turn off the ventilating fans, supply air, and exhaust air while listening to the chest. There is a pathognomonic test for pneumothorax which is available in the hyperbaric chamber and not available elsewhere. If the patient's respiratory distress worsens during decompression, but improves immediately on recompression, the diagnosis is made. Treatment is to insert a needle between the second and third or the third and fourth interspace on the affected side with a three-way stopcock and a large syringe. Gas can then be released from the chest and a Heimlich valve applied. Alternatively, continuous suction via a 30-cm water seal may be started. When this has been accomplished, decompression can be continued.

The situation is much more difficult in the monoplace chamber, both from the standpoint of diagnosis and management. Obviously, it will be impossible to listen for breath sounds, and one must rely on the patient's description of his/her symptoms, tracheal deviation if any, differences in movement between the two sides of the chest during breathing, and, finally, the pathognomonic decompression/compression test. Once it has been determined that a pneumothorax does indeed exist, and its side has been ascertained, the patient should be held at a comfortable pressure until a full management team can be assembled. This would ideally consist of a thoracic surgeon, an anesthesiologist, intubation equipment, a full thoracentesis set, and suction. When all preparations have been made, the necessary drugs drawn up in syringes with needles attached, and all instruments made ready, the patient is quickly decompressed, usually taking no more than one minute. Immediately, the patient is withdrawn from the chamber and a needle inserted in the affected side. Over-pressure in the thorax must be exhausted quickly to allow venous return to the heart and to re-establish circulation. When this has been accomplished, the usual surgical management of pneumothorax is carried out.

## Cardiac Arrest

Cardiac arrest is a rarity in the chamber, as most arrhythmias seem to improve under hyperbaric conditions. Anecdotally, it can be noted that one patient with a myocardial infarction, who was being treated with hyperbaric oxygen as part of a research study, suffered 30 cardiac arrests during the 48 hours he was being treated with the chamber. The schedule being followed called for two hours at pressure in the chamber followed by one hour on the surface. This cycle was repeated for two days. It can be seen that the patient spent only 1/3 of his time breathing air on the surface. During the study, the patient suffered 28 cardiac arrests while breathing air on the surface, but only two arrests while at pressure in the chamber. The patient eventually recovered and returned to work. (Thurston, J. Westminster Hosp, London, Personal Communication, 1973.)

In the multi-place chamber, CPR can be initiated immediately by the inside tender, and a full cardiac arrest code can be called. The resuscitation from cardiac arrest can be carried out in the chamber, including defibrillation, as long as certain precautions are taken. The availability of high partial pressures of oxygen may be of value in restarting the patient's heart. It is probably better not to administer intracardiac drugs percutaneously. These drugs can normally be introduced intratracheally. Alternatively, if the cardiac arrest team does not wish to, or cannot, enter the chamber under pressure, the patient can be emergently decompressed to the surface and standard cardiac resuscitation carried out. Because of the number of people involved in the typical cardiac arrest code, it is probably the better part of valor to decompress the patient immediately and turn a hyperbaric emergency into a normobaric one. If cardiac arrest occurs in the monoplace chamber, the patient must be removed in order to proceed with cardiopulmonary resuscitation. The emergency button can be used, being sure that the patient is not trapping air. This is unlikely if the patient is indeed totally flaccid and unconscious. The patient can normally be removed from the chamber in less than a minute, but it must be remembered that in any case of hyperbaric cardiac arrest, the arrest will have occurred while that patient's arterial $pO_2$ was of the order of 1,200 mmHg or greater. Thus, there is a grace period of several minutes before CPR need be established. Once the patient has been removed from the chamber, standard cardiac resuscitative procedures can be used. In tests carried out by the author, when the chamber door is opened, the oxygen within the chamber has been demonstrated, to diffuse to the floor, as it is cold and heavier than ambient air. There is literally no rise in ambient oxygen at the level of the patient's chest outside the chamber. Within 30 to 40 seconds, all of the oxygen issuing from the chamber will have dissipated in the room and will not be measurable. For this reason, defibrillation should carry no added risk of fire.

## Omitted Decompression for the Inside Attendant

In the event it that a patient treatment must be aborted due to a cardiac arrest or any other cause, it is important to be sure that the inside tender has had adequate decompression. If required decompression has been missed, the inside tender must be immediately recompressed, as soon as the patient is evacuated from the chamber. The U.S. Navy guidelines for missed decompression are as follows (5):

### Emergency ascent from 20 feet (6 meters) or shallower

If the inside tender surfaces from 20 feet or shallower, indicates that he/she is well, and can be returned to his/her stop within one minute, the normal decompression stop(s) can be completed. The decompression stop from which ascent occurred is lengthened by one minute. If the one-minute surface interval is exceeded, and the tender remains asymptomatic, return the tender to the stop from which he/she ascended, and multiply the 20- and/or 10-foot stop times by 1.5. My recommendation is that oxygen be breathed at all times, and that the tender should be taking a 2-minute stop 10 feet (3 meters) deeper than specified in the table written for air. See the chapter by Hart entitled "The Monoplace Chamber."

### *Emergency ascent from deeper than 20 feet (6 meters)*

Standard Navy procedure requires treatment on Table 5 or Table 6 if more that 30 minutes of decompression has been missed. This is probably excessive after aborting most of the profiles used in the treatment of clinical HBO patients. Since oxygen will be breathed by the inside tender instead of air during his/her recompression, the Navy rule for air recompression of the asymptomatic diver in the water will usually suffice. Use the following schedule (which was written for air breathing) with one minute between stops:

- At 40 feet (12 meters) remain for one-fourth of the 10-foot (3 meter) stop time.
- At 30 feet (9 meters) remain for one-third of the 10-foot stop time.
- At 20 feet (6 meters) remain for one-half of the 10-foot stop time.
- At 10 feet (3 meters) remain for one and one-half times the scheduled 10 foot stop time.

Oxygen breathing instead of air is used in the above schedule for added safety.

Another option is to use the U.S. Navy surface decompression table using oxygen if the tender can be returned to forty feet (12 meters) within 5 minutes. In such a case it would be a good idea to pad the stop times by at least 25 percent.

The above guidelines are for aborting typical profiles for HBO patients, which will usually not be deeper than 66 feet (3 ATA). In the rare event that the tender is surfaced precipitously from a depth greater than 66 feet (20 meters), or immediately has symptoms of DCS or AGE on surfacing, recompress to 165 feet (50 meters) and treat on Table 6A with mixed gas or on the Lee Table. See the chapter by Elliott entitled "Decompression Sickness."

## CONCLUSION

Complications are rare in hyperbaric treatment compared with other forms of therapy applied to patients in the clinical setting. This must never lull the hyperbaric physician or technician into a state of inattentiveness, however, as the consequences of improper management of these emergencies can be serious indeed.

## REFERENCES

1. Atkinson JR. "Experimental air embolism." Northwest Medicine. 1963;62:699-703.

2. Carlson, S, J Jones, M Brown and C Hess. "Prevention of hyperbaric-associated middle ear barotrauma." Annals of Emerg. Med. 1992; 21(12):70-72.

3. Dutka AJ, Polychronidis J, Mink RB, Hallenbeck JM. "Head-down position after air embolism impairs recovery of brain function as measured by the somatosensory evoked response in canines." Undersea Biomedical Research. 1990;17(Suppl):64.

4. Gorman DF, Edmonds CW, Parsons DW, Beran RG, Anderson TA, Green RD, Loxton MJ, Dillon TA. "Neurologic Sequelae of Decompression Sickness: A Clinical Report." In: (Bove, AA, Bachrach AJ, Greenbaum LJ, Jr. Eds.) Underwater and Hyperbaric Physiology IX, Undersea and Hyperbaric Medical Society, Inc., Bethesda. 1987; pp. 993-998.

5. U.S. Navy Diving Manual, Revision 5, Volume 5 U.S. Naval Sea Systems Command 2005

CHAPTER 14

# HYPERBARIC MEDICINE IN PEDIATRIC PRACTICE

## CHAPTER FOURTEEN OVERVIEW

# Hyperbaric Medicine in Pediatric Practice

*Paul A. Thombs, Robert C. Borer, Jr., Frank J. Martorano*

## INTRODUCTION

Clinical and basic science investigations have revealed many of the biological actions of breathing oxygen at partial pressures greater than atmospheric. Some of these actions include: restoration of normal tissue oxygen gradients, enhancement of neutrophil function, suppression of clostridial toxin production, changes in systemic and cerebral vascular tone, reduction in tissue gas phase size, enhanced excretion of inert gas, prevention or amelioration of reperfusion injuries, and modification of the host inflammatory response. While all these mechanisms of hyperoxygenation apply to the entire spectrum of age, there are some recently recognized biological actions, which have special relevance to the pediatric patient.

The pediatric age patient is unique when compared to the adult or aging patient in that both growth and development are dominant phenomena. From the newly born infant through adolescence, there is a continuum of change in which cell proliferation and maturation is occurring. Associated with this growth is a complex array of intracellular and extracellular signals, which modulate cellular proliferation. It is becoming clear that intermittent hyperoxygenation potentiates the protein extracellular ligands known as growth factors. The action of vascular endothelial growth factor in stimulating capillary proliferation is synergistically enhanced by hyperbaric oxygen exposure in a dose-dependent manner (2). Similarly, fibroblastic replication is increased by hyperbaric oxygen (13, 33). The specific mechanism by which hyperbaric oxygen accomplishes this is not clear but there is a suggestion that the intracellular flux of reactive oxygen and reactive nitrogen species may function as second intracellular messengers (17). Hydrogen peroxide has been shown to be an essential requirement for vascular smooth-muscle cell proliferation, mediated by platelet-derived growth factor (31). The levels and distribution of growth factors of various tissues decreases with age. With an abundance of growth factors, the younger patients are in an optimal position, compared to adults, for favorable clinical responses to hyperbaric oxygen therapy in situations where cellular proliferation is important. Fewer hyperbaric treatments may be required for a specific clinical outcome. A review of the number of treatments required for hypoxic non-healing wounds associated with cyanotic congenital heart disease in the neonate (35) and for radiation-induced tissue injury in children (3) shows that fewer treatments are required than commonly described for similar conditions in adults. Recent studies have also shown that hyperbaric oxygen can mobilize stem cells (35 ).

Another feature of increasing age is the intracellular accumulation of unstable modified proteins, which impede normal homeostasis (30). Dermal derived cells, fibroblasts, and keratinocytes from the young, which are important in wound healing have energy-efficient catabolic processes to remove these ineffectual proteins, when compared to the adult (12). All of these age-dependent cellular differences provide a rationale for a rapid clinical response to hyperbaric oxygen therapy in the pediatric patient.

There are no significant differences in side effects or morbidity with hyperbaric oxygen treatments for children compared to adults (19, 26). This suggests that the customary adult dose of oxygen is tolerated by the growing and developing postnatal human organism, as well as being sufficient to achieve the desired clinical effect.

## INDICATIONS

Generally, the indications for the use of hyperbaric oxygen in pediatric practice are very similar to those in adult practice. Children, like adults, are subject to accidents producing ischemia/reperfusion injuries (29, 39) and open fractures subject to chronic, non-hematogenous osteomyelitis (8). Children, too, undergo intense immunosuppression for the treatment of malignancies and the prevention of rejection of transplanted organs, thereby increasing their risks of developing rapidly progressive, necrotizing, soft tissue infections or life threatening infections such as brain abscess and rhinocerebral Zygomycetes (5, 10, 15, 22, 24, 36, 37, 42). Congenital immunodeficiency frequently presents during childhood as an overwhelming infection (28). Ionizing radiation remains a mainstay in the treatment of certain pediatric malignancies, setting the stage for hard-and soft-tissue radiation necrosis (16). Atherosclerotic peripheral vascular disease is not a pediatric malady, but children do develop acute peripheral arterial insufficiency from purpura fulminans (25, 38). They may also suffer the aftereffects of accidental, intra-arterial infusion of medication or extravasations of irritant solutions. Children may undergo extensive and repeated reconstructive surgeries for the correction of congenital malformations. Nonhealing wounds and compromised flaps may result (9, 34).

A significant number of serious burns occur in the pediatric age group (6). Accidental and intentional carbon monoxide poisoning remains common in the pediatric age group (7, 11, 14). Children also undergo the same invasive medical procedures that occasionally result in iatrogenic cerebral gas embolism (20, 41).

The distribution of trauma, sites of tumors requiring radiation therapy and structures subject to developing necrotizing infections may be different. Hence the circumstances that lead to these medical problems may be different, but, in the end, the pathophysiologic result is the same.

The field of investigation of the unique physiologic effects of hyperbaric oxygen in pediatric and adult medicine is not static. For example, recent published studies include successful treatment of bone marrow edema and aseptic necrosis in children with malignancies after receiving hyperbaric oxygen (40). At least one study has attempted to answer the question of the use of hyperbaric oxygen in the treatment of anoxic brain injury (43).

The process of making a decision to use hyperbaric oxygen is the same in adults and children. Two questions must be answered. First, are the effects of hyperbaric oxygen likely to favorably influence the pathophysiological state leading to decreased morbidity and mortality? Second, do the benefits outweigh the risks? The literature affirms the former question, but does not directly address the latter issue.

## RISK AND BENEFIT

Studies suggest that normobaric, 100% oxygen significant has significant physiologic effects on term and pre-term infants at birth. These include reduced cerebral blood flow, alteration in tidal volume and alteration of reduced to oxidized glutathione ratio. Animal models using normobaric, 100% oxygen versus air for resuscitation have shown an even wider array of changes (44). Application of this data to infants receiving hyperbaric oxygen, outside of the immediate perinatal period, must be done with great caution.

One published report has systematically explored the occurrence of side effects in children treated with oxygen greater than 1.0 ATA. In 153 patients reviewed over a 20-year period, a 1.7% incidence of side effects and complications occurred that is similar to that in adults (26). Middle-ear barotrauma was the most frequently seen problem (6.0%) and showed a higher frequency in 11 to 16-year-olds than in younger patients. Central nervous system oxygen toxicity (0.7%) occurred only in critically ill patients who were unconscious and ventilator dependent. No evidence suggests that the dose-response curve for hyperbaric oxygen versus neurologic or pulmonary toxicity is different for term infants or older children. In children, as in adults, reducing the incidence of otic barotrauma seems to depend both on patient education and screening for Eustachian tube dysfunction. Undiagnosed, congenital malformations of the lung can lead to air trapping and pulmonary over-inflation with its sequelae of alveolar rupture, pneumothorax, and potential air embolism. A chest radiograph should be obtained in infants and children prior to treatment, as clinical presentation of the underlying malformation may be delayed.

Three special risks should be addressed when considering the use of hyperbaric oxygen in preterm infants or neonates. Exposure to elevated partial pressures of oxygen had been associated with retinopathy of prematurity (ROP), formerly known as retrolental fibroplasia. Recent studies have shown that other risk factors are important, and, indeed, ROP has occurred in term infants and in preterm infants not exposed to elevated partial pressures of oxygen (18, 23, 45). A careful examination of the retina to ascertain the degree of vascular maturity may be helpful in assessing risk. A preliminary report of necrotizing enterocolitis in three premature infants, treated with 2.0 ATA oxygen for 45 minutes (as two 20-minute periods separated by a five-minute air break) is encouraging since there was complete resolution of peritoneal sepsis without retinal abnormality. These infants required only one to four adjunctive treatments to alter a deteriorating clinical course (27). No further clinical information has been published regarding this issue. Further elucidation of the differences in the pharmacology of hyperbaric oxygen versus normobaric oxygen, particularly with respect to nitric oxide production and function, may help answer this clinically important question.

Bronchopulmonary dysplasia (BPD) is a common and serious sequel of barotrauma associated with the use of mechanical ventilation and elevated inspired partial pressures of oxygen in the treatment of respiratory distress syndrome. The mechanisms are not completely clear, but likely include some, if not all, of the mechanisms of pulmonary oxygen toxicity in adults. The addition of hyperbaric oxygen to the care regimen of a preterm infant already receiving assisted ventilation with high partial pressures of oxygen is likely to accelerate this process. English language literature in this matter is nonexistent.

Oxygen is a potent stimulus for closure of the ductus arteriosus. Studies on pregnant ewes have shown that the ductal flow was significantly reduced during HBO. Total aortic flow was preserved due to increased transpulmonic flow and this transitional type of circulation disappeared promptly, post HBO (4). This does not represent a problem for HBO in pregnancy, but it does represent a potential problem for ductal-dependent congenital heart disorders. In the setting of severe congenital pulmonic outflow obstruction, the flow of blood to the systemic circulation may depend on persistent ductal patency. The increase in blood oxygen tension with hyperbaric oxygen could result in a sudden and catastrophic decrease in cardiac output due to ductal constriction. This is a rare constellation of events, but the possibility should be kept in mind if treating an infant with complex congenital heart disease. This risk is excluded by an adequate physical examination, chest radiograph, and, if indicated, echocardiography.

What of the benefits of hyperbaric oxygen treatment in infants, children, and adolescents? These are similar to those in adults. The benefit obtained in children in preventing permanent neurological disability, as in carbon monoxide poisoning, or preventing the need for ablative surgery, as in necrotizing infections, is measured in decades of preserved function, not just in months or years.

## PRACTICAL CONSIDERATIONS IN THE TREATMENT OF CHILDREN

Successful treatment of children must take into account the physiological and psychological changes of maturation. In administering hyperbaric oxygen, these axioms apply to the physical environment of the chamber, oxygen administration devices, middle-ear physiology, psychological preparation and support, dealing with parent-child interactions, and medical support. No one method will work for every child; personnel, equipment availability, and, of course, the patients themselves seem to represent an approximation of infinity. Problem prevention and solutions may be quite different, depending upon whether one uses a monoplace or multiplace chamber. Including pediatricians on the hyperbaric medicine treatment team and pretreatment planning make the task easier.

### Thermal Protection

The ratio of body surface to mass increases with decreasing age, resulting in a greater relative heat loss for infants. Core temperature maintenance is a biological priority and calories will be diverted to preserve it. An ill and anorectic child cannot afford to lose these calories. Additionally, the body's ability to generate heat is finite. Adiabatic cooling on chamber decompression further increases convective and conductive losses. Ventilation of the chamber imposes an added stress by increasing evaporative heat loss. Hypothermia is, therefore, a real concern in the treatment of infants.

Special attention must be directed to detecting and preventing heat loss. By the time a child has developed language skills sufficient to express the concept of being cold, the body mass to surface area has tipped away from potentiating the rapid, dangerous losses. Physical assessment of the skin, looking for piloerection (goosebumps), shivering, cool skin or mottling, identifies the problem when it is already present and potentially harmful.

Regular monitoring of core temperature is the most sensitive method for early detection of significant losses, and affords the opportunity for prevention. It should be utilized for all infants to establish, at a minimum, that heat loss is not a significant problem. If supplementary warming is needed, continued assessment of temperature must be carried out to insure that the plan for thermal regulation is working. Use of continuously-reading cutaneous, rectal, and vascular or urinary bladder probes is likely to be needed during monoplace operations where patient access is limited once the hatch is sealed. Intermittent rectal, cutaneous, or otic monitoring, using a hyperbaric-environment compatible thermometer, may be sufficient during multiplace operations. Once monitoring has identified that the temperature is being maintained, further monitoring may not be necessary if the treatment environment is reproducible, and major changes in caloric intake or heat loss do not occur.

The requirement for preventing excessive heat loss and reduction of evaporative, conductive, and convective losses is the same in monoplace and multiplace chambers. They are somewhat different in practice. In both chamber types, the use of blankets decreases evaporative losses by preventing exposure of the skin to air currents, as well as limiting convective and conductive losses through their insulating effects. In small infants (< 2,500 gm), the ability to generate metabolic heat is extremely limited. In the face of a relatively large radiating surface, or where mild hypothermia is already present, heat must be added to the environment through the use of external warmers such as hot water bottles or pre-warmed blankets. Radiant heaters or devices heated by an electrical resistor are not safe in either the monoplace or multiplace environment. Experience has shown the fire hazard of using blankets warmed in a microwave oven (21). In profound hypothermia, external warming alone will be insufficient and core warming via heated respiratory gases or cavity lavage will be needed.

In the monoplace chamber, devices that act as heat reservoirs must provide a sufficient heat gradient during the entire treatment, without inflicting a thermal injury early in the course of the exposure. Additionally, the heat must be sufficient to offset increased heat losses during decompression due to adiabatic cooling. In multiplace chambers equipped with a medical transfer lock, heat sources may be replaced as needed.

## Psychological Preparation and Support

For both medical and ethical reasons, patients should not be subjected to excessive anxiety; yet, anxiety is a classical human response to the unknown.

For young children with limited life experience nearly every situation is likely to hold some degree of the unknown. The combination of illness, a novel environment such as a hyperbaric chamber, and separation from the most constant factor in their lives, parents, can produce profound anxiety or fear. Addressing these issues beforehand will make treatment much less stressful for the patient and staff.

Illness in children usually causes regression in behavior and the ability to reason is likely to be the first casualty. Appealing to a child's logic is unlikely to be a useful tactic. It is appropriate to explain to children beyond the age of 3 to 4 years, in simple terms, that the treatment is to make them better. The next task is to make the treatment as nonstressful as possible. To be effective, measures to achieve this must take into account the developmental age of the patient.

Make the environment less novel. When the initial treatment is elective, pretreatment teaching, like preoperative teaching, using pictures, dolls, models, and child-oriented stories provides facts and dispels fears. Child Life Education specialists can help by making the format and content of the presentation age-appropriate. In non-emergent situations with children, preschool age and older, examining the facility and equipment prior to treatment, with a parent present, also makes the environment less anxiety provoking. If possible, the staff member carrying out the orientation should also carry out the first treatments, either as the inside tender in multiplace operations, or as the operator in monoplace chamber. Consistency of procedure is also important in reducing novelty. In emergent or semi-emergent situations, this orientation will need to be truncated or skipped.

Distraction during treatment is another method for making the hyperbaric environment less novel. In elective, as well as emergent situations, distraction during treatment is a valuable tool for stress avoidance. Distraction methods will vary with chamber types and staffing availability. The 100% oxygen atmosphere of a monoplace chamber significantly limits the type of items that can be placed in the chamber with the child. In multiplace chambers, the range of items that can be safely introduced for distraction and play is wider. The advantage of the monoplace chamber with an acrylic hull is that it makes video a powerful agent of distraction. The use of video images in multiplace chamber treatment is also possible, but not as simple. Reading to a child during treatment can also be an excellent distraction, and can be accomplished in either chamber type.

Two caveats must be kept in mind when selecting methods of distraction: 1) Items used in a chamber must not represent a safety hazard – common sense will need to be the guide, as few things are labeled as "intrinsically safe." Toys should be incapable of producing sparks, and any fabrics incorporated in them must not produce static electricity. 2) Items used must be age-appropriate to be effective – the child's parents and Child Life Educators are excellent sources of information.

Pediatric procedures that are painful or frightening should be performed under carefully-controlled sedation. The use of sedation allows the procedure to be done in the shortest time possible and avoids making repetition of the therapy impossible. In hyperbaric oxygen treatment, when psychological preparation and distraction alone are insufficient in preventing significant anxiety, sedation is indicated. The touch of another human can also be a sedative, and its value should not be underestimated. A variety of agents are available, each with different potential strengths and weaknesses. For each patient in need of it, a plan for sedation should be developed taking into account the severity of anxiety, the degree of sedation needed to carry out the treatment safely, and provides the ability to monitor and control the level of sedation. For patients requiring minimal sedation to fall asleep, an antihistamine such as diphenhydramine (Benadryl) may be all that is needed. It should be kept in mind that paradoxically, some children develop increased activity when given antihistamines, hence a history regarding reactions to over-the-counter cold medications should be elicited prior to using them. If antihistaminic medications provide insufficient sedation, benzodiazepines provide an alternative that can be administered either orally or intravenously. If given intravenously, appropriate monitoring of heart rate, respiratory rate, and, if possible, blood pressure should be carried out. Hypoxemia during HBO is unlikely, but hypercarbia can occur. For patients with pain requiring intravenous treatment, the combination of smaller doses of a benzodiazepine or Propofol and a narcotic provide ideal sedation, pain relief, and a degree of retrograde amnesia. With this combination, respiratory depression is a possibility, but can easily be reversed with naloxone .

Continued efforts at pretreatment psychological preparation are warranted, even if the initial attempts meet with limited success and sedation is required. Ongoing reassurance and familiarization may decrease the need for sedation, making the treatment less complicated.

Physical restraint is often required in the practice of pediatric medicine to prevent the removal of needed medical devices such as IV access, nasogastric or endotracheal tubes or simply to prevent escape, an event more common in pediatrics than adult medicine. Likewise, physical restraint may be required in either the monoplace or the multiplace chamber. In multiplace chambers, restraint can be carried out using the same techniques as used in the pediatric ward setting, swaddling for infants, a papoose board for toddlers, or loose restraint of the hands, to prevent them from reaching the face or other vital areas. These methods can be carried out in monoplace chambers, but care must be taken to insure that the airway will not become compromised; as for example, following emesis as during treatment, the child cannot immediately be repositioned. Immobility is as frustrating for a child as it is for an adult. Therefore, thought should be given to some degree of sedation to make this process less onerous for the child.

What role should parents play in making the environment seem less threatening? At a minimum, parents must be supportive of the treatment with a positive and reassuring attitude. Parents should be instructed to tell the child that the treatment is necessary and that they expect the child to cooperate. The child should not see a parent as being able to delay or cancel therapy. Done even once, a recurring power struggle is nearly inevitable. Including parents in pretreatment orientation is a must. A parent may have special insights regarding unexpressed fears, or questions that a child has, but will not ask.

Parents have fears as well. With the exception of emergent treatment, obtaining informed consent from parents to treat their children is mandatory. This is an excellent time to address questions and concerns parents may have.

For all children, parents represent a refuge from frightening events. Therefore, it is not surprising that a child would want either or both parents physically present, nearby, or in the chamber. Parents will frequently raise this issue as well. The staff must answer two questions in their own minds to give the child and parent an adequate answer. For multiplace operations, where having a parent in the chamber is not impossible, do the psychological benefits to the child outweigh the risks of barotrauma, oxygen toxicity, and decompression sickness to the parent? For both multiplace and monoplace settings, is the proximity of the parent actually going to be a calming influence or a source of conflict over treatment requirements? Experience has shown that children can successfully be treated in the absence of their parents without permanent psychological injury. The hyperbaric facility staff should feel comfortable excluding parents from any phase of treatment, if they feel the parents' absence complicates therapy.

## MIDDLE-EAR EQUALIZATION

Equalization of the middle-ear and paranasal sinuses is no different in children than in adults. Freedom from ear discomfort is perhaps even more important for children than for adults. An adult may be able to rationalize some discomfort if, in the long term, they will benefit. Children find this much more difficult, and one painful experience may make further treatment impossible. The process is complicated by two factors. A certain level of cognitive function is required to understand the need to equalize pressure, to follow instructions, and to carry out the procedure. Secondly, Eustachian-tube dysfunction is common in children, and, at times, prohibits even cooperative children from successfully equalizing.

At approximately 4 to 6 years, a child may be able to focus his or her attention sufficiently to be taught to clear via Valsalva or Frenzel maneuver, or via other eustachian-tube stretching exercises, yawning, swallowing or gum chewing. Phenylephrine nosedrops (0.125% for ages 2-6 years and 0.25-0.5% beyond 6 years), may be helpful. Paradoxically, sucking, as from a baby bottle nipple, may lead to eustachian tube opening, presumably from a Frenzel-type maneuver. As in adults, performing a Valsalva or Frenzel maneuver while breathing 80/20 heliox may be more effective, as flow through a tight Eustachian-tube orifice may be enhanced. Screaming or crying at times also produces Eustachian-tube opening, but is difficult for those involved in the child's care to tolerate, and could just as well be a sign of excruciating pain. Extremely slow compression rates may be effective in the monoplace setting. In multiplace operations, prolonged descents increase inert gas accumulation for inside attendants, and decompression schedules may need to be altered accordingly.

The sequelae of barotrauma are the same for children as in adults. Middle-ear effusions may, in fact, take longer to resolve in children, and are more likely to lead to bacterial otitis media. Myringotomy must be considered for every toddler or infant, as their preverbal status slows our recognition of their otic pain. The myringotomy, for treatments over a 1-3 day period, may not require insertion of a ventilating tube. It will likely require sedation for pain control, and to insure that movement of the child's head does not occur, and cause middle-ear ossicular injury. In infants and toddlers, the external auditory canal is narrower, necessitating the use of a smaller speculum. As speculum diameter decreases, the instrument used for puncture obscures the view of the tympanum, making precise placement more difficult. Use of a thin-walled speculum and magnification makes the task easier. When treatment is expected to continue for more than three days, myringotomy and tube insertion are indicated and should be performed by an otolaryngologist.

If hyperbaric treatment is to begin or continue in the post-operative period following gaseous anesthesia by endotracheal tube, strong consideration should be given to tube placement during the operation, as post intubation nasopharyngeal edema is likely to severely compromise eustachian-tube function. Myringotomy is highly desirable for intubated and/or unconscious patients, unless a resulting delay would compromise the outcome.

As in adults, equalization of paranasal sinus pressure is not commonly a problem nor, when it occurs, is it any easier to deal with. Topical vasoconstrictors,or oral sympathomimetics may improve sinus ventilation temporarily. Intranasal corticosteroids may be of value if the edema is caused by allergic rhinitis. Chronic bacterial sinusitis does occur in children and should be considered as a possible etiology for failure to equalize paranasal sinus pressure.

## OXYGEN ADMINISTRATION TECHNIQUES

Administration of 100% oxygen to children too young to willingly cooperate in their own care can be a challenge. For non-intubated children requiring little direct, hands-on care, the oxygen-compressed monoplace chamber is ideal, as they cannot avoid constant 100% oxygen. The same can be said for the administration of 100% oxygen via endotracheal tube in the multiplace setting, where a ventilator appropriate for the pulmonary requirements of children can be used. The majority of children fall outside these categories, and some ingenuity is required to accomplish the mission.

### Multiplace Operations

Nonintubated patients must submit to the nasopharynx or head being surrounded by oxygen. Most children dislike having objects placed on the face, which they cannot remove at their pleasure, or that impede placing the fingers and hands in the mouth. Commercially available oronasal masks frequently are too large for children under the age of 5-6 years. Alternative strategies are available. Anesthesia masks with appropriate head straps are made that fit all facial sizes and require minimal alteration to fit most in-chamber gas delivery systems. Hand restraint and/or sedation may be needed to keep the mask in place.

The hood and neckdam appliance is a versatile piece of equipment. Unmodified it will fit children above approximately 3-4 years of age. Below this age, an alternative is to widely open the neckdam and pull the dam down to the waist level. This allows the child's hands to be free inside the hood, reducing anxiety, but doesn't permit the child access to supply and exhaust hoses. Frequently, this method is well tolerated, and it can be used to administer oxygen to a child with a tracheostomy. A variation of this theme is to use a neckdam ring with the rubber dam cut away to connect two hoods, making a capsule. This is an ideal size for an infant up to approximately 6-9 months of age. A tape-on Duke Hood can also be joined to another similar hood to form a treatment capsule (1). Flows must be sufficient to keep the hoods well inflated and to prevent carbon dioxide accumulation. Respiratory rate must be closely monitored, if the $CO_2$ level itself is not.

## Monoplace Operations

The monoplace chamber is ideal for children not requiring ventilatory assistance—no oronasal mask or hood is required. The most commonly used monoplace chamber, the Sechrist, currently utilizes a mechanical ventilator that is poorly adapted for pediatric use. At low tidal volumes needed for infants and small children, the delivered volume is not constant during compression and decompression. An attendant lying next to the child in the chamber and utilizing a positive pressure bag has ventilated infants.

## Oxygen Administration Schedules

Detailed studies have clearly defined the safe limits of exposure to hyperbaric oxygen for adults. As yet, no such study has been carried out to delineate these limits for all age groups. Based on the literature describing the hyperbaric treatment of children, as well as practical experience, they do not in general, appear to be at increased risk for developing pulmonary or neurological oxygen toxicity. Therefore, oxygen administration schedules do not need to be routinely altered for the treatment of children.

Seizure with fever is a common phenomenon in early childhood. The threshold for evoking cortical irritation sufficient to produce seizure seems to be lowered during this period of development. The dose of oxygen required to produce seizures may be lower for a febrile child who has previously had seizures with fever. In this setting, the dose of oxygen may be altered by adding extra air breathing periods, or treating at a lower pressure.

Two specific groups of children appear to be at risk for oxygen toxicity while breathing 100% oxygen at ambient pressure. In infants with immature retinal vasculature, oxygen appears to play a role in developing retinopathy of prematurity. Preterm infants with pulmonary surfactant deficiency, who incur respiratory distress syndrome and require supplemental oxygen, may develop a chronic form of obstructive pulmonary disease. The chances of this are enhanced if mechanical ventilation is required. In these two specific populations, it is prudent to avoid the use of hyperbaric oxygen until further data are available.

## PREPARATION FOR TREATING PEDIATRIC PATIENTS

As the use of hyperbaric oxygen increases in clinical practice, the likelihood of being asked to treat children grows. The chance of a facility needing to treat children with carbon monoxide poisoning emergently is virtually 100%. Being prepared for this eventuality will improve patient safety and reduce stress on the staff. All units should have skilled, experienced personnel and suitable equipment available for advanced life support, in-chamber oxygen administration, and ventilation. A prior working relationship with a pediatrician is obviously a great help.

# REFERENCES

1. Aguiluz L, Hill RK Jr. "Alternate method of oxygen delivery for neonatal use." J Hyperbaric Med. 1990;5:259-261.

2. Angeles A, Gibson J, Cianci P and Hunt TK. "Hyperbaric oxygen and angiogenesis." (1997) Undersea and Hyperbaric Medicine 24(Suppl):31.

3. Ashamalla HL, Thom SR and Goldwein, JW. " Hyperbaric oxygen therapy for the treatment of radiation-induced sequelae in children." (1996) Cancer 77:2407- 2412.

4. Assali NS, Kirschbaum TH, Dilts PV Jr. "Effects of hyperbaric oxygen on uteroplacental and fetal circulation." Circulation Research. 1968;22:573-588.

5. Chu DZJ, Fainstein V, Bodey GP, Hopfer RL, Luna MA, Hickey RC. "Necrotizing gas-forming infections in cancer patients." Southern Med J. 1989;82:860-863.

6. Cianci P, Williams C, Leuders H, Lee H, Shapiro R, Sexton J, Sato R. "Adjunctive hyperbaric oxygen in the treatment of thermal burns. An economic analysis." J Burn Car Rehabil. 1990;11:140-143.

7. Crawford R, Campbell DGD, Ross R. "Carbon monoxide poisoning in the home: recognition and treatment." Br Med J. 1990;301:977-979.

8. Davis JC, Heckman JD, DeLee JC, Buckwold FJ. "Chronic non-hematogenous osteomyelitis treated with adjuvant hyperbaric oxygen." J Bone Joint Surg. 1986;68-A:1210-1217.

9. Dillon BT, Warford LR, Vogel RG. "Hyperbaric oxygen therapy in a newborn infant: A case presentation." J Arkansas Med Soc. 1987;83:325-326.

10. Ferguson BJ, Mitchell TG, Moon R, Camporesi EM, Farmer J. "Adjunctive hyperbaric oxygen for treatment of rhinocerebral mucormycosis." Rev Infect Dis. 1988;10:551-559.

11. Gemelli F, Cattani R. "Carbon monoxide poisoning in childhood." Br Med J. 1985;291:1197.

12. Gracy RW, Yuksel U, Jacobson TM, et.al. "Cellular models and tissue equivalent systems for evaluation the structures and significance of age-modified proteins." (1991) Gerontology 37:113-127.

13. Hehenberger K, Brismar K, Lind F and Kratz G. "Dose-dependent hyperbaric oxygen stimulation of human fibroblast proliferation." (1997) Wound Rep Reg 5:147-50.

14. Kim JK, Coe CJ. "Clinical study on carbon monoxide intoxication in children." Yonsei Med J. 1987;28:266-273.

15. Kirk CR, Dorgan JC, Hart CA. "Gas gangrene: A cautionary tale." Br Med J. 1988;296:1236-1237.

16. Kveton JF. "Surgical management of osteoradionecrosis of the temporal bone." Otolaryngol Head Neck Surg. 1988;98:231-234.

17. Lander HM. "An essential role for free radicals and derived species in signal transduction." (1997) FASEB 11:118-124.

18. Lucey JF, Dangman B. "A reexamination of the role of oxygen in retrolental fibroplasia." Pediatrics. 1984;76:339-344.

19. Martorano FJ, Hoover D. "The child patient." J Hyperbaric Med. 1986;1:15-21.

20. Massey EW, Moon RE, Shelton D, Camporesi EM. "Hyperbaric oxygen therapy of iatrogenic air embolism." J Hyperbaric Med. 1990;5:15-21.

21. PRESSURE, Newsletter of the Undersea and Hyperbaric Medical Society, Inc., Bethesda. Page 3, May/June, 1989.

22. Radaelli F, Volpe AD, Colombi M, Bregani P, Polli EE. "Acute gangrene of the penis and scrotum in four hematologic patients." Cancer. 1987;7:1462-1464.

23. Ricci B, Calogero G. "Oxygen-induced retinopathy in newborn rats: Effects of prolonged normobaric and hyperbaric oxygen supplementation." Pediatrics. 1988;82:193-198.

24. Riseman JA, Zamboni WA, Curtis A, Graham DR, Konrad HR, Ross DS. "Hyperbaric oxygen therapy for necrotizing fasciitis reduces mortality and the need for debridements." Surgery. 1990;108:847-850.

25. Rosenthal E, Benderly A, Monies-Chass I, Fishman J, Levy J, Bialik V. "Hyperbaric oxygen in peripheral ischaemic lesions in infants." Arch Dis Child. 1985;60:372-374.

26. Sanchez EC, Myers RAM. "Hyperbaric oxygen therapy in the pediatric patient, a 20 year experience." (1992) Undersea Biomedical Res. 19(Suppl.):109.

27. Sanchez EC. "Case presentations". (Sept.12-15,1988) National Meeting of Pediatric Critical Care, Veracruz, Mexico.

28. Seidel M, Weiss M, Nicolai T, Roos R, Grantzow R, Belohradsky BH. "Gas gangrene and congenital agranulocytosis." Pediatr Infect Dis J. 1990;9:437-440.

29. Shupak A, Gozal D, Ariel A, Melamed Y, Katz A. "Hyperbaric oxygenation in acute posttraumatic ischemia." J Hyperbaric Med. 1987;2:7-14.

30. Stadtman ER. "Protein oxidation and aging." (1992) Science 257:1220-1224.

31. Sundaresan M, Yu Z, Ferrans VJ, Irani K and Finkel T. "Requirement for generation of H2O2 for platelet-derived growth factor signal transduction." (1995) Science 270:296-299.

32. Thom SR, Lauermann MW and Hart GB. "Intermittent hyperbaric oxygen therapy for reduction of mortality in experimental polymicrobial sepsis." (1986) J of Infectious Dis. 154:504-510.

33. Tompach PC, Lew D and Stoll JL. "Cell response to hyperbaric oxygen treatment." (1997) Int J Oral Maxillofac Surg 26:82-86. 34.

34. Vazquez RL and Spahr RC. "Hyperbaric oxygen use in neonates, A report of four patients." (1990) AJDC 144:1022-1024.

35. Thom, SR, Bhopale VM, Velazquez OC, Goldstein LJ, Thom LH, Buerk DG. "Stem cell mobilization by hyperbaric oxygen." (2006) Am J Hear Circ Physiol 290(4)1378-1386.

36. Garcia-Covarrubia SL. "Invasive aspergillosis treated with adjunctive hyperbaric oxygen: a retrospective clionical series at a single institution." (2002) South Med J 95(4)450-456.

37. John BV, Chamilos G, Kontoyiannis DP. "Hyperbaric oxygen as an adjunctive treatment for zygomycosis" (2005) Clin Microbiol Infect 11:515-517.

38. Krzelj V, Petri NM, Mestrovic J, Andric D, Biocic M. "Purpura fulminans successfully treated with hyperbaric oxygen- a report of 2 cases." (2005) Pediatr Emerg Care 21(1):31-34.

39. Rapley JH, Lawrence WT, Witt PD. "Composite grafting and hyperbaric oxygen therapy in pediatric nasal tip reconstruction after avulsive dog bite injury." (2001) Ann Plast Surg 46(4)434-438.

40. Bernbeck B, Christaras A, Krauth K, Lentrodt S, Strelow H, Schaper J, Janssen G, Modder U, Gobel U. "Bone marrow oedema and aseptic osteonecrosis in children and adolescents with acute lymphoblastic leukaemia or non-hodgkins lymphoma treated with hyperbaric oxygen therapy (HBO) an approach to cure?" (2001) Klin Padiatr 216(6) 370-378.

41. LeDez K, Zbitnew G. "Hyperbaric treatment of cerebral air embolism in an infant with cyanotic congenital heart disease." (2005) Can J Anesth 52:4 403-408.

42. Kurschel S, Mohia A, Weigel V, Eder HG. (2006) "Hyperbaric oxygen in the treatment of brain abscess in children." Childs Nerv Syst 22(1):38-42.

43. Collet JP, Vanasse M, Marois P, Amar M, Goldberg J, Lambert J, Lassonde M, Hardy P, Fortin J, Tremblay SD, Montgomery D, Lacroix J, Robinson A, Majnemer A. "Hyperbaric oxygen for children with cerebral palsy: a randomized multicentre trial. HBO-CP research Group." (2001) Lancet 357(9256)582-586.

44. Richmond S, Goldsmith JP. "Air or 100% oxygen for neonatal resuscitation?" (2006) Clin Perinatol 33: 11-27.

45. Higgins, RD. "50 years ago in the Journal of Pediatrics: incidence of retrolentaql fibroplasias: past and present." (2006) J Pediatr. 148(6).

# NOTES

CHAPTER 15

# WOUND HEALING AND HYPERBARIC OXYGENATION

## CHAPTER FIFTEEN OVERVIEW

# WOUND HEALING AND HYPERBARIC OXYGENATION

*Michael L. Gimbel, Thomas K. Hunt*

## INTRODUCTION

Wound repair consists of an exquisitely regulated orchestration of molecular and cellular instruments which act in concert to restore the local tissue environment to pre-wound conditions. Metabolic imbalances in the wound milieu conduct this orchestration, and continue to direct it until healing resolves the mechanical and metabolic problems. Rapidly progressing research has shed new light on many of the components of wound repair. The purpose of this chapter is to review the basic tenants of the wound healing response and to present recent ideas and data that are modifying the understanding of this critical biological system.

## WOUND PHYSIOLOGY

### Early Events

Tissue injury profoundly disrupts the tissue microenvironment and sets into motion a cascade of events that combine to reestablish something resembling a status quo. Disrupted blood vessels fill the wound space with red blood cells and plasma. Injured cells release factor III (thromboplastin) that accelerates the clotting cascade (1). Clotting factors in the plasma are activated to form thrombin and eventually fibrin. Simultaneously, the complement system activates and produces chemoattractive protein fragments. Platelets, activated by thrombin and exposed collagen, release a number of growth factors and cytokines (2). Traumatized vessels contract in response to both direct physical stimulation (mediated by the autonomic nervous system) and prostaglandins released by platelets (3). Soon thereafter intact local microvasculature vasodilates and leaks plasma in response to inflammatory mediators such as histamine, kinins, and serotonin (2). These early events, and others, establish hemostasis and inflammation. See Figure 1.

### Platelets

Platelet activation initiates the first major escalation in the inflammatory response. Within minutes, platelets release a number of signaling molecules from their $\mu$-granules, including platelet-derived growth factor (PDGF), insulin-like growth factor binding protein-3 (IGFBP-3), and platelet factor 4 (PF-4). These macromolecules, along with other chemotactic factors (C5f, C3f, kallikrein, tissue plasminogen activator, fibrinopeptide B,

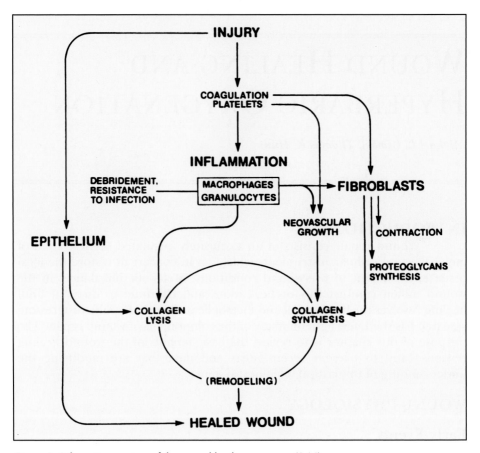

*Figure 1. Schematic overview of the wound healing response (144).*

elastin, collagen, and fibronectin), attract macrophages, polymorphonuclear cells (PMN), fibroblasts, and vascular endothelial cells (1, 4-6).

PDGF is particularly important in these processes is an attractant for multiple cell lines, a powerful mitogen for fibroblasts and smooth muscle cells, and a stimulant for increased collagen synthesis and angiogenesis (6). For these reasons, PDGF has been the subject of several clinical wound healing trials and is approved for topical use in the treatment of diabetic ulcers (7-11).

## Granulocytes

Early events contribute to edema and tissue debris. Within a few hours of injury, PMNs and macrophages marginate, invade the wound space and begin to remove tissue debris, coagulation proteins, and bacteria. They do so in part by releasing degradative enzymes such as collagenases and elastases that remove connective tissue to make way for repair, and oxidases and hydroxylases that condition the environment to produce new blood vessels and matrix molecules. PMNs dominate during the first few days (12).

Neutrophils also constitute the primary defense against contaminating organisms which have breached the epithelial barrier. PMNs and macrophages, in concert with the complement system, form the basis of "natural" or "nonspecific" immunity, that is, microbial resistance which is immediate, innate, and independent of previous exposure to a specific organism. Microorganisms are opsoninized by immunoglobulins and complement proteins which bind to PMN membrane receptors, thereby allowing neutrophil recognition and phagocytosis (13). This process is the most important defense against wound infection and will be discussed later. In particular, oxygen plays perhaps its most important role in immunity.

## Microbial Killing Mechanisms

Neutrophils must kill offending microorganisms after ingesting them. There are two systems for bacterial killing within granulocytes. One system requires oxygen, while the other does not. The oxygen-independent system was first demonstrated by Hirsch (14), who noted that both Gram positive and Gram negative organisms were killed when exposed to a protein fraction extracted from PMNs. Further investigations found that cytoplasmic granules in neutrophils contain a number of antibacterial enzymes that kill microbes when phagosomes containing organisms fuse with lysosomes that contain these bactericidal enzymes (2, 14). This oxygen-independent system is very important, and, fortunately, rarely deficient.

Despite the efficiency of the oxygen-independent bacterial killing system, it is by itself insufficient to rid the wound of all pathogens, as evidenced by studies that show decreased bacterial killing under hypoxic conditions (15, 16). The oxygen-dependent system is required for adequate antibacterial activity in granulocytes and monocytes. This system requires the consumption of large amounts of molecular oxygen immediately after phagocytosis in a process called the "respiratory" or "oxidative" burst. See Figure 7. Abnormalities of this oxygen-dependent system result in a dramatic reduction in immunity. An experiment of nature, chronic granulomatous disease (CGD), demonstrates this mechanism. CGD is caused by the inability of leukocytes to mount a burst of oxygen consumption ("oxidative burst") due to gene deficiencies of the NADPH-linked oxidase a highly complex enzyme that normally produces reactive oxygen species (ROS). The disease is characterized by profound susceptibility to bacterial and fungal infections resulting in multiple abscesses and granulomas (17, 18). Absence of the substrate for this enzyme (i.e. hypoxia) produces an identical and clinically important vulnerability (19). See below for further discussion of the role of oxygen in bacterial resistance.

If there is no infection or foreign material, the neutrophil population quickly diminishes while macrophages continue to amass. This event is associated with lessened scar formation.

## Monocytes/Macrophages

Like neutrophils, monocytes marginate on capillary endothelial cells in response to chemoattractants such as bacterial components, complement proteins, transforming growth factor-β(TGF-β), PDGF, PF-4, vascular endothelial growth factor (VEGF), and fibrin degradation products. Issekutz et al. (12) showed that monocyte/macrophage accumulation in wounds is substantial as early as one hour after injury, with maximum accumulation rate occurring at three to four hours. They become the major populant by the third day after injury and dominate the wound region for days to weeks. Macrophages are thought to be the "masterminds" behind the complicated and finely tuned array of repair events which characterize the proliferative phase of healing. These versatile cells assume several functions.

Newly arrived macrophages are activated to produce many of these functions by some of the same products that initially attracted them. Like neutrophils, activated macrophages continue the task of wound debridement, employing similar processes of phagocytosis and bacterial killing, both oxygen-dependent and oxygen-independent. Phagocytosis activates oxidant production. Cytokines and lactate accumulation activate growth factor production. Macrophages lead the characteristic procession of new tissue into the wound dead space. Immature, replicating fibroblasts follow the macrophages. Mature fibroblasts then advance into the wound space and are, in turn, followed by newly forming capillary buds, the last cells in the procession. These relationships become clear when the wound repair module is forced to grow across a narrow space, i.e. the so-called "rabbit ear chamber," that facilitates both *in vivo* and histologic analysis, as shown in Figure 2 (20).

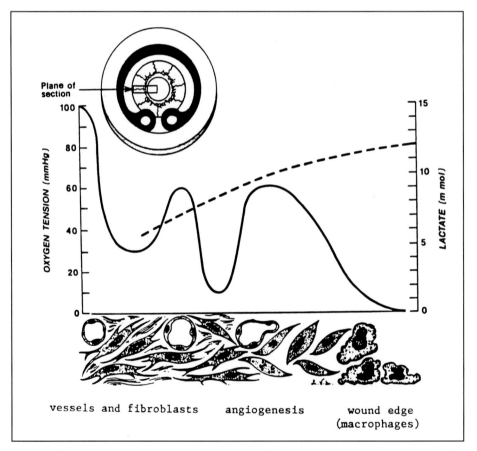

*Figure 2. The wound module. Schematic cross-section of the wound module in a rabbit ear chamber (left upper corner of diagram). Note that pO$_2$ (solid line above the histologic cross-section) is highest next to vessels, and approaches zero at the wound edge. Lactate concentration (dashed line) is high in the dead space and lower (but still higher than plasma) toward the neovasculature (145).*

Macrophages are a rich source of degradative enzymes that process the extracellular matrix (ECM) to make room for remodeling. These enzymes, including collagenases, tissue plasminogen activator, and urokinase plasminogen activator, are capable of digesting almost all of the ECM components (21). Macrophages also direct the control system for these enzymes through synthesis of tissue inhibitors of metallo- and serine-proteases (22). These enzymes are responsible for "separation" of burn wound eschars, for instance.

Over the last decade, intense research has been directed at a dozen or more signaling products that activated macrophages secrete into the wound environment. See Table 1. Tightly coordinated release of the many growth factors, colony stimulating factors, interleukins, interferons, and cytokines gives macrophages their ability to regulate migration, proliferation, and specific protein synthesis in several cell types. Before these effector cell lines are considered, the metabolic conditions of the wound microenvironment must first be addressed. These conditions provide macrophages with the information they need to instruct fibroblasts and endothelial cells.

## WOUND ENVIRONMENT

### Metabolic Conditions

As previously mentioned, injury perturbs the microenvironment and leads to the auto-amplifying inflammatory phase. As a result of these processes, the environment becomes hypoxic, acidotic, and hyperlactated (23). Hypoxia is caused by the initial vascular damage, coagulation, and vasoconstriction as well as by vastly increased local oxygen consumption due to leukocyte accumulation. In fact, the leukocyte respiratory burst may increase oxygen consumption by an estimated fifty-fold. Oxygen tension then plummets in wounded tissue. This drop was directly measured in 1968 by Remensnyder and Majno (24). See Figure 3.

## TABLE 1. MACROPHAGE DERIVED ANGIOMODULATORS (150)

| Factor | Stimulates migration of endothelial cells (E.C.) | Stimulates mitosis of EC. | Promotes differentiation of capillary tubes | Inhibits migration or proliferation of E.C. |
|---|---|---|---|---|
| bFGF | + | + | + | - |
| GM-/G-CSF | + | + | + | - |
| VEGF/VPF | + | + | - | - |
| IL-8 | + | + | - | - |
| Substance P | + | + | - | - |
| Angiotropin | + | - | + | - |
| HAF | + | - | - | - |
| PDGF | + | + | - | - |
| IL-6 | + | - | - | + |
| IL-1 | + | + | - | + |
| TGF-beta | + | + | - | + |
| TNF-alpha | + | - | - | + |
| TGF-alpha | - | + | - | - |
| IGF-I | - | + | - | - |
| Interferon-α | - | - | + | + |
| Interferon-γ | - | - | + | + |

Adapted with permission from: Sunderkotter, C., Steinbrink, K., Goebeler, M., Bhardwaj, R., and Sorg, C. Macrophages and angiogenesis. Journal of Leukocyte Biology, 1994; 55: 410-22.

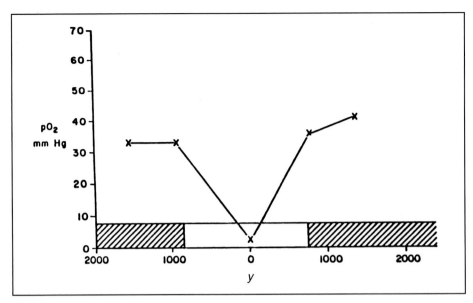

*Figure 3. Topography of oxygen tensions found in a four-day-old rat cremaster muscle wound. The wound is represented on the x axis, clear area representing the avascular center, and hatched areas representing surrounding tissue. Distances from the center of the wound are measured in microns. Oxygen tension at each measuring position (center-edge-tissue) is plotted on the y axis in mmHg. Note the steep oxygen gradient from center to edge (146).*

Acidosis arises partially due to the imbalance of decreased oxygen supply in the face of increased oxygen demand. Some local cells resort to anaerobic glycolysis for energy production, leading to the accumulation of lactate. More importantly, leukocytes, as well as fibroblasts and endothelial cells, contain relatively few mitochondria and therefore normally rely on glycolysis and the hexose monophosphate shunt for ATP production, even in conditions of plentiful oxygen (aerobic glycolysis). Therefore, the energy derived for leukocyte oxidant production results in lactate accumulation. Contrary to what might be expected, accumulation of lactate under aerobic circumstance does not cause significant acidosis. Thus, leukocytes actively maintain the high lactate concentrations (5 to 15 mM) in wounds (20, 25-27). Lactate accumulation in the presence of oxygen may be the central event at this stage of healing.

## ADPR/pADPR System

The high lactate concentration and hypoxia in wounded cells are accompanied by the reduction of NAD+ to NADH (28). The NAD+ /NADH pools within cells reflect their redox state. Lactate converts NAD+ to NADH, thereby lowering the NAD+ pools.

There is at least one biochemical pathway by which low redox potential can signal cells to take biologic action — the adenosine diphosphoribose (ADPR) system. This pathway, first reported independently in the mid 1960s by both Hayaishi (29, 30) and Chambon (31, 32), was originally thought to be involved exclusively with DNA strand break repair. Loetscher et al. suggested that ADP-ribosylation might represent the link between cell energy status and cell phenotype (33). We now know that the system instigates post-translational modification of many specific proteins, thereby altering their protein structure and function. Mono and poly (ADP-ribose) reversibly regulate the activities of many enzymes. The enzyme ADPR transferase mediates these ribosylations in the cytoplasm of cells, while poly (ADPR) synthetase mediates them within the nucleus.

Specifically, recent evidence has shown that alterations of pADPR affect regulation of collagen and vascular endothelial growth factor (VEGF) transcription. The extent to which both types of ADPR reactions occur is limited by the availability of NAD+, the substrate for the reactions. Adenosine diphosphoribose is formed as a result of removing the nicotine (N) group from NAD+ (but not NADH). When NAD+ is abundant, ADPR reactions are driven forward and many cellular proteins are affected. When NAD+ is scarce, as in hyperlactated wound conditions, ADP ribosylations are inhibited and these cellular protein alterations are reversed (34). See Figure 4. Thus, the metabolic (redox) state, which is so deranged in the wound microenvironment, is intimately linked to altered cellular function, leading to "reparative" cell phenotypes. Furthermore, the most potent stimulus to pADPR synthetase activity is oxidant damage to DNA. The oxidants that are produced by inflammatory cells, therefore, appear to strongly influence this regulatory mechanism as well. The question now arises as to how the NAD+ and ADPR/pADPR pathways specifically affect fibroblasts, macrophages, and endothelial cells in wounds.

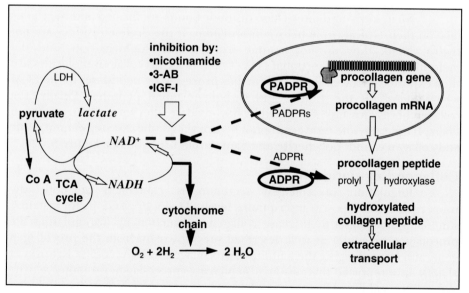

Figure 4. Regulation of collagen synthesis by ADP-ribosylation. As lactate concentration increases, NAD+ is converted to NADH, thereby decreasing ADP/pADP-ribosylation reactions in the nucleus and cytoplasm. Decreased ribosylation releases the collagen gene from transcriptional inhibition and releases prolyl hydroxylase from enzymatic activity suppression (dashed lines represent inhibition). The pathway from NAD+ to ADPR/pADPR is also inhibited by nicotinamide, 3-aminobenzamide (3-AB), and insulin-like growth factor-1 (IGF-I). Abbreviations: poly(ADP-ribose) synthetase, (pADPRs); ADP-ribose transferase, (ADPRt); lactate dehydrogenase, (LDH); coenzyme A, (CoA); tricyclic acid cycle, (TCA cycle) (147).

## Fibroblasts/Collagen Synthesis

After inflammation has begun, fibroblasts are attracted by many stimuli, and then proliferate and migrate into the site of injury (35). One of their less appreciated functions is to assist macrophages in degrading the existing ECM for repair and remodeling by releasing collagenases and tissue inhibitors of matrix metalloproteinases (TIMP). Macrophage-derived basic fibroblast growth factor (bFGF) increases fibroblast collagenase release, while TGF-β lessens this effect and stimulates secretion of TIMP (36).

## Collagen Synthetic Pathway

Fibroblasts are the major producers of collagen in the repair response. ADPRibosylations in the context of a normal tissue environment suppress collagen gene transcription and post-translational modification and thus collagen deposition. However, in the context of an oxidative environment such as a wound, diminution of ADP ribosylations reduces the normal repression of collagen synthesis and deposition and stimulates them instead. Lactate accumulation suppresses ADPRibose and thus plays a role in collagen synthesis.

After gene transcription, procollagen peptides are assembled and delivered into the endoplasmic reticulum, where prolyl- and lysyl-hydroxylase enzymes post-translationally modify the pro-α-chains by adding hydroxyl groups to proline and lysine residues. The substrate for this important reaction is molecular oxygen. Cofactors are ascorbate, α-ketoglutarate, and ferrous ion (37-42).

Next, intra- and inter-chain disulfide bonds are formed and the chains take on their typical triple helix conformation. If the proline residues are not hydroxylated, they do not assume triple helical conformation, and the molecule remains nonfunctional (41). Triple helix procollagen molecules are then exported extracellularly and further processed by peptidases in the ECM which cleave off the amino- and carboxy-terminal peptides. Finally, the collagen fibrils crosslink. Catalyzed by lysyl-oxidase, they form mature collagen fibers. If critical lysine residues are not hydroxylated, this last step cannot occur and collagen cannot polymerize and gain tensile strength. See Figure 5.

## Collagen Regulation

Regulation of collagen secretion is controlled at both the transcriptional and post-transcriptional levels (34, 43-45). TGF-β , for instance, stimulates fibroblasts to increase collagen production by upregulating the procollagen promoter at well described sites upstream from the procollagen gene, and by prolonging the half-life of procollagen mRNA (46-50). Krupsky et al. (50) have reported that insulin also increases procollagen promoter activity and mRNA stability. Glucocorticoids decrease promoter activity by inhibiting both the glucocorticoid response element and the TGF-β response element in the procollagen promoter. Both tumor necrosis factor-α (TNFα) and interferon-γ reduce procollagen promoter activity (51). A reduction of inflammation and lactate production might also contribute.

Ghani and colleagues (34) recently linked redox state to transcriptional control of collagen synthesis. In their study, fibroblasts exposed to pADPR synthetase inhibitors (lactate, 3-aminobenzamide, and

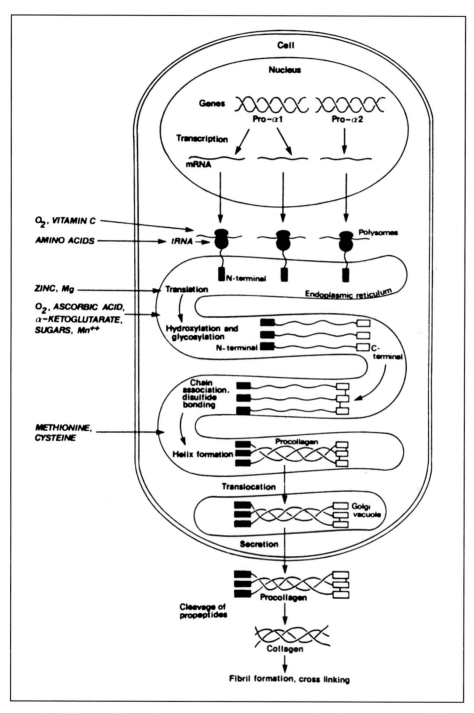

Figure 5. Collagen synthesis pathway. Procollagen genes are translated into procollagen mRNA. mRNA strands are translated in rough endoplasmic reticulum into procollagen peptides. Peptides undergo hydroxylation (via prolyl- and lysyl-hydroxylase) and glycosylation, as well as disulfide bonding. Triple helix conformation is attained and procollagen is secreted extracellularly, where it is further cleaved and cross-linked to form mature collagen fibrils. Cofactors of specific steps are indicated to the left of schematic (148).

nicotinamide) were found to have increased levels of procollagen mRNA. In fact, the stimulatory effect of insulin-like growth factor-I on collagen synthesis appears to operate through pADPR synthetase inhibition. Conversely, fibroblasts exposed to the pADPR substrate NAD+ contained significantly decreased levels of procollagen mRNA. These findings strongly implicate the pADPR pathway in the up- and down-regulation of the procollagen gene promoter. Existing evidence supports this line of thought, as investigators have shown that the redox environment biochemically alters many transcriptional factors and activators (52). Lactate also decreases the activity of ADPR transferase in the cytoplasm. Prolyl-hydroxyls is inhibited by ADP ribosylation. Predictably, the high lactate concentration in wounds reduces ADP ribosylation, and stimulates prolyl-hydroxyls function, thereby upregulating post-translational control of both types I and III collagen synthesis. These two types of collagen predominate in scars (28, 53).

## The Role of Oxygen in Collagen Deposition

Hypoxia has various effects on fibroblasts including decreased IGF-I production (54), increased TGF-β production (55), increased procollagen mRNA levels (56), and increased fibroblast proliferation (156). Numerous studies have proved, however, that wound collagen deposition is greatly increased in well-oxygenated wounds (57-59).

Molecular oxygen is important in many biological processes other than aerobic respiration. Enzymes which harness oxygen may be divided into three groups: monooxygenases, intermolecular deoxygenates, and intermolecular deoxygenates. Mono-oxygenases (or mixed-function oxygenases) add one atom from $O_2$ to an organic molecule, and donate the other molecule to form $H_2O$. Intermolecular dioxygenases catalyze the incorporation of one atom of oxygen into each of two separate products. Intramolecular dioxygenases catalyze the incorporation of both atoms from $O_2$ into the same organic product (60).

As noted earlier, mature collagen synthesis depends on the action of prolyl- and lysyl-hydroxylase as well as lysyl-oxidase. Prolyl-hydroxylase activity is particularly sensitive to oxygen concentration ($pO_2$). The $KmO_2$ of prolyl-hydroxylase is 20 $mmHgpO_2$. In other words, prolyl-hydroxylase functions at half-maximal rate at a $pO_2$ of 20 mmHg. Compare this to the $KmO_2$ of oxidative phosphorylation, which is between 0.1 and 1 $mmHgpO_2$ (61). The $pO_2$ of wounded tissue ranges from 0 to 30 mmHg (20, 62). Clearly, energy metabolism is first priority. In profoundly hypoxic conditions, use of oxygen for procollagen hydroxylation is a luxury that cells cannot afford. Thus, although hypoxia may signal fibroblasts to begin collagen assembly, the cells cannot produce and deposit mature collagen unless adequate oxygen concentrations are present. Michaelis-Menton kinetics dictate that if all other substrates are present in excess, the rate of collagen hydroxylation will vary with changes in within the range of zero to approximately ten times the $KmO_2$. Because the $KmO_2$ is approximately 20 $mmHgpO_2$, the Vmax of prolyl-hydroxylase therefore occurs at around 200 $mmHgpO_2$. This calculation predicts that raising tissue $pO_2$ to superphysiologic levels will increase the collagen production rate to above that of normal, healthy tissue in room air conditions. Years of clinical experience with supplemental normobaric and hyperbaric $O_2$ confirm this prediction, and experimental data supports it.

The effects of increased oxygen do not conflict with the proposed role of lactate. Supplemental oxygen breathing only slightly lowers wound lactate concentration. Both lactate and growth factors serve as sufficient signals for initiation of fibroblast collagen synthesis in the absence of low oxygen tension. See Figure 6.

Adding oxygen at ambient atmospheric pressure increases collagen production in animals and humans. Polyvinyl sponges were implanted in rabbits exposed continuously to either 50% $O_2$ or 21% $O_2$ (room air) for seven days. Sponges from the 50% $O_2$ group accumulated 20% more collagen than those from the room air group. A similar study with implanted wire mesh wound chambers showed a two- to three-fold difference (63). Conversely, animals living in hypoxic conditions demonstrated less collagen deposition in wound models (64). Human studies have corroborated these findings. When subcutaneous tissue oxygen tension and wound collagen deposition were measured in postoperative surgical patients, collagen deposition was directly and significantly proportional to tissue oxygen tension. These changes were of the same magnitude as those found in animals (57).

## Tissue $O_2$ Concentration vs. Blood $O_2$ Content

In order to put this information to work, one must realize that the dependence on oxygen by the collagen synthetic mechanism is related to oxygen concentration ($pO_2$), not blood oxygen content. For years surgeons have recognized the poor wound healing properties of ischemic tissue. Only in more recent decades has this observation been refined with the demonstration that arterial hypoxemia retards repair even in the presence of adequate blood

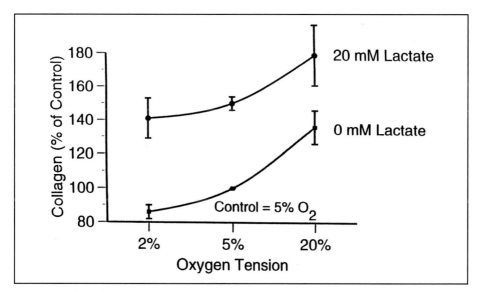

Figure 6. Effect of oxygen tension and lactate concentration on collagen synthesis. Fibroblasts incubated in various combinations of lactate concentrations and $pO_2$ were pulsed with tritiated proline. Secretion of hydroxylated collagen into the cell-conditioned medium was enhanced by both lactate and oxygen (149).

flow and hematocrit (i.e., even when the oxygen transport system is preserved). Unfortunately, many surgeons continue to recommend that hemoglobin should be maintained at ≥ 10 g/dL for reasons of providing adequate oxygen content for wound healing. This policy loses credence when two facts are understood. First, the rate of collagen synthesis is dependent upon the partial pressure of oxygen at the level of the fibroblast. This point has already been discussed. The second fact is that actual oxygen consumption in collagen-producing tissue is low. Normal wound tissue $O_2$ extraction is 0.7 ml $O_2$/100 ml blood. This rate corresponds to only 3% of the perfusing blood oxygen content and can be met without a large $pO_2$ drop along the capillary (65, 66). High hematocrit is, therefore, not required to meet this small demand, even if subjects breathe room air. High blood $pO_2$, however, accelerates collagen deposition in conditions of both normal and low hemoglobin concentration, as long as tissue perfusion is adequate. Given a moderate hemoglobin, $pO_2$ and perfusion are the quantities that mainly should concern surgeons who wish to reduce wound infection and support healing.

## Angiogenesis

Angiogenesis refers to the complex chain of events by which the cellular metabolic need (or as in some tumors, the feigned need) translates into mature vessel ingrowth. Vital links in this chain include angiogenic signal generation and reception, cell proliferation and migration, extracellular matrix degradation and reconstruction, and capillary tube formation. It is extremely important to distinguish between angiogenic factor production and actual neovascularization. Blood vessel growth cannot proceed without collagen deposition and collagen deposition cannot occur without oxygen, regardless of the amount of stimulating cytokines present (168).

Activated macrophages produce many factors which both directly and indirectly stimulate angiogenesis (22, 67, 68). See Table 1. Clark et al. (69) injected autologous wound macrophages into rabbit corneas to stimulate neovascularization. Polverini et al. (70) found that activated peritoneal macrophages induced more vessel growth than nonactivated macrophages in the corneal angiogenesis assay. Thakral et al. (71) noted that macrophages harvested from established wounds and then injected into ear chambers accelerated new vessel ingrowth. Clearly macrophages are vital players in the angiogenic response. Later, Jensen et al. (72) demonstrated that acellular macrophage-conditioned media alone was sufficient to cause angiogenesis, underscoring the likelihood of a secreted angiogenic factor. In 1989, investigators Ferrara and Connolly each independently isolated and characterized that substance, coining the term vascular endothelial growth factor (73, 74). VEGF is a particulary intriguing molecule in that unlike all other angiogenic factors, its receptors reside exclusively on endothelial cells. Despite these fascinating advances, the source of signals that cause macrophage angiogenic factor production were yet to be elucidated. The question remained, "Why is VEGF secreted?"

## The Metabolic Basis of Angiogenesis

Just as a stressed metabolic state (low redox potential, but not necessarily hypoxia) stimulates collagen production, so does it ignite the angiogenesis cascade. A flurry of recent studies has proved that low $O_2$ tension triggers angiogenic growth factor production *in vitro* (75-80). Even before VEGF had been characterized, Knighton et al. showed that media conditioned by macrophages grown at 15 mmHgp$O_2$ actively stimulated angiogenesis, while media conditioned by macrophages grown at 38 mmHg (normoxic tissue p$O_2$) or 76 mmHg (normal arterial p$O_2$) did not (80). Drawing on the knowledge that hypoxia upregulates transcription of the erythropoietin gene, several investigators proposed a similar mechanism for VEGF regulation. Their studies showed that low $O_2$ tension caused increases in VEGF promoter activity, gene transcription, and mRNA stability (75, 77-79). This activity is driven by hypoxia inducible factor-1 ($\alpha$) (HIF-1($\alpha$)), a factor that has been shown to be upregulated in hypoxic conditions (170). In addition, hypoxia has been reported to upregulate VEGF receptors on endothelial cells (81).

While these findings strongly suggest a role for hypoxia in VEGF signaling, low p$O_2$ actually diminishes angiogenesis both clinically and in animal wound models (158). Neovascularization requires endothelial cells for tube formation and fibroblasts for collagenous mechanical support (168). Both of these effector cells require substantial amounts of oxygen to perform their angiogenic functions – fibroblasts for collagen deposition and endothelial cells for energy-consuming proliferation. Thus, a paradox is born. If angiogenesis requires appreciable oxygen levels, how can hypoxia be the biologically operative stimulus for VEGF production? The existence of another metabolic indicator separate from hypoxia solves this conundrum.

The parsimony of biological systems suggests that because fibroblasts and macrophages are exposed to the same wound environment, the trigger for angiogenesis is likely to be the same as the trigger for collagen synthesis. In fact, growing vessels depend on the mechanical support afforded by collagen for architectural guidance and strength. In a clever experiment, Bornstein and Sage transfected an $\alpha$1(I)-procollagen promoter/marker gene construct into endothelial cells exhibiting one of two phenotypes–capillary tube-forming cells or quiescent cells. They found that the collagen promoter activity was upregulated by seven-fold in tube-forming cells compared to quiescent cells. They concluded that transcriptional activation of the collagen gene is closely linked to the phenotypic alterations which accompany the transition of endothelial cells from the quiescent to the angiogenic state. Clinically we know from scurvy, in which ascorbate deficiency leads to inadequate collagen synthesis, that angiogenesis without collagen support results in pathologically fragile capillaries.

Guided by this knowledge, the authors hypothesized that the metabolic stimulus for angiogenesis is, again, lactate and the signal pathway is, again, the ADPR/pADPR system. To this end, Zabel et al. (82) cultured macrophages in either 0 or 15 mM lactate and measured NAD+ and poly (ADP-ribose) concentrations. Cells incubated with lactate showed 40% lower NAD+ levels and 40% less poly (ADP-ribose) synthesis. Simultaneous addition of oxamate, which competes with lactate on lactate dehydrogenase and inhibits it, abolished the observed reductions. Constant et al. measured VEGF levels in media conditioned by macrophages grown in normoxia, hypoxia, 15mM lactate, or hypoxia and lactate together. Both hypoxia and lactate alone stimulated increased VEGF levels. The highest concentration occurred with the combination of lactate and hypoxia (23). Furthermore, the upregulation of VEGF by lactate probably occurs, at least in part, at the level of transcription, as VEGF mRNA levels are elevated in lactate-treated macrophages (169). It appears, then, that lactate does indeed stimulate angiogenesis though the pADPR system.

How else does lactate work? Lactate is a part of a homeostatic mechanism that regulates oxidant balance. When it rises in a wound (as discussed earlier), it chelates to iron in the endoplasmic reticulum. In the presence of hydrogen peroxide, hydroxyl radical then passes into the endoplasmic reticulum where it then facilitates the translocation of HIF-1($\alpha$) from the endoplasmic reticulum into the nucleus, whereupon VEGF transcription is then stimulated (171, 172). So lactate may drive the sequence of events that results in HIF-1($\alpha$) mediated VEGF expression.

As mentioned earlier, ADP-ribosylation post-translationally modifies proteins. Feng et al. (83) combined this concept with the known angiogenic potential of VEGF, and hypothesized that post-translational changes in the VEGF protein may regulate its activity. They took media conditioned by macrophages grown in the presence of lactate, and then ADP-ribosylated its proteins with cholera toxin A subunit, a known ADP-ribosylating agent. A portion of this media was then incubated with hydroxylamine to reverse the ribosylation. The ADP-ribosylated media produced significantly less angiogenesis than both the non-ADP-ribosylated-media and the hydroxylamine-treated media. These results suggest that post-translational ADP-ribosylation of VEGF regulates VEGF activity and, therefore, angiogenesis. In other words, metabolic stress seems to command its own resolution.

## Oxygen and Angiogenesis

Oxygen is required for angiogenesis to proceed. But how much oxygen is necessary? Does more oxygen result in heartier angiogenesis? Cho, Hunt, and Hussain exposed macrophages to hydrogen peroxide and showed a dose-dependent increase in VEGF mRNA, an effect mediated by upregulation of the VEGF gene promoter (157). Thus, oxidants appear to be involved in the early events of angiogenesis *in vitro*.

Physicians have observed for years that poorly healing wounds often respond to hyperbaric oxygen treatments by forming new granulation tissue. Marx et al irradiated the mandibles of rabbits and allowed the animals to develop the typical hypovascular, hypoxic radiation changes. At six months post-treatment, one group of rabbits began hyperbaric hyperoxia treatments, while another group began normobaric hyperoxia treatments. The control group breathed room air. Post-therapeutic microangiograms indicated significantly greater vascular networks in the hyperbaric group compared to the other two groups (84). Gibson et al. (85) and Hopf et al. (158) reported that 100% oxygen administered at 1 to 3 atmospheres of pressure in mice implanted with Matrigel® plugs significantly improved *in vivo* angiogenesis over controls breathing room air at one atmosphere. The response was dose dependent. Furthermore, they showed that addition of anti-VEGF antibody to the Matrigel® inhibited this angiogenic response. These results suggest that hyperoxia acts by either increasing VEGF release or enhancing its activity. A similar *in vivo* study by Mechine et al. (159) corroborated the enhancement of angiogenesis by hyperbaric oxygenation. In another animal wound model Sheikh et al. (160) also showed a direct relationship between wound VEGF levels and inspired $FiO_2$. Feng and colleagues measured VEGF protein levels in macrophage cultures exposed to various levels of oxygen tension, from hypoxic to hyperoxic. They discovered that, while only hypoxic macrophages ($pO_2$ = 15 mmHg) increased VEGF levels at 12 hours post-treatment, both hypoxic and hyperoxic ($pO_2$ = 300 mmHg) cells secreted greater amounts of VEGF at 24 hours. Thus, hyperoxia appears to act through a separate mechanism from that of hypoxia in stimulating VEGF release (Feng, J.J., unpublished data). Despite all of this evidence suggesting the role of VEGF in HBO-related angiogenesis, Lin et al. (161) did not find increased VEGF expression in endothelial cells treated with HBO. They did, however, show that HBO increased angiopoeitin-2 protein and mRNA levels, an effect apparently mediated by endothelial nitric oxide synthase (eNOS).

Does this angiogenic stimulation by hyperoxia lead to improved blood flow to wounds, or is it merely an interesting finding? Sheikh (162) measured blood flow in dermal wounds in rats over the course ten days post-operatively using the scanning laser Doppler technique. Rats exposed to hyperbaric oxygenation treatment during the post-operative period showed 20% more blood flow to the wound bed than control animals.

It is possible that hyperoxia may also work via intranuclear protein pADP-ribosylations. Interest in ADP-ribosylation first developed over its role in repairing DNA strand breaks. DNA damage stimulates pADPR synthetase activity. With this stimulation, NAD+ pools tend to be depleted because pADPR synthetase uses NAD+ for substrate. Depleted NAD+ pools might then cause the intracellular and intranuclear protein alterations needed for VEGF transcriptional modulation, just as they are implicated in the collagen synthesis pathway. Hyperoxia might trigger this pathway by causing the initial DNA strand breaks. This theory suggests that oxidants other than high $pO_2$ may also harbor angiogenic potential. This avenue of investigation is currently being actively pursued. Despite the great strides which have been made towards understanding neovascularization, further research is required to elucidate the driving mechanisms.

## Epithelization

Our knowledge about epithelization is relatively sparse. Epidermal cells are attracted to the healing wound by the same cytokines which attract fibroblasts (86). In addition, at least one growth factor, epidermal growth factor (EGF), is more specific for epithelial cells. EGF is a small polypeptide that circulates systemically in inactive form. Peptidases released from inflammatory cells inactivate the growth factor (87). EGF stimulates epithelial proliferation (88). TGF-β on the other hand, retards epithelial regeneration in split-thickness porcine skin wounds (89) and inhibits keratinocyte proliferation in culture (90, 91). More recently TGF-β application has been shown to delay epithelization in organotypic cultures (92).

Oxygen is also important for wound epithelization. Medawar observed that hypoxic epidermal cells exhibited poor movement and mitosis (93). Bullough and Johnson confirmed that squamous cell mitosis rate was oxygen dependent throughout a wide range of oxygen tensions (94). Winter and others have reported that wounds covered with an oxygen-permeable dressing epithelized faster than wounds covered with an oxygen-impermeable dressing (95, 96). Winter and Perrins demonstrated accelerated epithelization with hyperbaric oxygen treatments (97). Pai and Hunt showed that not only did increased oxygen tension increase collagen production, it also increased epithelization in a rat model. Wound contraction, on the other hand, was not affected by oxygen levels (98). In a living skin equivalent model, Dimitrijevich (163) found dramatically increased keratinocyte differentiation and epidermopoiesis with hyperbaric treatment. The mechanism of improved epithelization due to oxygen appears to involve increased cell proliferation. Part of the effect may also be related to improved basement membrane production (type IV collagen) resulting in better epithelial cell anchorage.

Cells migrate more effectively through a moist environment, partially because ambient oxygen diffuses far more readily through wet rather than dry tissue. This concept is especially important for epithelization, a process dependent upon cell movement and coverage. If eschar forms over a wound, epithelial cells migrate beneath it, extending "tongues" of cells which digest tissue in anticipation of advancing epithelium. When wound dressings are allowed to dry, epithelial cells are deprived of a humid environment. Also, when dry dressings are removed, both dead and healthy tissue alike are stripped off. Dressings should always remain moist. The idea of a "wet-to-dry" dressing is imprecise and archaic. If this term refers to dressings which are allowed to dry out in order to debride adherent tissue, it is a prescription for damage. If it refers to dressings which have a moist inner layer and a dry outer layer, it means merely that dressings must be changed more often. Simple, less wasteful methods exist for maintaining a moist wound environment.

## Dressings

Major advances in dressings have been made in the last decade. There is logic in this change despite the confusing number of commercial offerings. The principles are the following:

1. Wounds must be kept moist. Allowing wounds to dry is harmful, even if debridement is the object. Drying increases the amount of tissue that needs to be debrided, and retards healing.
2. Dressings should protect from physical injury.
3. Dressings should separate pus from the wound, but not necessarily remove uninfected wound fluid (which has healing properties). These types of absorbent dressings are plentiful.
4. Dressings should retain warmth, if possible. Usually warmth is achieved by preventing evaporation, but preventing radiation loss is also useful.

In general, hydrogels absorb water yet maintain a moist environment. Alginates and pectins absorb pus and probably stimulate healing. Particulates, such as starch granules, separate pus and can be impregnated with medication (e.g., vitamin A or iodine). If infection is controlled, some dressings can be kept in place for up to a week. This advantage is enormously important to patients who have painful wounds, or who cannot change dressings due to arthritis or other debility. Moisture-retaining dressings can reduce pain remarkably.

## OXYGEN AND RESISTANCE TO INFECTION

Healthy wounds in well-vascularized tissues are extremely resistant to infection. Ischemic wounds, however, are highly susceptible. Although this concept has been a part of surgical dogma for centuries, the underlying reasons have only recently been uncovered. The importance of the oxygen-dependent branch of nonspecific immunity has already been presented. The ability to influence this system through oxygen tension manipulation will now be examined.

The respiratory burst first involves the reduction of molecular oxygen ($O_2$) to superoxide anion ($O_2$-) by the NADPH oxidase system, a network of flavoproteins which resides in and around the phagosomal membrane, and which transports electrons across the membrane (99). Superoxide has potent microbicidal activity. Superoxide dismutase (SOD) catalyzes the interaction of two superoxide molecules to form $O_2$ and hydrogen peroxide ($H_2O_2$), another bactericidal oxidant. Myeloperoxidase (MPO), which is released by the azurophilic granules of the neutrophil, facilitates the reaction between $H_2O_2$ and iodide, bromide, or chloride to form halide oxidation products. Hypochlorous acid (HOCl) and its salt, hypochlorite are the major products, and are potent oxidants which attack membrane proteins in bacteria (2, 99). See Figure 7.

Phagocytes engulf bacteria and subject them to antimicrobial enzymes and reactive oxygen species. Inhibitors of oxidative pathways, such as cyanide and hypoxia, do not inhibit phagocytosis *in vitro*, but greatly impair leukocyte

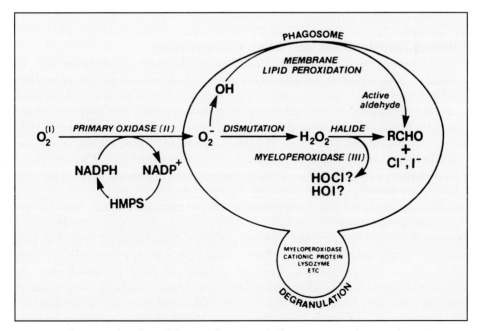

*Figure 7. Schematic of oxidative killing mechanism and relation to nonoxidative pathway (151).*

migration rate and microbial killing (100). The ability to produce oxygen radicals and to kill via oxidative mechanisms is directly proportional to local oxygen tension in the wound environment (16, 101). Reactions resulting in superoxide production are vulnerable to hypoxia over a wide range. Allen et al. found that half-maximal superoxide production ($KmO_2$) by neutrophils occurs in the range of 45 to 80 $mmHgpO_2$. Tissue oxygen tension in wounds is certainly within this range, indicating that suboptimal microbial killing is a common problem. This range predicts that maximal production is not reached until $pO_2$ is greater than 300 mmHg (102). Even minor wounds may contain areas with oxygen tension as low as 15mmHg. Given a mean wound tissue $pO_2$ of 15 mmHg, and using calculations made from the results of Allen et al. (102), bactericidal activity in wounds would rise three- to four-fold by raising tissue $pO_2$ to 100 mmHg, a level which is usually attainable with optimized perfusion and supplemental oxygen.

Hypoxia favors growth of anaerobes and suppresses killing of aerobes. It is significant that almost all of the frequent wound-infecting organisms and some of the less frequent are susceptible mainly to oxidative killing. Many studies have demonstrated the correlation between oxygenation and resistance to bacteria. *Pseudomonas aeruginosa* bacterial counts in inoculated wire mesh wound chambers were shown to decrease significantly in animals receiving high fractions of inspired oxygen at ambient pressure, compared to those breathing room air (15). Knighton et al. later showed that when guinea pigs received dermal inoculations of *Escherichia coli*, the number and sizes of the resulting necrotic skin lesions varied inversely with $FiO_2$ (19). *Staphylococcus aureus* inoculation of random pattern skin flaps versus musculocutaneous flaps in dogs caused much more necrosis in the less well-perfused and oxygenated random flaps (103, 104). From these studies it becomes apparent that oxygen tension is the single most important local factor affecting oxidative leukocyte killing.

## Clinical Implications of Tissue Oxygenation

Human studies confirm the laboratory findings. High tissue $pO_2$ is associated with reduced infection rate. Hopf et al. measured perioperative subcutaneous $pO_2$ and compared the measurements to the subsequent incidence of surgical wound infection. Subcutaneous $pO_2$ was found to be an accurate predictor of wound infection, better than other current risk assessment strategies (105). See Figure 8. However, there are currently no noninvasive means of obtaining accurate, direct measurements of wound $pO_2$. Transcutaneous $pO_2$ ($TcpO_2$) electrodes have been very useful in determining risk of poor healing and in deciding the appropriate level of amputation in ischemic limbs (106-110). Unfortunately, $TcpO_2$ measurements suffer from the classic problem of the measuring device which alters the measurement. Oxygen diffusion through the skin is very poor. Skin must be heated to the point of erythema to obtain measurable oxygen concentrations. The temperature increase causes major alterations in local perfusion due to autonomic vasodilation. The instrument, therefore, tends to overestimate tissue oxygenation because the effect of heat on blood flow is greater than the effect of heat on oxygen consumption. Also, the heat causes changes in skin lipid structure and oxygen-hemoglobin dissociation characteristics, thereby

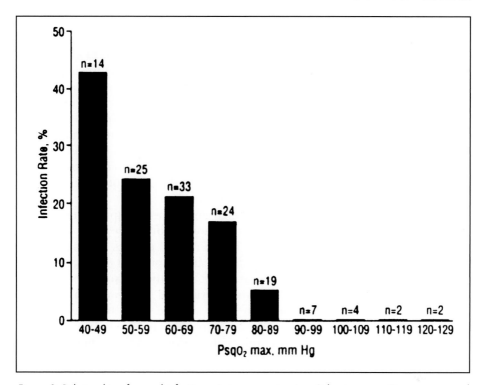

Figure 8. Relationship of wound infection rate to oxygen tension. Subcutaneous $pO_2$ was measured in patients undergoing various general surgery procedures. Subsequent wound infection rate was found to be inversely proportional to maximum subcutaneous wound $pO_2$ (PsqO_2 max) (p<0.01) (152).

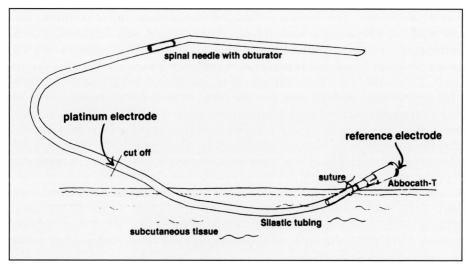

Figure 9. Silastic tonometer. Subcutaneous placement of the tonometer is achieved utilizing a needle with obturator. An oxygen probe is passed into the silastic tube in the subcutaneous tissue space, while a temperature probe is placed in the opposite end. Both oxygen and temperature measurements are acquired continuously (153).

further skewing measurements (65). A mildly invasive technique exists for assessing tissue $pO_2$ directly. Gottrup et al. described the placement of a Clark-type electrode under the skin to directly measure subcutaneous $pO_2$ (65). See Figure 9. Chang and Goodson correlated subcutaneous $pO_2$ with adequacy of post-operative resuscitation. Their conclusion was based on a simple line of logic. Because subcutaneous tissue vessels are extraordinarily sensitive to vasoconstrictive influences, they constrict quickly in response to mild hypovolemia. These vessels are the first to clamp down in blood-volume deficit and the last to relax with resuscitation. Subcutaneous oxygen tension reliably reflects local blood flow and falls dramatically with local vasoconstriction. Subcutaneous $pO_2$ is, therefore, a sensitive indicator not only of local perfusion, but also of total body perfusion (111, 112).

Traditional criteria, of which patellar and glabellar capillary refill, skin turgor, and eye globe pressure are the most informative, are useful in determining adequacy of resuscitation in the clinical setting. Unfortunately, these signs are sometimes equivocal. Of all the clinical signs of perfusion, urine output is the most misleading. In one study, directly measured $pO_2$ levels were found to more accurately detect peripheral vasoconstriction than experienced physicians who tended to judge volume status by urine output (113). Subcutaneous oximetry has its own problems, however. In particular, the devices are delicate, costly, and require considerable knowledge to operate. Improved technology should solve these problems. Improvements are clearly needed in direct tissue $pO_2$ analysis methods which can be performed at the bedside. Fortunately, a number of noninvasive oximetry technologies are being developed. As direct tissue $pO_2$ measurement becomes simpler and more common, the use of hyperbaric oxygen treatment will become more precise.

In a landmark article, Greif with the Outcomes Research Group examined the effects of supplemental perioperative oxygen on surgical wound infection. The group compared the postoperative surgical site infection rates between a study group that received 80% inspired oxygen perioperatively and a control group that received 30% oxygen. The 80% group developed half the postoperative infection rate than the 30% group (164). The authors advocate the use of supplemental oxygen in all patients who are deemed at high risk for infection, who are undergoing surgical procedures, or who are in the acute recovery phase following injury. It must be stressed, however, that increased $FiO_2$ and the resulting increased arterial $pO_2$ do not equate to increased tissue $pO_2$. They can never substitute for adequate perfusion. Blood flow must be optimized in any treatment involving supplemental oxygen in order to minimize vasoconstriction and improve wound $pO_2$. The most important causes of vasoconstriction are dehydration, cold, pain, tobacco use, medications, and fear (114, 115). All of these influences can be controlled. The essential point is that all of these factors must be corrected at the same time, because any one of them alone may result in maximal vasoconstriction.

Wounds are often located in cold locations on the body–the extremities. The arms and legs are, by nature, colder than the trunk due to large surface area/volume ratios and environmental exposure. Peripheral vascular disease only worsens this temperature differential. Unfortunately, the extremities are also the most frequently traumatized regions. Providing exogenous heat maximizes blood flow to these poorly perfused wounds by inducing local vasodilation.

Warmth in the acute setting of surgery has been shown to have benefits. In a large prospective, double-blind study, abdominal surgery patients were randomized to either the hypothermia group (routine intraoperative care) or the normothermia group (additional intraoperative warming to approach core and surface temperatures of 36.5°C). The normothermia group had one-third the number of wound infections, faster healing wounds, and twenty percent shorter hospital stays than the hypothermia group. These margins all reached statistical significance (116). In this trial, pain and hypovolemia were minimized by the protocol. Correcting these factors and others, such as smoking and nonessential vasoconstrictive drugs, undoubtedly achieves even better results. Perfusion may also be improved through the use of alpha receptor antagonists to counteract catecholamine driven vascular tone. Although clinical experience suggests that treatment with clonidine transdermal patches may improve peripheral perfusion in this way, no trial has yet been attempted.

## HYPERBARIC OXYGEN

### Rationale for Hyperbaric Oxygen Therapy in Problem Wounds

The arguments for the use of hyperbaric oxygen treatment (HBO) in wounds are based on all of the research regarding oxygen and wound healing presented earlier in this chapter. Oxygen tension is a major controlling factor in bacterial killing, resistance to infection, collagen synthesis, angiogenesis, and epithelization. In the presence of tissue hypoxia, some or all of these processes are impaired. Even if the central determinants of tissue perfusion are optimized, tissue hypoxia may persist due to macrovascular or microvascular disease. In this situation, hyperbaric oxygen therapy may be useful in improving wound-tissue oxygenation, as long as the tissue is receiving at least

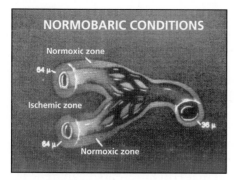

Figure 10a. Illustration of a typical pattern (light shading) of normal oxygen diffusion in pre-capillary arteriolar vessels at one atmosphere. Note adjacent zone of ischemia between converging arterioles (154).

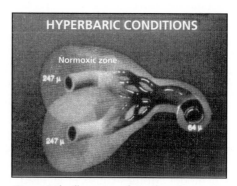

Figure 10b. Illustration of significantly increased pattern of oxygen diffusion during hyperbaric treatment at three atmospheres of pressure. Note absence of prior ischemic zone because of overlapping oxygen diffusion patterns of converging arterioles (155).

some blood flow. At supraphysiologic oxygen tensions, these problems may not only be corrected, but wound healing and resistance to infection may actually be enhanced beyond normal. In compromised wounds at normobaric conditions, watershed areas of ischemic tissue exist between individual blood vessels. With hyperbaric oxygenation, these hypoxic regions are reduced because the diffusion pattern of oxygen is greatly increased (117). See Figures 10a and 10b.

Mader et al. showed that HBO was at least as effective as antibiotic therapy in the treatment of osteomyelitis in an animal model (118). Tompach et al. found that HBO stimulated the proliferation of fibroblasts and endothelial cells in culture; this effect persisted for at least 72 hours post-treatment (119). Marx et al. demonstrated significantly improved angiogenesis *in vivo* in irradiated tissue treated with hyperbaric hyperoxia compared to normobaric hyperoxia (84). These data confirmed the idea of an oxygen gradient stimulus for angiogenesis, a theory first proposed by Remensnyder (24) in 1968, and championed by Knighton, Silver, and Hunt in later years (120). The theory states simply that central wound hypoxia stimulates initiation of angiogenesis while peripheral wound hyperoxia drives the process to completion, thereby obliterating the oxygen gradient (120). However, the oxygen gradient theory fails to account for the importance of lactate in angiogenesis. Mustoe reasoned that HBO contributes to wound healing not only by providing needed nutrition, but also via a signal pathway (121). Feng et al. support this idea, reporting that when cultured macrophages are exposed to oxygen at high tension (levels similar to tissue treated with HBO) they increase production of VEGF (Feng, J J, unpublished data). Ongoing investigations point to the participation of oxidants in a positive-regulatory pathway for VEGF secretion. These studies all suggest that the increased levels of tissue oxygen seen with HBO therapy boost the multifaceted wound healing response.

## Indications for Hyperbaric Oxygen Use with Wounds

Despite the fact that HBO therapy has been in our therapeutic arsenal for more than fifty years, controversy exists regarding its indications for use in wounds. Although many clinical studies have been performed, very few large, prospective, double-blind, randomized, clinical trials of HBO have been undertaken. However, given the previously outlined mechanisms of oxygen, the case is clear that increasing oxygen tension in wounds is important, regardless of the means of oxygen delivery, whether it be sea level oxygen supplementation, hyperbaric oxygenation, or surgical revascularization.

HBO therapy is beneficial in many partially ischemic wounds, including some diabetic ulcers (122, 123). Uhl et al. (124) reported that HBO treatment resulted in significantly shorter healing time in an ischemic mouse ear model. Monies-Chass et al. (125) found that HBO prevented gangrene in seven vascular trauma patients who had persistent limb ischemia, even after successful vessel repair.

Baroni et al. (123) performed a prospective trial of HBO therapy in patients with diabetic foot ulcers. In this study, the HBO treated patients were significantly less likely to undergo leg amputation than the non-HBO treated patients (8% vs. 40%, respectively). In a larger study by some of the same authors, Faglia et al. (126) performed a prospective, non-blind, randomized trial examining the use of HBO in the treatment of diabetic foot ulcers. They found that 8.6% of the patients in the HBO group went on to major amputation, compared to 33.3% in the control group. They also reported that at time of discharge, the patients in the HBO group had significantly higher dorsal foot $TcpO_2$ measurements than the controls, despite no difference in Tc $pO_2$ prior to treatment. $TcpO_2$ measurements, before and after oxygen challenges, have been used as guidelines in determining which patients will benefit from HBO therapy. Many criteria have been suggested (127-129), but the method is still undergoing evaluation, and will likely continue to evolve. However, no transcutaneous oximetry protocol will ever fully replace experienced clinical expertise in assessing $TcpO_2$ results. In a small, non-blind prospective randomized trial, Kessler found faster reduction of open wound area in the HBO group at two weeks. However, the control and HBO groups achieved similar results at four weeks (165). In another small, prospective trial the HBO patients enjoyed 76% healed wounds and 12% below-knee amputations at three years in comparison to 48% healed in the non-HBO group with 33% below-knee amputations (166).

The first prospective, randomized, double-blind study evaluating the benefits of HBO in the treatment of chronic wounds was performed by Hammarlund and Sundberg (130). While this study found marked wound size improvement in patients receiving HBO compared to those receiving pressurized air, individuals with diabetes or large vessel disease were specifically excluded. Thus, their conclusions do not necessarily apply to these patient groups. In a more recent prospective, randomized, double-blind study Abidia et al compared eight patients receiving hyperbaric 100% oxygen (HBO) to eight patients receiving hyperbaric air (HBA). At six weeks after treatment, five of eight HBO patients were completely healed while only one of eight HBA patients were healed. Amputation rates and healing at six months were similar in the two groups (167).

Perhaps the least disputed indication for hyperbaric oxygenation is the treatment of wounds in irradiated tissue. Upon exposure to radiation, some cells die immediately, while others are damaged to the extent that they cannot reproduce. Rapidly dividing cells, such as skin or gut epithelium, exhibit this damage early with sloughing and break down. Expression of damage in more slowly renewing tissues, such as connective tissues, requires longer periods of time, often years. Slowly progressing vascular damage causes endarteritis, thrombosis, and fibrosis over months to years. Osteoradionecrosis is often the end result (132). The poor wound healing qualities of irradiated tissue were recognized early in the use of radiation treatment (XRT) for malignancy (133). Discussions of this problem and its treatment have been particularly prominent among reconstructive surgeons (134-137). Before the use of HBO in this capacity, Marchetta et al. compared the outcomes of head and neck reconstructions between XRT recipients and non-recipients. XRT treated patients had a 30% infection rate and 43% complication rate, compared to 22% and 10%, respectively, in the non-recipients. Greenwood and Gilchrist (138) first described the use of hyperbaric oxygenation in post-irradiation head and neck surgery in 1973, finding that HBO treatment improved wound healing. Neovius et al. (139) reviewed the literature and reported unanimously positive evaluations of the use of HBO in irradiated head and neck wounds. The same authors also performed their own retrospective study and found an 80% healing rate in HBO treated patients compared to 58% in the reference group.

Prior to the use of HBO in previously irradiated mandible reconstructions the complication rate was as high as 70%, with 25% failure rate (140, 141). Marx (142) achieved drastically improved results by employing pre- and post-operative HBO. He reported a surgical success rate of 94%. Using a similar HBO protocol for patients undergoing tooth extractions from previously irradiated mandibles, Marx et al. were also able to reduce the incidence of osteoradionecrosis by almost 25% (143). That hyperbaric oxygen therapy has earned a role in the treatment of wounds in radiation-damaged tissues is no longer disputable.

## CONCLUSION

Wound healing is a complicated process performed by troops of cells which communicate not only with each other, but also with the wound environment. The normal host requires two basic staples to support an effective healing effort–adequate perfusion and sufficient oxygen supply. Basic science and clinical research have guided us to the many modalities at our disposal to satisfy these needs. Diligent examination and careful intervention are required, however, to detect and correct deficiencies. Investigators must continue to pursue well-designed studies to further the understanding of the molecular basis of repair and the usefulness of current and future treatments.

# REFERENCES

1. Michaeli D, Hunt, TK, and Knighton, DR. The role of platelets in wound healing: Demonstration of angiogenic activity. In: T. Hunt, Heppenstall, RB, Pines, and Rovee, D, ed. Soft and Hard Tissue Repair. New York: Praeger: 380-94.

2. Hunt TK. The physiology of wound healing. Ann Emerg Med 1988; 17:1265-73.

3. Knighton D. Mechanisms of wound healing. In: E. Kindwall, ed. Hyperbaric medicine practice. Vol. 1. Flagstaff, AZ: Best Publishing, 1994;119-39.

4. Deuel TF, Senior RM, Chang D, Griffin GL, Heinrikson RL and Kaiser ET. Platelet factor 4 is chemotactic for neutrophils and monocytes. Proc Natl Acad Sci U S A 1981; 78:4584-7.

5. Deuel TF, Senior RM, Huang JS and Griffin GL. Chemotaxis of monocytes and neutrophils to platelet-derived growth factor. J Clin Invest 1982; 69:1046-9.

6. Knighton DR, Hunt TK, Thakral KK and Goodson WH, 3rd. Role of platelets and fibrin in the healing sequence: an *in vivo* study of angiogenesis and collagen synthesis. Annals of Surgery 1982; 196:379-88.

7. Steed DL, Donohoe D, Webster MW and Lindsley L. Effect of extensive debridement and treatment on the healing of diabetic foot ulcers. Diabetic Ulcer Study Group. Journal of the American College of Surgeons 1996; 183: 61-4.

8. Steed DL. Clinical evaluation of recombinant human platelet-derived growth factor for the treatment of lower extremity diabetic ulcers. Diabetic Ulcer Study Group. Journal of Vascular Surgery 1995; 21:71-8; discussion 9-81.

9. Robson MC, Phillips LG, Thomason A, Robson LE and Pierce GF. Platelet-derived growth factor BB for the treatment of chronic pressure ulcers. Lancet 1992; 339:23-5.

10. Robson MC, Phillips LG, Thomason A, Altrock BW, Pence PC, Heggers JP, Johnston AF, McHugh TP, Anthony MS, Robson LE and et al. Recombinant human platelet-derived growth factor-BB for the treatment of chronic pressure ulcers [see comments]. Annals of Plastic Surgery 1992; 29:193-201.

11. Mustoe TA, Cutler NR, Allman RM, Goode PS, Deuel TF, Prause JA, Bear M, Serdar CM and Pierce GF. A phase II study to evaluate recombinant platelet-derived growth factor-BB in the treatment of stage 3 and 4 pressure ulcers. Archives of Surgery 1994; 129:213-9.

12. Issekutz TB, Issekutz AC and Movat HZ. The *in vivo* quantitation and kinetics of monocyte migration into acute inflammatory tissue. Am J Pathol 1981; 103:47-55.

13. Dunphy JE and Hunt TK. Fundamentals of wound management. New York: Appleton Century Crofts, 1979:xi, 612.

14. Hirsch JG. [The lysosomes in phagocytic cells]. Nouvelle Revue Francaise D Hematologie 1965; 5:553-8.

15. Hunt TK, Linsey M, Grislis H, Sonne M and Jawetz E. The effect of differing ambient oxygen tensions on wound infection. Annals of Surgery 1975; 181:35-9.

16. Hohn DC, MacKay RD, Halliday B and Hunt TK. Effect of $O_2$ tension on microbicidal function of leukocytes in wounds and *in vitro*. Surgical Forum 1976; 27:18-20.

17. Hunt TK and Minnesota Mining and Manufacturing Company. Wound healing and wound infection : theory and surgical practice. New York: Appleton-Century-Crofts, 1980:xii, 303 ,.

18. Nemet K, Fekete G, Schuler D, Kiss E, Meszner Z, Krivan G, Kardos G, Galantai I, Poder G, Kalmar A, Boer M and Roos D. Chronic granulomatous disease: Dysfunction of the phagocyte NADPH-oxydase enzyme. Orvosi Hetilap 1997; 138:397-401.

19. Knighton DR, Halliday B and Hunt TK. Oxygen as an antibiotic. The effect of inspired oxygen on infection. Arch Surg 1984; 119:199-204.

20. Hunt TK, Banda MJ and Silver IA. Cell interactions in post-traumatic fibrosis. Ciba Foundation Symposium 1985; 114:127-49.

21. Werb Z and Gordon S. Secretion of a specific collagenase by stimulated macrophages. Journal of Experimental Medicine 1975; 142:346-60.

22. Sunderkotter C, Steinbrink K, Goebeler M, Bhardwaj R and Sorg C. Macrophages and angiogenesis. J Leukoc Biol 1994; 55:410-22.

23. Constant J, Suh, DY, Hussain, MZ, and Hunt, TK. Wound healing angiogenesis: The metabolic basis of repair. In: M. E. Maragoudakis and North Atlantic Treaty Organization. Scientific Affairs Division, eds. Molecular, cellular, and clinical aspects of angiogenesis. New York: Plenum Press, 1996:ix, 298.

24. Remensnyder JP and Majno G. Oxygen gradients in healing wounds. American Journal of Pathology 1968; 52:301-23.

25. Im MJ and Hoopes JE. Enzyme activities in the repairing epithelium during wound healing. Journal of Surgical Research 1970; 10:173-9.

26. Im MJ and Hoopes JE. Energy metabolism in healing skin wounds. Journal of Surgical Research 1970; 10:459-64.

27. Caldwell MD, Shearer J, Morris A, Mastrofrancesco B, Henry W and Albina JE. Evidence for aerobic glycolysis in lambda-carrageenan-wounded skeletal muscle. Journal of Surgical Research 1984; 37:63-8.

28. Hussain MZ, Ghani QP and Hunt TK. Inhibition of prolyl hydroxylase by poly(ADP-ribose) and phosphoribosyl-AMP. Possible role of ADP-ribosylation in intracellular prolyl hydroxylase regulation. Journal of Biological Chemistry 1989; 264:7850-5.

29. Nishizuka Y, Ueda K, Nakazawa K and Hayaishi O. Studies on the polymer of adenosine diphosphate ribose. I. Enzymic formation from nicotinamide adenine dinuclotide in mammalian nuclei. Journal of Biological Chemistry 1967; 242:3164-71.

30. Reeder RH, Ueda K, Honjo T, Nishizuka Y and Hayaishi O. Studies on the polymer of adenosine diphosphate ribose. II. Characterization of the polymer. Journal of Biological Chemistry 1967; 242:3172-9.

31. Chambon P, Weill J and Mandel P. Nicotinamide mononucleotide activation of a new DNA-dependent polyadenylic acid synthesizing nuclear enzyme. Biochemical and Biophysical Research Communications 1963; 11:38-43.

32. Chambon P, Weill J, Dory J, Strosser M and Mandel P. The formation of a novel adenylic compound by enzymatic extracts of liver nuclei. Biochemical and Biophysical Research Communications 1966; 25:638.

33. Loetscher P, Alvarez-Gonzalez R and Althaus FR. Poly(ADP-ribose) may signal changing metabolic conditions to the chromatin of mammalian cells. Proceedings of the National Academy of Sciences of the United States of America 1987; 84:1286-9.

34. Ghani Q, Hussain, MZ, Zhang, J, and Hunt, TK. Control of procollagen gene transcription and prolyl hydroxylase activity by poly(ADP-ribose). In: G. G. Poirier and P. Moreau, eds. ADP-ribosylation reactions. New York: Springer-Verlag, 1992:xxxvi, 410.

35. Grotendorst GR, Martin GR, Pencev D, Sodek J and Harvey AK. Stimulation of granulation tissue formation by platelet-derived growth factor in normal and diabetic rats. Journal of Clinical Investigation 1985; 76:2323-9.

36. Chua CC, Chua BH, Zhao ZY, Krebs C, Diglio C and Perrin E. Effect of growth factors on collagen metabolism in cultured human heart fibroblasts. Connect Tissue Res 1991; 26:271-81.

37. Bates CJ, Prynne CJ and Levene CI. Ascorbate-dependent differences in the hydroxylation of proline and lysine in collagen synthesized by 3T6 fibroblasts in culture. Biochim Biophys Acta 1972; 278:610-6.

38. Hutton JJ, Jr. and Udenfriend S. Soluble collagen proline hydroxylase and its substrates in several animal tissues. Proceedings of the National Academy of Sciences of the United States of America 1966; 56:198-202.

39. Hutton JJ, Jr., Trappel AL and Udenfriend S. Requirements for alpha-ketoglutarate, ferrous ion and ascorbate by collagen proline hydroxylase. Biochemical and Biophysical Research Communications 1966; 24:179-84.

40. Hutton JJ, Jr., Kaplan A and Udenfriend S. Conversion of the amino acid sequence gly-pro-pro in protein to gly-pro-hyp by collagen proline hydroxylase. Archives of Biochemistry and Biophysics 1967; 121:384-91.

41. Prockop DJ, Kivirikko KI, Tuderman L and Guzman NA. The biosynthesis of collagen and its disorders first of two parts. N Engl J Med 1979; 301:13-23.

42. Prockop DJ, Kivirikko KI, Tuderman L and Guzman NA. The biosynthesis of collagen and its disorders second of two parts. N Engl J Med 1979; 301:77-85.

43. Hasegawa T, Takeuchi A, Miyaishi O, Isobe K and de Crombrugghe B. Cloning and characterization of a transcription factor that binds to the proximal promoters of the two mouse type I collagen genes. Journal of Biological Chemistry 1997; 272:4915-23.

44. Rippe RA, Lorenzen SI, Brenner DA and Breindl M. Regulatory elements in the 5'-flanking region and the first intron contribute to transcriptional control of the mouse alpha 1 type I collagen gene. Molecular and Cellular Biology 1989; 9:2224-7.

45. Boast S, Su MW, Ramirez F, Sanchez M and Avvedimento EV. Functional analysis of cis-acting DNA sequences controlling transcription of the human type I collagen genes. Journal of Biological Chemistry 1990; 265:13351-6.

46. Ritzenthaler JD, Goldstein RH, Fine A and Smith BD. Regulation of the alpha 1(I) collagen promoter via a transforming growth factor-beta activation element. Journal of Biological Chemistry 1993; 268:13625-31.

47. Jimenez SA, Varga J, Olsen A, Li L, Diaz A, Herhal J and Koch J. Functional analysis of human alpha 1(I) procollagen gene promoter. Differential activity in collagen-producing and -nonproducing cells and response to transforming growth factor beta 1. Journal of Biological Chemistry 1994; 269:12684-91.

48. Greenwel P, Inagaki Y, Hu W, Walsh M and Ramirez F. Sp1 is required for the early response of alpha2(I) collagen to transforming growth factor-beta1. Journal of Biological Chemistry 1997; 272:19738-45.

49. Falanga V, Tiegs SL, Alstadt SP, Roberts AB and Sporn MB. Transforming growth factor-beta: selective increase in glycosaminoglycan synthesis by cultures of fibroblasts from patients with progressive systemic sclerosis. J Invest Dermatol 1987; 89:100-4.

50. Krupsky M, Fine A, Kuang PP, Berk JL and Goldstein RH. Regulation of type I collagen production by insulin and transforming growth factor-beta in human lung fibroblasts. Connective Tissue Research 1996; 34:53-62.

51. Higashi K, Kouba DJ, Song YJ, Uitto J and Mauviel A. A proximal element within the human alpha 2(I) collagen (COL1A2) promoter, distinct from the tumor necrosis factor-alpha response element, mediates transcriptional repression by interferon-gamma. Matrix Biology 1998; 16:447-56.

52. Sun Y and Oberley LW. Redox regulation of transcriptional activators. Free Radical Biology and Medicine 1996; 21:335-48.

53. Levene C, Aleo J, Prynne C et al. The activation of protocollagen proline hydroxylation by ascorbic acid in cultured 3T6 fibroblasts. Biochem Biophys Acta 1974; 338:29.

54. Dinkins GA, Scheuenstuhl H, Hussain MZ, Spencer EM and Hunt TK. The effect of oxygen tension on insulin-like growth factor production by fibroblasts. Surgical Forum 1995; 46:676-8.

55. Falanga V, Qian SW, Danielpour D, Katz MH, Roberts AB and Sporn MB. Hypoxia upregulates the synthesis of TGF- eta 1 by human dermal fibroblasts. J Invest Dermatol 1991; 97:634-7.

56. Falanga V, Martin TA, Takagi H, Kirsner RS, Helfman T, Pardes J and Ochoa MS. Low oxygen tension increases mRNA levels of alpha 1 I procollagen in human dermal fibroblasts. J Cell Physiol 1993; 157:408-12.

57. Jonsson K, Jensen JA, Goodson WHd, Scheuenstuhl H, West J, Hopf HW and Hunt TK. Tissue oxygenation, anemia, and perfusion in relation to wound healing in surgical patients. Annals of Surgery 1991; 214:605-13.

58. Hunt TK and Pai MP. The effect of varying ambient oxygen tensions on wound metabolism and collagen synthesis. Surgery, Gynecology and Obstetrics 1972; 135:561-7.

59. Shandall A, Lowndes R and Young HL. Colonic anastomotic healing and oxygen tension. British Journal of Surgery 1985; 72:606-9.

60. Stryer L. Biochemistry. New York: W.H. Freeman, 1995:xxxiv, 1064.

61. Denison D. Oxygen supply and uses in tissues. In: K. Reinhart and K. Eyrich, eds. Clinical aspects of O*-transport and tissue oxygenation. Berlin ; New York: Springer-Verlag, 1989:xiii, 511.

62. Hunt T, Twomey P and Zederfeldt B. Respiratory gas tensions in healing wounds. American Journal of Surgery 1967; 114:302-7.

63. Niinikoski J, Hunt, TK, Dunphy, JE. Oxygen supply in healing tissue. American Journal of Surgery 1972; 123:247-52.

64. Goodwin C and Heppenstall R. The effect of chronic hypoxia on wound healing. Advances in Experimental Med Biol 1977; 94:669-72.

65. Gottrup F, Firmin R, Chang N, Goodson WHd and Hunt TK. Continuous direct tissue oxygen tension measurement by a new method using an implantable silastic tonometer and oxygen polarography. Am J Surg 1983; 146:399-403.

66. Gottrup F, Firmin R, Rabkin J and al e. Directly measured tissue oxygen tension and arterial oxygen tension assess tissue perfusion. Critical Care Medicine 1987; 15:1030-6.

67. Phillips G, Stone A, Schultz J, Jones B, Goodkin M, Lisowski M, Whitehead R, Fiegel V and Knighton D. Do growth factors stimulate angiogenesis? A comparison of putative angiogenesis factors. Wounds: A compendium of clinical research and practice 1997; 9:1-14.

68. Knighton DR, Phillips GD and Fiegel VD. Wound healing angiogenesis: indirect stimulation by basic fibroblast growth factor. Journal of Trauma 1990; 30:S134-44.

69. Clark RA, Stone RD, Leung DY, Silver I, Hohn DC and Hunt TK. Role of macrophages in wound healing. Surgical Forum 1976; 27:16-8.

70. Polverini PJ, Cotran PS, Gimbrone MA, Jr. and Unanue ER. Activated macrophages induce vascular proliferation. Nature 1977; 269:804-6.

71. Thakral KK, Goodson WHd and Hunt TK. Stimulation of wound blood vessel growth by wound macrophages. Journal of Surgical Research 1979; 26:430-6.

72. Jensen JA, Hunt TK, Scheuenstuhl H and Banda MJ. Effect of lactate, pyruvate, and pH on secretion of angiogenesis and mitogenesis factors by macrophages. Laboratory Investigation 1986; 54:574-8.

73. Keck PJ, Hauser SD, Krivi G, Sanzo K, Warren T, Feder J and Connolly DT. Vascular permeability factor, an endothelial cell mitogen related to PDGF. Science 1989; 246:1309-12.

74. Leung DW, Cachianes G, Kuang WJ, Goeddel DV and Ferrara N. Vascular endothelial growth factor is a secreted angiogenic mitogen. Science 1989; 246:1306-9.

75. Levy AP, Levy NS and Goldberg MA. Hypoxia-inducible protein binding to vascular endothelial growth factor mRNA and its modulation by the von Hippel-Lindau protein. Journal of Biological Chemistry 1996; 271:25492-7.

76. Levy AP, Levy NS and Goldberg MA. Post-transcriptional regulation of vascular endothelial growth factor by hypoxia. Journal of Biological Chemistry 1996; 271:2746-53.

77. Minchenko A, Salceda S, Bauer T and Caro J. Hypoxia regulatory elements of the human vascular endothelial growth factor gene. Cellular and Molecular Biology Research 1994; 40:35-9.

78. Finkenzeller G, Technau A and Marmé D. Hypoxia-induced transcription of the vascular endothelial growth factor gene is independent of functional AP-1 transcription factor. Biochemical and Biophysical Research Communications 1995; 208:432-9.

79. Goldberg MA and Schneider TJ. Similarities between the oxygen-sensing mechanisms regulating the expression of vascular endothelial growth factor and erythropoietin. Journal of Biological Chemistry 1994; 269:4355-9.

80. Knighton DR, Hunt TK, Scheuenstuhl H, Halliday BJ, Werb Z and Banda MJ. Oxygen tension regulates the expression of angiogenesis factor by macrophages. Science 1983; 221:1283-5.

81. Ferrara N and Davis-Smyth T. The biology of vascular endothelial growth factor. Endocr Rev 1997; 18:4-25.

82. Zabel DD, Feng JJ, Scheuenstuhl H, Hunt TK and Hussain MZ. Lactate stimulation of macrophage-derived angiogenic activity is associated with inhibition of Poly ADP-ribose synthesis. Lab Invest 1996; 74:644-9.

83. Feng J, Ghani Q, Ledger G, Barkhordar R, Hunt T and Hussain M. Modulation of vascular endothelial growth factor angiogenic activity by ADP-riboxylation. In: M. E. Maragoudakis and North Atlantic Treaty Organization. Scientific Affairs Division., eds. Molecular, cellular, and clinical aspects of angiogenesis. Vol. 298. New York: Plenum Press, 1998:ix, 298.

84. Marx RE, Ehler WJ, Tayapongsak P and Pierce LW. Relationship of oxygen dose to angiogenesis induction in irradiated tissue [see comments]. Am J Surg 1990; 160:519-24.

85. Gibson JJ, Angeles AP and Hunt TK. Increased oxygen tension potentiates angiogenesis. Surgical Forum 1997; 48:696-9.

86. Duell E and Voorhees J. Control of epidermal growth. In: L. A. Goldsmith, ed. Biochemistry and physiology of the skin. New York: Oxford University Press, 1983:2 v. (xx, 1323 ).

87. Hollenberg MD. Epidermal growth factor-urogastrone, a polypeptide acquiring hormonal status. Vitamins and Hormones 1979; 37:69-110.

88. Brown GL, Nanney LB, Griffen J, Cramer AB, Yancey JM, Curtsinger LJd, Holtzin L, Schultz GS, Jurkiewicz MJ and Lynch JB. Enhancement of wound healing by topical treatment with epidermal growth factor [see comments]. New England Journal of Medicine 1989; 321:76-9.

89. Quaglino D, Jr., Nanney LB, Kennedy R and Davidson JM. Transforming growth factor-beta stimulates wound healing and modulates extracellular matrix gene expression in pig skin. I. Excisional wound model. Laboratory Investigation 1990; 63:307-19.

90. Sarret Y, Woodley DT, Grigsby K, Wynn K and O'Keefe EJ. Human keratinocyte locomotion: the effect of selected cytokines. Journal of Investigative Dermatology 1992; 98:12-6.

91. Shipley GD, Pittelkow MR, Wille JJ, Jr., Scott RE and Moses HL. Reversible inhibition of normal human prokeratinocyte proliferation by type beta transforming growth factor-growth inhibitor in serum-free medium. Cancer Research 1986; 46:2068-71.

92. Garlick JA and Taichman LB. Effect of TGF-  eta 1 on re-epithelialization of human keratinocytes *in vitro*: an organotypic model. J Invest Dermatol 1994; 103:554-9.

93. Medawar P. The cultivation of adult mammalian skin epithelium. Q. J. Micr. Sci. 1948; 89:187.

94. Bullough W and Johnson M. Epidermal mitotic activity and oxygen tension. Nature 1957; 167:488.

95. Winter GD. A note on wound healing under dressings with special reference to perforated-film dressings. Journal of Investigative Dermatology 1965; 45:299-302.

96. Alvarez OM, Mertz PM and Eaglstein WH. The effect of occlusive dressings on collagen synthesis and re-epithelialization in superficial wounds. Journal of Surgical Research 1983; 35:142-8.

97. Winter G and Perrins D. Effects of hyperbaric oxygen treatment on epidermal regeneration. In: T. Iwa and J. Wada, eds. Proceedings of the fourth international congress on hyperbaric medicine. Tokyo: Igaku Shoin, Ltd, 1970:x, 555.

98. Pai MP and Hunt TK. Effect of varying oxygen tensions on healing of open wounds. Surg Gynecol Obstet 1972; 135:756-8.

99. Klebanoff S. Phagocytic cells: products of oxygen metabolism. In: J. I. Gallin, I. M. Goldstein and R. Snyderman, eds. Inflammation : basic principles and clinical correlates. New York: Raven Press, 1988:xvii, 995.

100. Klebanoff S. Oxygen metabolism and the toxic properties of phagocytes. Annals of Internal Medicine 1980; 93:480-89.

101. Rabkin J and Hunt T. Infection and oxygen. In: J. Davis and T. Hunt, eds. Problem Wounds: The Role of Oxygen. New York: Elsevier, 1988:1-16.

102. Allen D, Maguire J, Mahdavian M, Wicke C, Marcocci L, Scheuenstuhl H, Chang M, Le A, Hopf H and Hunt T. Wound hypoxia and acidosis limit neutrophil bacterial killing mechanisms. Archives of Surgery 1997; 132:991-6.

103. Chang N and Mathes SJ. Comparison of the effect of bacterial inoculation in musculocutaneous and random-pattern flaps. Plast Reconstr Surg 1982; 70:1-10.

104. Gottrup F, Firmin R, Hunt TK and Mathes SJ. The dynamic properties of tissue oxygen in healing flaps. Surgery 1984; 95:527-36.

105. Hopf H, Hunt T, West J, Blomquist P and al e. Wound tissue oxygen tension predicts the risk of wound infection in surgical patients. Archives of Surgery 1997; 132:997-1005.

106. Reiber GE, Pecoraro RE and Koepsell TD. Risk factors for amputation in patients with diabetes mellitus. A case-control study [see comments]. Ann Intern Med 1992; 117:97-105.

107. Oishi CS, Fronek A and Golbranson FL. The role of non-invasive vascular studies in determining levels of amputation. J Bone Joint Surg [Am] 1988; 70:1520-30.

108. Harward TR, Volny J, Golbranson F, Bernstein EF and Fronek A. Oxygen inhalation—induced transcutaneous $pO_2$ changes as a predictor of amputation level. J Vasc Surg 1985; 2:220-7.

109. Dowd GS, Linge K and Bentley G. Measurement of transcutaneous oxygen pressure in normal and ischaemicischemic skin. J Bone Joint Surg [Br] 1983; 65:79-83.

110. Pecoraro RE, Ahroni JH, Boyko EJ and Stensel VL. Chronology and determinants of tissue repair in diabetic lower-extremity ulcers. Diabetes 1991; 40:1305-13.

111. Chang N, Goodson WHD, Gottrup F and Hunt TK. Direct measurement of wound and tissue oxygen tension in postoperative patients. Ann Surg 1983; 197:470-8.

112. Knudson MM, Bermudez KM, Doyle CA, Mackersie RC, Hopf HW and Morabito D. Use of tissue oxygen tension measurements during resuscitation from hemorrhagic shock. J Trauma 1997; 42:608-14; discussion 14-6.

113. Jensen J, Riggs K, Vaconez L and al e. Clinical assessment of postoperative perfusion. Surgical Forum 1987; 38:66-7.

114. Rabkin J and Hunt T. Local heat increases blood flow and oxygen tension in wounds. Archives of Surgery 1987; 122:221-5.

115. Jensen J, Goodson W, Hopf H and Hunt T. Cigarette smoking decreases tissue oxygen. Archives of Surgery 1991; 126:1131-4.

116. Kurz A, Sessler D, Lenhardt R and Group TSoWIaT. Perioperative normothermia to reduce the incidence of surgical-wound infection and shorten hospitalization. The New England Journal of Medicine 1996; 334:1209-15.

117. Williams RL. Hyperbaric oxygen therapy and the diabetic foot. Journal of the American Podiatric Medical Association 1997; 87:279-92.

118. Mader JT, Guckian JC, Glass DL and Reinarz JA. Therapy with hyperbaric oxygen for experimental osteomyelitis due to Staphylococcus aureus in rabbits. J Infect Dis 1978; 138:312-8.

119. Tompach PC, Lew D and Stoll JL. Cell response to hyperbaric oxygen treatment. International Journal of Oral and Maxillofacial Surgery 1997; 26:82-6.

120. Knighton DR, Silver IA and Hunt TK. Regulation of wound-healing angiogenesis-effect of oxygen gradients and inspired oxygen concentration. Surgery 1981; 90:262-70.

121. Siddiqui A, Davidson JD and Mustoe TA. Ischemic tissue oxygen capacitance after hyperbaric oxygen therapy: a new physiologic concept. Plastic and Reconstructive Surgery 1997; 99:148-55.

122. Davis JC. The use of adjuvant hyperbaric oxygen in treatment of the diabetic foot. Clin Podiatr Med Surg 1987; 4:429-37.

123. Baroni G, Porro T, Faglia E, Pizzi G, Mastropasqua A, Oriani G, Pedesini G and Favales F. Hyperbaric oxygen in diabetic gangrene treatment. Diabetes Care 1987; 10:81-6.

124. Uhl E, Sirsjö A, Haapaniemi T, Nilsson G and Nylander G. Hyperbaric oxygen improves wound healing in normal and ischemic skin tissue. Plastic and Reconstructive Surgery 1994; 93:835-41.

125. Monies-Chass I, Hashmonai M, Hoere D, Kaufman T, Steiner E and Schramek A. Hyperbaric oxygen treatment as an adjuvant to reconstructive vascular surgery in trauma. Injury 1977; 8:274-7.

126. Faglia E, Favales F, Aldeghi A, Calia P, Quarantiello A, Oriani G, Michael M, Campagnoli P and Morabito A. Adjunctive systemic hyperbaric oxygen therapy in treatment of severe prevalently ischemic diabetic foot ulcer. A randomized study. Diabetes Care 1996; 19:1338-43.

127. Brakora MJ and Sheffield PJ. Hyperbaric oxygen therapy for diabetic wounds. Clinics in Podiatric Medicine and Surgery 1995; 12:105-17.

128. Magnant CM, Milzman DP and Dhindsa H. Hyperbaric medicine for outpatient wound care. Emergency Medicine Clinics of North America 1992; 10:847-60.

129. Wyss CR, Harrington RM, Burgess EM and Matsen FAd. Transcutaneous oxygen tension as a predictor of success after an amputation. Journal of Bone and Joint Surgery. American Volume 1988; 70:203-7.

130. Hammarlund C and Sundberg T. Hyperbaric oxygen reduced size of chronic leg ulcers: a randomized double-blind study. Plast Reconstr Surg 1994; 93:829-33; discussion 34.

132. Marx RE and Johnson RP. Studies in the radiobiology of osteoradionecrosis and their clinical significance. Oral Surg Oral Med Oral Pathol 1987; 64:379-90.

133. Powers WE, Ogura JH and Palmer LA. Radiation therapy and wound healing delay. Animals and man. Radiology 1967; 89:112-5.

134. Kiener JL, Hoffman WY and Mathes SJ. Influence of radiotherapy on microvascular reconstruction in the head and neck region. Am J Surg 1991; 162:404-7.

135. Nemiroff PM, Merwin GE, Brant T and Cassisi NJ. Effects of hyperbaric oxygen and irradiation on experimental skin flaps in rats. Otolaryngol Head Neck Surg 1985; 93:485-91.

136. Granstrom G, Tjellstrom A, Branemark PI and Fornander J. Bone-anchored reconstruction of the irradiated head and neck cancer patient. Otolaryngol Head Neck Surg 1993; 108:334-43.

137. Granstrom G. Hyperbaric oxygen therapy as a stimulator of osseointegration. Adv Otorhinolaryngol 1998; 54:33-49.

138. Greenwood TW and Gilchrist AG. Hyperbaric oxygen and wound healing in post-irradiation head and neck surgery. Br J Surg 1973; 60:394-7.

139. Neovius EB, Lind MG and Lind FG. Hyperbaric oxygen therapy for wound complications after surgery in the irradiated head and neck: a review of the literature and a report of 15 consecutive patients. Head Neck 1997; 19:315-22.

140. Adamo AK and Szal RL. Timing, results, and complications of mandibular reconstructive surgery: report of 32 cases. J Oral Surg 1979; 37:755-63.

141. Komisar A. The functional result of mandibular reconstruction. Laryngoscope 1990; 100:364-74.

142. Marx RE and Ames JR. The use of hyperbaric oxygen therapy in bony reconstruction of the irradiated and tissue-deficient patient. J Oral Maxillofac Surg 1982; 40:412-20.

143. Marx RE, Johnson RP and Kline SN. Prevention of osteoradionecrosis: a randomized prospective clinical trial of hyperbaric oxygen versus penicillin. J Am Dent Assoc 1985; 111:49-54.

144. Levenson S, Seifter E, Van Winkle E Jr. "Nutrition," in Hunt TK Dunphy JE (eds): Fundamentals of Wound Management, NY. Appleton-Century-Crofts, 1979, 286-363. Modified with permission.

145. Silver, IA. "The physiology of wound healing," in Hunt, Tk (ed): Wound Healing and Wound Infection: Theory and Surgical Practice, NY. Appleton-Century-Crofts, 1980, 30 Figure6). Modified with permission.

146. Remensnyder JP, and Majno G. "Oxygengradients in healing wounds." American Journal of Pathology, 1968, 52: 308 Figure 4). Modified with permission.

147. Ghani Q, Hussain MZ, Zhang J, and Hunt TK. "Control of procollagen gene transcription and prolyl hydroxylase activity by poly(adp-ribose)." In: Poirer GG and Moreau, P (eds). ADP-ribosylation Reactions. New York: Springer-Verlag, 1992. Modified with permission.

148. No References

149. Skover GR. "Cellular and biochemical dynamics of wound repair: wound environment in collagen regeneration." Clinics in Podiatric Medicine and Surgery, 1991; 8: 723-56. Modified with permission.

150. Sunderkotter C, Steinbrink K, Goebeler M, Bhardwaj R., and Sor C. "Macrophages and angiogenesis." Journal of Leukocyte Biology, 1994; 55: 410-22. Modified with permission.

151. Hunt TK, and Van Winkle E Jr., "Normal Repair," in Hunt, TK, Dunphy. JE (eds): Fundamentals of Wound Management, NY. Appleton-Century-Crofts, 1979, 85. Modified with permission.

152. Hopf HW, Hunt TK, West JM, Blomquist P, et al. "Wound tissue oxygen tension predicts the risk of wound infection in surgical patients." Archives of Surgery, 1997: 1342: 997-1005. Copyright 1997, American Medical Associtation. Modified with permission.

153. Hopf HW, Hunt TK. "The role of O$_2$ in wound repair and wound infection." In: Esterhai, J Gristina, A, Poss, R (eds). Musculoskeletal Infection. Rosemont, IL: American Academy of Orthopedic Surgeons, 1992; 333 (figure 3). Modified with permission.

155. Boykin JV Jr. "Hyperbaric oxygen therapy: a physiological approach to selected problem wound healing." Wounds, 1996; 8(6): 183-198. Copyright © 1996 by Health Management Publications, Inc. Modified with permission.

156. Tompach PC, Lew D, and Stoll JL, "Cell response to hyperbaric oxygen treatment." Int. J. Oral Maxillofac. Surg., 1997; 26: 82-6.

157. Cho, M., T. K. Hunt, et al. (2001). "Hydrogen peroxide stimulates macrophage vascular endothelial growth factor release." Am J Physiol Heart Circ Physiol 280(5): H2357-63.

158. Hopf, H. W., J. J. Gibson, et al. (2005). "Hyperoxia and angiogenesis." Wound Repair Regen 13(6): 558-64.

159. Mechine, A., S. Rohr, et al. (1999). "Wound healing and hyperbaric oxygen. Experimental study of the angiogenesis phase in the rat." Ann Chir 53(4): 307-13.

160. Sheikh, A. Y., J. J. Gibson, et al. (2000). "Effect of hyperoxia on vascular endothelial growth factor levels in a wound model." Arch Surg 135(11): 1293-7.

161. Lin, S., K. G. Shyu, et al. (2002). "Hyperbaric oxygen selectively induces angiopoietin-2 in human umbilical vein endothelial cells." Biochem Biophys Res Commun 296(3): 710-5.

162. Sheikh, A. Y., M. D. Rollins, et al. (2005). "Hyperoxia improves microvascular perfusion in a murine wound model." Wound Repair Regen 13(3): 303-8.

163. Dimitrijevich, S. D., S. Paranjape, et al. (1999). "Effect of hyperbaric oxygen on human skin cells in culture and in human dermal and skin equivalents." Wound Repair Regen 7(1): 53-64.

164. Greif, R., O. Akca, et al. (2000). "Supplemental perioperative oxygen to reduce the incidence of surgical-wound infection. Outcomes Research Group." N Engl J Med 342(3): 161-7.

165. Kessler, L., P. Bilbault, et al. (2003). "Hyperbaric oxygenation accelerates the healing rate of nonischemic chronic diabetic foot ulcers: a prospective randomized study." Diabetes Care 26(8): 2378-82.

166. Kalani, M., G. Jorneskog, et al. (2002). "Hyperbaric oxygen (HBO) therapy in treatment of diabetic foot ulcers. Long-term follow-up." J Diabetes Complications 16(2): 153-8.

167. Abidia, A., G. Laden, et al. (2003). "The role of hyperbaric oxygen therapy in ischaemic diabetic lower extremity ulcers: a double-blind randomised-controlled trial." Eur J Vasc Endovasc Surg 25(6): 513-8.

168. Berthod F, Germain L, Tremblay N, Auger F. Extracellular matrix deposition by fibroblasts is necessary to promote capillary-like tube formation *in vitro*. J Cell Physiol. 2006 May;207(2):491-8.

169. Constant JS, Feng JJ, Zabel DD, Yuan H, Suh DY, Scheuenstuhl H, Hunt TK, Hussain MZ. Lactate elicits vascular endothelial growth factor from macrophages: a possible alternative to hypoxia. Wound Repair Regen. 2000 Sep-Oct;8(5):353-60.

170. Semenza GL. HIF-1: using two hands to flip the angiogenic switch. Cancer Metastasis Rev. 2000;19(1-2):59-65

171. Liu Q, Berchner-Pfannschmidt U, Moller U, Brecht M, Wotzlaw C, Acker H, Jungermann K, Kietzmann T. A Fenton reaction at the endoplasmic reticulum is involved in the redox control of hypoxia-inducible gene expression. Proc Natl Acad Sci U S A. 2004 Mar 23;101(12):4302-7.

172. Ali MA, Yasui F, Matsugo S, Konishi T. The lactate-dependent enhancement of hydroxyl radical generation by the Fenton reaction. Free Radic Res. 2000 May;32(5):429-38.

# NOTES

CHAPTER 16

# CHRONIC WOUND MANAGEMENT: PRACTICE GUIDELINES FOR THE HYPERBARIC SPECIALIST

## CHAPTER SIXTEEN OVERVIEW

# Chronic Wound Management: Practice Guidelines for the Hyperbaric Specialist

*Jeffrey A. Niezgoda, Diane L. Krasner, R. Gary Sibbald*

## INTRODUCTION

Management of chronic wounds is an evolving process. Best-practice models for achieving optimal outcomes are commonly based on a multidisciplinary team approach. This team is centered around the patient and guided by the decisions of the patient's primary care provider. The other members of the team providing advanced wound healing include the hyperbaric physician, wound care nurses and technicians, and possibly additional providers such as the dietitian, infectious disease specialist, pedorthist, orthotist, physical therapist, endocrinologist, general and vascular surgeon and the plastic surgeon. Patient's family members and caregivers also play an integral part in developing individualized goals and the treatment plan. These goals and outcomes must be realistic and not idealistic for the treatment setting and resource availability. Standards of care, guidelines, and algorithms are useful, but must be interpreted and implemented based on local expertise, resource availability, and the individualized patient plan of care. This is referred to as Advanced Wound Caring (29), and can be implemented to optimize healing outcomes and improve the quality of life for people with non-healing wounds.

In addition, the wound care team must focus their attention on the medical management of underlying chronic conditions, such as control of diabetes and hypertension, stabilization of peripheral vascular problems, and interventions to minimize risk factors. Requests for subspecialty consultations are often based on specific management goals and are typically required for specific times and tasks, such as surgery for debridement, infectious disease consultation for decisions about invasive or deep infections, physiatrists for rehabilitation and off-loading recommendations, and dietary for nutritional interventions. Appropriate patient referrals can optimize the outcomes associated with timely accurate interventions. Excellent communication and interaction are paramount to ensure success of the team approach and to enhance overall patient optimization and wound-specific therapies.

Over the past decade or two, there has been a paradigm shift in the treatment of chronic wounds (33). Best practice interventions incorporate maintenance of a moist wound environment (23, 67-69) and address etiology-specific needs. These interventions include pressure reduction/relief for pressure ulcers, graduated compression for venous insufficiency ulcers, and off-loading of plantar diabetic foot ulcers. Treating the needs of the patient, not just the wound, means that nutrition, pain management, infection control, and quality of life are addressed in the hyperbaric plan of care. The science behind the interventions drive the decision making process of providing best practice advanced wound care and hyperbaric medicine. Expert practitioners hone their skills by becoming proficient at chronic wound assessment, which then helps them to tailor their treatment decisions to the wound, the patient, and the setting (35).

Over the past thirty years, dressing technologies have evolved from passive plug and conceal methods to the use of interactive and bioactive materials (23, 33, 39, 62). While research is uncovering new knowledge and defining effective treatments almost daily, this chapter is aimed to present the most current and successful methods of wound management and will describe best practice wound care interventions.

## WOUND CLASSIFICATION

Classifying or categorizing a wound by underlying cause (Etiology) or the presenting characteristics (Appearance) can guide the practitioner in making appropriate decisions related to treatment and management (See Figures 1-12). The etiology of a wound provides an algorithm or strategy for the global management of the patient, with the ultimate goal of achieving wound healing. Etiologic categories include pressure ulcers, venous ulcers, diabetic or neuropathic ulcers, surgically created wounds, and ischemic or arterial ulcers. Similarly, the general appearance of the wound guides the wound care management regarding the use of topical treatment and appropriate dressing regimen. The general appearance categories include necrotic, infected, draining, and granular wounds.

## Etiology

*Pressure Ulcers:* Pressure ulcers are the result of a mechanical force creating enough pressure on the vasculature to disrupt the blood supply to soft tissues, usually between a bony prominence and a supporting surface (34). The resulting ischemia sets up a domino effect of events. Cellular hypoxia leads to cellular stress which increases the metabolic needs of the tissues that may already have a compromised blood supply. Depending on the depth of penetration, the angle, and the duration of the pressure, the tissue damage may be either easily reversed or it can result in a partial or full thickness wound involving fascia, muscle, tendon and bone (66).

*Venous Ulcers:* Venous insufficiency ulcers affect the lower legs. These are the most common type of ulcer reported. The mechanical force leading to venous ulcerations is increased hydrostatic pressure within the compartment of the lower leg. Varicosities, deep vein thromboses, calf muscle pump failure, obesity, surgical interruption of the venous system, and incompetent perforator valves from the deep to superficial venous system are the most

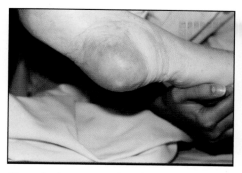

Figure 1. Assessment of etiology: pressure ulcer of the heel, stage 1.

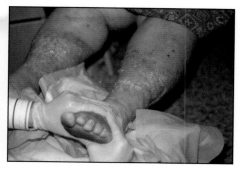

Figure 2. Assessment of perfusion in a person with bilateral venous ulcers.

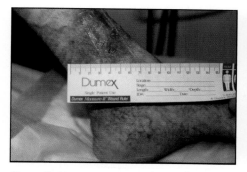

Figure 3. Measuring venous ulcer surface with a paper ruler.

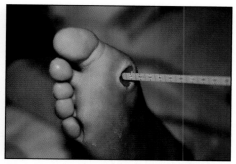

Figure 4. Measuring depth with a plastic depth guide on a diabetic foot ulcer over the first metatarsal head.

often cited precursors to venous disease. The increased hydrostatic pressure results in edema, induration, dilated superficial veins, change in skin pigmentation related to hemosiderin extravasation, and a predisposition for cellulitis. The venous ulcer is typically shallow, often beginning as an irregularly shaped blister, which is highly exudative, painful, and develops adherent fibrin at the base (55).

*Diabetic Ulcers:* Diabetic/neuropathic ulcers are the result of the effects of uncontrolled or poorly controlled diabetes mellitus (70). The microvascular effects of diabetes result in neurologic damage causing a polyneuropathy. This combination of autonomic, motor, and sensory neuropathies culminate in an insensate foot with altered mechanics of weight bearing, resulting in deformity and a blunted immune and vascular response. The diabetic ulcer characteristically occurs on the plantar aspect of the foot and is usually accompanied by callus formation in response to the repeated trauma (60).

*Surgical Wounds:* Surgically created or traumatic wounds are acute in nature and should follow the normal wound healing trajectory when closed by primary intention. If there is an underlying factor that alters the progress of the normal healing cascade, dehiscence, partial wound healing or infection may ensue.

*Arterial Ulcers:* Arterial or ischemic ulcers develop due to disruption or blockage of arterial blood vessels (3). Causes of blockage include the

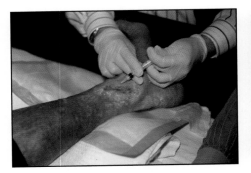

Figure 5. Infiltration of local anesthetic to reduce pain prior to biopsy.

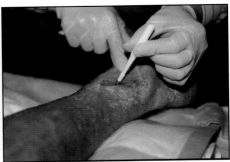

Figure 6. Punch biopsy to rule out cancer (Marjolin's ulcer) in a chronic leg wound.

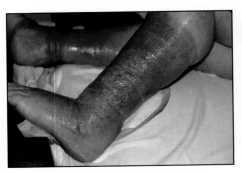

Figure 7. Edematous limb due to venous disease.

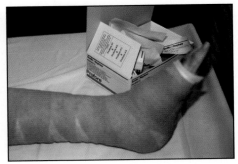

Figure 8. Four layer compression bandaging to control edema due to venous disease.

arterial occlusive diseases such as arteriosclerosis and autoimmune inflammatory disorders such as vasculitis. Local tissue does not receive adequate blood supply and the tissue dies. Ischemic ulcers tend to be very painful, occur at locations distal on the extremity, and may be over a bony area (the lateral malleolus is a frequent site). The wound bed is typically pale, dry, and has a punched out appearance. The extremity may show signs of slowed cellular growth exhibited as thickened brittle nails, thin dry skin and decreased or no hair growth. Oftentimes pulses are not palpable, and elevation of the limb causes pain and pallor. Individuals with this condition will sit at the bedside or in a chair with the feet in a dependent position to alleviate the discomfort (24).

## Appearance

*Necrotic Wounds:* Necrotic tissue is often referred to as fibrinous slough when it is moist and eschar when dry. Slough is soft, moist, fibrinous tissue that may be tan, yellow or gray in color. It can present stringy and loose, or dense and adherent to the wound bed. Eschar is desiccated, dark brown to black and leather-like. It may present as a large "scab" covering the entire wound or as a percentage of the tissue on the wound surface. Eschar and slough can obscure visualization of the true wound bed. Necrotic tissue is the ideal medium for bacterial growth and impedes the healing process. To decrease the

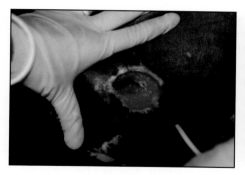

Figure 9. Stage four pressure ulcer with drainage.

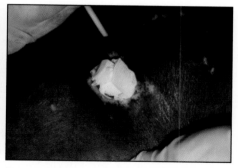

Figure 10. Same ulcer as in Figure 9 packed with hypertonic gauze for exudate absorption.

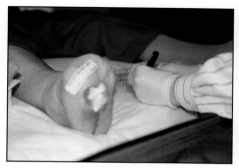

Figure 11. Calcium alginate rope dressing used post debridement for hemostasis in a diabetic foot ulcer.

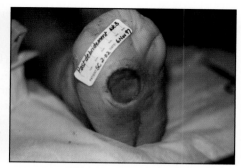

Figure 12. Human skin equivalent (skin substitute) (Dermagraf®) in place on a diabetic foot ulcer.

risk of infection and prepare the wound bed for granulation the devitalized tissue must be removed, or debrided.

*Infected Wounds:* Infection involving the wound bed and surrounding tissue may present much like the inflammatory phase following injury. All open wounds are considered contaminated with resident flora from the surrounding skin of the host. Colonization occurs when the pathogens begin to proliferate on the surface of the wound without causing a tissue or host response. Critical colonization is that point when the multiplying bacteria begin to compete with the wound bed cells for nutrients and the superficial wound bed is compromised and healing does not progress. The host response may include increased exudate, mild to moderate odor, lack of or poor quality friable granulation tissue growth. The patient may experience an increase in pain. Wounds will not improve in the presence of an overwhelming bacterial load and so there is a recession in the rate of healing. Intervention with topical anti-microbials may be helpful in the management of excess bioburden, but localized infection and cellulitis are best addressed systemically.

*Draining Wounds:* The amount and character of drainage exuding from the wound provides the clinician with clues regarding wound status. Healthy proliferating granulation tissue is slightly moist and glistening. The theory behind moist wound healing is to maintain the ambient moisture inherent in normal tissue, bathing the wound in naturally occurring proteins and nutrients. The moisture also enables the epithelial cells to migrate across the granulation tissue unimpeded rather than borrow under a dry wound bed or necrotic eschar. An ischemic wound with inadequate blood flow will present as dry and desiccated. A sudden increase in the amount of exudate and change in the drainage characteristics from clear or serous to cloudy or purulent may be an indicator of increasing bacterial proliferation or impending infection.

*Granular Wounds:* When chronic wounds heal by secondary intention, there is creation and deposition of new tissue to fill the defect. This new substrate is not a regrowth of the previous tissue type, but in effect is a filler called granulation tissue. Granulation tissue is the hallmark of healing. It is usually described as beefy red or pearly pink tissue with a cobblestone appearance. The tiny mounds of tissue are comprised of angiocytes and fibroblasts created during the proliferative phase. These elements form the new capillaries and the extracellular collagen matrix. Several variations of granulation tissue can be seen. If there is an increased bacterial load, granulation tissue may become dark red-brown, friable or malodorous. Hypergranulation tissue or exuberant tissue lacks the firm composition of healthy granular tissue and mounds above the level of the surrounding intact skin. In many cases hypergranulation requires removal or reduction in volume to facilitate re-epithelialization. A wound bed that is pale or dusky and dry may indicate poor perfusion. Dark red-brown or purple granulation may signal injury by repeated trauma or pressure such as failure to offload the wounded area or from matted gauze or inappropriate dressing application.

## FACTORS COMPROMISING WOUND HEALING

Factors that impair wound healing are often overlooked, but play a major role in wound chronicity. Evaluation of the wound patient must begin with a complete history and head to toe physical examination. The history can provide valuable insight into the mechanism of injury or onset of the wound, prior complications and infections, and subjective findings suggesting the presence of underlying disease processes, and other factors that are contributing to compromised healing. A detailed history can also begin to formulate the management plan by identifying prior wound care strategies, diagnostic testing and therapeutic interventions to further identify and correct compromising factors.

For example, altered tissue perfusion starves the tissue of essential oxygen and nutrients. In addition there is a build up of waste products in the cells and the interstitium. Oxygen is a critical component in the development of mature collagen in the formation and maintenance of granulation tissue (30).

Tissue perfusion can be hampered by a variety of conditions including:

- Arterial occlusive disease
- Collagen vascular disorders
- Internal compression and cellular distancing created by the edema of venous insufficiency and lymphedema
- Cardiovascular and pulmonary disorders

Examination findings of diminished pulses, dependent rubor and elevation pallor, combined with a report of symptoms consistent with claudication would support a diagnosis of an arterial etiology prompting aggressive vascular evaluation.

Infection is one of the most common complications of chronic wounds. Infection increases the metabolic needs of the tissues, initiates or perpetuates the inflammatory response, increases pain, and places the patient at risk for extended tissue necrosis, limb loss or death. Critical colonization of the wound bed by bacteria competes with the granulation tissue for oxygen. In the face of frank infection, the metabolic demands and oxygen requirements of tissue can increase by a factor of 20 or more (30). Bacteria and other pathogens produce toxins and inflammatory mediators. Colonization denotes replication of bacteria on the surface of the wound. Cellulitis or "locally infected" periwound tissue occurs when bacteria migrate into the surrounding tissue and create a host response, typically redness, swelling, heat, pain, and increased wound drainage. Development of infection is dependent on many factors including chronic medical conditions such as diabetes, obesity, edema forming states (CHF, ESRD, hepatic failure).

Mechanical forces such as pressure, friction, and shear can cause significant negative impact on wound healing. These forces must be recognized and managed with appropriate pressure redistribution devices. Other external mechanical forces also play a role in initiating or perpetuating a pressure ulcer, for example, altered gait placing strain on the mid foot bony structures, dermatitis and pruritus leading to incessant scratching of the skin, and the weight of body parts of obese individuals creating traction on wounds opposing the contractile forces present during the proliferative phase also deserve consideration.

Cellular factors that compromise wound healing include an altered immune response related to uncontrolled hyperglycemia, renal and hepatic failure, and thyroid or adrenal diseases. Nutritional deficiencies are primarily manifest at the macronutrient level with protein and calorie deficiencies, but micronutrient deficiencies of vitamins, essential fatty acids and minerals also play a role. Some medication regimens can inhibit healing. Even when medications are appropriate as indicated for co-morbid conditions, they may have deleterious effects. Diuretics can lead to hypotension and decreased perfusion of at risk tissues. The necessary inflammatory phase can be suppressed if the patient is receiving corticosteroids or non-steroidal anti-inflammatory medications. Anti-neoplastic drugs, anticoagulants, anti-prostaglandins, and immune system modulators may retard the entire healing process. The diabetic patient with a non-healing wound requires monitoring and control of blood glucose levels. Daily finger stick blood sugar checks should be implemented if they are not currently monitoring blood sugar levels. A diary or journal recording the values helps to determine patterns. Overall blood sugar control should be monitored every 3 months with a glycosylated hemoglobin A1C. If the Hgb A1C is over 7% there is impairment of healing and the host response to infection. The ADA recommends maintaining the Hgb A1C as close to normal as possible without causing medically significant hypoglycemia (4).

Conducting a detailed history and physical examination of the patient is critical to identify these and other compromising factors. The plan of care created by the wound care team must include interventions to attempt to ameliorate the detrimental effects of these compromising factors on the goal of wound healing.

# WOUND MANAGEMENT CONSIDERATIONS, TECHNIQUES, AND TECHNOLOGIES

## Infection

Wound infection is also one of the most controversial areas of practice and experts continue to debate best practices for obtaining wound cultures and using systemic antibiotics, topical antibiotics and antimicrobials. Providers are generally in agreement that devitalized tissue must be removed in a timely manner to reduce the metabolic and bioburden to control infection, and enable progression through the phases of regeneration or repair. The exception to this rule is dry gangrene to the distal aspect of an extremity without enough blood supply to heal. It should not be debrided or subjected to moist interactive healing that will just result in a larger wound (66).

The longer the wound is present, the more likely the surrounding tissue will acquire an increased bacterial load. Local signs and symptoms of infection may be masked in immunocompromised patients, such as those who have a history of poorly controlled diabetes or have been treated with chemotherapeutic agents, radiation therapy, or immune system modulators. Increased bacterial bioburden can significantly delay wound healing when they compete for the oxygen and nutrients supplied to the wound area. Local signs of infection may include increased discharge, frank purulence, necrotic tissue and malodor. The surrounding tissue may become indurated, exhibiting edema, erythema, and pain. An analysis of a series of quantitative bacterial biopsies shows the average number of organisms found is as high as 4.8 species per ulcer (56). This polymicrobial result is a typical finding in diabetic foot ulcers and warrants the use of broad-spectrum antibiotics.

A wound that probes to bone is almost universally considered empirical evidence of osteomyelitis (20). A bone scan under these circumstances to "diagnose" osteomyelitis is almost always an unnecessary expense. In the patient with a diabetic foot ulcer, it is particularly ominous if the erythema around the ulcer extends more than 2 cm, the patient exhibits systemic signs of infection such as fever, chills, and malaise, or there is a worsening of his or her diabetic control (12). Routine x-rays are often initially negative due to relative osteopenia in the neurotrophic foot; however, x-rays still have clinical utility because they may demonstrate foreign bodies, fractures associated with a Charcot foot, or gas in the tissue. A follow-up x-ray 2 to 4 weeks later may demonstrate the bony erosion of osteomyelitis or periosteal new bone formation associated with healing. Routine bone scans are expensive and only helpful if positive, but are often negative. MRI or other specialized tests, when available, may have greater diagnostic accuracy.

Some clinicians suggest that the use of an infrared thermometry device may help diagnostically (7, 43). The thermometer should be used in four quadrants surrounding the ulcers and compared to the opposite foot in the same locations. In the diabetic foot, differences of three degrees Fahrenheit or more suggest infection.

Surface bacterial cultures of the wound are often misleading and may not represent the organisms invading the underlying tissue of the wound. While the "gold standard" is a punch or tissue biopsy, these approaches are invasive and specialized microbiological processing is not always available. A culturing method should be chosen which samples the exudate expressed from the intact tissue only after cleansing and removal of necrotic debris avoiding sampling of frank collections of pus.

## Diagnosis and Treatment of Peripheral Arterial Disease

Even in patients with predominantly small vessel disease, the large vessels supplying the area must carry sufficient blood to ensure healing. HBOT does not have any significant effect on large vessels significantly diseased by peripheral arterial disease (PAD), so one must first determine if there is adequate large vessel patency before beginning hyperbaric treatment. When a patient presents with a non healing wound of the distal extremity or a wound with ischemic characteristics suggestive of underlying PAD, additional vascular evaluation is mandatory. Referral to the Vascular Center can be invaluable.

The Vascular Center is an integrated, multidisciplinary program that comprises a variety of subspecialties including, vascular medicine internists, vascular surgeons, vascular interventionalist, and cardiologists. The vascular consultation consists of an in-depth clinical and imaging evaluation in order to determine the best treatment options and to ascertain the best possible intervention for patients who suffer from nonhealing ischemic wounds. In many patients who suffer from claudication and the lesser manifestations of PAD, conservative management is the best option; this treatment is coordinated and provided by the vascular internist. Management may consist of pharmacological therapy and risk factor and behavior modification. However, in patients who actually have nonhealing wounds, clinicians will aggressively promote healing by enhancing arterial flow to the ischemic wound. This can be achieved with an endovascular procedure such as angioplasty or stint, surgical revascularization, or a combined surgical endovascular procedure. The vascular medicine specialist provides the initial Vascular Center consultation (51).

*Ankle Brachial Index:* The traditional noninvasive screening vascular test is the ankle-brachial index (ABI). The ABI is a simple yet sensitive test used to determine the presence of occlusions and/or stenoses in the arterial vascular system of the lower extremity. Calculation of the ABI begins by measuring the systolic blood pressure in both arms (the brachial pressure) and the systolic pressure in each ankle. The ABI is calculated by dividing the ankle pressure by the brachial pressure. If the ABI is 1 or normal, the pressure at the level of the arm and the ankles are equal; therefore, no obstructing lesions are present between the aorta and the right or left foot. An ABI of less than 1 strongly suggests the presence of PAD. Patients with an ABI of less than 0.9 should receive additional evaluation and close follow up. An ABI of less than 0.5 will usually correlate with the presence of ischemic rest pain or tissue ischemia and necrosis.

| ABI Value | Interpretation |
|-----------|----------------|
| > 0.95 | Normal |
| 0.80 – 0.95 | Mild Disease (Presence of PAD) |
| 0.50 – 0.80 | Moderate Disease (Ulceration, Intermittent Claudication) |
| 0.30 – 0.50 | Moderate to Severe Disease |
| < 0.30 | Severe Disease (Rest Pain, Gangrene, Threat of Limb Loss) |

The ABI also can be measured after exercising the patient using a protocol that controls the speed and elevation of the treadmill device. This test is primarily performed on patients who suffer from claudication; typically, it would not be performed on patients suffering from ischemic rest pain or ischemic ulcerations. The post exercise ABI measurement will be categorized as abnormal if a decrease of more than 20% occurs from the baseline pre-exercise pressures.

Frequently patients with diabetes are found to have non-compressible vessels as a result of medial wall calcification. If the artery is calcific and incompressible, the derived ABI is inaccurate and likely to be falsely elevated. When this occurs, obtaining digital pressures is advised. Toe pressures are particularly useful in diabetes, because the medial calcific sclerosis that confounds occlusive blood pressure determination at higher levels in the limb rarely occurs in the digital arteries. However, Doppler is usually not sensitive enough to detect flow in the digital arteries, so photoplethysmography (PPG) is commonly utilized to obtain digital pressures. Systolic toe pressures of less than 30 mmHg are usually associated with decreased wound healing. One study indicated a 29% ulcer healing rate at this pressure, while toe pressures greater than 30 mmHg were associated with approximately 92% ulcer healing rate. It should also be noted that 66% of patients with toe pressures less than 30 mmHg went on to amputation (10).

The use of segmental blood pressure determination has become widespread as a noninvasive attempt to localize the level of arterial narrowing in the lower extremities. Occlusion pressures are measured at multiple levels (thigh, the upper calf, the ankle, and sometimes around the foot and the toes). The highest thigh cuff should be 30 mmHg higher than the highest brachial value. From there down, a drop of 30 mmHg between any two cuffs signifies significant arterial disease within that segment.

*Duplex Ultrasonography:* Duplex ultrasonography or color duplex ultrasound is an important tool for both the preoperative and postoperative evaluation of patients who have had any type of vascular reconstruction or endovascular intervention. The two general categories of ultrasound-derived information are imaging and Doppler-derived waveform – when combined this is called "duplex" testing. This direct noninvasive imaging tool consists of a color-coded blood flow image superimposed on a gray-scale image. The physics are derived from the Doppler shift methods that allow clinicians to measure peak systolic velocities and wave forms at different points through an interrogated blood vessel and determine with high sensitivity and high specificity whether occlusions and/or stenoses are present. The examination identifies stenotic lesions of 50% to 99% when peak systolic velocity increases by more than 100% as compared to the arterial flow velocity found in the more normal proximal segments. Additionally, distal to significant narrowing, the "pulsatility" of the waveform typically decreases, becoming monophasic rather than the normal biphasic or triphasic (40).

Initial Doppler waveform information can usually be obtained easily at bedside with the continuous-wave Doppler device during the physical exam. Listening to each of the pedal pulses for a biphasic or triphasic waveform is a very good screening test, as normal pulsatility essentially rules out significant arterial disease. Higher level and more detailed duplex information can be provided by the Vascular Center.

The duplex examination has important clinical utilization before and after endovascular intervention. For instance, in patients with claudication, it provides an anatomical roadmap for the interventionalist to determine whether a lesion in the superficial femoral artery would better be served with angioplasty or bypass. It is also utilized after an endovascular treatment therapy to assess residual stenosis in an artery after angioplasty. In addition, it is used to determine the durability of endovascular as well as surgical interventions, particularly for patients who have been reconstructed with an infra-femoral bypass graft. Graft surveillance technique is widely used to determine if reconstruction is at risk of becoming occluded or at risk of failing (15).

*Plethysmography:* Plethysmography is the measurement of volume changes or blood flow within an organ. Of interest to us is plethysmographic measurement of lower extremity arterial blood flows. Already mentioned above is the use of photoplethysmography (PPG) as an endpoint detector for detecting pulsatile flow in measuring toe pressure. This uses an infrared LED and a detector to measure bulk flow in the tissue within several centimeters of the probe. Laser Doppler velocimetry is a related technique, but measures flow only within the dermal layers. Both these techniques can be used to determine occlusion pressure endpoints, but the PPG electrode is simpler and the one ordinarily chosen.

Pneumoplethysmography uses detection of a pressure wave within an air cuff around an extremity to measure pulsatility. The most common use is in automated blood pressure cuffs. This is also the technique employed in the "pulse volume recording," which is a graphic trace of the pressure wave in the cuff at a defined inflation pressure. This is frequently reported in conjunction with segmental blood pressures. As in Doppler testing, the waveform provides additional information to the detection of occlusion pressure.

*Magnetic Resonance Angiography:* Magnetic resonance angiography (MRA) uses the radio frequency oscillation of hydrogen nuclei in a strong magnetic field to produce an image of the arterial lumen. When accomplished by experienced technicians this study correlates well with the image produced by angiography. Although some centers perform peripheral bypass procedures based on the results of MRA, most surgeons still prefer invasive angiography.

MRA cannot be used in patients with implanted pacemakers, defibrillators, or other metallic objects that would present a danger if placed in a strong magnetic field. In addition, implanted metallic objects produce image artifacts that limit the usefulness of the study. MRA is also limited in its intra-operative utility because of the bulky equipment and patient preparation required.

In the evaluation of lower extremity wounds, the primary use of MRA is in those patients at risk from iodinated radiographic contrast material. MRA can define the arterial anatomy to help decide if invasive angiography is warranted in such patients and so that the subsequent dose of contrast material can be reduced.

*Vascular Intervention (Arteriography):* Arteriography is an invasive procedure that remains the gold standard diagnostic test for surgical or endovascular intervention. The indications for vascular intervention include intermittent claudication, ischemic leg pain, ischemic ulceration, and gangrene. Arteriography requires the intra-arterial injection of iodinated contrast material, with risk of renal failure or allergic reaction. Other risks include bleeding, clotting, distal embolization of atheroma material, or pseudoaneurysm formation and thus angiography should be reserved for those patients who may benefit from either endovascular or surgical revascularization. In the setting of an ischemic ulcer with absent or decreased pulses, or evidence of stenosis on non-invasive testing, it is an absolute requirement to evaluate and treat the patient with correctable lesions before embarking on a course of hyperbaric management.

The angiographic acquisition is multilevel and includes the infra-renal aorta, the iliac arteries and the infra-inguinal vessels, the profunda femoris, the superficial femoral artery, the popliteal artery and the trifurcating tibial arteries below the knee. The angiogram can be utilized to diagnose and grade the severity of lesions, to allow for endovascular corrections or to provide a "roadmap" for surgical correction. For instance, the short focal lesion that is amenable to an angioplasty would be the treatment of choice in a patient with claudication. On the other hand, with a longer, more complicated lesion, angioplasty alone traditionally has not provided successful outcomes. In patients with nonhealing wounds, a stint may be in order, particularly in patients who may not have any surgical options due to their co-morbidities or the lack of vein conduit to provide a surgical bypass.

At the time of the angiogram certain lesions may be amenable to correction with endovascular intervention. The two primary endovascular methods commonly utilized include balloon angioplasty, which basically compresses and cracks the peripheral vascular plaque; and vascular stinting, which uses a metallic device, such as a balloon expandable stint or self-expanding stint, to maintain the vessel patency. Endovascular techniques have evolved over the past few years. Devices have become smaller with lower profiles and are much easier to manipulate and deliver in an area remote from the access site. For example, in a patient being treated for a distal (below knee) stenosis, the device can be manipulated and deployed if needed as far down as the dorsalis pedis artery in the foot.

Because numerous options for vascularization are available, controversy among sub-specialists occurs, not only as to the technical aspect (which reconstruction is best) but also regarding competition between the surgical and the endovascular methods of revascularization. The role of the Vascular Center is to eliminate competing pressures and provide the patient with the best option for optimal revascularization, one that is tailored to the individual anatomy of the patient and his/her risks (42, 52).

Close follow up and surveillance is important in maintaining optimal long term results. Adjunctive therapies such as hyperbaric oxygen can be utilized and often are necessary to complement and enhance outcomes following endovascular intervention and revascularization procedures.

## Transcutaneous Oxygen Assessment

The use of the periwound $TcPO_2$ determination has become the sine qua non for deciding whether a patient with critical peripheral ischemia will benefit from hyperbaric oxygen treatment. Despite great care in the manufacture and use of these instruments, the readings can never be 100% reliable. The technician carrying out the measurements should be well trained in the use of the $TcPO_2$ meter, and preferably should have formal training for certification. Even with exacting standards for measurement, there will be the occasional patient who is rejected for HBO treatment when he or she could have benefited and visa versa. Nevertheless, it is a practical requirement that arbitrary limits be set to minimize inappropriate use of the chamber and meet the needs of insurers. The parameters given below are based on extensive clinical experience and were reported in the Proceedings of the European Consensus Conference on Hyperbaric Oxygen in the Treatment of Foot Lesions in Diabetic Patients (London in December of 1998/sponsored by the European Committee for Hyperbaric Medicine) (8, 17, 50).

If the periwound $TcPO_2$ is less than 30 mmHg, it can be assumed that the wound will not heal without the oxygen deficit being corrected. If nothing more can be done from the standpoint of a vascular procedure or smoking cessation, the patient becomes a potential candidate for hyperbaric oxygen treatment on the basis of critical ischemia. To determine if HBO will be of value, the patient is given an "oxygen challenge." This consists of breathing oxygen while the $TcPO_2$ is re-measured. If the patient breathes 100% oxygen at one atmosphere via a tight-fitting mask and the periwound $TcPO_2$ rises above 100 mmHg within about 20 minutes, the patient should respond to HBO, and he or she can be accepted for HBO treatment. Ideally the mask used should be a tight-fitting demand mask or an anesthesia mask with a 5-liter breathing bag (31).

If the oxygen challenge at one atmosphere yields a value less than 100 mmHg, the patient is placed in the hyperbaric chamber and taken to 2.0-2.5 ATA breathing 100% oxygen. At pressure, the $TcPO_2$ should rise to greater than 200 mmHg. If it fails to do so within about 20 minutes, the patient should be rejected for hyperbaric treatment, in the absence of infection. It is important not to place the electrode over a vein, or bony prominence. All measurements must be made with the patient either supine or prone, and the patient must be in the same position when repeat measurements are made. It is critically important that repeat measurements be made at exactly the same site as the initial measurement; a shift of only a few millimeters will give a spurious comparative result. It is helpful to mark the electrode placements with semi-permanent ink that resists repeated washings. Unfortunately, accurate readings cannot be made on the plantar aspect of the foot, as the readings, if made there, will produce paradoxical results. Readings should be made only when the foot has warmed up if the patient has come from the outside when temperatures are low.

When treating patients for radiation injury, the $TcPO_2$ is not routinely measured, at least initially, as it is known to be low and the values do not influence choice of therapy.

If the patient is being treated for critical ischemia with hyperbaric oxygen, it is vitally important that the transcutaneous $PO_2$ be followed at least on a weekly basis. It is measured with the patient breathing air at least 12 hours after the most recent HBO treatment. If the $TcPO_2$ is not seen to rise significantly (secondary to neovascularization) during the first 14 treatments, further treatment is discontinued in the absence of infection. Occasionally the $TcPO_2$ may fall, which may be due to reinfarction or new infarction. Periodic monitoring will pick up such an event, which, if it cannot be rectified, will prevent lengthy, expensive and futile HBO treatment. When the periwound $TcPO_2$ rises to 40 mmHg or above, in the absence of infection, HBO treatment is stopped, even if the wound is not healed. With transcutaneous tissue $PO_2$ readings of 40 mmHg or better at all points around the ulcer, the patient becomes "host-competent" and should be able to heal spontaneously with attention to good wound care and other host factors alone.

## Wound Cleansing and Irrigation

Cleansing and irrigation are used to remove surface debris and exudate, allowing for proper assessment of the wound base and facilitating wound healing. Removal of debris decreases the bacterial load and reduces the inflammatory response. Complete cleansing of the wound bed allows visualization of subtle signs of wound infection or other significant changes in wound status (56).

In the past, foot soaks were a common practice for diabetic foot care. Current thought is that foot soaks may cause over-hydration, which can lead to maceration, particularly at the toe webs, nail folds and heel tissues. Repetitive soaking and drying of the skin decreases the barrier function of the keratin layer and create fissures between the epidermal plates. The seeded bacteria in these sites then have an entry point due to impaired skin integrity and may lead to cellulitis. The presence of exposed bone, joints, or deep sinuses is an absolute contraindication for foot soaks or other immersion therapies.

For the majority of chronic wounds, saline is the cleansing solution of choice. The use of tap water is controversial, especially in immuno-compromised patients. It may be contraindicated because of the possibility of introducing unwanted pathogens. Individual assessment of the patient, the environment, and the water source is warranted prior to the use of tap water for cleansing chronic wounds (37). The use of commercial wound cleansers is also highly controversial. Most experts agree that non-ionic surfactants do the least harm. Rodeheaver et al. measured the toxicity indexes for a number wound or skin cleansers which can provide direction for clinical practice (56). All commercial cleansers have a greater toxicity than saline.

Cleansing is usually accomplished by one of the following methods:

- Wetting with saline-soaked gauze compresses.
- Rinsing by pouring the solution over the wound.
- Irrigating with minimal force with a piston or bulb syringe.

Pressure exerted on a surface is measured in PSI (pounds per square inch). The recommended wound cleansing pressure is between 5 and 8 PSI. For those wounds containing necrotic tissue (slough or eschar) or requiring removal of thick exudate or debris, irrigation may be selected instead of simple cleansing. Irrigation involves the delivery of a directed stream of solution at higher pressures, usually 8 to 15 PSI. Pressures over 15 PSI may be harmful, causing tissue destruction and edema (56).

Irrigation is usually accomplished by one of the following methods:

- 30 cc syringe with 18-20 gauge Angiocath®.
- Commercial wound irrigation kit.
- Pulsed lavage.

When cleansing or irrigating a wound, protect the patient and the provider from overspray, splashing or air borne mist containing blood or body fluids by implementing standard precautions and donning protective equipment appropriate to the procedure.

## Debridement

Wound management is often complicated by the presence of necrotic tissue or bone. Steed et al. demonstrated that aggressive, ongoing surgical debridement converts a chronic non-healing ulcer into an acute, healing wound (59). Adequate debridement of necrotic tissue is needed before adequate assessment and staging can be accomplished. Debridement of non-viable tissue is necessary in order for wounds to progress through the phases of wound healing to closure. Debridement lessens the chance of infection, as necrotic tissue is a prime growth medium for pathogens. Debridement may result in a wound that appears larger than it originally appeared. Patients should be made aware of this when treatment begins. Methods of debridement include: surgical, sharp, conservative sharp, ultrasonic, mechanical, enzymatic, and autolytic (65).

Debridement is accomplished via a continuum of techniques, from flushing away debris with low-pressure irrigation to wide excision. The following factors must be taken into consideration when selecting a method of debridement:

- Amount and extent of necrotic tissue to be removed.
- Pain.
- Presence of infection (local, advancing, or systemic).
- Vascular status.
- Coagulation status.
- Facility resources and setting.

A thorough assessment, history, and physical and vascular work-up should be completed prior to initiating any form of wound debridement. Caution must be exercised when debriding leg and/or foot ulcers secondary to arterial disease or occlusion. If an area with a poor blood supply is debrided, one is often left with an even larger wound which will not heal. Ischemic wounds with stable eschar and no signs or symptoms of infection may best be served by being left open to the air, protected and allowed to dry out.

*Sharp Debridement:* Sharp debridement is performed with scissors, scalpel or curette to remove grossly necrotic or tightly adherent fibrinous exudates. This method is immediate and reduces the volume of devitalized tissue present in the wound bed. Wide excision to a healthy tissue margin is considered an invasive procedure. It is important that the surgical debridement remove all overhanging edges so that the epithelium can be seen in contact with the granulation tissue base. All sinuses or tracts should be opened or marsupialized to allow healing from the edges. Exposed bone often requires local surgical removal of the infected focus to promote healing. The availability of surgical debridement may depend on qualified health care professionals and an appropriate practice setting. Conservative sharp debridement removes necrotic tissue bulk without excising to a bleeding base.

*Ultrasonic Wound Debridement:* Ultrasonic wound debridement and treatment utilizes low frequency (20-25 kHz) pulsed ultrasound applied directly to the wound surface and surrounding tissues. The ultrasound waves create microcavitations, cyclically imploding gas bubbles which penetrate tissue, releasing energy, and shearing bacterial and viral cell walls killing the microbe.

The results of this form of ultrasonic debridement are as immediate as sharp or surgical debridement – creating a wound bed devoid of slough and necrotic tissue allowing the stages of wound healing to proceed uninterrupted. With a portable unit, procedures can be performed at the bedside in the acute and immediate care setting as well as in the operating room at the time of surgery to provide adjunctive therapy during incision and drainage procedures. Ultrasonic energy induced mechanisms of action involve vasodilatation and resolution of vasospasm, both of which produce increased blood flow (thermal effect); fibrinolytic division and debridement of denatured proteins; decreased bacterial load and stimulation of fibroblasts, macrophages and endothelial cells.

*Hemostasis Following Debridement:* Bleeding is often desirable after surgical debridement of chronic wounds because it indicates a viable wound base. Hemorrhage needs to be contained to avoid local hematoma, eschar, and underlying inflammatory response. Local pressure and elevation may be supplemented by application of calcium alginates that possess hemostatic properties. The alginates donate calcium to facilitate local hemostasis and in turn accept sodium, converting a calcium alginate fiber into a sodium alginate gel. Other forms of hemostasis include silver nitrate, electrocautery, absorbable gelatin sponge (Gelfoam®) or chemical cautery. Caution is to be used; some of these methods may damage underlying granulation tissue or cause pain.

*Enzymatic Debridement:* Enzymatic debridement involves the use of commercially available products which contain enzymes. The enzymes will denature the proteins of the necrotic tissue, essentially liquefying the semisolid mass. Each product has a different mode of action and product-specific instructions must be adhered to or the enzyme will be inactivated. Enzymatic debridement results are slower than sharps or mechanical debridement. Sharp debridement in conjunction with enzymatic debriders speeds the process. Historically, enzymes (collagenase, papain, urokinase, etc.) have been used as debriding agents for slough and eschar. Enzymatic debriders are selective and affect only necrotic tissue.

*Autolytic Debridement:* Autolytic debridement is selective and liquefies slough and eschar as well as promotes granulation tissue formation (27). Autolytic debridement utilizes the body's natural proteases, macrophages, and immune complement present in the tissue fluid to break down necrotic tissue. The accumulation of this fluid can be enhanced with the use of occlusive dressings, hydrogels, calcium alginates, etc. This method is usually the least expensive and least painful of the three methods discussed; however, it may be the slowest.

*Mechanical Debridement:* Mechanical debridement may be accomplished with wet to dry gauze dressings, irrigation, or hydrotherapy (pulsatile lavage) (27, 68). These methods are the least selective of all methods of debridement and are potentially damaging to healthy granulation tissue and new epithelium. Wet to dry dressings are often used to pack large necrotic wounds. Mechanical debridement utilizes external forces to remove devitalized tissue and wound exudates. Pulsed lavage uses the mechanical force of pulsating fluid to cleanse and irrigate. Scrubbing the wound surface or utilizing the wet to dry gauze method will also remove waste materials and tissue non-selectively. This form of debridement is often painful and detrimental to the healing process.

## Topical Antimicrobial Therapy

There is a lack of consensus on the use of topical antibacterial therapy for local wound care. If a wound has associated signs of infection (septicemia, osteomyelitis, cellulitis) systemic antibacterials should be used. If increased local discharge and odor are present without skin surface temperature change, a short course of a topical antibacterial agent can be instituted with careful monitoring of the wound for signs of infection. Still other wounds may have an increased bacterial burden (greater than or equal to $1.0 \times 10^6$ organisms per gram of tissue) without any localized symptoms or signs. These wounds may also benefit from a short course of topical or systemic antibacterials.

The ideal topical antibacterial agent:

- Has a broad spectrum of antibacterial coverage.
- Allows good penetration of the topical agent.
- Is not used systemically.
- Is not a contact allergen (sensitizer).
- Is wound friendly promoting moist interactive healing.

Antibiotics applied topically may lead to antibiotic resistant organisms. With increased, sometimes unwarranted or oversealous antibiotic use, the emergence of methicillin resistant *Staphylococcus aureus* (MRSA) and other multi-antibiotic resistant organisms is a concern (61). Mupirocin is effective against MRSA and some institutions are restricting this agent for resistant *staphylococcus* including MRSA. Topical antibacterials may provide good local penetration of agents. The use of these agents can decrease bacterial burden, exudate, or wound odor. Topical antibacterial agents should be reviewed at regular intervals. A suggested review time would be every two weeks. Prolonged use of these agents can lead to the emergence of resistant strains both in the laboratory and in clinical practice, although laboratory resistance does not always equate with the clinical ineffectiveness of these agents. Topical antibacterial agents have a definite indication in chronic wounds, but their indiscriminate use and lack of close monitoring is to be discouraged. They do not act as a substitute for systemic antibiotics and should be discontinued when bacterial balance has been established.

Sensitization is common from topical preparations. The skin processes antigens through sensitized Langerhans cells migrating to regional lymph nodes. Common allergens are neomycin, lanolin, and fragrances. Neomycin contains two allergens: the neosamine sugar and the deoxystreptomine backbone. The deoxystreptomine backbone is also part of the aminoglycoside group that includes gentamicin. Sensitization to the aminoglycosides eliminates a very important class of systemic antibiotics.

In lieu of topically applied antibiotic preparations there are several broad spectrum antimicrobial substances that have been found to be effective against common skin and soft tissue specific bacteria. These antimicrobials either kill or inhibit the growth of bacteria, viruses, and fungal components without the risk of increasing resistance to antibiotics. Cadexomer iodine is a slow-release elemental iodine product available in a paste or wafer (5). The product absorbs wound exudate forming a protective gel that is non-occlusive and non-adherent. Ionic silver coated dressings provide a slow release of silver imparting a broad spectrum antibacterial coverage as well (71). Other antimicrobial substances include sodium hypochlorite, acetic acid, methylene blue, gentian violet, chlorhexadine, and betadine.

## Wound Dressings

Research of the late 1950s and early 1960s demonstrated that a moist wound environment provides the best microenvironment for wound regeneration and repair and optimizes wound healing (23, 67, 68, 69). Since then, hundreds of wound care products have become available that promote moist wound healing (24, 35). While many of these advanced wound care products are appropriate for chronic wound management, it remains true that many conventional dressings are efficient and cost-effective as well. The abundance of wound dressings for wound management can be daunting. The explosion of materials that have been developed in the past 20 years has brought wound care to the level of an art as well as a science (63).

Dressings have four basic functions:

- Protect the wound from contamination and trauma.
- Promote wound cleansing and debridement of necrotic tissues.
- Absorb excess tissue fluid and wound exudates.
- Maintain a moist environment for healing.

Since none of the common dressing products contain cytokines or growth factors, they do not "accelerate" healing, but merely allow healing to take place as well as the patient's immune system and nutritional state will support. Wounds are dynamic and their characteristics will change as the wound progresses, and so will the needs for the dressing management, based on the current wound assessment (58).

The five basic categories of primary (in contact with the wound bed) dressings are listed below:

- Transparent films
- Hydrocolloids
- Alginates/Hydrofibers
- Hydrogels
- Foams

*Transparent Film Dressings:* These are thin, polyurethane or polyethylene sheets, which are transparent and self adhering to the surrounding skin without adhesion to a moist wound bed. They are routinely used for IV insertion sites. Films are semi-permeable membranes which allow for transmission of oxygen and water vapor yet are waterproof and provide a barrier from contaminants. The film dressing is indicated for shallow wounds with little to no exudate. They have no absorptive qualities. Other functions include protection of intact skin against friction, autolytic debridement, and maintenance of a moist wound bed. The transparent film dressing is available in various sizes and thicknesses. For the best results, the dressing should cover at least a 1-inch margin around the wound. The wear time of the dressing will vary depending on the wound type and location, but can be left in place up to 7 days. Films are also commonly used as a waterproof cover dressing.

*Hydrocolloid Dressings:* Hydrocolloid dressings are a solid wafer-type dressing composed of gelatin or pectin, carboxymethyl cellulose for absorption, and adhesive components. They were one of the first so called advanced wound care dressings. They evolved from ostomy wafer materials. Dressings vary in thickness, and have a film or thin foam surface. The adhesive wafer and film covering provides an occlusive environment impermeable to fluids and bacteria. They can be used for partial- to shallow full-thickness wounds. Functions of the dressings include absorption of light to moderate exudate, autolytic debridement, maintenance of a moist environment, and can be used as a preventative dressing to relieve friction. The dressings can be worn for up to 7 days, although they rarely last so long in high trauma areas such as the sacrum, coccyx and ischium. Use in infected or unstable wounds should be avoided or used cautiously due to the occlusive and opaque nature of the dressing. There are also complimentary pastes and powders available to fill small amounts of space.

*Alginates:* Alginates are absorbent dressings composed of fibers spun from calcium salts of alginic acid (brown seaweed) and compressed into sheets. When exposed to wound exudate, calcium and sodium ions are exchanged, and the end product, sodium alginate, becomes a gel. Alginates are capable of absorbing large amounts of wound exudate and are most often the dressing of choice for moderately to copiously draining pressure ulcers. They can be used in the presence of infection, and are generally changed daily, extending to every 2-3 days as exudate diminishes. The dressing should be discontinued when there is inadequate exudate to hydrate the dressing between changes. Alginates are available in a variety of forms and sizes, flat sheets, ribbons, and ropes for packing wounds. They are a softer, much more absorbent alternative to gauze for packing deeper pressure ulcers. Alginates differ in form, some pull apart like "angel hair" and others maintain their integrity when saturated with wound fluid. A high integrity alginate should be used when packing tunnels or undermining to reduce the chance of leaving fibers behind. A cover dressing will be required.

*Hydrogel Dressings:* The hydrogels are a group of polymers with added water and other ingredients such as glycerin to reduce evaporation and increase moisture and viscosity. They are available in an amorphous form provided in a tube or foil pack, impregnated into gauze and packing ribbon, or cross-linked into sheets. The hydrogel is used to hydrate the wound surface, enable or enhance autolytic debridement, or to maintain a wound that is moist, but not exudating. The amorphous form is generally changed daily and requires a cover dressing. The sheet form can be used for superficial wounds such as skin tears or connected strands can be used to pack deeper areas. Sheet hydrogels can generally be left in place for 3-5 days. Some hydrogel include an adhesive border eliminating the need for a cover dressing.

*Foams:* This category includes polyurethane and polyvinyl alcohol foam dressings which come in a variety of sizes and thicknesses and may have a film surface to prevent strike-through. They can be used as standalone dressings to absorb exudate and maintain a moist wound surface or as a secondary dressing for padding and increased absorbency over another type of wound filler. They also are available with adhesive surfaces intended to adhere to the peri-wound skin while not adhering or traumatizing the moist wound surface. One such group utilizes soft silicone as the adhesive, which provides non-traumatic removal from the skin and wound surface, which reduces the pain of dressing changes for the patient.

*Gauze:* Gauze can no longer be considered a primary dressing. Instead it should be utilized primarily as a sponge in cleansing the wound, as a delivery device for pastes and enzymatic debriding agents, and as a wrap to secure other dressings. The use of fluffed gauze as a wound filler has been tempered by its propensity to matt into a hard mass and cause repetitive injury to the granulation tissue. In addition, the cotton fibers have been found to initiate a foreign body reaction when shreds of gauze are enveloped by granulation tissue, extending the inflammatory phase leading to chronicity. Iodoform-impregnated and other antiseptic products should be reserved for use with wounds demonstrating clinical signs of infection or increased bacterial burden and only for a short course of treatment, because these agents have been shown to be cytotoxic *in vitro* to healing cells, such as fibroblasts (68).

It is important to note that there is a wide range in effective performance within categories: a hydrocolloid is not a hydrocolloid is not a hydrocolloid. Generally speaking, the advanced dressings should maintain an ideal moist wound environment by either absorbing exudate (e.g., foams, alginates, collagen, or hydrocolloids) or donating or maintaining moisture (e.g., hydrogels or films) (35, 62).

The traditional distinction between primary dressings (that fill or touch the wound) and secondary dressings (that secure the primary dressing) still apply (16).

- Primary wound care products are those that are intended to be in contact with the wound bed.
- Secondary products are largely for absorption of wound exudates.
- Cover dressings secure the other layers in place.

Each layer is chosen based on characteristics of the wound itself, the integrity of the surrounding skin and the anatomic location. Some products combine all three functions into a single dressing type, such as a bordered hydrocolloid dressing, or combine features, such as an "island dressing," which is composed of an absorptive material backed by an adherent occlusive layer.

Primary wound care products pose the most variability and widest selection. The clinician must characterize the wound bed and determine the best products to bring about cleansing, debridement, the growth of granulation tissue, and wound contraction. For debridement of eschar or slough, one could consider an enzymatic agent; for a dry wound bed, a hydrogel; for wounds where there is a suspicion of superficial bacterial overload, a product containing heavy metal ions, such as silver or iodine, or an antimicrobial preparation; and for a healthy clean wound, a minimally adherent product that will not traumatize the granulation tissue, such as a hydrocolloid.

The secondary, or absorptive, layer has fewer choices, which can readily be stratified by their capacity to contain tissue exudates, and therefore the amount of drainage drives the product selection. Gauze pads are the standard, and the newer products are often compared to their absorptive capacity in relation to an equal weight of cotton gauze. The simplest is to add an internal absorptive layer of cotton or cellulose fibers, while others use a strategy akin to diapers with a non-adherent layer encasing a fiber pad. Alginates have an absorptive capacity nearly eight times that of cotton gauze and have the additional advantage of turning into an easily cleansed gel rather than a matted mass. Foam dressings are equally absorptive to alginates, remain soft and pliable, and are nontraumatic to remove and remain intact. Finally, an important point is to avoid excessively absorptive materials in minimally to moderately exudative wounds, as the product competes with the granulation tissue for moisture and may desiccate the new tissue.

The cover layer holds the other layers in place, contains any excess tissue fluid, maintains a moist environment, and protects the wound from contamination and further trauma when the patient is incontinent or moved. There are two factors that are not usually considered in the choice of these products. The first is the permeability of the outer layer to evaporation of the tissue fluid. Polyurethane is fluid retentive and minimally gas permeable, which may lead to maceration. Products that allow gas permeability, such as polyethylene plastics, are less likely to lead to maceration, but more likely to lead to a dry dressing and the release of noxious anaerobic gases. The second is the adhesiveness of the bordered area on the intact skin. Too strong an adhesion and the patient may suffer skin tears with dressing changes and increased chances of skin irritation that leads to pruritis and dermatitis; too loose and the dressing loses its integrity.

The previous categories are broad and do not encompass all of the products available for wound management. There are other unique wound fillers, contact layers, composite and island dressings, advanced and active materials that contribute to achieving an environment most conducive to achieving wound healing.

Dressings that combine properties from more than one category can go a long way towards protecting the skin and managing the exudate. A fundamental understanding of the basic categories will allow the practitioner to prescribe dressings based on their function and the current wound status. Another confounding factor is that within the categories there are numerous brands. Some brand names have become synonymous with the product type. Choice of brand is often dictated by contracts, cost and availability in a certain area. Other factors in the final selection must also be considered, such as ease of use, frequency of change, shelf-life and storage, patient comfort and quality of materials.

While the advanced dressing products may seem more costly at face value, they provide an enhanced wound environment and extended wear times reduces the frequency of dressing changes. Dressings can be obtained through the home care agency, if one is involved in the patient's case, through local medical supply distributors, as well as mail order. Those patients who have Medicare Part B (and some private insurance patients) will be eligible to have their dressings sent directly to their home, if the patient is living independently and is not receiving services from a home health agency.

## Nutritional Considerations

"Wounds heal from the inside, out." Nutritional repletion of calorie and protein stores is arguably the most important intervention for patients with wounds, especially those with multiple co-morbid conditions that may compromise their healing potential. Activation of the wound healing cascade induces a systemic hypermetabolic state necessitating increased energy production as well as a catabolic state due to the requirement for increased protein synthesis needed for local tissue repair. Wound healing therefore increases the nutritional demands of any patient; even those with adequate nutritional stores initially will require additional nutritional support for healing. Malnourished patients are also at increased risk for cardiac and respiratory failure, infection, and deep venous thrombosis, as well as peri-operative mortality (14).

*Nutritional Assessment:* When managing wounded patients, it is important to identify those patients at high risk for malnutrition and those who have depleted their nutritional reserves through an acute phase reaction to the mass of necrosis in deep tissue injury. The evaluation begins with a systematic series of screening questions about involuntary weight loss and decreased appetite. A nutritionally targeted physical examination is completed including height and weight, an assessment of muscle mass, adequacy of subcutaneous fat, and hydration status. If this screen raises suspicion for malnutrition, laboratory assessment may be considered, which typically includes prealbumin, albumin, CBC and total lymphocyte count. For diabetic patients hemoglobin A1C may also be obtained. Other findings that may corroborate the loss of visceral proteins are an unexpectedly low serum creatinine or urea nitrogen, or an elevated INR (2).

*Laboratory Testing:* Prealbumin has a half-life of two days and is not significantly affected by hydration status. Prealbumin levels typically respond to nutritional interventions in approximately 7 days and are a better predictor of the visceral protein response to nutritional intervention than other available lab tests. Normal values are 16-30 mg/dl, with values of 10-15 mg/dl reflecting mild depletion and <7 mg/dl indicating severe depletion.

Corticosteroid treatment and renal insufficiency can falsely elevate prealbumin levels. Albumin levels have a half-life of 20 days are very sensitive to hydration status, may be decreased in renal disease and liver disease, but is often a better predictor of outcome. A normal albumin level is greater than or equal to 3.5 g/dl. Changes in albumin generally lag behind the actual nutritional state by several weeks.

Total cholesterol levels are indicative of fat reserves, and should be greater than 160 mg/dl; lesser values are correlated with poor wound healing outcomes. Total lymphocyte count (TLC) is calculated from the results of a complete blood count (CBC). The percentage of lymphocytes is multiplied by the total white count in cubic millimeters. The normal TLC is 2500 $mm^3$ (mild depletion <1,500 $mm^3$; moderate depletion <1,200 $mm^3$ and severe depletion <800 $mm^3$). Protein–calorie malnutrition compromises the immune system thus reducing the number of white blood cells and depressing the TLC.

Unfortunately, many of these laboratory findings can reflect the effects of an acute systemic inflammatory response depleting the nutritional stores rather than a prolonged period of inadequate intake, and therefore can be misleading when used to assess the adequacy of long term nutritional status. Body habitus can also be misleading. In the event of an acute physiologic stress and inadequate protein-calorie intake, the body will preferentially derive its energy from muscle tissue, not fat. Therefore, patients that were obese before becoming ill may continue to appear grossly overweight, yet be gravely undernourished. Treatment should be directed at reducing the underlying inflammatory state and restoring the nutritional reserves, not at reducing body fat.

*Bioelectric Impedance Analysis:* To compliment the laboratory testing, a simple, inexpensive bedside assessment device that may be used in the hospital, clinic or home is bioelectric impedance analysis (BIA), can be performed to analyze body composition and give the provider a snapshot of the patient's nutritional status at that moment. BIA is a noninvasive measurement of electrical properties of tissues and fluids which is a superior technique to monitor the body's response to stress (infection, wounds, malignancy, trauma, etc), recovery, and stabilization. The three compartments analyzed are body cell mass (BCM), extra-cellular mass (ECM) and adipose. BIA assessment is based on the principle that lean body mass conducts electricity better than adipose tissue (13).

Body cell mass is compromised of muscle and organ tissues. These tissues are metabolically active and required for wound healing and other metabolic processes such as medication metabolism. For the body to function efficiently it requires 100% of the expected level of body cell mass for a given individual. BCM below 95% of the expected level indicates functional compromise, which can predispose to poor wound healing, despite aggressive advanced wound care interventions. When BCM declines to 55% or less of the expected level, death may be imminent, it is imperative that aggressive nutritional interventions be initiated, or arrangements made for end-of-life care. ECM on the other hand is comprised of bone, collagen, and fluid tissues around cells. ECM and adipose are less metabolically active and therefore do not require significant calories, but the function of these tissues can be compromised by malnutrition.

*Nutritional Intervention:* After identifying the patient at risk for protein-energy malnutrition and compromised wound healing, consultation with a registered dietician can clarify the individual's nutritional requirements, with adjustments to accommodate other co-morbidities, as well as provide recommendations regarding dietary modification and supplementation to meet the various nutrient and caloric requirements for wound healing.

## Maintaining a Moist Wound Healing Environment

Chronic wounds are prone to infection and many chronic wound patients are immunocompromised. They may not muster a visible immune response. Many wound care experts avoid using occlusive dressings (e.g. films, hydrocolloids, ointments) with wounds in immunocompromised or diabetic patients or with wound infection, unless they are reasonably certain that they are being monitored frequently by a knowledgeable wound care provider (25). Occlusion refers to the relative inability of a wound dressing to transmit water vapor and gases from the wound surface into the environment. The rationale for this caution about occlusion is that exudates typically will pool in the wound bed in an occlusive environment and can become a breeding ground for microorganisms. As mentioned previously, Robson has concluded that tissue organism loads in excess or equal to $1.0 \times 10^6$ colony-forming units per gram of tissue can impair healing (54).

Some other research suggests that occlusive environments do not negatively impact on the healing of certain chronic dermal wounds. In pressure and venous ulcers, where bacterial counts of 106 to 108 organisms per gram of tissue and a shift to gram negative flora was observed, the wounds did not show clinical signs of infection and continued to heal at an apparently normal rate (54). The final word on occlusive versus nonocclusive environments is not yet in. In the meantime, we suggest following this advice from The Diabetic Foot (3): "Occlusion . . . must be carefully controlled." In diabetic patients, it should be limited to the management of superficial wounds or full-thickness wounds that exhibit healthy granulation tissue. Diabetic patients whose foot ulcers are managed with occlusive dressings need to be followed closely (at least once weekly) and with more frequent dressing changes (at least once daily). The same environment that enhances healing may enhance pathogenic growth. Thus, occlusion is contraindicated in infected and draining wounds. The benefits and potential dangers of occlusive wound therapies are listed below.

### *Advantages of moisture retentive dressings:*
- Reduced pain.
- Rapid healing.
- Selective autolytic debridement.
- Increased granulation and epithelialization.
- Reduced friction and shear.

### *Disadvantages:*
- Increased potential for periwound maceration.
- Accumulation of wound exudates on the wound surface.

- If adhesive, adherence to healthy/new granulation tissue with potential for harm.
- Increased numbers of microorganisms on the wound surface.

## ADJUNCTIVE THERAPIES

A number of adjunctive therapies are currently being utilized for care of chronic wounds. Much benefit can be realized with the utilization of advanced modalities, especially when standard and basic wound care has failed to produce evidence of wound healing. These include electrical stimulation, topical oxygen, Ultrasound Assisted Wound therapy (UAW), Vacuum-Assisted Closure (VAC), Pulsed Electromagnetic Therapy (PEMT) and biological skin substitutes. Each of these therapies will be briefly addressed below.

## Electrical Stimulation

Electrical stimulation is usually considered a physical therapy modality in North America. Claims have been made for its efficacy in decreasing wound bioburden, debridement, and promoting granulation tissue formation, improving tensile strength and reducing pain (11, 28). While the body of research to support the use of electrical stimulation for wound healing is growing (19), there is no consensus to date as to which voltages, currents, wave forms or polarities produce which effects. Electrode placement is also an area of debate.

## Topical Oxygen

Topical oxygen therapy is the topical application of oxygen to a wound. It should not be confused with systemic hyperbaric oxygen therapy, in which the patient breathes 100% oxygen while they are inside of a monoplace or multiplace chamber under greater-than-normal atmospheric pressure. Topical oxygen is frequently (and inappropriately) called "topical hyperbaric oxygen." Use of this term simply adds confusion and is a misapplication of the word hyperbaric. Hyperbaric oxygen as defined by the Undersea and Hyperbaric Medical Society is the inhalation of 100% oxygen while the entire patient is enclosed within a chamber at pressures of at least 1.4 atmospheres absolute or greater. Advocates claim that topical oxygen dissolves in tissue fluids, is bacteriostatic and stimulates angiogenesis and wound healing (22). Clinical trials comparing topical oxygen and hyperbaric oxygen have been undertaken in centers in the United States. However, there are only two quantitative studies involving topical oxygen which have been reported in the literature, one controlled and the other using electron microscopy to assess results. Both show an impediment to healing (21, 38).

## Pulsed Electromagnetic Therapy (PEMT)

Various types of growth factors are involved in signaling pathways for cell growth and proliferation. Based on the hypothesis that defects in growth factor signaling contribute to the development or deterioration of pressure ulcers, correction of these defects and normalization of these signaling pathways should promote wound healing. PEMT is the application of a specific spatial-temporal low level, nonthermal, confined high frequency electromagnetic field to the wound bed and subjacent tissues. This therapy has been shown to promote the release of endogenous growth factors, which in turn stimulates a cascade of secondary messengers, resulting in increases in cell growth and proliferation and increases in the number of fibroblasts progressing through the cell cycle.

A RCT has been conducted to assess the clinical efficacy of PEMT on the rate of wound closure for pressure ulcers in long term patients. Patients with Stage II or III pressure ulcers were randomized to receive PEMT, administered twice daily or placebo therapy with a sham device. The study was conducted for 12 weeks. At 6 weeks, 100% of the patients with Stage II wounds treated with PEMT healed, versus only 36% of the control patients (p< 0.005). At 12 weeks, 50% of the patients with Stage III wounds treated with PEMT were healed, versus on 14% of the controls (p<0.01) (53).

## Vacuum-Assisted Closure (V.A.C.®)

Vacuum-assisted closure, represented in the marketplace by the KCI company's V.A.C.®, is a method for applying negative pressure via suction to chronic wounds (6). It provides an alternative to traditional wound closure with sutures, skin grafts, and flaps or by secondary intention. It can also serve as a tool for patients who are not surgical candidates and as a means to help prepare and fill in a wound so that definitive procedures, such as grafts and flaps, can be performed with a greater chance of take, smaller procedure, or a better cosmetic outcome. This form of therapy has been shown in the laboratory and clinically to enhance granulation tissue formation, to reduce bioburdens and edema (41). V.A.C.® is also credited with enhancing cellular migration, promoting moist wound healing, and increasing blood flow and oxygenation to the area (41). The therapy is particularly useful for large chronic, exudative wounds, but it has been used successfully in diabetic foot ulcers and in preparing foot ulcer beds for flap closure. It is contraindicated with fistulas to organs or body cavities, necrotic tissue, untreated osteomyelitis and malignancy. V.A.C.® system includes a powered therapy unit (a rental item), a collection canister, a sponge dressing that is cut to fit the wound bed and film drape. One possible problem is that some patients have reported this form of therapy to be too painful to tolerate.

When HBOT is utilized in the management of a wound that is also being treated with negative pressure wound therapy (NPWT), the combined approach is synergistic and results in improved wound healing. Modifications to the hyperbaric chamber can be made to facilitate maintaining the NPWT dressing and continuing application of negative pressure to the wound bed. Negative pressure wound therapy and HBOT implemented simultaneously, maintaining negative pressure to the wound bed during hyperbaric therapy, has been reported to result in higher healing outcomes than each modality did independently. Comparative analysis of a population of twenty patients with compromised post surgical wounds or wounds secondary to arterial insufficiency, matched for age and co-morbid disease factors, treated with NPWT alone (10 patients) or with NPWT and HBOT together (10 patients) was conducted. One hundred percent wound granulation was used as a study endpoint. When combined modalities were used the granulation endpoint was achieved in 28 days (versus 58 days with NPWT alone) (46).

Practitioners interested in obtaining more information regarding hyperbaric oxygen therapy, including clinical practice standards, regulatory, billing and coding issues can contact the American College of Hyperbaric Medicine (www.ACHM.org). This is a professional society organized in support of US hyperbaric physicians, and is dedicated to enhancing the practice of clinical hyperbaric medicine.

## Biological Skin Substitutes

Recent advances in tissue culture techniques have made it possible to culture cells from human foreskin donors. Donated newborn foreskins are used to extract epidermal precursor cells and fibroblasts to a master cell bank. Both the cells and mothers are extensively and repeatedly screened for possible infectious agents. Very few donors are needed because these cells are transferred to working cell banks and can produce enough skin substitute to cover four to six football fields.

Skin substitutes are defined as synthetic counterparts of skin grafts (without the pain and challenges of harvesting procedures) along with the added convenience of availability and applicability in any setting. Designing a successful tissue engineered skin substitute is dependent on three elements: cell source, matrix, and tissue-differentiation inducers. The ideal skin substitute continues to elude the bioengineering expert. The ultimate skin substitute would quickly adhere to the wound, approximate and simulate the physiology and function of the skin, avoid rejection by the recipient, be capable of promoting wound healing and restoration, and also be affordable. There are a variety of commercial products that have been developed (e.g. Apligraft, Dermagraft®) and these have achieved some success in creating a dermal replacement for the treatment of burns, diabetic ulcers and even rare conditions like epidermolysis bullosa.

Clinical trials thus far have demonstrated encouraging results with the use of various skin substitutes, but much remains to be understood at the molecular and cellular level. If products comprised of proteins such as growth factors are definitively linked to generating enhanced outcomes and clinical efficacy, then efforts should be geared towards the genetic over-expression of precursor cytokines and chemokines. Eventually this approach is expected to have a significant positive impact in chronic non-healing wounds.

Dermagraft® (Advanced BioHealing/La Jolla CA) is an *in vitro* bioengineered dermal skin construct consisting of a bioabsorbable polyglactin mesh (Vicryl®, Ethicon Inc.) and seeded fibroblasts. The seeded fibroblasts proliferate and spread through the mesh, producing cytokines (growth factors), glycosaminoglycans (GAGs) and other matrix proteins, including collagen, fibronectin, and tenascin (47). After the construct has matured, it is cryopreserved to –70 degrees centigrade in a bioreactor and then thawed prior to patient application. In the rat aorta ring assay, enhancement of wound tissue expansion and angiogenesis was linked to Hepatocyte Growth Factor/Scatter Factor produced by the cells (26).

A pilot study protocol in non-healing diabetic neuropathic foot ulcers implanted Dermagraft® weekly for 8 weeks. There was a 12-week healing rate of 50 percent, compared to 8 percent in the control group (18). In a follow-up, multi-center study, there were 129 patients in the control group and 109 in the

Dermagraft® group (19). At the interim analysis, it was discovered that the therapeutic range for Dermagraft® should be narrower than the original release criteria. Testing pre-and post-cryopreservation was performed to determine a therapeutic range. The MTT (3-[4,5,-dimethylthiazol-2-y-l] - 2,5, diphenyltetrazolium bromide) assay result was compared to healing rates post application and it was found that both very low and very high levels inhibited healing (45). The 12-week healing rate of all Dermagraft® in the multi-center study was 38.5 percent (40/109), but increased to 50.8 percent (31/61) if therapeutic range product was given for the majority of applications, compared to control 31.7 percent (p=0.007) (49). Complete healing at week 32 for all Dermagraft® patients was 57.5 percent; therapeutic range patients only, 57.7 percent; and control, 42.4 percent (p=0.022 and 0.39 respectively). This study is now being repeated with the more precise therapeutic range release criteria for Dermagraft®.

Apligraf™ (Human Skin Equivalent, Organogenesis, Canton, MA) is a skin substitute composed of an epidermis (epidermal cells, stratum corneum) and dermis (bovine collagen, dermal fibroblasts) (57). In this construct, bovine collagen is acid dissociated and added to a transwell with fibroblasts from newborn donors. After 5 to 6 days, epidermal cell precursors are added and when 3 to 5 layers of epithelium are formed, the construct is raised to the air-liquid interface to facilitate the production of a stratum corneum. This skin equivalent is also currently being tested for non-healing diabetic foot ulcers. Besides knowing the technology, we also need to determine the optimal clinical technique to use these products and if bacterial burden of the wound needs to be corrected for optimal results.

In the future, many new generations of skin substitutes will become available. The dermis can be manipulated with glycosaminoglycans (GAGs) that can enhance wound healing and the transplanted cells can be transfected with extra copies of genes that promote the wound healing process such as platelet derived growth factor. For widespread use, however, these products not only have to demonstrate clinical effectiveness, but cost-effectiveness.

## AREAS OF SPECIAL CONSIDERATION

### Wound Classification and Staging

There are general and disease-specific tools for grading or staging chronic wounds. Staging or grading systems can be useful for initial assessment of the chronic wound, such as the National Pressure Ulcer Advisory Panel/Agency for Healthcare Policy and Research staging system for pressure ulcers (9, 36, 48). The Wagner scale is commonly used for ulcers of the diabetic foot (64).

### Documentation

Optimal management of the non-healing wound requires on-going, consistent assessment and documentation of the patient's condition and the wound status. Close monitoring leads to early identification of complications and affords for prompt and appropriate management.

Describe the precise location of the wound and document using anatomical descriptions, or mapped on a body diagram. Wound tracings and photography help the provider and patient to monitor changes in the wound. Wound area is approximated by measurement of length and the maximum width (in centimeters) at right angles to each other. Length multiplied by width equals surface area. Measure the maximum depth with a probe (cotton tipped applicator, sterile swab or sterile plastic depth guide). Wound volume can be obtained by filling the defect with fluid and obtaining the measurement in cubic centimeters or milliliters. Assess and document wound characteristics such as undermining and tunneling. Location of these defects can be described using the clock face for orientation. Describe wound characteristics in detail and document clearly, preferably using a flow chart to easily follow healing progress. Include the condition of the base of the wound. Necrotic tissue may present as hard black or soft brown eschar, loosely or densely adherent yellow or tan fibrinous slough. In order to fully assess the wound base or stage a pressure ulcer, the necrotic tissue must be removed to reveal the true depth of tissue damage.

Digital photography is a useful tool for recording the progression of wound healing. Computer programs are available to enhance digital photographs with planimetry and quantification of tissue types. The digital camera combined with the electronic medical record provides the clinician with the ability to store, retrieve and share data regarding wound care outcomes. This tool can also connect providers in the field, in real time, to specialist's miles away through the concept of telemedicine. In a sense, this facilitates a long-distance consultation.

## Clean vs. Sterile Technique

While the research base to support a decision regarding clean or aseptic technique versus sterile wound care is shaky at best (37), we believe that best practice at this time involves the use of sterilized products and sterilized solutions. This point is self-evident when treating immunocompromised patients.

The potential for increased bacterial load when using products, especially gauze products, that have not been sterilized does not warrant the pennies saved in our opinion. It is standard of care to accomplish dressing changes and to perform wound debridement using aseptic technique with sterile products and instruments. Until research studies are published and replicated that show identical outcomes in all settings for all patient populations, following the gold standard of using sterile wound care products and instruments is the reasonably prudent thing to do.

## Pain

Wound pain should be routinely assessed and documented using the patient's own self-report. The 10-cm visual analogue scale is the "gold standard" for quantitative pain assessment (32). The patient is asked to grade his or her pain by placing a mark along a 10-cm line where zero is no pain and the 10-cm mark represents the worst pain ever experienced. In addition to the degree of pain experienced, the quality or type of pain felt helps to distinguish the causative agent or factors. Neurologic pain is experienced differently than traumatic or inflammatory pain. Interventions that relieve the pain can also provide clues to the cause. If pain increases in the lower extremity when it is elevated versus decreased pain with elevation the source may be decreased arterial perfusion. New onset or increased severity of pain in the chronic wound patient often signals complications such as infection, a Charcot arthropathy, or vascular compromise.

## Issues Unique to the Hyperbaric Environment

This section will address several wound management issues of particular concern for the hyperbaric practitioner, including the timing of treatments, the use of certain types of dressings and pressure reduction/relief in the hyperbaric chamber. Many wound management protocols are based on traditional practice and are not evidence-based. This is true for many general wound management interventions as well as hyperbaric-specific ones.

The timing of wound management treatments is still very much an art and not an exact science. For example, how often a dressing should be changed—daily, every other day, every third day and so on—is based on a clinical assessment of the status of the wound, with special consideration of the amount of exudate. Certainly it can safely be stated as a rule that all occlusive dressings should be changed whenever they are leaking and no longer occlusive, thereby providing an entry point for microorganisms. Most wound experts believe that the longer you can leave a healing wound undisturbed the better.

Whether dressings should be regularly changed before or after hyperbaric treatments is a matter of debate. Another consideration involves the timing and frequency of debridement and the resulting possibility of perfusion/reperfusion injury.

The following practical issues should be considered. Is documentation of the wound status prior to and/or after the hyperbaric treatment required (either by the institution or the payer)? Will the presence of a particular type of dressing material or device interfere with the hyperbaric treatment? Most institutions accomplish dressing changes and provide wound care using the same protocol and frequency as appropriate to meet the needs of the individual patient and/or wound regardless of whether the patient is receiving HBOT or not.

Traditionally, many hyperbaric practitioners have avoided the use of certain types of dressings in the chamber because of concerns that these dressings might represent a fire hazard. These include gauze dressings impregnated with oil-based products (such as petrolatum based gauze and ointment) and gauze dressings that are not 100% cotton. In many institutions in the United States and throughout the world, these restrictions have not been followed and there have been no fires or other consequences attributed to wound dressings. Metal external fixation devices are permitted in the monoplace chamber, but they should be padded to avoid scratching the plastic walls. Fiberglass casts are also permitted.

The science to support the ban on these dressings and splints is totally lacking. While the 1970 NFPA regulations considered the hyperbaric atmosphere an explosive atmosphere, the 1999 NFPA guidelines correctly recognize the chamber as a hazardous atmosphere, not an explosive one (44). Therefore, traditional practices of excluding certain types of dressings should be revisited. Vaseline® gauze dressings are permitted in the monoplace chamber and have been used for many years without incident. A good practice is simply to cover them during treatment. If a patient with severe psoriasis, for example, requires a lotion or cream with a petroleum base to control the skin eruption, it is counter-productive and harmful to the patient to scrub away the entire medicament on a daily basis prior to HBO treatment. Simply cover the treated areas.

All chamber fires to date, save one, have been caused by the purposeful or inadvertent introduction of an ignition source, or the creation of an ignition source within the chamber due to fault or misuse of chamber equipment. Of the fire triad, oxygen is de facto not removable and fuel is always present. The only element of which the operator has absolute control is ignition. It is in this area that there must be meticulous and obsessive oversight for each and every hyperbaric exposure, with careful examination of any object or process that can provide ignition.

Pressure reduction or relief can be an important issue for patients with pressure ulcers or at risk for pressure ulcers who must spend extended periods of time in a chamber. The use of air-filled pressure relieving products such as mattresses is not effective in either monoplace or multiplace chambers. Use of gel or water-filled pressure relieving or reducing products is a reasonable option. The best products reduce tissue interface pressures to below capillary closure pressures.

## Evaluating the Ability to Heal

The plan of care for each patient is individualized and incorporates the assessment, diagnosis, treatment plan, interventions, and follow-up evaluations of progress. In order to monitor progress a set of goals and expected outcomes are determined. The identification of goals and outcomes should be a joint venture of the provider team, the patient, and his or her family. While healing is the ideal outcome that everyone would like to achieve, healing is not always possible. If the underlying causes are addressed and best wound management practices are implemented for the patient who is expected to heal, evidence of healing should be noted in two to four weeks. If there is no forward progress or deterioration is noted, it is appropriate to consider other alternatives or modification of goals.

The capacity of the body to heal a chronic wound depends on the condition of the host. In some patients, the chronic wound is a result of or is secondary to a primary health condition that cannot be corrected or improved. In patients with inadequate blood supply, gross deformity, persistent infections (especially chronic osteomyelitis), or an underlying terminal condition, healing may not be a realistic outcome. In this case the best management may be to transition to palliative wound care efforts. This assessment should be carefully documented and supported by appropriate investigations and colleague opinion. The conclusion should be shared diplomatically with the patient and his or her family. When cure is not the goal, there are interventions, goals, and outcomes that are appropriate for this patient population. These may include palliative interventions such as amputation, preventing infection, reducing systemic complications, and controlling pain.

Dressings and treatments that might not be used when healing is the expected outcome, may be appropriately utilized for these patients to control bacterial load. These include antiseptics that are cytotoxic to viable healing cells: povidone-iodine, hydrogen peroxide, and sodium hypochlorite. Aggressive debridement of these wounds may lead to larger non-healing wounds. Dry gangrene may be best left to demarcate and auto-amputate; in these cases avoiding debridement and the autolytic activity of moist interactive dressings is the best approach.

It is important that care be patient-focused. Quality of life tools, both general and disease-specific, help us to adequately address the fears, concerns, and everyday issues of the chronic wound patient and the family. The use of quality of life tools has to date been predominantly a research activity, but it needs to become part of everyday, routine practice. Measuring the activities of the patient lets the wound care specialist follow progress towards the stated goals and achieves the best possible outcomes.

## CONCLUSION

Chronic wound care is a challenge for both providers and patients. An interdisciplinary team approach based on best practices is necessary to identify and treat general medical conditions and to provide local wound management. A holistic approach to the assessment and management of chronic wounds is needed to optimize care. As a member of the team, the hyperbaric practitioner offers one special tool in an entire toolbox of options.

With an aging population and more and more chronic illnesses, the incidence of chronic wounds is expected to rise. It is important to optimize holistic care of chronic wound patients in order to improve outcomes. Despite correction of the underlying causes and best-practice wound care, a proportion of these wounds will not heal in a timely manner. The wound care specialist provides expertise in wound management and skill in the deployment of advanced technologies including hyperbaric oxygen therapy, biological alternatives, negative pressure wound therapy, and advanced debridement modalities. As a key member of the multidisciplinary wound care team the wound care expert can contribute significantly in the effort to heal refractory wounds, preventing limb loss and improve the quality of life.

# A QUICK REFERENCE GUIDE TO WOUND CARE PRODUCT CATEGORIES*

## January 1999

This listing of wound care products highlights the importance of generic product categories. Under each generic product category, up to four product examples are given (a mix of old and new products), to help familiarize the reader with each category. No endorsement of any product or manufacturer is intended. Within each category, products must be individually evaluated. All products within a category do not necessarily perform equally. Combination products may be listed in more than one category. Refer to manufacturers' instructions for specifics regarding product usage.

## 1. Antimicrobial Dressings

| Product | Manufacturer |
|---|---|
| Acticoat™ | Westaim Biomedical |
| Arglaes® Film/Island | Medline Industries |
| Iodosorb® Gel | Healthpoint |
| Iodoflex™ Gel Pad | Healthpoint |

## 2. Alginate Dressings

| Product | Manufacturer |
|---|---|
| Cutinova® alginate | Beiersdorf-Jobst |
| Restore CalciCare | Hollister |
| Seasorb™ | Coloplast Sween |
| Sorbsan™ | Dow Hickam Pharmaceuticals |

## 3. Biosynthetic Dressings

| Product | Manufacturer |
|---|---|
| BiobraneII® | Dow Hickam Pharmaceuticals |
| Silon® | BioMed Sciences |

## 4. Cleansers

| Product | Manufacturer |
|---|---|
| a. Saline | Multiple |
| b. Skin Cleansers | |
| Peri-Wash® | Sween |
| Sensi-Care™ | ConvaTec |
| Skin Cleanser | Mentor |
| Prevacare™ | Johnson & Johnson Medical |
| c. Wound Cleansers | |
| Clinical Care® | Care-Tech Laboratories |
| Curasol™ | Medical |
| Dermagran® Spray | Derma Sciences |
| RadiaCare™ Klenz | Carrington Laboratories |

* All product names should be considered copyrighted or trademarked regardless of the absence of an ® or ™.

## 5. Collagen Dressings

| Product | Manufacturer |
|---|---|
| BGC Natrix (Collagen/Beta-glucan) | Brennen Medical |
| ChroniCure™ | Derma Sciences |
| Fibracol® (Collagen/Alginate) | Johnson & Johnson Medical |
| Medifil™/SkinTemp® | BioCore |

## 6. Composite Dressings

| Product | Manufacturer |
|---|---|
| Alldress® | SCA Mölnlycke |
| CombiDERM™ ACD™ | ConvaTec |
| CovaDerm™/CovaDerm™ Plus | DeRoyal |
| OsmoCyte® Island | ProCyte Corporation |

## 7. Compression Bandages/Wraps

| Product | Manufacturer |
|---|---|
| Coban® | 3M Health Care |
| Dome Paste® | Miles |
| Elastoplast® | Beiersdorf-Jobst |
| Setopress® | ConvaTec |

### Multi-Layered Systems

| Product | Manufacturer |
|---|---|
| Circulon™ System | ConvaTec |
| Dyna-Flex™ | Johnson & Johnson Medical |
| Profore® | Smith & Nephew |
| Unna-Pak | Glenwood |

## 8. Conforming/Wrapping Bandages

| Product | Manufacturer |
|---|---|
| Dutex/Duform | Dumex Medical |
| Elastomull® | Beiersdorf-Jobst |
| Kerlix® Lite | Kendall Healthcare |
| SOF-KLING™ | Johnson & Johnson Medical |

## 9. Contact Layers

| Product | Manufacturer |
|---|---|
| Mepitel® | SCA Mölnlycke |
| Profore® | Smith & Nephew |
| Tegapore | 3M Healthcare |
| Ventex™ Vented Dressing | Kendall Healthcare |

## 10. Creams/Oils

| Product | Manufacturer |
|---|---|
| Biafine® | KCI® |
| Decubitene™ Oxygenated Oil | Ferndale Labs |
| Eucerin Cream | Beiersdorf-Jobst |
| Sween Cream® | Coloplast Sween |

## 11. Devices

| Product | Manufacturer |
|---|---|
| THBO™ (topical hyperbaric oxygen) | GWR Medical LLP |
| V.A.C. | KCI® |
| Warm-Up"™ | Augustine Medical |

## 12. Enzymes/ Debriding Agents

| Product | Manufacturer |
|---|---|
| Accuzyme™ (Papain-Urea) | Healthpoint |
| Elase® (Fibrinolysin/ desoxyribonuclease) | Fugisawa |
| Panifil® Ointment (Papain) | Rystan |
| Santyl (Collagenase) | Knoll Pharmaceuticals |

## 13. Foam Dressings

| Product | Manufacturer |
|---|---|
| Allevyn® | Smith & Nephew |
| Flexzan™/thin | Dow Hickam Pharmaceuticals |
| Lyofoam®/Lyofoam® C/Lyofoam® T | ConvaTec |
| PolyMem® | Ferris Manufacturing |

## 14. Gauze Dressings (see also Composite Dressings)

| Product | Manufacturer |
|---|---|
| a. Woven | Multiple |
| b. Non-woven | |
|    EXCILON® | Kendall Healthcare |
|    NATURALON™ | Kendall Healthcare |
|    NU GAUZE General Use | Johnson & Johnson Medical |
|    SOF-WICK™ | Johnson & Johnson Medical |
| c. Packing/Packing Strips (Non-impregnated) | |
|    Dumex Pak-Its | Dumex Medical |
|    Kerlix® | Kendall Healthcare |
|    NU-BREDE™ | Johnson & Johnson Medical |
|    TENDERSORB® | Kendall Healthcare |
| d. Debriding | |
|    NU-BREDE™ | Johnson & Johnson Medical |
|    TENDERSORB® | Kendall Healthcare |
| e. Impregnated - Sodium Chloride | |
|    Mesalt® | SCA Mölnlycke |
|    Thalafix® | Dumex Medical |
| f. Impregnated - Other | |
|    Dermagran™ Wet Dressing (Saline) | Derma Sciences |
|    Dumex Wet Dressings (Saline) | Dumex Medical |
|    Dumex Pak-It Hydrogel | Dumex Medical |
|    Gentell™ Hydrogel Dressing | MKM Healthcare |
| g. Non-adherent gauze | |
|    Primapore® | Smith & Nephew |
|    Release® | Johnson & Johnson Medical |
|    Telfa® | Kendall Healthcare |

h. Specialty Absorptive Gauze

| | |
|---|---|
| EXU-DRY® | Smith & Nephew |
| SURGIPAD® Combine Dressings | Johnson & Johnson Medical |
| TENDERSORB® Wet-Pruf Abdominal Pad | Kendall Healthcare |
| TOPPER™ | Johnson & Johnson Medical |

## 15. Growth Factors

| Product | Manufacturer |
|---|---|
| Procuren (autologous) | Curative Health Services |
| Regranex® Gel (becaplermin 0.01%) | Ortho-McNeil Pharmaceutical |

## 16. Human Skin Equivalents (HSE)/Skin Substitutes

| Product | Manufacturer |
|---|---|
| Apligraf™ (Graftskin) | Organogenesis/Novartis |
| Dermagraft | Advanced Tissue Sciences/ Smith & Nephew |

## 17. Hydrocolloid Dressings

| Product | Manufacturer |
|---|---|
| DuoDERM®/CGF/Extra Thin | ConvaTec |
| Hydrocol® | Dow Hickam Pharmaceuticals |
| Restore™/CX/Extra Thin | Hollister |
| Tegasorb™/Extra Thin | 3M Healthcare |

## 18. Hydrogel Dressings  (see also Impregnated Gauze Dressings)

| Product | Manufacturer |
|---|---|
| **SHEET** | |
| CarraSorb™ M | Carrington Laboratories |
| Elasto-Gel™ | Southwest Technologies |
| Gentell™ | MKM |
| Vigilon® | Bard |
| **AMORPHOUS** | |
| Carrington Gel Wound Dressing™ | Carrington Laboratories |
| Confeel® Purilon™ Gel | Coloplast |
| DuoDERM® Hydroactive Gel (Hydrogel/Hydrocolloid) | ConvaTec |
| IntraSite® Gel | Smith & Nephew |

## 19. Skin Sealants

| Product | Manufacturer |
|---|---|
| Preppies™ | Kendall Healthcare |
| Skin Prep™ | Smith & Nephew United |
| Skin Shield® | Mentor |
| 3M No Sting Skin Protectant | 3M |

## 20. Transparent Film Dressings

| Product | Manufacturer |
| --- | --- |
| BIOCLUSIVE™/MVP | Johnson & Johnson Medical |
| Flexfilm™ | Dow Hickam Pharmaceuticals |
| OpSite®/Flexifix/Flexigrid/3000 | Smith & Nephew |
| Tegaderm™/HP | 3M Health Care |

## 21. Wound Fillers: Pastes, Powders, Beads, Strands

| Product | Manufacturer |
| --- | --- |
| AcryDerm® Strands™ | AcryMed |
| Bard® Absorption Dressing | Bard |
| OsmoCyte™ Pillow Wound Dressing | Procyte |
| Multidex | DeRoyal Industries |

## 22. Wound Pouches

| Product | Manufacturer |
| --- | --- |
| Wound Drainage Collector | Hollister |
| Wound Manager™ | ConvaTec |
| **ADULT AND PEDIATRIC SIZED** | |
| Ostomy Pouches | Multiple |

## PRODUCT CATEGORIES NOT OTHERWISE CLASSIFIED (NOC)

23. **Adhesives**
24. **Adhesive Removers**
25. **Adhesive Skin Closures**
26. **Adhesive Tapes**
27. **Antibiotics**
28. **Antimicrobials**
29. **Antiseptics**
30. **Bandages**
31. **Dressing Covers**
32. **Healthcare Personnel Handrinses**
33. **Lubricating/Stimulating Sprays**
34. **Moisture Barrier Ointments/Creams/Skin Protectant Pastes**
35. **Moisturizers**
36. **Ointments**
37. **Perineal Cleansing Foams**
38. **Sterile Fields**
39. **Surgical Scrubs**
40. **Surgical Tapes**
41. **Miscellaneous**

# REFERENCES

1. Allie DE, Hebert CJ, Lirtzman MD. Critical limb ischemia: A global epidemic. A critical analysis of current treatment unmasks the clinical and economic costs of CLI. Eurointervention, 1 (1):60-69, 1995.

2. Abu-Rumman P, Armstrong D, Nixon B. Use of clinical lab parameters to evaluate wound healing potential in Diabetes Mellitus. Journal of the American Podiatric Medical Association 2002; 92(1):38-47.

3. Alvarez OM, Gilson G, and Auletta MJ. Local aspects of diabetic foot ulcer care: Assessment, dressings, and topical agents, pp. 265-266. In Levin ME, O'Neal LW, Bowker, JH: The Diabetic Foot (5th ed), St. Louis, MO, 1993, Mosby Year Book.

4. American Diabetes Association http://www.diabetes.org.

5. Apelqvist J, Ragnarson R, and Tenvall G. Cavity foot ulcers in diabetic patients: a comparative study of cadexomer iodine ointment and standard treatment. An economic analysis alongside a clinical trial. Acta Derm Venereol 76(3):231-235, 1996.

6. Argenta LC, and Morykwa, MJ. Vacuum-assisted closure: A new method for wound control and treatment: Clinical experience. Annals of Plastic Surgery 38: 563-576, 1997.

7. Armstrong DG, Lavery LA, Liswood PL, and Todd WF. Infrared dermal thermometry of the high risk diabetic foot. Diabetologia 39(supp):1013:A266, 1996.

8. Ballard JL, Eke CC, Bunt, TJ, Killen JD. A prospective evaluation of transcutaneous oxygen measurements in the management of diabetic foot problems. J. Vasc. Surg. 1995: 5-492.

9. Bergstrom N, Bennett MA, Carlson CE, et al. Treatment of pressure ulcers. Clinical Practice Guideline, No 15. Rockville, MD: U.S. Department of Health and Human Services. Public Health Service, Agency for Healthcare Policy and Research. AHCPR Publication No. 95-0652. December 1994.

10. Bowers BL, Valentine RJ, Myers SI, et al. The Natural History of Patients with Claudication with Toe Pressures of 40 mmHg or Less. J. Vasc Surg. 1993; 18506-11.

11. Brown M. Electrical stimulation for wound management. In PP Gogia. Clinical Wound Management, pp. 175-184, Thorofare NJ, 1995, SLACK Incorporated.

12. Caputo GM, Cavanagh PR, Ulbrecht JS, Gibbons GW, and Karchmer AW. Assessment and management of foot disease in patients with diabetes. NEJM. 854-860, 1994.

13. Collins N. Assessment and treatment of involuntary weight loss and protein-calorie malnutrition. Advances in Skin and Wound Care 2000;13(Supplement 1):4-10.

14. Demling RH. Involuntary weight loss, protein-energy malnutrition, and the impairment of cutaneous wound healing. Wounds Supplement D 2001; 13(4):3D-21D.

15. Deweese Ja, Leather R, Porter J, Practice Guidelines: Lower Extremity Revascularization. J. Vasc Surg. 1993; 18280-93.

16. Elliott IMZ. A Short History of Surgical Dressings. London, Pharmaceutic Press, 1964.

17. Fife CE, Buyukcakir C, Otto GH, Sheffield PJ, Warriner RA, Love TL, Mader J. The predictive value of transcutaneous oxygen tension measurement in diabetic lower extremity ulcers treated with hyperbaric oxygen therapy: a retrospective analysis of 1,144 patients. Wound Repair Regen. 2002 Jul-Aug;10(4):198-207.

18. Gentzkow GC, Iwasaki SD, Hershon KS, et al. Use of Dermagraft®, a cultured human epidermis, to treat diabetic foot ulcers. Diabetes Care 4:350-354, 1996.

19. Gogia PP. Physical therapy intervention in wound management. In Krasner D, and Kane D. Chronic Wound Care: A Clinical Source Book for Healthcare Professionals, pp. 251-259. Wayne, PA, 1997, Health Management Publications, Inc.

20. Grayson LM, Gibbons GW, Balosh K, Levine E, Karchmer AW. Probing to bone in infected pedal ulcers. JAMA 1995: 273(9) 721-723.

21. Heng, MCY and Kloss, SG. Endothelial Cell Toxicity in Leg Ulcers Treated with Topical Hyperbaric Oxygen. Am. J. Dermatopath 8(5):403-410, 1986.

22. Heng MCY. Topical hyperbaric therapy for problem skin wounds. J Dermatol Surg Oncol 19:784-793, 1993.

23. Hinman CD, and Maibach HI. Effect of air exposure and occlusion on experimental human skin wounds. Nature 200:377-378, 1963.

24. Hopf HW, Ueno C, Aslam R, et al. Guidelines for the treatment of arterial insufficiency ulcers. Wound Rep Reg. 14: 693-710, 2006.

25. Hutchinson JJ. Prevalence of wound infection under occlusive dressings: A collective survey of reported research. WOUNDS, 1(2): 123-133, 1989.

26. Jiang WG, and Harding K. Enhancement of wound tissue expansion and angiogenesis by matrix-embedded fibroblast (Dermagraft®), a role of hepatocyte growth factor/scatter factor. International Journal of Molecular Medicine, 2:203-210, 1998.

27. Kennedy KL, and Tritch DL. Debridement. In Krasner D, and Kane D, editors. Chronic Wound Care: A Clinical Source Book for Healthcare Professionals, ed 2, pp. 227-235, Wayne, PA, 1997, Health Management Publications, Inc.

28. Kloth LC, and Feedar JA. Electrical stimulation in tissue repair. In Kloth LC, McCulloch JM, and Feedar JA. Wound Healing: Alternatives in Management pp. 221-256. Philadelphia, 1990, F. A. Davis.

29. Kane D, and Krasner D. Wound healing and wound management. In Krasner D, and Kane D, editors. Chronic Wound Care: A Clinical source book for healthcare professionals, ed 2, pp 1-4, Wayne, PA, 1997, Health Management Publications, Inc.

30. Kindwall EP, Niezgoda JA. Hyperbaric Medicine Procdures: The Kindwall HBO Handbook. ed 9, pp 12-15. 2006. Aurora St. Lukes Medical Center, Milwaukee, WI.

31. Kindwall EP, Niezgoda JA. Hyperbaric Medicine Procdures: The Kindwall HBO Handbook. ed 9, pp 42. 2006. Aurora St. Lukes Medical Center, Milwaukee, WI.

32. Krasner, D. Chronic Wound Pain. In: Krasner D, and Kane D, eds. Chronic Wound Care: A Clinical Source Book for Healthcare Professionals, ed 2, pp 336-343, Wayne, PA, 1997, Health Management Publications, Inc.

33. Krasner D. Dressing decisions for the twenty-first century: on the cusp of a paradigm shift. In Krasner D, and Kane D, editors: Chronic Wound Care: A Clinical Source Book for Healthcare Professionals, ed 2, pp. 139-151, Wayne, PA, 1997, Health Management Publications, Inc.

34. Krasner, D. Pressure Ulcers: Assessment, Classification and Management. In: Krasner D, and Kane D, eds. Chronic Wound Care: A Clinical Source Book for Healthcare Professionals, ed 2, pp 152-157, Wayne, PA, 1977, Health Management Publications, Inc.

35. Krasner D: Resolving the dressing dilemma: Selecting wound dressings by category. Ostomy/Wound Management, 35:62-70, 1991.

36. Krasner D, and Sibbald RG(eds). Moving beyond the AHCPR guidelines: Wound care evolution over the last five years. WOUNDS 11:January Suppl, 1S-120S, 1999.

37. Krasner D, et al. Sterile versus Nonsterile Wound Care: An Interactive Monograph for Healthcare Professionals. Toronto: Dumex Medical Surgical Products Ltd., 1998.

38. Leslie, CA, Sapico FL, Ginunas, VJ and Adkins, RH. Randomized Control Trial of Topical Hyperbaric Oxygen for Treatment of Diabetic Foot Ulcers. Diabetes Care 11:111-115, 1988.

39. Majno G. The Healing Hand. Cambridge, MA. The Harvard University Press, 1975.

40. Mehta et al.Fallibility of Doppler Ankle Pressures in Predicting Healing of Transmetatarsal Amputation, J. Surg Res, 28:466-470, 1980.

41. Morykwas MJ, Argenta LC, Shelton-Brown EI, and McGuirt W. Vacuum-assisted closure: A new method for wound control and treatment: Animal studies and basic foundation. Annals of Plastic Surgery 38:553-562, 1997.

42. Moss SE, Lein R, Klein Bek, The Prevalence and Incidence of Lower Extremity Amputation in a Diabetic Population. Arch. Intern. Med. 1992; 152:610-16.

43. Murff RT, Armstrong DG, Lanctot D, Lavery LA, and Athanasiou KA. How effective is manual palpation in detecting subtle temperature differences. Clinics in Pod Med and Surg. 15(1):151-154, 1998.

44. National Fire Protection Association. NFPA 53 Guide on Fire Hazards in Oxygen-Enriched Atmospheres. 1994 Edition. NFPA, Quincy, MA 1994.

45. Naughton G, Mansbridge J, and Gentzkow G. A Metabolically Active Human Dermal Replacement for the Treatment of Diabetic Foot Ulcers. Artificial Organs 21(11):1203-1210, 1997.

46. Niezgoda JA: Combining negative pressure wound therapy with other wound management modalities. PUBLISHED, February 2005 OSTOMY WOUND MANAGEMENT (Ostomy Wound Manage. 2005 Feb;51(2A Suppl):36S-38S).

47. Ovington LG. The well-dressed wound: an overview of dressing types. WOUNDS 10 Supplement A:1A-11A, 1998.

48. Panel for the Prediction and Prevention of Pressure Ulcers in Adults. Pressure Ulcers in Adults: Prediction and Prevention. Clinical Practice Guideline, Number 3. AHCPR Publication No. 92-0047. Rockville, MD: Agency for Health Care Policy and Research, Public Health Service, U.S. Department of Health and Human Services. May 1992.

49. Pollak RA, Edington H, and Jensen JJ. A Human Dermal Replacement for the Treatment of Diabetic Foot Ulcers. WOUNDS, 9(1):175-183, 1997.

50. Proceedings of the ECHM Consensus Conference on the Hyperbaric Treatment of Foot Lesions in Diabetic Patients, 1999; European Committee for Hyperbaric Medicine, London.

51. Raines, et. al. Vascular Lab Criteria for Management of PVD of Lower Extremities, Surg. 1976.

52. Reiber GE, Boyko EJ, Smith DG. Lower extremity foot ulcers and amputations diabetics. In: Diabetes in America, 2nd ed. National Diabetes Data group.

53. Ritz MC. Provant Wound Closure System accelerates closure of pressure wounds in a randomized, double-blinded, placebo controlled trial. Annals of NY Academy of Sciences, Vol 1247, Reparative Medicine and Growing Tissues, Editors: Sipe, Kelly & McNichol, 2002.

54. Robson MC. Wound infection. A failure of wound healing caused by an imbalance of bacteria. Surg Clin North Am 77(3):637-650, Jun 1997.

55. Robson MC, Cooper DM, Aslam R, et al. Guidelines for the treatment of venous ulcers. Wound Rep Reg. 14: 649-662, 2006.

56. Rodeheaver, GT. Wound cleansing, wound irrigation, wound disinfection. In: Krasner D, and Kane D, eds. Chronic Wound Care: A Clinical Source Book for Healthcare Professionals, ed 2, pp 97-108, Wayne, PA, 1997, Health Management Publications, Inc.

57. Sabolinski ML, Alverez O, Auletta M, et al. Cultured skin as a 'smart' material for healing wounds: experience in venous ulcers. Biomaterials 17:311-320, 1996.

58. Steed DL. Diabetic wounds: assessment, classification and management. In: Krasner D, and Kane D, eds. Chronic Wound Care: A Clinical Source Book for Healthcare Professionals, ed 2, pp 172-177, Wayne, PA, 1997, Health Management Publications, Inc.

59. Steed DL, Donohoe D, Webster MW, and Lindsley L. Effect of extensive debridement and treatment on the healing of diabetic foot ulcers. Diabetic Ulcer Study Group. Journal of the American College of Surgeons, 183(1):61-64, 1996.

60. Steed DL, Attinger C, Colaizzi T, et al. Guidelines for the treatment of diabetic ulcers. Wound Rep Reg. 14: 680-692, 2006.

61. Stevens DL, Bisno AL, Chambers HF, et al. Practice guidelines for the diagnosis and management of skin and soft tissue infections. Clin Infect Dis 2005; 41:1373-1406.

62. Turner TD. The development of wound management products. In Krasner D, and Kane D, editors. Chronic Wound Care: A Clinical Source Book for Healthcare Professionals, ed 2, pp 124-138, Wayne PA, 1997, Health Management Publications, Inc.

63. van Rijswijk L, and Beitz J. The traditions and terminology of wound dressings: food for thought. Journal of WOCN 25(3):116-122, 1998.

64. Wagner FW. The dysvasular foot: a system for diagnosis and treatment. Foot Ankle 2:64-122 1998.

65. Weir D, Scarbourough P, Niezgoda J. Wound Debridement. In: Krasner DL, Rodeheaver GT, Sibbald RG, eds. Chronic Wound Care: A Clinical Source Book for Healthcare Professionals. 4th Edition. Malvern PA, HMP Communications, 2007, 335-347.

66. Whitney J, Phillips L, Aslam R, et al. Guidelines for the treatment of pressure ulcers. Wound Rep Reg. 14: 663-679, 2006.

67. Winter GD. Formation of the scab and the rate of epithelisation of superficial wounds in the skin of the young domestic pig. Nature 193:293-294, 1962

68. Winter GD. Healing of skin wounds and the influence of dressings on the repair process. In Harkiss KJ, editor. Surgical Dressings and Wound Healing, pp. 46-60, London, 1971, Crosby Lockwood.

69. Winter GD, and Scales JT. Effect of air drying and dressings on the surface of a wound. Nature 197:91-92, 1963.

70. Wiseman DM, Rovee DT, and Alverez OM. Wound dressings: design and use. In Cohen IK, Diegelmann RF, Lindblad WJ. Wound Healing: Biochemical & Clinical Aspects, pp 562-580, Philadelphia, 1992,W.B. Saunders Co.

71. Wright JB, Hansen DC, Burrell RE. The comparitive efficacy of two antimicrobial barrier dressings; *in vitro* examination of two controlled release silver dressings. Wounds 1998; 10(6): 179-188.

CHAPTER 17

# CARBON MONOXIDE AND CYANIDE POISONING

## CHAPTER SEVENTEEN OVERVIEW

# CARBON MONOXIDE AND CYANIDE POISONING

*Stephen R. Thom, Roy A.M. Myers, Eric P. Kindwall*

## INTRODUCTION

Carbon monoxide (CO) is one of the leading causes of injury and death by poisoning worldwide. Approximately 10,000 people in the United States per year seek medical attention for CO exposure and an average of 3,800 people die from CO poisoning: 1,500 due to accidents and the rest from suicide (32, 52, 132, 135, 219). Because CO is colorless, odorless, tasteless, and nonirritating, its presence is difficult to detect. It is produced as a consequence of incomplete combustion of carbon-containing materials. The major source remains fire; therefore, CO presents an occupational hazard to fire fighters (180). CO exposure from automobile exhaust is also common, the internal combustion engine accounts for 75% of all CO generated by pollution-generating human activities (44). CO levels of more than 5% have been measured in nonsmokers exposed to engine exhaust on freeways (9). Another major source of CO is cigarette smoking. Stewart et al. documented carboxyhemoglobin levels (COHb) above 9% in heavy cigarette smokers (198). In the home and industrial settings, exhaust fumes also produce CO poisoning. Similarly, inadequate ventilation in conjunction with the use of fuels for home heating and cooking, such as wood, gas, and Sterno® blocks (83, 93), can elevate CO levels. In rural Korea, charcoal briquettes are used for home heating, with the heated air passing in ducts under the floor boards. Leaks through the ducts produce major problems with CO poisoning. In industry, the major factor is inadequate ventilation where propane-powered vehicles (e.g., forklifts) that transport and stack materials produce significant amounts of CO, as does the machinery for clearing ice rinks during hockey games (108). Other work environments that produce large amounts of CO, and therefore heighten the risk of poisoning, are the steel industry, due to coke ovens, and the paint industry, in which inhaled methylene chloride (dichloromethane) breaks down in the body to CO (173, 175). These environmental and occupational exposures to CO have been a point of increasing concern, as numerous investigations have linked ambient CO concentrations to morbidity and mortality related to cardiovascular and pulmonary diseases (29, 136, 137, 185).

Other than a raised COHb level and a history of exposure, there are no truly specific findings from CO poisoning. Thus, it is a great mimic, with diverse and nonspecific clinical symptoms and signs (70). As many as 30% of the victims of CO poisoning may be undiagnosed (13). Therefore, to ensure good clinical outcome and reduce neurologic sequelae, clinicians must be well attuned to the various presentations of CO poisoning, and to the need for its early diagnosis and treatment. In marginal cases the index of suspicion must be high to make the diagnosis.

Numerous factors may cloud the presentation and diagnosis of CO poisoning. In structural fires, toxins produced by combustion of building materials may affect the body. Among these substances are hydrogen cyanide and sulfide, which are chemical asphyxiants. The chemical by-products of combustion include acrolein, ammonia, benzene, and other aromatic compounds, carbon dioxide, chlorine, formaldehyde, methane, metallic oxides, carbonyls, nitrates and nitrites, phosgene, and sulfur dioxide (163).

## SPECIFIC CARBON MONOXIDE EFFECTS

### Fetal Toxicity

A pregnant woman exposed to CO usually has a 10 to 15% lower level of COHb than does her fetus. This difference arises following diffusion of maternal blood-borne CO into fetal blood (66, 116). Fetal hemoglobin has a higher affinity for CO than does hemoglobin in the adult. As fetal weight increases with gestational age, so does placental CO diffusion (24). Transplacental diffusion occurs at a slow, steady state: the fetal COHb level exceeds the maternal level after 10 hours of exposure (115). Thus, the fetal hemoglobin saturation is dependent on the duration of exposure and the concentration of CO to which the mother is exposed. The fetal $PaO_2$ is usually 20 to 30 mmHg lower than the normal maternal $PaO_2$. This level falls in the fetal blood in direct proportion to the increasing COHb concentrations in both the fetal and maternal blood. The normal fetal oxyhemoglobin-dissociation curve is to the left of the adult curve, allowing discharge of oxygen at lower oxygen tensions in fetal tissue. Exposure to CO results in a further leftward shift in both maternal and fetal oxyhemoglobin curves, decreasing oxygen release from the mother to the fetus, and from fetal hemoglobin to fetal tissue. Phillips, in 1924 (162), was the first to describe the classic red tingeing of the skin in the macerated fetus exposed to a lethal dose of CO. A further eight cases were reported in a literature review by Muller and Graham (138). The neonates showed a range of psychomotor disturbances from mental retardation to idiocy, with hypotonia of extremities and the neck. In 15 other incidences, the fetuses died as a result of CO exposure in utero.

It is common for the mother to survive exposure to CO levels that are lethal for the fetus. Should the treating physician have greater sensitivity for the fetus than the mother exposed to CO? Cramer (48) reported a fetal death occurring as a result of accidental maternal CO poisoning. The mother's highest recorded COHb level was 23.7%. In the same exposure, the father had a COHb level of 45%. Both mother and father were treated with 100% oxygen via normal rebreathing mask for 8 hours. After that treatment, their COHb levels were below 3%. Within 48 hours of discharge, the mother returned to the hospital, reporting loss of fetal movement. Sonography confirmed intrauterine death, and after induction of labor, a stillborn male was delivered. The fetus showed the classic signs of cherry red lips and pink nail beds and skin in the non-macerated areas. A right ventricle sample of blood indicated a 25% COHb level. Higher levels of COHb (35.1%) were found on analysis of the liver and spleen. The difference in level between right ventricular and tissue levels may reflect peripheral vascular shunting/stasis or tissue absorption/deposition of CO.

## Neuropathologic Lesions

Cerebral metabolism is adversely affected by reduction in the oxygen supply to the tissue, as occurs with CO poisoning. Numerous mechanisms have been postulated as causing the neurologic tissue damage: arterial hypoxemia (189), direct cellular toxicity of CO (33, 84, 94), and reduction of cerebral blood flow (56, 170). MacMillan (118) showed that animals exposed to 1% CO (10,000 ppm) for periods up to 60 minutes did not exhibit loss of consciousness or a change in cerebral energy status. When 2% CO was used for 30 minutes, however, the animals became unresponsive during exposure. Cerebral energy homeostasis was maintained until perfusion decreased and, concurrent with hypoperfusion, cerebral adenosine triphosphate (ATP) decreased, there were increases in adenosine diphosphate (ADP) and adenosine monophosphate (AMP), and depletion of tissue citrate and oxyglutarate. Similar metabolic responses to both CO and hypoxia were noted in the brain with regard to intermediary metabolites, high energy phosphates, intracellular pH, and cytoplasmic redox state. When cerebral homeostasis was disrupted, hypotension was a major factor, soon followed by cardiovascular collapse. Thus, depressed cardiovascular function induced by CO, and a limited cerebral blood flow, may be major factors leading to neurologic cellular damage from CO poisoning (118).

Survivors of serious CO poisoning may develop neurological and psychiatric sequelae such as dementia, Parkinsonism, amnesia, and depression. Neuropathology may include demyelination of cerebral cortex and neuronal death in the cortex, hippocampus, substantia nigra and globus pallidus (111). Evidence of tissue damage varies from acute coagulation necrosis with petechial hemorrhages or congestion to delayed neuronal degeneration (64, 147). Early investigators who studied CO pathophysiology remarked that demyelination occurred in a perivascular distribution, and that the blood-brain barrier was disturbed (47, 129, 171). Acute vascular and perivascular changes have been found in brains of experimental animals (58, 153, 154). Clinical pathology examiners have stressed the extent of vascular disorders (111). Using traditional neuro-imaging techniques, such as computed tomography and magnetic resonance imaging, brain lesions have been detected sporadically in severely poisoned patients (182, 218, 221). The primary shortcoming with these imaging techniques is their limited sensitivity; hence, neuro-imaging has not yet provided a reliable method for assessing the severity of CO poisoning. However, Bianco et al. (20) and Silverman et al. (191) hypothesized that the initial site of injury by CO may be the vasculature, based on detection of hemosiderin deposits on magnetic resonance imaging. These deposits are thought to be the result of focal hemorrhages.

Recently, more sophisticated neuro-imaging techniques have been used to detect abnormalities in patients who, in some cases, exhibited only subtle neurological impairments. Abnormalities in resting cerebral blood flow

(121, 190), and abnormalities in cerebral vasoactivity to carbon dioxide (54) have been detected by single-photon emission computed tomography (SPECT). Changes have also been detected which suggest that CO causes a disturbance in coupling between neuronal $O_2$ demand and blood flow. DeReuck et al. (54) examined 7 patients between 5 and 7 days after CO poisoning, using positron emission tomography (PET) with (15 Isotope) $O_2$. They found a global increase in cerebral $O_2$ extraction along with regional areas of diminished blood flow, especially in the frontal and temporal lobes.

## CLINICAL PRESENTATION

Many factors impinge on the actual clinical presentation; the concentration of CO to which a patient is exposed, the duration of that exposure, the rate and depth of breathing, the heart rate, and, most importantly, the time between discovery of the patient after the exposure, and arrival at a hospital emergency department. Fortunately for the patient, today's pre-hospital care providers administer high oxygen concentrations as part of the resuscitation and treatment of the CO victim, at the scene and during transport.

In 1930, Sayers and Davenport (183) described the classic symptomatology. Minimal symptoms were present at levels of COHb of less than 10%. Tightness across the forehead and headache were experienced at levels between 10% and 20%. Levels of 20% to 30% resulted in a throbbing headache in the temporal regions. Levels of 30% to 40% produced severe headache, generalized weakness, visual changes, dizziness, nausea and vomiting, and ultimate collapse. As the levels increased to 40% to 50%, syncope, tachycardia, and tachypnea occurred. Levels of over 50% were associated with coma and intermittent convulsions. Above 60%, death occurred due to cardiac depression and respiratory failure.

In our experience, and that reported by most investigators, the carboxyhemoglobin (COHb) level is only an indicator of exposure to CO; the level does not correlate well with symptoms or with outcome (38, 60, 141, 214, 232). Therefore, other tools are needed to prospectively evaluate the severity of CO poisoning. We have developed some psychometric tools for the determination of central nervous system involvement (128, 143). Because CO poisoning is known to be a great imitator of other illnesses (70, 79), including presenting as flu-like symptoms (12, 52), delays in the recognition and treatment of CO poisoning are frequent.

The physical findings also vary greatly in CO-poisoned patients. They depend on the time between exposure and presentation at the hospital, as well as the duration of exposure and concentration of CO. The most common physical findings include tachycardia and tachypnea. There may be mild hypotension, with systolic blood pressures in the range of 100 mmHg, or hypertension (231). Pre-existing heart disease may severely aggravate the symptomatology at lower levels of COHb. In our experience, many patients who die at the scene, or immediately on reaching the hospital, do so with a cardiac problem, which may be arrhythmias or hypotension with severe tissue perfusion impairment. Marek observed at autopsy that 45% of 265 patients who died of acute CO poisoning showed signs of acute circulatory failure. Histologically there was evidence of hyperemia of the myocardial stroma, muscle fiber damage with swelling, and loss of cross striation. Potassium levels in the myocardium were also lower than in victims not poisoned by CO (119). Anderson demonstrated the development of angina pectoris, arrhythmias, or infarction in patients with preexisting heart disease (4). Aronow et al. (6, 8) and Mofenson et al. (132) documented that COHb levels above 15% increased the risk for myocardial infarction. A 9% COHb level lowers the ventricular fibrillation threshold (52), and also causes intermittent claudication in patients with peripheral vascular disease (7). Allred et al. (3) studied patients with atherosclerotic cardiovascular disease exposed to low concentrations of carbon monoxide while undergoing exercise on a treadmill. Their changes, documented electrocardiographically, showed a significant dose-response relationship with the length of time to the ST endpoint (P<0.0001), and change in the "length of time until the onset of angina" (P=0.02) on the treadmill. They concluded that low levels of COHb exacerbated myocardial ischemia during graded exercise (3).

Occupational exposure of patients with coronary artery disease to CO exacerbates the clinical problems, even to the extent of causing death. Atkins and Baker described two workers dying from CO exposure with COHb levels in the 20 to 30% range; preexisting heart disease and atherosclerosis were documented at autopsy (11). It was felt that the COHb level alone was insufficient to produce death from central nervous system toxicity, and that the cardiac arrhythmia was the major factor. The authors recommended that the working environment should be better controlled to prevent sudden death in patients with coronary artery disease, rather than requiring pre-placement examination of all people entering the work force. Thus, occupational exposure to CO is an area for much concern. Emergency physicians should consider this type of poisoning when treating patients with myocardial infarctions or angina (11). There is also a concern that exposure to CO may accelerate atherosclerotic vascular disease (43, 73, 80, 107, 136, 158, 159, 197). However, significant gaps in our understanding of this association persist (85, 103).

Hammond (76) showed that men between the ages of 40 and 49, smoking 40 cigarettes per day, had a five times greater risk of dying from ischemic heart disease than nonsmokers. Doll and Hill showed that smoking more than 15 cigarettes a day tripled the risk of dying from ischemic heart disease in men aged 45 to 55 (53). Wald et al. showed that people with COHb levels of 5% or more were 21 times more likely to have atherosclerotic diseases, including ischemic heart disease, than similar aged and sexed people with COHb levels less than 3% (223). In 2006, Henry et al. published a report which surprisingly showed that following an acute CO poisoning with apparent complete recovery with HBO treatment, myocardial infarction rates were several times that of controls when followed up for 10 years or more (79A).

Pre-existent chronic obstructive pulmonary disease can also reduce exercise tolerance in patients with COHb levels as low as 9%. This may result in acute pulmonary decompensation (133). Heavy smokers may reduce their exercise tolerance with COHb levels as low as 9% (31).

It is extremely rare to find the cherry red color that is classically described in CO poisoning. This sign represents a true soaking of the tissues with CO over a significant length of time. Thus it is a classical finding at autopsy, but contrary to popular belief, is not a clinical presentation. Any evidence of smoke or toxic-gas inhalation, and a history of exposure to a fire resulting in soot in the nasal or upper airways, singed nasal hair, and voice changes must be considered as an indicator of exposure to CO. Another uncommon finding is rhabdomyolysis (168), which can lead to acute tubular necrosis and renal failure (19). Skin lesions may present with superficial blisters similar to those seen in burns (140). This, however, like rhabdomyolysis, is rare and relates to severe CO poisoning. Ophthalmologic manifestations include retinal hemorrhages, papilledema, blindness, homonymous hemianopsia, and paracentral scotomata (50, 100). Damage to the labyrinth, eighth nerve, or brain stem nuclei results in loss of balance, ataxia, nystagmus, hearing loss, and tinnitus (132).

## NEUROPSYCHIATRIC PRESENTATIONS

Neuropsychiatric manifestations of CO poisoning include non-focal alterations in mental status, seizures, amnesia, apraxia, agnosia, Parkinsonism, cortical blindness, incontinence, and peripheral neuropathy (60). The first major follow-up evaluation of unconscious CO victims was by Smith and Brandon (193). They documented, on a 3-year follow-up, a 33% personality deterioration, and a 43% memory impairment. These deficits were directly related to the level of consciousness on admission. A further eight patients showed gross neuropsychiatric damage.

Central nervous system morbidity is most often subtle, and nearly always overlooked in the normal situation (96). Traditionally, the method of assessing the neurologic normality of a patient is the use of the Glasgow Coma Scale and general orientation questions. The normal routine is to question the patient for his or her name, age, address, and present date. Unless the personal information is corroborated by a friend or family member, the clinician may never know the true answers. If the patient's response is rapid, it is assumed to be correct. Errors are invariably overlooked in favor of the patient, and the environmental tensions induced by the emergency department. In reality, abnormal responses may represent neurologic involvement from CO poisoning. A short neuropsychometric screening battery, as that first developed at the Maryland Institute for Emergency Medical Services Systems (MIEMSS), can be administered in an emergency setting (128). The battery has the following components: General Orientation to establish a rapport with the patient and develop an informal assessment of mental status; the Digit Span, assessing short-term memory and ability to maintain attention and function; Trail Making tests A & B, testing visual discrimination and temporospatial orientation; Digit Symbols, assessing visuomotor coordination and visual discrimination; Aphasia Screening, evaluating a variety of language and praxic functions; and the Block Design test, assessing visuospatial function (1, 17, 63, 229). Recently, using another battery of tests, CO-poisoned patents were shown to have impaired context-aided memory, and to have improved function after hyperbaric oxygen therapy (125). The test batteries described above appear to be helpful in determining subtle dysfunction.

# DELAYED NEUROPSYCHIATRIC PRESENTATION

Patients may appear to recover from acute CO poisoning, and then develop abnormalities from 1 to 21 days later (230, 235). Included in the presentation of the delayed syndrome may be aphasia, apraxia, apathy, disorientation, hallucinations, nuchal rigidity, gait disturbances, fecal and urinary incontinence, and bradykinesia. Cognitive and neurologic deficits may also be present, as can be personality changes with impulsiveness, violence, verbal aggressiveness, and mood changes. The reported incidence of this syndrome ranges from 3 to 47% (38, 193, 235). The true incidence of delayed presentation may be higher, because personality and pathologic changes are often subtle and overlooked (230). There are no clinical indicators that will predict the occurrence of this syndrome, but psychometric testing may allow earlier detection of the problem. It is prudent for patients to be followed closely for a minimum of 10 days, following CO exposure, to rule out these subtle neurologic changes. The mechanism for this delayed neuropsychiatric deterioration has always been puzzling. It is hard to understand how a CO-poisoned neuron can appear to recover completely, function normally for days to weeks and then precipitously fail to function. Several investigators have looked at this phenomenon and on the basis of brain biopsies and histologic studies it appears that the oligodendroglia could be a root cause. There is no question that myelin in the white matter is severely attacked by CO and CT scans, MRIs, and autopsy findings amply bear this out. Myelin is produced by the oligodendrocytes in fetal life and it is maintained by these same cells in adult life. The oligodendroglias are extremely sensitive to CO and in acute CO poisoning they are quickly killed. The myelin continues to function normally for several days to weeks, but eventually as it is supposed to be recycled and replaced, the oligodendrocytes are not there to accomplish it. Electron microscopy reveals the neurofibrils to be entirely intact, but the myelin supporting structures are severely damaged or absent (100A).

# CARBON MONOXIDE POISONING IN CHILDREN

Ninety percent of children presenting with CO poisoning have their exposure in the home (49). Gastrointestinal disturbances (nausea, vomiting, and diarrhea) occur early and the COHb levels at presentation may be lower than those in the adult. The diagnosis is often overlooked or incorrect (61). Lethargy and syncope are the most important symptoms in children (49).

The handling of a child in a hyperbaric environment may be complex. In a 22-year period at the Shock Trauma Center in Baltimore, 88 pediatric patients with CO poisoning were managed. Thirty-two of the children required myringotomies and three required pressure-equalizing tubes. Five of these patients (5.6%) developed middle ear barotrauma and two (2.2%) developed convulsions from oxygen toxicity. Both of these patients were unconscious and on ventilators and receiving 3 atmospheres of absolute (ATA) oxygen. Twenty-four of the children (27.2%) required endotracheal tubes and/or ventilation. Eighty-one of the 88 patients (92%) had a favorable outcome, with a return to normal at the end of the treatment. In 6 patients (6.9%) there was no change; all suffered cardiac arrest at the scene, and arrived unconscious with fixed pupils. In essence, they were considered brain dead before arriving in the chamber. It was felt that at least one treatment should be undertaken to be sure that the patient's status could not be changed. An additional patient was determined to be dead on arrival, having been in full arrest at the scene. If the seven patients who were considered dead before treatment are removed from this series, the outcome is 100% favorable in these children. The low complication rate enables us to conclude that there is no contraindication to treating children with CO poisoning with hyperbaric oxygen.

## DIAGNOSIS

A high index of suspicion of CO poisoning must be maintained at all times. Diagnosing the acute exposure is relatively simple if the patient has been in a fire, a known exhaust situation, or an industry where the possibility of CO generation is high. In the home, exposure to CO may be more subtle; the source of the poison may not be recognized as the furnace or blocked flues. In this situation, findings such as the development of flu-like symptoms in many members of the family, or even problems with pets, must make the physician consider CO as a potential source of the problems. The general clinical presentation in the early phase is nausea, vomiting, mental confusion, dizziness, and periods of unconsciousness. A compounding factor is the frequency with which alcohol is involved and, consequent to alcohol and smoking, fires.

Whenever the diagnosis is considered, certain investigative steps must be undertaken. The simplest, most conclusive test for the presence of CO in the body is determination of the COHb level. This measures the load of CO present in red blood cells, but does not assess consequent cellular CO-associated effects that may be involved with injuries in the myocardium and brain. Either an arterial or a venous blood sample may be used to measure COHb, because the levels are the same. In using an arterial blood gas, one must not attempt to extrapolate an oxygen partial pressure level as reflecting the non-saturating component equilibrating to COHb levels. Most blood gas analyzers use the $PaO_2$ value to calculate the total oxygen content and hemoglobin saturations, which are not, measured levels. When they are specifically measured, they may reflect the loading of CO onto red cells. To measure the blood COHb level, a CO oximetric determination must be made. More recently, specific finger tip detectors that look like pulse oximeters have been introduced using lasers producing 7 different wavelengths. specifically tuned to frequencies that reflect CO and methemoglobin (Masimo Corporation, Irvine, CA www.masimo.com). The ordinary pulse oximeter cannot distinguish between oxyhemoglobin and carboxyhemoglobin. Using this new instrument one can get an instant CO saturation level without having to send a blood sample to the lab. In general, the arterial blood gases demonstrate nonspecific changes, but metabolic acidosis may indicate a more severe CO poisoning. A weak correlation exists between the actual pH and the COHb level in the initial arterial gas. With hypoxia and acidosis, there is a stronger correlation between high COHb levels and acidosis. It must be stressed, however, that in our experience (142), at COHb levels ranging from below 10% to 62%, patients have presented with acidosis, alkalosis, or normal blood gases and have equally severe neurologic symptoms. We have found greater correlation between abnormal psychometric test results and COHb levels, than between abnormal psychometric results and blood gases. Electrocardiographic abnormalities, with nonspecific ST wave changes and dysrhythmias have been used as evidence of CO poisoning in the past, as have computed tomography and magnetic resonance imaging. Electroencephalography may show diffuse frontal slow wave activity consistent with metabolic encephalopathy. This too has been used to infer CO poisoning. In essence, the only specific test for CO poisoning is COHb levels; unfortunately, the ability to perform this test is not present in every emergency department. CO levels in expired alveolar air may be used as another indicator of poisoning.

Once CO has been detected in the system, the effect of the CO on the patient must be determined. The two areas most commonly assessed are the myocardial status and the neurologic status. Chest radiographs are nonspecific, but are valuable in determining a baseline appearance, if smoke-inhalation injury has occurred. Changes may not be evident in the first 6 to 12 hours following exposure. Assays of the blood levels of lactate, creatinine kinase, and lactate dehydrogenase, as well as the serum levels of alanine transferase and aspartate transferase may be useful, although elevations are themselves nonspecific. Drug screening is carried out on the usual indications. Hyperglycemia is nonspecific, but may indicate an extreme degree of CO involvement of other systems such as internal organs and muscle. A lactate level above 10 mmol/liter may be a reliable, relatively rapid way to determine the presence of cyanide poisoning (14).

## PROGNOSTIC FACTORS

It is difficult to determine a prognosis for patients with mild to moderate exposure to CO poisoning, primarily because the COHb level is not a true indicator of severity of neurologic or cardiac involvement. For severely affected persons, poor prognostic indicators are prolonged coma; CT or magnetic resonance imaging abnormalities, particularly in the basal ganglion region (87, 182); and predisposing factors, such as heart disease and age. Until we are better able to do controlled comparative trials of various treatments, it will be difficult to predict outcomes. Long-term and severe psychiatric sequelae are also difficult to measure and compare. The writings describing these various conditions tend to be in earlier literature, that from the 1940s, 1950s, and 1960s, when the system for retrieval of patients from the scene and delivery to the hospital was radically different, and did not include oxygen as part of rescue resuscitation therapy. In today's world, there are rapid response times to fires and other emergencies, and early application of oxygen is a standard treatment modality. These interventions, though often life-saving, cloud the clinical presentation, affect the COHb level, and may alter the body's response to CO poisoning. The half-life of CO is rapidly reduced by higher oxygen concentrations; in 3 atmospheres of hyperbaric oxygen, the half-life is 23 minutes versus 320 minutes on air. However, there is great variation in the individual half-life, whether on air, 100% oxygen, or hyperbaric oxygen (142, 144, 235).

## PATIENT MANAGEMENT

### At the Scene

Today's pre-hospital care providers retrieving a person from a CO exposure would, in essence, clear the victim's airway, and then provide as high an oxygen concentration as they could with the available equipment, and commensurate with their level of training. The equipment may range from nasal prongs to facemasks to intubation and ventilation. The highest oxygen concentration possible can be achieved with endotracheal intubation, or with a reservoir oxygen bag in-line, with a tight fitting face mask firmly applied to the patient's face. The rigid plastic mask commonly used clinically in emergency rooms provides only 55 to 60 % oxygen when flow is set on flood. A good "test" for tightness is to ask oneself if the patient could breathe from the mask lying on his back under water. An IV line is established to obtain a blood sample measurement of COHb, and to be able to administer drugs, should cardiac arrhythmias develop. All of the accepted advanced cardiac and trauma life support (2) protocols should be followed to ensure safe stabilized transport of the patient. Unconscious patients, or patients showing evidence of respiratory distress, should be intubated as early as possible. If intubation is done in the field, it is followed by ventilation with an Ambu or Laerdal bag until arrival at the hospital, where the patient would be switched to a ventilator.

### Hospital Treatment

Unconscious patients need to be examined to exclude other causes of unconsciousness, and to identify associated injuries that might have been sustained in the traumatic event. It is essential to do a full work-up of the patient, as advocated in the Advanced Trauma Life Support course (2). A detailed neurologic assessment must be undertaken. Patients who present with hypotension or arrhythmias may require fluid resuscitation and the use of lidocaine and dopamine. An EKG is most helpful in ruling out myocardial infarction; this is particularly important in patients with known coronary artery disease who are exposed to CO. Routine blood tests should be done, particularly for COHb levels, but also for the previously mentioned substances, such as agents measuring muscle breakdown.

The critical determination is the severity of the poisoning. In general, patients who should be observed in the emergency department or admitted to the hospital are those with the following problems:

1. COHb levels greater than or equal to 25%.
2. History of ischemic heart disease and COHb level greater than 15%.
3. COHb levels greater than 10% in a pregnant woman, leading to concern about the effects of CO on the fetus.
4. Ischemic chest pains and/or electrocardiographic evidence of ischemia.
5. Metabolic acidosis.
6. Abnormal psychometric testing.
7. History of unconsciousness.

8. Patients who remain symptomatic following 4 hours of 100% oxygen treatment.

9. Those patients arriving moderately symptomatic, but conscious, and with suspected CO poisoning at a hospital that lacks the ability to test COHb.

The majority of patients seen in emergency departments have a mild exposure to CO and become asymptomatic after receiving 100% oxygen for 3 to 4 hours. In this situation, the asymptomatic patient may then be sent home with the admonition to return should there be any recurrence of symptomatology within the next 7 to 10 days. In general, this type of patient may rapidly return to normal activity after a 24-hour layoff. It is also important to determine the source of CO in the home or industrial setting, and control it. Our policy has been to follow patients after discharge from the emergency department or hyperbaric chamber facility with a phone call between 7 and 10 days after the episode. The patients are also advised in writing that, if they have any symptoms, including neurologic deterioration, headaches, nausea, confusion, irritability, or personality change, they should contact us immediately for reassessment. We have noted that 12% to 23% of patients treated with surface oxygen develop delayed or recurrent sequelae between 1 and 21 days after their original exposure (141, 214).

## Oxygen Treatment

Until recently, controversy existed as to the optimal method of treatment of CO poisoning; using 100% surface oxygen as opposed to hyperbaric oxygen at 2.8 atmospheres of pressure. An historical review of treatment theory and practice was compiled by Youngberg (235). Youngberg's review of the literature dated from 1857 and included pathophysiologic theories, relationship to current standards of clinical practice, and the major case series where treatment, using either surface or hyperbaric oxygen, was tabulated. The difficulty in drawing direct conclusions from this work stems from the wide variability in the manner with which authors assessed severity of primary exposure, and methods used to determine morbidity (particularly neurological disturbances). These difficulties persist in modern investigations, as well.

Essential for assessment of treatment efficacy is the incidence of complications of care occurring both with hyperbaric oxygen and surface oxygen as a component of the total outcome. The types of complications seen with hyperbaric oxygen include oxygen tonic seizures, nausea, vertigo, visual problems, barotrauma, and claustrophobia. It is difficult to ascertain from the literature the total number of oxygen complications. At the Shock Trauma Center in Baltimore, from 1978 to 1983, 891 patients underwent 14,966 treatments at depths ranging from 2 to 3 ATA. Oxygen toxicity occurred in 0.92% of treatments, and seizures in 0.21%. Other symptoms, including nausea, vomiting, muscle twitching, anxiety, respiratory changes, vertigo, behavior changes, visual changes, sweating, and auditory changes, occurred during the treatment. No patients had any permanent sequelae, and the majority of these complications occurred within the first 10 treatments in the patients' exposure to oxygen. Between July 1988 and January 1989, 4,110 patient treatments were done, with 20 complications. Three patients had oxygen toxicity in the form of seizures in two, and sweating in one. Thus, the incidence of oxygen toxicity is thus 0.07% of total treatments given. Two other patients had visual disturbances after 60 treatments, with complete resolution of the visual problems after cessation of therapy. One case of claustrophobia was reported, and one case of pneumothorax, unrelated to hyperbaric therapy treatment, was noted. Fourteen patients had ear and sinus barotrauma, which resolved without significant treatment. The total complication rate in the 7-month period was 0.4% with no permanent sequelae. From this experience and other published reports (86), it can be seen that problems encountered during hyperbaric oxygen treatment for all conditions are relatively small and infrequent. Similarly, a detailed summary of the management of critically ill children in hyperbaric chambers shows that, although complications do occur, most can be managed easily by a skilled clinical team (99).

Complications among patients treated with surface oxygen present a different picture. Krantz and colleagues (106), describing a series of 79 patients, found that 24 had direct care complications contributive to their long and serious coma, which was caused by CO poisoning. At their facility, treatment was on surface oxygen, and the complication rate was 30.4%, which is higher than what we experienced, or has been seen by others. Min et al. (131) had 24 surface-oxygen-treated patients with decubitus ulcers, 8 with pneumonias, and 3 with sepsis directly related to the long hospital stay. The complication rate was 4.9% among 738 patient admissions. These complications arise due to prolonged coma, which, based on the previously discussed figures, is higher by 5 to 30-fold than in hyperbaric-treated patients.

Since 1960, hyperbaric oxygen has been used with increasing frequency for severe CO poisoning, as clinical recovery has appeared to be improved beyond that expected with ambient pressure oxygen therapy (68, 122, 124, 141, 194, 214). However, the first prospective clinical trial involving hyperbaric oxygen therapy failed to find it to be superior to ambient pressure treatment (172). This study has been criticized because the authors used a low oxygen partial pressure 2 ATA versus the more usual protocols with 2.5 to 3 ATA), and because, in nearly half of the study population hyperbaric treatments were initiated more than 6 hours after patients were discovered (164). In 1969, a retrospective study indicated that hyperbaric oxygen reduced mortality and morbidity, only if administered within 6 hours after CO poisoning (69).

At the Shock Trauma Center in Baltimore, 1,271 carbon-monoxide-poisoned patients were treated between 1967 and 1993. Our experience indicates clinical benefit of hyperbaric oxygen therapy over surface oxygen (e.g., lower rates of complications and subsequent neurologic sequelae). Of 1,271 patients, 822 were treated with hyperbaric oxygen, and 449 with surface oxygen. Psychometric testing was employed, after 1978 (the year the test was developed), to evaluate cognitive function (128). The tests could not be administered to patients who were unconscious, intubated, or otherwise unable to cooperate.

The patients' average age was 36.3 years (range, 0.25 to 92 years). Most patients were 20 to 40 years of age, followed by the 41- to 50-year-old group, and the 11- to 20-year-old group. Fifty-nine percent of the patients were male. More patients were seen during the winter months (November through March) than at other times of year. Eleven percent of the patients were children, 9% had attempted suicide, and 2% were pregnant women. Records of presenting signs and symptoms were available for 809 patients. The most common were loss of consciousness (n=569), headache (n=294), nausea and vomiting (n=255), dizziness (n=126), lightheadedness (n=74), shortness of breath (n=72), weakness (n=45), and blurred vision (n=14). Thirty patients were asymptomatic.

Sources of carbon monoxide included the following: house fires (46%), malfunctioning home furnace (24%), automobile exhaust (16%), work equipment (9%), work fire (3%), and other (2%). Among the 646 patients whose records indicated exposure only to carbon monoxide, 449 were treated with hyperbaric oxygen and 197 with surface oxygen. Of the 608 smoke inhalation victims, 360 received hyperbaric oxygen and 248 received surface oxygen.

The average COHb level for the 809 hyperbaric oxygen-treated patients was 29.8 at the scene (range, 0.5 to 75) and 15.2 on admission to hospital (range, 0.4 to 79). For the 445 treated with surface oxygen, the average on-scene level was 16.1 (range, 0.5 to 54.1) and the average level at admission was 6.6 (range, 0.1 to 37.4). The admission pH level for the hyperbaric oxygen-treated group was 7.36 (range, 6.73 to 7.73) and, for the surface-oxygen-treated group, 7.4 (range, 7.16 to 7.67). The time between exposure and treatment averaged 12 hours (range, 2 to 60).

The patients exposed only to CO averaged two hyperbaric oxygen treatments (range, 1 to 34). The smoke-inhalation group received an average of 3.5 treatments, with a range of 1 to 49. Eighty percent of the patients received 36% of all treatments.

During 2,184 treatments, there were 36 episodes of barotrauma and 17 of central nervous system oxygen toxicity, yielding a total complication rate of 2.4%. Two hundred thirty-four patients (29%) required pressure-equalizing tubes (grommets) or myringotomy.

Of the surface-oxygen-treated group, 428 patients recovered completely. Symptoms recurred (without re-exposure to carbon monoxide) in 17 patients (3.8%). Eleven patients were referred for hyperbaric oxygen, and 47 had an unclear outcome.

In the hyperbaric-oxygen-treated group, recurrent symptoms requiring re-treatment emerged in only two patients (0.2%). Ninety-two percent of the HBO-treated patients returned to normal levels. Improvement was seen in 12 patients, and 18 interrupted their treatments. Twelve patients (2.4%) showed no change in mental status, and 33 patients (5%) were declared dead. For non-survivors, the average pH was 7.29 (range, 6.73 to 7.62). The Glasgow Coma Scale score was <6 in 94% of cases, and all 33 were ventilated at arrival. Seventy-nine percent of the patients who were declared dead, or who had no change in status, had a full cardiopulmonary arrest.

In our experience, the CONSB neuropsychometric test (128) remains the most sensitive indicator of central nervous system dysfunction, following carbon monoxide poisoning. We are in the process of shortening the 25-

minute test to one requiring only 10 minutes. Preliminary results suggest that the shortened version remains sensitive to cognitive dysfunction and thus may further simplify evaluation of carbon monoxide poisoned patients.

No definition has been established for staging the severity of CO poisoning. Therefore, it remains difficult to evaluate patients in a prospective manner or compare the efficacy of different treatments. Current recommendations for hyperbaric oxygen therapy are based on an aim to treat those with the greatest mortality and morbidity risks. This includes patients who have suffered some interval of unconsciousness due to CO (86). Some centers have proposed using a psychometric screening test to identify patients with subtle neurological compromise and as a method to identify patients needing hyperbaric oxygen therapy. We recently published a prospective, randomized investigation involving 60 patients. These patients appeared to suffer from mild to moderately severe poisoning, they had symptoms such as headache, nausea, and lethargy, but none of the signs or symptoms presumed to be associated with severe poisoning, such as ischemic changes on electrocardiogram or a history of unconsciousness (214). Delayed neurological sequelae were defined as development of new neurological symptoms, and also as reductions from original scores on the standardized psychometric battery developed at MIEMSS. The initial test scores were not helpful in identifying those who went on to suffer delayed sequelae. Twenty-three percent of patients (7 of 30) treated with ambient pressure oxygen developed neurological sequelae 6+1(SE) days after poisoning and sequelae persisted for 41+8 days. No patients (0 of 30) [p<0.05] treated with hyperbaric oxygen (2.8 ATA) developed sequelae.

Hyperbaric oxygen therapy was also found to have a significant benefit in another prospective, randomized trial (54). Twenty-six patients were hospitalized within 2 hours of discovery, and they were equally divided between two treatment groups: Ambient pressure oxygen, or 2.5 ATA O2. Three weeks later, patients treated with hyperbaric oxygen had significantly fewer abnormalities on electroencephalogram, and SPECT scans showed that cerebral vessels had nearly normal reactivity to carbon dioxide, in contrast to diminished reactivity in patients treated with ambient pressure oxygen. Scheinkestel et al. (184) reported no benefit from hyperbaric oxygen therapy in a prospective trial of 179 patients. Unfortunately, the mean delay to treatment was 9.3 hours, only 42% of patients who entered the study were assessed to determine treatment efficacy, and the study design may have caused a false-positive rate of up to 33%. These issues severely diminish potential impact of the investigation.

Mathieu et al. (123) reported a much larger trial of hyperbaric oxygen therapy for patients with acute symptoms, including transient loss of consciousness (n=575 patients). Patients who were not treated with hyperbaric oxygen had a higher incidence of delayed sequelae, 15% versus 9.5%, among patients treated with hyperbaric oxygen. The differences between groups were statistically significant at interval examinations done at 3 and 6 months, but the difference was no longer significant at the 1 year follow-up examination. Slow recovery of cortical function in half, or more, of all patients has been described in studies going back to Shillito et al. from

1936 (187). Therefore, whereas the question of clinical efficacy for hyperbaric oxygen therapy may have been answered, it has been replaced with a more modern concern related to cost versus benefit.

In October 2002, in what appears to be a definitive paper, published in the ***New England Journal of Medicine*** by Weaver, et al., a new standard of care for CO patients is described (228A). The study design was a randomized (allocation concealed), blinded, (patients, outcome assessors and statisticians) controlled trial with follow-up at 6 weeks, 6 months and one year. One hundred and fifty two patients (mean age 36 yr, 62% male) with documented or obvious exposure to CO and any of 11 predetermined symptoms were treated. Patients excluded were those less than 16 years old, moribund or pregnant or if greater than 24 hours had elapsed since exposure. Follow-up at 6 weeks was 97%.

### Treatment protocol:

All patients had 3 hyperbaric chamber sessions at intervals of 6 to 12 hours within 24 hours after carbon monoxide exposure. Non-intubated patients received oxygen, 15 liters/min via a non-rebreathing face mask. Intubated patients were mechanically ventilated with 100% oxygen. Seventy-six patients were allocated to HBO and exposed to 100% oxygen at 3 atmospheres and then 2 atmospheres absolute during the first chamber session. One hundred percent oxygen was given at 2 atmospheres absolute for sessions 2 and 3. Seventy-six patients were allocated to normobaric oxygen and exposed to ambient pressure at one atmosphere absolute (sea level pressure) in the chamber for all three sessions.

### Main outcome measures:

Cognitive sequelae at 6 weeks were assessed using a battery of neuropsychological tests and were considered present if any subtest score was >=2 standard deviations (SDs) below the mean of demographically corrected standardized scores or if >=2 scores were 1 SD below the mean.

### Main results:

Analysis was by intention to treat. The trial was stopped early after 3 of 4 planned interim analyses were completed. At 6 weeks, 6 months and one year, patients in the hyperbaric group had fewer cognitive sequelae than did patients in the normobaric group. The analysis was adjusted for cerebellar dysfunction because it was not equally distributed (4 HBO vs. 15 normobaric group patients), with no change in results.

| Outcomes: | HBO Patients | Normobaric Patients |
|---|---|---|
| Neurologic sequelae at 6 wks | 25% | 46% |
| Neurologic sequelae at 6 mo | 25% | 46% |
| Neurologic sequelae at 1 yr | 18% | 44% |

## *Details of HBO Treatment Protocol:*

First HBO Treatment:

>Pressurization to 3 ATA over 15 minutes. Two 25-minute oxygen breathing periods separated by a 5-minute air break. Then one more 5-minute air break at 3 ATA followed by two 30-minute oxygen breathing periods at 2 ATA separated by a 5-minute air break. Return to surface over 15 minutes breathing oxygen.

Chamber Sessions 2 and 3:

>Pressurization to 2 ATA over 10 minutes. Three 30-minute oxygen breathing periods separated by two 5-minute air breaks. Return to surface over 10 minutes breathing oxygen.

One must remember that until reliable diagnostic tests are identified to prospectively determine the relative risk of carbon monoxide poisoning, a conservative treatment plan is likely to be in the patient's best interest. In other words, when in doubt it is better to treat with HBO than not.

Below you will see Dr. Weaver's treatment profiles in graphic form. Dr. Weaver started pressurization commencing at 0.85 ATA instead of 1 ATA (Figure 1). This is because Salt Lake City, where the study was carried out, is at high altitude and not at sea level. Dr. Weaver compensated for this in treating his patients so that they got an identical amount of oxygen as those treated at sea level.

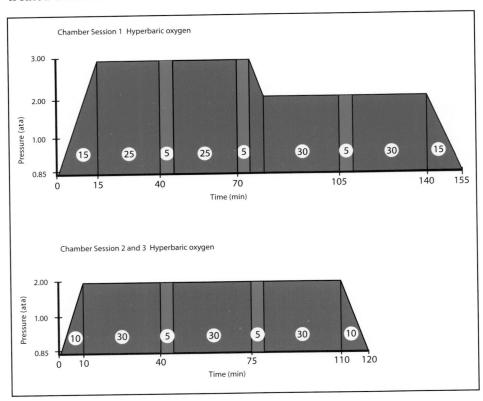

Figure 1. Weaver protocol for treatment of acute CO poisoning.

For patients who were  controls  treated with oxygen at one ATA, the chamber pressure was slightly increased from 0.85 ATA to 1 ATA. The total treatment time was 2 hours (120 minutes) with 5-minute airbreaks at 40 and 80 minutes. This would correspond to normobaric oxygen treatment at sea level.

## CONCLUSION

The ultimate decision for the use of surface oxygen versus hyperbaric oxygen treatment should be based on neurologic presentation, rather than the COHb level alone. There is overwhelming evidence to support the use of hyperbaric oxygen in CO poisoning when there is a risk of mortality or morbidity. In terms of defining clear guidelines for referral for hyperbaric oxygen treatment, however, the major dilemma appears to be in establishing a threshold for poisoning severity below which clinical outcomes are not favorably affected by hyperbaric oxygen (e.g., reference 94). There is little doubt that patients should be referred for emergency treatment when they are comatose or have suffered an interval of unconsciousness. Some centers regularly prescribe hyperbaric oxygen therapy for patients with neurologic impairment documented by psychometric testing or other means of neuropsychological assessment; patients with COHb levels over 40%; patients who are pregnant and have COHb levels over 15% (assuming that the fetus is being treated); patients with a history of ischemic heart disease and a COHb level of 20% or above; patients who have been treated with surface oxygen and develop recurrent symptomatology up to 3 weeks after the original treatment, and patients whose symptoms do not resolve after 4 to 6 hours of continuous 100% oxygen. Separate from the question of hyperbaric therapy, serious consideration should be given to close monitoring of patients with cardiovascular involvement, including angina, ischemic ECG changes, cardiac arrhythmias, and a history of carbon monoxide exposure.

With the present-day advanced cardiac-life-support systems available for transportation, the hazards of transporting patients from a hospital without a hyperbaric facility to one with a chamber have been reduced dramatically. It is understood that all necessary intervention will be done, and that the patient will be stabilized as much as possible prior to transportation. This includes airway management, IV line placement, infusion of medications and, when necessary, ventilators. It is essential that patients with cardiac arrhythmias, or previous cardiac arrest, will be stabilized first and then transferred at a later time, even though their carbon monoxide level has dropped.

Experience in Milwaukee with helicopter transport of CO patients from 1984 to 1989, consisted of 59 patients transported with a mean Glasgow Coma Scale (GCS) of 12.8. Sixteen patients were intubated with a mean GCS of 6.4. Four patients later died who had a mean GCS of 3.7 during flight. No patients died during helicopter flight. In severe poisonings it is both advantageous and safe to transport patients by helicopter for hyperbaric treatment (110A).

The ultimate decision to treat a patient with 100% oxygen at a local hospital, or to transfer that patient to a hyperbaric facility, will remain a difficult one to make. The community, transportation problems, available staff, and severity of symptoms must be considered. Each area should establish its own specific criteria, prior to a CO emergency, to determine which patients will be transferred. Information about the location of hyperbaric facilities in the continental United States and Canada is available from the Diver's Alert Network (DAN) at Duke University in Durham, North Carolina (919-684-8111). DAN operates a 24-hour service so that anyone exposed to CO can be sent for therapy in a hyperbaric facility if required.

## MECHANISMS OF ACTION

### CO Uptake and $O_2$ Transport

The portal of entry for CO into the body is the alveolar-capillary membrane; CO binding to hemoglobin follows. Because the relative affinity of CO for hemoglobin is approximately 200-fold greater than that of $O_2$, this is a central aspect to the dissemination of CO throughout the body. The dynamics of CO movement across the lung boundary are well described mathematically (e.g. Coburn-Forster-Kane equation) (40). Movement is influenced by the CO and $O_2$ partial pressures in inspired gas, the content of these two gases in the blood, pulmonary CO diffusivity, alveolar ventilation, the duration of exposure, and pulmonary perfusion.

Hypoxia is the most clearly recognized aspect of CO pathophysiology. Deprivation of $O_2$ to cells occurs by several mechanisms. Arterial blood $O_2$ content is decreased directly due to carboxyhemoglobin (COHb), since CO renders the involved hemoglobin unable to bind $O_2$. During the later stages of CO exposure, alveolar $O_2$ content, and hence arterial $O_2$ tension, can decrease as a result of respiratory suppression. The hypoxic stress is worsened indirectly due to a leftward shift of the oxyhemoglobin dissociation curve. This shift occurs primarily because of the presence of COHb in erythrocytes. Early in the course of CO exposure, a small contribution to the leftward shift arises due to hyperventilation-induced respiratory alkalosis.

### Blood Flow, Cardiac Effects, and Extravascular CO Binding

Organ blood flow rises within minutes following exposure to CO. For example, brain perfusion increases 47% above normal in lambs exposed to 1,000 ppm CO (104). Exposure to 3,000 ppm CO can cause brain blood flow to rise 450% in cats (196). A dose/response relationship has been observed in rats, with increases in brain flow of 200 to 400% occurring due to exposures to 5,000 to 20,000 ppm CO (117). Vasodilation in response to high concentrations of CO is linked to extravascular acidosis, and hypoxic stimulation of the carotid bodies (109, 117). However, cerebral blood flow will increase with CO exposure, even in situations where brain tissue exhibits no metabolic irregularities, including hypoxia. Recent studies indicate that cerebral vasodilation, early during CO exposure is mediated through the release of the free radical, nitric oxide [NO] (124, 126, 127).

Although local tissue blood flow is markedly elevated early during exposure to CO, animals sustain a temporary drop in systemic blood pressure as time of exposure becomes prolonged. This change appears to be accentuated in some vascular beds. For example, Song et al. studied the cardiovascular responses of cats to 3,000 ppm CO for 90 to 193 minutes (196). Brain blood flow increased 200% within minutes while mean systemic blood pressure decreased somewhat, from 150 to 100 mmHg. The animals tolerated this state for approximately 2 hours, and then blood pressure dropped to about 70 mmHg. Although systemic pressure dropped only approximately 30%, blood flow in several areas of the brain dropped by 100% (back to the normal blood flow rate from the previous, two-fold increase). The sudden relative drop in local blood flow correlated with development of pathology in the globus pallidus. Development of brain pathology in several other animal models has also been associated with exposures that terminated with systemic hypotension and metabolic acidosis (64, 153).

When there is a period of hypotension that need last only seconds, lipid peroxidation of cell membranes may ensue. It has been shown that the products of lipid peroxidation will continue to rise even as the carbon monoxide levels fall. Lipid peroxidation is not inhibited by normobaric oxygen, but is dramatically inhibited at 3 ATA of oxygen. Clinically, anyone who has had even a brief period of syncope can be presumed to have had an episode of hypotension and consequent initiation of lipid peroxidation. This finding alone would indicate mandatory hyperbaric treatment.

The precipitous drop in blood pressure in animal studies is associated with electrocardiographic evidence of myocardial compromise (e.g. ventricular dysrhythmias, ST segment evaluation, inverted or bi-phasic T-waves). Several investigators have suggested that myocardial compromise may be related to CO binding to myoglobin (39, 64, 200). As myoglobin is an intracellular protein which facilitates $O_2$ transport from hemoglobin to mitochondria, abnormal functioning of the protein is most likely to be seen in muscles with high metabolic demand—hence the myocardium. Loading of myoglobin with CO is quite feasible from a biochemical perspective, as its affinity for CO is 40 times greater than for $O_2$. Coburn estimated that myoglobin may be the principal protein responsible for extravascular CO binding, which accounts for 10 to15% of the total body burden (39).

CO binding to extravascular proteins in addition to myoglobin is possible, particularly during hypoxic conditions. Binding to cytochrome P450 has been observed, although no pathophysiological significance for this has been found (176). CO can also bind to cytochrome c oxidase (28, 33). Hypotension and hypoxia augment this process *in vivo* (41, 42). Brown and Piantadosi have shown experimentally that during exposure to 5,000 to 10,000 ppm CO, as the COHb level rises and hypotension occurs, some binding of CO to cytochrome c oxidase can be detected (27). This binding may cause cellular stress.

## CO Pathophysiology, the Likelihood for Overlapping Cascades

The mechanism of acute injuries from CO appears to be based on CO-mediated hypoxia; severe CO poisoning causes both mitochondrial dysfunction and oxidative stress in the central nervous system. Acute impairment of mitochondrial electron transport is caused by deficient $O_2$ delivery from the elevated COHb level and to CO binding by cytochromes. Mitochondrial dysfunction inhibits ATP synthesis and causes mitochondria to generate hydroxyl-like radicals (28, 165). Energy production and mitochondrial function are restored after COHb levels decrease (28). In contrast, the mechanisms associated with delayed neurological injuries appear to be more complex, as they have not been found to be correlated with elevated COHb levels (28, 60, 141, 214, 232).

As was discussed above, clinical reports have frequently noted vascular insults to precede or coincide with neurological deficits. At least one biochemical mechanism by which CO can damage vascular endothelium is via .NO. Exposure to CO at concentrations as low as 50 ppm causes systemic vascular oxidative stress (207, 210, 213). CO enhances the rate of release of NO from both platelets and endothelial cells (215, 211), animals exposed to CO exhibit increases in the concentration of .NO in both lung and brain, based on electron paramagnetic resonance spectroscopy (88, 213). At CO concentrations less than 3,000 ppm, nitric oxide synthase activity is unchanged from control, but CO competes with .NO for intracellular hemoprotein binding sites (211, 213, 215). Therefore, the steady state concentration of .NO rises and allows for alternative reactions, including the reaction between superoxide anion ($O_2.-$) and .NO to yield the potent oxidizing and nitrating agent, peroxynitrite. Nitrotyrosine, the product of protein tyrosine nitration by peroxynitrite, is increased in aorta, lung, and brain after exposure to CO, and it is found closely associated with the vascular endothelium (88, 210, 213).

Endothelial .NO-mediated changes are a prerequisite for leukocyte adherence to the cerebral microvasculature following CO poisoning. Leukocyte adherence occurs after animals are removed from the CO-contaminated environment (88, 208). However, .NO-mediated oxidative stress alone is not sufficient to cause leukocyte sequestration. There must also be a change in cerebral blood flow. When rats are exposed to sufficient CO to cause unconsciousness, they invariably sustain a period of hypotension that is presumably mediated by cardiac hypoxic stress (124). Cerebral blood flow, which initially is above normal due to .NO-mediated vasodilation as well as CO-induced hypoxia, decreases to its baseline value or, in other studies, to about 50 % below normal for a period of 4 to 6 minutes when rats lose consciousness (124, 126, 196). It appears that the sudden alteration in microvascular flow causes leukocytes to adhere to endothelium. The factors responsible for initial adherence have not been identified, but beta-2 integrin adhesion molecules are required for subsequent leukocyte activation and progression of the oxidative stress cascade (88, 208).

Leukocyte activation occurs as beta-2 integrins interact with their endothelial (intercellular adhesion molecule; ICAM) counter-receptors (222). This occurs after experimental animals are removed from CO, based on the inhibitory potential of monoclonal antibodies to beta-2 integrins (208). Once leukocytes are adherent and activated, they liberate proteases and reactive $O_2$ species that cause conversion of endothelial xanthine dehydrogenase to xanthine oxidase, and xanthine oxidase activity is required for subsequent brain lipid peroxidation (88, 204, 205, 208). Whereas brain histology appears to be normal immediately after CO poisoning, studies have documented both impaired learning and localized areas with metabolic defects in the basal ganglia and hippocampus three weeks after poisoning (207, 216).

CO poisoning causes elevations of glutamate, norepinephrine, and dopamine in brains of experimental animals and in human fatalities (10, 89, 90, 147, 148, 149, 167). Enzymatic breakdown, as well as auto-oxidation of the monoamine neurotransmitters, will generate reactive oxygen species (21). Free radical production in brains of CO-poisoned rats can be reduced by inhibiting monoamine oxidase-B, an enzyme principally localized to microglia (166, 174). Based on the effects of agents that block the N-methyl-D-aspartate (NMDA) receptor, elevations of glutamate in experimental CO poisoning have been linked to delayed amnesia, but not acute amnesia, to the loss of CA1 neurons in the hippocampus of mice, and to the loss of glutamate-dependent cochlear ganglion cells of rats (89, 90, 112, 147, 148). Antioxidants can protect against CO-mediated cytotoxicity of glutamate-dependent nerve cells (57). Mechanisms of glutamate neurotoxicity include excessive calcium influx, free radical-mediated injury, which may include $Ca++$-calmodulin dependent activation of cytosolic nitric oxide synthase, and lipid peroxidation. Moderate stimulation by excitatory amino acids may cause mitochondrial dysfunction with impaired ATP synthesis, and production of reactive $O_2$ species (16). Cell death can be through necrosis or programmed cell death, depending on the intensity of the stimulus (72, 167). There may also be a synergistic injury with other forms of oxidative stress because reactive $O_2$ species can intensify excitotoxicity (26, 161). Glutamate can also injure cells in the central nervous system that do not have NMDA receptors by competing for cysteine uptake, which inhibits synthesis of glutathione (113, 139, 152).

Hemodynamic compromise and hypoxia precede the development of CO-mediated neuropathology (64, 82, 153). Particularly with regard to brain injury, the similarities are striking between CO poisoning and post-ischemic reperfusion injury, so-called post-anoxic encephalopathy. A common mechanistic basis has been hypothesized for these and several other forms of brain injury (146, 188). Indeed, brain lesions similar to those caused by CO poisoning occur under conditions of nitrogen hypoxia followed by cerebral ischemia (146). Findings such as these offer valuable insight into CO pathophysiology. However, these observations do not dismiss the possibility that there may be peculiar toxicological attributes to CO. In this regard, CO-mediated primary vascular effects, concurrent hypoxic stress, and excitotoxicity that may be linked to blood flow changes in brain, may all work in concert to precipitate one or more of the clinical manifestations of delayed neurological sequelae.

## Mechanisms of Action of Hyperbaric Oxygen in CO Poisoning

A major impediment to establishing the mechanism for the clinical benefit for hyperbaric oxygen has been, not surprisingly, our ignorance regarding CO pathophysiology. Based on current knowledge, reviewed in the previous section, there are at least three possible levels where hyperbaric oxygen may be acting.

Based on the law of mass action, elevated partial pressures of $O_2$ will accelerate the rate of CO dissociation from hemoglobin. Thus, COHb half-life can be decreased from approximately 5.5 hours when breathing air, and to approximately 23 minutes when breathing $O_2$ at 3 ATA (155). Indeed, this was the reasoning behind the first clinical implementation of hyperbaric oxygen therapy for CO poisoning (194). The efficacy of hyperbaric oxygen in clinical CO poisoning is discussed elsewhere in this chapter. As it does not appear that the COHb level is associated with clinical risk, it is hard to accept that a more rapid dissociation of CO from hemoglobin could be the central factor for the benefit of hyperbaric oxygen. A fraction of the acute mortality from CO is due to hypoxia, however, and in this regard, prompt removal of CO from hemoglobin will be of benefit (62). Peirce et al. demonstrated that hyperbaric oxygen significantly improved early survival in dogs subjected to severe CO poisoning (160). Restoration of consciousness and a hastened removal of CO from animals by hyperbaric oxygen was demonstrated in the classic studies of End and Long (55).

CO may bind to cytochrome c oxidase, particularly when the COHb level exceeds 40 to 50% (27). This may have an adverse effect on cellular oxidative metabolism. Depending upon the degree of electron transport chain branching, cytochrome oxidase inhibition may also enhance $O_2$ radical production by mitochondria (25). Brown and Piantadosi (27) demonstrated that hyperbaric oxygen at 3 ATA markedly accelerates the dissociation of CO from cytochrome oxidase, and hence would be expected to relieve whatever compromise in oxidative phosphorylation is caused by CO binding to cytochrome oxidase.

The third level of action of hyperbaric oxygen is related to the cascade of vascular injury triggered by CO poisoning (88, 204, 205, 209). Hyperbaric oxygen was found to be effective for preventing brain oxidative injury in animals because it inhibited leukocyte adherence to the vasculature that was mediated by beta-2 integrins (206). The mechanism appears to be associated with denaturation of a membrane-associated guanylate cyclase that plays a role in coordinating the elevated affinity of beta-2 integrins expressed on the cell surface (15, 33). Hyperbaric oxygen at partial pressures of 2.8 to 3 ATA inhibits beta-2 integrin function in human polymorphonuclear leukocytes, and the effect persists for approximately 12 hours after a 45-minute oxygen exposure (212). Given that vascular changes are prominent in clinical CO poisoning, it is feasible that neurological sequelae in patients may involve a perivascular injury mediated by leukocyte sequestration and activation, as was found in animals (88, 208). Hence, timely administration of hyperbaric oxygen may ameliorate the cascade leading to brain injury by inhibiting leukocyte sequestration.

## Cyanide Poisoning and Treatment

Cyanide produces an intracellular hypoxic poisoning due to the binding of cyanide anion to the ferric iron of mitochondrial cytochrome oxidase. Impaired oxidative phosphorylation results in the depletion of cellular high energy phosphate stores and lactic acidosis. The rapidity of cellular dysfunction and death are determined by the rate of entry of cyanide into the body. Thus, inhalation of a high concentration of hydrogen cyanide gas (e.g. 270 ppm) is immediately fatal to man (whole blood cyanide levels of approximately 3.0 ug/ml). Ingestion of cyanide-containing salts are less rapidly fatal. At lower doses, cyanide may cause symptoms such as tachycardia and depression in the level of consciousness (e.g., whole blood cyanide levels of 0.5 to 2.5 ug per ml) (46).

Specific treatment of cyanide poisoning traditionally has been aimed at dissociating cyanide from cytochrome oxidase by instilling into the circulation an agent which has a higher affinity for cyanide than does the ferrous iron moiety of cytochrome oxidase. The Lilly Cyanide Antidote Kit is currently the only specific cyanide antidote available in the United States. It contains amyl nitrite perles for inhalation, as well as vials of 10% sodium nitrite and 25% sodium thiosulfate for intravenous administration. Administration of nitrite by inhalation, and then intravenously (usual dose, 0.33 ml/kg of 10% sodium nitrite), is used to produce methemoglobin. The ferric iron of the heme moiety will bind cyanide, and thus free cytochrome oxidase to function in the respiratory chain. Sodium thiosulfate (usual dose, 1.65 ml/kg of 25% solution) is infused to provide sulfur for the enzyme, rhodanase. As cyanide dissociates from methemoglobin, rhodanase combines the cyanide with sulfur to form thiocyanate. Thiocyanate has very low toxicity and is excreted in the urine. This combination of agents was first proposed for treating cyanide poisoning by Chen et al. in 1930 (35), and it has been shown to be effective in both animal experiments and human poisonings (36, 114). It should be noted, however, that at least one report suggests that sodium nitrite therapy may not be based on the mechanism described above. Way et al. (227, 228) pretreated cyanide-poisoned animals with methylene blue to prevent subsequent methemoglobin formation by sodium nitrite. Nitrite therapy was equally effective whether or not methylene blue was introduced into the animals. The authors could not explain this result, but they suggested that a local vasodilation caused by nitrites might, somehow, influence the toxicity of cyanide.

Alternative antidotes to nitrite/thiosulfate are available in Europe. The motive for considering alternative therapies stems from the risk of nitrite toxicity. Too rapid administration can cause extreme vasodilatation and hypotension (36). Excessive methemoglobin formation, rendering a large fraction of hemoglobin unable to carry oxygen, can be fatal (18). Administration of a single therapeutic dose should produce a methemoglobin level of approximately 20% (36). It is generally recommended that methemoglobin levels be maintained at less than 40% (177).

Dicobalt-EDTA (Kelocyanor) binds with cyanide to form cobalticyanide, and is used for treatment in Britain and France (98). However, there is a risk of profound hypertension and cardiac dysrhythmias if this agent is administered mistakenly in the absence of cyanide. Given that the clinical detection methods for cyanide are relatively slow, these toxic effects are a legitimate concern. Hydroxocobalamin (vitamin B12a) appears to have almost no toxic effects and has been used clinically in France for more than 15 years. Hydroxocobalamin is infused to chelate cyanide, and sodium thiosulfate is administered to provide sulfur for rhodanase, just as it is with the Lilly Cyanide Antidote Kit (23, 233).

Antidote therapy and supporting vital signs are standard measures in the management of cyanide poisoning. Provision of supplemental oxygen is an additional treatment, and its importance cannot be overemphasized (45).

Ventilation with an oxygen-enriched gas mixture significantly decreases cyanide toxicity. Oxygen administration at ambient pressure diminishes sensitivity to low doses of cyanide in animal and human experiments (45, 46). Paulet investigated the effect of oxygen on the sensitivity of anesthetized dogs infused with a dose of sodium cyanide just sufficient to produce apnea (157). He found that even slight increases in oxygen partial pressure, to 1.03 ATA, improved respiratory function, compared with results with 1.0 ATA $O_2$, as well as the results with air. The slight excess oxygen pressure in this study was achieved with continuous positive airway pressure. Hyperbaric oxygen at 2.0 to 2.8 ATA decreases mortality from even high doses of cyanide in comparison with ambient pressure oxygen treatment (92, 192).

Compared with antidote treatment (nitrite/thiosulfate), oxygen treatment (100% at 1 ATA) by itself has no greater benefit, and often is less effective in maintaining aerobic metabolism and survival after cyanide poisoning. Combined nitrite/thiosulfate and oxygen treatments result in benefits significantly greater than when they are used individually (30, 91, 186, 226). Therefore, the practical consideration from these studies is that in the standard clinical setting, antidote therapy plus oxygen provides the greatest chance for therapeutic success. In the absence of antidote treatment, hyperbaric oxygen is of greater benefit than oxygen at 1 atmosphere pressure. While it seems reasonable that hyperbaric oxygen may have an even greater effect on survival versus ambient pressure oxygen, when combined with nitrite treatment, this was not found in a study by Way et al. (228). It is unclear, however, whether this observation may be related to the extraordinary oxygen pressure utilized (4 ATA for 2 hours). Experience with the current clinical recommendations for the use of hyperbaric oxygen, in cases refractory to standard management, is discussed elsewhere in this chapter.

Although one might debate the merit of hyperbaric oxygen versus ambient pressure oxygen, in conjunction with antidote therapy, the single greatest question with this subject is just what oxygen is doing to modify cyanide toxicity under any circumstances. When Warburg reported on his discovery of the "respiratory enzyme" (cytochrome oxidase) in 1926, he also described its inhibition by cyanide (224). The following year, he showed that inhibition by cyanide was independent of the partial pressure of oxygen (225). Paulet suggested that oxygen may be acting to increase respiration involving electron passage to alternative cytochromes (157). Cyanide-insensitive respiration has never been convincingly demonstrated in man. Takano et al. (201) have shown, however, that hyperbaric oxygen, more so than 1 ATA $O_2$, will maintain mitochondrial redox potential (i.e. electron transport function) despite the presence of cyanide administered at a lethal, "critical" level. They interpreted their data as being consistent with the so-called "branching" or "cushioning" in mitochondria that is preserved in the presence of high partial pressures of oxygen. Branching is a protective process whereby a constant electron flux can be maintained through cytochrome chains by allowing multiple chains to transfer electrons to whatever few cytochrome oxidase molecules still function, despite the presence of an inhibitor (e.g., cyanide). This interpretation is consistent with virtually all of the data on oxygen treatment. Moreover, the negative result of Way et al. (226) may be explainable by a related mechanism. Hyperbaric oxygen inhibits nicotine adenine dinucleotide (NAD) reduction. This effect is extremely small at partial pressures less than 3 ATA $O_2$, but quite prominent at 4 ATA $O_2$ or more (34).

## Combined Carbon Monoxide and Cyanide Exposure

Concurrent poisoning with carbon monoxide and cyanide is a relevant clinical problem in the treatment of patients suffering from smoke inhalation (22, 77, 117, 134, 99). Carbon monoxide and cyanide have been shown to be synergistic in producing lethality in a mouse model (151), which may explain a fraction of the mortality seen in smoke inhalation victims who die despite what might be considered sub-lethal carboxyhemoglobin levels (5, 134, 202). Beyond the arguments for utilization of hyperbaric oxygen for CO or CN, described above, additional issues exist regarding combined poisonings. Central to the treatment of cyanide poisoning is formation of methemoglobin, which normally is not a major cardiovascular stress at levels of between 20 and 40%. However, when there is concurrent carboxyhemoglobin, the added functional anemia caused by methemoglobin formation may have a severe adverse effect. Hypoxia caused by methemoglobinemia can be ameliorated with hyperbaric oxygen (67).

## CONCLUSION

Although hyperbaric oxygen therapy of CO poisoning was originally applied only to shorten the half life of carboxyhemoglobin and provide immediate oxygenation of the tissues, more recent research has revealed that the intra-cellular effects are paramount. Still further work is required to elucidate the exact mechanisms of how CO disrupts intra-cellular metabolism and, especially, the reasons for the "lucid interval" and the "late syndrome."

# REFERENCES

1. Adjutant General's Office: "The Trail Making Test, Parts A and B." U.S. Army, War Department. Washington, D.C., 1944.

2. "Advanced Trauma Life Support'" Committee on Trauma of the American College of Surgeons. 1988.

3. Allred EN, Bleecker ER, Chaitman BR, Dahms TE, Gottlieb SO, et al. "Short-term effects of carbon monoxide exposure on the exercise performance of subjects with coronary artery disease." N Engl J Med. 1989;321(210);1426-1432.

4. Anderson EW, Andelman RJ, Strauch JM, et al.: "Effect of low level carbon monoxide exposure on onset and duration of angina pectoris." Ann Intern Med. 1973;79:46-50.

5. Anderson, RA and Harland WA. "Fire deaths in the Glasgow area III: The role of hydrogen cyanide." Med Sci Law. 1982;22:35-39.

6. Aronow WS, Isbell MW. "Carbon monoxide effect on exercise-induced angina pectoris." Ann Intern Med. 1973;79:392.

7. Aronow WS, Stemmer EA, Isbell MW. "Effects of carbon monoxide exposure on intermittent claudication." Circulation. 1974;49:416.

8. Aronow WS, Cassidy J. "Effect of carbon monoxide on maximal treadmill exercise: A study in normal persons." Ann Intern Med. 1975;83:496.

9. Aronow WS, Harris CN, Isbell MW, et al. "Effect of freeway travel on angina pectoris." Ann Intern Med. 1972;77:669-676.

10. Arranz B, Blennow K, Eriksson A, Mansson JE, and Marcusson J. "Serotonergic, noradrenergic, and dopaminergic measures in suicide brains." Biol Psychiatry. 1997;41:1000-1009.

11. Atkins EH, Baker EL. "Exacerbation of coronary artery disease by occupational carbon monoxide exposure: A report of two fatalities and a review of the literature." Am J Ind Med. 1985;7:73-79.

12. Baker MD, Henretig FM, and Ludwig S. "Carboxyhemoglobin levels in children with nonspecific flu-like symptoms." J Pediat. 1988;113:501-504.

13. Barret L, Danel V, Faure J. "Carbon monoxide poisoning, a diagnosis frequently overlooked." Clin Toxicol. 1985;23:309.

14. Baud FJ, Barriot P, Toffis V, Riou B, Vicaut E, Lecarpentier Y, Bourdon R, and Astier A. "Elevated blood cyanide concentrations in victims of smoke inhalation." N Engl J Med. 1991;325:1761-1766.

15. Banick PD, Chen Q, Xu YA, and Thom SR. "Nitric oxide inhibits neutrophil bo2 integrin function by inhibiting membrane-associated cycle GMP synthesis." J Cell Physiol. 1997;172:12-24.

16. Beal MF. "Does impairment of energy metabolism result in excitotoxic neuronal death in neurodegenerative illness." Ann Neurol. 1992;31:119-130.

17. Benton AL. "Benton visual retention test: Clinical and experimental applications, 4th Ed." The Psychological Corp. New York, 1974.

18. Berlin Jr. CM. "The treatment of cyanide poisoning in children." Pediatrics. 1970;46:793-796.

19. Bessoudo R, Gray J. "Carbon monoxide poisoning and non-oliguric renal failure." Can Med Assoc J. 1978;119:41-44.

20. Bianco F, and Floris R. "Transient disappearance of bilateral low-density lesions of the globi pallidi in carbon monoxide intoxication and MRI." J Neuroradiol. 1988;15:381-385.

21. Bindoli A, Rigobello MP, Deeble DJ. "Biochemical and toxicological properties of the oxidation products of catecholamines." Free Rad Biol Med. 1992;13:391-404.

22. Birky MM and Clarke FB. "Inhalation of toxic products from fires." Bull NY Acad Med. 1981;57:997-1013.

23. Bismuth C, Cantineau JP, Pontal P. "Priorité de l'oxygenation dans l'intoxication cyanhydrique." J Toxicol Med. 1984;4:107-121.

24. Bissonnette JM, Wickham WK, Drummond WH. "Placental diffusing capacities at various carbon monoxide tensions." J Clin Invest. 1977;59:1038.

25. Boveris A, and Cadenas E. "Mitochondrial production of superoxide anions and its relationship to the antimycin insensitive respiration." FEBS Lett. 1975;54:311-314.

26. Bridges RJ, Koh JY, Hatalski CG, and Cotman CW. "Increased excitotoxic vulnerability of cortical cultures with reduced levels of glutathione." Eur J Pharmacol. 1991;192:199-200.

27. Brown SD and Piantadosi CA. "*in vivo* binding of carbon monoxide to cytochrome C oxidase in rat brain." J Appl Physiol. 1990;68:604-610.

28. Brown SD and Piantadosi CA. "Reversal of carbon monoxide-cytochrome C oxidase binding by hyperbaric oxygen *in vivo*." Adv Exp Biol Med. 1989;248:747-754.

29. Burnett RT, Dales RE, Brook JR, Raizenne ME, and Krewski D. "Association between ambient carbon monoxide levels and hospitalizations for congestive heart failure in the elderly in 10 Canadian cities." Epidemiology 1997;8:162-167.

30. Burrous GE and Way JL. "Cyanide intoxication in sheep: Therapeutic value of oxygen or cobalt." Am J Vet Res. 1977;38:223-227.

31. Caverley PMA, Leggett RJE, Flenley DC. "Carbon monoxide and exercise tolerance in chronic bronchitis and emphysema." Br Med J. 1981;283:875.

32. Centers for Disease Control, Mortality Morbidity Weekly Report. Carbon monoxide intoxication-A preventable environmental health hazard. 1982;31:529-531.

33. Chance B, Erecinska M, Wagner M. "Mitochondrial responses to carbon monoxide toxicity." Ann NY Acad Sci. 1970;174:193.

34. Chance B, Jamieson D, and Williamson JR. "Control of the oxidation-reduction state of reduced pyridine nucleotides *in vivo* and *in vitro* by hyperbaric oxygen." In: (Brown, IW and Cox BG, Eds.) Proceedings of the 3rd International Conference on Hyperbaric Medicine. National Academy of Science. 1966;14-41.

35. Chen KK, Rose CC, and Cloes GHA. "Methylene blue, nitrites and sodium thiosulfate against cyanide poisoning." Proc Soc Exp Biol Med. 1933;31:250-252.

36. Chen KK and Rose CL. "Nitrite and thiosulfate therapy in cyanide poisoning." JAMA. 1952;149:113-119.

37. Chen Q, Banick PD, and Thom SR. "Functional inhibition of rat polymorphonuclear leukocyte B2 integrins by hyperbaric oxygen is associated with impaired cGMP synthesis." J Pharmacol Expt'l Therap. 1996;276:929-933.

38. Choi IS. "Delayed neurologic sequelae in carbon monoxide intoxication." J Toxicol Clin Toxicol. 1982;19:297.

39. Coburn RF. "The carbon monoxide body stores." Ann NY Acad Sci. 1970;174:11-22.

40. Coburn RF, Forster RE, and Kane PB. "Considerations of the physiological variables that determine the blood carboxyhemoglobin concentration in man." J Clin Invest. 1965;44:1899-1910.

41. Coburn RF, Ploegmakers F, Gondric P et al. "Myocardial myoglobin oxygen tension." Am J Physiol. 1979;236:H307-H313.

42. Coburn RF, Wallace HW and Abboud R. "Redistribution of body carbon monoxide after hemorrhage." Am J Physiol. 1971;220:868-874.

43. Cohen SI, Deane M, and Goldsmith JR. "Carbon monoxide and survival from myocardial infarction." Arch Environ Health 1969;19:510-517.

44. Committee on Medical and Biologic Effects of Environmental Pollutants: Carbon Monoxide." National Research Council, National Academy of Sciences. Washington, D.C. 1977;28-37.

45. Cope C. "The importance of oxygen in the treatment of cyanide poisoning." JAMA. 1961;175:109-112.

46. Cope C and Abramowitz S. "Respiratory responses to intravenous sodium cyanide, a function of the oxygen cyanide relationship." Am Rev Respir Dis. 1960;81:321-328.

47. Courville CB. "The process of demyelination in the central nervous system." J Nerv Ment Dis 1957;125:504-546.

48. Cramer CR. "Fetal death due to accidental maternal carbon monoxide poisoning." J Toxicol Clin Toxicol. 1982;19(3);297.

49. Crocker PJ and Walker JS. "Pediatric carbon monoxide poisoning." J Emerg Med. 1986;2:443.

50. Dempsey L, O'Donnell JJ, Hoff JT. "Carbon monoxide retinopathy." Am J Ophthalmol. 1976;82:692.

51. DeReuck J, Decoo D, Lemahieu I, Strijckmans K, Boon P, Van Maele G, Buylaert W, Leys D, and Petit H. "A positron emission tomography study of patients with acute carbon monoxide poisoning treated by hyperbaric oxygen." J Neurol 1993;240:430-434.

52. Dolan MC. "Carbon monoxide poisoning." Can Med Assoc J. 1985;133:392.

53. Doll R and Hill AB. "The mortality of doctors in relation to their smoking habits: A preliminary report." Br Med J. 1954;1:1451-1455.

54. Ducasse JL, Celsis P, and Marc-Vergnes JP. "Non-comatose patients with acute carbon monoxide poisoning: hyperbaric or normobaric oxygenation?" Undersea and Hyperbaric Med. 1995;22:9-15.

55. End E, and Long CW. "Oxygen under pressure in carbon monoxide poisoning." J Ind Hyg Toxicol. 1942;24:302-306.

56. Eos G, Priestman G. "Cerebral vascular changes in carbon monoxide poisoning." J Neuropath Exp Neurol. 1942;1:158.

57. Fechter LD, Liu Y, and Pearce TA. "Cochlear protection from carbon monoxide exposure by free radical blockers in the guinea pig". Toxicol Appl Pharmacol. 1997;142:47-55.

58. Funata N, Okeda R, Takano T, Miyazaki Y, Higashino F, Yokoyama K, Manabe M, "Electron microscopic observations of experimental carbon monoxide encephalopathy in the acute phase.: Acta Pathol Jpn. 1982;32:219-229.

59. Furchgott RF and Jothianandan D. "Endothelium-dependent-and independent vasodilation involving cyclic GMP: Relaxation induced by nitric oxide, carbon monoxide and light." Blood Vessels. 1991;28:52-61.

60. Garland A and Pearce J. "Neurological complications of carbon monoxide poisoning." Q J Med. 1967;36(144):445.

61. Gemelli F and Cattani R. "Carbon monoxide poisoning in childhood." Br Med J. 1985;26:291.

62. Geyer RP. "Review of perfluorochemical-type blood substitutes." In Proceedings of the Tenth International Congress for Nutrition: Symposium on Perfluorochemical Artificial Blood. Kyoto 1975. Igakushobo, Osaka, Japan.

63. Ginsberg MD. "Delayed neurological deterioration following hypoxia." In: (Fahn S, Davis HN, Rowland LP Eds.) Advances in Neurology Vol 26. 1979;21-43.

64. Ginsberg MD, Myers RE and McDonagh BF. "Experimental carbon monoxide encephalopathy in the primate. II. Clinical aspects, neuropathology, and physiologic correlation." Arch Neurol. 1974;30;209-216.

65. Ginsberg MD, Hedley-White ET, Richardson EP Jr. "Hypoxic-ischemic leukoencephalopathy in man." Arch Neurol. 1976;33:5-14.

66. Ginsberg MD and Myers RE. "Fetal brain damage following maternal carbon monoxide intoxication: An experimental study." Acta Obstet Gynaecol Scan. 1974;53:309.

67. Goldstein GM and Doull J. "The use of hyperbaric oxygen in the treatment of p-aminopropiophenone-induced methemoglobinemia." Toxicol Appl Pharmacol. 1973;26:247-252.

68. Gorman DF, Clayton D, Gilligan JE and Webb RK. "A longitudinal study of 100 consecutive admissions for carbon monoxide poisoning to the Royal Adelaide Hospital." Anaesth Intens Care. 1992;20:311-316.

69. Goulon M, Barios A, and Rapin M. "Carbon monoxide poisoning and acute anoxia due to breathing coal gas and hydrocarbons." Ann Med Interne (Paris) 1969;120:335-349.

70. Grace TW and Platt FW. "Subacute carbon monoxide poisoning. Another great imitator." JAMA. 1981;246:1698-1700.

71. Graser T, Vedernikov YP and Li DS. "Study on the mechanism of carbon monoxide induced endothelium-independent relaxation in porcine coronary artery and vein." Biochem Biochim Acta. 1990;4:293-296.

72. Gwag BJ, Lobner D, Koh JT, Wie MB, and Choi DW. "Blockade of glutamate receptors unmasks neuronal apoptosis after oxygen-glucose deprivation *in vitro*." Neuroscience. 1995;68:615-619.

73. Hadley M. "Coal-gas poisoning and cardiac sequelae." Br Heart J. 1952;14:534-536.

74. Hallenbeck JM and Dutka AJ. "Background review and current concepts of reperfusion injury." Arch Neurol. 1990;47:1245-1254.

75. Halpin B, Fisher RS, Caplan YH. "Fire Fatality Study, International Symposium on Toxicity and Physiology of Combustion Products." University of Utah, Salt Lake City, Utah, March 22-26, 1976.

76. Hammond EC. "Proceedings of the second world conference on smoking and health." London, 1971. Richardson, RG. London, Pittman, 1972.

77. Hart GB, Strauss MB, Lennon PA, Whitcraft DD. "Treatment of smoke inhalation by hyperbaric oxygen." J Emerg Med. 1985;3:211-215.

78. Hatchen JD, Chiu LK, Jennings DB. "Anemia as a stimulus to aortic and carotid chemoreceptors in the cat." J Appl Physiol. 1978;44:696-702.

79. Heckerling PS, Leikin JB, Maturen A. "Occult carbon monoxide poisoning: validation of a prediction model." Am J Med. 1988;84:251-256.

79A. Henry C, Satran D, Lindgren B, Adkinson CD, et al. "Myocardial Injury and Long-tern Mortality Following Moderate to Severe Carbon Monoxide Poisoning" JAMA, 295(4):398-402, 2006.

80. Hexter AC, and Goldsmith JR. "Carbon monoxide association of community air pollution with mortality." Science. 1971;172: 265-267.

81. Hiramatsu M, Yokoyama S, Nabeshima T, and Kamneyama T. "Changes in concentrations of dopamine, serotonin, and their metabolites induced by carbon monoxide in the rat striatum as determined by *in vivo* microdialysis." Pharmacol Biochem and Behavior 1994;48:9-15.

82. Horita N, Ando S, Hagiwara I. "Experimental carbon monoxide leukoencephalopathy in the cat." J Neuropath Exp Neurol. 1980;39:197-211.

83. Horvath SM, Dahms TE, O'Hanlon JF. "Carbon monoxide and human vigilance." Arch Environ Health. 1971;23(5):343-347.

84. Hsu YK, Cheng YL. "Cerebral subcortical myelinopathy in carbon monoxide poisoning." Brain. 1938;61:384.

85. Hugod C, Hawkins L, Kjeldson K., et al. "Effect of carbon monoxide exposure on aorta and coronary intimal morphology in the rabbit. A revaluation." Atherosclerosis. 1978;30:333-342.

86. Hyperbaric Oxygen Therapy, A Committee Report (E.M. Camporesi, ed). Undersea and Hyperbaric Medical Society. 1996.

87. Ikeda T, Kondo T, Mogami H, et al. "Computerized tomography in cases of acute carbon monoxide poisoning." Med J Osaka Univ. 1978;29(3-4):253.

88. Ischiropoulos H, Beers MF, Ohnishi ST, Fisher D, Garner SE, and Thom SR. "Nitric oxide and perivascular tyrosine nitration following carbon monoxide poisoning in the rat." J Clin Invest. 1996;97:2260-2267.

89. Ishimaru H, Katoh A, Suzuki H, Fukuta T, Kameyama T, Nabeshima T. "Effects of N-methyl-D-aspartate receptor antagonists on carbon monoxide-induced brain damage in mice." J Pharmacol Exp Therap. 1992;261:349-352.

90. Ishimaru H, Nabeshima T, Katoh A, Suzuki H, Fukuta T, Kameyama T. "Effects of successive carbon monoxide exposures on delayed neuronal death in mice under the maintenance of normal body temperature." Biochem Biophys Res Comm. 1991;179:836-840.

91. Isom GE and Way JL. "Effect of oxygen on cyanide intoxication. VI. Reactivation of cyanide inhibited glucose metabolism." J Pharmacol Exp Ther. 1974;89:235-243.

92. Ivanov KP. "Effect of increased oxygen pressure on animals poisoned with potassium cyanide." Farmakol. Toksik. 1959;22:468-479.

93. Jackson DL and Menges H. "Accidental carbon monoxide poisoning." JAMA 1980;243:772.

94. Jakob A. "Ober die diffuse hemispherenmarkerkrankung nach Kohlenoxydvergiftung bei fallen mit klinisch intervallerer Verlaufsform. Zeitschrift For die Gesamte Neurologie und Psychiatrie, 1939;167:161-164.

96. Jefferson J."Subtle neuropsychiatric sequelae of carbon monoxide intoxication: Two case reports." Am J Psychiatry. 1976;133(8);961.

97. Johnson JW and Ascher P. "Glycine potentiates the NMDA response in cultured mouse brain neurons." Nature 1987;325:529-531.

98. Jougland J, Nava G, and Botta A. "Apropos d'une intoxication aique par le cyanure traite par l'hydroxocobalamine." Marseille Medicale. 1974;12:617-624.

99. Keenan HT, Bratton SL, Norkool DM, Brogan TV, and Hampson NB. "Delivery of hyperbaric oxygen therapy to critically ill, mechanically ventilated children." J Crit Care 1998;13:7-12.

100. Kelley JS, Sophocleus GH. "Retinal hemorrhages in subacute carbon monoxide poisoning." JAMA. 1978;239:1515.

100A. Kindwall EP, "Delayed sequelae in carbon monoxide poisoning and their probable mechanism." In: Carbon Monoxide: An Old Foe Revisited (Penney DG, Ed.) New York, CRC Press 1996.

101. Kinuta Y, Kimura M, Itokawa Y, Ishikawa M, Kiknchi H. "Changes in xanthine oxidase in ischemic rat brain." J Neurosurg. 1989;71:417-420.

102. Kinuta Y, Kikuchi H, Ishikawa M, Kimura M, and Itokawa Y. "Lipid peroxidation in focal cerebral ischemia." J Neurosurg. 1989;71:421-429.

103. Kjeldson K, Astrup P, Wanstrup J. "Ultrastructural intimal changes in the rabbit aorta after a moderate carbon monoxide exposure." Atherosclerosis. 1972;16:67-82.

104. Koehler RC, Jones MD Jr., Traystman RJ. "Cerebral circulatory response to carbon monoxide and hypoxic hypoxia in the lamb." Am J Physiol. 1982;243:H27-H32.

105. Kontos HA. "Oxygen radicals in CNS damage." Chem Biol Interactions. 1989;72:229-255.

106. Krantz T, Thisted P, Strom J, Sorrenson MB. "Acute carbon monoxide poisoning." Acta Anaesthesiol Scan. 1988;32:278-282.

107. Kuller LH, Radford EP, Swift D, Perper JA, and Fisher R. "Carbon monoxide and heart attacks." Arch Environ Health 1975;30:477-482.

108. Kwok PW. "Evaluation and control of carbon monoxide exposure in indoor skating arenas." Can J Public Health. 1983;74:261-265.

109. Lahiri S, Mulligan E, Nishino T, Mokashi A, Davies RV. "Relative responses of aortic body and carotid body chemoreceptors to carboxyhemoglobin." J Appl Physiol. 1981;50:580-586.

110. Lambertsen CJ, Kough RH, Cooper DY, Emmel GL, Loeschcke HH, Schmidt CF. "Oxygen toxicity. Effects in man of oxygen inhalation at 1 and 3.5 atmospheres upon blood gas transport, cerebral circulation and cerebral metabolism." J Appl Physiol. 1953;5:471-486.

110A. Lambrecht, CJ, Mateer JR, Kindwall, EP, Olson DW, Cisek JE and Stuven HA "Air Medical Transport for HBOT" Travel Medicine International, 10:51-56 1992.

111. LaPresle J, Fardeau M. "The central nervous system and carbon monoxide poisoning." in Progress in Brain Research (Bahr, H., Ledingham, I.M. Eds.)), Elsevier, Amsterdam, 1967;24:31-74.

112. Lin Y, Fechter LD. "MK-801 protects against carbon monoxide induced hearing loss." Toxicol Appl Pharmacol 1995;132:196-202.

113. Lipton SA, Kim WK, Choi YB, Kumar S, D'Emila DM, Rayudu PV, Arnelles DR, and Stamler JS. "Neurotoxicity associated with dual actions of homocysteine at the N-methyl-D-aspartate receptor." Proc Natl Acad Sci USA 1997;94:5923-5928.

114. Litovitz TL, Larkin RF, Myers RAM. "Cyanide poisoning treated with hyperbaric oxygen." Am J Emerg Med. 1983;1:94-101.

115. Longo LD and Chin KS. "Placental diffusing capacity for carbon monoxide and oxygen in unanesthetized sheep." J Appl Physiol. 1977;43:885.

116. Longo LD. "The biological effects of carbon monoxide on the pregnant woman, fetus and newborn infant." Am J Obstet Gynecol. 1977;129:69.

117. MacMillan V. "Regional cerebral blood flow of the rat in acute carbon monoxide intoxication." Can J Physiol Pharmacol. 1975;53:644-650.

118. MacMillan V. "The effects of acute carbon monoxide intoxication on the cerebral energy metabolism of the rat." Can J Pharmacol. 1975;53:354.

119. Marek Z and Piejko M. "Circulatory failure in acute carbon monoxide poisoning." Forensic Sci. 1972;1:419.

120. Martz D, Rayos G, Schielke GP, Betz AL. "Allopurinol and dimethylthiourea reduce brain infarction following middle cerebral artery occlusion in rats." Stroke. 1989;20:488-494.

121. Maeda Y, Kawasaki Y, Jibiki I, Yamaguchi N, Matsuda H, and Hisada K. "Effect of therapy with oxygen under high pressure on regional cerebral blood flow in the interval form of carbon monoxide poisoning: Observation from subtraction of technetium-99m HMPAO SPECT brain imaging." Eur Neurol. 1991;31:380-383.

122. Mathieu D, Nolf M, Durocher A, Saulnier F, Frimat P, Furon D, and Wattel F. "Acute carbon monoxide poisoning risk of late sequelae and treatment by hyperbaric oxygen." Clin Toxicol. 1985;23:315-324.

123. Mathieu D, Wattel F, Mathieu-Nolf M, Durak C, Tempe JP, Bouachour G, and Sainty JM. "Randonized prospective study comparing the effect of HBO versus 12 hours NBO in non-comatose CO poisoned patients." Undersea Hyperbaric Med. 23(suppl.): 7, 1996.

124. Mayevsky A, Meilin S, Rogatsky GG, Zarchin N, and Thom SR. "Multiparametric monitoring of the awake brain exposed to carbon monoxide." J Appl Physiol. 1995;78:1188-1196.

125. McNulty JA, Maher BA, Chu M, and Sitnikova T. "Relationship of short-term verbal memory to the need for hyperbaric oxygen treatment after carbon monoxide poisoning." Neuropsychiatr Neuropsychol Behavioral Neurol. 1997;10:174-179.

126. Meilin S, Rogatsky GG, Thom SR, Zarchin N, Guggenheimer-Furman E, and Mayevsky A. "Effects of carbon monoxide on the brain may be mediated by nitric oxide." J Appl Physiol. 1996;81:1078-1083.

127. Meilin S, Sonn J, Zarchin N, Rogatsky G, Guggenheimer-Furman E, and Mayevsky A. "Responses of rat brain to induced spreading depression following exposure to carbon monoxide." Brain Res. 1998; 780: 323-328.

128. Messier LD and Myers RAM. "A neuropsychological screening battery for emergency assessment of carbon-monoxide-poisoned patient." J Clin Psychol. 1991;47(5):675-684.

129. Meyer A. "Experimentelle erfahrungen uber die kohlenoxyverguftung des zentralnervens system." Zeitschrift fur die Ges. Neurol Psychiatr. 1928;112:187-212.

130. Mickel HS, Vaishnav YN, Kempski O, Lubitz DV, Weiss JF, Fauerstein G. "Breathing 100% oxygen after global brain ischemia in Mongolian gerbils results in increased lipid peroxidation and increased mortality." Stroke. 1987;18:426-430.

131. Min SK. "A brain syndrome associated with delayed neuropsychiatric sequelae following acute carbon monoxide poisoning." Acta Psychiatr Scan. 1986;73:80-86.

132. Mofenson HC, Caraccio TR, Brody GM. "Carbon monoxide poisoning." Am J Emerg Med. 1984;2:254.

133. Mogielnicki KRP and Chandler JE. "Association of the frequency of acute cardiorespiratory complication with ambient levels of carbon monoxide." Chest. 1978;74:10.

134. Mohler SR. "Air crash survival: Injuries and evacuation toxic hazards." Aviat Space Environ Med. 1975;46:86-88.

135. Moolenaar RL, Etzel RA, and Parrish RG. "Unintentional deaths from carbon monoxide poisoning in New Mexico, 1980 to 1988. A comparison of medical examiner and national mortality data." Western J Med. 1995;163:431-434.

136. Morris RD and Naumova EN. "Carbon monoxide and hospital admissions for congestive heart failure: Evidence of an increased effect at low temperature." Environ Health Perspect. 1998;106:649-653.

137. Morris RD, Naumova EN, and Munasinghe RL. "Ambient air pollution and hospitalization for congestive heart failure among elderly people in seven large US cities." Am J Public Health 1995;85:1361-1365.

138. Muller GL, Graham S. "Intrauterine death of the fetus due to accidental carbon monoxide poisoning." N Engl J Med. 1955;252:1075.

139. Murphy TH, Miyamoto M, Sastre A, Schnaar RL, and Coyle JT. "Glutamate toxicity in a neuronal cell line involves inhibition of cystine transport leading to oxidative stress." Neuron 1989;2:1547-1558.

140. Myers RAM, Snyder SK, Majerus TC. "Cutaneous blisters and carbon monoxide poisoning." Ann Emerg Med. 1985;14:603.

141. Myers RAM, Snyder SK, Emhoff TA. "Subacute sequelae of carbon monoxide poisoning." Ann Emerg Med. 1985;14:1163-1167.

142. Myers RAM. "Do arterial blood gases have value in prognosis and treatment decisions in carbon monoxide poisoning?" Crit Care Med. 1989;1720:139-142.

143. Myers RAM, Messier LD, Jones DW, Cowley RA. "New direction in the research and treatment of carbon monoxide exposure." Am J Emerg Med. 1983;2:226.

144. Myers RAM, Jones DW, Britten JS. "Carbon monoxide half life study." Proceedings of the Eighth International Congress on Hyperbaric Medicine, E. Kindwall, (Ed.) pp. 263-265, Best Publishing, Flagstaff, AZ, 1987.

145. Myers RAM. "Hyperbaric oxygen therapy for gas gangrene and carbon monoxide poisonings." Trauma: Emergency Surgery and Critical Care. Siegel JH (Ed.) Churchill Livingstone, New York. 1987;1133-1169.

146. Myers RE. "A unitary theory of causation of anoxic and hypoxic brain pathology." Adv Neurol. 1979;26:195-213.

147. Nabeshima T, Katoh A, Ishimaru H, Yoneda Y, and Ogita K. "Carbon monoxide-induced delayed amnesia, delayed neuronal death and change in acetylcholine concentration in mice." J Pharm Exp Therap. 1991;256:378-384.

148. Nabeshima T, Yoshida S, Morinaka H, Kameyama T, Thurkauf A, Rice KC, and Jacobson AE. "MK-801 ameliorates delayed amnesia, but potentiates acute amnesia induced by CO." Neurosci Let. 1990;108:321-327.

149. Newby MB, Roberts RJ, and Bhatnagar RK. "Carbon monoxide and hypoxia-induced effects on catecholamines in the mature and developing rat brain." J Pharmacol Exp Ther 1978;206:61-68.

150. Norkool DM, Kirkpatrick JN. "Treatment of acute carbon monoxide poisoning with hyperbaric oxygen: A review of 115 cases." Ann Emerg Med. 1985;14:1168-1171.

151. Norris JC, Moore SJ, Hume AS. "Synergistic lethality induced by the combination of carbon monoxide and cyanide." Toxicology. 1986;40:121-129.

152. Oka A, Belliveau MJ, Rosenberg PA, and Volpe JJ. "Vulnerability of oligodendroglia to glutamate: Pharmacology, mechanisms, and prevention." J Neurosci 1993;13:1441-1453.

153. Okeda R, Funata N, Takano T, Miyazaki Y, Higashino F, Yokoyama K, Manabe M. "The pathogenesis of carbon monoxide encephalopathy in the acute phase physiological morphological correlation." Acta Neuropath. 1981;54:1-10.

154. Okeda R, Funata N, Song SJ, Higashino F, Takano T, and Yokoyama K. "Comparative study on the pathogenesis of selective cerebral lesions in carbon monoxide and nitrogen hypoxia in cats." Acta Neuropathol. 1982;56:256-272.

155. Pace N, Strajman E, Walker EL. "Acceleration of carbon monoxide elimination in man by high pressure oxygen." Science. 1950;111:652-654.

156. Patt A, Harken AH, Burton LK, Rodell TC, Piermattei D, Schorr WJ, Parker NB, et al. "Xanthine oxidase-derived hydrogen peroxide contributes to ischemia reperfusion-induced edema in gerbil brains." J Clin Invest. 1988;81:1556-1562.

157. Paulet G. "Value and mechanisms of action of oxygen therapy in the treatment of hydrogen cyanide poisoning." Arch Internat Physiol Biochim. 1955;63:340-360.

158. Penn, A. "Determination of the atherosclerotic potential of inhaled carbon monoxide". HEI Report. Montpelier, VT: Capital City Press, 1993.

159. Penn A, and Snyder CA. "Inhalation of sidestream cigarette smoke accelerates development of arteriosclerotic plaques." Circulation 1993;88(part 1):1820-1825.

160. Peirce EC, Zacharias A, Alday JM Jr., Hoffman BA, Jacobson JH. "Carbon monoxide poisoning: Experimental hypothermic and hyperbaric studies." Surgery. 1972;72:229-237.

161. Pellegrini-Giampietro DE, Cherici G, Alesiani M, Carla V, and Moroni F. "Excitatory amino acid release and free radical formation may cooperate in the genesis of ischemia-induced neuronal damage." J Neuroscience 1990;10:1035-1041.

162. Phillips P. "Carbon monoxide poisoning during pregnancy." Br Med J. 1924;1:14.

163. Piantadosi CA. "The role of hyperbaric oxygen in carbon monoxide, cyanide, and sulfide intoxication." Problems in Respiratory Care. Moon RE and Camporesi EM (Eds.) Lippincott, Philadelphia, June 1991;4(2):215-231.

164. Piantadosi CA, and Brown SD. "Hyperbaric oxygen for carbon monoxide poisoning." Lancet II: 1989;1032.

165. Piantadosi CA, Tatro L, and Zhang J. "Hydroxyl radical production in the brain after CO hypoxia in rats." Free Rad Biol Med 1995;18:603-609.

166. Piantadosi CA, Zhang J, and Demchenko IT. "Production of hydroxyl radical in the hippocampus after CO hypoxia and hypoxic hypoxia in the rat." Free Rad Biol and Med. 1997;22:725-732.

167. Piantadosi CA, Zhang J, Levin ED, Folz RJ, and Schmechel DE. "Apoptosis and delayed neuronal damage after carbon monoxide poisoning in the rat." Exp Neurol. 1997;147:103-114.

168. Pinley J, VanBeek A, and Glover GL. "Myonecrosis complicating carbon monoxide poisoning." J Trauma. 1977;17:536-540.

169. Ponte J and Purues MJ. "The role of the carotid body chemoreceptors and carotid sinus baroreceptors in the control of cerebral blood vessels." J Physiol. (London) 1973;237:P215-340.

170. Preziosi TJ, Lindenberg R, Levy D, Christenson M. "An experimental investigation in animals of the functional and morphologic effects of single and repeated exposures to high and low concentrations of carbon monoxide." Ann NY Acad Sci. 1970;174:369.

171. Putnam TJ, McKenna JB, and Morrison LR "Studies in multiple sclerosis." JAMA 1991;97:1591-1596.

172. Raphael JC, Elkharrat D, Guincestre MCJ, Chastang C, Vercken JB, Chasles V, and Gajdos P. "Trial of normobaric and hyperbaric oxygen for acute carbon monoxide intoxication. " Lancet 1989;1:414-419.

173. Ratney RS, Wegman DH, Wilkins HB. "in vivo conversion of methylene chloride to carbon monoxide." Arch Environ Health. 1974;28:223.

174. Reiderer P, Pintar JE, and Breakfield XO. "Immunocytochemical demonstration of monoamine oxidase B in brain astrocytes and serotonergic neurons." Proc Natl Acad Sci USA 1982:79:6385-6389.

175. Rioux JP, Myers RAM. "Methylene chloride poisoning: A paradigmatic review." J Emerg Med. 1988;6:227-238.

176. Roth RA Jr. and Ruben RJ. "Role of blood flow in carbon monoxide - and hypoxic hypoxia-induced alterations in hexobarbital metabolism in rats." Drug Metab Dispos. 1976;4:460-467.

177. Rumak BA. "Cyanide poisoning." Newball, HH (Ed.) Respiratory Care of Chemical Casualties. Proceedings of the Symposium on Respiratory Care of Chemical Casualties. US Army Medical Research and Development Command. McLean, VA 1983.

178. Sakamoto A, Ohnishi ST, Ohnishi T, Ogawa R. "Protective effect of a new anti-oxidant on the rat brain exposed to ischemia-reperfusion injury: Inhibition of free radical formation and lipid peroxidation." Free Radical Biol Med. 1991;11:385-391.

179. Sakamoto A, Ohnishi ST, Ohnishi T, Ogawa R. "Relationship between free radical production and lipid peroxidation during ischemia-reperfusion injury in the rat brain." Brain Res. 1991;554:186-192.

180. Sammons JH, Coleman RL. "Firefighters' occupational exposure to carbon monoxide." J Occup Med. 1974;16:543.

181. Santiago TV and Edelman NH. "Mechanism of ventilatory response to carbon monoxide." J Clin Invest. 1976;57:977-986.

182. Sawada Y, Ohashi N, Maemura K, et al. "Computerized tomography as an indication of long term outcome after acute carbon monoxide poisoning." Lancet. 1980;1:783.

183. Sayers PR, Davenport SJ. "Review of carbon monoxide poisoning." Public Health Bulletin 195. U.S. Government Printing Office, Washington, DC. 1930.

184. Scheinkestel CD, Jones K, Cooper DJ, Millar I, Tuxen DV, and Myles PS. "Interim analysis- controlled clinical trial of hyperbaric oxygen in acute carbon monoxide poisoning." Undersea Hyperbaric Med. 1996;23(suppl.): 7.

185. Schwartz J, and Morris RD. "Cardiovascular disease and airborne particulate levels in Detroit, Michigan." Am. J. Epidemiol. 1995;142:23-35.

186. Sheehy M, Way JL. "Effect of oxygen on cyanide intoxication. III. Mithridate." J Pharmacol Exp Ther. 1968;161:163-168.

187. Shillito FH, Drinker CK, and Shaughnessey TJ. "The problem of nervous and mental sequelae in carbon monoxide poisoning." JAMA 1936;106:669-674.

188. Siesjö BK. "Carbon monoxide poisoning. Mechanism of damage, late sequelae and therapy." Clin Toxicol. 1985;23:247-248.

189. Siesjö BK, Nilsson L. "The influence of arterial hypoxemia upon labile phosphates and upon extracellular lactate and pyruvate concentrations in the rat brain." Scand J Clin Lab Invest. 1971;27:83.

190. Shimosegawa E, Hatazawa J, Nagata K, Okudera T, Inugami A, Ogawa T, Fujita H, Itoh H, Kanno I, and Uemura K. "Cerebral blood flow and glucose metabolism measurements in a patient surviving one year after carbon monoxide intoxication." J Nucl Med 1992;33:1696-1698.

191. Silverman CS, Brenner J, and Murtagh FR. "Hemorrhagic necrosis and vascular injury in carbon monoxide poisoning: MR demonstration." Am J Neuroradiol. 1993;14:168-170.

192. Skene WG, Norman JN, Smith G. "Effect of hyperbaric oxygen in cyanide poisoning." Brown I and Cox B (Eds.) Proceedings of the Third International Congress on Hyperbaric Oxygen. Washington, DC, National Academy of Science, NRC, 1966;705-710.

193. Smith JS and Brandon S. "Morbidity from acute carbon monoxide poisoning at three year follow up." Br Med J. 1973;1:318.

194. Smith G and Sharp GR. "Treatment of carbon-monoxide poisoning with oxygen under pressure." Lancet. 1960;1:905-906.

195. Sokal JA and Kralkowska E. "The relationship between exposure duration, carboxyhemoglobin, blood glucose, pyruvate and lactate and the severity of intoxication in 39 cases of acute carbon monoxide poisoning in man." Arch Toxicol. 1985;57:196-199.

196. Song SY, Okeda R, Funata N Higashino F. "An experimental study of the pathogenesis of the selective lesion of the globus pallidus in acute carbon monoxide poisoning in cats." Acta Neuropathol. 1983;61:232-238.

197. Stern FB, Lemen RA, and Curtis RA. "Exposure of motor vehicle examiners to carbon monoxide: A historical prospective mortality study." Arch Environ Health 1980;36:59-66.

198. Stewart RD, Bartetta ED, Plate LR, et al. "Carboxyhemoglobin levels in American blood donors." JAMA. 1974;229:1187-1195.

199. Symington IS, Anderson RA, Oliver JS, Thomson I, Harland WA, Kerr JW. "Cyanide exposure in fires." Lancet. 1978;91-92.

200. Takano T, Miyazaki Y, Shimoyama H, Maeda H, Okeda R. "Direct effect of carbon monoxide on cardiac function." Int Arch Occup Environ Health. 1981;49:35-40.

201. Takano T, Myazaki Y, Nashimoto I, and Kobayashi K. "Effect of hyperbaric oxygen on cyanide intoxication: In situ changes in intracellular oxidation reduction." Undersea Biomed Res. 1980;7:191-197.

202. Teige B, Lundevall J, Fleischen E. "Carboxyhemoglobin concentrations in fire victims and in cases of fatal carbon monoxide poisoning." Z Rechtsmed. 1977;8:17-21.

203. Thom SR. "Antagonism of carbon monoxide-mediated brain lipid peroxidation by hyperbaric oxygen." Toxicol Appl Pharmacol. 1990;105:340-344.

204. Thom SR. "Carbon monoxide-mediated brain lipid peroxidation in the rat." J Appl Physiol. 1990;68:997-1003.

205. Thom SR. "Dehydrogenase conversion to oxidase and lipid peroxidation in brain after carbon monoxide poisoning." J. Appl. Physiol. 1992;73:1584-1589.

206. Thom SR. "Functional inhibition of leukocyte B2 integrins by hyperbaric oxygen in carbon monoxide-mediated brain injury in rats." Toxicol Appl Pharmacol. 1993;123:248-256.

207. Thom SR. "Learning dysfunction and metabolic defects in globus pallidus and hippocampus after CO poisoning in a rat model." Undersea Hyperbaric Med. 1997;23(suppl.):20.

208. Thom SR. "Leukocytes in carbon monoxide-mediated brain oxidative injury." Toxicol Appl Pharmacol. 1993;123:234-247.

209. Thom SR and Elbuken ME. "Oxygen-dependent antagonism of lipid peroxidation." Free Rad Biol Med. 1991;10:413-426.

210. Thom SR, Fisher D, Xu YA, Garner S, and Ischiropoulos H. "Role of nitric oxide-derived oxidants in vascular injury from carbon monoxide in the rat." Am J Physiol in press, 1998a.

211. Thom SR, Kang M, Fisher D, and Ischiropoulos H. "Release of glutathione from erythrocytes and other markers of oxidative stress in carbon monoxide poisoning." J Appl Physiol. 1997;82:1424-1432.

212. Thom SR, Mendiguren I, Hardy KR, Bolotin T, Fisher D, Nebolon M, and Kilpatrick L. "Inhibition of human neutrophil beta 2 integrin-dependent adherence by hyperbaric oxygen," Am j Physiol (Cell Physiology) 1997;272:C770-C777.

214. Thom SR, Taber RL, Mendiguren II, Clark JM, Hardy KR, and Fisher AB. "Delayed neuropsychological sequelae following carbon monoxide poisoning and its prophylaxis by treatment with hyperbaric oxygen." Ann Emerg Med. 1995;25:474-480.

215. Thom SR, Xu YA, and Ischiropoulos H. "Vascular endothelial cells generate peroxynitrite in response to carbon monoxide exposure." Chem Res Toxicol 1997;10:1023-1031.

216. Tomaszewski C, Rudy J, Wathen J, Brent J, Rosenberg N, and Kulig K. "Prevention of neurologic sequelae from carbon monoxide by hyperbaric oxygen in rats." Ann Emerg Med. 1992;21:631-632.

217. Turrens JF, Crapo JD, Freeman BA. "Protection against oxygen toxicity by intravenous injection of liposome-entrapped catalase and superoxide dismutase." J Clin Invest. 1984;73:87-95.

218. Uchino A, Hasuo K, Shida K, Matsumoto S, Yasumori K, and Masuda K. "MRI of the brain in chronic carbon monoxide poisoning." Neuroradiol.1994;36:399-401.

219. U.S. Public Health Service: Vital Statistics of the United States, Washington, DC, Government Printing Office, 1976.

220. Utz J and Ullrich V. "Carbon monoxide relaxes ileal smooth muscle through activation of guanylate cyclase." Biochem Pharmacol. 1991;41:1195-1201.

221. Vierregge P, Klostermann W, Blumm RG, and Borgis KJ. "Carbon monoxide poisoning: clinical, neurophysiological, and brain imaging observations in acute disease and follow-up." J Neurol. 1989;236:478-481.

222. Von Andrian UH, Chambers JD, McEvoy LM, Bargatze RF, Arfors KE, and Butcher EC. "Two-step model of leukocyte-endothelial cell interaction in inflammation: Distinct roles for LECAM-1 and the leukocyte $O_2$ integrins *in vivo*." Proc Natl Acad Sci USA 1991; 88: 7538-7542.

223. Wald N, Howard S, Smith, Kjeldsen K. "Association between atherosclerotic diseases and carboxyhemoglobin levels in tobacco smokers." British Medical Journal. 1973;1:761-765.

224. Warburg O. "Uber die wirkung des kohlenoxyds auf den stoffwechsel der Hefe." Biochem Zeitschrift. 1926;177:471-486.

225. Warburg O. "Uber die wirkung von kohlenoxyd und stickoxyd auf atmung und gËrung." Biochem Zeitschrift. 1927;189:354-380.

226. Way JL, Gibbon SL, Sheehy M. "Effect of oxygen on cyanide intoxication. I. prophylactic protection." J Pharmacol Exp Ther. 1966;153:381-385.

227. Way JC, Sylvester D, Morgan RL. "Recent perspectives on the toxicodynamic basis of cyanide antagonism." Fund Appl Toxicol. 1984;4:S231-S239.

228. Way JL, End E, Sheehy MH, Demiranda P, Feitknecht UF, Bachand R, Gibbon SL, Burrows GE. "Effect of oxygen on cyanide intoxication." Toxicol Appl Pharmacol. 1972;22:415-421.

228A. Weaver, LK, Hopkins RO, Chan KJ, Churchill S, Ellott, C. et al. "Hyperbaric Oxygen for Acute Carbon Monoxide Poisoning" New Eng J. Med. 347(14):1057-1067 Oct 3, 2002.

229. Wechsler D. "The Wechsler Adult Intelligence Scale." The Psychological Corp., New York, 1955.

230. Werner B, Beck W, Kerblom H, et al. "Two cases of acute carbon monoxide poisoning with delayed neurological sequelae after a 'free' interval." Clin Toxicol. 1985;23:249.

231. Whorton MD. "Carbon monoxide intoxication: A review of 14 patients." J Am Coll Emerg Physicians. 1976;5:505.

232. Winter PM and Miller JN. "Carbon monoxide poisoning." JAMA 1976;236: 1502-1504.

233. Yacoub M, Faur J, Morera H. "L'intoxication cyanhydrique aique. Donnes actuelles sur le metabolism du cyanure et le traitement par hydroxocobalamine." J Eur Toxicol. 1974;7:22-29.

234. Yoshida S, Inoh S, Asano T, Sano K, Kubota M, Shimazaki H, Ueta N. "Effect of transient ischemia on free fatty acids and phospholipids in the gerbil brain." J Neurosurg. 1980;53:323-331.

235. Youngberg JT, Myers RAM. "Use of hyperbaric oxygen in carbon monoxide, cyanide, and sulfide intoxication." Hyperbaric Oxygen Therapy, A Critical Review. Camporesi EM and Barker AC (Eds.) Undersea and Hyperbaric Medical Society, 1991:23-53.

# NOTES

# SECTION II
# DISORDERS APPROVED FOR HYPERBARIC TREATMENT

CHAPTER **18**

# DECOMPRESSION SICKNESS

## CHAPTER EIGHTEEN OVERVIEW

# DECOMPRESSION SICKNESS

*David H. Elliott, Eric P. Kindwall*

## INTRODUCTION

Decompression sickness (DCS) is considered as that type of decompression illness (DCI) which arises from the presence of bubbles formed from gases that have been dissolved in the tissues of the body during a sojourn at raised environmental pressure. Not all such bubbles lead to illness. Some can be detected by Doppler in the venous system and, if not too many, these venous gas emboli remain symptomless ('silent') while returning to the lungs where their gas is excreted. There are a number of clinical syndromes which are considered to be typical of DCS but there is also some overlap of manifestations between DCS and other decompression pathologies. In particular this may occur with arterial gas embolism (AGE; see the chapter by Kindwall entitled "Gas Embolism") which is a form of DCI that is secondary to decompression damage of the lungs (pulmonary barotrauma, PB) causing intravascular bubbles of alveolar gas.

The clinical picture of DCI is occasionally rendered yet more complex if it is due to both DCS and AGE pathologies at the same time. One example is a "biphasic DCI" in which some bubbles of AGE may then precipitate a secondary form of DCS when they pass through tissues loaded with dissolved gas after a no-stop or decompression dive that is considered safe and would not normally cause DCS.

Another example, in as many as one third of the population, is associated with the presence of a very small hole-in-the-heart that should have closed naturally at birth, the patent foramen ovale (PFO). In such persons there is a small risk that some of the silent venous bubbles may be diverted through a PFO (or other right-to-left shunt) into the arterial circulation. Some of these arterial gas emboli may lead to manifestations of AGE and/or, as they pass through tissues loaded with dissolved gas, cause DCS manifestations. These pathological mechanisms are complex and the manifestations can be ambiguous.

## HISTORY

An understanding of decompression sickness in its various forms and the evolution of treatment by recompression is best gained from a summary of its history. Even though some cases may have arisen in previous decades, the first published report was in 1845 by Triger (49), who reported that one compressed-air worker in a French mine had suffered sharp pain in the left arm, and that another had pain in the knees and left shoulder after emerging from a 7-hour exposure at an unspecified pressure, probably between 2.4 and 4.2 atmospheres absolute (240 and 420 kPa). The men were affected one-half hour after returning to normal pressure. Triger wrote, "Rubbing with spirits of wine soon relieved this pain in both men and they kept working on the following days." Pol and Watelle a few years later noted that they were "justified in hoping that a sure and prompt means of relief would be to recompress immediately, then decompress very carefully" (40), but they never actually returned anyone to pressure for this purpose. The use of compressed air increased rapidly throughout the 1850s and 1860s, but there is no written account of any cases of DCS on those projects being treated with recompression.

Dr. Jaminet, the project physician for the Eads Bridge in St. Louis, spent two hours and 45 minutes at a pressure equal to 97 feet (29 meters) of water and was decompressed in three and a half minutes. He suffered severe spinal cord decompression illness, but was never recompressed and apparently made a slow recovery. The total number of workmen employed on that project was 352, of whom 30 were seriously injured and 12 died (22). Washington A. Roebling, son of the designer, John Augustus Roebling, and the chief engineer for the Brooklyn Bridge project was a victim of "spinal cord bends" and directed the remainder of the bridge construction from a sick bed overlooking the work site (30).

It was from the Brooklyn Bridge Project that the term "bends" for decompression sickness was coined. An affected style of walking used by fashionable women of the era was called "the Grecian Bend," "Sandhogs," as the compressed-air caisson workers were called, adopted the term to lend a touch of humor in describing the antalgic gait seen in those suffering from musculoskeletal decompression sickness. Soon it was shortened to "the bends" and the term "bent" became recognized by colloquial usage.

Many physicians at the time felt that the extreme chill experienced in the decompression lock during decompression was in some way responsible for causing the disease. For this reason, steam heat was installed in the decompression locks on the Brooklyn Bridge job to prevent chilling, but there was no recompression chamber. Dr. Andrew Smith, an ear, nose, and throat specialist, was engaged to look after the men working in compressed air, and logged 110 cases of DCS serious enough to come to his attention. He also considered recompression and made the observation that the caisson workers had relief of symptoms on being returned to pressure. However, he called this treatment "the heroic mode" and never used it (45). Paul Bert (1878) had later demonstrated in animals that the cause of DCS was dissolved nitrogen becoming gaseous during decompression, and that this bubble formation was responsible for "bends." He also noted that, in rapidly decompressed animals, asphyxial death could be prevented if the animals were given surface oxygen to breathe; however, the breathing of oxygen without the addition of pressure failed to cure spinal cord paralysis (6).

Ernest W. Moir (1889), a British engineer, was the first to apply recompression to relieve DCS. At the time he took over as superintendent of the construction of the Hudson River tunnel, death due to decompression sickness occurred in 25% of the men employed. Possibly these men died asphyxial deaths from the "chokes" or of bends shock. After he installed a recompression chamber, during the next 15 months only two deaths (1.66%) occurred among the 120 men employed.

*"With a view to remedying the state of things (that is, the serious mortality), an air compartment like a boiler was made in which the men could be treated homeopathically, Bende treatment or re-immersed in compressed air. It was erected near the top of the shaft, and when a man was overcome or paralyzed, as I have seen them often, completely unconscious and unable to use their limbs, they were carried into the compartment and the air pressure raised to about one-half to two-thirds of that in which they had been working, with immediate improvement. The pressure was then lowered at the very slow rate of one pound per minute or even less. The time allowed for equalization being from 25 to 30 minutes, and even in severe cases the men went away quite cured"* (33).

## ETIOLOGY OF DECOMPRESSION SICKNESS

While at pressure, the respiratory gases of a diver or compressed-air worker are being dissolved in the blood and tissues and in a prolonged exposure this would continue to occur until equilibrium is achieved ("saturation"). The body comprises a mathematical spectrum of fast and slow compartments ("tissues") in some of which, for practical purposes, saturation with dissolved gas occurs in just a few minutes and in others some 12 to 36 hours. When a diver or compressed-air worker leaves maximum pressure, he may not have been there long enough to absorb sufficient gas to provide a clinical risk of significant bubble formation, and he can make a direct ascent safely from what is thus termed a "no-stop dive". Beyond a threshold determined by various combinations of depth and duration, there is a greater absorption of dissolved gas and so a direct ascent to the surface is no longer safe. In these circumstances a slow ascent, usually by means of prescribed "stops" at progressively shallower depths, is required in order to allow time for the dissolved gas to be exhaled. Many versions of these diving tables are available and have been based upon mathematical models and modified by experience (5). Some divers carry personal computers which, with a pressure transducer, use similar models during the dive to provide an on-line display of their predicted decompression profile.

There are many factors that can contribute to individual susceptibility. Certainly there is more needed than mere biological variation around a central mathematical model of decompression to explain the variability between individuals. Indeed, in the construction of the Dartford tunnel around 50% of the "bends" were experienced by just some 4% of the compressed-air workers (17). Some degree of adaptation may arise from regular decompressions by compressed-air workers and divers, seemingly permitting them to shorten their predicted decompression times safely. However such "acclimatization" may quickly be lost during a few days break from regular daily work, after which resumption of the same pattern of diving has been associated for a while with a higher bends-rate until immunity returns.

In contrast, there seems to be a tendency among sport divers when making several dives daily during a one-week vacation, to become symptomatic about the fourth or fifth day. This may be because dissolved gas loads in the slowest tissues may not have been entirely eliminated before the next day's diving, even though the table or computer has not predicted the presence of any residual gas.

Another disconcerting observation is that of the occasional untoward effect of an additional quick dive at the end of a full day's diving. A mere breath-hold dive to retrieve an anchor after completing an appropriate decompression for a compressed-air dive has led to sudden death on more than one occasion (31). A speculative explanation is that the second dive reduced the diameter of silent venous gas emboli sufficient for them to slip through the pulmonary filter and into the arterial distribution.

Various factors predispose an individual to DCI and include dehydration, hangovers, heavy physical exercise at depth, environmental hot water at depth and cold exposure during decompression. A recent injury may cause localized bubble formation with symptoms. Exercise or having a hot shower after surfacing has also been associated with the onset of DCS.

Thus, the theoretical basis for calculating safe decompression procedures is subject to so many other influences that, while a small number of decompression incidents may be regarded as unavoidable, the general success of the published diving tables can be considered as a remarkable achievement. Assessing the apparent success or otherwise of a particular decompression table is based upon knowing the number of cases of decompression sickness that arise from it in relation to the total number of dives that have been made without incident. Too often these data are not available and, when they are, they may not tell the whole story because:

- Individuals vary in their threshold for reporting symptoms.
- No objective criteria exist to confirm the diagnosis.
- Those assessing divers for recompression vary in their interpretations.

Decompression illness can occur after compliance with a "safe" decompression profile and is not confined to those who fail to follow the decompression tables. Many explanations tend to oversimplify the etiology of DCS but there is a great profusion of possible pathways in its causation and development. No simple description can account for all the observations. At the same time it is necessary to keep in mind the aetiology of PB and AGE (described in the next chapter) which can follow any dive and has been reported after just one breath of gas at an ambient pressure less than 2 meters (6.56 feet) of seawater may be sufficient (3). This broader awareness is essential because the manifestations of AGE and DCS can exist concurrently in one patient.

## PATHOLOGY OF DECOMPRESSION SICKNESS

The excess of dissolved gas which can form bubbles during decompression may occur in one or more of several bodily tissues, depending on many factors including the profile of the dive and its decompression. Bubbles may be formed extravascularly or intravascularly and their subsequent distribution can be widespread (20). However, the pathology of acute decompression sickness in man is not fully known simply because the condition is usually transient, is not accurately reproducible in animals, and also because many of the bubbles found at autopsy are post-mortem artifacts.

For the purposes of the subsequent clinical description, the following overview provides a working hypothesis and, for a more scientific review, the reader is referred to other texts such as Francis and Mitchell (15).

The bubble may cause its effects by simple mechanical expansion or by surface activity at the blood-gas interface. A bubble in the region of a musculo-tendinous insertion may, by pressure on nerve endings, be responsible for the local sharp pain of some cases of "limb-bends". The stimulation of platelet aggregation and release is just one example of the effect of the electrokinetic forces at the surface of an intravascular bubble. Activation of complement, Hageman factor, and of enzyme groups are other mechanisms that, by one pathway or another, lead to consequences such as rheological changes and the hypovolemic shock of serious decompression illness. Embolic bubbles (whether of DCS or AGE) may cause neurological dysfunction as a result of mechanical vascular obstruction, but the mere passage of bubbles through a vessel without lodgment can cause endothelial and subsequent circulatory disturbances there.

## MANIFESTATIONS OF DECOMPRESSION SICKNESS

The traditional classification of DCS into Type 1 ("pain-only") and Type 2 ("serious symptoms") was introduced by those concerned with decompression sickness among compressed-air workers. A similar distinction had been made previously in the treatment protocols published in the United States Navy Diving Manual. The attraction of such an approach when cases must be treated immediately without a medical officer present is simplicity for the divers present. However this is far from foolproof not merely because the severe pain of a "mild" manifestation may cause a concurrent "serious" deficit to be overlooked but also because the diagnostic distinction between DCS and AGE is not always obvious. Traditionally the distinction was important because the treatment algorithms were different. Gorman, Des in treating "pain-only" decompression sickness successfully with modern oxygen treatment tables found that one week later, despite normal neurologic exams and cortical evoked potentials, 60% of the patients had abnormal psychological testing, 40% had abnormal EEGs and 10% had abnormal brain scans. One month later the psychological testing had all reverted to normal and the EEGs showed only a 20% abnormality (18). Thus with today's broader perspective of the decompression disorders and with a common algorithm in the *USN Diving Manual* (51) one must respect those traditional descriptions but be careful to consider additional diagnostic options.

### Cutaneous Decompression Sickness

Itching, *"les puces"* or "divers lice", may occur in those parts of the skin that have been exposed to compressed air during the pressure exposure, but not in those parts that were immersed. This uncommon manifestation is not a serious condition, but is associated with compressed-air exposures of marginal safety. They usually vanish in 20 to 30 minutes. No specific treatment is required, but the individual should be advised to proceed to the vicinity of a recompression chamber in case other manifestations follow.

A blotchy red or purple rash, termed *"cutis marmorata"*, is usually over the upper trunk, and may be due to the superficial vasodilatation and stasis.

This rash blanches under direct local pressure. Though mild in itself, this condition may be associated with the subsequent onset of a more serious condition and, if recompression facilities are readily available, treatment not only resolves this condition but may be prophylactic therapy against any later manifestations. Thus for a person presenting with such a rash, arrangements should be prepared for transfer to a recompression chamber.

The lymphatic form of decompression illness, *"peau d'orange"*, is not truly cutaneous but is thought to be due to bubbles blocking the lymphatics and the lymphatic glands. It is usually seen in the limbs but the edema has also appeared in the parotid and mammary regions. The condition is itself not serious but if the patient is recompressed for some other manifestation, the edema also resolves.

## Musculoskeletal Pain

Musculo-skeletal pain is less ambiguous than the term *"bends"* which, though given first to the most widely known manifestation of decompression sickness, limb pain, has since been applied more generally. In some papers it has been even used for neurological fatalities and so it should be avoided. Interestingly joint pain does not occur in those who do not have a significant gas load, such as submarine escape trainees who are usually diagnosed with AGE. In both recreational and working compressed-air divers, limb pain is more common in the shoulders whereas in compressed-air workers and saturation divers, limb pain is more common in the knees and lower legs.

However musculo-skeletal pain can occur in almost any synovial joint (only the tempero-mandibular joint seeming to be immune). Joint pain may be the presenting symptom in as many as 90% of compressed-air workers and naval divers but in less than 25% of recreational divers (2) and is certainly not present in all DCS cases. One important feature is that limb pain has been associated with a less obvious, but more serious, neurological manifestation in as many as a third of presentations (2).

The pain can be discrete or diffuse, mild or intense, steady or fluctuating. It may be possible to distinguish between cases with sharp, localized and superficial pain, and those with a more dull, diffuse and deeper pain. The pain may be in a single joint, flitting, or in multiple sites. Sometimes there may be associated redness, edema or some limitation of movement. If mild and not treated by recompression, the pain may rapidly regress (a *"niggle"*) or more usually slowly resolve over some days or even weeks.

## Constitutional Manifestations

Fatigue disproportionate to the amount of preceding activity, malaise and anorexia are each an early manifestation of DCI. If they occur alone, recompression is not necessarily required, but may quickly give the patient much relief if applied. Their presence must be regarded as a warning that further manifestations may soon develop because they later become a common accompaniment to DCI.

## Cardiopulmonary Decompression Sickness

Respiratory manifestations (*"chokes"*) represent a severe form of DCS thought to be due to a build-up of venous gas emboli and the associated vasoactive products of surface activity in the pulmonary circulation.

Cardiopulmonary DCS been associated with deep dives of short duration and also with some slow decompressions of compressed-air workers. It is relatively rare in professional diving but in recreational divers it tends to arise among those who exceed the recommended limits of the principal training agencies. Rivera found it in 2% of U.S. Navy divers (42) and Kindwall estimates it to be about 6% in compressed-air workers (24). Pulmonary DCS has not been reported among submarine escape trainees but they do get the pulmonary manifestations of pulmonary barotrauma (see the chapter by Kindwall, "Gas Embolism").

The onset of a retro-sternal pain which limits deep inspiration may be the first symptom of "chokes". A dry cough and shallow, rapid respirations may mark the onset of circulatory collapse. Milder presentations may occur, but all are potentially lethal. A possible differential diagnosis is ARDS due to salt water inhalation and the two conditions may be concurrent (13).

## Bends Shock

Although rare, bends shock can be rapidly fatal. Survival hinges on the rapid infusion of IV fluids. Kindwall treated a case where 5 liters of Dextran 40, Dextran 80, and plasmanate were administered over a 6-hour period, while the hematocrit continued to rise from 51% to 62%. The vascular system opens up and leaks copious fluids into the "third space." Ouabain was used to control heart rate and restore blood pressure. The patient survived with plus 4 edema of the soles of his feet, before he diuresed 10 days later.

## Neurological Decompression Illness

Almost any neurological manifestation can follow a dive associated with sufficient gas-loading but many such manifestations are also found among submarine-escape trainees who have no significant dissolved gas. With the possibility of minor AGE precipitating DCS in supersaturated tissues that, until the arrival of the gas emboli, were safely decompressing, and also with the other pathway of venous gas emboli passing through a PFO to supersaturated tissues, it follows that it is not always possible to diagnose neurological DCS or neurological AGE with certainty. Any neurological symptom or deficit after a dive should be considered to be a manifestation of decompression illness until proven otherwise and must be managed accordingly. Whereas the classic presentation of AGE due to PB is an immediate loss of consciousness on surfacing and often leads rapidly to death, hemiplegia, monoplegia or vertigo, the classic neurological presentation of DCS is an ascending paraplegia. The colloquial term *"spinal bends"* is used but a fuller description is needed.

The onset of tingling or woolliness of the feet ascending in minutes or maybe over an hour or so, into complete paraplegia is the classic presentation of "spinal decompression sickness." Less commonly a sudden onset of unilateral or bilateral girdle pain of the trunk may be associated with an almost immediate paraplegia below that level. Pathology demonstrates that the lesions at this stage are usually multiple, discrete, and multilevel. Thus, almost any peripheral neurological deficit can occur.

Paradoxical interpretation of hot and cold and a diminished vibration sense may be detected at the early stages of "spinal bends." Impairment of the bulbo-cavernous reflex and of anal sphincter tone are early signs possibly leading to retention of urine, rectal incontinence, and impotence.

Quadriplegia, with the patient having only the phrenic nerves for respiration, marks a limit of survivable decompression illness, but it must be understood that many minor cases do not progress and that a number have recovered spontaneously.

Cerebral dysfunction of DCS and AGE can take the form of a feeling of "spaciness," a detachment from reality, dysarthria, visual disturbances or, occasionally, a psychosis. The vertiginous form of decompression illness must be distinguished from aural barotrauma and may be associated with nausea, vomiting and ipsilateral deafness. It has also been suggested that, after the acute phase of cerebral decompression illness, some are at risk from the development of a "dysexecutive syndrome," a delayed manifestation that seems analogous to a post-concussional syndrome.

## Latency

Loss of consciousness or stroke-like manifestations on arriving at the surface from a relatively rapid ascent, are characteristic of the immediacy of conditions associated with arterial gas embolism (see the chapter by Kindwall entitled "Gas Embolism"). A delay of some minutes may occur before the onset of lesser neurological deficits such as weakness or disorientation, but a delay longer than this is not characteristic of presentations in those whose prior exposure was too brief to acquire a significant gas load (14).

The onset of limb pain is not associated with brief exposures. It occurs only after dives in which there has been sufficient time to dissolve a significant mass of gas in the tissues. In compressed-air workers and divers, a latency of as long as 24 hours is possible, though the onset is usually sooner. In saturation divers the onset of limb pain and other manifestations of DCS may appear to have no latency because they arise during a multi-day decompression to the surface. They can also arise at the living or "storage" depth of saturation divers following an excursion to a deeper working depth.

Apparent latencies longer than 24 hours after surfacing may be due to the diver failing to recognize or to report earlier symptoms, but usually some 85% of neurological manifestations present within an hour of surfacing (2, 14).

## DIAGNOSIS

Any symptom or sign arising within 24 hours of a decompression should be considered to be DCI if there is no other obvious cause and must be managed accordingly. Failure to do so can lead to delay in treatment and that would permit a progression of the underlying condition that will render it less responsive to treatment.

The diagnosis can often be made from the history alone and while an examination may demonstrate physical signs, these are not always present.

There is a natural tendency for individuals to deny their problems or to seek some other explanation for their manifestations. For instance, a knee injury sustained while getting into a boat may cause pain but the pain may be due to bubbles at that joint.

Those complaining of limb pain only, however, are not often urgent but must be examined meticulously prior to recompression in order to discover any unsuspected neurological deficit. However, it is important to keep in mind that untreated bends or missed decompression may result in eventual dysbaric osteonecrosis if not recompressed within about 6 hours.

Deterioration and the need for immediate treatment may justify a foreshortening of the examination in some cases, but the full examination should be conducted as soon as time permits. If a compression chamber is on site, the examination of neurological or cardiopulmonary illness may be conducted at depth after treatment has begun. This is effective emergency treatment and establishes a baseline of any residual manifestations against which subsequent progress can be judged. If there is no chamber on site, time for the full examination and supplementary investigations may be available while waiting for transport. In all cases, the desire to complete the examination should be balanced against the greater need to minimize delay before definitive treatment can be started. Supplementary investigations are not always done, perhaps because of the need for immediate treatment or when the chamber is at a remote location, perhaps at sea.

There may often be a delay of many hours before the patient can be brought to a recompression chamber. In these circumstances a chest x-ray and blood for a hematocrit may be appropriate. The use of ultrasound to detect bubbles has no place in the management of persons who already have symptoms.

## THE DEVELOPMENT OF TREATMENT PROTOCOLS

It was long recognized that a return to pressure would ameliorate the symptoms of decompression sickness but a reason for the great reluctance of physicians to use recompression was that this constituted a "homeopathic treatment." Homeopathy implies giving in minute doses a drug (in this case, compressed air), which is capable of producing symptoms in healthy people similar to those of the disease to be treated.

Despite the view that returning an individual with DCS to compressed air might be scientific nonsense, not only did the caisson workers themselves recognize that symptoms could disappear but also that then one could often decompress without the symptoms reappearing. It was simply a matter of decompressing slowly enough so that the additional uptake of nitrogen would not cause a recurrence. Moir, an engineer, became the first man intentionally to recompress a victim of DCS for the purpose of treatment, even though he himself called his treatment "homeopathic" (33). Perhaps, not being a physician, he was not worried about being stigmatized for applying a homeopathic treatment and the effectiveness of his mechanical recompression of bubbles cannot be denied.

Air recompression became firmly established as the *sine qua non* for the treatment of DCS but its acknowledged effectiveness was bought at a considerable price because of the quantities of additional nitrogen that are dissolved in the tissues. This was later exemplified by the USN Treatment Table 4 with decompressions from 165 feet (50 m) of 38 hours or more.

It has always been difficult to know which procedure will be most successful in treating a particular case of DCI and, with insufficient cases at any one location for a powerful statistical analysis, management has necessarily remained more of an art than evidence-based. Early physicians have treated bends in accordance with their own experience, and some may still be so influenced today.

At first, Moir recommended that victims be recompressed to an air pressure of one-half to two-thirds of that at which they had been working. This indicates that, from the start, he was aware of the hazard of adding too much iatrogenic nitrogen. For those afflicted immediately on leaving the tunnels, this prompt recompression seemed to work. The pressure was then lowered at the rate of one pound per minute, or more slowly (33). Subsequent experience, probably with patients treated with more delay, showed that greater pressure was required for resolution. The recommendation was then made to return to the original working pressure and when this proved inadequate, the recommendation was made to go to the depth of relief. Thus as recompression depth increased the subsequent decompressions became longer.

Although Haldane introduced a rational approach to the development of decompression tables in 1908, little was done to codify treatment procedures. By and large, diving supervisors or tunnel superintendents had their own schemes for treatment, based more or less on personal experience. In 1924, the U.S. Navy introduced a set of treatment tables, but these ultimately proved to have a 50% failure rate. By 1945, the depth of relief was no longer considered adequate for treatment because it was realized that even then, bubbles persist. As one descends or increases the pressure in the chamber, spherical bubbles become smaller and smaller, but never disappear, as their volume approaches an asymptote and so it was felt that pressurization should be to the depth of relief plus at least one atmosphere. In 1945, Tables 1 to 4 were developed at the U.S. Navy's Experimental Diving Unit that embodied the concept of going to depth of relief plus one atmosphere with a maximum pressure of six atmospheres thus avoiding the problems of nitrogen narcosis for the inside tender. The procedure was viewed as a compromise between recompressing the offending bubbles and the prolongation of the subsequent decompression.

U.S. Navy Tables 1 to 4 were never tested on actual cases of DCS prior to their promulgation, but were simply designed to be safe for use following a previous dive. In testing, divers were taken to 130 feet (39 m) for an hour and then decompressed on a standard table. After a 30 to 60 min surface interval, they were then recompressed according to one of these experimental treatment tables. Only 84 manned dives were made and they were considered successful. Although these air treatment tables were primitive, at the time of their development they represented a 9-fold improvement over all previous recompressions. Despite their great length, Tables 1 to 4 became the standard of the world for some 20 years and, with small modifications, are still available for use in certain circumstances today.

A disconcerting trend then emerged. In 1946 the Tables 1 to 4 had only a 6% failure rate but by 1963 the failure rate in serious cases on initial recompression had climbed to 46% and by 1964 to 47.1%. A reason for the increasing failure of these Tables was that recreational scuba divers were being treated in increasingly greater numbers. These divers had often failed to follow any established decompression procedure, had often made multiple dives and typically presented only after much delay. This meant that a paralyzed diver could lie helpless in a cramped cylinder for 36 hours while experiencing no relief of his distress.

Oxygen seemed a logical option. In 1937, Behnke and Shaw had experimented with oxygen in the treatment of DCS by first taking bends victims to 165 feet (50 m; 6 bar, atmospheres absolute) on air for a brief period and then to 60 feet (18 m; 2.8 bar) to continue treatment at on oxygen. (4) Their results were excellent, but the U.S. Navy considered that oxygen treatments were too hazardous. Oxygen fires were greatly feared and oxygen-breathing under pressure was known also to produce occasional seizures, so Behnke and Shaw's work was not pursued further.

By 1964, circumstances required that the Navy reinvestigate oxygen treatment once again and Goodman and Workman of the USN Experimental Diving Unit began to investigate alternative modes of treatment. (16) Oxygen treatment has more than one advantage. Most importantly, when the patient is breathing oxygen, the "oxygen window" is enlarged and nitrogen faces no resistance to washout. This accounts for the oxygen tables' brevity compared to air treatments. Treatment does not end when maximum pressure is reached, as is the case for homeopathic air treatment, and thus the time to relief was viewed as having the same importance as had the depth of relief previously. Also of importance is the amelioration of DCS-induced blood sludging when oxygen is breathed (47). White cells become more flexible (39) and HBO inactivates the leukocyte adhesion molecule which is responsible for leukocyte stickiness and the no-reflow phenomenon (48).

Goodman and Workman experimented with various oxygen protocols, ranging in pressure from 2.0 to 2.8 atmospheres absolute (200 to 280 kPa). After 79 patients had been treated under these protocols, they chose 50 cases whom they felt had received "minimally adequate therapy". This they defined as oxygen breathing for at least 30 min at a maximum depth of 60 feet (18 m) followed by a total oxygen-breathing time of 90 minutes, the remainder at lesser depths. "Minimally adequate therapy" produced in those 50 cases a failure rate of only 3.6% as compared to the 47% currently being experienced on Table 4. In their report (16), they stated that the experimental caseload "is composed of older divers who have been exposed for longer bottom time durations and at greater depths. The incidence of 'serious' cases exceeds that of the comparative group..." In the appendix to their report, however, it should be noted that 84% of their cases were treated within six hours of symptom onset, and thus the effects of delayed treatment were not assessed. Despite this fact, the background statement included in the Navy promulgation instruction for the new tables stated: "Tables 5 and 6 have now been shown to be both safe and effective, especially for those severe injuries in which treatment has been delayed..."

The new treatment schedules, Tables 5 and 6, had been derived by multiplying minimally adequate therapy time by ratios of approximately 1.5 and 3 respectively. Table 5 provided for two hours of oxygen breathing, with 40 min of that oxygen time being spent at 2.8 bar and was for pain-only decompression sickness that cleared within 10 min at 60 feet (18 m). Table 6 embodied four hours of oxygen breathing, with one hour of that being spent at 60 feet (18 m) and was for serious symptoms, pain-only cases which did not clear completely in ten minutes, and recurrences. These new tables were promulgated to the fleet in 1967.

At the same time, Waite at the USN Submarine Medical Center had been experimenting with short treatment tables for air embolism. At that time, air embolism was treated on Table 3 (22 h) or Table 4 (38 h) because embolism always produced "serious symptoms." In dogs embolized with air through the carotid arteries, Waite found that a bounce dive to 165 feet (50 m) followed by standard decompression (on the 170 foot (52 m table) for 10 min provided a cure (52). He saw through a cranial window that all the superficial air bubbles disappeared as the pressure passed 80 feet (24 m). Despite the fact that Waite saw no physiologic reason for going deeper than 80 feet to clear the bubbles, he selected 165 feet (50 m) for 30 min on air before ascending in four min to 60 feet (18 m) and continuing on the new Tables 5 or 6. Waite felt that his new table would be more acceptable to traditionalists if it went to maximum pressure (53).

Thus the new embolism table was a combination of the older homeopathic approach of Moir and the more modern oxygen-washout protocol. A short embolism Table 5A was adopted initially for those with full resolution within 15 min at 165 feet. This and Table 6A (with 30 min at maximum depth) were promulgated at the same time as Tables 5 and 6 and eagerly accepted by the diving navy. Their success rate appeared to be high and the time that had to be spent in the chamber for serious cases was reduced from 38 to less than 5 hours. As experience was gained, modifications were made. For cases which did not respond immediately to Table 6, extensions at 60 and 30 feet (18 and 9 m) were provided. Table 5A was eventually abandoned as recurrences were encountered.

It should be noted that Table 6A for air embolism was intended for use solely in submarine escape training, i.e. when the victims of air embolism had no significant nitrogen load. This was the reason why Waite was able to specify a rapid (4 min) decompression to 60 feet (18 m). It was later used for divers who had embolized in the open sea and sometimes after dives during which substantial amounts of nitrogen had been absorbed. What was not realized at that time was that, while the 4 min decompression from 165 feet to 60 feet (50 m to 18 m) presented little risk to those without a significant nitrogen-load in their tissues, it was too precipitous for those who did have a prior gas load. Until very recently, nitrox was the only mixed gas used for treatment. Some Navy facilities do not have nitrox available to treat decompression sickness, but continue to use air at 165 feet (50 m) on Table 6A.

An attempt to solve this problem was provided by Comex Table 30 (Cx 30), developed by Fructus in the early 70s from the French Navy's 30 m tables (19) which used 40% or 60% nitrox at depth. Cx 30 called for an initial recompression to 30 m (100 feet), breathing 50/50 nitrox or heliox for those stops deeper than 18 m (60 feet). The entire table takes about 7½ hours. The 50/50 nitrox was breathed for almost two hours at depths greater than 60 feet (18 m). This table had great success and is used extensively in North Sea operations. Others then adopted 50/50 nitrox for the deep portion of Table 6A thus producing an inspired partial pressure of 3.0 bar of oxygen. This made an excursion to high pressure more acceptable when treating air embolism in divers who had a significant gas load.

In treating 140 cases of decompression sickness in Milwaukee compressed-air tunnel workers, Kindwall relied almost entirely on USN Tables 5 and 6 (24). He believed, as did most of the diving medical community, that low-pressure oxygen was superior in such cases than going to higher pressures. Dr. Edgar End of Milwaukee (who had produced the first successful heliox table and a world-record dive of 420 feet in 1937) reasoned that treating caisson workers with oxygen at 30 psig (3 atmospheres absolute) made much more sense than taking them deep and absorbing more nitrogen. He treated over 200 cases of DCS using only oxygen at pressures no greater than 30 psig with great success from 1947 onward, but he never published them. A factor towards success of low-pressure oxygen treatment is that caisson workers usually work at modest pressures e.g. 35 psig (80 feet, 24 m, 3.4 bar) for a whole shift. Almost all Kindwall's cases were treated within 2 to 5 hours of onset and resolved completely. Neurological cases that were delayed did not fare as well, but all patients returned to full-time heavy manual labor.

As illustrated by the following case, before mixed gas was available, treatment was not always straightforward (24).

*The patient had been working a split shift at 24 psig (1.63 bar) with only 20 to 30 min decompression after each 3 h exposure. He had tried self-treatment in the muck lock with air recompression for 75 min followed by a 30 min decompression that only worsened his symptoms. He presented with pain-only DCS in the hip and failed to get resolution after 20 min at 60 feet (18 m) on Table 6. With the patient breathing air, the pressure was increased to 100 feet (30 m) and there was a dramatic relief of symptoms. Because Kindwall was convinced of the superiority of oxygen treatment over compressed air, the patient was decompressed to 60 feet (18 m) and resumed on Table 6. However, on decompression to 30 feet (9 m) the pain worsened. Even after extensions and the addition of extra 20 minutes oxygen back at 60 feet (18 m), the pain was not resolved completely. The fact that symptoms had been originally relieved completely by the sudden increase in pressure to 100 feet (30 m) led to a reconsideration of the wisdom of remaining at 60 feet (18 m) for every case.*

In a series as large as 140 cases, it is ra.re to have no one with permanent incapacitating sequelae and all these compressed-air workers returned to work. The success of treatment Tables 5 and 6 was possibly due to the fact that none of them had been exposed to pressures greater than 100 feet (30 m) (24). Gary Beyerstein (1) suggested that "bubbles have a memory" for the depths at which they originated. For this reason, dives which have exceeded 100 feet (30 m) would be less responsive to treatment at 60 feet (18 m) despite oxygen breathing. The U.S. Navy treatment algorithm ignores the history of the air dive (except for treatment of blow-up) and does not consider delay before treatment when choosing a recompression protocol.

In the 2005 revision of their Diving Manual, U.S. Navy treatment for AGE and serious DCS starts out on Table 6 and requires assessment of the patient within 20 min. If unchanged or worsening the patient is compressed to depth of relief or significant relief not exceeding 165 feet (50 m) on Table 6A with the option of an oxygen-enriched mixture. The long-serving Table 4 is available in this algorithm in case more time at depth is required but at depth is on air. The optional oxygen extensions for Table 6 at 60 and 30 feet (18 and 9 m) are found in the algorithm for symptom recurrence (51).

If symptoms persist following the initial recompression, serial treatments on Table 6 can be given daily (or Tables 5 or 9 twice daily) for up to 14 days. However, if the working diver is not to be medically disqualified and become unemployed, the essential need is to achieve a full clinical recovery. A more aggressive approach to achieving full recovery in the initial recompression is needed. The earlier use of pressures greater than 60 feet (18 m) and other tables, especially if the victim was diving deeper than 100 feet (30 m), or if treatment has been delayed and/or the patient deteriorating, are found in non-military algorithms.

Four studies of the treatment of air embolism in dogs (29) have tended to repudiate the advantages of pressure. Using cortical evoked potentials as measurement of the effect of treatment, they found no difference between dogs treated at 60 feet (18 m) on Table 6 and those treated at 165 feet (50 m) on Table 6A. Additionally, they found at autopsy that the spinal cords of the dogs treated at 165 feet (50 m) had been embolized by nitrogen. Intracranial pressure was found to rise and remain high for over 90 min when air was breathed at 165 feet (50 m). Based on their results and other data, the Navy now permits the initial treatment of AGE at 60 feet (18 m). However, normal or improved cortical evoked potentials are not really adequate indices of success in clinical bends treatment (18). Given the fact that most Navy cases were treated early, that the published work for oxygen treatment was largely favorable, and that cases treated at pressures greater than 60 feet (18 m) were very few in number, there was little interest in going to higher pressures.

Beckman and Overlock experimented with higher pressures and brought into routine use in Hawaii the initial deep treatment of DCS at depths as deep as 230 feet (70 m). Their rationale was that they were crushing bubble nuclei and at depths greater than 60 feet (18 m) they used nitrox with 35% oxygen (37). However, the results of their few cases cannot be compared with other series because, using a grading system they devised, they reported only changes in clinical status from one grade to another. An analysis of true recovery is not available. This form of treatment has not been used elsewhere.

Meanwhile, Lee and others at the Tsoying Naval Hospital in Taiwan, were faced with a formidable problem. Frequently they were called on to treat DCS in Chinese fishermen divers with severe neurologic symptoms, often delayed many hours or days (28). Their training had been provided by the U.S. Navy and they adhered to U.S. Navy rules. They knew that some kinds of decompression sickness did not respond readily to oxygen treatment, as witnessed by a little-known article by Workman in 1968, which reported a 41.2% failure rate in the initial treatment of 34 civilian cases (54). The experiences of Lee et al. using Table 6 were even more dismal. In 36 consecutive cases of Type II DCS treated before 1982, Table 6 achieved a cure rate of only 8.3%. Knowing that additional measures were necessary, they began methodically exploring alternatives. They first chose Table 6A, using air breathing at 165 feet (50 meters). Between 1982 and 1986, using 6A, they increased their cure rate for 31 cases to 67.7%. However, five of those patients suffered recurrences during the very fast ascent from 165 feet to 60 feet (50 to 18 m). As a result they shifted to Table 4 in such cases. Niu modified Table 6A to stretch out the decompression time between 165 and 60 feet, making stops at 120, 80 and 70 feet (36, 24, and 21 m) making it suitable for patients with a nitrogen load. The time spent between 165 and 60 feet (50 and 18 m) was increased tenfold, from 4 to 40 min. A further modification was to use nitrox with 40% oxygen on the same lengthened table at depths greater than 60 feet (18 m). In terms of pulmonary oxygen toxicity, UPTD scores were calculated and found to be within acceptable limits.

Between 1986 and 1989, the Tsoying Naval Hospital facility carried out a study involving 374 cases of Type II decompression sickness comparing Table 6A, the lengthened version termed 6A1, breathing air, and the mixed gas version, labeled 6A1M. Each of these were difficult cases in which one would not expect to effect an easy cure and 75% had been delayed more than 48 hours (range 2 to 96 h). In that study, Table 6A produced a 51% cure rate; Table 6A1, the lengthened table using air, achieved an almost 60% cure rate; whereas the lengthened table using mixed gas (Table 6A1M) had a 70.7% cure rate (26). All the patients not cured were improved. Comparison of the results between the tables showed that the percentages were real, with a p-value of < 0.05. This is the only paper in the literature to give a statistical validation of its success rates.

Despite research efforts and clinical observations, the mechanisms of DCS are not fully known. There are many hypothetical pathways for the processes of decompression pathology and none are mutually exclusive. This means that several mechanisms may be operating at the same time and doing so to a varying and undetermined degree. There are many uncertainties.

It is not known how long bubbles persist following an episode of decompression sickness, but there seems to be some clinical evidence that they last for a while that may measured in days, despite the inherent unsaturation of the body with nitrogen. The fact that the addition of high pressure alone, after long delay, can produce relief tends to substantiate this.

However, acute decompression sickness affecting the spinal cord has been demonstrated to produce flame hemorrhages in some cases. These may represent those who fail to respond to recompression.

The spinal cord appears to be amazingly resilient to bubble injury in which the lesions are multiple, discrete, and multilevel, as opposed to other forms of traumatic spinal cord damage, in which a transection may occur at a single level. Treatment with pressure and oxygen can produces remission some days following paralysis which suggests that the local pathology may have vastly diminished the oxygen supply to neurons but not necessarily killed them. If bubble formation and blockage of the circulation produced neuronal-cell death within minutes, as is seen in other forms of circulatory arrest, recompression hours or days later would have no effect. This implies that there must be neurons which are alive but which do not have sufficient blood supply to function. This accords with the concept of the "ischemic penumbra" in some forms of stroke.

Physical therapists like to work with paralyzed divers because the prognosis, in general, is a great deal better than when treating similar symptoms following the trauma of a motor vehicle or horse riding accident.

## The Use of Helium/Oxygen

From 1958 to 1973, the U.S. Navy diving manual gave the option of using the mixture of 80% helium and 20% oxygen instead of air at any time on any treatment table. In fact, in Goodman and Workman's report on the development of Tables 5 and 6, they state "80/20 helium/oxygen can be breathed in lieu of chamber air during the air intervals and for several minutes after surfacing" (10, 54).

When helium became available to Kindwall at a large community hospital, he substituted it for air when going to 6 atmospheres in order to avoid introducing more nitrogen. Heliox was used with success in the treatment of air embolism and there were no counter-diffusion problems. Kindwall first used helium/oxygen for DCS in 1969:

*A patient, who had been working a split shift at 1.72 ATA, presented with severe shoulder pain. This patient had also tried air recompression as self-treatment, working an additional shift in order to get rid of his pain. However, after decompressing from the third shift, the patient was suffering excruciating pain and reported for chamber treatment. Because the patient had only minimal relief after two 20-minute oxygen periods at 60 feet, he was compressed to 165 feet (50 m). On reaching maximum depth, the patient noted that the pain shifted from his shoulder to his left elbow, but did not completely disappear. The patient was held at maximum pressure for 90 min, but a residual soreness persisted. Because of the length of his exposure, the patient was decompressed on a US Navy Table 4 to the 60-foot level, but breathing 20% heliox, from a depth of 140 feet (42 m). The delay in using helium until 140 feet was operational and unavoidable. The patient continued heliox until 60 feet (18 m). At 60 feet, he was shifted to an extended Table 6. The patient left the chamber with only residual soreness after a stay of eleven hours. It is believed that this was the first time a patient was shifted from a Table 4 to a Table 6 at the 60-foot (18 meters) level. No counter-diffusion problems occurred, despite the fact that heliox was given not at maximum depth but begun during decompression.*

## Counter-Diffusion

In 1972, Lambertsen and Idicula reported severe problems with counter-diffusion when neon was substituted, as a breathing gas by mask, while the subjects were immersed in a helium atmosphere at high pressure (27). In 1974, Richard Strauss described isobaric bubble formation in a gelatin block, when the gas surrounding the gelatin was changed from nitrogen to helium (46). The implication was that helium diffused into the gelatin faster than nitrogen diffused out and that, for a time, the sum of their partial pressures exceeded ambient pressure, causing bubbles to form. Because of these observations, efforts to use helium as a treatment gas were abandoned and the US Navy removed the option of its use from the diving manual. Encouraged by the adverse medico-legal climate in which all medicine functions, it was felt that helium posed too many risks, despite the fact that it had been used clinically in the past.

However, those in commercial diving began to use helium/oxygen for treatment when it was realized that, when it had been used, no one had experienced problems clinically. The French began using 50/50 heliox with the Comex 30 Table in place of the original 50/50 nitrox and it is now standard. The Israeli Navy now routinely uses helium oxygen at treatment pressures greater than 18 m (60 ft) (26). The US Navy manual reinstated the option of using 79% helium / 21% oxygen in place of air on the air treatment tables, but offered no detailed instructions. Table 8 includes the use of helium/oxygen for recompression beyond 165 feet (50 m) (50).

In 1994, Philip James (21) reviewed the physics of helium diffusion and cases where the substitution of heliox appeared life-saving in divers who were deteriorating during treatment on air. Although helium diffuses faster in blood, he pointed out that it is less soluble than nitrogen and will therefore cause a reduction in the size of bubbles. Most importantly, he noted that there have been no adverse effects clinically when heliox has been breathed during treatment following an air dive. Even if bubbles were to grow briefly in the pulmonary circulation, as shown by Catron et al. (7) when helium is breathed following supersaturation of the tissues in nitrogen, helium breathing in recompression is accompanied by a large increase in pressure when the patient is taken to depths beyond 60 feet (18 m). Thus, even if bubbles were initially to grow before beginning to disappear rapidly, in no way would they approach their original size seen on the surface. In the future, higher pressures may be used more frequently, especially in the treatment of delayed cases, with helium as the only logical diluent gas following air dives. Pressure can solve many problems, especially in delayed cases, but its use should not include a return to the homeopathic air recompression with its greater nitrogen uptake.

The final point to make is that the physician must ensure that his chamber facility is prepared in advance to treat difficult cases. This means procuring the necessary mixed gas and having it readily available before any need to use it arises.

## IMMEDIATE TREATMENT

Where no chamber is readily available, there are a number of measures that should begin immediately at the surface.

- The first priority is 100% oxygen by close-fitting mask and is essential in all cases. Sufficient oxygen should be available to last until the casualty reaches the chamber.
- If serious symptoms are present, an intravenous drip should be set up with isotonic saline or Ringer's solution; in milder cases, oral fluids should be pushed until the urine is pale and copious. A fluid balance chart should be started.

- Catheterization may be required. Attention should be given to the pressure points of a paralyzed patient, with the affected limbs regularly put through their full range of passive movement.
- In rare cases, pleurocentesis may be required for a pneumothorax due to pulmonary barotrauma.

In cases of severe limb pain, the use, during transport, of nitrous oxide analgesic mixtures which are available in some ambulances should be discouraged because the nitrous oxide is known to enlarge bubble size by counter diffusion, albeit temporarily.

The patient should be transferred to a recompression chamber as soon as possible and, if by air, at an altitude of less than 1,000 ft (300 m) above ground level. If available, a pressurized aircraft should be used and some can maintain sea level pressure up to an altitude of 23,000 ft (6970 m). Travel over a mountain range by road may exacerbate symptoms and in such areas a monoplace chamber has been used not for treatment at pressure but simply to maintain ground-level pressure during transfer.

## DCS ANCILLARY TREATMENT

Ancillary treatments are important and, depending on circumstances such as the absence of immediate recompression, it may be appropriate to start them immediately.

### Hydration

Hydration is the most important ancillary treatment in DCS. Blood sludging was first described by Swindle in 1937 (47) and is a significant adverse factor in DCS by retarding circulation. To counter the Hemoconcentration of DCS, the immediate rehydration of the patient can aid a more rapid elimination of inert gas and improve the manifestations even before reaching the chamber. Patients should drink water if they can and produce a clear urine flow of at least 50 ml per hour, preferably more.

Intravenous fluids should be used for those who cannot drink. If the DCS patient is in severe shock, fluid replacement is an absolute requirement for survival. The *UHMS Guidelines for Adjunctive Therapy* (34) suggests that lactated Ringers solution or other glucose-free isotonic crystalloid is selected for neurological DCS but that efficacy is less well established in AGE or "chokes".

### Steroids

Steroids have been used expectantly in spinal cord DCS where it is assumed that edema is present. To be effective, they would probably have to be given in massive doses similar to those in traumatic spinal cord injury. but there have been no controlled trials. There is a negative study showing that steroids have not been effective in treatment of air embolism (11).

### Lidocaine

There is insufficient evidence to support the regular use of this in DCI and it does have some significant side effects. Researchers at the Naval Medical Research Institute found that in a cat model, lidocaine has a considerable protective effect in air embolism. It is given in anti-arrhythmic dosage. Thus, the side effects are no more that would be expected in myocardial infarction patients. However, its effects have not yet been demonstrated in humans.

## Diazepam

The use of diazepam can be effective in the symptomatic relief of vertigo, nausea, and vomiting, in vestibular DCS, but the suppression of obvious symptoms should not influence or shorten the subsequent recompression management of the underlying pathology (23).

## Glycerol

Glycerol given orally can be effective in reducing spinal cord edema in humans and has been found to be more effective than mannitol or urea. Its therapeutic onset is quicker than mannitol (44). It has been reported, anecdotally, to be helpful in spinal cord DCS. The hourly dosage is one gram (0.8 ml) per kilogram of body weight mixed half and half with water or lemonade. It is unpalatable, so if it causes retching it can be given via N.G. tube.

## Digitalis, in DCS

Digitalis can be life-saving in DCS shock. Kindwall had one patient who was in shock, had pulmonary edema, and was on 10cm of PEEP, the blood pressure was 70 over unobtainable and the heart rate was 140 despite massive fluid replacement. A dose of Deslanoside 0.4 mg IV dropped his heart rate to 120 and his blood pressure came up to nearly normal. Digitalization was then continued with digitoxin.

## Other Drugs

There are a number of drugs which have been used in the past, but some of which await additional human study before definite conclusions can be made. These include:

- Heparin in low sub-anticoagulant doses for which there are a number of anecdotal reports where the results of treatment were better than expected a animal studies (8, 38), but no controlled human study, and one study in dogs (41) that found it of no benefit in mild to moderate bends.
- Aspirin for its inhibition of platelet aggregation must be balanced against the risk of enhancing hemorrhage in the CNS or an inner ear already damaged by bubbles. Nevertheless it has been recommended in French DCS algorithms in an intravenous form.

# RECOMPRESSION, DCS

When choosing a recompression scheme, it is imperative to consider the dive profile, the nature of the symptoms and signs, the time of symptom onset, the duration of delay before treatment and whether there is continuing deterioration (43).

The early return of the stricken diver or compressed-air worker to raised environmental pressure often provides an immediate and complete resolution of the illness. The subsequent therapeutic decompression is designed to be sufficiently slow to prevent a relapse. The tables and algorithms which can be followed during recompression are well established. Most chambers are run on site by personnel trained for the task and with the support of a nominated diving doctor experienced in such therapy.

Controversies exist (35, 36) concerning what the optimum treatment might be, especially in unresponsive or deteriorating cases. The following account will describe one aggressive algorithm that allows maximum theoretical washout of nitrogen combined with early and efficient bubble compression. It is based on published work and experience gained in clinical treatment of commercial, as well as sport divers. The choice of treatment table utilizes the factors of the dive profile and its depth, as well as the factor of delay in treatment, in addition to symptoms and signs. For simplicity it incorporates published tables.

Where a recompression chamber is available, the nature of the recompression therapy will be determined by several factors:

- Assessment of the patient.
- Pressure capability of the chamber.
- Availability of oxygen and other gases.
- A lock for access to the patient by medical personnel.
- Training, experience and availability of the staff.
- Availability of ICU support if needed.

Common to all chamber systems is the need for recompression without undue delay. Immediate recompression and examination at depth is the accepted procedure with submarine-escape training, where the patient is within a minute of the chamber. At the other extreme, where the transfer of the patient may have taken 12 or more hours, clinical examination, hematocrit, an intravenous drip, catheterization, CXR and pleurocentesis, as appropriate, can precede a fairly prompt recompression.

While as many as 85% of cases may turn out to have been relatively mild and may have made a full recovery, the remaining 15%, whatever their treatment (40), develop a serious illness and may deteriorate rapidly, requiring prompt and aggressive treatment. In the early phase, the difficulty is not being able to predict how a particular case may develop. Features that are associated with a potentially poor outcome include those cases arising after a deep dive:

- An early onset of symptoms.
- The presence of pulmonary manifestations.
- Objective evidence of sensory change.
- Subjective symptoms of motor impairment.
- Any cranial nerve or cerebral involvement.
- Deterioration and delay before recompression.

These guidelines are not all-inclusive. Severe cases can arise following an apparently "safe" dive conducted within the appropriate procedures and decompression tables.

A positive approach to the restoration of function is to be aware that traditional decision points in some treatment algorithms are based on the presence or absence of life-threatening and other serious manifestations. While this is indeed extremely important, it is no longer enough. Any residual neurological sign, no matter how mild, may be sufficient to medically disqualify a working diver from returning to work. Also, for the recreational diver, nothing more than an impaired sensation of the finger tips could mean the end of a violinist's career. The so-called "minor" neurological manifestations deserve additional commitment by the HBO team towards attaining the best possible result during the first recompression.

Sometimes a patient presents initially with serious neurological signs such as paralysis but then seems to make a spontaneous recovery. One must not be caught out by this because it is not rare for the symptoms to recur later when they can be refractory to treatment. So it is important to recompress such patients even in the absence of their original symptoms. The alternative, which is to wait and observe, could lead to a medico-legal outcome. When summoned to the emergency room to attend a stricken diver, no matter how mild the case be described, do so without delay as there may be severe medico-legal liability if the outcome is less than perfect. "I'll see the patient as soon as I finish rounds" is no longer acceptable.

## Monoplace Chambers

Monoplace chambers are becoming more commonplace in hospitals as wound care centers find them to be a useful adjunct to wound healing. Almost universally, they are limited to a 2 bar (3 ATA, 66 ft, 20 m) pressure capability. All are equipped to deliver 100% oxygen to the patient, but some do not have masks to deliver air to the patient for the air breathing periods used by standard Navy recompression tables. If the chamber is equipped with a mask, the conscious patient can cooperate by holding the tight-fitting air mask in place for the required "air breaks" of a USN Table 6. Compressed air from a standard cylinder next to the chamber can be directed into the chamber via a reducing valve through a modified port in the chamber door or the end frame. Most demand masks require the air to be delivered at 50 psig (3.4 Kg/cm$^2$) over chamber pressure and thus the pressure reducing valve should be set at a minimum of 80 psig (5.2 Kg/cm$^2$).

If a demand mask supplied with air is not available or if the patient is not able to cooperate with his treatment, a treatment schedule can be used which incorporates the "minimal adequate treatment" described by Goodman and Workman (16). The patient is taken to 60 feet (18 m) in the oxygen-filled chamber as rapidly as tolerated, and he is held there for 30 min. Decompression to 30 feet (9 m) is then carried out over 30 min. The patient is held there for 60 min and decompressed to the surface over 30 min. This provides the same amount of oxygen (i.e. 2 h) as USN Table 5. If a monoplace chamber is available immediately with an adequate staff, it may be best to use it if getting to a multiplace chamber would involve significant delay. If symptoms persist after this protocol, it may be repeated after a 30-min surface interval if the patient cannot be transferred to a multiplace chamber for treatment at greater pressure. In monoplace chambers not equipped with demand air masks, oxygen time (4 h) equivalent to that provided in USN Table 6 cannot be given because of the risk of oxygen toxicity. The ability to handle acute emergencies such as pneumothorax, respiratory or cardiac arrest, or vomiting and aspiration that can occur in the chamber is also made more difficult as the patient will have to be decompressed to the surface for prompt alleviation of the problem. (See the chapter by Kindwall entitled "Management of Complications in Hyperbaric Treatment.")

The Divers Alert Network compiled the 90-day outcomes for patients treated in monoplace chambers compared to those treated in multiplace units; the results are surprising (35). For "Pain only" or Type I cases, the percentage of patients with residuals at 90 days was 5.9% for multiplace units, and 7.7% for patients receiving monoplace treatment. Typically the residuals were neurological symptoms which were missed initially or which appeared later. Type II cases were divided into "mild" and "severe." Severe cases were those which involved motor weakness, loss of consciousness, speech and gait problems, bladder or bowel incontinence, or convulsions. Everything else was classified as "mild" neurological. For these, the cases with residuals were 16.2% for the multiplace, and 16.1% for the monoplace units. For severe neurological patients, 21.2% had residuals when treated in multiplace units, versus 24.3% when treated in a monoplace unit. These comparative results may reflect early referral to monoplace chambers, or the lack of more aggressive treatment in multiplace units. Air embolism patients, with an undefined loading of dissolved nitrogen, did not appear to fare nearly as well; 58.3% of the patients had residuals when given monoplace treatment compared to 19.4% treated in the multiplace chamber (35) but conclusions about outcome in air embolism were not statistically significant as only 12 patients received monoplace treatment, compared to 232 receiving treatment in the multiplace chambers.

Used in places where no other chamber is readily available, a one-compartment chamber has no facility to allow a doctor to "lock in" to visit the patient. The management of neurological deterioration or a tension pneumothorax during decompression becomes very difficult if no physician is present inside. In such an event, a monoplace chamber, in which there is the patient on oxygen but no air-breathing attendant, could be surfaced rapidly and, after the medical crisis has been dealt with, returned to depth. One-man chambers which are transportable, and which can be mated onto a larger pressure chamber elsewhere, are used successfully in some parts of the world. Other one-man chambers, inflatable and easily transported when empty, can be taken to a remote project site by the diving expedition as an emergency resource.

A two-compartment recompression chamber, capable of taking the patient to an equivalent pressure of 165 fsw (50 m) and providing oxygen-enriched mixtures or pure oxygen by means of a built-in breathing system (BIBS), is always to be preferred.

## TEST OF PRESSURE

Sometimes it may not be clear if the patient's musculo-skeletal pain or other symptoms are due to DCS. To clarify this doubt a test of pressure may be considered because an injury should not be affected by compression. The patient is taken to 60 feet (18 m) and given 100% oxygen for 20 min. If there is absolutely no change in the nature, quality, position, character or intensity of the symptom by the end of 20 min, an experienced diving doctor may conclude that it is not DCI and will decompress and offer other treatment. Should the symptoms improve on recompression, it may be DCI and treatment should continue accordingly. If the pain *worsens* on recompression, it is termed a "bone bubble" and also implies a positive test of pressure. No one knows the aetiology of the "bone bubble" but some have postulated that it is due to a bubble under the periosteum (*Vide infra*). If no experienced diving doctor is available and in commercial diving, where divers are not likely to have a doctor on site, a test of pressure comprises a full U.S. Navy Table 6.

## TREATMENT TABLE CHOICE

Assuming that one has a two-compartment chamber with at least a 6 ATA (50 m) pressure capability and with mixed gas and oxygen each available, one can then choose an appropriate treatment protocol that is based on the clinical assessment of the patient, but DCI is not a common condition. For treating it there are many algorithms in use around the world and, at each location, various recompression tables are available. With the relatively thin distribution of cases associated with a wide variety of clinical presentations, the majority of treatment centers can report on the experience they have had with a series of cases but evidence of treatment effectives rarely goes beyond a consensus of experts. The authors have each had a lifetime of experience in this field and are not satisfied that the ideal protocol has been defined. We expect each reader first to follow the algorithm adopted by their own treatment centre and then to begin the quest for improvement. Worldwide the basic HBO treatment is very similar to USN Table 6, or, and this usually works. The constant discussion is about the difficult case that does not respond as hoped. Perhaps one of the most useful diagnostic and management aids is the telephone because among the international network of diving medical physicians there will be someone competent to review a problem and offer advice at that critical time.

Decompression sickness is a dynamic condition. An important feature in the management of all cases is a constant awareness of the possibility of sudden or, more difficult to assess, insidious deterioration (43). The patient should never relapse during treatment without further immediate recompression to alleviate such symptoms. At depth and during the ascent phases of any treatment table, the patient must be carefully examined and monitored by the inside tender. The patient must be advised to report any deterioration because subjective changes usually precede physical signs.

The shorter oxygen table, USN Table 5 (Figure 1), was intended for use only in cases of limb pain and for that it is effective. The fact that some 30% of persons presenting with limb pain already have or shortly develop neurological manifestations has led to the practical view that where no doctor is present to conduct a neurological examination, all cases of limb pain should be treated on USN T6 as a minimum. This is now the rule in commercial diving. USN T5 is also used in the prevention of DCS in symptom-free divers who have surfaced but who have omitted or compromised their appropriate decompression stops.

If the patient has been diving to depths less than 100 feet (30 m) and presents within 6 or 8 h of symptom onset, USN T6 (Figure 2) will probably be effective in achieving resolution. When using USN T6, even with no extensions, the inside tender should breathe oxygen during the last half hour because DCS has been reported, rarely, in the inside tender on USN T6 where he/she breathes air at all times.

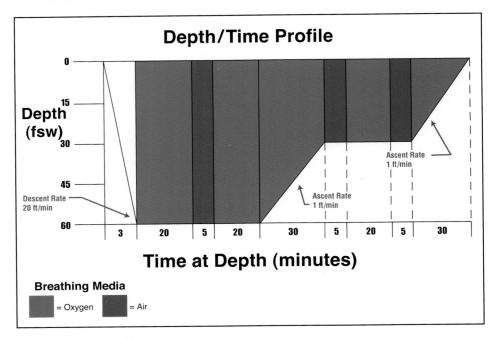

Figure 1. Treatment Table 5.

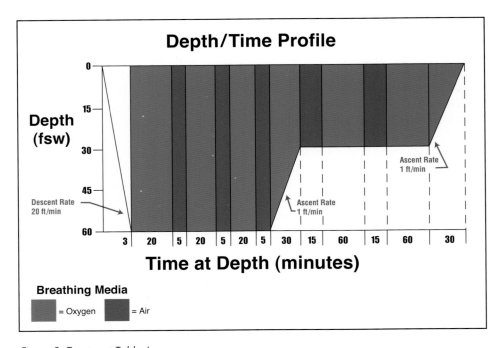

Figure 2. Treatment Table 6.

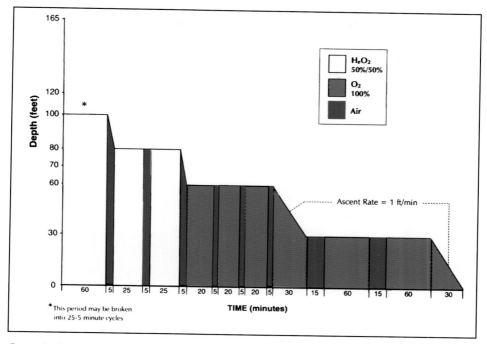

Figure 3. Comex 30 (Modified) patient shifted Table 6 at 60 ft used for dives in excess of 100 ft.

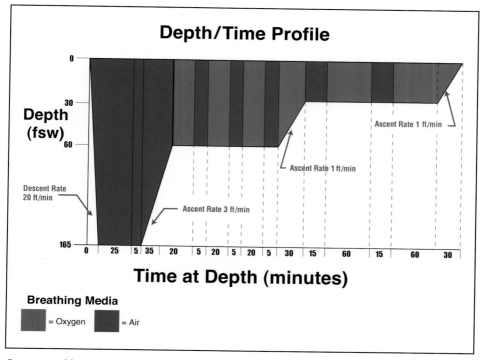

Figure 4. Table 6A, patient has obvious case of severe bends with long delay before treatment.

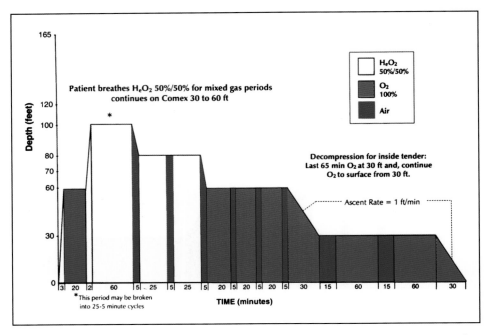

Figure 5. Patient fails to show the desired improvment after 20 minutes breathing oxygen at 60 ft. on Table 6. Patient then shifted to Comex Table 30 breathing heliox.

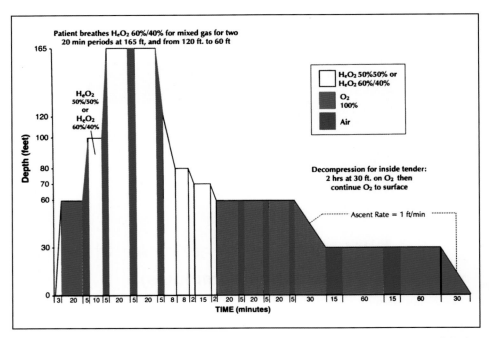

Figure 6. Patient fails to improve significantly at 60 ft on Table 6 after 20 minutes. Patient shifted to Comex Table 30. No significant improvement after 10 minutes on heliox at 100 ft. (30 m). Patient shifted to Lee Table 6A1M (Modified).

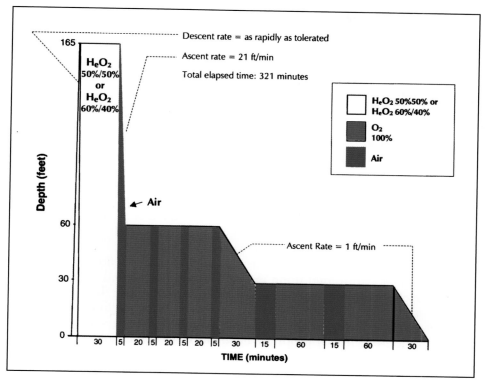

Figure 7. Table 6A for Air Embolism (Modified with mixed gas).

If the patient has been diving to depths in excess of 100 feet (30 m), a Modified Comex 30 (Figure 3) with 50/50 heliox would be a better initial choice. Animals with DCS at 132 feet (40 m) have shown resolution of bubbles in the pulmonary artery as measured with Doppler twice as fast when treated with Comex 30 on heliox, compared to USN T6. As shown in the figure, the patient's decompression is continued on Table 6 when he/she reaches the 60 foot (18 m) level. This is a modification of the Table Cx 30 which is used regularly in commercial diving.

For patients with severe symptoms and signs, such as paralysis, and for whom the delay to treatment has been many hours, the Lee Table 6A1M (Figure 4) with initial compression to 165 feet (50 m) breathing 40/60 oxy-helium and continuing on that mix until decompressed to 60 feet (18 m), can be recommended. An aggressive and early use of pressure and mixed gas has been advocated in the U.S. commercial diving industry (1). Under-treatment is a major error in diving medicine because there is never a second chance to intervene early with sufficient pressure.

If USN T6 was initially chosen but the patient is not rapidly improving after the first 20 minute oxygen period, a viable option is to compress to 100 feet (30 m) and continue on a Modified Comex 30 table with heliox (Figure 5). If the progress was not seen in 20 min at 60 feet (18 m) and again no progress is seen after 10 min at 100 feet (30 m), further recompression is indicated. One option is to compress to 165 feet (50 m) and continue on Table 6A (Figure 6).

Cases in which AGE is suspected are treated in a similar manner but, as discussed in the next chapter, they should begin their recompression with a brief excursion on mixed gas to 165 feet (50 m) on USN T6A (Figure 7). However, in those cases where the patient may have a significant nitrogen gas load in his tissues from diving, Table 6A1M should be used (Figure 4). The use of 50/50 or 40/60 oxy-helium to breathe at that depth (or, if not available, an oxy-nitrogen mixture) is now routine. Because air may be breathed at maximum depth on USN T6A, the USN now recommends a 35-min ascent from 165 to 60 feet (50 to 18 m).

Some centers prefer to treat the air embolism case initially with USN T6 and compress to 165 ft (50 m) only if there has been little response by the end of the first oxygen-breathing period. Although the US Navy approves this procedure, the authors do not recommend this approach if mixed gas is available. If mixed gas is not available and also if the case is delayed, a trial at 60 feet (18 m) may be considered. To go deep immediately with mixed gas costs little compared with the possible gains.

Conclusive data between the use of nitrox and heliox have not yet been published (10). Based upon animal studies, helium has been shown to have a beneficial effect upon bubble size following air diving, but this opinion is not universally accepted. A consensus view is that helium, in place of nitrogen, does no harm and the option of using the heliox version of the tables can be considered if the appropriate heliox mixture is available.

Other recompression tables are available and effective. For example, in one Caribbean island, the chamber attendants are all volunteers who, whenever a patient needs to be treated, have to take time off from work. The procedure was modified to allow each attendant to limit their time under pressure by locking a new tender into, and the previous one out from the chamber at predetermined points in the profile.

Recompression is not always successful and a life-threatening condition can arise quickly. Based on experience gained initially by a need to reduce oxygen percentages and thereby to try and reverse pulmonary oxygen toxicity in a prolonged treatment of neurological decompression sickness, various "saturation" treatments have been introduced and subsequently used as a definitive option for treatment at Duke University (32). In difficult circumstances, a simpler recommendation is to use USN Table 7. This permits an indefinite duration at 60 ft (18 m) on air, thus providing a period of stability for resuscitation and rest, without the hazard of gas expansion by continuing the decompression until later. However, there is risk in committing the patient and inside tender to saturation, as a failure in air supply can have grave consequences. It also ties up the chamber and staff for many hours that can stretch into days, so a large staff to man the necessary shifts is a requirement.

Other authorities and other countries routinely use other algorithms for these cases. In the hands of those trained and experienced with them, these also work well. Also, for those diving with a recompression chamber at the diving site and particularly for saturation divers, there are other specific management protocols, but for those whose clinical responsibilities are confined to divers who are transported to a hospital-based chamber, it is necessary only to be aware that there are other valid protocols successfully in use elsewhere.

## Decompression of a Tender

There have been occasions when an aborted treatment schedule, a prolonged exposure associated with resuscitation, an unplanned multilevel dive, or a forced repetitive use of the same inside tender on the same day have led to difficulties in ensuring the safe return to atmospheric pressure of a tender.

The current revision of the *US Navy Diving Manual* (51) and/or the *Canadian DCIEM Diving Manual* (9) should be a standard work of reference at all HBO units and provides tables that can be guides to decompression, but are helpful together with relevant safety procedures and precautions. If the tender breathes 100% oxygen from a tight-fitting demand mask with air breaks, instead of continuous air, for much of the decompression time shallower than 60 feet (18 m), one automatically adds a significant safety factor.

From deeper depths an oxy-nitrogen mix within oxygen toxicity limits can be used. Any time at the shallowest (10 foot; 3 m) stop should be made for a minimum of 10 min on oxygen if a longer time is not specified.

The U.S. Navy tables when used as written are not satisfactory. The Navy schedules were written to ensure no more than a 5% bends rate. If one were to use them without modification one would theoretically be facing having to treat one of the chamber staff for DCS once every two weeks if carrying out two chamber dives a day. For example, the U.S. Navy schedule for a 110 minute exposure at 45 ft (14 m), a typical hyperbaric treatment protocol, is a three minute stop at 10 feet (3m) breathing air. Kindwall reports that using that table he has seen cases of DCS in multiple joints, spinal cord DCS and vestibular DCS.

His own preference for such an exposure is decompress the tender to 20 feet (6m) for a 2-minute stop on oxygen and then to 10 feet (3m) for an additional 10 minutes, all on oxygen. Alternatively, the entire 12-minute decompression time can take place at 20 feet breathing oxygen. This scheme has worked effectively for twenty years with only one case of DCS reported. In hyperbaric practice, the inside tender always breathes oxygen instead of air at stops less than 50 feet and then with generous "padding" of the written table. Based on research by both Behnke and Kindwall (7, 25), nitrogen elimination is more efficient at the deeper stops. If you have a problem with decompression of the inside tender, the telephone line to a centre of expertise is another useful emergency resource.

## Decompression Schedules for Inside Tender when using Lee Table 6A1M or Combinations of Table 6, Comex 30 and Table 6A1M

Scenario 1. Patient has obvious case of severe bends with long delay before treatment. See Figure 8.

Scenario 2. Patient fails to show the desired improvement afer 20 minutes at 60 feet on Table 6. Patient is then shifted to Comex Table 30. See Figure 9.

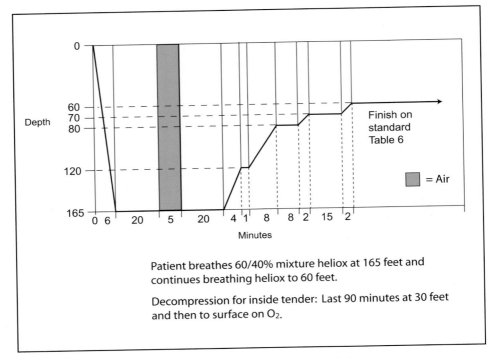

Patient breathes 60/40% mixture heliox at 165 feet and continues breathing heliox to 60 feet.

Decompression for inside tender: Last 90 minutes at 30 feet and then to surface on $O_2$.

Figure 8. Patient has obvious case of severe bends with long delay before treatment.

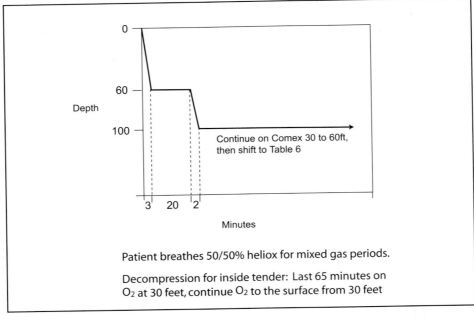

Patient breathes 50/50% heliox for mixed gas periods.

Decompression for inside tender: Last 65 minutes on $O_2$ at 30 feet, continue $O_2$ to the surface from 30 feet

Figure 9. Patient fails to show the desired improvement afer 20 minutes at 60 feet on Table 6. Patient is then shifted to Comex Table 30.

# EMERGENCY NUMBERS FOR DIVING AND DECOMPRESSION ACCIDENTS

The best place to call in a diving emergency or an in-house emergency with a tender, is the Diver's Alert Network (DAN) where one can get clinical advice. Emergency numbers are as follows:

DAN United States: +1-919-684-4326. Collect calls accepted.
DAN Latin America: +1-919-684-9111. Collect calls accepted in most areas.
DAN Europe: +39-06-4211-8685.
DAN Japan: +81-3-3812-4999.
DAN Southern Africa
    (within South Africa): +0800-020-111.
    (outside South Africa): +27-11-254-1112. Collect calls accepted.
DAN South East Asia-Pacific region
    Diving Emergency Services (DES)
        DES Australia
            (within Australia):+1-800-088-200. Toll free.
            (outside Australia): + 61-8-8212-9242
        DES New Zealand: + 0800-4-DES-111
    Singapore Naval Medicine and Hyperbaric Center: 67-58-1733
DAN Asia-Pacific
    DAN Philippines: + 02-632-1077
    DAN Malaysia: + 05-939-4114
    DAN Korea: +(010) 4500-9113

# RECOMPRESSION – PAIN WORSENING

As noted above, occasionally a diver may complain that his pain symptoms become worse as pressure in the chamber increases. It has been suggested that this occurrence could be explained by the presence of a small bubble in a bone, perhaps under the bone periosteum, and that during recompression it is "squeezed," a form of barotrauma causing the pain to worsen. Recompression can be slowed, but it should not be halted until the desired treatment depth has been reached. The pain will eventually disappear as any offending bubble is resorbed. The mechanism remains conjectural but the treating physician should not halt treatment should this symptom occur, as it will resolve.

# RECOMPRESSION ON SITE

There should be no place in professional or sport diving for dressing the diver in his equipment again and sending him down while breathing compressed air for recompression in the water. The difficulties are obvious:

- The patient may not be able to support himself physically.
- Difficult to monitor progress or deterioration.
- Poor communications.
- Difficult to maintain fluid balance.

- Inaccessible to medical intervention if needed.
- Limitations of gas supply.
- Need to maintain thermal balance at rest.
- Not possible to comply with any proven air-recompression table.

Many heroic attempts to alleviate decompression illness by returning the diver to depth in the water have not succeeded; indeed, some patients have been made worse.

The only time that a diver can be returned to the water breathing air is immediately after surfacing if the diver has omitted some or all of the planned decompression. On surfacing he should be symptom free and he needs to be returned to depth within 5 minutes to complete predetermined stops. The whole protocol can be considered analogous to the routine and safe operational procedure of surface decompression. It is not to be used if there are any symptoms.

The only in-water recompression is where an oxygen-breathing procedure has been agreed before diving begins. This technique was introduced by Edmonds (12). Subject to careful risk analysis this may be the only practical solution for some remote scientific expeditions where evacuation is not a realistic option. The team must have special equipment and appropriate training to use it: a full face mask, or preferably an open helmet, at least two large (240 cubic foot) "H" cylinders of oxygen (welding oxygen is acceptable) providing at least 3 standard cubic feet a minute flow though the helmet. The treatment site should be carefully chosen in 30 feet (9 m) of water a sheltered bay or lagoon. This enables oxygen recompression to 30 feet (9 m) for 30 to 60 minutes. An assisting diver breathing air, must accompany the patient but as it is only nine meters, he does not risk bends Additional air tanks can be supplied to the tender. Its reputed success may be due to the promptness of intervention. With suitable thermal protection the in-water oxygen treatment table has been used by the Australian Antarctic Survey team and Kindwall has taught it to the Indonesian Navy. Normally its use is possible only in warm tropical waters because of heat loss considerations.

Another on-site option accepted by several navies is an inflatable monoplace chamber that is fully capable of a USN T6, but no deeper and subject to appropriate risk analysis and acceptance, can be taken by divers to wherever they are diving.

## NEUROLOGICAL RESIDUALS

Should neurological manifestations persist on return to the surface after the completion of the maximal recommended recompression appropriate to the circumstances, daily hyperbaric oxygen may be given for as long as there is continuing improvement. There is no universal procedure for this but there are some specific tables such as USN Treatment Table 9 (90 minutes of oxygen at 45 feet (2.4 atmospheres), once or twice a day, or USN Treatment Table 5 once a day is commonly used. A shallower depth for recompression has also been used by some with the intention of minimising vasoconstriction during oxygen breathing. Whatever regimen is adopted, it is generally agreed that daily recompression should be continued for as long as the patient reports subjective improvement or for at least 5, and up to 14 days.

An additional consideration for those with paraplegia is the prevention of deep vein thrombosis.

## PROGNOSIS

The majority of cases, particularly those treated soon after the onset of manifestations, appear to make a full recovery, many immediately, and most within 24 hours. Those with only limb pain may return to diving some 24 hours after full recovery. A number fail to respond in spite of the best of treatment and may suffer permanent neurological residuals. A spontaneous functional improvement of decompression paraplegia tends to occur over subsequent weeks and months and perhaps this is a reflection of the multiple discrete lesions of spinal decompression sickness in contrast to the permanent nature of a cord transection. There is no evidence of subsequent neurological deterioration. An individual should not return to diving if neurological residuals can be detected. The argument for this is the evidence that, while functional recovery may be excellent, the scars of the original lesion in the spinal cord remain and there is less neurologic reserve.

After the treatment of severe cerebral decompression illness, successful or otherwise, one should beware of the delayed onset of memory loss, an inability to make decisions, and a circumscribed collection of other symptoms described by psychiatrists as a "dysexecutive syndrome." Because this syndrome was not manifest and capable of being diagnosed at the time of treatment, the only defense against subsequent litigation is to demonstrate that the treatment of the overt cerebral manifestations was full and rigorous.

Flying after recompression for neurological decompression illness should be avoided for at least 5 days and some authorities recommend longer. The marginally viable neurological tissues in an ischemic penumbra may respond adversely to altitude hypoxia and promote a relapse which, hopefully, may be only temporary. Some airline medical departments will provide, upon request, sufficient oxygen for a constant flow to keep the patient at a ground level $pO_2$ throughout an intercontinental flight.

## CONCLUSION

In summary, early treatment with complete resolution of all detectable neurological manifestations within 24 hours is considered compatible with continued diving after a layoff of some six weeks and reassessment by a diving medical officer. In patients who have suffered vestibular decompression sickness, a disparity of more than 30% between the two sides in the electronystagmogram on specialist review is among the residua that may be considered permanently disqualifying. The diver should be offered echocardiography to detect the presence of a right to left intracardiac shunt if the neurological episode was "undeserved" (i.e. after compliance with the dive's decompression requirements) or if the individual has had at least one neurological episode previously. However, though such a shunt may be a contributory factor in some, the prevalence of patent foramen ovale in the diving population far exceeds those requiring recompression for neurological manifestations.

Equally difficult is any decision on the prognosis of an individual after pulmonary barotrauma. While a full clinical recovery is the general rule, the individual's lungs are considered to be at greater risk of damage during some future decompression. At present, for professional divers, the Diving Medical Advisory Committee recommends a minimum of 3 months before specialist review of pulmonary barotrauma prior to any resumption of diving. Advice to sport divers should be even more cautious.

## THE U.S. NAVY AIR DECOMPRESSION TABLES

Included below are the U.S. Navy Standard Air Decompression Tables, the Exceptional Exposure Air Tables, and the Repetitive Dive Tables (Figures 10-14). They are included in this text as a rough guide to decompression for use at those facilities with multiplace chambers where inside tenders breathe air. Their use as written requires great caution, as they can produce up to a 5% incidence of decompression sickness. This was known and accepted at the time they were promulgated, as the Navy was willing to accept that low incidence operationally. Navy master divers routinely "pad" the decompression times specified by "pretending" the time was for the next greater time shown in the tables; in addition, they very often will decompress on the next table deeper than the one required.

### Unlimited/No-Decompression Limits and Repetitive Group Designation Table for Unlimited/No-Decompression Air Dives–1999

| Depth (feet) | (meters) | No-Decompression Limits (min) | A | B | C | D | E | F | G | H | I | J | K | L | M | N |
|---|---|---|---|---|---|---|---|---|---|---|---|---|---|---|---|---|
| 10 | 3.0 | unlimited | 60 | 120 | 210 | 300 | 797 | ★ | | | | | | | | |
| 15 | 4.6 | unlimited | 35 | 70 | 110 | 160 | 225 | 350 | 452 | ★ | | | | | | |
| 20 | 6.1 | unlimited | 25 | 50 | 75 | 100 | 135 | 180 | 240 | 325 | 390 | 917 | ★ | | | |
| 25 | 7.6 | 595 | 20 | 35 | 55 | 75 | 100 | 125 | 160 | 195 | 245 | 315 | 361 | 540 | 595 | |
| 30 | 9.1 | 405 | 15 | 30 | 45 | 60 | 75 | 95 | 120 | 145 | 170 | 205 | 250 | 310 | 344 | 405 |
| 35 | 10.7 | 310 | 5 | 15 | 25 | 40 | 50 | 60 | 80 | 100 | 120 | 140 | 160 | 190 | 220 | 270 |
| 40 | 12.2 | 200 | 5 | 15 | 25 | 30 | 40 | 50 | 70 | 80 | 100 | 110 | 130 | 150 | 170 | 200 |
| 50 | 15.2 | 100 | | | 10 | 15 | 25 | 30 | 40 | 50 | 60 | 70 | 80 | 90 | 100 | |
| 60 | 18.2 | 60 | | | 10 | 15 | 20 | 25 | 30 | 40 | 50 | 55 | 60 | | | |
| 70 | 21.3 | 50 | | 5 | 10 | 15 | 20 | 30 | 35 | 40 | 45 | 50 | | | | |
| 80 | 24.4 | 40 | | 5 | 10 | 15 | 20 | 25 | 30 | 35 | 40 | | | | | |
| 90 | 27.4 | 30 | | 5 | 10 | 12 | 15 | 20 | 25 | 30 | | | | | | |
| 100 | 30.5 | 25 | | 5 | 7 | 10 | 15 | 20 | 22 | 25 | | | | | | |
| 110 | 33.5 | 20 | | | 5 | 10 | 13 | 15 | 20 | | | | | | | |
| 120 | 36.6 | 15 | | | 5 | 10 | 12 | 15 | | | | | | | | |
| 130 | 39.6 | 10 | | | 5 | 8 | 10 | | | | | | | | | |
| 140 | 42.7 | 10 | | | 5 | 7 | 10 | | | | | | | | | |
| 150 | 45.7 | 5 | | | 5 | | | | | | | | | | | |
| 160 | 48.8 | 5 | | | | | 5 | | | | | | | | | |
| 170 | 51.8 | 5 | | | | | 5 | | | | | | | | | |
| 180 | 54.8 | 5 | | | | | 5 | | | | | | | | | |
| 190 | 59.9 | 5 | | | | | 5 | | | | | | | | | |

★Highest repetitive group that can be achieved at this depth regardless of bottom time

Figure 10. US Navy Standard Air Decompression Table 3.

## Residual Nitrogen Timetable for Repetitive Air Dives – 1999

Locate the diver's repetitive group designation from his previous dive along the diagonal line above the table. Read horizontally to the interval in which the diver's surface interval lies.

Next read vertically downward to the new repetitive group designation. Continue downward in this same column to the row which represents the depth of the repetitive dive. The time given at the intersection is residual nitrogen time, in minutes, to be applied to the repetitive dive.

\* Dives following surface intervals of more than 12 hours are not repetitive dives. Use actual bottom times in the Standard Air Decompression Tables to compute decompression for such dives.

\*\* If no Residual Nitrogen Time is given, then the repetitive group does not change.

*Repetitive group at the beginning of the surface interval*

Surface interval ranges (top value = start, bottom value = end) by repetitive group:

| Group | Surface intervals |
|---|---|
| A | 0:10 / 12:00* |
| B | 0:10–3:20, 3:21–12:00* |
| C | 0:10–1:39, 1:40–4:49, 4:50–12:00* |
| D | 0:10–1:09, 1:10–2:38, 2:39–5:48, 5:49–12:00* |
| E | 0:10–0:54, 0:55–1:57, 1:58–3:24, 3:25–6:34, 6:35–12:00* |
| F | 0:10–0:45, 0:46–1:29, 1:30–2:28, 2:29–3:57, 3:58–7:05, 7:06–12:00* |
| G | 0:10–0:40, 0:41–1:15, 1:16–1:59, 2:00–2:58, 2:59–4:25, 4:26–7:35, 7:36–12:00* |
| H | 0:10–0:36, 0:37–1:06, 1:07–1:41, 1:42–2:23, 2:24–3:20, 3:21–4:49, 4:50–7:59, 8:00–12:00* |
| I | 0:10–0:33, 0:34–0:59, 1:00–1:29, 1:30–2:02, 2:03–2:44, 2:45–3:43, 3:44–5:12, 5:13–8:21, 8:22–12:00* |
| J | 0:10–0:31, 0:32–0:54, 0:55–1:19, 1:20–1:47, 1:48–2:20, 2:21–3:04, 3:05–4:02, 4:03–5:40, 5:41–8:50, 8:51–12:00* |
| K | 0:10–0:28, 0:29–0:49, 0:50–1:11, 1:12–1:35, 1:36–2:03, 2:04–2:38, 2:39–3:21, 3:22–4:19, 4:20–5:48, 5:49–8:58, 8:59–12:00* |
| L | 0:10–0:26, 0:27–0:45, 0:46–1:04, 1:05–1:25, 1:26–1:49, 1:50–2:19, 2:20–2:53, 2:54–3:36, 3:37–4:35, 4:36–6:02, 6:03–9:12, 9:13–12:00* |
| M | 0:10–0:25, 0:26–0:42, 0:43–0:59, 1:00–1:18, 1:19–1:35, 1:36–2:05, 2:06–2:34, 2:35–3:08, 3:09–3:52, 3:53–4:49, 4:50–6:18, 6:19–9:28, 9:29–12:00* |
| N | 0:10–0:24, 0:25–0:39, 0:40–0:54, 0:55–1:11, 1:12–1:30, 1:31–1:53, 1:54–2:18, 2:19–2:47, 2:48–3:22, 3:23–4:04, 4:05–5:03, 5:04–6:32, 6:33–9:43, 9:44–12:00* |
| O | 0:10–0:23, 0:24–0:36, 0:37–0:51, 0:52–1:07, 1:08–1:24, 1:25–1:43, 1:44–2:04, 2:05–2:29, 2:30–2:59, 3:00–3:33, 3:34–4:17, 4:18–5:16, 5:17–6:44, 6:45–9:54, 9:55–12:00* |
| Z | 0:10–0:22, 0:23–0:34, 0:35–0:48, 0:49–1:02, 1:03–1:18, 1:19–1:36, 1:37–1:55, 1:56–2:17, 2:18–2:42, 2:43–3:10, 3:11–3:45, 3:46–4:29, 4:30–5:27, 5:28–6:56, 6:57–10:05, 10:06–12:00* |

**NEW GROUP DESIGNATION — Residual Nitrogen Times (Minutes)**

| Repetitive Dive Depth feet / meters | Z | O | N | M | L | K | J | I | H | G | F | E | D | C | B | A |
|---|---|---|---|---|---|---|---|---|---|---|---|---|---|---|---|---|
| 10 / 3.0 | ** | ** | ** | ** | ** | ** | ** | ** | ** | ** | ** | 797 | 279 | 159 | 88 | 39 |
| 20 / 6.1 | ** | ** | ** | ** | ** | ** | 917 | 399 | 279 | 208 | 159 | 120 | 88 | 62 | 39 | 18 |
| 30 / 9.1 | † | † | † | 349 | 279 | 229 | 190 | 159 | 132 | 109 | 88 | 70 | 54 | 39 | 25 | 12 |
| 40 / 12.2 | 257 | 241 | 213 | 187 | 161 | 138 | 116 | 101 | 87 | 73 | 61 | 49 | 37 | 25 | 17 | 7 |
| 50 / 15.2 | 169 | 160 | 142 | 124 | 111 | 99 | 87 | 76 | 66 | 56 | 47 | 38 | 29 | 21 | 13 | 6 |
| 60 / 18.2 | 122 | 117 | 107 | 97 | 88 | 79 | 70 | 61 | 52 | 44 | 36 | 30 | 24 | 17 | 11 | 5 |
| 70 / 21.3 | 100 | 96 | 87 | 80 | 72 | 64 | 57 | 50 | 43 | 37 | 31 | 26 | 20 | 15 | 9 | 4 |
| 80 / 24.4 | 84 | 80 | 73 | 68 | 61 | 54 | 48 | 43 | 38 | 32 | 28 | 23 | 18 | 13 | 8 | 4 |
| 90 / 27.4 | 73 | 70 | 64 | 58 | 53 | 47 | 43 | 38 | 33 | 29 | 24 | 20 | 16 | 11 | 7 | 3 |
| 100 / 30.5 | 64 | 62 | 57 | 52 | 48 | 43 | 38 | 34 | 30 | 26 | 22 | 18 | 14 | 10 | 7 | 3 |
| 110 / 33.5 | 57 | 55 | 51 | 47 | 42 | 38 | 34 | 31 | 27 | 24 | 20 | 16 | 13 | 10 | 6 | 3 |
| 120 / 36.6 | 52 | 50 | 46 | 43 | 39 | 35 | 32 | 28 | 25 | 21 | 18 | 15 | 12 | 9 | 6 | 3 |
| 130 / 39.6 | 46 | 44 | 40 | 38 | 35 | 31 | 28 | 25 | 22 | 19 | 16 | 13 | 11 | 8 | 6 | 3 |
| 140 / 42.7 | 42 | 42 | 40 | 38 | 35 | 32 | 29 | 26 | 23 | 20 | 18 | 15 | 12 | 10 | 7 | 2 |
| 150 / 45.7 | 40 | 40 | 38 | 35 | 32 | 30 | 27 | 24 | 22 | 19 | 17 | 14 | 12 | 9 | 7 | 2 |
| 160 / 48.8 | 37 | 38 | 36 | 33 | 31 | 28 | 26 | 23 | 20 | 18 | 16 | 13 | 11 | 9 | 6 | 2 |
| 170 / 51.8 | 35 | 34 | 34 | 31 | 29 | 26 | 24 | 22 | 19 | 17 | 15 | 12 | 10 | 8 | 6 | 2 |
| 180 / 54.8 | 32 | 32 | 31 | 29 | 27 | 25 | 22 | 20 | 18 | 16 | 14 | 11 | 10 | 8 | 6 | 2 |
| 190 / 59.9 | 31 | 31 | 30 | 28 | 26 | 24 | 21 | 19 | 17 | 15 | 13 | 10 | 10 | 8 | 6 | 2 |

† Read vertically downward to the 40/12.2 (feet/meter) repetitive dive depth. Use the corresponding residual nitrogen times (minutes) to compute the equivalent single dive time. Decompress using the 40/12.2 (feet/meter) standard air decompression table.

*Figure 11. US Navy Standard Air Decompression Table 4.*

## U.S. Navy Standard Air Decompression Table – 1999

| Depth feet/meters | Bottom time (min) | Time first stop (min:sec) | Decompression stops (feet/meters) | | | | | Total decompression time (min:sec) | Repetitive group |
|---|---|---|---|---|---|---|---|---|---|
| | | | 50 15.2 | 40 12.1 | 30 9.1 | 20 6.0 | 10 3.0 | | |
| **40** **12.1** | 200 | | | | | | 0 | 1:20 | * |
| | 210 | 1:00 | | | | | 2 | 3:20 | N |
| | 230 | 1:00 | | | | | 7 | 8:20 | N |
| | 250 | 1:00 | | | | | 11 | 12:20 | O |
| | 270 | 1:00 | | | | | 15 | 16:20 | O |
| | 300 | 1:00 | | | | | 19 | 20:20 | Z |
| | *Exceptional Exposure* | | | | | | | | |
| | 360 | 1:00 | | | | | 23 | 24:20 | ** |
| | 480 | 1:00 | | | | | 41 | 42:20 | ** |
| | 720 | 1:00 | | | | | 69 | 70:20 | ** |
| **50** **15.2** | 100 | | | | | | 0 | 1:40 | * |
| | 110 | 1:20 | | | | | 3 | 4:40 | L |
| | 120 | 1:20 | | | | | 5 | 6:40 | M |
| | 140 | 1:20 | | | | | 10 | 11:40 | M |
| | 160 | 1:20 | | | | | 21 | 22:40 | N |
| | 180 | 1:20 | | | | | 29 | 30:40 | O |
| | 200 | 1:20 | | | | | 35 | 36:40 | O |
| | 220 | 1:20 | | | | | 40 | 41:40 | Z |
| | 240 | 1:20 | | | | | 47 | 48:40 | Z |
| **60** **18.2** | 60 | | | | | | 0 | 2:00 | * |
| | 70 | 1:40 | | | | | 2 | 4:00 | K |
| | 80 | 1:40 | | | | | 7 | 9:00 | L |
| | 100 | 1:40 | | | | | 14 | 16:00 | M |
| | 120 | 1:40 | | | | | 26 | 28:00 | N |
| | 140 | 1:40 | | | | | 39 | 41:00 | O |
| | 160 | 1:40 | | | | | 48 | 50:00 | Z |
| | 180 | 1:40 | | | | | 56 | 58:00 | Z |
| | 200 | 1:20 | | | | 1 | 69 | 72:00 | Z |
| | *Exceptional Exposure* | | | | | | | | |
| | 240 | 1:20 | | | | 2 | 79 | 83:00 | ** |
| | 360 | 1:20 | | | | 20 | 119 | 141:00 | ** |
| | 480 | 1:20 | | | | 44 | 148 | 194:00 | ** |
| | 720 | 1:20 | | | | 78 | 187 | 267:00 | ** |
| **70** **21.3** | 50 | | | | | | 0 | 2:20 | * |
| | 60 | 2:00 | | | | | 8 | 10:20 | K |
| | 70 | 2:00 | | | | | 14 | 16:20 | L |
| | 80 | 2:00 | | | | | 18 | 20:20 | M |
| | 90 | 2:00 | | | | | 23 | 25:20 | N |
| | 100 | 2:00 | | | | | 33 | 35:20 | N |
| | 110 | 1:40 | | | | 2 | 41 | 45:20 | O |
| | 120 | 1:40 | | | | 4 | 47 | 53:20 | O |
| | 130 | 1:40 | | | | 6 | 52 | 60:20 | O |
| | 140 | 1:40 | | | | 8 | 56 | 66:20 | Z |
| | 150 | 1:40 | | | | 9 | 61 | 72:20 | Z |
| | 160 | 1:40 | | | | 13 | 72 | 87:20 | Z |
| | 170 | 1:40 | | | | 19 | 79 | 100:20 | Z |

\* See no Decompression Table for repetitive groups
\*\* Repetitive dives may not follow exceptional exposure dives

Figure 12a. US Navy Standard Air Decompression Table 5.

## U.S. Navy Standard Air Decompression Table – 1999 (Continued)

| Depth feet/meters | Bottom time (min) | Time first stop (min:sec) | Decompression stops (feet/meters) | | | | | Total decompression time (min:sec) | Repetitive group |
|---|---|---|---|---|---|---|---|---|---|
| | | | 50 15.2 | 40 12.1 | 30 9.1 | 20 6.0 | 10 3.0 | | |
| **80** **24.3** | 40 | | | | | | 0 | 2:40 | * |
| | 50 | 2:20 | | | | | 10 | 12:40 | K |
| | 60 | 2:20 | | | | | 17 | 19:40 | L |
| | 70 | 2:20 | | | | | 23 | 25:40 | M |
| | 80 | 2:00 | | | | 2 | 31 | 35:40 | N |
| | 90 | 2:00 | | | | 7 | 39 | 48:40 | N |
| | 100 | 2:00 | | | | 11 | 46 | 59:40 | O |
| | 110 | 2:00 | | | | 13 | 53 | 68:40 | O |
| | 120 | 2:00 | | | | 17 | 56 | 75:40 | Z |
| | 130 | 2:00 | | | | 19 | 63 | 84:40 | Z |
| | 140 | 2:00 | | | | 26 | 69 | 97:40 | Z |
| | 150 | 2:00 | | | | 32 | 77 | 111:40 | Z |
| | | | | | *Exceptional Exposure* | | | | |
| | 180 | 2:00 | | | | 35 | 85 | 122:40 | ** |
| | 240 | 1:40 | | | 6 | 52 | 120 | 180:40 | ** |
| | 360 | 1:40 | | | 29 | 90 | 160 | 281:40 | ** |
| | 480 | 1:40 | | | 59 | 107 | 187 | 355:40 | ** |
| | 720 | 1:20 | | 17 | 108 | 142 | 187 | 456:40 | ** |
| **90** **28.7** | 30 | | | | | | 0 | 3:00 | * |
| | 40 | 2:40 | | | | | 7 | 10:00 | J |
| | 50 | 2:40 | | | | | 18 | 21:00 | L |
| | 60 | 2:40 | | | | | 25 | 28:00 | M |
| | 70 | 2:20 | | | | 7 | 30 | 40:00 | N |
| | 80 | 2:20 | | | | 13 | 40 | 56:00 | N |
| | 90 | 2:20 | | | | 18 | 48 | 69:00 | O |
| | 100 | 2:20 | | | | 21 | 54 | 78:00 | Z |
| | 110 | 2:20 | | | | 24 | 61 | 88:00 | Z |
| | 120 | 2:20 | | | | 32 | 68 | 103:00 | Z |
| | 130 | 2:00 | | | 5 | 36 | 74 | 118:00 | Z |
| **100** **30.4** | 25 | | | | | | 0 | 3:20 | * |
| | 30 | 3:00 | | | | | 3 | 6:20 | I |
| | 40 | 3:00 | | | | | 15 | 18:20 | K |
| | 50 | 2:40 | | | | 2 | 24 | 29:20 | L |
| | 60 | 2:40 | | | | 9 | 28 | 40:20 | N |
| | 70 | 2:40 | | | | 17 | 39 | 59:20 | O |
| | 80 | 2:40 | | | | 23 | 48 | 74:20 | O |
| | 90 | 2:20 | | | 3 | 23 | 57 | 86:20 | Z |
| | 100 | 2:20 | | | 7 | 23 | 66 | 99:20 | Z |
| | 110 | 2:20 | | | 10 | 34 | 72 | 119:20 | Z |
| | 120 | 2:20 | | | 12 | 41 | 78 | 134:20 | Z |
| | | | | | *Exceptional Exposure* | | | | |
| | 180 | 2:00 | | 1 | 29 | 53 | 118 | 204:20 | ** |
| | 240 | 2:00 | | 14 | 42 | 84 | 142 | 285:20 | ** |
| | 360 | 1:40 | 2 | 42 | 73 | 111 | 187 | 418:20 | ** |
| | 480 | 1:40 | 21 | 61 | 91 | 142 | 187 | 505:20 | ** |
| | 720 | 1:40 | 55 | 106 | 122 | 142 | 187 | 615:20 | ** |

\* See no Decompression Table for repetitive groups
\** Repetitive dives may not follow exceptional exposure dives

Figure 12b. US Navy Standard Air Decompression Table 5 Continued.

## U.S. Navy Standard Air Decompression Table – 1999 (Continued)

**Depth 110 feet/meters 33.1**

| Bottom time (min) | Time first stop (min:sec) | 50 15.2 | 40 12.1 | 30 9.1 | 20 6.0 | 10 3.0 | Total decompression time (min:sec) | Repetitive group |
|---|---|---|---|---|---|---|---|---|
| 20 | | | | | | 0 | 3:40 | * |
| 25 | 3:20 | | | | | 3 | 6:40 | H |
| 30 | 3:20 | | | | | 7 | 10:40 | J |
| 40 | 3:00 | | | | 2 | 21 | 26:40 | L |
| 50 | 3:00 | | | | 8 | 26 | 37:40 | M |
| 60 | 3:00 | | | | 18 | 36 | 57:40 | N |
| 70 | 2:40 | | | 1 | 23 | 48 | 75:40 | O |
| 80 | 2:40 | | | 7 | 23 | 57 | 90:40 | Z |
| 90 | 2:40 | | | 12 | 30 | 64 | 109:40 | Z |
| 100 | 2:40 | | | 15 | 37 | 72 | 127:40 | Z |

**Depth 120 feet/meters 36.5**

| Bottom time (min) | Time first stop (min:sec) | 70 21.3 | 60 18.2 | 50 15.2 | 40 12.1 | 30 9.1 | 20 6.0 | 10 3.0 | Total decompression time (min:sec) | Repetitive group |
|---|---|---|---|---|---|---|---|---|---|---|
| 15 | | | | | | | | 0 | 4:00 | * |
| 20 | 3:40 | | | | | | | 2 | 6:00 | H |
| 25 | 3:40 | | | | | | | 6 | 10:00 | I |
| 30 | 3:40 | | | | | | | 14 | 18:00 | J |
| 40 | 3:20 | | | | | | | 25 | 34:00 | L |
| 50 | 3:20 | | | | | | 15 | 31 | 50:00 | N |
| 60 | 3:00 | | | | | 2 | 22 | 45 | 73:00 | O |
| 70 | 3:00 | | | | | 9 | 23 | 55 | 91:00 | O |
| 80 | 3:00 | | | | | 15 | 27 | 63 | 109:00 | Z |
| 90 | 3:00 | | | | | 19 | 37 | 74 | 134:00 | Z |
| 100 | 3:00 | | | | | 23 | 45 | 80 | 152:00 | Z |
| *Exceptional Exposure* | | | | | | | | | | |
| 120 | 2:40 | | | | 10 | 19 | 47 | 98 | 178:00 | ** |
| 180 | 2:20 | | | 5 | 27 | 37 | 76 | 137 | 286:00 | ** |
| 240 | 2:20 | | | 23 | 35 | 60 | 97 | 179 | 398:00 | ** |
| 360 | 2:00 | | 18 | 45 | 64 | 93 | 142 | 187 | 553:00 | ** |
| 480 | 1:40 | 3 | 41 | 64 | 93 | 122 | 142 | 187 | 656:00 | ** |
| 720 | 1:40 | 32 | 74 | 100 | 114 | 122 | 142 | 187 | 775:00 | ** |

**Depth 130 feet/meters 39.6**

| Bottom time (min) | Time first stop (min:sec) | 70 | 60 | 50 | 40 | 30 | 20 | 10 | Total decompression time (min:sec) | Repetitive group |
|---|---|---|---|---|---|---|---|---|---|---|
| 10 | | | | | | | | 0 | 4:20 | * |
| 15 | 4:00 | | | | | | | 1 | 5:20 | F |
| 20 | 4:00 | | | | | | | 4 | 8:20 | H |
| 25 | 4:00 | | | | | | | 10 | 14:20 | J |
| 30 | 3:40 | | | | | | 3 | 18 | 25:20 | M |
| 40 | 3:40 | | | | | | 10 | 25 | 39:20 | N |
| 50 | 3:20 | | | | | 3 | 21 | 37 | 65:20 | O |
| 60 | 3:20 | | | | | 9 | 23 | 52 | 88:20 | Z |
| 70 | 3:20 | | | | | 16 | 24 | 61 | 105:20 | Z |
| 80 | 3:00 | | | | 3 | 19 | 35 | 72 | 133:20 | Z |
| 90 | 3:00 | | | | 8 | 19 | 45 | 80 | 156:20 | Z |

* See no Decompression Table for repetitive groups
** Repetitive dives may not follow exceptional exposure dives

*Figure 12c. US Navy Standard Air Decompression Table 5 Continued.*

## U.S. Navy Standard Air Decompression Table – 1999 (Continued)

| Depth feet/meters | Bottom time (min) | Time first stop (min:sec) | 90 27.4 | 80 24.3 | 70 21.3 | 60 18.2 | 50 15.2 | 40 12.1 | 30 9.1 | 20 6.0 | 10 3.0 | Total decompression time (min:sec) | Repetitive group |
|---|---|---|---|---|---|---|---|---|---|---|---|---|---|
| **140 42.6** | 10 | | | | | | | | | | 0 | 4:40 | * |
| | 15 | 4:20 | | | | | | | | | 2 | 6:40 | G |
| | 20 | 4:20 | | | | | | | | | 6 | 10:40 | I |
| | 25 | 4:00 | | | | | | | | 2 | 14 | 20:40 | J |
| | 30 | 4:00 | | | | | | | | 5 | 21 | 30:40 | K |
| | 40 | 3:40 | | | | | | | 2 | 16 | 26 | 48:40 | N |
| | 50 | 3:40 | | | | | | | 6 | 24 | 44 | 78:40 | O |
| | 60 | 3:40 | | | | | | | 16 | 23 | 56 | 99:40 | Z |
| | 70 | 3:20 | | | | | | 4 | 19 | 32 | 68 | 127:40 | Z |
| | 80 | 3:20 | | | | | | 10 | 23 | 41 | 79 | 157:40 | Z |

Exceptional Exposure

| Depth feet/meters | Bottom time (min) | Time first stop (min:sec) | 90 27.4 | 80 24.3 | 70 21.3 | 60 18.2 | 50 15.2 | 40 12.1 | 30 9.1 | 20 6.0 | 10 3.0 | Total decompression time (min:sec) | Repetitive group |
|---|---|---|---|---|---|---|---|---|---|---|---|---|---|
| | 90 | 3:00 | | | | | 2 | 14 | 18 | 42 | 88 | 168:40 | ** |
| | 120 | 3:00 | | | | | 12 | 14 | 36 | 56 | 120 | 242:40 | ** |
| | 180 | 2:40 | | | | 10 | 26 | 32 | 54 | 94 | 168 | 388:40 | ** |
| | 240 | 2:20 | | | 8 | 28 | 34 | 50 | 78 | 124 | 187 | 513:40 | ** |
| | 360 | 2:00 | | 9 | 32 | 42 | 64 | 84 | 122 | 142 | 187 | 686:40 | ** |
| | 480 | 2:00 | 31 | 44 | 59 | 100 | 114 | 122 | 142 | 187 | | 803:40 | ** |
| | 720 | 1:40 | 16 | 56 | 88 | 97 | 100 | 114 | 122 | 142 | 187 | 926:40 | ** |

| Depth feet/meters | Bottom time (min) | Time first stop (min:sec) | 90 27.4 | 80 24.3 | 70 21.3 | 60 18.2 | 50 15.2 | 40 12.1 | 30 9.1 | 20 6.0 | 10 3.0 | Total decompression time (min:sec) | Repetitive group |
|---|---|---|---|---|---|---|---|---|---|---|---|---|---|
| **150 45.7** | 5 | | | | | | | | | | 0 | 5:00 | C |
| | 10 | 4:40 | | | | | | | | | 1 | 6:00 | E |
| | 15 | 4:40 | | | | | | | | | 3 | 8:00 | G |
| | 20 | 4:20 | | | | | | | | 2 | 7 | 14:00 | H |
| | 25 | 4:20 | | | | | | | | 4 | 17 | 26:00 | K |
| | 30 | 4:20 | | | | | | | | 8 | 24 | 37:00 | L |
| | 40 | 4:00 | | | | | | | 5 | 19 | 33 | 62:00 | N |
| | 50 | 4:00 | | | | | | | 12 | 23 | 51 | 91:00 | O |
| | 60 | 3:40 | | | | | | 3 | 19 | 26 | 62 | 115:00 | Z |
| | 70 | 3:40 | | | | | | 11 | 19 | 39 | 75 | 149:00 | Z |
| | 80 | 3:20 | | | | | 1 | 17 | 19 | 50 | 84 | 176:00 | Z |

| Depth feet/meters | Bottom time (min) | Time first stop (min:sec) | 90 27.4 | 80 24.3 | 70 21.3 | 60 18.2 | 50 15.2 | 40 12.1 | 30 9.1 | 20 6.0 | 10 3.0 | Total decompression time (min:sec) | Repetitive group |
|---|---|---|---|---|---|---|---|---|---|---|---|---|---|
| **160 48.7** | 5 | | | | | | | | | | 0 | 5:20 | D |
| | 10 | 5:00 | | | | | | | | | 1 | 6:20 | F |
| | 15 | 4:40 | | | | | | | | 1 | 4 | 10:20 | H |
| | 20 | 4:40 | | | | | | | | 3 | 11 | 19:20 | J |
| | 25 | 4:40 | | | | | | | | 7 | 20 | 32:20 | K |
| | 30 | 4:20 | | | | | | | 2 | 11 | 25 | 43:20 | M |
| | 40 | 4:20 | | | | | | | 7 | 23 | 39 | 74:20 | N |
| | 50 | 4:00 | | | | | | 2 | 16 | 23 | 55 | 101:20 | Z |
| | 60 | 4:00 | | | | | | 9 | 19 | 33 | 69 | 135:20 | Z |

Exceptional Exposure

| Depth feet/meters | Bottom time (min) | Time first stop (min:sec) | 90 27.4 | 80 24.3 | 70 21.3 | 60 18.2 | 50 15.2 | 40 12.1 | 30 9.1 | 20 6.0 | 10 3.0 | Total decompression time (min:sec) | Repetitive group |
|---|---|---|---|---|---|---|---|---|---|---|---|---|---|
| | 70 | 3:40 | | | | | 1 | 17 | 22 | 44 | 80 | 169:20 | ** |

\* See no Decompression Table for repetitive groups
\*\* Repetitive dives may not follow exceptional exposure dives

Figure 12d. US Navy Standard Air Decompression Table 5 Continued.

## U.S. Navy Standard Air Decompression Table – 1999 (Continued)

| Depth feet/meters | Bottom time (min) | Time first stop (min:sec) | 110 33.5 | 100 30.4 | 90 27.4 | 80 24.3 | 70 21.3 | 60 18.2 | 50 15.2 | 40 12.1 | 30 9.1 | 20 6.0 | 10 3.0 | Total decompression time (min:sec) | Repetitive group |
|---|---|---|---|---|---|---|---|---|---|---|---|---|---|---|---|
| **170** **51.8** | 5 | | | | | | | | | | | | 0 | 5:40 | D |
| | 10 | 5:20 | | | | | | | | | | | 2 | 7:40 | F |
| | 15 | 5:00 | | | | | | | | | | 2 | 5 | 12:40 | H |
| | 20 | 5:00 | | | | | | | | | | 4 | 15 | 24:40 | J |
| | 25 | 4:40 | | | | | | | | | 2 | 7 | 23 | 37:40 | L |
| | 30 | 4:40 | | | | | | | | | 4 | 13 | 26 | 48:40 | M |
| | 40 | 4:20 | | | | | | | | 1 | 10 | 23 | 45 | 84:40 | O |
| | 50 | 4:20 | | | | | | | | 5 | 18 | 23 | 61 | 112:40 | Z |
| | 60 | 4:00 | | | | | | | 2 | 15 | 22 | 37 | 74 | 155:40 | Z |
| | Exceptional Exposure | | | | | | | | | | | | | | |
| | 70 | 4:00 | | | | | | | 8 | 17 | 19 | 51 | 86 | 186:40 | ** |
| | 90 | 3:40 | | | | | | 12 | 12 | 14 | 34 | 52 | 120 | 249:40 | ** |
| | 120 | 3:00 | | | | 2 | 10 | 12 | 18 | 32 | 42 | 82 | 156 | 359:40 | ** |
| | 180 | 2:40 | | | 4 | 10 | 22 | 28 | 34 | 50 | 78 | 120 | 187 | 538:40 | ** |
| | 240 | 2:40 | | | 18 | 24 | 30 | 42 | 50 | 70 | 116 | 142 | 187 | 684:40 | ** |
| | 360 | 2:20 | | 22 | 34 | 40 | 52 | 60 | 98 | 114 | 122 | 142 | 187 | 876:40 | ** |
| | 480 | 2:00 | 14 | 40 | 42 | 56 | 91 | 97 | 100 | 114 | 122 | 142 | 187 | 1010:40 | ** |
| **180** **54.8** | 5 | | | | | | | | | | | | 0 | 6:00 | D |
| | 10 | 5:40 | | | | | | | | | | | 3 | 9:00 | F |
| | 15 | 5:20 | | | | | | | | | | 3 | 6 | 15:00 | I |
| | 20 | 5:00 | | | | | | | | | 1 | 5 | 17 | 29:00 | J |
| | 25 | 5:00 | | | | | | | | | 3 | 10 | 24 | 43:00 | L |
| | 30 | 5:00 | | | | | | | | | 6 | 17 | 27 | 56:00 | N |
| | 40 | 4:40 | | | | | | | | 3 | 14 | 23 | 50 | 96:00 | O |
| | 50 | 4:20 | | | | | | | 2 | 9 | 19 | 30 | 65 | 131:00 | Z |
| | 60 | 4:20 | | | | | | | 5 | 16 | 19 | 44 | 81 | 171:00 | Z |
| **190** **57.9** | 5 | 5:40 | | | | | | | | | | | 0 | 6:20 | D |
| | 10 | 5:40 | | | | | | | | | | 1 | 3 | 10:20 | G |
| | 15 | 5:40 | | | | | | | | | | 4 | 7 | 17:20 | I |
| | 20 | 5:20 | | | | | | | | | 2 | 6 | 20 | 34:20 | K |
| | 25 | 5:20 | | | | | | | | | 5 | 11 | 25 | 47:20 | M |
| | 30 | 5:00 | | | | | | | | 1 | 8 | 19 | 32 | 66:20 | N |
| | 40 | 5:00 | | | | | | | | 8 | 14 | 23 | 55 | 106:20 | O |
| | Exceptional Exposure | | | | | | | | | | | | | | |
| | 50 | 4:40 | | | | | | | | 4 | 13 | 22 | 33 | 72 | 150:20 | ** |
| | 60 | 4:40 | | | | | | | 10 | 17 | 19 | 50 | 84 | 186:20 | ** |

\* See no Decompression Table for repetitive groups
\*\* Repetitive dives may not follow exceptional exposure dives

Figure 12e. US Navy Standard Air Decompression Table 5 Continued.

## U.S. Navy Standard Air Decompression Table – 1999 (Continued)

*Exceptional Exposure* (all depths below)

| Depth feet/meters | Bottom time (min) | Time first stop (min:sec) | 130 / 39.6 | 120 / 36.5 | 110 / 33.5 | 100 / 30.4 | 90 / 27.4 | 80 / 24.3 | 70 / 21.3 | 60 / 18.2 | 50 / 15.2 | 40 / 12.1 | 30 / 9.1 | 20 / 6.0 | 10 / 3.0 | Total decompression time (min:sec) |
|---|---|---|---|---|---|---|---|---|---|---|---|---|---|---|---|---|
| 200 / 60.9 | 5 | 6:20 | | | | | | | | | | | | | 1 | 7:40 |
| | 10 | 6:00 | | | | | | | | | | | | 1 | 4 | 11:40 |
| | 15 | 5:40 | | | | | | | | | | | | 4 | 10 | 21:40 |
| | 20 | 5:40 | | | | | | | | | | | 1 | 7 | 27 | 43:40 |
| | 25 | 5:40 | | | | | | | | | | | 7 | 14 | 25 | 52:40 |
| | 30 | 5:20 | | | | | | | | | | 2 | 9 | 22 | 37 | 76:40 |
| | 40 | 5:00 | | | | | | | | | 2 | 8 | 17 | 23 | 59 | 115:40 |
| | 50 | 5:00 | | | | | | | | | 6 | 16 | 22 | 39 | 75 | 164:40 |
| | 60 | 4:40 | | | | | | | | 2 | 13 | 17 | 24 | 51 | 89 | 202:40 |
| | 90 | 3:40 | | | | | | | 2 | 12 | 12 | 30 | 38 | 74 | 134 | 327:40 |
| | 120 | 3:20 | | | | 1 | 10 | 10 | 12 | 24 | 28 | 40 | 64 | 98 | 180 | 476:40 |
| | 180 | 2:40 | | 1 | 10 | 10 | 18 | 24 | 24 | 42 | 48 | 70 | 106 | 142 | 187 | 688:40 |
| | 240 | 2:40 | | 6 | 20 | 24 | 24 | 36 | 42 | 54 | 68 | 114 | 122 | 142 | 187 | 845:40 |
| | 360 | 2:20 | 12 | 22 | 36 | 40 | 44 | 56 | 82 | 98 | 100 | 114 | 122 | 142 | 187 | 1061:40 |
| 210 / 64.0 | 5 | 6:40 | | | | | | | | | | | | | 1 | 8:00 |
| | 10 | 6:20 | | | | | | | | | | | | 2 | 4 | 13:00 |
| | 15 | 6:00 | | | | | | | | | | | 1 | 5 | 13 | 26:00 |
| | 20 | 6:00 | | | | | | | | | | | 4 | 10 | 23 | 44:00 |
| | 25 | 5:40 | | | | | | | | | | 2 | 7 | 17 | 27 | 60:00 |
| | 30 | 5:40 | | | | | | | | | | 4 | 9 | 24 | 41 | 85:00 |
| | 40 | 5:20 | | | | | | | | | 4 | 9 | 19 | 26 | 63 | 128:00 |
| | 50 | 5:20 | | | | | | | | 1 | 9 | 17 | 19 | 45 | 80 | 178:00 |
| 220 / 67.0 | 5 | 7:00 | | | | | | | | | | | | | 1 | 8:20 |
| | 10 | 6:40 | | | | | | | | | | | | 2 | 5 | 14:20 |
| | 15 | 6:20 | | | | | | | | | | | 2 | 5 | 16 | 30:20 |
| | 20 | 6:00 | | | | | | | | | | 1 | 3 | 11 | 24 | 46:20 |
| | 25 | 6:00 | | | | | | | | | | 3 | 8 | 19 | 33 | 70:20 |
| | 30 | 5:40 | | | | | | | | | 1 | 7 | 10 | 23 | 47 | 95:20 |
| | 40 | 5:40 | | | | | | | | | 6 | 12 | 22 | 29 | 68 | 144:20 |
| | 50 | 5:20 | | | | | | | | 3 | 12 | 17 | 18 | 51 | 86 | 194:20 |

* See no Decompression Table for repetitive groups
** Repetitive dives may not follow exceptional exposure dives
12f

*Exceptional Exposure* (230, 240)

| Depth feet/meters | Bottom time (min) | Time first stop (min:sec) | 130 / 39.6 | 120 / 36.5 | 110 / 33.5 | 100 / 30.4 | 90 / 27.4 | 80 / 24.3 | 70 / 21.3 | 60 / 18.2 | 50 / 15.2 | 40 / 12.1 | 30 / 9.1 | 20 / 6.0 | 10 / 3.0 | Total decompression time (min:sec) |
|---|---|---|---|---|---|---|---|---|---|---|---|---|---|---|---|---|
| 230 / 70.1 | 5 | 7:20 | | | | | | | | | | | | | 2 | 9:40 |
| | 10 | 6:20 | | | | | | | | | | | 1 | 2 | 6 | 16:40 |
| | 15 | 6:20 | | | | | | | | | | | 3 | 6 | 18 | 34:40 |
| | 20 | 6:20 | | | | | | | | | | 2 | 5 | 12 | 26 | 52:40 |
| | 25 | 6:20 | | | | | | | | | | 4 | 8 | 22 | 37 | 78:40 |
| | 30 | 6:00 | | | | | | | | | 2 | 8 | 12 | 23 | 51 | 103:40 |
| | 40 | 5:40 | | | | | | | | 1 | 7 | 15 | 22 | 34 | 74 | 160:40 |
| | 50 | 5:40 | | | | | | | | 5 | 14 | 16 | 24 | 51 | 89 | 206:40 |
| 240 / 73.1 | 5 | 7:40 | | | | | | | | | | | | | 2 | 10:00 |
| | 10 | 7:00 | | | | | | | | | | | 1 | 3 | 6 | 18:00 |
| | 15 | 7:00 | | | | | | | | | | | 4 | 6 | 21 | 39:00 |
| | 20 | 6:40 | | | | | | | | | | 3 | 6 | 15 | 25 | 57:00 |
| | 25 | 6:20 | | | | | | | | | | 4 | 9 | 24 | 40 | 86:00 |
| | 30 | 6:20 | | | | | | | | 1 | 4 | 8 | 15 | 22 | 56 | 113:00 |
| | 40 | 6:00 | | | | | | | | 4 | 8 | 15 | 22 | 39 | 75 | 171:00 |
| | 50 | 5:40 | | | | | | | 1 | 8 | 15 | 16 | 29 | 51 | 94 | 222:00 |

*Exceptional Exposure* (250)

| Depth feet/meters | Bottom time (min) | Time first stop (min:sec) | 200 / 60.9 | 190 / 57.9 | 180 / 54.8 | 170 / 51.8 | 160 / 48.7 | 150 / 45.7 | 140 / 42.6 | 130 / 39.6 | 120 / 36.5 | 110 / 33.5 | 100 / 30.4 | 90 / 27.4 | 80 / 24.3 | 70 / 21.3 | 60 / 18.2 | 50 / 15.2 | 40 / 12.1 | 30 / 9.1 | 20 / 6.0 | 10 / 3.0 | Total decompression time (min:sec) |
|---|---|---|---|---|---|---|---|---|---|---|---|---|---|---|---|---|---|---|---|---|---|---|---|
| 250 / 76.2 | 5 | 7:40 | | | | | | | | | | | | | | | | | | | 1 | 2 | 11:20 |
| | 10 | 7:20 | | | | | | | | | | | | | | | | | | 1 | 4 | 7 | 20:20 |
| | 15 | 7:00 | | | | | | | | | | | | | | | | | 1 | 4 | 7 | 22 | 42:20 |
| | 20 | 7:00 | | | | | | | | | | | | | | | | | 4 | 7 | 17 | 27 | 63:20 |
| | 25 | 6:40 | | | | | | | | | | | | | | | | 2 | 7 | 10 | 24 | 45 | 96:20 |
| | 30 | 6:40 | | | | | | | | | | | | | | | | 6 | 7 | 17 | 23 | 59 | 120:20 |
| | 40 | 6:20 | | | | | | | | | | | | | | | 5 | 9 | 17 | 19 | 45 | 79 | 182:20 |
| | 60 | 5:20 | | | | | | | | | | | | 4 | 10 | 10 | 10 | 12 | 22 | 36 | 64 | 126 | 302:20 |
| | 90 | 4:20 | | | | | | | | | | | 8 | 10 | 10 | 10 | 28 | 28 | 44 | 68 | 98 | 186 | 518:20 |
| | 120 | 3:40 | | | | | | | 5 | 10 | 10 | 10 | 10 | 16 | 24 | 24 | 36 | 48 | 64 | 94 | 142 | 187 | 688:20 |
| | 180 | 3:00 | | | | 4 | 8 | 8 | 10 | 10 | 22 | 24 | 24 | 32 | 42 | 44 | 60 | 84 | 114 | 122 | 142 | 187 | 935:20 |
| | 240 | 3:00 | | | | | 9 | 14 | 21 | 22 | 22 | 40 | 40 | 42 | 56 | 76 | 98 | 100 | 114 | 122 | 142 | 187 | 1113:20 |

* See no Decompression Table for repetitive groups
** Repetitive dives may not follow exceptional exposure dives
12g

Figure 12f and 12g. US Navy Standard Air Decompression Table 5 Continued.

## U.S. Navy Standard Air Decompression Table – 1999 (Continued)

Exceptional Exposure (applies to each depth group below)

| Depth feet/meters | Bottom time (min) | Time first stop (min:sec) | 200/60.9 | 190/57.9 | 180/54.8 | 170/51.8 | 160/48.7 | 150/45.7 | 140/42.6 | 130/39.6 | 120/36.5 | 110/33.5 | 100/30.4 | 90/27.4 | 80/24.3 | 70/21.3 | 60/18.2 | 50/15.2 | 40/12.1 | 30/9.1 | 20/6.0 | 10/3.0 | Total decompression time (min:sec) |
|---|---|---|---|---|---|---|---|---|---|---|---|---|---|---|---|---|---|---|---|---|---|---|---|
| **260 / 79.2** | 5 | 8:00 | | | | | | | | | | | | | | | | | | | 1 | 2 | 11:40 |
| | 10 | 7:40 | | | | | | | | | | | | | | | | | | 2 | 4 | 9 | 23:40 |
| | 15 | 7:20 | | | | | | | | | | | | | | | | | | 4 | 10 | 22 | 46:40 |
| | 20 | 7:00 | | | | | | | | | | | | | | | | 1 | 4 | 7 | 20 | 31 | 71:40 |
| | 25 | 7:00 | | | | | | | | | | | | | | | | 3 | 8 | 11 | 23 | 50 | 103:40 |
| | 30 | 6:40 | | | | | | | | | | | | | | | 2 | 6 | 8 | 19 | 26 | 61 | 130:40 |
| | 40 | 6:20 | | | | | | | | | | | | | | 1 | 6 | 11 | 16 | 19 | 49 | 84 | 194:40 |
| **270 / 82.3** | 5 | 8:20 | | | | | | | | | | | | | | | | | | | 1 | 3 | 13:00 |
| | 10 | 8:00 | | | | | | | | | | | | | | | | | | 2 | 5 | 11 | 27:00 |
| | 15 | 7:40 | | | | | | | | | | | | | | | | | 3 | 4 | 11 | 24 | 51:00 |
| | 20 | 7:20 | | | | | | | | | | | | | | | | 2 | 3 | 9 | 21 | 35 | 79:00 |
| | 25 | 7:00 | | | | | | | | | | | | | | | 2 | 3 | 8 | 13 | 23 | 53 | 111:00 |
| | 30 | 7:00 | | | | | | | | | | | | | | | 3 | 6 | 12 | 22 | 27 | 64 | 143:00 |
| | 40 | 6:40 | | | | | | | | | | | | | | 5 | 6 | 11 | 17 | 22 | 51 | 88 | 209:00 |
| **280 / 85.3** | 5 | 8:40 | | | | | | | | | | | | | | | | | | | 2 | 2 | 13:20 |
| | 10 | 8:00 | | | | | | | | | | | | | | | | | 1 | 2 | 5 | 13 | 30:20 |
| | 15 | 7:40 | | | | | | | | | | | | | | | | 1 | 3 | 4 | 11 | 26 | 54:20 |
| | 20 | 7:40 | | | | | | | | | | | | | | | | 3 | 4 | 8 | 23 | 39 | 86:20 |
| | 25 | 7:20 | | | | | | | | | | | | | | | 2 | 5 | 7 | 16 | 23 | 56 | 118:20 |
| | 30 | 7:00 | | | | | | | | | | | | | | 1 | 3 | 7 | 13 | 22 | 30 | 70 | 155:20 |
| | 40 | 6:40 | | | | | | | | | | | | | 1 | 6 | 6 | 13 | 17 | 27 | 51 | 93 | 223:20 |
| **290 / 88.4** | 5 | 9:00 | | | | | | | | | | | | | | | | | | | 2 | 3 | 14:40 |
| | 10 | 8:20 | | | | | | | | | | | | | | | | | 1 | 3 | 5 | 16 | 34:40 |
| | 15 | 8:00 | | | | | | | | | | | | | | | | 1 | 3 | 6 | 12 | 26 | 57:40 |
| | 20 | 8:00 | | | | | | | | | | | | | | | | 3 | 7 | 9 | 23 | 43 | 94:40 |
| | 25 | 7:40 | | | | | | | | | | | | | | | 3 | 5 | 8 | 17 | 23 | 60 | 125:40 |
| | 30 | 7:20 | | | | | | | | | | | | | | 1 | 5 | 6 | 16 | 22 | 36 | 72 | 167:40 |
| | 40 | 7:00 | | | | | | | | | | | | | 3 | 5 | 7 | 15 | 16 | 32 | 51 | 95 | 233:40 |
| **300 / 91.4** | 5 | 9:20 | | | | | | | | | | | | | | | | | | | 3 | 3 | 16:00 |
| | 10 | 8:40 | | | | | | | | | | | | | | | | | 1 | 3 | 6 | 17 | 37:00 |
| | 15 | 8:20 | | | | | | | | | | | | | | | | 2 | 3 | 6 | 15 | 26 | 62:00 |
| | 20 | 8:00 | | | | | | | | | | | | | | | 2 | 3 | 7 | 10 | 23 | 47 | 102:00 |
| | 25 | 7:40 | | | | | | | | | | | | | | 1 | 3 | 6 | 8 | 19 | 26 | 61 | 134:00 |
| | 30 | 7:40 | | | | | | | | | | | | | | 2 | 5 | 7 | 17 | 22 | 39 | 75 | 177:00 |
| | 40 | 7:20 | | | | | | | | | | | | | 4 | 6 | 9 | 15 | 17 | 34 | 51 | 90 | 236:00 |
| | 60 | 6:00 | | | | | | | | 4 | 10 | 10 | 10 | 10 | 10 | 10 | 14 | 28 | 32 | 50 | 90 | 187 | 465:00 |
| | 90 | 4:40 | | | | | 3 | 8 | 8 | 10 | 10 | 10 | 10 | 16 | 24 | 24 | 34 | 48 | 64 | 90 | 142 | 187 | 698:00 |
| | 120 | 4:00 | | | 4 | 8 | 8 | 8 | 8 | 10 | 14 | 24 | 24 | 24 | 34 | 42 | 58 | 66 | 102 | 122 | 142 | 187 | 895:00 |
| | 180 | 3:30 | 6 | 8 | 8 | 8 | 14 | 20 | 21 | 21 | 28 | 40 | 40 | 48 | 56 | 82 | 98 | 100 | 114 | 122 | 142 | 187 | 1173:00 |

\* See no Decompression Table for repetitive groups
\*\* Repetitive dives may not follow exceptional exposure dives

Figure 12h. US Navy Standard Air Decompression Table 5 Continued.

## Surface Decompression Table Using Oxygen

| Depth feet meters | Bottom time (min) | Time to first stop or surface (min:sec) | Time (min) breathing air at water stops (feet/meters) | | | | Surface Interval | Time at 40-foot chamber stop (min) on oxygen | Surface | Total decompression time (min:sec) |
|---|---|---|---|---|---|---|---|---|---|---|
| | | | 60 18.2 | 50 15.2 | 40 12.1 | 30 9.1 | | | | |
| **70** **21.3** | 52 | 2:20 | | | | | | | | 2:20 |
| | 90 | 2:20 | | | | | | 15 | | 22:40 |
| | 120 | 2:20 | | | | | | 23 | | 30:40 |
| | 150 | 2:20 | | | | | | 31 | | 43:40 |
| | 180 | 2:20 | | | | | | 39 | | 51:40 |
| **80** **24.3** | 40 | 2:40 | | | | | | | | 2:40 |
| | 70 | 2:40 | | | | | | 14 | | 22:00 |
| | 85 | 2:40 | | | | | | 20 | | 28:00 |
| | 100 | 2:40 | | | | | | 26 | | 34:00 |
| | 115 | 2:40 | | | | | | 31 | | 44:00 |
| | 130 | 2:40 | | | | | | 37 | | 50:00 |
| | 150 | 2:40 | | | | | | 44 | | 57:00 |
| **90** **27.4** | 32 | 3:00 | | | | | | | | 3:00 |
| | 60 | 3:00 | | | | | | 14 | | 22:20 |
| | 70 | 3:00 | | | | | | 20 | | 28:20 |
| | 80 | 3:00 | | | | | | 25 | | 33:20 |
| | 90 | 3:00 | | | | | | 30 | | 38:20 |
| | 100 | 3:00 | | | | | | 34 | | 47:20 |
| | 110 | 3:00 | | | | | | 39 | | 52:20 |
| | 120 | 3:00 | | | | | | 43 | | 56:20 |
| | 130 | 3:00 | | | | | | 48 | | 61:20 |
| **100** **30.4** | 26 | 3:20 | | | | | | | | 3:20 |
| | 50 | 3:20 | | | | | | 14 | | 22:40 |
| | 60 | 3:20 | | | | | | 20 | | 28:40 |
| | 70 | 3:20 | | | | | | 26 | | 34:40 |
| | 80 | 3:20 | | | | | | 32 | | 45:40 |
| | 90 | 3:20 | | | | | | 38 | | 51:40 |
| | 100 | 3:20 | | | | | | 44 | | 57:40 |
| | 110 | 3:20 | | | | | | 49 | | 62:40 |
| | 120 | 2:20 | | | | 3 | | 53 | | 69:20 |
| **110** **33.5** | 22 | 3:40 | | | | | | | | 3:40 |
| | 40 | 3:40 | | | | | | 12 | | 21:00 |
| | 50 | 3:40 | | | | | | 19 | | 28:00 |
| | 60 | 3:40 | | | | | | 26 | | 35:00 |
| | 70 | 3:40 | | | | | | 33 | | 47:00 |
| | 80 | 2:40 | | | | 1 | | 40 | | 55:00 |
| | 90 | 2:40 | | | | 2 | | 46 | | 62:00 |
| | 100 | 2:40 | | | | 5 | | 51 | | 70:00 |
| | 110 | 2:40 | | | | 12 | | 54 | | 80:00 |

Surface Interval column: TOTAL TIME FROM LAST WATER STOP TO FIRST CHAMBER STOP NOT TO EXCEED 5 MINUTES

Surface column: 1-MINUTE 20 SECOND ASCENT FROM 40 FEET IN CHAMBER TO SURFACE

*Figure 13a. US Navy Surface Decompression Table Using Oxygen.*

## Surface Decompression Table Using Oxygen (Continued)

| Depth feet / meters | Bottom time (min) | Time to first stop or surface (min:sec) | 60 / 18.2 | 50 / 15.2 | 40 / 12.1 | 30 / 9.1 | Surface Interval | Time at 40-foot chamber stop (min) on oxygen | Surface | Total decompression time (min:sec) |
|---|---|---|---|---|---|---|---|---|---|---|
| 120 / 36.5 | 18 | 4:00 | | | | | | | | 4:00 |
| | 30 | 4:00 | | | | | | 9 | | 18:20 |
| | 40 | 4:00 | | | | | | 16 | | 25:20 |
| | 50 | 4:00 | | | | | | 24 | | 33:20 |
| | 60 | 3:00 | | | | 2 | | 32 | | 48:20 |
| | 70 | 3:00 | | | | 4 | | 39 | | 57:20 |
| | 80 | 3:00 | | | | 5 | | 46 | | 65:20 |
| | 90 | 3:00 | | | 3 | 7 | | 51 | | 72:20 |
| | 100 | 3:00 | | | 6 | 15 | | 54 | | 83:20 |
| 130 / 39.6 | 15 | 4:20 | | | | | | | | 4:20 |
| | 30 | 4:20 | | | | | | 12 | | 21:40 |
| | 40 | 4:20 | | | | | | 21 | | 30:40 |
| | 50 | 3:20 | | | | 3 | | 29 | | 41:40 |
| | 60 | 3:20 | | | | 5 | | 37 | | 56:40 |
| | 70 | 3:20 | | | | 7 | | 45 | | 66:40 |
| | 80 | 3:00 | | | 6 | 7 | | 51 | | 78:40 |
| | 90 | 3:00 | | | 10 | 12 | | 56 | | 92:40 |
| 140 / 42.6 | 13 | 4:40 | | | | | | | | 4:40 |
| | 25 | 4:40 | | | | | | 11 | | 21:00 |
| | 30 | 4:40 | | | | | | 15 | | 25:00 |
| | 35 | 4:40 | | | | | | 20 | | 30:00 |
| | 40 | 3:40 | | | | 2 | | 24 | | 36:00 |
| | 45 | 3:40 | | | | 4 | | 29 | | 43:00 |
| | 50 | 3:40 | | | | 6 | | 33 | | 54:00 |
| | 55 | 3:40 | | | | 7 | | 38 | | 60:00 |
| | 60 | 3:40 | | | | 8 | | 43 | | 66:00 |
| | 65 | 3:20 | | | 3 | 7 | | 48 | | 73:00 |
| | 70 | 3:00 | | 2 | 7 | 7 | | 51 | | 82:00 |
| 150 / 45.7 | 11 | 5:00 | | | | | | | | 5:00 |
| | 25 | 5:00 | | | | | | 13 | | 23:20 |
| | 30 | 5:00 | | | | | | 18 | | 28:20 |
| | 35 | 4:00 | | | | 4 | | 23 | | 37:20 |
| | 40 | 3:40 | | | 3 | 6 | | 27 | | 46:20 |
| | 45 | 3:40 | | | 5 | 7 | | 33 | | 60:20 |
| | 50 | 3:20 | | 2 | 5 | 8 | | 38 | | 68:20 |
| | 55 | 3:00 | 2 | 5 | 9 | 4 | | 44 | | 79:20 |
| 160 / 48.7 | 9 | 5:20 | | | | | | | | 5:20 |
| | 20 | 5:20 | | | | | | 11 | | 21:40 |
| | 25 | 5:20 | | | | | | 16 | | 26:40 |
| | 30 | 4:20 | | | | 2 | | 21 | | 33:40 |
| | 35 | 4:00 | | | 4 | 6 | | 26 | | 47:40 |
| | 40 | 3:40 | | 3 | 5 | 8 | | 32 | | 63:40 |
| | 45 | 3:20 | 3 | 4 | 8 | 6 | | 38 | | 74:39 |
| 170 / 51.8 | 7 | 5:40 | | | | | | | | 5:40 |
| | 20 | 5:40 | | | | | | 13 | | 24:00 |
| | 25 | 5:40 | | | | | | 19 | | 30:00 |
| | 30 | 4:20 | | | 3 | 5 | | 23 | | 42:00 |
| | 35 | 4:00 | | 4 | 4 | 7 | | 29 | | 55:00 |
| | 40 | 3:40 | 4 | 4 | 8 | 6 | | 36 | | 74:00 |

Surface Interval column (note): TOTAL TIME FROM LAST WATER STOP TO FIRST CHAMBER STOP NOT TO EXCEED 5 MINUTES

Surface column (note): 1-MINUTE 20 SECOND ASCENT FROM 40 FEET IN CHAMBER TO SURFACE

Figure 13b. US Navy Surface Decompression Table Using Oxygen Continued.

## Surface Decompression Table Using Air

### 14a

| Depth feet / meters | Bottom time (min) | Time to first stop or surface (min:sec) | Water stop 30 / 9.1 | Water stop 20 / 6.0 | Water stop 10 / 3.0 | Surface Interval | Chamber 20 / 6.0 | Chamber 10 / 3.0 | Total decompression time (min:sec) |
|---|---|---|---|---|---|---|---|---|---|
| 40 / 12.1 | 230 | 1:00 | | | 3 | | | 7 | 16:20 |
| | 250 | 1:00 | | | 3 | | | 11 | 20:20 |
| | 270 | 1:00 | | | 3 | | | 15 | 24:20 |
| | 300 | 1:00 | | | 3 | | | 19 | 28:20 |
| 50 / 15.2 | 120 | 1:20 | | | 3 | | | 5 | 14:40 |
| | 140 | 1:20 | | | 3 | | | 10 | 19:40 |
| | 160 | 1:20 | | | 3 | | | 21 | 30:40 |
| | 180 | 1:20 | | | 3 | | | 29 | 38:40 |
| | 200 | 1:20 | | | 3 | | | 35 | 44:40 |
| | 220 | 1:20 | | | 3 | | | 40 | 49:40 |
| | 240 | 1:20 | | | 3 | | | 47 | 57:40 |
| 60 / 18.2 | 100 | 1:40 | | | 3 | | | 14 | 24:00 |
| | 140 | 1:40 | | | 3 | | | 39 | 49:00 |
| | 180 | 1:40 | | | 3 | | | 56 | 66:00 |
| 70 / 21.3 | 70 | 2:00 | | | 3 | | | 14 | 24:20 |
| | 90 | 2:00 | | | 3 | | | 23 | 33:20 |
| | 110 | 1:40 | | 3 | | | 3 | 41 | 54:50 |
| | 130 | 1:40 | | 3 | | | 6 | 52 | 68:50 |
| | 150 | 1:40 | | 3 | | | 9 | 61 | 10:50 |
| | 170 | 1:40 | | 3 | | | 19 | 79 | 108:50 |
| 80 / 24.3 | 50 | 2:20 | | | 3 | | | 10 | 20:40 |
| | 60 | 2:20 | | | 3 | | | 17 | 27:40 |
| | 70 | 2:20 | | | 3 | | | 23 | 33:40 |
| | 80 | 2:00 | | 3 | | | 3 | 31 | 44:40 |
| | 90 | 2:00 | | 3 | | | 7 | 39 | 56:40 |
| | 100 | 2:00 | | 3 | | | 11 | 46 | 67:40 |
| | 110 | 2:00 | | 3 | | | 13 | 53 | 76:40 |
| | 120 | 2:00 | | 3 | | | 17 | 56 | 83:40 |
| | 130 | 2:00 | | 3 | | | 19 | 63 | 92:40 |
| | 140 | 2:00 | | 26 | | | 26 | 69 | 128:40 |
| | 150 | 2:00 | | 32 | | | 32 | 77 | 148:40 |

Surface Interval note: TOTAL TIME FROM LAST WATER STOP TO FIRST CHAMBER STOP NOT TO EXCEED 5 MINUTES

### 14b

| Depth feet / meters | Bottom time (min) | Time to first stop or surface (min:sec) | Water stop 30 / 9.1 | Water stop 20 / 6.0 | Water stop 10 / 3.0 | Surface Interval | Chamber 20 / 6.0 | Chamber 10 / 3.0 | Total decompression time (min:sec) |
|---|---|---|---|---|---|---|---|---|---|
| 90 / 27.4 | 40 | 2:40 | | | 3 | | | 7 | 18:00 |
| | 50 | 2:40 | | | 3 | | | 18 | 29:00 |
| | 60 | 2:40 | | | 3 | | | 25 | 36:00 |
| | 70 | 2:20 | | 3 | | | 7 | 30 | 48:30 |
| | 80 | 2:20 | | 13 | | | 13 | 40 | 74:30 |
| | 90 | 2:20 | | 18 | | | 18 | 48 | 92:30 |
| | 100 | 2:20 | | 21 | | | 21 | 54 | 104:30 |
| | 110 | 2:20 | | 24 | | | 24 | 61 | 117:30 |
| | 120 | 2:20 | | 32 | | | 32 | 68 | 140:30 |
| | 130 | 2:00 | 5 | 36 | | | 36 | 74 | 159:30 |
| 100 / 30.4 | 40 | 3:00 | | | 3 | | | 15 | 26:20 |
| | 50 | 2:40 | | 3 | | | 3 | 24 | 38:50 |
| | 60 | 2:40 | | 3 | | | 9 | 28 | 48:50 |
| | 70 | 2:40 | | 3 | | | 17 | 39 | 67:50 |
| | 80 | 2:40 | | 23 | | | 23 | 48 | 102:50 |
| | 90 | 2:20 | 3 | 23 | | | 23 | 57 | 114:50 |
| | 100 | 2:20 | 7 | 23 | | | 23 | 66 | 127:50 |
| | 110 | 2:20 | 10 | 34 | | | 34 | 72 | 158:50 |
| | 120 | 2:20 | 12 | 41 | | | 41 | 78 | 180:50 |
| 110 / 33.5 | 30 | 3:20 | | | 3 | | | 7 | 18:40 |
| | 40 | 3:00 | | 3 | | | 3 | 21 | 35:40 |
| | 50 | 3:00 | | 3 | | | 8 | 26 | 45:40 |
| | 60 | 3:00 | | 18 | | | 18 | 36 | 80:40 |
| | 70 | 2:40 | 1 | 23 | | | 23 | 48 | 103:40 |
| | 80 | 2:40 | 7 | 23 | | | 23 | 57 | 118:40 |
| | 90 | 2:40 | 12 | 30 | | | 30 | 64 | 144:40 |
| | 100 | 2:40 | 15 | 37 | | | 37 | 72 | 169:40 |

Surface Interval note: TOTAL TIME FROM LAST WATER STOP TO FIRST CHAMBER STOP NOT TO EXCEED 5 MINUTES

Figure 14a and 14b. US Navy Surface Decompression Table Using Air.

## Surface Decompression Table Using Air (Continued)

| Depth feet meters | Bottom time (min) | Time to first stop or surface (min:sec) | 50 15.2 | 40 12.1 | 30 9.1 | 20 6.0 | 10 3.0 | Surface Interval | 20 6.0 | 10 3.0 | Total decompression time (min:sec) |
|---|---|---|---|---|---|---|---|---|---|---|---|
| **120 35.5** | 25 | 3:40 | | | | | 3 | TOTAL TIME FROM LAST WATER STOP TO FIRST CHAMBER STOP NOT TO EXCEED 5 MINUTES | | 6 | 18:00 |
| | 30 | 3:40 | | | | | 3 | | | 14 | 26:00 |
| | 40 | 3:20 | | | | 3 | | | 5 | 25 | 42:30 |
| | 50 | 3:20 | | | | 15 | | | 15 | 31 | 70:30 |
| | 60 | 3:00 | | | 2 | 22 | | | 22 | 45 | 100:30 |
| | 70 | 3:00 | | | 9 | 23 | | | 23 | 55 | 119:30 |
| | 80 | 3:00 | | | 15 | 27 | | | 27 | 63 | 141:30 |
| | 90 | 3:00 | | | 19 | 37 | | | 37 | 74 | 176:30 |
| | 100 | 3:00 | | | 23 | 45 | | | 45 | 80 | 202:30 |
| **130 39.6** | 25 | 4:00 | | | | | 3 | | | 10 | 22:20 |
| | 30 | 3:40 | | | | 3 | | | 3 | 18 | 33:20 |
| | 40 | 3:40 | | | | 10 | | | 10 | 25 | 53:20 |
| | 50 | 3:20 | | | 3 | 21 | | | 21 | 37 | 91:20 |
| | 60 | 3:20 | | | 9 | 23 | | | 23 | 52 | 116:20 |
| | 70 | 3:20 | | | 16 | 24 | | | 24 | 61 | 134:20 |
| | 80 | 3:00 | | 3 | 19 | 35 | | | 35 | 72 | 173:20 |
| | 90 | 3:00 | | 8 | 19 | 45 | | | 45 | 80 | 206:20 |
| **140 42.6** | 20 | 4:20 | | | | | 3 | | | 6 | 18:40 |
| | 25 | 4:00 | | | | 3 | | | 3 | 14 | 29:40 |
| | 30 | 4:00 | | | | 5 | | TOTAL TIME FROM LAST WATER STOP TO FIRST CHAMBER STOP NOT TO EXCEED 5 MINUTES | 5 | 21 | 40:40 |
| | 40 | 3:40 | | | 2 | 16 | | | 16 | 26 | 69:40 |
| | 50 | 3:40 | | | 6 | 24 | | | 24 | 44 | 107:40 |
| | 60 | 3:40 | | | 16 | 23 | | | 23 | 56 | 127:40 |
| | 70 | 3:20 | | 4 | 19 | 32 | | | 32 | 68 | 164:40 |
| | 80 | 3:20 | | 10 | 23 | 41 | | | 41 | 79 | 203:40 |
| **150 45.7** | 20 | 4:20 | | | | | 3 | | 3 | 7 | 23:00 |
| | 25 | 4:20 | | | | | 4 | | 4 | 17 | 35:00 |
| | 30 | 4:20 | | | | | 8 | | 8 | 24 | 50:00 |
| | 40 | 4:00 | | | 5 | 19 | | | 19 | 33 | 86:00 |
| | 50 | 4:00 | | | 12 | 23 | | | 23 | 51 | 119:00 |
| | 60 | 3:40 | | 3 | 19 | 26 | | | 26 | 62 | 146:00 |
| | 70 | 3:40 | | 11 | 19 | 39 | | | 39 | 75 | 193:00 |
| | 80 | 3:20 | 1 | 17 | 19 | 50 | | | 50 | 84 | 231:00 |
| **160 48.7** | 20 | 4:40 | | | | | 3 | | 3 | 11 | 27:20 |
| | 25 | 4:40 | | | | | 7 | | 7 | 20 | 44:20 |
| | 30 | 4:20 | | | 2 | 11 | | | 11 | 25 | 59:20 |
| | 40 | 4:20 | | | 7 | 23 | | | 23 | 39 | 102:20 |
| | 50 | 4:00 | | 2 | 16 | 23 | | | 23 | 55 | 129:20 |
| | 60 | 4:00 | | 9 | 19 | 33 | | | 33 | 69 | 173:20 |
| | 70 | 3:40 | 1 | 17 | 22 | 44 | | | 44 | 80 | 218:20 |

*Figure 14c. US Navy Surface Decompression Table Using Air Continued.*

***Surface Decompression Table Using Air (Continued)***

| Depth feet meters | Bottom time (min) | Time to first stop or surface (min:sec) | Time (min) at water stops (feet/meters) 50 15.2 | 40 12.1 | 30 9.1 | 20 6.0 | 10 3.0 | Surface Interval | Chamber stops (air) (min) (feet/meters) 20 6.0 | 10 3.0 | Total decompression time (min:sec) |
|---|---|---|---|---|---|---|---|---|---|---|---|
| 170 51.8 | 15 | 5:00 | | | | 3 | | TOTAL TIME FROM LAST WATER STOP TO FIRST CHAMBER STOP NOT TO EXCEED 5 MINUTES | 3 | 5 | 21:40 |
| | 20 | 5:00 | | | | 4 | | | 4 | 15 | 33:40 |
| | 25 | 4:40 | | | 2 | 7 | | | 7 | 23 | 49:40 |
| | 30 | 4:40 | | | 4 | 13 | | | 13 | 26 | 66:40 |
| | 40 | 4:20 | | 1 | 10 | 23 | | | 23 | 45 | 112:40 |
| | 50 | 4:20 | | 5 | 18 | 23 | | | 23 | 61 | 140:40 |
| | 60 | 4:00 | 2 | 15 | 22 | 37 | | | 37 | 74 | 197:40 |
| | 70 | 4:00 | 8 | 17 | 19 | 51 | | | 51 | 86 | 242:40 |
| 180 54.8 | 15 | 5:20 | | | | 3 | | | 3 | 6 | 23:00 |
| | 20 | 5:00 | | | 1 | 5 | | | 5 | 17 | 39:00 |
| | 25 | 5:00 | | | 3 | 10 | | | 10 | 24 | 58:00 |
| | 30 | 5:00 | | | 6 | 17 | | | 17 | 27 | 78:00 |
| | 40 | 4:40 | | 3 | 14 | 23 | | | 23 | 50 | 124:00 |
| | 50 | 4:20 | 2 | 9 | 19 | 30 | | | 30 | 65 | 166:00 |
| | 60 | 4:20 | 5 | 16 | 19 | 44 | | | 44 | 81 | 220:00 |
| 190 57.9 | 15 | 5:40 | | | | 4 | | | 4 | 7 | 26:20 |
| | 20 | 5:20 | | | 2 | 6 | | | 6 | 20 | 45:20 |
| | 25 | 5:20 | | | 5 | 11 | | | 11 | 25 | 63:20 |
| | 30 | 5:00 | | 1 | 8 | 19 | | | 19 | 32 | 90:20 |
| | 40 | 5:00 | | 8 | 14 | 23 | | | 23 | 55 | 134:20 |
| | 50 | 4:40 | 4 | 13 | 22 | 33 | | | 33 | 72 | 188:20 |
| | 60 | 4:40 | 10 | 17 | 19 | 50 | | | 50 | 84 | 241:20 |

*Figure 14d. US Navy Surface Decompression Table Using Air Continued.*

As written, the Exceptional Exposure Air Decompression Table is particularly dangerous, as it was tested only at the 140-foot level. On each test there were no more than six men in the dry chamber and on every occasion at least one individual suffered DCS, and sometimes two. For this reason, the Navy maintains it for emergency use only, typically for situations where a diver is fouled on the bottom and cannot be surfaced within the time constraints of a standard table.

The limits for "no decompression" dives are also too great. For example, the 50-foot for 100 minute dive is considered a "no decompression" dive with ascent permitted directly to the surface at a rate of 30 feet per minute. When pushed to a full 100 minutes at 50 feet, I (EPK)have seen inside tenders sustain vestibular DCS, spinal cord paralysis, and pain at multiple sites. Safe, routine decompression of inside tenders is covered elsewhere. (See the chapter by Kindwall entitled "The Multiplace Chamber.")

However, if one is faced with an unusual dive profile for the inside tender which may arise from an aborted treatment schedule, an unplanned multilevel dive, or a forced repetative use of the same inside tender on the same day, the U.S. Navy Air Decompression Tables can give one a framework on which to construct a safe decompression schedule. If one has the tender breathe 100% oxygen from a tight-fitting demand mask, instead of air, for most of the decompression time, one automatically adds a theoretical five-to-one safety factor. This is true for single dives as well as repetitive dives. Then, the addition of a two-minute stop (on oxygen) 10 feet (3 meters) deeper than called for in the schedule will add extra safety. Any time at the shallowest 10-foot (3 meters) stop should be made a minimum of 10 minutes on oxygen if a longer time is not specified.

## GENERAL TREATMENT INFORMATION

This section contains the diving accident treatment flow charts and a number of U.S. Navy Treatment Tables used to recompress divers who have experienced decompression sickness or arterial gas embolism as a result of their diving activities. The information in this section reflects treatment procedures recommended by the NOAA Diving Program and taught in the NOAA training program. All of the tables in this section have been widely used in the field and have been shown to be safe and effective.

### Diving Accident Treatment Flow Charts

The flow charts shown are decision trees designed to aid dive supervisors, diving physicians, Diving Medical Technicians, chamber operators, and other health care professionals who must decide how best to treat stricken divers. Use of the decision tree requires only that the diver's condition be observed; a medical diagnosis is not required for treatment to begin. These flow charts are used by the US Navy and NOAA but are not used in the commercial diving arena, as they are considered archaic. See treatment schemes on preceeding pages.

## RECOMPRESSION TREATMENT TABLES

The recompression treatment tables recommended by NOAA are explained on the following pages. Instructions for the use of these tables appear with each table and should be followed precisely.

### Recompression Treatments when Chamber is Available

Oxygen Treatment Tables are more effective and, therefore, preferable over Air Treatment Tables. Treatment Table 4 can be used with or without oxygen but should always be used with oxygen if it is available.

### Symptoms During Decompression and Surface Decompression

If symptoms of decompression sickness occur in the water during decompression, follow Flow Chart 1. After completing recompression treatment, observe the diver for at least 6 hours. If any symptoms recur, treat as a recurrence of Type II symptoms. As an option, the on-site Diving Supervisor may elect not to recompress the diver 10 feet in the water, but to remove the diver from the water when decompression risks are unacceptable and treat him in the chamber. When this is done, the surface interval should be 5 minutes or less, with the diver always treated as having Type II symptoms.

### Treatment of Symptoms During Sur-D Surface Interval

If surface decompression procedures are used, symptoms of decompression sickness may occur during the surface interval. Because neurological symptoms cannot be ruled out during this short period, the symptomatic diver is treated as having Type II symptoms, even if the only complaint is pain.

### Treating for Exceeded Sur-D Surface Interval

If the prescribed surface interval is exceeded but the diver remains asymptomatic, the diver is treated with Treatment Table 5, or Treatment

Table lA if no oxygen is available. If the diver becomes symptomatic, the diver is treated as if Type II symptoms were present. Any symptoms occurring during the chamber stops are treated as recurrences in accordance with Flow Chart 3.

## Recompression Treatments when Oxygen is not Available

If no oxygen is available, select the appropriate Air Treatment Table in accordance with Table 1A, Table 2A, Table 3, and Table 4.

Use Table 1A if pain is relieved at a depth less than 66 feet. If pain is relieved at a depth greater than 66 feet, use Table 2A. Table 3 is used for treatment of serious symptoms where oxygen cannot be used. Use Table 3 if symptoms are relieved within 30 minutes at 165 feet. If symptoms are not relieved in less than 30 minutes at 165 feet, use Table 4.

## Descent/Ascent Rates for Air Treatment Tables

The Air Treatment Tables (lA, 2A, 3, and 4 using air) are used when no oxygen is available. They are not as effective as the Oxygen Treatment Tables. The descent rate is 20 feet per minute; the ascent rate is not to exceed 1 foot per minute.

## Recompression Treatments when Oxygen is Available

Use Oxygen Treatment Tables 5, 6, 6A, 4, or 7, according to Flow Charts 2, 3, and 4. The descent rate is 20 feet per minute. Upon reaching treatment depth not to exceed 60 fsw, place the patient on oxygen. For depth deeper than 60 fsw, use treatment gas if available. Additional guidelines for each treatment table are given below.

## Treatment Table 5

Treatment Table 5 may be used for the following:

- Type I (except for cutis-marmorata) symptoms when a complete neurological examination has revealed no abnormality.
- Asymptomatic omitted decompression of shallow surfacing (20 fsw or less).
- Asymptomatic omitted decompression of rapid ascent (from deeper than 20 fsw) if the missed decompression is less than 30 minutes.
- Asymptomatic divers who have exceeded surface interval limits following a Sur-D dive.
- Treatment of resolved symptoms following in-water recompression
- Follow-up treatments for residual symptoms.

## Performance of Neurological Exam at 60 fsw

After arrival at 60 fsw a neurological exam shall be performed to ensure that no overt neurological symptoms (e.g., weakness, numbness, incoordination) are present. If any abnormalities are found, the stricken diver should be treated using Treatment Table 6.

## Extending Oxygen Breathing Periods on Treatment Table 5

Treatment Table 5 may be extended by two oxygen breathing periods at 30 fsw. Air breaks are not required prior to an extension, between extensions, or prior to surfacing. In other words, the Diving Supervisor may have the diver breathe oxygen continuously for 60 minutes at 30 fsw and travel to the surface while breathing oxygen. If the Diving Supervisor elects to extend this treatment table, the tender does not require additional oxygen breathing than currently prescribed.

## When Use of Treatment Table 6 is Mandatory

- Type I pain is severe and immediate recompression must be instituted before a neurological examination can be performed, or
- A complete neurological examination cannot be performed, or
- Any neurological symptom is present.

These rules apply no matter how rapidly or completely the symptoms resolve once recompression begins.

Complete Relief after 10 Minutes: If complete relief of Type I symptoms is not obtained within 10 minutes at 60 feet, Table 6 is required.

## Musculoskeletal Pain Due to Orthopedic Injury

Symptoms of musculoskeletal pain that have shown absolutely no change after the second oxygen breathing period at 60 feet may be due to orthopedic injury rather than decompression sickness. If, after reviewing the patient's history, the Diving Medical Doctor feels that the pain can be related to specific orthopedic trauma or injury, Treatment Table 5 may be completed. If no Diving Medical Doctor is on site, Treatment Table 6 shall be used.

> Note: *Once recompression to 60 feet is done, Treatment Table 5 shall be used even if it was decided symptoms were probably not decompression sickness. Direct ascent to the surface is done only in emergencies.*

## Treatment Table 6

Treatment Table 6 is used for the following:

- Type I symptoms where relief is not complete within 10 minutes at 60 feet or where a neurological exam is not complete.
- Type II symptoms.
- Cutis marmorata.
- Arterial gas embolism.
- Symptomatic uncontrolled ascent.
- Asymptomatic divers with omitted decompression greater than 30 minutes.
- Treatment of unresolved symptoms following in-water treatment
- Recurrence of symptoms shallower than 60 fsw.

## Treating Arterial Gas Embolism

Arterial gas embolism is treated by initial compression to 60 fsw. If symptoms are improved within the first oxygen breathing period, then treatment is continued using Treatment Table 6. Treatment Table 6 may be extended for two oxygen breathing periods at 60 fsw (20 minutes on oxygen, then 5 minutes on air, then 20 minutes on oxygen) and two oxygen breathing periods at 30 fsw (15 minutes on air, then 60 minutes on oxygen, then 15 minutes on air, then 60 minutes on oxygen). If there has been more than one extension, the tenders' oxygen breathing period is extended 60 minutes at 30 feet.

## Treatment Table 6A

Arterial gas embolism or severe decompression symptoms are treated by initial compression to 60 fsw. If symptoms improve, complete Treatment Table 6. If symptoms are unchanged or worsen, assess the patient upon descent and compress to depth of relief (significant improvement), not to exceed 165 fsw. Once at the depth of relief, begin treatment gas ($N_2O_2$, $HeO_2$) if available. Stay there for 30 minutes. A breathing period of 25 minutes on treatment gas, interrupted by 5 minutes of air, is recommended at depth to simplify time keeping. The patient may remain on treatment gas during ascent from treatment depth to 60 fsw since the $PO_2$ will continually decrease during ascent. Decompress to 60 fsw at a travel rate not to exceed 3 ft/min. Upon arrival at 60 fsw, complete Treatment Table 6. Consult with a Diving Medical Doctor at the earliest opportunity. The Diving Medical Doctor may recommend a Treatment Table 4. Treatment Table 6A may be extended for two oxygen breathing periods at 60 fsw and two oxygen breathing periods at 30 fsw. If deterioration is noted during ascent to 60 feet, treat as a recurrence of symptoms (Flow Chart 4).

## Treatment Table 4

If a shift from Treatment Table 6A to Treatment Table 4 is contemplated, a Diving Medical Doctor shall be consulted before the shift is made. Treatment Table 4 is used when it is determined that the patient would receive additional benefit at depth of significant relief, not to exceed 165 fsw. The time at depth shall be between 30 to 120 minutes, based on the patient's response.

## Recurrence of Symptoms

If deterioration is noted during ascent to 60 feet, treat as a recurrence of symptoms (Flow Chart 4).

## Oxygen Breathing Periods

If oxygen is available, the patient should begin oxygen breathing periods immediately upon arrival at the 60-foot stop. Breathing periods of 25 minutes on oxygen, interrupted by 5 minutes of air, are recommended. This simplifies timekeeping. Immediately upon arrival at 60 feet, a minimum of four oxygen breathing periods (for a total time of 2 hours) should be administered. After that, oxygen breathing should be administered to suit the patient's individual needs and operational conditions. Both the patient and tender must breathe oxygen for at least 4 hours (eight 25-minute oxygen, 5-minute air periods), beginning no later than 2 hours before ascent from 30 feet is begun. These oxygen-breathing periods may be divided up as convenient, but at least 2 hours' worth of oxygen breathing periods should be completed at 30 feet.

## Treatment Table 7

Treatment Table 7 is considered an heroic measure for treating non-responding severe gas embolism or life-threatening decompression sickness. Committing a patient to Treatment Table 7 involves isolating the patient and having to minister to his medical needs in the recompression chamber for 48 hours or longer. Experienced diving medical personnel must be available before committing to Treatment Table 7.

## Considerations

A Diving Medical Doctor shall be consulted before shifting to a Treatment Table 7 and careful consideration shall be given to life support capability. In addition, it must be realized that the recompression facility will be committed for 48 hours or more.

## Indications

Treatment Table 7 is an extension at 60 feet of Treatment Tables 6, 6A, or 4 (or any other nonstandard treatment table). This means that considerable treatment has already been administered. Treatment Table 7 is not designed to treat all residual symptoms that do not improve at 60 feet and should never be used to treat residual pain. Treatment Table 7 should be used only when loss of life may result if the currently prescribed decompression from 60 feet is undertaken.

## Time at Depth

When using Treatment Table 7, a minimum of 12 hours should be spent at 60 feet, including time spent at 60 feet from Treatment Table 4, 6, or 6A. Severe Type II decompression sickness and/or arterial gas embolism cases may continue to deteriorate significantly over the first several hours. This should not be cause for premature changes in depth. Do not begin decompression from 60 feet for at least 12 hours. At completion of the 12-hour stay, the decision must be made whether to decompress or spend additional time at 60 feet. If no improvement was noted during the first 12 hours, benefit from additional time at 60 feet is unlikely and decompression should be started. If the patient is improving but significant residual symptoms remain (e.g., limb paralysis, abnormal or absent respiration), additional time at 60 feet may be warranted. While the actual time that can be spent at 60 feet is unlimited, the actual additional amount of time beyond 12 hours that should be spent can only be determined by a Diving Medical Doctor (in consultation with on-site supervisory personnel), based on the patient's response to therapy and operational factors. When the patient has progressed to the point of consciousness, can breathe independently, and can move all extremities, decompression can be started and maintained as long as improvement continues. Solid evidence of continued benefit should be established for stays longer than 18 hours at 60 feet. Regardless of the duration at the recompression below 60 feet, at least 12 hours must be spent at 60 feet and then Table 7 followed to the surface. Additional recompression below 60 feet in these cases should not be undertaken unless adequate life support capability is available.

## Decompression

When using Treatment Table 7, tenders breathe chamber atmosphere. Chamber oxygen should be kept above 19% and carbon dioxide below 1.5% surface equivalent (sev) (11.4 mmHg). Decompression on Treatment Table 7 is begun with an upward excursion at time zero from 60 to 58 feet. Subsequent 2-foot upward excursions are made at time intervals appropriate to the rate of decompression:

| Depth | Rate/Time | Interval |
|---|---|---|
| 58-40 feet | 3 ft/hr | 40 min |
| 40-20 feet | 2 ft/hr | 60 min |
| 20-4 feet | 1 ft/hr | 120 min |

## Preventing Inadvertent Early Surfacing

Upon arrival at 4 feet, decompression should be stopped for 4 hours. At the end of 4 hours at 4 feet, decompress to the surface at 1 foot per minute. This procedure prevents inadvertent early surfacing.

## Time Intervals

The travel time between subsequent stops is considered as part of the time interval for the next shallower stop. The time intervals shown above begin when ascent to the next shallower stop has begun.

## Oxygen Breathing

On a Treatment Table 7, patients should begin oxygen breathing periods as soon as possible at 60 feet. Oxygen breathing periods of 25 minutes on 100% oxygen, followed by 5 minutes breathing chamber atmosphere, should be used. Normally, four oxygen breathing periods are alternated with 2 hours of continuous air breathing. In conscious patients, this cycle should be continued until a minimum of eight oxygen breathing periods have been administered (previous 100% oxygen breathing periods may be counted against these eight periods). Beyond that, oxygen breathing periods should be continued as recommended by the Diving Medical Doctor, as long as improvement is noted and the oxygen is tolerated by the patient. If oxygen breathing causes significant pain on inspiration, it should be discontinued unless it is felt that significant benefit from oxygen breathing is being obtained. In unconscious patients, oxygen breathing should be stopped after a maximum of 24 oxygen breathing periods have been administered. The actual number and length of oxygen breathing periods should be adjusted by the Diving Medical Doctor to suit the individual patient's clinical condition and response to oxygen toxicity.

## Sleeping, Resting, and Eating

At least two tenders should be available when using Treatment Table 7, and three may be necessary for severely ill patients. Not all tenders are required to be in the chamber, and they may be locked in and out as required following appropriate decompression tables. The patient may sleep anytime except when breathing oxygen deeper than 30 feet. While asleep, the patient's pulse, respiration, and blood pressure should be monitored and recorded at intervals appropriate to the patient's condition. Food may be taken at any time and fluid intake should be maintained.

## Ancillary Care

Patients on Treatment Table 7 requiring intravenous and/or drug therapy should have these administered in accordance with a Diving Medical Doctor.

## Abort Procedures

In some cases, a Treatment Table 7 may have to be terminated early. If extenuating circumstances dictate early decompression and less than 12 hours have elapsed since treatment was begun, decompression may be accomplished using the appropriate 60–foot Air Decompression Table as modified. The 60–foot Air Decompression Tables may be used even if time was spent between 60 and 165 feet (e.g., on Table 4 or 6A), as long as at least 3 hours have elapsed since the last excursion below 60 feet. If less than 3 hours have elapsed, or if any time was spent below 165 feet, use the Air Decompression Table appropriate to the maximum depth attained during treatment. All stops and times in the Air Decompression Table should be followed, but oxygen-breathing periods should be started for all chamber occupants as soon as a depth of 30 feet is reached. All chamber occupants should continue oxygen-breathing periods of 25 minutes on 100% oxygen, followed by 5 minutes on air, until the total time breathing oxygen is one-half or more of the total decompression time.

If more than 12 hours have elapsed since treatment was begun, the decompression schedule of Treatment Table 7 shall be used. In extreme emergencies, the abort recommendations may be used if more than 12 hours have elapsed since beginning treatment.

## Treatment Table 8

Treatment Table 8 is an adaptation of a Royal Navy Treatment Table 65 mainly for treating deep uncontrolled ascents when more than 60 minutes of decompression have been missed. Compress symptomatic patient to depth of relief not to exceed 225 fsw. Initiate Treatment Table 8 from depth of relief. The Table 8 schedule from 60 feet is the same as Treatment Table 7.

## Treatment Table 9

Treatment Table 9 is a hyperbaric oxygen treatment table using 90 minutes of oxygen at 45 feet. This table is recommended by the Diving Medical Doctor cognizant of the patient's medical condition. Treatment Table 9 is used for residual symptoms from AGE/DCS

This table may also be recommended by the cognizant Diving Medical Doctor when initially treating a severely injured patient whose medical condition precludes long absences from definitive medical care.

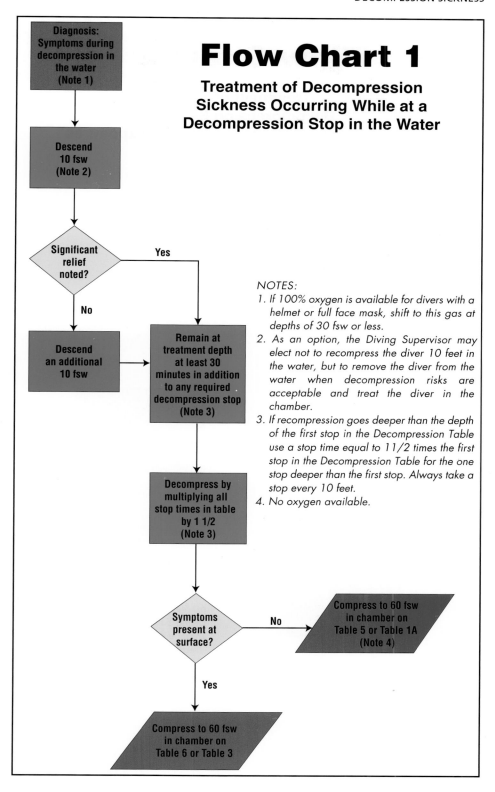

# Flow Chart 1
## Treatment of Decompression Sickness Occurring While at a Decompression Stop in the Water

NOTES:
1. If 100% oxygen is available for divers with a helmet or full face mask, shift to this gas at depths of 30 fsw or less.
2. As an option, the Diving Supervisor may elect not to recompress the diver 10 feet in the water, but to remove the diver from the water when decompression risks are acceptable and treat the diver in the chamber.
3. If recompression goes deeper than the depth of the first stop in the Decompression Table use a stop time equal to 11/2 times the first stop in the Decompression Table for the one stop deeper than the first stop. Always take a stop every 10 feet.
4. No oxygen available.

# Flow Chart 2

## Treatment of Type I
## Decompression Sickness
## Treatment from Diving or Altitude Exposures

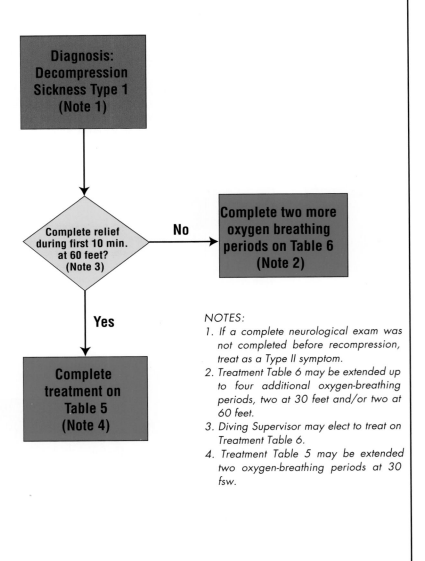

**Diagnosis:**
**Decompression**
**Sickness Type 1**
**(Note 1)**

**Complete relief during first 10 min. at 60 feet? (Note 3)**

**No** → **Complete two more oxygen breathing periods on Table 6 (Note 2)**

**Yes**

**Complete treatment on Table 5 (Note 4)**

NOTES:
1. If a complete neurological exam was not completed before recompression, treat as a Type II symptom.
2. Treatment Table 6 may be extended up to four additional oxygen-breathing periods, two at 30 feet and/or two at 60 feet.
3. Diving Supervisor may elect to treat on Treatment Table 6.
4. Treatment Table 5 may be extended two oxygen-breathing periods at 30 fsw.

# Flow Chart 3

## Treatment of Arterial Gas Embolism or Decompression Sickness

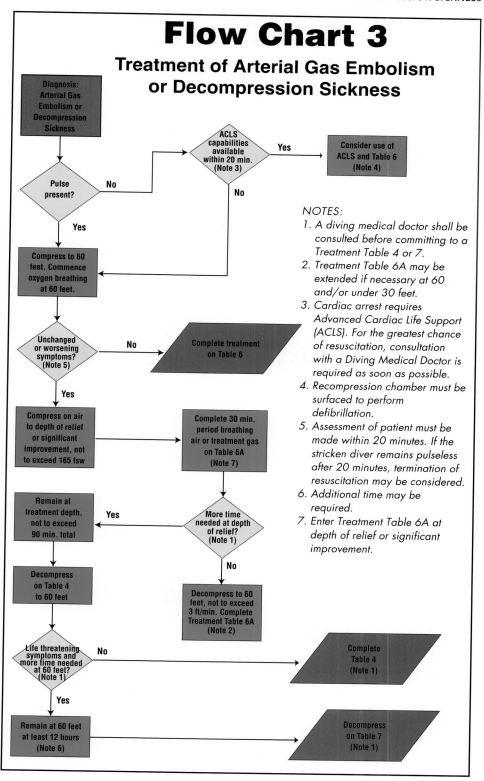

NOTES:
1. A diving medical doctor shall be consulted before committing to a Treatment Table 4 or 7.
2. Treatment Table 6A may be extended if necessary at 60 and/or under 30 feet.
3. Cardiac arrest requires Advanced Cardiac Life Support (ACLS). For the greatest chance of resuscitation, consultation with a Diving Medical Doctor is required as soon as possible.
4. Recompression chamber must be surfaced to perform defibrillation.
5. Assessment of patient must be made within 20 minutes. If the stricken diver remains pulseless after 20 minutes, termination of resuscitation may be considered.
6. Additional time may be required.
7. Enter Treatment Table 6A at depth of relief or significant improvement.

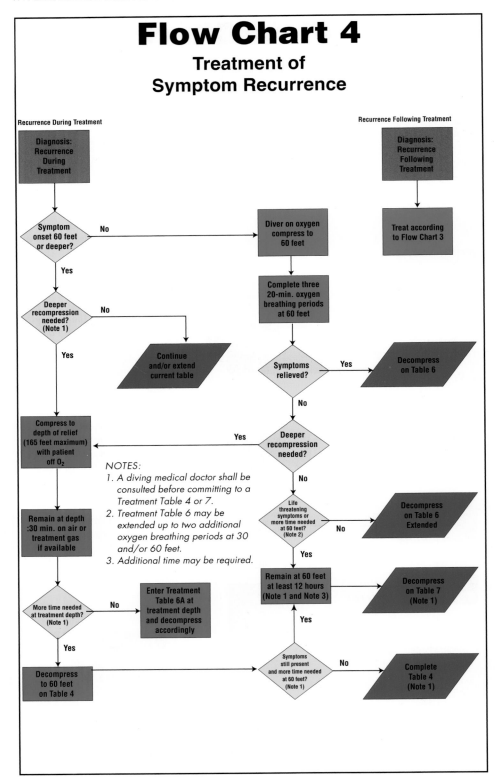

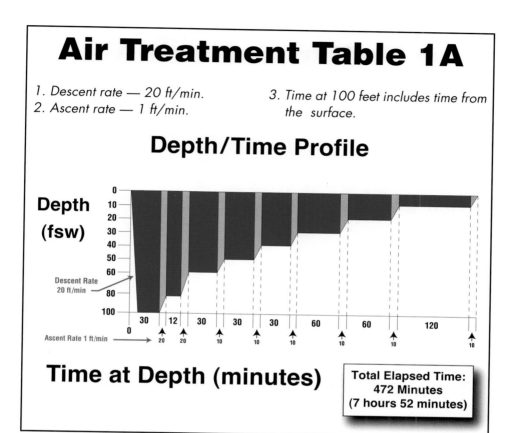

# Air Treatment Table 1A

1. Descent rate — 20 ft/min.
2. Ascent rate — 1 ft/min.

3. Time at 100 feet includes time from the surface.

## Depth/Time Profile

**Time at Depth (minutes)**

Total Elapsed Time:
472 Minutes
(7 hours 52 minutes)

| Depth (feet) | Stop Time (minutes) | Ascent Time (minutes) | Breathing Media | Total Elapsed Time (hrs:min.) |
|---|---|---|---|---|
| 100 | 30 | | Air | 0:30 |
| 80 | 12 | 20 | Air | 1:02 |
| 60 | 30 | 20 | Air | 1:52 |
| 50 | 30 | 10 | Air | 2:32 |
| 40 | 30 | 10 | Air | 3:12 |
| 30 | 60 | 10 | Air | 4:22 |
| 20 | 60 | 10 | Air | 5:32 |
| 10 | 120 | 10 | Air | 7:42 |
| 0 | | 10 | Air | 7:52 |

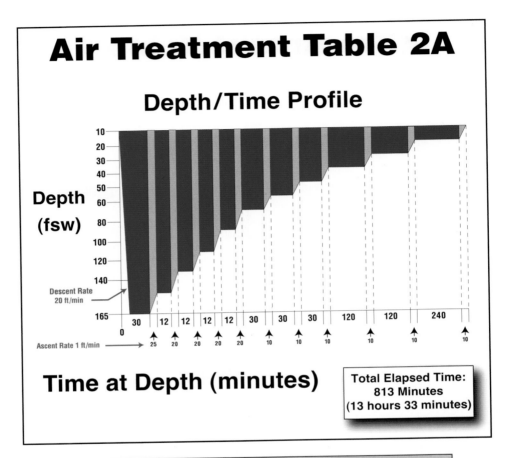

| Depth (feet) | Stop Time (minutes) | Ascent Time (minutes) | Breathing Media | Total Elapsed Time (hrs:min.) |
|---|---|---|---|---|
| 165 | 30 | | Air | 0:30 |
| 140 | 25 | 25 | Air | 1:07 |
| 120 | 20 | 20 | Air | 1:39 |
| 100 | 20 | 20 | Air | 2:11 |
| 80 | 20 | 20 | Air | 2:43 |
| 60 | 20 | 20 | Air | 3:33 |
| 50 | 10 | 10 | Air | 4:13 |
| 40 | 10 | 10 | Air | 4:53 |
| 30 | 10 | 10 | Air | 7:03 |
| 20 | 10 | 10 | Air | 9:13 |
| 10 | 10 | 10 | Air | 13:23 |
| 0 | | 10 | Air | 13:33 |

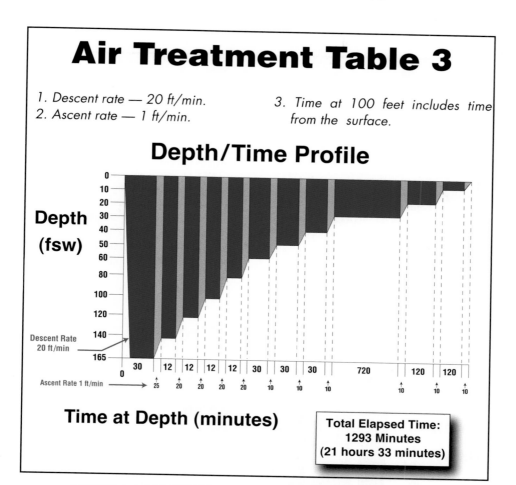

# Air Treatment Table 3

1. Descent rate — 20 ft/min.
2. Ascent rate — 1 ft/min.

3. Time at 100 feet includes time from the surface.

## Depth/Time Profile

Depth (fsw)

Descent Rate 20 ft/min

Ascent Rate 1 ft/min

## Time at Depth (minutes)

**Total Elapsed Time:
1293 Minutes
(21 hours 33 minutes)**

| Depth (feet) | Stop Time (minutes) | Ascent Time (minutes) | Breathing Media | Total Elapsed Time (hr:min.) |
|---|---|---|---|---|
| 165 | 30 | | Air | 0:30 |
| 140 | 12 | 25 | Air | 1:07 |
| 120 | 12 | 20 | Air | 1:39 |
| 100 | 12 | 20 | Air | 2:11 |
| 80 | 12 | 20 | Air | 2:43 |
| 60 | 30 | 20 | Air | 3:33 |
| 50 | 30 | 10 | Air | 4:13 |
| 40 | 30 | 10 | Air | 4:53 |
| 30 | 720 | 10 | Air | 17:03 |
| 20 | 120 | 10 | Air | 19:13 |
| 10 | 120 | 10 | Air | 21:23 |
| 0 | | 10 | Air | 21:33 |

# Treatment Table 4

1. Descent rate — 20 ft/min.
2. Ascent rate — 1 ft/min.
3. Time at 165 feet includes time from the surface.
4. If only air is available, decompress on air. If oxygen is available, patient begins oxygen breathing upon arrival at 60 feet with appropriate air breaks. Both tender and patient breathe oxygen beginning two hours before leaving 30 feet.
5. Ensure life support considerations can be met before committing to Table 4. Internal chamber temperature should be below 85°F.

6. If oxygen breathing is interrupted, no compensatory lengthening of the table is required.
7. If switching from Treatment Table 6A or 3 at 165 feet, stay a maximum of two hours at 165 feet before decompressing.
8. If the chamber is equipped with a high-$O_2$ treatment gas, it may be administered at 165 fsw, not to exceed 2.8 ata $O_2$. Treatment gas is administered for 25 minutes interrupted by 5 minutes of air.

## Depth/Time Profile

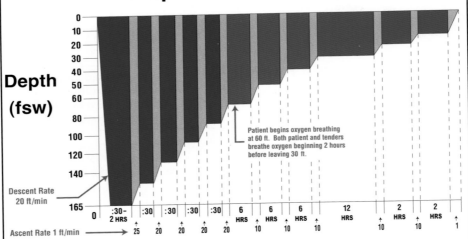

**Time at Depth (minutes)**

Total Elapsed Time:
39 Hours 6 Minutes
(30 minutes at 165 fsw)
to 40 hours 36 minutes
(2 hours at 165 fsw)

# Treatment Table 5

1. Descent rate — 20 ft/min.
2. Ascent rate — Not to exceed 1 ft/min. Do not compensate for slower ascent rates. Compensate for faster rates by halting the ascent.
3. Time on oxygen begins on arrival at 60 feet.
4. If oxygen breathing must be interrupted because of CNS Oxygen Toxicity, allow 15 minutes after the reaction has entirely subsided and resume schedule at point of interruption. *
5. Treatment Table may be extended two oxygen-breathing periods at the 30-foot stop. No air break required between oxygen-breathing periods or prior to ascent.
6. Tender breathes 100% O$_2$ during ascent from the 30-foot stop to the surface. If the tender had a previous hyperbaric exposure in the previous 12 hours, an additional 20 minutes of oxygen breathing is required prior to ascent.

## Depth/Time Profile

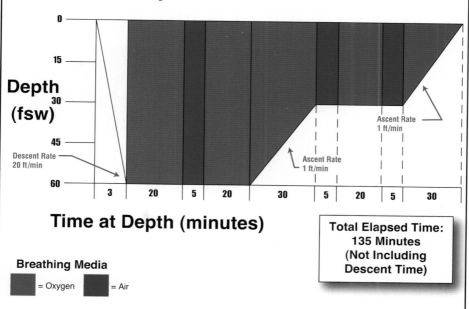

**Depth (fsw)**

Descent Rate 20 ft/min

Ascent Rate 1 ft/min

Ascent Rate 1 ft/min

0 — 15 — 30 — 45 — 60

### Time at Depth (minutes)

3 | 20 | 5 | 20 | 30 | 5 | 20 | 5 | 30

**Total Elapsed Time: 135 Minutes (Not Including Descent Time)**

**Breathing Media**

= Oxygen    = Air

*Procedures In the Event of Oxygen Toxicity. At the first sign of CNS oxygen toxicity, the patient should be removed from oxygen and allowed to breathe chamber air. Oxygen breathing may be restarted 15 minutes after all symptoms have subsided. If symptoms of CNS oxygen toxicity develop again, interrupt oxygen breathing for another 15 minutes. If CNS oxygen toxicity develops a third time, contact a Diving Medical Doctor as soon as possible to modify oxygen breathing periods to meet requirements.

# Treatment Table 6

1. Descent rate — 20 ft/min.
2. Ascent rate — Not to exceed 1 ft/min. Do not compensate for slower ascent rates. Compensate for faster rates by halting the ascent.
3. Time on oxygen begins on arrival at 60 feet.
4. If oxygen breathing must be interrupted because of CNS Oxygen Toxicity, allow 15 minutes after the reaction has entirely subsided and resume schedule at point of interruption. *
5. Table 6 can be lengthened up to two additional 25–minute periods at 60 feet (20 minutes on oxygen and five minutes on air),

or up to two additional 75–minute periods at 30 feet (15 minutes on air and 60 minutes on oxygen), or both.
6. Tender breathes 100% $O_2$ during the last 30 minutes at 30 fsw and during ascent to the surface for an unmodified table or where there has been only a single extension at 30 or 60 feet. If there has been more than one extension, the $O_2$ breathing at 30 feet is increased to 60 minutes. If the tender has had a hyperbaric exposure within the past 12 hours, an additional 60–minute $O_2$ period is taken at 30 feet.

## Depth/Time Profile

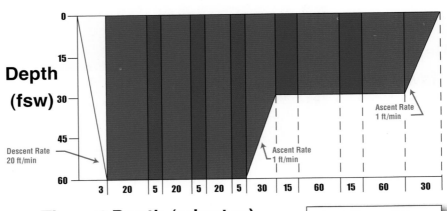

Total Elapsed Time:
285 Minutes
(Not Including
Descent Time)

Breathing Media

■ = Oxygen   ■ = Air

*Procedures In the Event of Oxygen Toxicity. At the first sign of CNS oxygen toxicity, the patient should be removed from oxygen and allowed to breathe chamber air. Oxygen breathing may be restarted 15 minutes after all symptoms have subsided. If symptoms of CNS oxygen toxicity develop again, interrupt oxygen breathing for another 15 minutes. If CNS oxygen toxicity develops a third time, contact a Diving Medical Doctor as soon as possible to modify oxygen breathing periods to meet requirements.

# Treatment Table 6A

1. Descent rate — 20 ft/min.
2. Ascent rate — 165 fsw to 60 fsw, not to exceed 3 ft/min, 60 fsw and shallower, not to exceed 1 ft/min. Do not compensate for slower ascent rates. Compensate for faster rates by halting the ascent.
3. Time at treatment depth does not include compression time.
4. Table begins with initial compression to depth of 60 fsw. If initial treatment was at 60 feet, up to 20 minutes may be spent at 60 feet before compression to 165 fsw. Contact a Diving Medical Doctor.
5. If a chamber is equipped with a high-$O_2$ treatment gas, it may be administered at 165 fsw and shallower, not to exceed 2.8 ata O2. Treatment gas is administered for 25 minutes interrupted by five minutes of air. Treatment gas is breathed during ascent from the treatment depth to 60 fsw.
6. Deeper than 60 feet, if treatment gas must be interrupted because of CNS oxygen toxicity, allow

15 minutes after the reaction has entirely subsided and resume schedule at point of interruption. *
7. Table 6A can be lengthened up to two additional 25-minute periods at 60 feet (20 minutes on oxygen and five minutes on air), or up to two additional 75-minute periods at 30 feet (60 minutes on oxygen and 15 minutes on air), or both.
8. Tender breathes 100% oxygen during the last 60 minutes at 30 fsw and during ascent to the surface for an unmodified table or where there has been only a single extension at 30 or 60 fsw. If there has been more than one extension, the $O_2$ breathing at 30 fsw is increased to 90 minutes. If the tender had a hyperbaric exposure within the past 12 hours, an additional 60 minute $O_2$ breathing period is taken at 30 fsw.
9. If significant improvement is not obtained within 30 minutes at 165 feet, consult with a Diving Medical Doctor before switching to Treatment Table 4.

## Depth/Time Profile

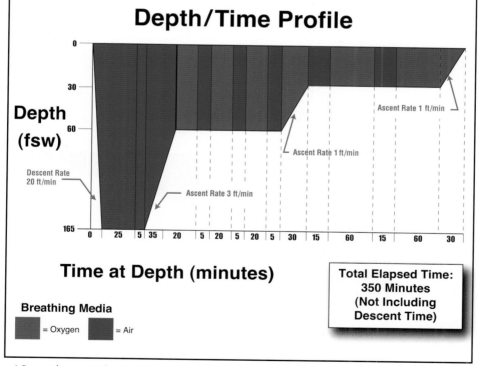

**Depth (fsw)**

Descent Rate 20 ft/min

Ascent Rate 3 ft/min

Ascent Rate 1 ft/min

Ascent Rate 1 ft/min

Time at Depth (minutes): 0 | 25 | 5 | 35 | 20 | 5 | 20 | 5 | 20 | 5 | 30 | 15 | 60 | 15 | 60 | 30

### Time at Depth (minutes)

**Total Elapsed Time: 350 Minutes (Not Including Descent Time)**

**Breathing Media**
= Oxygen    = Air

*Procedures In the Event of Oxygen Toxicity. At the first sign of CNS oxygen toxicity, the patient should be removed from oxygen and allowed to breathe chamber air. Oxygen breathing may be restarted 15 minutes after all symptoms have subsided. If symptoms of CNS oxygen toxicity develop again, interrupt oxygen breathing for another 15 minutes. If CNS oxygen toxicity develops a third time, contact a Diving Medical Doctor as soon as possible to modify oxygen breathing periods to meet requirements.

# Treatment Table 7

1. Table begins upon arrival at 60 feet. Arrival at 60 feet is accomplished by initial treatment on Table 6, 6A, or 4. If initial treatment has progressed to a depth shallower than 60 feet, compress to 60 feet at 20 ft/min to begin Table 7.
2. Maximum duration at 60 feet is unlimited. Remain at 60 feet a minimum of 12 hours unless overriding circumstances dictate earlier decompression.
3. Patient begins oxygen breathing periods at 60 feet. Tender should breathe only chamber atmosphere throughout. If oxygen breathing is interrupted, no lengthening of the table is required.
4. Minimum chamber $O_2$ concentration is 19%. Maximum $CO_2$ concentration is 1.5% SEV (11.4 mmHg). Maximum chamber internal temperature is 85°F.
5. Decompression starts with a 2-foot upward excursion from 60 to 58 feet. Decompress with stops every two feet for times shown in profile below. Ascent time between stops is approximately 30 seconds. Stop time begins with ascent from deeper to next shallower step. Stop at four feet for four hours and then ascend to the surface at 1 ft/min.
6. Ensure chamber life-support requirements can be met before committing to Treatment Table 7.
7. A Diving Medical Doctor shall be consulted before committing to this treatment table.

## Depth/Time Profile

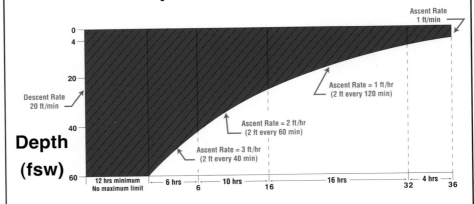

Time at Depth (hours)

# Treatment Table 8

1. Enter the table at the depth which is exactly equal to or next greater than the deepest depth attained in the recompression. The descent rate is as fast as tolerable.
2. The maximum time that can be spent at the deepest depth is shown in the second column. The maximum time for 225 fsw is 30 minutes; for 165 fsw, 3 hours. For an asymptomatic diver, the maximum time at depth is 30 minutes for depths exceeding 165 fsw and 2 hours for depths equal to or shallower than 165 fsw.
3. Decompression is begun with a 2-fsw reduction in pressure if the depth is an even number. Decompression is begun with a 3-fsw reduction in pressure if the depth is an odd number. Subsequent stops are carried out every two fsw. Stop times are given in column three. The stop time begins when leaving the previous depth. Ascend to the next stop in approximately 30 seconds.
4. Stop times apply to all stops within the band up to the next quoted depth. For example, for ascent from 165 fsw, stops for 12 minutes are made at 162 fsw, and at every two-foot interval to 140 fsw. At 140 fsw, the stop time becomes 15 minutes. When traveling from 225 fsw, the 166-foot stop is 5 minutes; the 164–foot stop is 12 minutes. Once begun, decompression is continuous. For example, when decompressing from 225 feet, ascent is not halted at 165 fsw for 3

hours. However, ascent maybe halted at 60 fsw and shallower for any desired period of time.
5. While deeper than 165 fsw, a helium-oxygen mixture with 16–21% oxygen shall be breathed by mask to reduce narcosis. At 165 fsw and shallower, a heliox mix with a $PO_2$ not to exceed 2.8 ata may be given to the diver as a treatment gas. At 60 fsw and shallower, pure oxygen may be given to the diver as a treatment gas. For all treatment gases ($HeO_2$, $N_2O_2$, and $O_2$), a schedule of 25 minutes on gas and 5 minutes on chamber air should be followed for a total of four cycles. Additional oxygen may be given at 60 fsw after a 2-hour interval of chamber air. See Treatment Table 7 for guidance.
6. A high-$O_2$ treatment mix can be used at treatment depth and during decompression. If high $O_2$ breathing is interrupted, no lengthening of the table is required.
7. To avoid loss of the chamber seal, ascent may be halted at four fsw and the total remaining stop time of 240 minutes taken at this depth. Ascend directly to the surface upon completion of the required time.
8. Total ascent time from 225 fsw is 56 hours, 29 minutes. For a 165-fsw recompression, total ascent time is 53 hours, 52 minutes, and for a 60-fsw recompression, 36 hours, 0 minutes.

| DEPTH (FSW) | MAX TIME AT INITIAL TREATMENT DEPTH (HOURS) | 2-FSW STOP TIMES (MINTES) |
|---|---|---|
| 225 | 0.5 | 5 |
| 165 | 3 | 12 |
| 140 | 5 | 15 |
| 120 | 8 | 20 |
| 100 | 11 | 25 |
| 80 | 15 | 30 |
| 60 | Unlimited | 40 |
| 40 | Unlimited | 60 |
| 20 | Unlimited | 120 |

# Treatment Table 9

1. Descent rate — 20 ft/min.
2. Ascent rate — 20 ft/min. Rate may be slowed to 1 ft/min depending upon the patient's medical condition.
3. Time at 45 feet begins on arrival at 45 feet.
4. If oxygen breathing must be interrupted because of CNS Oxygen Toxicity, oxygen breathing may be restarted 15 minutes after all symptoms have subsided. Resume schedule at point of interruption. *

5. Tender breathes 100% $O_2$ during last 15 minutes at 45 feet and during ascent to the surface regardless of ascent rate used.
6. If patient cannot tolerate oxygen at 45 feet, this table can be modified to allow a treatment depth of 30 feet. The oxygen breathing time can be extended to a maximum of three to four hours.

## Depth/Time Profile

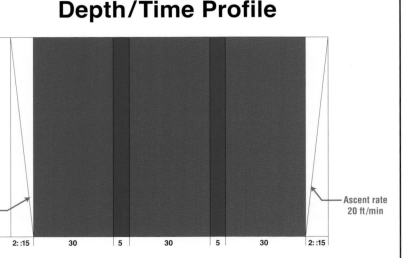

Depth (fsw)

0
15
30
45

Descent Rate 20 ft/min

Ascent rate 20 ft/min

2: :15    30    5    30    5    30    2: :15

## Time at Depth (minutes)

**Total Elapsed Time: 102 Minutes 15 Seconds (Not Including Descent Time)**

**Breathing Media**

■ = Oxygen    ■ = Air

*Procedures in the Event of Oxygen Toxicity. At the first sign of CNS oxygen toxicity, the patient should be removed from oxygen and allowed to breathe chamber air. Oxygen breathing may be restarted 15 minutes after all symptoms have subsided. If symptoms of CNS oxygen toxicity develop again, interrupt oxygen breathing for another 15 minutes. If CNS oxygen toxicity develops a third time, contact a Diving Medical Doctor as soon as possible to modify oxygen breathing periods to meet requirements.*

# REFERENCES

1. Association of Diving Contractors. "Guidelines for Treatment of Decompression Incidents." 1994, New Orleans.

2. Bennett, P. B., Dovenbarger, J. and Corson, K. "Etiology and treatment of air diving accidents." Diving Accident Management. Bennett, P. B., Moon, R. E. (Eds.) Bethesda: Undersea and Hyperbaric Medical Society. 1990;12-22.

3. Benton P. J., Woodfine J. D., Westwood P. R. "Arterial gas embolism following a 1-metre ascent during helicopter escape training: a case report." Aviat. Space Environ. Med. 1996; 67: 63-64.

4. Behnke, A. R., and Shaw, A. L. "The use of oxygen in the treatment of compressed-air illness." U.S. Naval Medical Bulletin. 36: 542-558, 1937.

5. Behnke, A. R. and T. L. Wilmon. Gaseous nitrogen and helium elimination from the body during rest and exercise. Am. J. Physiol. 131(3):369 1941.

6. Bert, P. "Barometric Pressure." Paris: Masson, 1878. [Translation by Hitchcock, M. A., Hitchcock, F. A. College Book Company, Columbus, Ohio, 1975; republished by Undersea Medical Society, Inc., Bethesda, Maryland, 1978.]

7. Catron, P. W., Thomas, L. B., Flynn, E. T., et al. "Effects of $HeO_2$ breathing during experimental decompression sickness following air dives." Undersea Biomedical Research. 14: 101-111, 1987.

8. Cockett, A.T.K., Pauley, S.M. and Roberts, A.P. Advances in the treatment of decompression treatment: An evaluation of heparin. Proc. 3rd Int. Conf. on Hyperbaric and Underwater Physiol. X. DOIN Editeurs, (Fructus Ed.) 1972.

9. Defence and Civil Institute of Environmental Medicine (now DRDC). "DCIEM Diving Manual" 1992 and 2nd edition update 1993. Universal Dive Techtronics: Richmond BC, Canada.

10. Drewry, A., and Gorman, D. F. "A progress report on the prospective randomized double-blind controlled study of oxygen and oxygen-helium in the treatment of air-diving decompression illness (DCI)." Undersea and Hyperbaric Medicine (Suppl.) 21:98, 1994. [Abstract only.]

11. Dutka, A.J., Mink, R.B., Pearson, R.R., et al. "Effects of treatment with dexamethasone on recovery from experimental cerebral arterial gas embolism" Undersea Biomedical Research. 19:131-141 1992.

12. Edmonds C., Lowry C., Pennefather J. and Walker R. "Diving and subaquatic medicine." 4th Edition. Hodder Arnold: London. 2002.

13. Francis, T. J. R. and Mitchell, S. J. "Manifestations of decompression disorders." p.585 in Bennett and Elliott's Physiology and Medicine of Diving. 5th Edition. Brubakk, A. O. and Neuman, T. S. (Eds.) Saunders: Edinburgh. 2003.

14. Francis, T. J. R., Pearson, R. R. P., Robertson, A. G., Hodgson, M., Dutka, A. J., Flynn, E. T. "Central Nervous System Decompression Sickness: Latency of 1070 Human Cases." Undersea Biomedical Research. 1988;15;403-418.

15. Francis, T. J. R. and Mitchell, D. F. "Pathophysiology of the decompression sickness." Pp.530-556 in Bennett and Elliott's Physiology and Medicine of Diving. 5th Edition. Brubakk, A. O. and Neuman, T. S. (Eds.) Saunders: Edinburgh. 2003.

16. Goodman, M. W. and Workman, R. D. "Minimal recompression, oxygen-breathing approach of treatment of decompression sickness in divers and aviators." BU-SHIPS Project SF0110605, Task 11513-2, Research Report 5-65, Washington, DC, Bureau of Medicine and Surgery, November, 1965.

17. Golding, F. C., Griffiths, P. D., Paton, W. D. M., Walder, D. N., Hempleman, H. V. "Decompression sickness during construction of the Dartford tunnel." Br. J. Ind. Med. 1960; 17: 167-180.

18. Gorman, D. F., Edmonds, C. W., Parsons, D. W., Beran, R. G., Anderson, T. A., Green, R. D., Coxton, M. J., Dillon, T. A. "Neurologic sequelae of decompression sickness: A clinical report." Underwater and Hyperbaric Physiology IX. Bove, A. A., Bachrach, A. J., and Greenbaum L. J, (Eds.) Bethesda, MD: Undersea and Hyperbaric Medical Society, 1987.

19. Groupes d'Études et Recherches Sousmarines. "Guide for diving with air: Part II. Genesis, signs and treatment for the accidents of diving." Toulon: GERS. 1968. U.S.NAVSHIPS translation No.1113.

20. Hallenbeck, J. M. and Anderson, J. C. "Pathogenesis of the decompression disorders." The Physiology and Medicine of Diving, 3rd Edition., Bennett, P. B. and Elliott, D. H., (Eds.) London: Bailliere Tindall. 1983;435-460.

21. James, P. B. "The use of heliox treatment tables." In: Proceedings of the First European Consensus Conference on Hyperbaric Medicine, Lille, France, September 19-21, 1994.

22. Jaminet A. "Physical effects of compressed air and of the causes of pathological symptoms produced on man, by increased atmospheric pressure employed for the sinking of piers in the construction of the Illinois and St. Louis bridge over the Mississippi River at St. Louis, Missouri." 1871 Quoted by Fryer, D. I., Subatmospheric Decompression Sickness in Man. Agardograph 125. Slough: Technivision, 1969.

23. Kidd, D. J. and Elliott, D. H. p.488 in "Decompression disorders in divers" The Physiology and Medicine of Diving", 2nd Edition., Bennett, P. B. and Elliott D. H. (Eds.) London: Bailliere Tindall, 1975; 471-495.

24. Kindwall, E. P. "Compressed air tunnelling and caisson work: Decompression procedures, development, problems and solutions". Undersea and Hyperbaric Med. 1997, 24(7):337-345.

25. Kindwall, E.P., A. Baz, E. Lanphier, E. Lightfoot, and A. Seireg. "Nitrogen Elimination in Man During Decompression" Undersea Biomedical Research. 2(4):285-297 1975.

26. Kol, S., Adir, Y., Gordon, C. I. and Melamed, Y. "Oxy-helium treatment of severe spinal decompression sickness after air diving." Undersea and Hyperbaric Medicine. 20: 147-154, 1993.

27. Lambertsen, C. J. and Idicula, J. "A new gas lesion syndrome in man, induced by isobaric gas counterdiffusion." Journal of Applied Physiology. 39:434-443, 1975.

28. Lee, H. C., Niu, K.C., Chen, S. H., et al. "Therapeutic effects of different tables on Type II decompression sickness." Journal of Hyperbaric Medicine. 6(1): 11-17, 1991.

29. Leitch, D. R., Greenbaum, L. J., and Hallenbeck, J. M. "Cerebral arterial air embolism I, II, III, IV." Undersea Biomedical Research. 11(3): 221-274, 1984.

30. McCullough, D. The Great Bridge, Simon & Schuster, Touchstone Edition, pages 309-312, 1982.

31. Melamed Y. Personal communication, 1990.

32. Miller, J. N., Fagreaus, L., Bennett P. B., Elliott, D. H., Shields, T. G. and Grimstad, J. "Nitrogen-oxygen saturation therapy in serious cases of compressed-air decompression sickness." Lancet. 1978; ii: 169-171.

33. Moir, E. W. "Tunnelling by compressed air." Journal of the Society of Arts, Vol. XLIV: 567-583, May 15, 1896.

34. Moon, R. E. (Editor). "Adjunctive Therapy for Decompression Illness." Report of the UHMS Adjunctive Therapy Committee. Bethesda, Maryland: UHMS. 2002.

35. Moon, R. E. and Sheffield, P. J. (Editors). "Workshop on Treatment of Decompression Illness." 45th Workshop of the Undersea and Hyperbaric Medical Society, June 1995 Publish 1996 pp122-126.

36. Moon, R.E. and Gorman, D. F. "Treatment of the decompression disorders." The Physiology and Medicine of Diving (4th Edition). Bennett, P. B. and Elliott, D. H., (Eds.) London: Saunders, 1993;506-541.

37. Overlock, R. K. and Arnold, A. A. "Dysbaric disease: A Hawaiian experience." Diving Accident Management. Bennett, P. B. and Moon, R. E. (Eds.) Bethesda, MD: Undersea and Hyperbaric Medical Society. 1990; 266-274.

38. Philp, R.B. "The ameliorated effects of heparin and depolymerized hyaluronate on decompression sickness in rats" Canad. J. Physiol. and Pharmacol.42:818-829 1964.

39. Pimlott, J., Ormsby, P. L. and Cross, M. R. "The effects of white cells on blood filterability at pressure." Proceedings of the Annual Meeting of the European Undersea Biomedical Society (Palermo), 1987.

40. Pol, M. and Wattelle, M. "Memoire sur des èffets de la compression de l'air appliqué au creusement des puits houille."  Annales Hygiéne Publique et de Medicine Légale. Second Series 1:241-249, 1854.

41. Reeves, E. and Workman, R.D. "Use of heparin for therapeutic/prophylactic treatment of decompression sickness." Aerospace Medicine. 42:20-23.

42. Rivera, J. C. "Decompression sickness among divers: An analysis of 935 cases." Milit. Med. 1964;129:314-334.

43. Ross J. A. "Clinical audit and outcome measures in the treatment of decompression illness in Scotland." Report to the National Health Services in Scotland. Department of Environmental and Occupational Medicine: University of Aberdeen. 2000.

44. Saper J.R. and Yosselson, S., "Raised intracranial pressure diagnosis and management." Postgraduate Medical J. 57:89-94 1975.

45. Smith, AH, The effects of high atmospheric pressure, including the caisson disease. Brooklyn , N.Y. The Eagle Press, 1873.

46. Strauss, R. H. "Bubble formation in gelatin: Implications for the prevention of decompression sickness." Undersea Biomedical Research. 1:169-174, June, 1974.

47. Swindle, P. F. "Occlusion of blood vessels by agglutinated red cells, mainly as seen in tadpoles and very young kangaroos." American Journal of Physiology. 120: 59-74, 1937.

48. Thom, S. R. "Hyperbaric oxygen inhibits neutrophil adherence to brain microvessels after carbon monoxide poisoning." Undersea and Hyperbaric Medicine 20. (Suppl): 16, 1993.

49. Triger M. "Letter to Monsieur Arago," Compte Rendus de l'Académie des Sciences. Paris. 1845;20:445-449.

50. U.S. Navy Diving Manual, Revision 3. Volume 1, Air Diving. US Naval Sea Systems Command. 2003.

51. U.S. Navy Diving Manual, Revision 5. Volume 5, Diving Medicine and Recompression Chamber Operations. US Naval Sea Systems Command. 2005.

52. Waite, C.L and W.F Mazone, et al. « Cerebral Air Embolism, I Basic studies. U.S. Naval Submarine Medical Center, Research Report 439. April 1967.

53. Waite, C.L Personal communication, 1972.

54. Workman, R. D. "Treatment of bends with oxygen at high pressure: Modern aspects of treatment of decompression sickness." Aerospace Medicine 39: 1076-1083, 1968.

CHAPTER 19

# GAS EMBOLISM

## CHAPTER NINETEEN OVERVIEW

# GAS EMBOLISM

*Eric P. Kindwall*

## INTRODUCTION

Gas embolism, or the presence of intravascular gas, varies widely; its consequences range from being undetectable to producing immediate and rapid death. Typically, gas on the arterial side is of much greater import than gas on the venous side. However, gas originating on the venous side may move by one of two mechanisms to the arterial side producing a so-called paradoxical embolism. Air entering the venous side is usually removed by the pulmonary filter without producing symptoms. Ilyin, quoted by Van Allen, Hrdina, and Clark, reported being able to give up to two liters of air intravenously to dogs at the rate of 30 cc a minute without producing symptoms (27). If, however, the amount of gas delivered in a bolus to the lung is extremely large, e.g., of the order of a liter or more, some gas may be forced through intrapulmonary shunts. With the rise in pulmonary artery pressure, the pressure in the right atrium may temporarily exceed that in the left atrium; this can cause the opening of a normally closed, probe-patent, intra-atrial septal defect.

Approximately 30% of the adult population of the United States carries a probe-patient septal opening between the right and left atria of the heart, which is normally closed. Under circumstances of raised, right-sided pressure, any gas bubbles present in the right atrium may be driven into the left side of the heart; from there they may be distributed intra-arterially (11). If death does not ensue immediately, arterial gas embolism typically targets the brain, producing a stroke-like syndrome. Immediate death may be the result of coronary artery embolization.

## CAUSES OF GAS EMBOLISM

### Commercial and Sport Diving

A diver working under water is typically supplied with compressed air as a breathing medium, although, for very deep work, exotic mixtures with other inert gases, such as helium, may be used. In any case, the mechanisms for gas embolism in diving are the same, regardless of the breathing gas used. In order for the diver to expand his lungs normally, the breathing medium must be supplied at a pressure equal to the water pressure at which the diver is working. If the diver holds his breath while ascending, the gas within his lungs expands, and the intrapulmonary pressure becomes greater than the surrounding water pressure. When this occurs, the alveolae dilate and rupture at a transpulmonic pressure of approximately 80 mmHg (22). This pressure change corresponds to a change in sea water depth of 3.47 feet (106 cm). This is often referred to as burst lung syndrome.

Following lung rupture, the gas may proceed centrally beneath the fascial coverings of the tracheobronchial tree to cause mediastinal emphysema, or it may rupture through the pleural lining to cause pneumothorax. The most serious consequence of burst lung is entrance of gas into the pulmonary venous system, resulting in subsequent arterial gas embolism.

Mediastinal emphysema, in the absence of neurologic signs, is usually benign. Air dissecting centrally along the perivascular sheath may cause pneumopericardium, but it is never responsible for tamponade. Air tends to migrate cephalad in the mediastinum; it may become palpable in the neck as subcutaneous emphysema above the clavicles and below the angle of the jaw. Occasionally, gas may impinge on the nerves which supply the larynx; this action causes a change in the tonal quality of the voice. In about one-third of the cases, mediastinal emphysema is noted in arterial gas embolism among sport divers, probably because there is delay in their presenting at a chamber. In gas embolism associated with submarine escape training, it is not seen, because treatment is immediate.

In examining any patient following a diving accident, it is important to first palpate the neck for the presence of subcutaneous emphysema to determine if lung rupture has occurred. The presence of subcutaneous crepitus is pathognomonic for ruptured lung, although its absence does not rule it out. In the absence of cerebral or other neurologic signs, treatment is simply bed rest, with or without the intermittent inhalation of 100% oxygen. The mediastinal gas usually resolves within three or four days.

## Case Report

*The patient was a 25-year-old male, diving to a depth of 120 feet to remove artifacts from a wreck. The patient had a bottom time of approximately 15 minutes. He surfaced without using the ascending line, while cradling a heavy wooden sheave from the wreck against his chest, using his left arm.*

*Approximately one-half hour after leaving the water, the patient noted the onset of chest pain, worsened by taking a deep breath. He also developed nausea and vomiting. The pain spread from the central part of his chest into his neck; the following morning, he noticed a change in the quality of his voice.*

*Because the pain in the neck and chest persisted, he consulted a local physician who diagnosed the problem as some sort of lung congestion and prescribed an antibiotic. Later in the day the patient consulted a fellow diver who suggested he contact a hyperbaric facility. The patient was flown at low altitude to the chamber.*

*On arrival at the chamber the patient was in no acute distress, but complained of chest pain on deep inspiration, pain bilaterally in his anterior neck, and a subjective voice change. A chest film showed normal-appearing lungs and no gross air visible in the mediastinum. Soft-tissue air was noted in the neck structures, however. Crepitus was palpable in the neck above the clavicles. Neurologic examination was completely negative, and the patient had no symptoms of decompression sickness. It was therefore elected not to treat the patient in the chamber, but to admit him to the hospital for observation.*

*By the following morning the patient's voice had improved markedly and the neck pain had eased, but he still complained of chest pain. By the third hospital day, the pain in the chest had completely disappeared, as well as all symptoms relating to voice timbre. On x-ray air was no longer demonstrable in the soft-tissues of his neck. Subcutaneous crepitus had disappeared. The patient was discharged on the third hospital day with instructions not to dive for at least one month, and to have a pressure test in another chamber before resuming diving.*

A factor which may have been crucial in this accident was that the patient ascended without the use of an ascending line, and carried a heavy weight. Because of the straining necessary to maintain a hold on the weight, he may have closed his glottis occasionally during ascent. This would be the most likely cause for his lung rupture. The final diagnosis was a lung over-pressure accident with mediastinal emphysema, subcutaneous emphysema, and impingement of air on the recurrent laryngeal nerves.

Fortunately, pneumothorax is rare, and typically occurs only when the pleural wall has a congenital or acquired weakness such as a pleural bleb. Air may then migrate laterally through the ruptured bleb, causing a pneumothorax. If pneumothorax is the only consequence, simple insertion of a thoracostomy tube and standard management will usually suffice. If the patient is simultaneously suffering from arterial gas embolism, insertion of the tube should be done before the patient is recompressed in the chamber. Patients suffering from pneumothorax, when recompressed, will have the pneumothorax diminish in size in accordance with Boyle's law. While at depth, if the patient breathes oxygen, the pneumothorax should decrease further in volume. During subsequent decompression, the pneumothorax will re-expand, but if nitrogen or other inert gas has diffused out of the pneumothorax while at depth, the pneumothorax will be smaller than it was on the surface. The danger, however, is that a tension pneumothorax may develop which will increase its volume at depth. It may then become impossible to decompress the patient without life-threatening pulmonary and cardiac distress. Also; blood return to the heart may be severely curtailed due to the dramatically increased intra-thoracic pressure, unless a thoracostomy tube is in place. For this reason, untreated pneumothorax is considered an absolute contraindication to recompression. This is particularly true in the monoplace chamber, where it is impossible to insert a tube prior to decompression.

As noted above, gas may leak out of the distended alveolae and invade the peri-alveolar capillaries; from there, it is carried to the pulmonary veins and the left heart. Leaving the left heart, it is usually pumped directly into the brain. As little as 0.5 milliliters of blood-air foam delivered to the medulla can be fatal. If the patient does not die, he/she will present a stroke-like picture, usually with symptoms of hemiparesis extending from the face to the toes. Symptoms may be bilateral. There is typically a loss or severe disturbance of consciousness.

Nitrogen bubbles form on the venous side during decompression from nearly every normal dive, but these bubbles are efficiently caught in the pulmonary filter and do not cause symptoms. Should a venous nitrogen bubble escape to the arterial circulation through a patent atrial septal defect or pulmonary shunt, it potentially becomes quite dangerous. Fortunately, these occurrences are relatively rare.

In any case, the definitive treatment is recompression in a hyperbaric chamber to reduce bubble size and restore circulation. If the patient survives to reach a chamber, the prognosis is usually excellent. Patients have made successful recoveries with no detectable residua, even when treated many hours after the embolism.

## Escape From a Submerged Vehicle

When a car falls into a river or lake and the victim continues to breathe, the air he breathes within the vehicle as it gradually floods is compressed as the water approaches the roof level. If the individual then takes a deep breath and exits by a window or door, he usually will reflexively hold his breath until he reaches the surface. This produces the same result as it would in a diver ascending with a closed glottis. The patient may subsequently be found unconscious in the water or on the river bank. The diagnosis of near drowning is usually entertained if the patient is found alive, and gas embolism may be easily overlooked. Localizing cerebral signs, such as unequal pupils, may be the key to diagnosis.

## Insufflation of Air into the Vagina During Pregnancy and Other Gynecologic Manipulation

During pregnancy, the vagina becomes quite distensible. On about a dozen occasions, the blowing of air into the vagina during sex play has been reported to produce cerebral gas embolism (9). Up to 1,000 or 1,500 milliliters of air may be blown into the vagina, whence it passes through the patent cervical os to dissect between the placental membranes and the uterine lining. Entering the uterine sinusoids, it is carried by the vena cava to the right heart and the lungs. A large bolus of greater than a liter of gas arriving at the lungs may overwhelm the pulmonary filter and cause leakage of some gas through the intrapulmonary shunts. Alternatively, the rise in pulmonary artery pressure may cause a back-up of pressure in the right heart forcing any gas bubbles in the right atrium through a probe-patent septal defect. The result is the same, causing cerebral gas embolism. When a previously healthy pregnant woman arrives in the emergency room after an apparent sudden intra-cerebral catastrophe, a high index of suspicion is necessary to make this diagnosis. It is often difficult to get an accurate history from the patient's partner. Historically, all such patients not treated in hyperbaric chambers have died. Two patients treated with recompression have survived (2, 3). Other causes of gas embolism include attempts to induce abortion, usually with a catheter. This also results in paradoxical embolism.

## Iatrogenic Gas Embolism

This is the most common cause of cerebral gas embolism seen in the hospital. Typically it results from air bubbles introduced into the arterial side from heart-lung machines, open central lines, percutaneous lung biopsy, (25) cardiac catheterization and renal dialysis. Head and neck surgery, with injection of air into the neck veins, may also produce symptoms. When the gas is first introduced on the venous side, but later becomes arterial, it is a case of paradoxical embolism. Definitive treatment is recompression in a hyperbaric chamber. Stoney has estimated that approximately 400 gas embolisms occur each year in the United States, an incidence of about one in 1,000 (23). There is a 33% fatality rate in those so afflicted. Unfortunately, the embolism is often unrecognized, left untreated or referred late, which often results in severe permanent deficits in the survivors.

## MECHANISM OF EMBOLISM INJURY

Classically, it was felt that all symptoms of cerebral gas embolism could be attributed to mechanical blockage of the arterial vessels with gas. If blockage due to the presence of gas bubbles could be ameliorated with simple recompression, this would be the end of the problem.

However, more recent work suggests that factors other than simple mechanical blockage of the vessels by bubbles may be at work. Air bubbles cause trauma and subtle damage to the endothelial lining of the vessels, as well as activation of platelets and alteration of white cells. Sludging of the formed elements plays a major role in the vessel occlusion. This all may contribute to the no-reflow phenomenon. Helps and Gorman have shown that the anticipated decline in cerebral blood flow caused by infusion of air into the internal carotid could not be reproduced in leucocytopenic rabbits (12). It is also probable that activated platelets cause sludging of formed elements of the blood.

It is clear that the mechanical effect of increased pressure reduces bubble size and helps to reestablish blood flow. The maximum effect is seen within the first few pounds of pressure. Leitch et al. have demonstrated in dogs that the maximal mechanical effect appears to be achieved within 2.8 atmospheres, or pressurization to 18 meters (60 FSW). The optimum mechanical effect is seen to take place within about eight minutes (18). However, hyperbaric oxygen also appears to play a prominent role. Swindle (24) and End (7) showed that raising the oxygen tension in blood decreased sludging of the formed elements following decompression sickness. Zamboni et al. have shown that HBO produces a sharp reduction in adherence of leukocytes in the venules in post-ischemic muscle (29). They believe that leukocytes play a major role in the ultimate production of the no-reflow phenomenon and that HBO may be beneficial in blocking leukocyte action.

## DIAGNOSIS

When a diver surfaces unconscious, it will not be immediately clear what is wrong with him, but gas embolism must be kept high on the list of possibilities. Immediate and sudden incapacitation within seconds of surfacing are usually hallmarks of gas embolism, and are rarely seen in decompression sickness, except following explosive decompression from extreme depth. In gas embolism, the sensorium is usually disturbed, or the patient is unconscious, which is uncommon in decompression sickness. Immediate brain symptomatology is much rarer in the diver with decompression sickness, where the spinal cord is typically the target. In gas embolism, the paralysis seen is usually on one side of the body, as opposed to the paraplegia typical of decompression sickness. Cranial nerve signs, such as unequal pupils and hemianopsia, may very well be present. If the patient has true vertigo, it may be difficult to distinguish inner-ear pathology secondary to barotrauma from true arterial embolism. Careful questioning of the patient (assuming he is conscious) may enable you to determine if he had problems with ear clearing during descent or ascent. Vestibular decompression sickness will be in the differential diagnosis, but this typically comes on later, not immediately. If the dive has been to a depth less than 10 meters, decompression sickness can be ruled out. It would be a rarity, but gas embolism may be delayed for 20 minutes to half an hour before its onset. This is very atypical, and in such cases, embolization is probably secondary to bubbles being dislodged after entrapment in the heart.

In post-surgical patients, the initial signs and symptoms of gas embolism are often masked by the after-effects of anesthesia. Simple thrombotic stroke must be ruled out, as well as the possibility of solid emboli, as seen in atrial fibrillation and after endarterectomy. Whether or not such patients are referred for hyperbaric treatment becomes a judgment call. If there is a suspicion or possibility of gas embolism, a trial of pressure is probably warranted. Being able to see "boxcars" caused by gas bubbles in the retinal vasculature is rare, but might be considered. In the diver, immediately palpate the neck for crepitus. Following any catheter procedures, particularly on the arterial side, any sudden alteration of consciousness with lateralizing signs should heighten one's suspicions. Occasionally, the only thing manifest following apparent "recovery" from gas embolism may be a subtle personality change. If this is present, and is confirmed by the victim's companions or family, it may be an indication for recompression, particularly in a diver who was previously well. When gas embolism is suspected, a complete mental status exam should be carried out which includes: fluency of spontaneous speech, comprehension, repetition, naming, reading, writing, immediate, recent, and remote memory, constructional ability, calculation and tests for apraxia, and right-left disorientation (20). Mottling of the tongue (Liebermeister's sign) is rare, but pathognomonic. This is caused by gas trapped within the highly vascular capillary bed of the tongue.

## TREATMENT

### Immediate Management of Embolism

I feel it is probably advisable to put the patient in an immediate steep Trendelenburg position following diagnosis of gas embolism. In primary venous embolism, the patient is positioned on the left side, but in arterial embolism this is not indicated. In 1963, Kruse observed that a scuba diver who was tilted head-down, momentarily, seemed to recover, and after being repeatedly rocked back and forth into the head down position became asymptomatic. Within a couple of hours recovery was complete (17). This observation prompted an experimental study by Atkinson with embolized cats. Atkinson produced a large cranial window in which he could observe the surface of the brain. He then created an overpressure in the lungs precipitating intra-arterial gas emboli. When the cerebral circulation had been blocked by bubbles, he tilted the animals steeply head-down between 30 and 60 degrees. He noted that within five minutes, blood flow was seen to be restored and the air had moved out of the arteries in the direction of arterial flow. Observation of one of these cats in a cage for an additional 14 hours showed no further deleterious change in the appearance of the brain (1).

Dutka, meanwhile, has done studies to show that when animals are continuously held head-down for an hour or more following embolization, their condition worsens, as compared to controls who have been held supine (6). This worsening is due to an increase in cerebral edema. For this reason, it is important never to hold a victim in the head-down position for more than a maximum of 10 minutes. Obviously, if the patient is pulseless or apneic, cardiopulmonary resuscitation takes precedence over positioning. The use of the head-down position is controversial; skeptics pointing out that spontaneous recovery often occurs, and that the head-down position may not be causal when the victim recovers.

However, I have seen quick recovery following head-down placement in at least three well-documented cases in the field. Critics say Trendelenburg placement may be applied inadvertently to bends victims, as many divers (as well as physicians) are unable to make a definitive diagnosis or distinguish between the two. Even if that were the case, a brief period of head-down positioning would not harm a bent diver, if other emergent care needs are being met. If the Trendelenburg position is not used, the victim should be kept supine. Under no circumstances should he/she be allowed to sit up before chamber treatment, even if an apparent complete recovery is seen.

## Case Report

*A 26-year-old sport diver descended to the wreck of a sunken freighter in 80 feet of water. On arrival at the bottom, the patient became entangled in some cables lying next to the wreck, and inadvertently triggered the $CO_2$ cartridge, inflating his buoyancy compensator vest. The patient started an uncontrollable ascent to the surface which became faster as he rose through the water. Undoubtedly, he struggled to stay down, or slow his ascent. On arrival at the surface, the patient cried out, and then became unresponsive. Two members of the support crew immediately dived into the water to retrieve him. He was unconscious and incapable of helping himself as he was removed from the water, but was placed in immediate steep head-down position. Within a few minutes, while the police boat was being summoned by radio, the patient gradually returned to normal. After being carried ashore by the police boat to a waiting ambulance, the patient was seen at the hyperbaric facility within an hour of having embolized. At that time, he appeared to be completely normal, and a meticulous neurologic exam failed to reveal any deficits. Because he had been unconscious, it was elected to treat him on Table 6 to remove any residual, silent air bubbles which might remain in his vasculature. The patient completed Table 6 uneventfully and was discharged home. However, within four hours, the patient returned to the hospital complaining of severe bilateral flank pain. Urinalysis revealed a 4+ proteinuria. The patient was admitted for diagnosis, but a thorough work-up failed to reveal any renal pathology. The flank pain and proteinuria cleared within three days and the patient was discharged with no further sequelae. In retrospect, it was felt that the extreme head-down position had helped to clear bubbles in the patient's brain, but that bubbles rising toward the kidneys, which were held superior to the heart, caused embolization and ischemia of the renal cortex.*

## Development of Recompression Treatment for Gas Embolism

Gas embolism in divers was first discovered to be a distinct disorder, different from decompression sickness, in the early 1930s, when submarine escape training was instituted at the Submarine Escape Training Tower at New London, Connecticut. Gas embolism was treated with recompression, as was decompression sickness. After 1945, with the promulgation of U.S. Navy Treatment Tables 1-4, gas embolism was always treated on Table 3 or Table 4, taking between 22 and 38 hours. This was because Tables 3 and 4 were designed for serious decompression sickness where the patient carries a heavy tissue-nitrogen load. These tables were for serious symptom cases. As gas embolism was always considered serious, it was automatically treated on Tables 3 and 4, with little regard for whether the patient was carrying excess tissue nitrogen from his dive. In 1966, Waite, Mazzone, and co-workers at the U.S. Navy Submarine Base, New London, Connecticut, investigated more rational treatment for gas embolism as it occurred in submarine escape training (28). They embolized dogs by injecting 5 ml of air into the carotid artery and then, through a cranial window, observed the spread of bubbles across the brain. Those dogs which were not immediately recompressed all died or were left with severe residual neurologic defects. Half of the animals were immediately recompressed to 6 ATA (50 meters) and then decompressed on the standard U.S. Navy table for 10 minutes exposure at that depth. They all made a complete recovery, except for one dog that developed a cerebral hemorrhage. This demonstrated that the long decompressions then used for treatment were unnecessary.

Waite also observed that the bubbles disappeared from the cerebral circulation, as seen through the calvarial window, by the time the dogs had reached 80 feet (3.42 ATA). However, he specified six ATA (50 meters), as the maximum treatment depth because of the known prejudices of the U.S. Navy Bureau of Medicine and Surgery, which held that a six ATA was a requirement (Waite CL. Personal Communication, 1972). It should be noted that there was no apparent physiologic basis for going to this pressure. In 1967, Waite proposed tables which embodied going to six ATA initially, followed by low pressure oxygen treatment from 2.8 atmospheres of pressure to the surface. He produced two tables, one for cases which were observed to clear within 15 minutes, and the other for those cases which took longer to resolve. These new tables were labeled 5A and 6A and promulgated on August 22, 1967 (26). Subsequently, Table 5A which mandated only a 15-minute stay, at six ATA followed by two hours of oxygen, was felt to be too short, as it produced inferior results. For this reason, it was dropped from the Navy's treatment schedules. In Waite's original dog studies, the animals were all recompressed within a couple of minutes of being embolized, so that brief recompression was adequate. In the clinical situation, the patient is usually referred after some delay, and seems to benefit more from the longer exposure to oxygen provided by Table 6A. Table 6A requires a 30-minute stay at 50 meters, followed by four hours of hyperbaric oxygen. Unfortunately, the U,S, Navy Diving Manual still states that if the patient is not symptom-free or rapidly improving after 30 minutes at 6 ATA (165 feet) the patient should be committed to the 38-hour Table 4. This makes no physiologic sense as Table 4 was designed to treat decompression sickness and is now an anachronism.

Meanwhile, Hart in 1974, reported on 30 patients treated for gas embolism, 18 from diving accidents, 11 from iatrogenic sources, and 1 from criminal means. One death occurred in the iatrogenic group and one in the criminal group. Four patients had permanent neurologic deficit. All patients were treated at a maximum depth of three ATA (20 meters) with 100% oxygen. The maximum time spent at 20 meters was 30 minutes and the maximum time for each treatment was 90 minutes (12). Kindwall, in 1990, reported on 32 cases of gas embolism treated at a maximum pressure of six atmospheres and had results in mortality which were not statistically different from the results Hart achieved at three atmospheres (16). However, careful comparison of neurologic function post treatment was not done.

Leitch et al. showed that treatment depths greater than 18 meters showed no advantage in dogs embolized with 0.4 milliliters of air injected into the right internal carotid artery. Measurements included somatosensory cortical evoked potentials, cerebral spinal fluid pressure, EEG, EKG, and blood pressure recordings. Cortical-evoked potentials recovered to 63% of base line in those animals treated at 18 meters, whereas those initially treated at 50 meters with compressed air showed a final value of 51% of base line. Their data also suggested that the clearance of gas is probably independent of pressure once past the threshold of 2.8 atmospheres, and that it is certainly hastened by oxygen. A time of about eight minutes is probably required to clear the embolism. All dogs exposed to air pressure and then surfaced, regardless of whether or not they were embolized, had an elevated cerebral spinal fluid (CSF) pressure. Because of this pressure rise there appeared to be a decreased cerebral blood flow. Only in the oxygen-treated dogs, where CSF pressure had returned to normal, was cerebral blood flow also returned to normal. Very deep, short exposures to eight atmospheres and deeper were found to cause a flow deficit in the lumbo-sacral spinal cord. There was also a tendency for this to occur in a less severe form after air treatment at six atmospheres for 10 minutes or longer (18). These findings raise the possibility of secondary cord-decompression sickness and offer a possible explanation for secondary deterioration. If one can extrapolate from this model to the clinical arena, it could be said that the majority of patients with severe arterial gas embolism will achieve maximum benefit from compression to 2.8 atmospheres while breathing oxygen. Leitch et al. could not demonstrate superiority of Table 6A (breathing air) over Table 6, using a dog model.

I feel, however, that treatment at 2.6 ATA (60 feet) is not optimal, but that the patient should be taken to at least four or preferably 6 ATA. This is because Waite did not see bubbles disappear until *80 feet* was reached. Leitch et al. used cortical evoked potentials to measure and compare neurologic function in the dogs treated on Table 6 at 60 feet and Table 6A at 165 feet. However, Gorman et al in treating pain-only bends in divers using Table 6 found that cortical evoked potentials and clinical neurologic exams were normal following successful treatment. However, 60% of the patients had abnormal psychological testing and 40% had abnormal EEGs. Ten percent had abnormal CAT scans. When examined again one month later, all the psychological exams were normal, 20% had abnormal EEGs and 20% had abnormal CAT scans, one showing brain atrophy (10). Cortical evoked potentials are not indicative of normal cortical function. If helium/oxygen is breathed at 6 ATA, nitrogen embolization of the spinal cord can be obviated.

## Current Recompression Treatment

Once the diagnosis of gas embolism has been definitely established or cannot be ruled out, recompression therapy is the only definitive treatment. Classically, if a multiplace chamber with a six atmosphere capability is available, its use is preferred. However, the use of 6 atmospheres pressure is no longer mandated by the U.S. Navy. Treatment at 2.8 ATA is acceptable. Six atmospheres can be used if prescribed by a medical officer.

If the patient is treated on Table 6A, it is recommended that the patient not breathe air at maximum depth, but breathe mixed gas. Acceptable mixtures include 40% oxygen-60% helium, 50%/50% helium/oxygen (heliox) or 50%/50% nitrogen/oxygen (nitrox). The advantage of using mixed gas is that it lowers or eliminates the amount of iatrogenic nitrogen that will be added to the patient's tissues during treatment and simultaneously supplies a high partial pressure of oxygen. Since approximately 79% of the intracranial bubbles consist of nitrogen, it is advisable to add as little additional nitrogen to the tissues as possible. Mixed gas provides a lesser gradient for the nitrogen in the intravascular bubbles to work against, and speeds nitrogen elimination, as well as providing 2.4 to 3 ATA of oxygen to counteract cerebral edema and oxygenate ischemic tissue. We have used both 80%/20% and 50%/50% helium oxygen with excellent clinical success on the physiological grounds that it provided a resistance-free gradient for nitrogen in the patient's intravascular bubbles to work against. This is despite the fact that there was a considerable controversy for some years as to the advisability of using helium, as it had been shown to diffuse into existing bubbles faster than nitrogen diffuses out (*in vitro* experiments). However, when using helium/oxygen immediately following recompression, bubble growth is so much reduced by a mechanical compression that counter-diffusion plays no clinical role. Helium/oxygen treatment has been used very successfully at pressures of 165 feet (50 m).

In the commercial diving arena, there have been no bad experiences reported using helium treatment following an air dive, but using air treatment following a helium dive can be dangerous. If the patient is taken to 165 feet (50 m) depth, the stay at that depth should be limited to no more than about 10 minutes; by that time, the maximal mechanical effects of recompression will have been realized. Decompression is begun after 10 minutes, even if there has been no apparent clinical improvement. This is particularly true in the post-surgical patient who may still be under the influence of anesthesia. The patient is decompressed over a 4- to 40-minute period, (depending on the gas load, if the patient is a diver) to 18 meters equivalent pressure (2.8 ATA) and oxygen is then given in accordance with U.S. Navy Table 6. If the patient has not completely responded within three oxygen periods at 18 meters, a fourth or even a fifth oxygen period may be added. An additional one-hour oxygen breathing extension may be made at 1.9 ATA (9 meters). If these tables are prolonged, however, it is important to keep track of the inside attendant's bottom time so that he or she can be given supplemental oxygen to avoid decompression sickness when subsequently decompressed to the surface. Although rare, cases of decompression sickness in the inside attendant have been reported on standard U.S. Navy Table 6 treatment schedules, even when they have not been prolonged. For this reason, it is a good idea to routinely offer oxygen breathing to the inside attendant for the last 30 minutes, or for a longer time, if the dive has been extended.

## Case Report

*The patient was a 32-year-old white male school custodian who was being operated on for a vein bypass graft to the left anterior descending artery, and closure of an atrial septal defect, five months after a myocardial infarction. After the patient was on bypass and the heart fibrillated, the right atrium was opened. Three minutes after the patient went on bypass, the sump of the heart-lung machine overflowed onto the floor and a large amount of air appeared in the arterial line. The EEG trace became flat, and the patient's pupils dilated and became fixed. The aorta was clamped and the right atriotomy was closed with a running suture. The aorta was opened for approximately 2 centimeters, and the heart was massaged in an attempt to remove air. Air issued from the open aorta and a second arterial line was placed in the right femoral artery. Air issued from the femoral arteriotomy.*

*Twenty-two minutes after embolization, cardiopulmonary bypass was re-established. Cold blood was infused, as the patient had been partially exsanguinated, and he was placed on a hypothermia blanket. On full bypass, the patient's pupils slowly constricted and began to react to light. Activity reappeared on the EEG monitor. After the septal defect was repaired and the coronary artery was opened to permit an anastomosis with a vein graft, air bubbles issued from the coronary arteriotomy. The patient came off the pump with a single defibrillation and was referred to the HBO chamber 3 hours and 17 minutes after the event.*

*While the patient was recompressed to 165 ft. (50 m), 80%/20% helium oxygen was delivered via a Mark 7 Bird respirator and a constant suction was applied to the chest tubes over a 20 cm water seal. The patient was held for 9 minutes at 6 ATA breathing helium/oxygen and decompressed to 60 ft. (2.8 ATA) over a 7-minute period. The remainder of treatment was in accordance with the U.S. Navy Table 6A. The patient began opening his eyes and responded to bilateral superficial pin prick by the time chamber treatment of 5 hours, 13 minutes had been completed. The pupils were regular and equal and reacted to light. The deep tendon reflexes were 2+ and equal bilaterally. Bilateral Babinski's were present, however, and he remained comatose.*

*Ten hours after leaving the chamber the patient experienced a grand mal seizure and his temperature rose to 103 degrees. He was treated with Dilantin and a hypothermia blanket. The patient had a series of convulsions the following day, despite anticonvulsant medication, and his temperature peaked at 105.4 degrees. Seizures were Jacksonian, but originated on both sides. Six days post embolism the patient could move all four extremities on verbal command and seemed to become aware of his surroundings. The patient could stand a week post surgery. The patient left the intensive care unit 12 days after embolism. A week after leaving the ICU the patient was found to be neurologically intact, except for a 2-year gap in memory and a mild right foot drop, which was diagnosed as a perineal nerve palsy. The patient could mentate well and talked without difficulty. Nine months following discharge from the hospital, the patient was working at his former job as a school custodian 6 hours a day, 5 days a week. His only difficulties were reported to be occasional, but minor, lapses in memory.*

Helium/oxygen was used to negate inert gas augmentation in the patient's tissues (Today the author would recommend 60%/40% heliox to more quickly deliver maximal oxygen tensions. The fact that the patient was heparinized probably contributed in a major way to his survival. In essence, because of a pump malfunction, he received an exchange transfusion of air.)

If gas embolism treatment has begun at 165 ft (50 m) and the patient has been held there for 30 minutes to two hours, with the expectation that he/she might improve, it is still possible to avoid the trap of having to use Table 4. Decompression may be started on the U.S. Navy Exceptional Exposure Air Decompression Table to a depth of 18 meters. This involves decompressing at a rate not to exceed 30 feet (9 m) a minute and stopping for two to four minutes at 80 feet (24 m), followed by a 10-minute stop at 70 feet (21 m). Decompression is then carried out to 60 feet (18 m), where Table 6 (low-pressure oxygen) is instituted with oxygen breathing for the attendant, and the patient to clear the iatrogenically-induced nitrogen. It would be wise to use a 20-minute extension at 60 feet (18 m), and a one-hour extension (on oxygen) at 30 feet (9 m), if this method is used. The U.S. Navy Exceptional Exposure Air Schedules are grossly inadequate when used in their entirety. At the deeper stops, however, they appear to prevent decompression sickness, if oxygen is used subsequent to arrival at 60 feet (2.8 ATA). One physician (Martin Nemiroff) successfully used this schedule after having been exposed to 165 feet (6 ATA) for 101 minutes. The embolism patient, who had been suffering from a dense right hemianopsia that failed to clear with pressurization alone, dramatically cleared within five minutes, when oxygen breathing was commenced at 2.8 ATA after decompression from 50 meters. Both the patient and the physician were symptom-free at the completion of the oxygen table with all its extensions. If, for some reason, a slow decompression is to be used from 60 feet (18 m) to the surface, U.S. Navy Table 7, a saturation treatment table, would have to be recommended. There is a great deal of controversy concerning the utility of air/oxygen saturation treatment in accomplishing complete relief of symptoms, as compared to daily repetitive treatments. No study has been done to establish clinically significant superiority of the former over the latter. My own opinion is that there have been insufficient data, and no physiologic basis demonstrated, to warrant the considerable expense and potential danger of saturation treatment at this time.

In the multiplace chamber, if the patient clearly is not doing well or is deteriorating at 60 feet (18 m), I feel it is mandatory to compress to 6 ATA on mixed gas. If only the monoplace chamber is available, it is recommended that the physician use the method first described by Hart (12). The patient is taken to three ATA (20 meters) and held at that pressure breathing 100% oxygen for 30 minutes. The patient is then decompressed to 2.5 ATA (15 meters) and allowed to continue breathing oxygen for an additional hour. If all symptoms have not resolved with the first treatment, the patient is placed in the chamber and treated again after an hour's surface interval. Treatment may be given as many as three times in the first 24 hours.

## The Use of Table 6 for Gas Embolism Treated with the Monoplace Chamber

In the standard monoplace chamber, the patient breathes 100% oxygen directly from the chamber atmosphere and does not wear a mask. Under such circumstances, with an unmodified chamber, it is not usually possible to give air breaks as specified when using U.S. Navy Tables 5 and 6; the time required to completely clear oxygen from the chamber, by switching to compressed air, is 15 minutes (Sechrist chamber). However, it is easily possible to modify the chamber by installing a demand regulator attached to a mask or mouthpiece from which the patient can breathe air (if he is conscious and cooperative) (21). A cylinder of compressed air is set up outside the chamber, and a pressure regulator is attached to the cylinder which reduces the air pressure to a level that will be accommodated by the demand regulator. Compressed air is introduced through a port in the chamber door with the use of an adaptor. When it comes time to take the 5-or 15-minute air breaks, the patient himself places the oro-nasal mask to his face and breathes air through the demand regulator. This method has been used successfully in the monoplace chamber to complete U.S. Navy Table 6 treatments. Studies in the author's laboratory have shown that oxygen levels in the chamber are restored to near 100% levels within a very short time after air breathing has ceased (21). The problem in severe air embolism, however, is that the patient may be too impaired to use a mask unaided. With a properly-modified Sechrist ventilator, air breaks can be instituted if the patient is intubated (see the chapter by Weaver entitled "Management of Critically Ill Patients in the Monoplace Hyperbaric Chamber").

The training and experience of the physician in managing the patient during treatment appears to be much more critical than the choice of chamber (15). No matter which type of chamber is used, if the patient has residual symptoms after the first day of treatment, daily re-treatment at 2.4 or 2.5 ATA for 90 minutes is recommended until symptoms either plateau or disappear. Daily treatment may be continued for up to 14 days.

## Treatment Ancillary to Recompression

Immediate, brief placement in steep Trendelenburg position has already been discussed. For some years, it was common to give steroids to the post-embolic patient in the hope that brain swelling and edema would be reduced. However, Dutka et al. have shown that dexamethasone is of no value in gas embolism when given after the event (5). In experiments with 37 dogs embolized by injecting air into the right internal carotid, they failed to show a difference in brain water among treated and control dogs. They concluded that dexamethasone does not prevent cerebral edema, and is not an effective adjunctive therapy for gas embolism unless given three hours prior to embolization. This, of course, is rarely possible clinically! On the other hand, Evans and McDermott have reported that lidocaine given in anti-arrhythmic dose has a protective effect in acute cerebral ischemia caused by gas embolism (8, 19). As opposed to steroids, it is clinically effective when given after embolization.

The use of heparin is controversial. Even though heparin has been shown to be helpful prior to embolization, there have been no studies to document its usefulness after the fact (4). Hart routinely gave heparin to patients suffering from embolism with no apparent ill effect (12). However, Waite documented an intracranial bleed in one of his embolized dogs which would, of course, be worsened by heparin. The author is aware of at least one probable clinical gas embolism in a diver which resulted in a small intracranial hemorrhage, demonstrated by computerized tomography; fortunately produced only a headache and no focal neurologic signs.

## RESULTS

The earlier the patient is received after embolization, the better the results tend to be. In a series of 32 cases treated by the author over a 20-year period at St. Luke's Hospital in Milwaukee, Wisconsin, all the air embolisms attendant to diving (11 in number) were treated within an average of 2.4 hours from the time of embolization. The longest delay was six hours. No patients in this group had known sequelae, and all recovered. The 20 iatrogenic cases had somewhat longer times between diagnosis and presentation (16).

Five of the 32 patients died. The survivors averaged 3.7 hours to treatment from the time of embolization, while those who died averaged 9.1 hours. Of the 27 survivors, three had minor sequelae which were limited to localized numbness or weakness. Of those cases stemming from heart/lung machine accidents, 4 out of 7 survived. The average time to treatment for the survivors was 8.6 hours, while the fatal cases averaged more than 14 hours delay. Nevertheless, one patient who embolized due to ventilator malfunction was received 14 hours after the event and one patient from cardiopulmonary bypass malfunction was treated 24 hours later. Both suffered no sequelae (16).

If the patient is heparinized at the time of embolization, there probably is a greater likelihood that the no-reflow phenomenon will be lessened (4). Table 4 is to be avoided and was never meant for the treatment of gas embolism. It never was a consideration for the author's team (16).

One of the major problems is timely referral of the iatrogenic case. In the current medico-legal climate in the United States, if a surgeon refers a patient for treatment of a possible or probable gas embolism secondary to a surgical procedure, a malpractice suit is almost unavoidable. For this reason, one can be assured that there are many instances where a surgeon may subconsciously ignore obvious or subtle signs of gas embolism, and may tend to favor a solid embolism because of the possibility of legal action. A possible solution to this problem is for the surgeon to acknowledge to the patient pre-operatively that arterial gas embolism is a known hazard of cardiopulmonary bypass or catheterization. Then, to underscore the fact that this is a rare hazard whose potential is unavoidable, the patient would give his or her permission for hyperbaric oxygen therapy in the event of a gas embolism as part of the informed surgical consent (16). Under such circumstances, chamber treatment would come as no surprise to the patient in the event of accident, and the chances of malpractice proceedings would be very much diminished.

# REFERENCES

1. Atkinson JR. Experimental air embolism. Northwest Medicine. Sept., 1963;62:699-703.

2. Bernhardt TL, Goldmann RW, Thombs PA, Kindwall EP. Hyperbaric oxygen treatment of cerebral air embolism from oro-genital sex during pregnancy. Critical Care Medicine. 1988;16(7):729-730.

3. Bray P, Meyers RAM, Cowley RA. Oro-genital sex as a cause of non-fatal air embolism in pregnancy. Obstetrics and Gynecology. 1983;61:653.

4. Crowell JW, Sharpe GP, Lambright RL, Read WL. The mechanism of death after resuscitation following acute circulatory failure. Surgery. 1955;38(4):696-702.

5. Dutka AJ, Mink R, Hallenbeck JM. Dexamethasone prevents secondary deterioration only when given three hours prior to cerebral air embolism. Undersea Biomedical Research. June, 1988;15(Suppl):14. (Abstract only)

6. Dutka AJ, Polychronidis J, Mink RB, Hallenbeck JM. Head-down position after air embolism impairs recovery of brain function as measured by the somatosensory evoked response in canines. Undersea Biomedical Research. 1990;17(Suppl):64-65.36. (Abstract only)

7. End E. The use of new equipment and helium gas in a world record dive. Journal of Industrial Hygiene. 1938;20:511.

8. Evans DE, Kobrine AI, LeGrys DC, Bradley ME. Protective effect of lidocaine in acute cerebral ischemia induced by air embolism. Journal of Neurosurgery. 1984;60:257-263.

9. Fyke EF, Kazmier FJ, Harms RW. Venous air embolism: life threatening complication of orogenital sex during pregnancy. American Journal of Medicine. 1985;78:333-336.

10. Gorman, DF, Edmunds CW et al. "Neurologic sequelae of decompression sickness: A clinical report." Underewater and Hyperbaric Physiology IX. Bove AA, Bachrach AJ and Greenbaum LJ (Eds) Bethesda, Maryland, Undersea and Hyperbaric Medical Society 1987.

11. Gronert JA, Messick JM, Cucchiaria RF, et al. Paradoxical air embolism from a patent foramen ovale. Anesthesia. 1979;50:548.

12. Hart GB. Treatment of decompression illness and air embolism with hyperbaric oxygen. Aerospace Medicine. 1974;45(10):1190-1193.

13. Helps SC, Gorman DF. The effect of air emboli on brain blood flow and function of leukocytopenic rabbits. Undersea Biomedical Research. 1990;17(Suppl):71-72. (Abstract only)

14. Kindwall EP. New treatment of air embolism - Avoiding the use of U.S. Navy Table IV. Proceedings of the Fifth International Hyperbaric Congress. WG Trapp, et al., (Eds.) Simon Frazier University, Burnaby, Canada. Volume 2. 1974;895-899.

15. Kindwall EP, Goldmann RW, Thombs PA. The use of the monoplace vs. multiplace chamber in the treatment of diving diseases. Journal of Hyperbaric Medicine. 1988;3(1):5-10.

16. Kindwall EP, Johnson JP. Outcome of hyperbaric treatment in 32 cases of air embolism. Undersea Biomedical Research. 1990;17(Suppl):90. (Abstract only)

17. Kruse CA. Air embolism and other skin diving problems. Northwest Medicine. July, 1963;62:525-529.

18. Leitch DR, Greenbaum LJ, Hallenbeck JM. Cerebral arterial air embolism I, II, III, IV. Undersea Biomedical Research. 1984;11(3):221-274.

19. McDermott JJ, Dutka AJ, Evans DE, Flynn ET. Effects of treatment with lidocaine and hyperbaric oxygen in experimental cerebral ischemia induced by air embolism. Undersea Biomedical Research. 1990;17(Suppl):35-36. (Abstract only)

20. Neuman TS, Hallenbeck JM. Barotraumatic cerebral air embolism and the mental status examination: A report of four cases. Annals of Emergency Medicine. 1987;16(2):220-222.

21. Raleigh GW. Air breaks in the Sechrist Model 2500-B monoplace hyperbaric chamber. Journal of Hyperbaric Medicine. 1988;3(1);11-14.

22. Schaefer KE, McNulty WP Jr., Carey C, Liebow AA. Mechanisms in the development of interstitial emphysema and air embolism on decompression from depth. Journal of Applied Physiology. 1958;13:15-29.

23. Stoney WS, Alford WC, Burros GR, Glassford DM, Jr., Thomas CS, Jr. Air embolism and other accidents using pump oxygenators. Annals of Thoracic Surgery. 1980;29(4):336-340.

24. Swindle PF. Occlusion of blood vessels by agglutinated red cells, mainly as seen in tadpoles and very young kangaroos. American Journal of Physiology. 1937;120:59-74.

25. Tolly TL, Feldmeier JE, Czarnecki D. Air embolism complicating percutaneous lung biopsy. American Journal of Radiology. 1988;150:555-556.

26. US Navy Bumed Instruction 6620.2 Bumed 74, Oxygen breathing treatment for decompression sickness and air embolism. Bureau of Medicine and Surgery. Washington, D.C., August 22, 1967.

27. Van Allen, CM, Hrdina LS, Clark J. Air embolism from the pulmonary vein. Archives of Surgery. 1929;19(4):567-599.

28. Waite CL, Mazzone LS, Greenwood ME, Larsen RT. Cerebral air embolism, Basic Studies. US Naval Submarine Medical Center Research Report #493. April 18, 1967.

29. Zamboni WA, Roth AC, Russell RC, Suchy H, Kuckan J. The effect of hyperbaric oxygen treatment on the microcirculation of ischemic skeletal muscle. Undersea Biomedical Research. 1990;17(Suppl):26. (Abstract only)

# EFFECTS OF HYPERBARIC OXYGEN IN INFECTIOUS DISEASES: BASIC MECHANISMS

## CHAPTER TWENTY OVERVIEW

# Effects of Hyperbaric Oxygen in Infectious Diseases: Basic Mechanisms

*Matthew K. Park, Charles C. Falzon, Harry T. Whelan*

## INTRODUCTION

This review will discuss the basic mechanisms of action of hyperbaric oxygen in infectious diseases. It will present the evidence for the bacteriostatic and bactericidal effects of hyperoxia and hyperbaric oxygen on microbial organisms *in vitro* and in *in vivo* models of infection. It will also examine the effects of oxygen on the activity of antimicrobial agents and on the function of immune defense mechanisms. For a broader review on the role of oxygen tensions in infections, the reader is referred to reference 157.

### Regulation of Oxygen Delivery to Tissues

Tissue oxygen tensions are affected mainly by the concentration of inspired oxygen, cardiac output, local blood flow, cellular metabolism and substrate availability (106, 173, 174). Different partial pressures of oxygen ($pO_2$) are normally found in various body compartments. The $pO_2$s range from approximately 100 mmHg within pulmonary alveoli to 15 mmHg in the liver parenchymal cells. In traumatized or septic tissues, $pO_2$s may be even lower. In bacterial osteomyelitis, the $pO_2$ of bone is lowered by 50%; in experimental abscesses, $pO_2$s may measure as low as 0 mmHg (87). Within individual cells, $pO_2$s are heterogeneous and are much lower than extracellular $pO_2$s. For example, $pO_2$s in mitochondria are less than 1 mmHg (201).

Normoxia (15%-21% $O_2$) is defined in this review as the fractional inspired oxygen ($FIO_2$) concentration necessary to maintain aerobic metabolism and homeostasis in the body. Oxygen tensions outside this normal range will be defined as follows: Anaerobiosis (less than 0.01% $O_2$), hypoxia (12% $O_2$ or less), hyperoxia (45%-100% $O_2$), and hyperbaric oxygen (any $O_2$ tension greater than 1 atmosphere absolute pressure (ATA) or 760 mmHg).

### General Mechanisms of Action of Oxygen in Infections

Hyperoxia and hyperbaric oxygen (HBO) increase oxygen tensions in tissues to levels that inhibit microbial growth by inhibiting various microbial metabolic reactions. Hyperoxia and HBO by themselves also exert direct bacteriostatic and bactericidal effects on selected microorganisms because of increased generation of reactive oxygen species or free radicals (99, 164).

Free radicals are lethal for microorganisms that either lack or possess limited antioxidant defenses. HBO is a unique antibacterial agent. At doses used clinically, HBO is usually bacteriostatic. Not all doses of HBO have an antibacterial effect. The use of HBO at pressures of 1.5 ATA or less promotes the growth of aerobic bacteria *in vitro* (153).

Hyperbaric oxygen also raises oxygen tensions in hypoxic tissues to levels necessary for the killing of bacteria by neutrophils (122). While phagocytosis remains unaffected by low oxygen tensions (104, 185), killing of microorganisms by the oxidative burst is dependent on oxygen tensions (6, 11, 86). Polymorphonuclear leukocytes (PMNs) from patients with chronic granulomatous disease lack the enzyme NADPH-oxidase necessary for oxygen-dependent killing of such pathogenic bacteria as *Pseudomonas aeruginosa* and *Staphylococcus aureus* (126).

Hyperoxia and HBO also influence the activity of selected antimicrobial agents belonging to the following categories: antimetabolites, protein synthesis inhibitors, and reduction-oxidation cycling agents. See Table 1. Oxygen tensions also influence the pharmacokinetics of antimicrobial agents. For example, hypoxemia (32 mmHg) prolongs (two-fold) the serum half-life of aminoglycosides (132). Hypoxemia affects both the absorption from muscle, as well as the elimination of these antimicrobials (132).

Hyperbaric oxygen can also affect the outcome of infections indirectly by influencing tissue repair and regeneration responses in infected necrotic tissues. For example, hypoxia (12% $O_2$ at 1 ATA) retards healing of skin

## TABLE 1. OXYGEN TENSIONS INFLUENCE THE ACTIVITY OF ANTIMICROBIAL AGENTS

| ANTIMICROBIAL | HYPEROXIA OR HYPERBARIC OXYGEN | ANOXIA |
|---|---|---|
| AMINOGLYCOSIDES | Postantibiotic Effect ↑(156) | cidal ↓(83, 151, 166, 183, 192) |
| ANTIMETABOLITES Sulfamethoxazole Sulfisoxazole Trimethoprim | static ↑(71,155) static ↑(193) | static (193) static ↓(83, 193) |
| CELL WALL INHIBITORS Vancomycin | | cidal and static ↓(151) |
| FLUOROQUINOLONES Ciprofloxacin | | cidal ↓(176) |
| REDOX-CYCLING AGENTS Nitrofurantoin Streptonigrin | static ↑(138) | static ↓(81) and cidal ↓(81) |

*Numbers in brackets refer to citations listed in the reference section. The arrows indicate increase (↑) or decrease (↓) in antimicrobial activity.*

wounds and thus probably favors bacterial growth (111). Hyperbaric oxygen (100% $O_2$ at 2 ATA, for 2 hours, twice daily) does not affect the healing of vascularized, full-thickness skin wounds, but, HBO does enhance wound closure in ischemic wounds (109).

Hyperbaric oxygen also influences the cardiac output and the perfusion of various tissues. For example, 100% $O_2$ at 2.8 ATA decreases the percent cardiac output and blood flow to splanchnic tissues of rats within 20 minutes of exposure (139). Similar decreases in blood flow also occur upon exposure to 100% $O_2$ at 1 ATA (95). Hyperbaric oxygen (100% $O_2$, between 2-5 ATA) decreases blood flows to liver, muscle, brain, and spinal cord (188). Blood flows are also significantly decreased in uninfected bone of rabbits after exposure to HBO (100% $O_2$ at 2 ATA) (122). The hemodynamic changes induced by hyperbaric oxygen may be the result of increased oxygen delivery to tissue. It is also possible that negative inotropic effects on myocardium play a role in these changes. As far as can be judged from work with a model of antibiotic-controlled sepsis, the presence of sepsis, per se, does not cause any hemodynamic change during exposure to HBO (139).

## BACTERIOSTATIC AND BACTERICIDAL EFFECTS OF HYPERBARIC OXYGEN

### Susceptibility of Anaerobic and Aerobic Bacteria to HBO

Pathogenic bacteria are classified in terms of the partial pressure of oxygen in which they grow. By definition, anaerobic bacteria cannot survive in normal oxygen tensions because they lack antioxidant defenses. As such, they are susceptible to HBO. For example, hyperbaric oxygen (3 ATA for 18 hours) is completely bactericidal for *Clostridium perfringens in vitro* (88). However, there are differences in susceptibility to oxygen among *Clostridium* species. Hyperbaric oxygen (100% $O_2$ at 2 ATA) blocks the germination of *C. perfringens* spores *in vitro*, but is not bactericidal for the spores (40). Facultative anaerobic bacteria are able to grow in normoxia and hyperoxia by increasing the synthesis of antioxidant enzymes (74).

The growth of some aerobic bacteria is enhanced by hyperoxia, but is inhibited by HBO. For example, oxygen tensions up to 1 ATA enhance the growth of *Escherichia coli*, whereas oxygen tensions greater than 2 ATA inhibit growth *in vitro* (153). Hyperoxia (100% $O_2$ at 1 ATA) enhances the growth of P. aeruginosa *in vitro* (156); hyperoxia (0.2 to 0.87 ATA) enhances the growth of *Corynebacterium diphtheriae in vitro* (71).

Prolonged *in vitro* exposure to oxygen tensions greater than 1.5 ATA inhibits the growth of several aerobic and facultative anaerobic bacteria. Hyperbaric oxygen (greater than 1.5 ATA) is bacteriostatic for *E. coli* (15, 20, 138, 153), *P. aeruginosa* (17, 138, 155), *C. diphtheriae*, and *Lactobacillus casei*, (71). However, a 1-hour intermittent exposure to HBO (100% $O_2$ at 2 ATA, every 8 hours) has no effect on the growth of *P. aeruginosa* or *S. aureus* (23). Prolonged *in vitro* hyperbaric oxygen exposure (2.9 ATA $O_2$, 24 hours) is also bacteriostatic for the following enteric bacteria: *Salmonella typhosa, S. schottmuelleri, S. paratyphi, Shigella dysenteriae, S. flexneri,* and *Proteus vulgaris* (17). The growth of *Streptococcus (Enterococcus) faecalis* is partially inhibited by 2.9 ATA $O_2$ (71). However, an alpha hemolytic strain of *Streptococcus* is not inhibited by HBO (71), possibly because of the presence of a hyaluronic acid-containing capsule (36).

Hyperbaric oxygen is bactericidal for aerobic and facultative anaerobic bacteria, usually only at pressures and/or durations that are greater than can be used clinically. For example, HBO is bactericidal for *P. aeruginosa*, *Proteus vulgaris*, and *S. typhosa* (17) at 3 ATA for 24 hours, and for *E. coli* at 20 ATA when treated for 6 hours.

## Mechanisms of Bacteriostatic Effects of HBO

HBO inhibits the growth of aerobic and facultative anaerobic bacteria by inducing a variety of metabolic effects involved with the synthesis of proteins, nucleic acids, and essential cofactors of metabolic reactions; membrane transport functions are also affected. These effects were achieved with the use of hyperbaric oxygen *in vitro*.

## Inhibition of Amino Acid and Protein Biosynthesis

Exposure of *E. coli* to hyperbaric oxygen (100% $O_2$ at greater than 3 ATA) causes a rapid inhibition of growth (20, 25) and respiration (20). The inhibitory effects of HBO are most likely caused by free radicals and other reactive oxygen-based molecules, because hyperoxia (100% $O_2$ at 1 ATA) inhibits growth of a superoxide dismutase-deficient double mutant of *E. coli*, *(sodA sodB)* (30). Free radicals inactivate bacterial dihydroxyacid dehydratase (24, 115), which catalyzes the formation of alpha-ketoisovalerate, an intermediate in the formation of valine and leucine. Hyperbaric oxygen (100% $O_2$, 4.2 ATA) decreases the specific activity of dihydroxyacid dehydratase by destroying the Fe-S cluster of this enzyme; however, this enzyme remains in a form that can be reactivated (55). The inhibition of amino acid biosynthesis by HBO eventually leads to increased levels of uncharged tRNA, which is responsible for inducing the stringency response (31, 172). The stringency response is characterized by increased levels of tetra- and penta-phosphorylated guanosine that inhibit bacterial carbohydrate, lipid, and nucleotide synthesis, and enhance proteolysis (31). The end result is cessation of bacterial growth.

The inhibition by HBO of protein synthesis in bacteria (Table 2) may also be caused by a free radical-induced block in the transport of substrates used in RNA transcription. Hyperoxia or the superoxide anion free radical inhibit the transport of lactose, guanosine, and methylglucopyranoside into *E. coli* (52). Hyperoxia also inhibits the transport of protons and the synthesis of ATP in bacterial membranes (200). However, it appears that the growth inhibition caused by HBO begins long before a drop in ATP levels occurs (127). The mechanism of the decreased transport caused by HBO is thought to be the oxidation of sulfhydryl-containing proteins involved in the transport of metabolic substrates. Free radicals are able to inactivate other bacterial proteins with key enzymatic functions by oxidizing sulfhydryl-containing amino acids such as methionine (19, 29). Bacterial enzymes that convert the oxidized methionine back to its reduced form (19, 50) play a key role in defending against this type of oxidative damage to proteins.

## TABLE 2. HYPEROXIA OR HYPERBARIC OXYGEN INFLUENCE THE SYNTHESIS OF PROTEIN BY *PSEUDOMONAS AERUGINOSA*

| $O_2$ | PROTEIN SYNTHESIS NO TREATMENT | TOBRAMYCIN |
|---|---|---|
| 21% $O_2$; 1 ATA (Control) | 415 + 185 | 16.7 + 6.5 |
| 100% $O_2$; 1 ATA (Hyperoxia) | 514 + 237 | 7.4 + 4.3 |
| 100% $O_2$; 2.8 ATA (HBO) | 202 + 52 | 0.0 |

*Bacteria in each of the experimental groups were maintained at the three oxygen tensions for 1 hour. Tobramycin was then removed and the bacteria were pulse-chased with 35 S-methionine to label proteins. Data are DPMs and are normalized for the number of colony-forming units. HBO decreases protein synthesis compared to controls. Table adapted from Park et al. (156).*

## Decreased Levels of Key Cofactors of Metabolic Reactions

Hyperbaric oxygen also inhibits bacterial growth by decreasing the levels of thiamine and the levels of both the reduced and oxidized forms of nicotinamide adenine dinucleotide (NAD, NADH) (21, 22). Thiamine pyrophosphate is an essential coenzyme in carbohydrate metabolism and NADPH production. NADH is a critical cofactor in a wide range of metabolic reactions. The mechanisms of the decrease in NAD is an inhibition of the de novo NAD synthesis pathway and possibly also an increase in catabolism of NAD (60).

## Decreased Synthesis and Increased Degradation of DNA and RNA

Hyperbaric oxygen can also inhibit bacterial growth by directly blocking RNA transcription and DNA synthesis. For example, HBO (4.2 ATA) inhibits RNA transcription and DNA synthesis in both stringent and relaxed strains of *E. coli* after a 30-minute exposure (21).

Electron microscopic studies show ultrastructural evidence of degradation of nucleic acids and ribosomal proteins in *P. aeruginosa*, after bacteriostasis induced by prolonged exposure to HBO (100% $O_2$ at 2.9 ATA) for 24 hours (35). *P. aeruginosa* undergo marked changes in morphologic appearance when exposed to oxygen at pressures that do not induce bacteriostasis (100% $O_2$ at 2 ATA). These abnormal shape changes are reversible (107).

Another important mechanism of oxygen-induced toxicity to bacteria is via injury to DNA. Production of the superoxide anion *in vitro* and *in vivo* has been linked to mutations in bacteria. HBO is mutagenic in *E. coli* (62). Treatment with 10 ATA oxygen for 15 to 30 minutes induced the reversion of a tryptophan auxotroph (*E. coli* WP 2 hcr-) to prototrophy. Hassan and Fridovich (85) reported that paraquat toxicity for *E. coli* is in large part due to superoxide radical production. Moody and Hassan (136) showed that paraquat is highly mutagenic for two strains of *S. typhimurium*. Both base-pair substitution and frameshift mutations were noted in DNA from the *Salmonella* strains. Cells containing high levels of SOD are more resistant to toxicity and mutagenicity than cells containing normal levels of this enzyme.

## Mechanisms of Bactericidal Effects of HBO with Special Reference to Free Radicals

The increase in oxidation-reduction potentials induced by elevated oxygen tensions is not the mechanism of the toxicity of oxygen for anaerobic bacteria (194). It is generally agreed that bacteria with inadequate defenses against toxic oxygen species are most susceptible to killing by elevated oxygen tensions. It appears therefore that injury by free radicals is the primary mechanism of bacterial killing by HBO.

## Cellular Utilization of Oxygen and Generation of Oxygen-Based Free Radicals

Oxygen normally undergoes a four-electron reduction to water that is catalyzed by mitochondrial oxidases. This reaction accounts for the greatest proportion of oxygen consumption in the cell. During normal aerobic metabolism, partially reduced oxygen species are also generated within cells. These highly reactive species of oxygen are known as free radicals. The levels of oxygen free radicals and other reactive oxygen molecules formed within cells increase during exposure to hyperoxia (99). These molecules are toxic to cells because they react with and damage cellular proteins, membrane lipids, and DNA (99).

Increased oxygen tensions cause an increase in the conversion of molecular oxygen ($O_2$) to the free radical superoxide anion ($O_2$-). Superoxide anion can be converted to another toxic oxygen species, namely hydrogen peroxide ($H_2O_2$); $H_2O_2$ in the presence of iron can react with $O_2$- to form another toxic molecule, the hydroxyl radical (OH.) (169).

## Cellular Sources of Free Radicals

The production of toxic oxygen species can occur in various cellular compartments (including the cytosol) by enzymatic and nonenzymatic reactions. Flavoproteins and cuproproteins generate $H_2O_2$, while several types of flavin-containing oxidoreductases can generate $O_2$- (102).

A cellular source of superoxide of particular relevance in infectious diseases is the NADPH oxidase located in the plasma membrane of polymorphonuclear leukocytes and macrophages. This enzyme converts oxygen to $O_2$- (6). Phagocytic stimuli induce production of $O_2$- by NADPH oxidase. The majority of oxygen free radicals produced are directed into the phagosome where they participate in bacterial killing. If the activated NADPH oxidase remains on the external surface of the cell, oxygen products are shed into the surrounding tissues. Soluble substances, such as immune complexes and chemotactic factors, stimulate superoxide anion release from human neutrophils (196). There are multiple pathways of activation of the NADPH oxidase (13). Chemotactic factors, arachidonic acid, and cell-surface binding lectins activate NADPH oxidase by different pathways and with additive effects.

From a quantitative standpoint, an important cellular source of superoxide is the nonenzymatic oxidation of cytochrome intermediates of the electron transport chain in mitochondria. Superoxide is also generated by the cytochrome-P-450 substrate-oxygen complexes in the endoplasmic reticulum. Another cellular organelle producing toxic oxygen species is the peroxisome. Here $H_2O_2$ production occurs by oxidation of substrates such as long-chain fatty acids. In all these cellular organelles, the generation of toxic oxygen species is dependent on tissue oxygen tensions (190). Xanthine oxidase is a major source of $O_2$- in ischemic and hypoxic tissues that undergo re-oxygenation by blood reflow (118). In summary, the presence of an adequate amount of molecular oxygen is necessary for oxygen-dependent killing by PMNs and macrophages to occur. A variety of enzymatic and nonenzymatic cellular reactions also normally result in the production of $O_2$- and $H_2O_2$. The production of these molecules is enhanced by increasing tissue-oxygen tensions. Free radicals are highly reactive and, if not removed by scavengers, may cause extensive cellular injury.

## Bacterial Defense Mechanisms Against Free Radicals

For protection against the free radicals generated during normal aerobic metabolism, cells have developed antioxidant defense mechanisms. Three main antioxidant enzymes are known. Superoxide dismutase (SOD) is an extremely efficient $O_2$- scavenger. Catalase is a hydrogen peroxide scavenger. Glutathione peroxidase (GSH peroxidase) catalyzes the reduction of hydrogen peroxide to water and dioxygen, and is capable of converting toxic lipid peroxides into nontoxic products.

Superoxide anion may undergo spontaneous dismutation to form hydrogen peroxide. The rate of reaction is enhanced markedly by the presence of superoxide dismutase (SOD). Dismutation of two $O_2$- radicals results in the formation of one hydrogen peroxide molecule. Catalase subsequently converts hydrogen peroxide to water and oxygen. The role of catalase is probably more important during hyperoxic conditions than in normoxic conditions. In the presence of trace amounts of transition metals, particularly iron, hydrogen peroxide may participate in the Fenton reaction. This reaction serves to produce the highly reactive OH. radical. Removal of $H_2O_2$ by catalase is important in order to prevent lipid peroxidation of membranes by OH. radical.

Free radicals may also be inactivated by reacting with low molecular weight substances located in the cellular membranes or in the cytosol. Tocopherol (vitamin E) is an antioxidant located in membranes. Ascorbate, beta-carotene and sulfhydryl-containing compounds such as cysteine, cysteamine, and glutathione are water soluble antioxidant compounds. Under normal metabolic conditions, these free radical scavengers neutralize oxygen free radicals before they can cause cellular injury. However, if host defense mechanisms are overwhelmed, damage to eukaryotic cells as well as procaryotic cells will occur (57, 79).

It is clear that the primary mechanism of toxicity of HBO for eukaryotic cells, and for microorganisms, is through the generation of free radicals and other toxic oxygen species. Mammalian cells have various antioxidant defenses, and utilize free radical reactions for bacterial killing.

Augmentation of endogenous host antioxidant defenses may permit use of higher doses of HBO than are currently possible in the treatment of infectious disease states. One of the rationales for using hyperbaric oxygen in infections is the potential to exploit the enhanced sensitivity of selected microorganisms to toxic oxygen molecules.

## Role of Superoxide and Hydrogen Peroxide in Bacterial Killing by Hyperoxia and Hyperbaric Oxygen

The superoxide anion radical appears to be particularly important in bacterial killing (74, 75, 76). Several *in vitro* studies have shown that the absence of the enzyme responsible for the detoxification of $O_2$-, namely superoxide dismutase (SOD), increases the susceptibility of many anaerobic and facultative anaerobic bacteria to oxygen (119, 168). On the other hand, by raising bacterial levels of SOD, the susceptibility of the bacteria to oxygen can be diminished *in vitro*. For example, SOD levels in *B. fragilis* can be raised five-fold by exposure to 2% $O_2$ (161). The increased SOD activity markedly reduces killing of these bacteria by HBO (161). Pre-exposure of *E. coli* to hyperoxia also increases SOD activity and protects against killing by HBO (75). Killing of *S. sanguis* can also be prevented by increasing SOD activity; dimethylsulfoxide (a permeable OH. scavenger) does not protect against free radical toxicity (42). Studies with SOD- and catalase-deficient mutants of *E. coli* confirm that SOD is more important than catalase in protecting against the growth inhibition caused by hyperoxia (171).

Bacteria such as *N. gonorrhoeae* are particularly susceptible to a different toxic-oxygen species, namely $H_2O_2$. In these bacteria, resistance to oxygen-induced killing is associated with high levels of catalase, the enzyme responsible for detoxification of $H_2O_2$. Additional antioxidant defenses, such as peroxidase and high levels of glutathione, also contribute to survival of these bacteria in aerobic conditions (3).

Work done by Beaman et al. (12) has shown that surface-associated SOD and high levels of catalase in *Nocardia asteroides* act together to resist oxygen-dependent microbicidal activity of human PMNs. Microorganisms with adequate antioxidant defenses are resistant to toxic actions of $O_2$-, and may use the production of toxic-oxygen species to injure host cells (67). For example, virulent strains of *Listeria monocytogenes* exhibit maximal production of $H_2O_2$ and $O_2$-. Virulence is correlated with survival of *L. monocytogenes* in macrophage monolayers. The exogenous $H_2O_2$ damages macrophages. An avirulent strain of *L. monocytogenes* does not release $H_2O_2$ or $O_2$- in significant amounts (67).

It is not clear if damage to the bacterial cytoplasmic membrane caused by HBO is significant enough to be considered an important mechanism of HBO-induced killing. In the case of *E. coli*, very few broken cells and no evidence of membrane lipid peroxidation are seen after the bacteria have been killed by HBO *in vitro* (82). However, the presence of a capsule appears to protect bacteria against oxygen-induced damage. In the case of *Streptococcus pyogenes* the presence of a hyaluronic acid capsule increases resistance to the bacteriostatic effects of oxygen (36). Removal of the capsule from an encapsulated *Streptococcus* strain, using hyaluronidase digestion, increases susceptibility of this bacterium to the toxic effects of oxygen (36).

## Genetic Mechanisms of Bacterial Resistance to Oxygen

Two regulatory genes responsible for the increased resistance of bacteria to hyperoxia have been identified as the soxR and oxyR regulons. Hyperoxia and superoxide induce the synthesis of 30 proteins; approximately 20 of these proteins are regulated by the soxR or the oxyR regulons (33, 73, 181, 195). Many of these bacterial proteins are enzymes involved in detoxification of free radicals and repair of free radical damage; examples are SOD, endonuclease IV, and glucose 6-phosphate dehydrogenase (73, 189). Examples of these proteins include the antioxidant enzymes hydroperoxidase I-catalase, NAD(P)H-dependent alkyl hydroperoxide reductase, and glutathione reductase (33, 98). Exposure to toxic-oxygen species induces the synthesis of several other protective proteins whose specific identity remains to be characterized (33, 41, 181, 195).

## Effects of Hyperbaric Oxygen in Experimental Bacterial Infections

Early studies using hyperbaric oxygen in the absence of antimicrobial treatment found beneficial effects in infections caused by anaerobic bacteria. Hill and Osterhout (89) examined the effects of HBO (100% $O_2$ at 2-3 ATA) in two *in vivo* murine models of *C. perfringens* infection. In the first model (agar disc implantation model), *C. perfringens* was completely killed by 48 hours post-infection in mice exposed to HBO (1.5 hours, 4 times during the first 48 hours post-infection), while *C. perfringens* grew in mice maintained in a normoxic environment. In the second model of *C. perfringens* infection (intramuscular injection of *C. perfringens* and epinephrine), the overall mortality was significantly decreased in mice receiving a rigorous HBO treatment regimen (7 exposures of 1.5 hours duration: 3 times on day 1, twice daily on days 2 and 3). Mice receiving a less rigorous treatment (5 exposures of 1.5 hours duration: once on day 1, twice daily on days 2 and 3) showed no difference in mortality from normoxia-maintained, infected mice. The most critical difference between the two regimens was attributed to the intensive treatment on day 1 of infection in the former (89).

Hirn et al. (90) compared the efficacy of HBO and surgery, with surgery alone in a rat model of *Clostridium perfringens* gas gangrene. The mortality of infected rats receiving HBO and surgical debridement (12.5%) was significantly less than rats treated with surgery (37.5%), or untreated controls (100%). More strikingly, 82.5% of animals in the HBO and surgery group healed their wounds and ambulated, compared to only 12.5% of animals treated with surgery alone (90). While HBO was demonstrated to be a useful adjunct to surgery when used 1 hour after infection, a more clinically relevant model would have also included an antibiotic treatment group. Several years ago, two studies (140, 180) examined the use of HBO alone, and in combination with antibodies in a murine model of *Clostridium* myonecrosis. Both studies demonstrated the lack of enhanced survival when HBO was used alone. The inoculum size of *C. perfringens* ranged from $10^7$ CFU to $10^{10}$ CFU. HBO was administered b.i.d. (100% $O_2$ at 3 ATA 90 minutes) (140) or t.i.d. on day 1, b.i.d. on day 2 and 3, and once on day 4 (100% $O_2$ at 2.8 ATA, for 60 minutes) (180). Furthermore, HBO did not enhance survival when used in combination with penicillin G, clindamycin, metronidazole, or imipenem compared to when antibiotics were administered alone (140). However, HBO significantly enhanced the survival of mice treated with penicillin G or metronidazole when administered immediately after infection (180). The explanation for the contradictory results is not obvious, aside from differences in genetic background, since the *C. perfringens* strain and dose of antibiotic used were identical in both studies. In fact, the duration of HBO treatment favored the study showing a lack of beneficial effect of HBO (140). Although possible, it is unlikely that a 30 minute delay between the time of infection and the first HBO, treatment (140) could account for the lack of observed benefit of HBO or survival in the antibiotic-treated groups. The concordant finding in both studies (140, 180) was that clindamycin and metronidazole significantly enhanced survival. Clindamycin was more efficacious at a higher inoculum (exceeding $10^9$ CFU/mL), compared to metron dazole or penicillin G (180).

In a polymicrobial rat model of gas gangrene where $10^7$ CFU of *C. perfringens*, *B. fragilis*, *E. coli*, and *E. faecalis* were injected into muscle, HBO did not significantly enhance survival (80%) over surgery alone; (65%) the survival rate in the control group was 40% (91). However, 84% of the survivors in the HBO and surgery group recovered completely, compared to 15% of the survivors in the surgery alone group (p < 0.001) (91).

In a murine model of *S. pyogenes* myositis, HBO was not beneficial in decreasing mortality or bacterial growth (202). HBO and penicillin G exerted additive effects in improving the mean survival of dogs and by decreasing the CFU in muscles, obtained on the day of death (202). A more recent *in vitro* study showed that a 90-min exposure to HBO significantly inhibited growth of both MRSA (25%) and MSSA (24%) when compared with both normobaric normoxia and hyperoxia, indicating that *S. aureus*, including resistant strains, is susceptible to oxygen stress. This study also investigated the effects of increasing oxygen tension on *E. coli*, and showed that neither normobaric nor hyperbaric hyperoxia inhibited its growth (206).

The effects of HBO have also been studied in two models of polymicrobial sepsis induced by implanting pooled fecal material contained in gelatin capsules into the peritoneal cavity of rats. Treatment with HBO alone (100% $O_2$ at 2 ATA for 1.5 hours, every 6 hours) appeared to reduce mortality to 8%, from the 100% mortality seen in animals maintained in a normoxic environment (186). In another experiment, known strains of *B. fragilis*, *E. coli*, and *S. faecalis* were introduced into the peritoneal cavity of rats. Mortality was 79% in untreated rats; treatment with HBO alone decreased mortality to 23%. Hyperoxia (100% $O_2$ at 1 ATA) had no effect on mortality in either model (186). However, a more recent study (137), showed that HBO (100% $O_2$ at 2.7 ATA) did not significantly decrease mortality in septic rats with a single large undrained intra-abdominal abscess containing *E. coli* and/or *B. fragilis*.

In a rabbit model of experimentally-induced peritonitis by cecal ligation and puncture without antibiotics (101), the mortality rate of rabbits that received 100% $O_2$ (3-5 mmHg) intraperitoneally was significantly lower (28%) than the group receiving air (50%). The size of the inner wall of the abscesses was significantly reduced in oxygen-treated rabbits (by a factor of 3) and the percent of organisms (*E. coli*, *E. faecalis*, *S. aureus*, and *C. perfringens*) recovered from the abscesses was significantly decreased in oxygen treated rabbits. While it seems that elevated $O_2$ tensions may play a role in controlling peritonitis when used alone, it remains unclear if hyperoxia would be of added benefit compared to the use of antibiotics in this model.

Interestingly, low inspired oxygen tensions appear to be beneficial in some pneumonias caused by aerobic bacteria. Continuous exposure to 12% $O_2$ prolonged the survival of mice infected with *D (Streptococcus) pneumoniae* (2). The explanation for these results may be that alveolar $pO_2$ is sufficiently elevated, even at 12% $O_2$, to ensure adequate oxygenation of pulmonary parenchymal cells. On the other hand, continuous hyperoxic exposure (75% $O_2$ at 1 ATA) shortened survival of infected mice without inducing pulmonary toxicity (2). One *in vivo* study showed that exposure to hyperoxic conditions during the evolution of pneumonia resulted in a marked increase in lethality in mice with *Legionella* pneumonia (203). The enhanced lethality was characterized by an increase in lung permeability, but not changes in either lung bacterial burden or leukocyte accumulation. The same group later showed that treating infected mice with greater than 50% $O_2$ reduced survival of *Legionella*-infected mice in an oxygen concentration and exposure time-dependent manner (204). The study also showed that the enhanced lethality was associated with an increase in total lung weight and apoptosis markers, but not with bacterial burden in the lungs (204). These findings are all in agreement with the increased incidence and more severe course of pneumonias in patients treated for respiratory failure with continuous high $FIO_2$s.

In a rabbit model of bacterial osteomyelitis, HBO (100% $O_2$ at 2 ATA) is as effective as the antibiotic cephalothin in the treatment of *S. aureus* (123). In addition, treatment with HBO (100% $O_2$ at 2.5 ATA for 1.6 hours twice daily) and tobramycin for *P. aeruginosa* osteomyelitis is superior to either tobramycin alone or HBO alone (124). HBO enhances antibacterial activity in infected bone by restoring oxygen tensions to levels necessary for aminoglycoside activity and oxygen-dependent killing by phagocytes (122).

In mice infected with *Mycobacterium ulcerans*, HBO (100% $O_2$ at 2.5 ATA for 1.25 hours, twice daily) decreased mortality by 50% (at 25 weeks post-infection) compared to normoxia-exposed controls (113). The twice daily exposures were essential in decreasing mortality since once daily treatments (100% $O_2$ at 2.5 ATA for 2 hours or at 2 ATA for 3.5 hours) were not effective. Adjunctive HBO therapy (100% $O_2$, 2.5 ATA, 1.5 hours twice daily) did not extend the survival of mice infected with *Mycobacterium ulcerans* over that of rifampin or heat treatment (114).

Spirochetes and mycoplasmas are deficient in some antioxidant enzymes. For example, the survival of *T. pallidum* in 3% $O_2$ *in vitro* is enhanced by the addition of catalase, histidine, and mannitol; however SOD is ineffective (179). *Mycoplasma pneumoniae* and other *Mycoplasma sp.* lack SOD and catalase, and yet are aerotolerant (117). These microorganisms do not appear to be susceptible to hyperoxia. For select organisms, hyperoxia or HBO can worsen the outcome of infections. Hyperbaric oxygen (100% $O_2$ at 3 ATA) increases the mortality in one-day old rats inoculated with *Spiroplasma mirum* (9). Hyperoxia (80% $O_2$) increases the percentage of lung cultures positive for *Ureaplasma urealyticum* and mortality in newborn mice (39).

In summary, the bacteriostatic and bactericidal effects of hyperbaric oxygen are mediated in large part by oxygen-based free radicals. Free radicals oxidize proteins and membrane lipids, damage DNA, and inhibit metabolic functions essential for growth. Strict anaerobic bacteria have deficient defenses against free radicals, and other oxidants, and are susceptible to killing by oxygen. In contrast, facultative anaerobes and obligate aerobes can detoxify free radicals and are resistant to hyperoxia. Hyperoxia (100% $O_2$, 1 ATA) enhances *in vitro* growth of facultative anaerobic and obligate aerobic bacteria, while hyperbaric oxygen (100% $O_2$ at 2 ATA) is bacteriostatic for these bacteria. However, *in vivo*, it appears that the beneficial effects of oxygen varies from harmful effects to significant benefits, depending upon the specific type of infectious disease model examined.

## EFFECTS OF HYPERBARIC OXYGEN IN PARASITIC INFECTIONS

The levels of antioxidant defenses are in general low in parasites. As a consequence, these microorganisms are very susceptible to HBO. It is noteworthy that the mechanism of action of several anti-parasitic drugs is also based on inducing oxidative stress and exploiting the reduced or absent levels of antioxidant enzymes in parasites (44, 45).

### Inhibition of Protozoan Growth by Oxygen

Physiologic oxygen tensions are sufficient to inhibit the growth of several parasites, most likely by inducing oxidative stress. *Plasmodium falciparum* has very low levels of endogenous superoxide dismutase and its growth *in vitro* is optimal at 3% $O_2$ (170), whereas growth is slightly reduced (by 15%) at 20% $O_2$ (34). Inhibitors of parasite and RBC catalase markedly reduced growth by as much as 30% (34). There is no evidence of ultrastructural differences in *P. falciparum* at 20% $O_2$ when compared to 5% $O_2$. Growth of *Entamoeba histolytica* trophozoites *in vitro* is inhibited by 10% $O_2$ (7). *E. histolytica* lacks catalase (128, 144, 198) and has low levels of glutathione peroxidase and superoxide dismutase (144). *Tritrichomonas foetus* fails to grow in normoxia, while the growth of *Trichomonas vaginalis* is slowed by *in vitro* exposure to normoxia (121).

### Lethal Effects of Oxygen on Protozoa

Inadequate antioxidant defenses appear to play an important role in the marked susceptibility of some parasites to killing by raised oxygen tensions. For example, *Giardia lamblia* does not contain any catalase or peroxidase (197) and is killed by normal oxygen levels *in vitro* (63). Several protozoans such as *E. histolytica* (61, 144), promastigotes of *Leishmania donovani* (165) and *L. tropica* (142) are relatively susceptible to $H_2O_2$. Exogenously-added catalase reduces killing (61, 142, 165) *L. donovani* and *L. tropica* promastigotes have high superoxide dismutase activity, but low catalase and glutathione peroxidase activity (131, 142). On the other hand, *Toxoplasma gondii* have atypically high activities of catalase and glutathione peroxidase (142, 147) and is consequently more resistant to killing by $H_2O_2$, but not by $O_2^-$ (146). The susceptibility of parasites to oxidative stress also varies depending upon the stage in the parasite life cycle. Different stages in parasite life cycles are also associated with shifts in levels of antioxidant enzymes. For example, compared to promastigotes, amastigotes of *L. donovani* are more resistant to oxidant-mediated killing by monocytes (145) because of a 3-fold higher activity of SOD (143).

A Brazilian group has done several studies on the role of oxygen tension and HBO therapy in *L. amazonensis* infection. In an *in vitro* study analyzing the effect of hypoxia on *L. amazonensis* infection in human and murine macrophages, this group showed a reduction in the percentage of infected cells and the number of intracellular parasites per cell (210) Observations on the kinetics of infection indicated that hypoxia did not depress *L. amazonensis* phagocytosis but did induce macrophages to reduce intracellular parasitism (210). Another study investigated the effects of standard HBO treatment protocols on the life cycle of *L. amazonensis*. HBO treatment induced irreversible metabolic damage to the parasite and affected its ability to transform from promastigote to amastigote, while the addition of an anti-oxidant, N-acetylcysteine (NAC), prevented some of these deleterious effects, indicating an increase in oxidative stress due to HBO exposure (211). In addition, HBO-exposed, *L. amazonensis*-infected macrophage cultures showed reduction of the percentage of infected cells and of the number of intracellular parasites per cell (211). This group's most recent study showed that mice infected with *L. amazonensis* that were exposed to HBO (2.5 ATA), one hour before parasite inoculation and subsequently for 20 days, showed significant delay in lesion development, reduction in lesion parasite burdens, and significantly elevated circulating levels of IFN-gamma and TNF-alpha compared with HBO-unexposed mice (212).

## Susceptibility of Helminths to Oxygen

As is the case for protozoans, the susceptibility of helminths such as *Schistosoma mansoni* and *Trichinella spiralis* to oxygen appears to be dependent upon the levels of antioxidant enzymes present in specific developmental stages (8, 105, 134, 135, 149). Adult schistosomes have higher levels of antioxidant enzymes than the larval stage (schistosomula) and are protected against killing by oxygen (134, 135, 149). *Schistosoma* eggs in liver tissue cultured in 21% $O_2$ are killed in four days (53). The addition of an SOD-like compound prevents killing of the schistosomes (53). Two non-pathogenic nematodes, *Turbatrix aceti* and *Caenorhabditis elegans* are killed by a prolonged exposure to HBO (3 ATA) *in vitro*; SOD and catalase inhibitors increase the lethality of oxygen (14).

## Effects of Oxygen in Experimental Models of Parasitic Infections

*In vivo* studies confirm that the viability of *Schistosoma* eggs depends on tissue oxygen tensions (53). *Schistosoma* eggs in liver tissue remain viable for at least 12 days after infection. However, *Schistosoma* eggs in the lungs do not survive longer than 6 days. The ability of the egg to survive in the liver may in part be due to the normally low oxygen tensions ($pO_2$ averaging 15 mmHg) in this organ (100).

*Chlamydia trachomatis*, an obligate intracellular parasite, is also susceptible to killing by hyperoxia. Hyperoxia (77% $O_2$) prevents mortality in mice infected with *C. trachomatis*, while a 65% mortality occurs in the infected, normoxia-exposed group (69). Infectious titers are at least 25-fold lower in hyperoxia-exposed mice compared to normoxic mice 9 to 11 days after the start of the infection.

In summary, most parasites have limited antioxidant enzyme defenses. Differences in the oxygen susceptibility of various developmental stages of the parasite appear to be caused by changes in the levels of antioxidant enzymes.

## EFFECTS OF HYPERBARIC OXYGEN IN FUNGAL INFECTIONS

### Fungistatic Effects of Oxygen

Hyperoxia inhibits the growth of some fungi. Exposure of *Schizosaccharomyces pombe* to hyperoxia (100% $O_2$ at 1 ATA) or hyperbaric oxygen (100% $O_2$ at 2 ATA) for 8 hours decreases the growth rate by 41% and 72%, respectively (191). The growth of *Candida albicans in vitro* is inhibited by prolonged exposure to hyperbaric oxygen (50% $O_2$ at 2.5 ATA) (77). This protocol was chosen to approximate the levels of oxygen found in tissues of patients treated with HBO. An intermittent exposure protocol (3 x 1.5 hours every 8 hours followed by 4 x 1.5 hours every 12 hours) is also fungistatic (28). However, the *in vitro* growth of *C. albicans* is not affected by treatment with hyperbaric oxygen three times daily at 2 ATA for 1 hour (23). *Rhizopus oryzae*, a fungus that commonly causes rhinocerebral mucormycosis, is more susceptible than *Candida sp.* to hyperoxia. The effects of pressure and oxygen are additive in inhibiting the growth of *R. oryzae in vitro* (54).

### Fungicidal Effects of Oxygen

Prolonged exposure to HBO (100% $O_2$ between 2.5 and 3 ATA) is fungicidal for *C. albicans* and several other *Candida sp* (16, 77). There is strong evidence indicating that *Pneumocystis carinii* is a fungus (48). *P. carinii* has low levels of antioxidant enzymes and is very susceptible to hyperoxia. A 10-minute exposure to 70% $O_2$ *in vitro* appears to be lethal for this microorganism (158).

### Mechanisms of Antifungal Effects of Oxygen

Oxygen-based free radicals are thought to be responsible for the fungistatic and fungicidal effects of hyperbaric oxygen because mutants lacking antioxidant enzymes are more susceptible to killing by HBO. For example, mutants of *Saccharomyces cerevisiae* with an inactivated SOD gene exhibited diminished growth under hyperoxic conditions (100% $O_2$ at 1 ATA) *in vitro* (59). On the other hand, induction of antioxidant enzymes may protect fungi from subsequent exposure to hyperoxia. Enzyme inactivation and damage to membrane transport systems induced by free radicals account for the reduced growth rate caused by hyperoxia in fungi. In *S. pombe* for example (191), hyperoxia (100% $O_2$ at 1 ATA) *in vitro* reduces protein synthesis by one-half and completely inhibits the uptake of glycine, leucine, and uracil in a noncompetitive manner (191). Killing of *S. cerevisiae* by HBO is reduced by inducing antioxidant enzymes before the HBO exposure (76).

The antifungal agent Amphotericin B can generate the superoxide anion by reduction-oxidation cycling reactions (78). Incubation in hypoxia or the addition of catalase protect fungal protoplasts against lysis by Amphotericin B (178). Hyperbaric oxygen in addition to direct fungicidal effects, may potentiate the antifungal activity of Amphotericin B. An additive antifungal effect of HBO (100% $O_2$ at 2.5 ATA, 1.5 hours) and Amphotericin B has been found *in vitro* against *C. albicans* (77).

## Clinical Studies

Studies with animal models of fungal infections are needed to further evaluate the antifungal effects of HBO. Two clinical reports have found hyperbaric oxygen to be a useful adjunctive therapy in mucormycosis infections. Price and Stevens (160) used HBO (100% $O_2$ at 2 ATA, twice daily for 2 days, then once daily, for 18 days) and Amphotericin B to treat a patient with fulminant mucormycosis. The patient eventually died of unrelated causes; lack of fungal growth was documented at autopsy. Couch et al. (37) used HBO to successfully treat a patient diagnosed with rhinocerebral mucormycosis. HBO (100% $O_2$ at 2.5 ATA for 90 minutes, 6 days a week) was used as an adjunctive treatment to surgical debridement and Amphotericin B and ketoconazole.

Ferguson et al. (54) performed a retrospective study of 13 patients with rhinocerebral mucormycosis. All patients were treated with Amphotericin B and underwent surgical debridement; 6 of these patients received HBO treatments (2 ATA $O_2$ for 2 hours, 2-11 times at 12-hour intervals, then 3-20 times at 24-hour intervals). Two out of 6 patients receiving HBO therapy died of non-fungus related causes. In contrast, 4 out of 7 patients not receiving HBO therapy died as a result of the mucormycosis infection (54).

A more recent randomized controlled trial in a murine model analyzing the efficacy of HBO as an adjunct for treating zygomycosis showed that the addition of hyperbaric oxygen (2.0 ATA) to Amphotericin B did not improve survival over that achieved with Amphotericin B and placebo air treatments (213). Another group examined the effects of transient hyperoxia in CD4+ depleted mice with Pneumocystis pneumonia where the mice were initially maintained in normoxia, then exposed to a hyperoxic treatment regimen (214). Despite no difference in organism burden between the two groups, CD4+ depleted mice with Pneumocystis pneumonia demonstrated significant mortality after transient exposure to hyperoxia while all uninfected control mice survived the stress (214).

In summary, hyperbaric oxygen within clinically achievable ranges is either fungistatic or fungicidal for *Pneumocystis carinii* and *Rhizopus oryzae*. In the case of *P. carinii*, as little as a 10-minute exposure to hyperoxia appears to be lethal. However, hyperoxia should not be substituted for current antimicrobial therapy in the treatment of patients infected with *P. carinii*. The mechanism of fungal killing by HBO appears to be caused by oxidative stress, which inhibits protein synthesis and decreases transport of amino acids across fungal membranes.

## INFLUENCE OF OXYGEN TENSIONS IN VIRAL INFECTIONS

Presently there is no evidence of direct beneficial effects of HBO in viral infections. However, it appears that oxygen tensions affect the growth and virulence of certain viruses. Hypoxia (3% $O_2$) causes marked alterations in growth characteristics of some viruses. Plaque diameter and plating efficiency of adenoviruses cultured under hypoxic conditions are markedly reduced (46). In contrast, polioviruses are not adversely affected by hypoxic conditions (46). Replication of rubella virus in hamster kidney cells was not altered during exposure to oxygen tensions ranging from 1 to 330 mmHg (108).

Reactive oxygen species cause single-strand breaks in DNA (97). Viral DNA may be particularly susceptible to oxidative damage because viruses lack antioxidants and DNA repair mechanisms. Exogenous SOD and catalase combine to confer protection against inactivation of viruses (51). Therefore, it is possible that antioxidants in the host cells may protect viruses against free radicals. Thus, exogenous antioxidants may account, at least in part, for the viral resistance to hyperoxia.

Effects of various oxygen tensions in murine models of viral infections have been examined. In a model of encephalomyocarditis caused by the MM virus, hypobaric hypoxia (21% $O_2$ at 0.5 ATA) significantly increased mortality as compared to normoxia (71). Exposure to hypobaric normoxia (100% $O_2$ at 0.2 ATA) also increased mortality in mice infected with influenza A virus (68). However, neither normobaric hypoxia (11% $O_2$ at 1 ATA) nor hyperoxia (77% $O_2$ at 1 ATA) altered mortality. Thus, it appears that decreased atmospheric pressure, rather than oxygen tension, influenced mortality due to influenza A virus in that study. In contrast, Ayers et al. (5) found that exposure to hyperoxia (99% $O_2$ at 1 ATA) resulted in influenza-infected mice dying 3 to 4 days earlier than normoxic controls. One possible explanation is the finding by Naldini et al. (148) that the antiviral activity of interferon-alpha (and interferon-gamma) is decreased *in vitro* under "normoxic" conditions (140 mmHg $O_2$) compared to "hypoxic" conditions (14 mmHg $O_2$). Exposure to hypoxia (11% $O_2$) increased mortality and viral titers in tissue of mice infected with Coxsackie B-1 virus (65). Interestingly, hypobaric hypoxia (21% $O_2$ at 0.5 ATA) increased viral titers, but not mortality (65). In addition, HBO (100% $O_2$ at 3 ATA) enhanced mortality in mice infected with Coxsackie B-1 virus (154). Pretreatment of mice with HBO significantly increased viral titers in heart muscle and brown fat by three days after inoculation of the virus (154). The effects of HBO may have been mediated through free radicals since, in another model of Coxsackie B3 myocarditis, polyethylene-conjugated SOD reduced cellular infiltration, myocardial necrosis, and calcification scores, compared to the control group at day 14, after intraperitoneal challenge in C3H/He mice (92). There were no differences in viral titers among the three groups at day 7 and viral titers were no longer detected by day 14 in any of the treatment groups (92).

Another recent study investigated the basis of treating chronic hepatitis with HBO and to compare the changes in hepatic function, immunity, pathologic morphology, ultrastructure and HBV in hepatic tissues before and after treatment. The experimental group was treated with six courses of HBO while the control group was treated for 60 days with standard therapy (215). There were significant differences between the experimental and control groups after treatment; for the experimental group, all markers of hepatic function and hepatocyte degeneration or necrosis were decreased, but the fibrosis and fat-storing cells in the liver were not reduced (215).

In summary, oxygen tensions appear to influence the outcome of viral infections in animal models. Hyperoxia appears to increase mortality in mice infected with influenza A virus or Cocksackie B-1 virus. Hypoxic conditions also increase mortality in Coxsackie B-1 infected mice. Treatment of chronic HBV with HBO appears to be effective, and should be considered as an adjunct to standard pharmacologic therapy. HBO has not been shown to be effective at reversing liver fibrosis.

## OXYGEN TENSIONS ALTER THE ACTIVITY OF CERTAIN ANTIMICROBIAL AGENTS

### Effects of Anaerobiosis on Antibacterial Agents

Minimal inhibitory concentrations (MIC) and minimal bactericidal concentrations (MBC) assays have been used to study the interactions between oxygen and antimicrobial agents *in vitro*. It is clear that the activity of several antibacterial agents is diminished (as evidenced by increased MICs and/or MBCs) in an anaerobic atmosphere. See Table 1. In anaerobic environments, the MICs of the aminoglycoside antibiotics (amikacin, gentamicin, kanamycin, and tobramycin) are significantly increased against *E. coli*, *Enterobacter*, *Klebsiella*, *Salmonella*, *Serratia*, *Staphylococcus*, and *Streptococcus sp*. See Tables 1 and 3 (27, 83, 151, 166, 183, 192). The decreased activity of aminoglycosides in an anaerobic atmosphere is associated with decreased rates of bacterial quinone redox cycling and low transmembrane potential (26). These changes are thought to decrease the transport of aminoglycosides into bacteria. One way to circumvent the redox-dependent transport of aminoglycosides is to

## TABLE 3. DECREASED EFFECTIVENESS OF GENTAMICIN UNDER ANAEROBIC CONDITIONS

| E. coli Strain | ZONES OF INHIBITION (mm) | | RATIO |
| | Aerobic | Anaerobic | Aerobic/Anaerobic |
|---|---|---|---|
| atcc 25922 | 22.9 | 12.5 | 1.83 |
| 0:18 | 25.5 | 13.0 | 1.96 |
| 1 | 23.3 | 12.4 | 1.88 |
| 3 | 22.0 | 11.5 | 1.91 |
| 5 | 23.7 | 11.6 | 2.04 |
| 8 | 23.1 | 9.6 | 2.41 |
| 9 | 24.6 | 12.8 | 1.92 |
| 11 | 22.1 | 11.3 | 1.96 |
| 12 | 22.6 | 10.6 | 2.13 |
| 13 | 21.7 | 11.9 | 1.82 |
| 15 | 21.3 | 11.1 | 1.92 |

Strains of Escherichia coli were seeded onto cation-supplemented Mueller Hinton agar plates and gentamicin-containing discs were placed on the agar surface. After 24 hours in anaerobiosis or normoxia, diameters of zone of inhibition were measured.

disrupt the bacterial cell wall. Cefotaxime was able to enhance tobramycin and amikacin uptake in the isolates of *E. coli* under anaerobic conditions, resulting in enhanced bactericidal activity (27).

The MBC of sulfamethoxazole (193) and trimethoprim (83, 193) against *S. aureus* increase markedly under anaerobic and hypoxic conditions. Both the MIC and MBC of vancomycin against *S. aureus* increase 4-fold and 8-fold, respectively, under anaerobic conditions (151). The MBC of fluoroquinolones (ciprofloxacin, ofloxacin, and norfloxacin) against *E. coli* increase under anaerobic conditions (176). The mechanism(s) of the decreased activities of the antimicrobials listed above are not known. Interestingly, the bacteriostatic effects of ciprofloxacin were unchanged under anaerobic conditions (176). In contrast, the bactericidal activity of metronidazole is optimal under anaerobic conditions, and is reduced or almost absent in aerobic conditions (184). Oxygen-dependent changes in redox potential affect the activation of this antimicrobial, and explain the loss of activity in aerobic conditions.

## Interactions Between Hypoxia and Normoxia with Antibacterial Agents

Alterations of oxygen tensions within the normal physiologic range seen in body tissues can also alter the activity of antibacterial agents. For example, ceftazidime *in vitro* showed greater bactericidal activity against *P. aeruginosa* at a $pO_2$ of 80 mmHg as compared to a $pO_2$ of 40 mmHg (10).

Adequate oxygen tensions are also essential for optimum activity of reduction-oxidation cycling antimicrobials. These antimicrobials transfer electrons to oxygen and generate superoxide anion. The production of superoxide is at least in part responsible for the bacteriostatic activity of reduction-oxidation cycling antimicrobials (138). Organisms grown under anaerobic conditions contain lower constitutive levels of antioxidant enzymes. Bacteria grown under anaerobic conditions, and subsequently exposed to redox cycling antimicrobials under normoxic conditions, exhibit greater susceptibility to these antimicrobials. Streptonigrin (81) and rifamycin SV (112) are two examples of redox-cycling antimicrobials that exhibit greater activity under normoxic conditions as compared to anoxia.

Recent work indicates that oxygen tensions influence the period of bacterial growth suppression after exposure to an antibiotic. This period of growth suppression is known as the post-antibiotic effect (PAE) (38, 120). More specifically, the PAE is defined as the time required for antimicrobial-treated bacteria to increase in numbers by 1 log10 CFU/mL after the removal of the drug (38). Bayer et al. (10) showed that the *in vitro* PAE for amikacin against *P. aeruginosa* was diminished by 50% when the $pO_2$ was increased from 40 mmHg to 80 mmHg. A more recent study showed that hypoxia ($pO_2 = 26$ mmHg) did not influence the PAE of another aminoglycoside (tobramycin) against *P. aeruginosa* (156).

## Interactions Between Hyperoxia and HBO with Antibacterial Agents

Elevated oxygen tensions may alter the activity of certain antimicrobial agents. We have recently determined that hyperoxia (100% $O_2$ at 1 ATA for 1 hour) prolongs the *in vitro* PAE of tobramycin in *P. aeruginosa* by two-fold, compared to normoxia. See Table 4 (156). However, bactericidal effects of tobramycin against *P. aeruginosa* and *E. coli* are not enhanced by hyperoxia (100% $O_2$ at 1 ATA) or HBO (100% $O_2$ at 2 ATA or 98% $O_2$ at 2% $CO_2$, 2.8 ATA) (23, 138, 156).

HBO also potentiates the activity of antimetabolite antimicrobials. See Table 1. In the case of two para-aminobenzoic acid (PABA) analogs, sulfisoxazole and mafenide, HBO enhances the bacteriostatic activity by two-fold against *P. aeruginosa* (155). HBO also increases the bactericidal activity of mafenide to the same extent (155). HBO (100% $O_2$ at 2.87 ATA) also enhances the bacteriostatic effect of sulfisoxazole (five- to ten-fold) and trimethoprim (two to four fold) against *Corynebacterium diphtheriae* (71). HBO (98% $O_2$ at 2% $CO_2$ at 2.8 ATA for 24 hours) *in vitro* significantly decreases both the MIC and MBC of trimethoprim by 50% against *E. coli*, as compared to normoxia (138). Interestingly, while HBO (100% $O_2$ at 1.87 ATA) does not enhance the activity of sulfamethoxazole or trimethoprim alone against *Branhamella (moraxella) catarrhalis*, it does act synergistically when given in combination with both antimicrobials (70). These studies support the hypothesis that HBO oxidizes enzymes or metabolic intermediates of the folate synthesis pathway in both gram-positive and gram-negative bacteria.

In addition, HBO enhances the activity of reduction-oxidation cycling antimicrobials such as nitrofurantoin. HBO (98% $O_2$ and 2% $CO_2$ at 2.8 ATA for 24 hours *in vitro*) significantly decreases the MIC of nitrofurantoin by a factor of 3 against *E. coli* as compared to normoxia (138). The enhanced bacteriostatic activity is most probably due to increased $O_2$- production, since nitrofurantoin can increase cyanide-resistant respiration in *E. coli* under normoxic conditions (138).

A German group has done several recent studies on treating osteomyelitis due to *S. aureus* in rats with HBO and antibiotics. The first study analyzed the use of HBO and parenteral cefazolin, individually and in

## TABLE 4. HYPEROXIA OR HYPERBARIC OXYGEN INFLUENCE THE REGROWTH OF *PSEUDOMONAS AERUGINOSA* AFTER EXPOSURE TO TOBRAMYCIN

| TIME (HOURS) REQUIRED FOR BACTERIA TO INCREASE 1 $\log_{10}$ CFU/ml | | | |
|---|---|---|---|
| $O_2$ | No treatment | Tobramycin | Treatment |
| 21%$O_2$ | 1 ATA Control) | 2.2 + 0.13 | 2.9 + 0.13 |
| 100%$O_2$ | 1 ATA (Hyperoxia) | 2.0 + 0.12 | 3.4 + 1.9 |
| 100%$O_2$ | 2.8 ATA (HBO) | 2.7 + 0.09[a] | 4.4 + 0.18[bc] |

Cultures of Pseudomonas aeruginosa were treated with trobramycin at 4 X MIC in one of three different oxygen tensions. After 1 hour, tobramycin was removed by filtration and bacterial regrowth was measured. Significant differences are as follows: a) different from untreated control; b) different from tobramycin-treated control; c) different from tobramycin and hyperoxia-treated group. Table adapted from Park et al. (156).

combination (207). Treatment with HBO alone reduced the colony-forming units (CFU) from 2.9 x $10^6$ CFU per gram of tibial bone, as demonstrated in the control group, to 6.2 x $10^5$ CFU/gram, cefazolin reduced this to 10.5 x $10^4$ CFU/gram, and the combination of HBO and cefazolin reduced the colony count to 2.7 x $10^3$ CFU/gram (207). In a more recent study, the rat model was used to compare the efficacy of treating *S. aureus*-induced osteomyelitis with HBO, a gentamicin-containing collagen sponge, or a combination of the two. In the control group, the infection was 4.9 x $10^6$ CFU/gram of tibial bone three weeks after inoculation, which decreased to 3.7 x $10^6$ CFU/gram by the end of the experiment after soft tissue debridement (208). In the treatment groups, HBO reduced the infection to 1.7 x $10^5$ CFU/gram and the gentamicin-collagen sponge reduced the organisms to 1.4 x $10^2$ CFU/gram, but with combination therapy, bacteria was no longer detectable from samples of the processed bone substance in 9 of the 11 subjects (208).

In a related study, this group also compared monotherapy with cefazolin, gentamicin-PMMA beads, or gentamicin-containing collagen sponge with the combination of local and systemic antibiotic treatment. Single-agent therapy with parenterally administered cefazolin reduced the severity of infection from 3.7 x $10^6$ CFU/gram to 2.9 x $10^4$ CFU/gram. With local antibiotic delivery, the gentamicin-PMMA beads reduced the infection to 9.8 x $10^2$ CFU/gram and the gentamicin-containing collagen sponge reduced the bacterial count to 1.4 x $10^2$ CFU/gram (209). The combination of gentamicin-containing collagen sponge and parenteral cefazolin produced the most profound effect since bacteria was not detected in samples of the processed bone substance in 9 of the 11 subjects (209). These studies not only demonstrate the effectivness of HBO as a monotherapy, but also that it may be as effective as an adjunctive therapy as adding a parenteral antibiotic, in this case, cefazolin, to an implanted antibiotic delivery device containing an aminoglycoside.

In summary, HBO has important influences on the activity of certain antimicrobial agents. These influences are specific for certain types of antimicrobials and for certain species of bacteria. As Table 1 indicates, anoxia decreases the activity of several antimicrobials. HBO may normalize the activity of these antimicrobials by raising the $pO_2$ of ischemic tissue to normoxic levels. In addition, HBO may potentiate the activity of certain antimicrobials by inhibiting biosynthetic reactions in bacteria. Finally, HBO may influence the activity of certain types of antimicrobial agents by influencing the rates of their metabolic activation. Examples of these mechanisms of action of HBO are shown in Table 5.

## Effects of Oxygen on the Activity of Antiparasitic Agents

HBO promotes the generation of reactive oxygen species and may interact with certain antimicrobials to kill parasites that lack adequate antioxidant defenses. Free radical mechanisms account for the cidal actions of many antiparasitic drugs such as antimalarials, quinones and nitro compounds (44).

Several investigators have studied the effects of decreased oxygen tensions on the *in vitro* activity of antiparasitic drugs; however, there have not been any studies that we know of on the effects of elevated oxygen tensions on

## TABLE 5. MECHANISMS BY WHICH HBO INFLUENCED THE ACTIVITY OF ANTIMICROBIAL AGENTS

1) Elevation of the $pO_2$ of ischemic tissue to levels required for optimal activity of certain antimicrobial agents. Examples are: aminoglycosides, certain sulfonamides, fluoroquinolones, trimethoprim, vancomycin.

2) Inhibition of bacterial biosynthetic reactions. Examples are the potentiation of the activity of sulfonamides, and the prolongation of the postantibiotic effect of aminoglycosides in *Pseudomonas* infections.

3) Altering of the oxidation-reduction potential in bacteria. Examples are increased production of reactive intermediates (nitrofurantion) and decreased activation of antimicrobial agents dependent on low redox potential (metronidazole).

this class of antimicrobial agents. For example, the dose of miconazole and ketoconazole required to inhibit *Plasmodium falciparum* by 50% is decreased at normal oxygen tensions (18% $O_2$), compared to hypoxia (3% $O_2$) (159). In addition, the activity of clindamycin, erythromycin, chloramphenicol, and tetracyclines were also enhanced under 15% $O_2$, compared to 1% $O_2$ (43). By contrast, the antiparasitic activity of metronidazole is decreased under normal oxygen tensions. Normoxia reduces the uptake of metronidazole by *Trichomonas vaginalis, Tritrichomonas foetus,* and *Entamaoeba invadens*; (141) the decrease in uptake was reversible upon re-exposure to anoxia. The LC50 of metronidazole against *Giardia lamblia* trophozoites increases from 2.8 ug/mL under hypoxic conditions, to 500 ug/mL under normoxic conditions (64).

## Effects of Oxygen on the Activity of Antifungal Agents

Only a few studies have described the effects of oxygen on the activity of antifungal agents. Amphotericin B-mediated killing of *Candida albicans* appears to be the result of increased oxidative damage (178). In addition, either hypoxia or catalase protect *C. albicans* protoplasts from Amphotericin B-induced lysis (178). HBO (100% $O_2$ at 2.5 ATA) enhances the activity of Amphotericin B against *C. albicans* in an additive manner. A lower dose of HBO (50% $O_2$ at 2.5 ATA) did not decrease the MIC or the minimal cidal concentration (MCC) of Amphotericin B, nystatin, clotrimazole, miconazole or 5-fluorocytosine against *C. albicans*, as compared to normoxic controls (77). Interestingly, HBO (50% $O_2$ at 2.5 ATA) increases both the MIC and MCC for ketoconazole against *C. albicans* more than 1000-fold, as compared to normoxic controls (77). The mechanism for the loss of ketoconazole activity is unknown; however, HBO treatment did not inactivate ketoconazole.

The addition of the reduction-oxidation cycling drug menadione to *Saccharomyces cerevisiae* cultures completely inhibited growth under normoxic conditions (32). However, menadione did not affect the growth of *S. cerevisiae* under anaerobic conditions. Exogenous superoxide dismutase abolished the cidal effects of menadione against *S. cerevisiae* (32).

## OXYGEN TENSIONS AND ACUTE AND CHRONIC INFLAMMATORY CELLS

### Decrease in Bacterial Numbers in Ischemic and Hypoxic Tissues Exposed to Hyperoxia

In addition to direct interactions with microorganisms and antimicrobial agents, HBO can also influence the outcome of infections by interactions with parenchymal cells and with inflammatory cells. In necrotizing infections, HBO augments tissue survival by sustaining cellular oxidative metabolism. The size of necrotizing skin lesions in guinea pigs inoculated subcutaneously with *E. coli* decreases in animals breathing 45% $O_2$, and increases in animals breathing 12% $O_2$ (110, 111). Hyperoxia decreases tissue necrosis by decreasing bacterial numbers, and by enhancing the survival of ischemic infected tissue (110). In dogs breathing 12% $O_2$, the necrosis of *S. aureus*-infected musculocutaneous and cutaneous flaps increases (103). Hunt et al. (96) found that oxygen tensions were lowered in rabbit subcutaneous tissues infected with *P. aeruginosa*. Hypoxic rabbits (12% $O_2$) had approximately 1-2 log10 more bacteria, whereas rabbits breathing 45% $O_2$ had 2 log10 less bacteria compared to controls breathing 21% $O_2$ (96). See Table 6. The increase in bacterial growth under 12% $O_2$ can be explained by decreased PMN function under low $pO_2$ (94).

Increasing the amount of oxygen that is delivered to ischemic tissue with HBO may lower bacterial counts in wounds and improve healing by mechanisms other than its bacteriostatic and bacteriocidal properties. Treatment with HBO (2.1 ATA) in a mouse model resulted in improved microvascular perfusion and angiogenesis as indicated by a 20% increase in wound blood flow over baseline using laser Doppler imaging on day 7 and 10 in the treatment group, but only on day 10 in the control group (219). Another group investigated the effect of an HBO regimen (2.1 ATA) on wound healing in rats by analyzing wound fluids for VEGF and lactate 2, 5, and 10 days after injury (218). This study showed that wound oxygen rose with HBO from nearly 0 mmHg to as high as 600 mmHg by the end of a single treatment, VEGF levels significantly increased with HBO by 40%, and

### TABLE 6. HYPEROXIA INHIBITS WHILE HYPOXIA ENHANCES THE GROWTH OF *PSEUDOMONAS AERUGINOSA* IN SUBCUTANEOUS TISSUE

|  | FiO$_2$ INSPIRED AIR | pO$_2$ ARTERIAL BLOOD | pO$_2$ TISSUE | BACTERIAL NUMBERS log$_{10}$ CFU/ml |
|---|---|---|---|---|
| Hypoxia | 12% | 39 | 6 | 5.2 |
| Normoxia | 21% | 69 | 11 | 3.6 |
| Hyperoxia | 45% | 191 | 14 | 1.2 |

Table adapted from (96) with permission from Annals of Surgery. The bacterial suspension was inoculated under the skin of rabbits; bacterial numbers were measured from aspirated tissue fluid.

wound lactate levels remain unchanged with HBO treatment (218). A general study on the benefits of therapeutic oxygen in wound healing showed that applying topical oxygen therapy on chronic, complex wounds resulted in the healing of thirty-eight wounds in 15 patients with no detrimental effects (217). Despite the evidence that using higher doses of therapeutic oxygen can improve blood flow and accelerate the wound healing process, a recent double-blind, randomized controlled trial was performed to determine whether the routine use of $O_2$ at higher doses during the perioperative period altered the incidence of surgical site infection (SSI) (216). The incidence of infection was significantly higher in the group receiving 80% $O_2$ than the group receiving 35% $O_2$ (25.0% vs 11.3%; P = 0.02), showing that the routine use of high perioperative $FIO_2$ in a general surgical population does not reduce the overall incidence of SSI (216).

## Influence of Oxygen on Phagocytosis and Killing of Microorganisms by Polymorphonuclear Leukocytes

Oxygen tensions also affect PMN and macrophage function. Physiologic functions (eg., phagocytosis) of PMNs are sustained in hypoxic or near anaerobic environments of infected tissues by anaerobic glycolysis (4, 185). Oxidant-mediated killing of bacteria by PMNs, albeit at reduced rates can still occur at very low $pO_2$s, such as 3%, the mean oxygen tension present in abscesses (87). However, under anaerobic conditions, no oxidative burst occurs and bacterial killing is diminished. Anaerobiosis (< 1% $O_2$) inhibits the killing of *Staphylococcus aureus*, *Escherichia coli*, *Serratia marcescens*, *Klebsiella pneumoniae*, *Proteus vulgaris*, and *Salmonella typhimurium* by PMNs (94, 125). Killing of *S. aureus* by rabbit PMNs under anaerobic conditions decreases by one-half (94). Under hypoxic conditions (12% $FIO_2$) *in vivo*, the phagocytic clearance of *S. aureus*, *E. coli*, and *K. pneumoniae* in lung tissues is impaired (84).

Studies *in vivo* have confirmed that hyperoxia and HBO can increase phagocytic killing of bacteria by raising tissue oxygen tensions. Optimal killing of *S. aureus* in subcutaneous lesions occurs when rabbits breathe 45% $O_2$ (94). Hyperbaric oxygen (100% $O_2$ at 2 ATA) increases the killing of *Staphylococcus aureus* by PMNs in osteomyelitis by increasing the $pO_2$ in infected bone from 21 mmHg to 104 mmHg (122). Increasing $pO_2$ from 45 mmHg to 150 mmHg increases the killing of *S. aureus* by PMNs *in vitro*. It is possible that HBO indirectly increases bacterial killing in bone by providing optimal oxygen tensions for the oxidative burst in PMNs (122), but there is still no definitive evidence for this specific hypothesis.

One study evaluating the effects of HBO (2.5 ATA) on human neutrophils showed no differences in either respiratory burst or phagocytic activity either before or after HBO therapy, regardless of short- or long-term exposure, indicating that hyperoxia does not impair these two aspects of the human innate host defense (221). PMNs obtained from the peritoneal exudates of mice exposed to hyperbaric oxygen twice daily for 8 days showed no difference in the ability to phagocytose *S. aureus* or to generate an oxidative burst (58). Likewise, exposure to HBO (100% $O_2$ at 2-3 ATA) for 2 hours did not decrease adherence or inhibit phagocytosis in mouse spleen macrophages (129). A two-hour exposure of *P. aeruginosa* and peritoneal exudate cells to

HBO resulted in increased bacterial clearance, compared to normoxia-maintained cultures (199).

Continuous prolonged exposure to high $FIO_2$s such as are required for severe respiratory failure, can inhibit PMN function (39, 47, 167). Prolonged *in vitro* exposure (greater than 24 hours) of macrophages to hyperoxia or hyperbaric oxygen reduces bacterial clearance by inhibiting phagocytosis, oxidant-mediated killing, cell locomotion, and DNA synthesis (18, 56, 150, 162, 163, 175, 182, 199). *In vivo* studies have confirmed that continuous, prolonged exposure of lung tissue to a high $pO_2$ (85% $O_2$ for 90 hours) decreases the chemotactic activity, adherence, phagocytosis, and bactericidal activity of alveolar macrophages, probably by depleting intracellular levels of the reduced form of glutathione, and by affecting microtubule formation (152, 167). Another group used human subjects to investigate the effects of hyperoxia on Mac-1 mediated neutrophil function, and showed that neutrophil adhesion was reduced by 50% two hours after treatment with HBO (3.0 ATA) (220).

There is evidence that sub-lethal hyperoxia causes impairment of macrophage function, as well. An *in vivo* study done in mice showed that hyperoxia leads to greatly reduced alveolar epithelial cell GM-CSF expression, a growth factor that is critically involved in the maintenance of normal alveolar macrophage function in mice that are infected with *K. pneumonia* (224). Systemic treatment of the these mice with recombinant murine GM-CSF during hyperoxia exposure preserved alveolar macrophage function, as indicated by cell surface Toll-like receptor expression and by inflammatory cytokine secretion following stimulation with lipopolysaccharide (224). In another study, transgenic over expression of GM-CSF enhanced survival of mice in hyperoxia. On histologic examination, the mutant mouse lungs had preserved alveolar epithelial barrier function and fluid clearance, which may be attributable to a reduction in hyperoxia-induced apoptosis of cells in the alveolar wall (225). Another study investigating the effects of hyperoxia and antioxidant enzymes on inflammation and clearance of *P. aeruginosa* in both adult and neonatal mononuclear cells found that hyperoxia significantly increased bacterial adherence while impairing function of mononuclear cells, with adult cells being more impaired than neonatal cells (223). Both manganese superoxide dismutase (MnSOD) and catalase reduced bacterial adherence and inflammation, but only MnSOD and improved bacterial phagocytosis in mononuclear cells in response to hyperoxia (223).

Treatment with antioxidants after either hypoxia or hyperoxia has demonstrated an impact on the preservation of function in both neutrophils and macrophages. One group used apnea divers as a human model of chronic hypoxia and re-oxygenation, and measured the effects of both repeated oxidative stress and treatment with Vitamin C on neutrophil antioxidant defenses, NO production, and redox status. Exposure to diving apnea caused an increase in several markers of both intra- and extra-cellular oxidative stress and initiated neutrophil reactions that resemble the acute-phase immune response by increasing myeloperoxidase activity (222). In the treatment group, Vitamin C reduced neutrophil catalase activity and levels and glutathione peroxidase activity after diving, along with lowering neutrophil iNOS levels and NO production after both diving and recovery (222). Hyperoxia has been shown to decrease the levels of the antioxidant glutathione (GSH) in the lungs of mice infected with *L. pneumophila*, while exogenous tumour necrosis factor-alpha (TNF-alpha) improved survival of these treatment subjects, suggesting that hyperoxia may inhibit the native immune response, including production of GSH, thereby exacerbating *L. pneumophila* pneumonia (204). Another study showed that phagocytosis of *P. aeruginosa* in macrophages was similarly reduced after exposure to both moderate- (65%) and high-dose (95%) hyperoxia in both *in vitro* and *in vivo* models (205). In addition, treatment with antioxidants, regardless of its timing, preserved actin cytoskeleton organization and phagocytosis of *P. aeruginosa*, suggesting that hyperoxia inhibits macrophage phagocytosis by altering actin function, which can be preserved by antioxidant treatment (205).

As in the case for bacteria, PMN and macrophages killed greater numbers of *Candida albicans* blastospores under aerobic conditions compared to anaerobic conditions (187). The use of hyperoxia [100% $O_2$ at 1 ATA] enhanced rat alveolar macrophage oxidative killing of opsonized *Neurospora crassa* by 52%, without affecting phagocytosis (177). Hyperoxia did not affect *conidia* viability in the absence of pulmonary alveolar macrophages.

Interestingly, in the case of *Mycobacterium tuberculosis* and *Mycobacterium avium*, both organisms grew significantly better in macrophages cultured *in vitro* at 140 mmHg $O_2$ than at 36 mmHg $O_2$ (130). Varying oxygen tensions did not affect extracellular growth of mycobacteria, thereby implying that oxygen tensions in tissues exposed to HBO may interfere with the mycobactericidal activity of macrophages.

## Influence of Oxygen on Lymphocyte Function

Resting T-lymphocytes are highly resistant to injury by either hypoxia or hyperoxia (1). However, mitogen-stimulated lymphocytes are markedly affected by tissue oxygen tensions. DNA synthesis by phytohemagglutinin-stimulated human lymphocytes is reduced or completely inhibited by exposure to hypoxia (3% $O_2$ - 9% $O_2$). Hyperoxia (70% $O_2$ or 100% $O_2$, for longer than 48 hours) also inhibits DNA synthesis in these stimulated lymphocytes (1, 116). The growth inhibition is slowly reversible when T-lymphocytes are returned to normoxia (116). In lymphocytes exposed to hyperoxia, RNA synthesis is inhibited even before DNA synthesis; a three-hour exposure to hyperoxia does not inhibit 3H-thymidine incorporation, but it is sufficient to inhibit 3H-uridine incorporation (93). The growth of unstimulated B-lymphocytes is also completely inhibited by hyperoxia (250 mmHg) (133).

Hyperoxia also inhibits the proliferation of T-lymphocytes *in vivo*. T-lymphocytes from mice exposed daily to 100% $O_2$ for eight days (2.4 ATA for 1.5 hours) show a 50% decrease in lymphocyte proliferation (58). Hyperbaric oxygen activates a sub-population of mitogen-stimulated CD8+ T-cells (LYT2/IL-2R) (58). Spleen cells isolated from mice exposed to hyperoxia for 72 hours also show decreased proliferation in response to stimulation by concanavalin A (72). Proliferation returns to normal in the presence of either an antioxidant (2-mercaptoethanol) or of macrophages. This suggests that hyperoxia may also inactivate critical macrophage functions necessary for the restoration of lymphocyte proliferation.

The effect of hyperbaric oxygen (100% $O_2$ at 2.5 ATA for 5 hours, daily) on T-lymphocytes has been studied using a model of contact sensitivity to the chemical dinitrofluorobenzene (DNFB) (80). Treatment with hyperbaric oxygen four days before and five days after DNFB sensitization, decreased the amount of tissue swelling compared to normoxia-exposed controls (80). Another study (49) examined the effect of hyperbaric oxygen treatment (1 to 3 ATA for 1 hour daily) five days before and four days after transgenic transfusion of red blood cells. In the treated animals, the immunohumoral responses to the incompatible transfusion (direct hemagglutination) were transiently decreased. The immunocellular response (delayed hypersensitivity reaction) was not affected. However, the number of HBO-treated animals that developed lymphocytic infiltrates was significantly decreased (49). It appears that hyperoxia and hyperbaric oxygen decrease DNA synthesis in T- and B-lymphocytes. The immunosuppressive effects caused by hyperbaric oxygen *in vivo* are, in most cases, associated with decreases in delayed-type hypersensitivity reactions, lymphocyte proliferation, and lymphocyte numbers.

## CONCLUSION

The mechanisms of action of hyperbaric oxygen in infectious diseases fall under three main categories. Namely, effects on: the growth and viability of microorganisms, the activity of antimicrobial agents, and the function of the immune system. Hyperbaric oxygen can be bactericidal for anaerobes primarily because of its ability to increase the production of free radicals and other toxic oxygen products. The lack of adequate antioxidant defenses in anaerobic microorganisms contributes to their susceptibility to HBO. HBO also potentiates the activity of selected antimicrobial agents. Most parasites are deficient in antioxidant defenses, particularly in early stages of their life cycle, and the efficacy of several antiparasitic drugs is dependent on this deficiency. These considerations suggest that parasites may be found to be more susceptible to HBO than we currently appreciate. HBO has various effects on immune cells. Anaerobiosis abolishes the oxidative burst of polymorphonuclear leukocytes. HBO facilitates the generation of the oxidative burst by restoring normal $pO_2$s in ischemic infected tissues. HBO treatment regimens in routine clinical use do not affect PMN and macrophage functions such as phagocytosis, superoxide production, and locomotion. Hyperoxia and hyperbaric oxygen decrease DNA synthesis in stimulated T-lymphocytes. These effects are associated with decreases in delayed-type hypersensitivity reactions, and in lymphocyte numbers.

**Disclaimer:** *The initial authors of the first edition of this review chapter were Matthew K. Park, Kenneth H. Muhvich, Roy A.M. Myers and Louis Marzella. Matthew K. Park is currently a clinical associate in the National Institute of Allergy and Infectious Diseases, NIH. This review chapter does not represent the views of the Laboratory of Clinical Investigation, NIAID, NIH, or the U.S Government.*

# REFERENCES

1. Andersen V, Hellung-Larsen P., Sørensen SF. "Optimal oxygen tension for human lymphocytes in culture." J Cell Physiol. 1968;72:149-152.

2. Angrick EJ, Somerson NL, Weiss HS. "Oxygen effects on mortality of mice infected with Diplococcus pneumoniae." Aerospace Med. 1974;45:730-734.

3. Archibald FS, Duong M-N. "Superoxide dismutase and oxygen toxicity defenses in the genus Neisseria." Infect Immun. 1986;51:631-641.

4. Axline SG. "Functional biochemistry of the macrophage." Semin Hematol. 1970;7:142-160.

5. Ayers LN, Tierney DF, Imagawa D. "Shortened survival of mice with influenza when given oxygen at one atmosphere." Am Rev Respir Dis. 1973;107:955-961.

6. Babior BM. "Oxygen-dependent microbial killing by phagocytes." New Engl J Med. 1978;298:659-668.

7. Band RN, Cirrito H. "Growth response of axenic Entamoeba histolytica to hydrogen, carbon dioxide, and oxygen." J Protozool. 1979;26:282-286.

8. Bass DA, Szejda P. "Mechanisms of killing of newborn larvae of Trichinella spiralis by neutrophils and eosinophils. Killing by generation of hydrogen peroxide *in vitro*. J Clin Invest. 1979;64:1558-1564.

9. Bastian FO, Jennings RA, Hoff CJ. "Effect of trimethoprim/ sulphomethoxazole and hyperbaric oxygen on experimental Spiroplasma mirum encephalitis." Res Microbiol. 1989;140:151-158.

10. Bayer AS, O'Brien T, Norman DC, Nast CC. "Oxygen-dependent differences in exopolysaccharide production and aminoglycoside inhibitory-bactericidal interactions with Pseudomonas aeruginosa- implications for endocarditis. J Antimicrob Chemother. 1989;23:21-35.

11. Beaman L, Beaman BL. "The role of oxygen and its derivatives in microbial pathogenesis and host defense." Ann Rev Microbiol. 1984;38:27-48.

12. Beaman BL, Black CM, Doughty F, Beaman L. "Role of superoxide dismutase nd catalase as determinants of pathogenicity of Nocardia asteroides: Importance in resistance to microbicidal activities of human polymorphonuclear neutrophils." Infect Immun. 1985;47:135-141.

13. Bender JG, Van Epps DE. "Stimulus interactions in release of superoxide anion ($O_2$-) from human neutrophils." Inflammation. 1985;9:67-79.

14. Blum J, Fridovich I. "Superoxide, hydrogen peroxide, and oxygen toxicity in two free-living nematode species." Arch Biochem. 1983;222:35-43.

15. Boehme DE, Vincent K, Brown OR. "Oxygen and toxicity inhibition of amino acid biosynthesis." Nature (Lond). 1976;262:418-420.

16. Bornside GH. "Quantitative cidal activity of hyperbaric oxygen for opportunistic yeast pathogens." Aviat Space Environ Med. 1978;49:1212-1214.

17. Bornside GH, Pakman LM, Ordoñez Jr AA. "Inhibition of pathogenic enteric bacteria by hyperbaric oxygen: enhanced antibacterial activity in the absence of carbon dioxide." Antimicrob Agents Chemother. 1975;7:682-687.

18. Bowles AL, Dauber JH, Daniele RP. "The effect of hyperoxia on migration of alveolar macrophages *in vitro*. Am Rev Respir Dis. 1979;120:541-545.

19. Brot N, Weissbach L, Werth J, Weissbach H. "Enzymatic reduction of protein-bound methionine sulfoxide." Proc Natl Acad Sci USA. 1981;78:2155-2158.

20. Brown OR. "Reversible inhibition of respiration of Escherichia coli by hyperoxia." Microbios. 1972;5:7-16.

21. Brown OR, Seither RL. "Oxygen and redox-active drugs: shared toxicity sites." Fundam Appl Toxicol. 1983;3:209-214.

22. Brown OR, Song C-S."Pyridine nucleotide coenzyme biosynthesis: a cellular site of oxygen toxicity." Biochem Biophys Res Commun. 1980;93:172-178.

23. Brown GL, Thomson PD, Mader JT, Hilton JG, Browne ME, Wells CH. "Effects of hyperbaric oxygen upon S. aureus, P. aeruginosa, and C. albicans." Aviat Space Environ Med. 1979;50:717-720.

24. Brown OR, Yein F. "Dihydroxyacid dehydratase: the site of hyperbaric oxygen poisoning in branched-chain amino acid biosynthesis." Biochem Biophys Res Commun. 1978;85:1219-1224.

25. Brunker RL, Brown OR. "Effects of hyperoxia on oxidized and reduced NAD and NADP concentrations in Escherichia coli." Microbios. 1971;4:193-203.

26. Bryan LE, Kwan S. "Mechanisms of aminoglycoside resistance of anaerobic bacteria and facultative bacteria grown anaerobically." J Antimicrob Chemother. 1981;8(Suppl)D:1-8.

27. Bryant RE, Fox K, Oh G, Morthland VH. "Beta-lactam enhancement of aminoglycoside activity under conditions of reduced pH and oxygen tension that may exist in infected tissues." J Infect Dis. 1992;165:76-82.

28. Cairney WJ. "Effect of hyperbaric oxygen on certain growth features of Candida albicans." Aviat Space Environ Med. 1978;49:956-958.

29. Caldwell P, Luk DA, Weissbach H, Broth N. "Oxidation of the methionine residues of Escherichia coli: ribosomal protein L 12 decreases the protein's biological activity." Proc Natl Acad Sci USA. 1978;75:5349-5352.

30. Carlioz A, Touati D. "Isolation of superoxide dismutase mutants in Escherichia coli: is superoxide dismutase necessary for aerobic life?" EMBO J. 1986;5:623-630.

31. Cashel M. "Regulation of bacterial ppGpp and pppGpp." Ann Rev Microbiol. 1975;29:301-318.

32. Chaput M, Brygier J, Lion Y, Sels A. "Potentiation of oxygen toxicity by menadione in Saccharomyces cerevisiae." Biochimie. 1983;65:501-512.

33. Christman MF, Morgan RW, Jacobson FS, Ames BN. "Positive control of a regulon fr defenses against oxidative stress and some heat-shock proteins in Salmonella typhimurium." Cell. 1985;41:753-762.

34. Clarebout G, Slomianny C, Delcourt P, Leu B, Masset A, Camus D, Dive D. "Status of Plasmodium falciparum towards catalase." Br. J Haematol. 1998;103:52-59.

35. Clark JM, Pakman LM. "Inhibition of Pseudomonas aeruginosa by hyperbaric oxygen.II. Ultrastructural changes." Infect Immun. 1971;4:488-491.

36. Cleary PP, Larkin A. "Hyaluronic acid capsule: strategy for oxygen resistance in group A Streptococci." J Bacteriol. 1979;140:1090-1097.

37. Couch L, Theilen F, Mader JT. "Rhinocerebral mucormycosis with cerebral extension successfully treated with adjunctive hyperbaric oxygen therapy." Arch Otolaryngeol Head Neck Surg. 1988;114:791-794.

38. Craig WA, Gudmundsson S. "The postantibiotic effect." In: (Lorian V, Ed.) Antibiotics in laboratory medicine, 2nd ed. Baltimore: Williams and Wilkins, 1986;515-536.

39. Crouse DT, Cassell GH, Waites KB, Foster JM, Cassady G. "Hyperoxia potentiates Ureaplasma urealyticum pneumonia in newborn mice." Infect Immun. 1990;58:3487-3493.

40. Demello FJ, Hashimoto T, Hitchcock CR, Haglin JJ. "The effect of hyperbaric oxygen on the germination and toxin production of Clostridium perfringens spores." In: Wada J, Iwa T, Eds. Proceedings of the Fourth International Congress on Hyperbaric Medicine. Tokyo: Igaku Shoin Ltd, 1970;276-281.

41. Demple B, Halbrook J. "Inducible repair of oxidative DNA damage in Escherichia coli." Nature (Lond). 1983;304:466-468.

42. DiGuiseppi J, Fridovich I. "Oxygen toxicity in Streptococcus sanguis. The relative importance of superoxide and hydroxyl radicals." J Biol Chem. 1982;257:4046-4051.

43. Divo AA, Geary TG, Jensen JB. "Oxygen- and time-dependent effects of antibiotics and selected mitrochondrial inhibitors on Plasmodium falciparum in culture." Antimicrob Agents Chemother. 1985;27:21-27.

44. Docampo R. "Sensitivity of parasites to free radical damage by antiparasitic drugs." Chem-Biol Interact. 1990;73:1-27.

45. Docampo R, Moreno SNJ. "Free-radical intermediates in the antiparasitic action of drugs and phagocytic cells." In: Pryor WA, Ed., Free Radicals in Biology. Academic Press, New York 1984;244-280.

46. Dubes GR, Al-Moslih MI, Sambol AR. "Differential effect of limitation in oxygen supply on plaquing and multiplication of adenovirus and poliovirus." Arch Virol. 1981;70:247-54.

47. Dunn MM, Smith LJ. "The effects of hyperoxia on pulmonary clearance of Pseudomonas aeruginosa. J Infect Dis. 1986;153:676-681.

48. Edman JG, Kovacs JA, Masur H, Santi DV, Elwood HJ, Sogin ML. "Ribosomal RNA sequence shows Pneumocystis carinii to be a member of the fungi." Nature. 1988;334:519-522.

49. Eiguchi K, Bertholds M, Grana D, Malateste C, Mareso E, Gomez E, Falasca CA. "Immunoregulatory effect of HBO on rats." J Hyperbaric Med. 1990;5:187-191.

50. Ejiri S-I, Weissbach H, Brot N. "The purification of methionine sulfoxide reductase from Escherichia coli." Annal Biochem. 1980;102:393-398.

51. Farr SB, Natvig DO, Kogoma T. "Toxicity and mutagenicity of plumbagin and the induction of a possible new DNA repair pathway in Escherichia coli." J Bacteriol. 1985;164:1309-1316.

52. Farr SB, Touati D, Kogoma T. "Effects of oxygen stress on membrane functions in Escherichia coli: role of HPI catalase." J Bacteriol. 1988;170:1837-1842.

53. Feldman GM, Dannenberg Jr AM, Seed JL. "Physiologic oxygen tensions limit oxidant-mediated killing of schistosome eggs by inflammatory cells in isolated granulomas." J Leukocyte Biol. 1990;47:344-354.

54. Ferguson BJ, Mitchell TG, Moon R, Camporesi EM, Farmer J. "Adjunctive hyperbaric oxygen for treatment of rhinocerebral mucormycosis." Rev Infect Dis. 1988;10:551-559.

55. Flint DH, Smyk-Randall E, Tuminello JF, Draczynska-Lusiak B, Brown OR. "The inactivation of dihydroxy-acid dehydratase in Escherichia coli treated with hyperbaric oxygen occurs because of the destruction of its Fe-S cluster, but the enzyme remains in a form that can be reactivated." J. Biol. Chem. 1993;268: 25547-25552.

56. Forman HJ, Williams JJ, Nelson J, Daniele RP, Fisher AB. "Hyperoxia inhibits stimulated superoxide release by rat alveolar macrophages." J Appl Physiol. 1982;53:685-689.

57. Freeman BA, Crapo JD. "Biology of disease. Free radicals and tissue injury." Lab Invest. 1982;47:412-426.

58. Gadd MA, McClellan DS, Neuman TS, Hansbrough JF. "Effect of hyperbaric oxygen on murine neutrophil and T-lymphocyte functions." Crit Care Med. 1990;18:974-979.

59. Galiazzo F, Schiesser A, Rotilio G. "Glutathione peroxidase in yeast. Presence of the enzyme and induction by oxidative conditions." Biochem Biophys Res Commun. 1987;147:1200-1205.

60. Gardner PR, Fridovich I. "Quinolinate phosphoribosyl transferase is not the oxygen-sensitive site of nicotinamide adenine dinucleotide biosynthesis." Free Rad Biol Med. 1990;8:117-119.

61. Ghadirian E, Somerfield SD, Kongshavn PAL. "Susceptability of Entamoeba histolytica to oxidants" Infect Immun. 1986;51:263-267.

62. Gifford GD. "Mutation of an auxotrophic strain of Escherichia coli by high pressure oxygen." Biochem Biophys Res Commun. 1968;33:294-298.

63. Gillin FD, Diamond LS. "Entamoeba histolytica and Giardia lamblia: effects of cysteine and oxygen tension on trophozoite attachment to glass and survival in culture media." Exp Parasitol. 1981;52:9-17.

64. Gillin FD, Reiner DS. "Effects of oxygen tension and reducing agents on sensitivity of Giardia lamblia to metronidazole *in vitro*." Biochem Pharmacol. 1982;31:3694-3697.

65. Gillmore JD, Gordon FB. "Parabarosis and experimental infection. 5. Effect of altered oxygen tension on Coxsackie B-1 infection in adult mice." Aerospace Med. 1974;45:840-842.

66. Giron DJ, Pindak FF, Schmidt JP. "Effect of hypobaric hypoxia on MM virus infection." Aerospace Med. 1970;41:854-855.

67. Godfrey RW, Wilder MS. "Generation of oxygen species and virulence of Listeria monocytogenes." Infect Immun. 1985;47:837-839.

68. Gordon FB, Gillmore JD. "Parabarosis and experimental infections. 1. Effect of varying $O_2$ tensions on influenza virus infection in mice." Aerospace Med. 1974;45:241-248.

69. Gordon FB, Gillmore JD. "Parabarosis and experimental infections. 4. Effect of varying $O_2$ tensions on chlamydial infection in mice and cell cultures." Aerospace Med. 1974;45:257-262.

70. Gottlieb SF. "Interaction of oxygen, temperature and drugs on two species of Neisseria as concerns the mechanism of oxygen toxicity." In: Wada J, Iwa T, Eds. Proceedings of the Fourth International Congress on Hyperbaric Medicine. Tokyo: Igaku Shoin Ltd., 1970;288-296.

71. Gottlieb SF, Solosky JA, Aubrey R, Nedelkoff DD. "Synergistic action of increased oxygen tensions and PABA-folic acid antagonists on bacterial growth." Aerospace Med. 1974;45:829-833.

72. Gougerot-Pocidalo M-A, Fay M, Pocidalo JJ. "*In vivo* normobaric oxygen exposure depresses spleen cell *in vitro* Con A response. Effects of 2-mercaptoethanol and peritoneal cells." Clin Exp Immunol. 1984;58:428-435.

73. Greenberg JT, Monach P, Chou JH, Josephy PD, Demple B. "Positive control of a global antioxidant defense regulon activated by superoxide-generating agents in Escherichia coli." Proc Natl Acad Sci USA. 1990;87:6181-6185.

74. Gregory EM, Fridovich I. "Induction of superoxide dismutase by molecular oxygen." J Bacteriol. 1973;114:543-548.

75. Gregory EM, Fridovich I. "Oxygen toxicity and the superoxide dismutase." J Bacteriol. 1973;114:1193-1197.

76. Gregory EM, Goscin SA, Fridovich I. "Superoxide dismutase and oxygen toxicity in a eukaryote." J Bacteriol. 1974;117:456-460.

77. Gudewicz TM, Mader JT, Davis CP. "Combined effects of hyperbaric oxygen and antifungal agents on the growth of Candida albicans." Aviat Space Environ Med. 1987;58:673-678.

78. Haido RMT, Barreto-Bergter E. "Amphotericin B-induced damage of Trypanosoma cruzi epimastigotes." Chem-Biol Interact. 1989;71:91-103.

79. Halliwell B, Gutteridge JMC. "Oxygen toxicity, oxygen radicals, transition metals and disease." Biochem J. 1984;219:1-14.

80. Hansbrough JF, Piacentine JG, Eiseman B. "Immunosuppression by hyperbaric oxygen." Surgery 1980;87:662-667.

81. Harley JB, Fetterolf CJ, Bello CA, Flaks JG. "Streptonigrin toxicity in Escherichia coli: oxygen dependence and the role of the intracellular oxidation-reduction state." Can J Microbiol. 1982;28:545-552.

82. Harley JB, Flaks JG, Bayer ME, Goldfine H, Rasmussen H. "Hyperbaric oxygen toxicity and ribosomal destruction in Excherichia coli K-12." Can J Microbiol. 1981;27:44-51.

83. Harrell LJ, Evans JB. "Effect of anaerobiosis on antimicrobial susceptibility of Staphylococci." Antimicrob Agents Chermother. 1977;11:1077-1078.

84. Harris GD, Johanson Jr WG, Pierce AK. "Determinants of lung bacterial clearance in mice after acute hypoxia." Am Rev Respir Dis. 1977;116:671-677.

85. Hassan HM, Fridovich I. "Superoxide radical and the oxygen enhancement of the toxicity of paraquat in Escherichia coli." J Biol Chem. 1978;253:8143-8148.

86. Hassett DJ, Cohen MS. "Bacterial adaptation to oxidative stress: implications for pathogenesis and interaction with phagocytic cells." FASEB J. 1989;3:2574-2582.

87. Hays RC, Mandell GL. "$pO_2$, pH, and redox potential of experimental abscesses." Proc Soc Exp Biol Med. 1974;147:29-30.

88. Hill GB, Osterhout S. "Experimental effects of hyperbaric oxygen on selected Clostridial species.I. *In vitro* studies." J Infect Dis. 1972;125:17-25.

89. Hill GB, Osterhout S. "Experimental effects of hyperbaric oxygen on selected Clostridial species.II. *In vivo* studies in mice." J Infect Dis. 1972;125:26-35.

90. Hirn M, Niinikoski J, Lehtonen O-P. "Effect of hyperbaric oxygen and surgery on experimental gas gangrene." Eur. Surg. Res. 1992;24:356-62.

91. Hirn M, Niinikoski J, Lehtonen O-P. "Effect of hyperbaric oxygen and surgery on experimental multimicrobial gas gangrene." Eur. Surg. Res. 1992;25:265-69.

92. Hiraoka Y, Kishimoto C, Takada H, Kurokawa M, Ochiai H, Shiraki K, Sasayama S. "Role of oxygen derived free radicals in the pathogenesis of coxsackie B3 myocarditis in mice." Cardiovasc Res 1993;27:957-961.

93. Hofert JF. "An acute effect of high oxygen tension on the uptake of 3H-deoxycytidine into thymocyte deoxyribonucleic acid." Biochem Pharmacol. 1974;23:3216-3218.

94. Hohn DC, MacKay RD, Halliday B, Hunt TK. "Effect of $O_2$ tension on microbicidal function of leukocytes in wounds and *in vitro*." Surg Forum. 1976;27:18-20.

95. Hordnes C, Tyssebotn I. "Effect of high ambient pressure and oxygen tension on organ blood flow in conscious trained rats." Undersea Biomed Res. 1985;12:115-128.

96. Hunt TK, Linsey M, Grislis G, Sonne M, Jawetz E. "The effect of differing ambient oxygen tensions on wound infection." Ann Surg. 1975;181:35-39.

97. Imlay J, Linn S. "DNA damage and oxygen radical toxicity." Science. 1988;240:1302-1309.

98. Jacobson FS, Morgan RW, Christman MF, Ames BN. "An alkyl hydroperoxide reductase from Salmonella typimurium involved in the defense of DNA against oxidative damage. Purification and properties." J Biol Chem. 1989;264:1488-1496.

99. Jamieson D, Chance B, Cadenas E, Boveris A. "The relation of free radical production to hyperoxia." Ann Rev Physiol. 1986;48:703-719.

100. Jamieson D, Van den Brenk HAS. "Electrode size and tissue $pO_2$ measurement in rats exposed to air or high pressure oxygen." J Appl Physiol. 1965;20:514-518.

101. Jarabek L, Bednarik M, Mochnac T. "Effect of intraperitoneal administration of oxygen on the course of experimentally induced peritonitis." Am J Surg 1991;162:228-230.

102. Jones DP. "The role of oxygen concentration in oxidative stress: hypoxic and hyperoxic models. In: Oxidative Stress (Sies H, Ed.) Academic Press London, 1985;151-195.

103. Jönsson K, Hunt TK, Mathes SJ. "Oxygen as an isolated variable influences resistance to infection." Ann Surg. 1988;208:783-787.

104. Karnovsky ML. "The metabolism of leukocytes." Semin Hematol. 1968;5:156-165.

105. Kazura JW, Meshnick SR. "Scavenger enzymes and resistance to oxygen mediated damage in Trichinella spiralis." Mol Biochem Parasitol. 1984;10:1-10.

106. Kehrer JP, Jones DP, Lemasters JJ, Farber JL, Jaeschke H. "Mechanisms of hypoxic cell injury. Summary of the symposium presented at the 1990 Annual Meeting of the Society of Toxicology." Toxicol Appl Pharmacol. 1990;106:165-178.

107. Kenward MA, Alcock SR, Brown MRW. Effects of hyperbaric oxygen on the growth and properties of Pseudomonas aeruginosa." Microbios. 1980;28:47-60.

108. Kilburn DG, Van Wezel AL. "Rubella virus replication at controlled dissolved oxygen tension." Biotech Bioengin. 1972;14:493-497.

109. Kivisaari J, Niinikoski J. "Effects of hyperbaric oxygenation and prolonged hypoxia on the healing of open wounds." Acta Chir Scan. 1975;141:14-19.

110. Knighton DR, Fiegel VD, Halverson T, Schneider S, Brown T, and Wells CL. "Oxygen as an antibiotic. The effect of inspired oxygen on bacterial clearance." Arch Surg. 1990;125:97-100.

111. Knighton DR, Halliday B, Hunt TK. "Oxygen as an antibiotic. A comparison of the effects of inspired oxygen concentration and antibiotic adminstration on *in vivo* bacterial clearance." Arch Surg. 1986;121:191-195.

112. Kono Y. "Oxygen enhancement of bactericidal activity of rifamycin SV on Escherichia coli and aerobic oxidation of rifamycin SV to rifamycin S catalyzed by manganous ions: the role of superoxide." J Biochem. 1982;91:381-395.

113. Krieg RE, Wolcott JH, Confer A. "Treatment of Mycobacterium ulcerans infection by hyperbaric oxygenation." Aviat Space Environ Med. 1975;46:1241-1245.

114. Krieg RE, Wolcott JH, Meyers WM. "Mycobacterium ulcerans infection: treatment with rifampin, hyperbaric oxygenation, and heat." Aviat Space Environ Med. 1979;50:888-892.

115. Kuo CF, Mashino T, Fridovich I."a, b dihydroxyisovalerate dehydratase. A superoxide-sensitive enzyme." J Biol Chem. 1987;262:4724-4727.

116. Lindahl-Kiessling K, Karlberg I. "High oxygen pressure inhibits DNA synthesis in mitogen-activated lymphocytes." Int Arch Allergy Appl Immun. 1979;60:97-100.

117. Lynch RE, Cole BC. "Mycoplasma pneumoniae: a prokaryote which consumes oxygen and generates superoxide but which lacks superoxide dismutase." Biochem Biophys Res Commun. 1980;96:98-105.

118. McCord JM. "Oxygen-derived free radicals in postischemic tissue injury." N Engl J Med. 1985;312:159-163.

119. McCord JM, Keele Jr BB, Fridovich I. "An enzyme-based theory of obligate anaerobiosis: the physiological function of superoxide dismutase." Proc Natl Acad Sci USA. 1971;68:1024-1027.

120. McDonald PJ, Craig WA, Kunin CM. "Persistent effect of antibiotics on Staphylococcus aureus after exposure for limited periods of time." J Infect Dis. 1977;135:217-223.

121. Mack SR, Müller M. "Effect of oxygen and carbon dioxide on the growth of Trichomonas vaginalis and Tritrichomonas foetus." J Parasitol. 1978;64:927-929.

122. Mader JT, Brown GL, Guckian JC, Wells CH, Reinarz JA. "A mechanism for the amelioration by hyperbaric oxygen of experimental staphylococcal osteomyelitis in rabbits." J Infect Dis. 1980;142:915-922.

123. Mader JT, Guckian JC, Glass DL, Reinarz JA. "Therapy with hyperbaric oxygenation for experimental osteomyelitis due to Staphylococcus aureus in rabbits." J Infect Dis. 1978;138:312-318.

124. Mader JT, Hicks CA, Calhoun J. "Bacterial osteomyelitis. Adjunctive hyperbaric oxygen therapy." Orthop Rev. 1989;18:581-585.

125. Mandell GL. "Bactericidal activity of aerobic and anaerobic polymorphonuclear neutrophils." Infect Immun. 1974;9:337-341.

126. Mandell GL, Hook EW. "Leukocyte bactericidal activity in chronic granulomatous disease: correlation of bacterial hydrogen peroxide production and susceptibility to intracellular killing." J Bacteriol. 1969;100:531-532.

127. Mathis RR, Brown OR. "ATP concentration in Escherichia coli during oxygen toxicity." Biochem Biophys Acta. 1976;440:723-732.

128. Mehlotra RK, Shukla OP. "Reducing agents and Entamoeba histolytica." Parasitol Today. 1988;4:82-83.

129. Mehm WJ, Pimsler M. "Effect of oxygen on phagocytic and adherence functions in mouse spleen macrophages." J Hyperbaric Med. 1986;1:223-231.

130. Meylan PRA, Richman DD, Kornbluth RS. "Reduced intracellular growth of mycobacteria in human macrophages cultured at physiologic oxygen pressure." Am Rev Respir Dis. 1992;145:947-953.

131. Meshnick SR, Eaton JW. "Leishmanial superoxide dismutase: a possible target for chemotherapy." Biochem Biophys Res Commun. 1981;102:970-976.

132. Mirhij NJ, Roberts RJ, Myers MG. "Effects of hypoxemia upon aminoglycoside serum pharmacokinetics in animals." Antimicrob Agents Chemother. 1978;14:344-347.

133. Mizrahi A, Vosseller GV, Yagi Y, Moore GE. "The effect of dissolved oxygen partial pressure on growth, metabolism and immunoglobulin production in a permanent human lymphocyte cell line culture." Proc Soc Exp Biol Med. 1972;139:118-122.

134. Mkoji GM, Smith JM, Prichard RK. "Antioxidant systems in Schistosoma mansoni: correlation between susceptibility to oxidant killing and the levels of scavengers of hydrogen peroxide and oxygen free radicals." Int J Parasitol. 1988;18:661-666.

135. Mjoki GM, Smith JM, Prichard RK. "Antioxidant systems in Schistosoma mansoni: evidence for their role in protection of the adult worms against oxidant killing." Int J Parasitol. 1988;18:667-673.

136. Moody CS, Hassan HM."Mutagenicity of oxygen free radicals." Proc Natl Acad Sci. 1982;79:2855-2859.

137. Muhvich KH, Myers RAM, Marzella L. "Effect of hyperbaric oxygenation, combined with antimicrobial agents and surgery, in a rat model of intra-abdominal infection." J Infect Dis. 1988;157:1058-1061.

138. Muhvich KH, Park MK, Myers RAM, Marzella L. "Hyperoxia and the antimicrobial susceptibility of Escherichia coli and Pseudomonas aeruginosa." Antimicrob Agents Chemother. 1989;33:1526-1530.

139. Muhvich KH, Piano MR, Piano G, Myers RAM, Ferguson JL, Marzella L. "Splanchnic blood flows in a rat model of antibiotic-controlled intra-abdominal abscess during normoxia and hyperoxia." Circ Shock. 1989;253-262.

140. Muhvich KH, Anderson LHG, Mehm WJ. Evaluation of antimicrobials combined with hyperbaric oxygen in a mouse model of Clostridium myonecrosis." J Trauma 1994;36:7-10.

141. Müller M, Lindmark DG. "Uptake of metronidazole and its effect on viability in trichomonads and Entamoeba invadens under anaerobic and aerobic conditions." Antimicrob Agents Chemother. 1976;9:696-700.

142. Murray HW. "Susceptibility of Leishmania to oxygen intermediates and killing by normal macrophages." J Exp Med. 1981;153:1302-1315.

143. Murray HW. "Cell-mediated immune response in experimental visceral leishmaniasis. II. Oxygen-dependent killing of intracellular Leishmania donovani amastigotes." J Immunol. 1982;129:351-357.

144. Murray HW, Aley SB, Scott WA. "Susceptibility of Entamoeba histolytica to oxygen intermediates." Mol Biochem Parasitol. 1981;3:381-391.

145. Murray HW, Cartelli DM. "Killing of intracellular Leishmania donovani by human mononuclear phagocytes." J Clin Invest. 1983;72:32-44.

146. Murray HW, Cohn ZA. "Macrophage oxygen-dependent antimicrobial activity. I. Susceptibility of Toxoplasma gondii to oxygen intermediates." J Exp Med. 1979;150:938-949.

147. Murray HW, Nathan CF, Cohn ZA. "Macrophage oxygen-dependent antimicrobial activity. IV. Role of endogenous scavengers of oxygen intermediates." J Exp Med. 1980;152:1610-1624.

148. Naldini A, Carraro F, Fleishmann WR, Bocci V. "Hypoxia enhances the antiviral activity of interferons."J Interferon Res 1993;13:127-132.

149. Nare B, Smith JM, Prichard RK. "Schistosoma mansoni: levels of antioxidants and resistance to oxidants increase during development." Exp Parasitol. 1990;70:389-397.

150. Nerurkar LS, Zeligs BJ, Bellanti JA. "Proliferation of alveolar macrophages in hyperoxia." Ann Allergy. 1988;61:344-347.

151. Norden CW, Shaffer M. "Treatment of experimental chronic osteomyelitis due to Staphylococcus aureus with vancomycin and rifampin." J Infect Dis. 1983;147:352-357.

152. Oliver JM, Albertini DF, Berlin RD. "Effects of glutathione-oxidizing agents on microtubule assembly and microtubule-dependent surface properties of human neutrophils." J Cell Biol. 1976;71:921-932.

153. Ollodart RM. "Effects of hyperbaric oxygenation and antibiotics on aerobic microorganisms." In: Brown Jr IW, Cox BG, Eds. Proceedings of the Third International Conference on Hyperbaric Medicine. Washington, DC: Natl Acad Sci, 1966;565-671.

154. Orsi EV, Mancini R, Barriso J. "Hyperbaric enhancement of Coxsackievirus infection in mice." Aerospace Med. 1970;41:1169-1172.

155. Pakman LM. "Inhibition of Pseudomonas aeruginosa by hyperbaric oxygen. I. Sulfonamide activity enhancement and reversal." Infect Immun. 1971;4:479-487.

156. Park MK, Muhvich KH, Myers RAM, Marzella L. "Hyperoxia prolongs the aminoglycoside-induced postantibiotic effect in Pseudomonas aeruginosa." Antimicrob Agents Chemother. 1991;35:691-695.

157. Park MK, Myers RAM, Marzella L. "Oxygen tensions and infections: Modulation of microbial growth, activity of antimicrobial agents, and immunologic responses." Clin Infect Dis 1992;14:720-740.

158. Pesanti EL. "Pneumocystis carinii: oxygen uptake, antioxidant enzymes, and susceptibility to oxygen-mediated damage." Infect Immun. 1984;44:7-11.

159. Pfaller MA, Krogstad DJ. "Oxygen enhances the antimalarial activity of the imidazoles." Am J Trop Med Hyg. 1983;32:660-665.

160. Price JC, Stevens DL. "Hyperbaric oxygen in the treatment of rhinocerebral mucormycosis." Laryngoscope. 1980;90:737-747.

161. Privalle CT, Gregory EM. "Superoxide dismutase and $O_2$ lethality in Bacteroides fragilis." J Bacteriol. 1979;138:139-145.

162. Raffin TA, Braun D, Simon L, Theodore J, Robin ED. "Dose-response relationship between $pO_2$ and impairment of phagocytosis and the lack of tolerance." Clin Res. 1977;25:134A.

163. Raffin TA, Simon LM, Braun D, Theodore J, Robin ED. "Impairment of phagocytosis by moderate hyperoxia (40 to 60 per cent oxygen) in lung macrophages." Lab Invest. 1980;42:622-626.

164. Raffin TA, Simon LM, Theodore J, Robin ED. "Effect of hyperoxia on the rate of generation of superoxide anions (SOA) in free solution and in a cellular {alveolar macrophage (AM)} system." Clin Res. 1977;25:134A.

165. Reiner NE, Kazura JW. "Oxidant-mediated damage of Leishmania donovani promastigotes." Infect Immun. 1982;36:1023-1027.

166. Reynolds AV, Hamilton-Miller JMT, Brumfitt W. "Diminished effect of gentamicin under anaerobic of hypercapnic conditions." Lancet. 1976;i:447-449.

167. Rister M. "Effects of hyperoxia on phagocytosis." Blut. 1982;45:157-166.

168. Rolfe RD, Hentges DJ, Campbell BJ, Barrett JT. "Factors related to the oxygen tolerance of anaerobic bacteria." Appl Environ Microbiol. 1978;36:306-313.

169. Rosen H, Klebanoff SJ. "Bactericidal activity of a superoxide anion-generating system. A model for the polymorphonuclear leukocyte." J Exp Med. 1979;149:27-39.

170. Scheibel LW, Ashton SH, Trager W. "Plasmodium falciparum: microaerophilic requirements in human red blood cells." Exp Parasitol. 1979;47:410-418.

171. Schellhorn HE, Hassan HM. "Response of hydroperoxidase and superoxide dismutase deficient mutants of Escherichia coli K-12 to oxidative stress." Can J Microbiol. 1988;34:1171-1176.

172. Seither RL, Brown OR. "Induction of stringency by hyperoxia in Escherichia coli." Cell Mol Biol. 1982;28:285-291.

173. Sheffield PJ. "Tissue oxygen measurements." In: (Davis JC, Hunt TK, Eds.) Problem Wounds. The Role of Oxygen. New York: Elsevier, 1988;17-51.

174. Silver IA. "Polarographic techniques of oxygen measurement." In: (Gottlieb SF, Longmuir IS, Totter JR, Eds.) Oxygen: An In-Depth Study of its Pathophysiology. Bethesda, MD: Undersea Medical Society, 1984;215-239.

175. Simon LM, Axline SG, Robin ED. "The effect of hyperoxia on phagocytosis and pinocytosis in isolated pulmonary macrophages." Lab Invest. 1978;39:541-546.

176. Smith JT, Lewin CS. "Chemistry and mechanisms of action of the quinolone antibacterials." In: (Andriole VT, Ed.) The Quinolones. New York: Acad Press, 1988;23-82.

177. Smith RM, Mohideen P. One hour in 1 ATA oxygen enhances rat alveolar macrophage chemiluminescence and fungal cytotoxicity." Am J Physiol 1991;260:L457-L463.

178. Sokol-Anderson ML, Brajtburg J, Medoff G. "Amphotericin B-induced oxidative damage and killing of Candida albicans." J Infect Dis. 1986;154:76-83.

179. Steiner B, Wong GHW, Graves S. "Susceptibility of Treponema pallidum to the toxic products of oxygen reduction and the non-treponemal nature of its catalase." Br J Vener Dis. 1984;60:14-22.

180. Stevens DL, Bryant AE, Adams K, Mader JT. "Evaluatiuon of therapy with hyperbaric oxygen for experimental infection with Clostridium perfringens." Clin Infect Dis 1993;17:231-237.

181. Storz G, Tartaglia LA, Ames BN. "The OxyR regulon." Antonie van Leeuwenhoek. 1990;58:157-161.

182. Suttorp N, Simon LM. "Decreased bactericidal function and impaired respiratory burst in lung macrophages after sustained *in vitro* hyperoxia." Am Rev Respir Dis. 1983;128:486-490.

183. Tack KJ, Sabath LD. "Increased minimum inhibitory concentrations with anaerobiasis for tobramycin, gentamicin, and amikacin, compared to latamoxef, piperacillin, chloramphenicol, and clindamycin." Chemother. 1985;31:204-210.

184. Tally FP, Sullivan CE. "Metronidazole: *In vitro* activity, pharmacology and efficacy in anaerobic bacterial infections." Pharmacother. 1981;1:28-38.

185. Thalinger KK, Mandell GL. "Bactericidal activity of macrophages in an anaerobic environment." J Reticuloendothel Soc. 1971;9:393-396.

186. Thom SR, Lauermann MW, Hart GB. "Intermittent hyperbaric oxygen therapy for reduction of mortality in experimental polymicrobial sepsis." J Infect Dis. 1986;154:504-510.

187. Thomson HL, Wilton JMA. "Interaction and intracellular killing of Candida albicans blastospores by human polymorphonuclear leukocytes, monocytes, and monocyte-derived macrophages in aerobic and anaerobic conditions." Clin Exp Immunol 1992;87:316-321.

188. Torbati D, Parolla D, Lavy S. "Organ blood flow, cardiac output, arterial blood pressure, and vascular resistance in rats exposed to various oxygen pressures." Aviat Space Environ Med. 1979;50:256-263.

189. Tsavena IR, Weiss B. "soxR, a locus governing a superoxide response regulon in Escherichia coli K-12." J Bacteriol. 1990;172:4197-4205.

190. Turrens JF, Freeman BA, Crapo JD. "Hyperoxia increases $H_2O_2$ release by lung mitochondria and microsomes." Arch Biochem Biophys. 1982;217:411-419.

191. Vaughan GL. "Oxygen toxicity in a fission yeast." J Cell Physiol. 1971;77:363-371.

192. Verklin Jr RM, Mandell GL. "Alteration of effectiveness of antibiotics by anaerobiosis." J Lab Clin Med. 1977;89:65-71.

193. Virtanen S. "Antibacterial activity of sulphamethoxazole and trimethoprim under diminished oxygen tension." J Gen Microbiol. 1974;84:145-148.

194. Walden WC, Hentges DJ. "Differential effects of oxygen and oxidation-reduction potential on the multiplication of three species of anaerobic intestinal bacteria." Appl Microbiol. 1975;30:781-785.

195. Walkup LKB, Kogoma T. "Escherichia coli proteins inducible by oxidative stress mediated by the superoxide radical." J Bacteriol. 1989;171:1476-1484.

196. Ward PA. "Role of toxic oxygen products from phagocytic cells in tissue injury." Adv Shock Res. 1983;10:27-34.

197. Weinbach EC. "Biochemistry of enteric parasitic protozoa." TIBS. 1981;6:254-257.

198. Weinbach EC, Diamond LS. "Entamoeba histolytica: aerobic metabolism." Exp Parasitol. 1974;35:232-243.

199. Weislow OS, Pakman LM. "Inhibition of Pseudomonas aeruginosa by hyperbaric oxygen: interaction with mouse peritoneal exudate cells." Infect Immun. 1974;10:546-552.

200. Wilson DM, Adlerete JF, Maloney PC, Wilson TH. "Proton motive force as the source of energy for adenosine 5'-triphosphate synthesis in Escherichia coli." J Bacteriol. 1976;126:327-337.

201. Wilson DF, Erecinska M. "The role of cytochrome c oxidase in regulation of cellular oxygen consumption." In: (Gottlieb SF, Longmuir IS, Totter JR, Eds.) Oxygen: An In-Depth Study of its Pathophysiology. Bethesda, MD: Undersea Medical Society, 1984;459-492.

202. Zamboni WA, Mazolewski PJ, Erdman D, Bergman BA, Hussman J, Cooper MD, Smoot EC, Russell RC. "Evaluation of penicillin and hyperbaric oxygen in the treatment of streptococcal myositis." Ann Plast Surg 1997;39:131-136.

203. Tateda K, Deng JC, Moore TA, Newstead MW, Paine R 3rd, Kobayashi N, Yamaguchi K, Standiford TJ. Hyperoxia mediates acute lung injury and increased lethality in murine Legionella pneumonia: the role of apoptosis. J Immunol. 2003 Apr 15;170(8):4209-16.

204. Nara C, Tateda K, Matsumoto T, Ohara A, Miyazaki S, Standiford TJ, Yamaguchi K. Legionella-induced acute lung injury in the setting of hyperoxia: protective role of tumour necrosis factor-alpha. J Med Microbiol. 2004 Aug;53(Pt 8):727-33.

205. Morrow DM, Entezari-Zaher T, Romashko J 3rd, Azghani AO, Javdan M, Ulloa L, Miller EJ, Mantell LL. Antioxidants preserve macrophage phagocytosis of Pseudomonas aeruginosa during hyperoxia. Free Radic Biol Med. 2007 May 1;42(9):1338-49. Epub 2007 Jan 23.

206. Tsuneyoshi I, Boyle WA 3rd, Kanmura Y, Fujimoto T. Hyperbaric hyperoxia suppresses growth of Staphylococcus aureus, including methicillin-resistant strains. J Anesth. 2001;15(1):29-32.

207. Mendel V, Reichert B, Simanowski HJ, Scholz HC. Therapy with hyperbaric oxygen and cefazolin for experimental osteomyelitis due to Staphylococcus aureus in rats. Undersea Hyperb Med. 1999 Fall;26(3):169-74.

208. Mendel V, Simanowski HJ, Scholz HCh. Synergy of HBO$_2$ and a local antibiotic carrier for experimental osteomyelitis due to Staphylococcus aureus in rats. Undersea Hyperb Med. 2004 Winter;31(4):407-16.

209. Mendel V, Simanowski HJ, Scholz HC, Heymann H. Therapy with gentamicin-PMMA beads, gentamicin-collagen sponge, and cefazolin for experimental osteomyelitis due to Staphylococcus aureus in rats. Arch Orthop Trauma Surg. 2005 Jul;125(6):363-8. Epub 2005 Apr 30.

210. Colhone MC, Arrais-Silva WW, Picoli C, Giorgio S. Effect of hypoxia on macrophage infection by Leishmania amazonensis. J Parasitol. 2004 Jun;90(3):510-5.

211. Arrais-Silva WW, Collhone MC, Ayres DC, de Souza Souto PC, Giorgio S. Effects of hyperbaric oxygen on Leishmania amazonensis promastigotes and amastigotes. Parasitol Int. 2005 Mar;54(1):1-7.

212. Arrais-Silva WW, Pinto EF, Rossi-Bergmann B, Giorgio S. Hyperbaric oxygen therapy reduces the size of Leishmania amazonensis-induced soft tissue lesions in mice. Acta Trop. 2006 May;98(2):130-6. Epub 2006 Apr 25.

213. Barratt DM, Van Meter K, Asmar P, Nolan T, Trahan C, Garcia-Covarrubias L, Metzinger SE. Hyperbaric oxygen as an adjunct in zygomycosis: randomized controlled trial in a murine model. Antimicrob Agents Chemother. 2001 Dec;45(12):3601-2.

214. Paine R 3rd, Preston AM, Wilcoxen S, Jin H, Siu BB, Morris SB, Reed JA, Ross G, Whitsett JA, Beck JM. Granulocyte-macrophage colony-stimulating factor in the innate immune response to Pneumocystis carinii pneumonia in mice. J Immunol. 2000 Mar 1;164(5):2602-9.

215. Liu W, Zhao W, Lu X, Zheng X, Luo C. Clinical pathological study of treatment of chronic hepatitis with hyperbaric oxygenation. Chin Med J (Engl). 2002 Aug;115(8):1153-7.

216. Pryor KO, Fahey TJ 3rd, Lien CA, Goldstein PA. Surgical site infection and the routine use of perioperative hyperoxia in a general surgical population: a randomized controlled trial. JAMA. 2004 Jan 7;291(1):79-87.

217. Kalliainen LK, Gordillo GM, Schlanger R, Sen CK. Topical oxygen as an adjunct to wound healing: a clinical case series. Pathophysiology. 2003 Jan;9(2):81-87.

218. Sheikh AY, Gibson JJ, Rollins MD, Hopf HW, Hussain Z, Hunt TK. Effect of hyperoxia on vascular endothelial growth factor levels in a wound model. Arch Surg. 2000 Nov;135(11):1293-7.

219. Sheikh AY, Rollins MD, Hopf HW, Hunt TK. Hyperoxia improves microvascular perfusion in a murine wound model. Wound Repair Regen. 2005 May-Jun;13(3):303-8.

220. Kalns J, Lane J, Delgado A, Scruggs J, Ayala E, Gutierrez E, Warren D, Niemeyer D, George Wolf E, Bowden RA. Hyperbaric oxygen exposure temporarily reduces Mac-1 mediated functions of human neutrophils. Immunol Lett. 2002 Sep 2;83(2):125-31.

221. Jüttner B, Scheinichen D, Bartsch S, Heine J, Ruschulte H, Elsner HA, Franko W, Jaeger K. Lack of toxic side effects in neutrophils following hyperbaric oxygen. Undersea Hyperb Med. 2003 Winter;30(4):305-11.

222. Sureda A, Batle JM, Tauler P, Aguiló A, Cases N, Tur JA, Pons A. Hypoxia/reoxygenation and vitamin C intake influence NO synthesis and antioxidant defenses of neutrophils. Free Radic Biol Med. 2004 Dec 1;37(11):1744-55.

223. Arita Y, Kazzaz JA, Joseph A, Koo HC, Li Y, Davis JM. Antioxidants improve antibacterial function in hyperoxia-exposed macrophages. Free Radic Biol Med. 2007 May 15;42(10):1517-23. Epub 2007 Feb 15.

224. Baleeiro CE, Christensen PJ, Morris SB, Mendez MP, Wilcoxen SE, Paine R 3rd. GM-CSF and the impaired pulmonary innate immune response following hyperoxic stress. Am J Physiol Lung Cell Mol Physiol. 2006 Dec;291(6):L1246-55. Epub 2006 Aug 4.

225. Paine R 3rd, Wilcoxen SE, Morris SB, Sartori C, Baleeiro CE, Matthay MA, Christensen PJ. Transgenic overexpression of granulocyte macrophage-colony stimulating factor in the lung prevents hyperoxic lung injury. Am J Pathol. 2003 Dec;163(6):2397-406.

# NOTES

CHAPTER 21

# GAS GANGRENE

## CHAPTER TWENTY-ONE OVERVIEW

# GAS GANGRENE

*Richard D. Heimbach, Valerie J. Bonne, Charles C. Falzon, Harry T. Whelan*

## INTRODUCTION

Gas gangrene is a fulminating myonecrotic infection caused by the clostridial species of bacteria that can result in a rapidly fatal outcome when untreated. Historically, the incidence of gas gangrene has paralleled that of armed combat, because of contaminated wounds on the battlefield, but in the last 30 years this historical correlation has become less distinct. In eight years of combat in Vietnam, only 22 cases of gas gangrene were recorded in American casualties while in a ten-year period in Miami, Florida, there were at least 27 cases of clostridial infection (20).

Accidental trauma continues to be the leading cause of gas gangrene (25, 31, 64, 72) with 50% of the cases arising as a consequence of contamination of traumatic wounds. Gas gangrene following surgery is an uncommon, but devastating complication. The number of major and minor procedures that precede development of gas gangrene is extensive. The disease has been reported following amputation for peripheral vascular disease (136), intramuscular injection (26, 52, 61, 82, 100, 113-115, 131, 153), abortion (24, 35, 101), femoral venipuncture (36), gastric surgery (53, 78), hernia repair (110), colon surgery (68, 98), gall bladder and common bile duct surgery (58, 89, 133), appendectomy (54, 118), total hip replacement (126), small bowel surgery (91), chemotherapy for choriocarcinoma (91), endoscopy (57), colonic polypectomy (183), hip nailing (44), and vaginal delivery (121). In addition, the disease has been reported in association with carcinoma of the cecum (51, 112), femoral neck fracture (161), thermal burns (109), dissection of the aorta (122), retroperitoneal rupture of the duodenum (163), rupture of the humeral artery (14), diabetes (5, 111), metastatic breast cancer (184), intracardiac thrombus (185), and perforation of the esophagus (108). Hitchcock, et al. comment that, compared with gas gangrene secondary to trauma, the disease secondary to elective surgery is usually less suspected, diagnosed later, and, therefore, associated with a higher mortality rate (70).

The use of hyperbaric oxygen in the treatment of gas gangrene was first reported by Brummelkamp and his associates in 1961 (23). In this initial series of 26 patients, hyperbaric oxygen was the sole treatment modality used. Clinical series reported later, including a follow-up report on 10 years experience by Brummelkamp's associates, emphasize the use of surgery, antibiotics and hyperbaric oxygen adjunctively (31, 64, 70, 72, 125). This has been shown experimentally by Demello, et al., who demonstrated greater survival in dogs with experimental gas gangrene when all three treatment modalities were used together as compared with the use of each treatment modality alone or in combinations of two (32).

## BACTERIOLOGY

Clostridial species are gram-positive, spore forming, non-motile, rod-shaped organisms. Although over 90 species of clostridial bacteria have been identified, only six have been implicated in gas gangrene in humans. *Clostridium perfringens* is the most common of these bacteria, being found in close to 80% of contaminated wounds (99). The other causative clostridial bacteria, in decreasing order of prevalence, in wounds of gas gangrene patients are: *C. oedematiens*, 40%; *C. septicum*, 20%; *C. histolyticum*, *C. bifermentans* and *C. fallux*, less than 10% taken together (162).

These six clostridial organisms produce over twenty exotoxins, six of which are known to be lethal (99, 162). The more severe pathologic scenarios are usually caused by vascular compromise due to local trauma, resulting in an anaerobic environment that fosters the elaboration of exotoxins by clostridial organisms. Since the ensuing inflammatory response is triggered by the elaboration of toxin rather than the bacterium itself, the clinical scenario may be better described as intoxication rather than infection. Despite their remarkable prevalence in contaminated wounds, invasive clostridial organisms stimulate a remarkably minor inflammatory response and produce draining wounds with non-purulent exudates. Barring super-infection with other organisms, the classic disease process produces a broad range of clinical scenarios, including simple wound contamination, anaerobic cellulitis, and myonecrosis (165).

As the most common cause of clostridial myonecrosis, which is commonly referred to as "gas gangrene," the *C. perfringens* species has been of interest to clinical investigators for several decades. Since it is not a strict anaerobe, it grows freely in oxygen tensions of 30 mmHg with restricted growth in oxygen tensions up to 70 mmHg, and is ubiquitous in nature, particularly in both the normal flora of the gastrointestinal tract and is found in soil throughout the world, except in the North African desert. *C. perfringens* has been identified as having 5 specific sub-types, A-E, of which type A has been shown to cause the majority of human infections. The species also produces several extracellular toxins, but only two of them are critical to inducing the pathologic state.

Alpha toxin is the defining component of its parent species' virulence, and its detection in tissue samples or blood cultures is ultimately diagnostic for *C. perfringens* infection (166). Alpha toxin is a phospholipase-C (PLC) compound, which allows it to catalyze the hydrolysis of phosphatidyl choline and sphingomyelin. The PLC activity is essential to the inhibition of the influx of polymorphonuclear leukocytes (PMNL) at the infected site and initiation of local microvascular thrombosis. This creates an environment favorable for tissue necrosis at the inoculation site, which is the hallmark of clostridial wound infections (165, 167, 168).

One study demonstrated that a *C. perfringens*-mutant lacking the ability to produce alpha toxin were non-virulent when injected into a mouse model. By complementing the chromosomal mutation with a recombinant plasmid that carried a wild-type PLC gene, the investigators were restored *C. perfringens'* ability to produce both alpha toxin and re-establish lethality in infected mice (165). Another study showed that vaccination with a part of the C-terminal domain of PLC protected mice from experimental *C. perfringens* infection (169, 170). Finally, intramuscular injection of PLC in experimental animals caused a rapid and irreversible decline in skeletal muscle blood flow due to the formation of intravascular aggregates of activated platelets, leukocytes, and fibrin, which primarily mediated by PLC activation of the platelet fibrinogen receptor gp-IIb/IIIa (171, 172).

Theta toxin, also known as perfringolysin O (PFO), has been shown in studies to have a synergistic effect on the degree of hemolysis, leukostasis, and necrosis induced by alpha toxin (189). Experimental models have shown that exposure to theta toxin increases production of several factors that induce vasodilation, including prostacyclin, platelet activating factor, and various lipid autocoids.(173). Upregulation of these native hematologic factors results in "warm shock," which is defined as a markedly reduced systemic vascular resistance combined with markedly increased cardiac output, and rapid expansion of the intravascular blood volume (174, 175).

While alpha toxin is the only truly lethal toxin produced in significant quantities by *C. perfringens*, its effects can be significantly augmented by the presence of other non-lethal toxins, including several varieties of hyaluronidases, hemolysins and elastases. Among this class of non-lethal, clostridial factors, kappa toxin has significant proteolytic activity. In addition, "circulating factor" inhibits phagocytosis, while Mu toxin, neuraminidase, and hemagglutinin function to modify DNA, destroy immunologic receptors, and inactivate group-A factor of erythrocytes (70). When these accessory toxins are elaborated by of the parent clostridial organisms, they act synergistically with alpha toxin to create a rapidly spreading liquefaction necrosis.

The destruction of tissue that characterizes gas gangrene depends upon the continuous production of alpha toxin by clostridial organisms at the site of infection. Even though the infected tissue succumbs to liquefaction necrosis, alpha toxin becomes tissue-fixed and neutralized into a non-toxic form within two hours of being produced (99). These factors can also be removed from the inoculation site through the bloodstream and transported to the liver and kidneys for detoxification. This means that the overall impact of a clostridial infection is attributable to the severity of the initiating injury and local levels of alpha toxin, which combine to create the increasingly hypoxic, avascular environment that is essential to the survival of *C. perfringens*.

## PATHOPHYSIOLOGY

Studies have shown that the mere presence of clostridial organisms is insufficient for gas gangrene to develop at the site of inoculation. While it has been estimated that 30% of traumatic wounds are contaminated with *C. perfringens* spores, clostridial myonecrosis develops in less than 3% of these wounds (99). DeHaven and Evarts suggested that gas gangrene could be thought of as a disease associated with a particular opportunity rather than with a specific organism (31). Consequently, two clinical conditions have been established as necessary for this disease to occur: 1) clostridial contamination, and 2) a decreased oxidation-reduction potential in the wound.

Since clostridial contamination of wounds is a fairly common event, establishing the necessary oxidation-reduction potential is likely the rate-limiting step in this process. Local circulatory failure at the wound site is the primary cause of below normal oxidation-reduction potentials, which establishes the ischemic, hypoxic conditions. This is most often caused by trauma to vessels from penetrating foreign bodies that introduce non-native bacteria and cause hemorrhage or edema. The situation can be exacerbated during the initial management of these patents by applying excessively tight tourniquets, casts, or dressings that create additional necrotic tissue.

Wounds caused by high-velocity missiles, such as bullet fragments and debris in motor vehicle accidents, result in the rapid transfer of high levels of kinetic energy when a projectile initially strikes the tissue. The penetrating object produces a relatively small, superficial entrance wound, while generating significantly more damage by transferring kinetic energy to internal structures as it slows along its path. While the projectile travels within the tissue planes, it forms large cavities by fracturing bones, shearing tissue, and severing blood vessels. Many muscles have small, well-defined arterial supplies with minimal collateral flow, so damage to these principle vessels may eliminate a significant percentage, if not all, of their vasculature. This compromised circulation immediately results in local ischemia and tissue hypoxia, and eventually causes necrosis of the affected muscle. The literature indicates that damage to vessels supplying the affected area is found in up to 75-85% of cases of gas gangrene following trauma (162).

Even under more controlled conditions, tissue hypoxia remains the primary cause of gas gangrene. In the surgical suite, where every effort is made to eliminate contamination and infection, post-operative clostridial infections following "clean" procedures are most frequently encountered in patients with atherosclerosis or diabetes mellitus (188). When the gastrointestinal tract is instrumented in patients with these pre-disposing conditions, gas gangrene of the trunk is seen as convincing evidence of a bowel leak. Post-injection gas gangrene is commonly associated with the use of epinephrine, whose vasoconstrictive properties can last as long as two hours (187). As a result, the use of epinephrine with local anesthetics is contraindicated during wound debridements and primary closure. Outside the hospital, many intravenous drug users are not educated in the principles of sterile technique, and have experienced infection and recurrent trauma at their injection sites. These injection sites contain fibrotic tissue that is relatively hypoxic, and predisposes these patients to developing clostridial infections (186).

It is important to note that not all cases of clostridial myonecrosis are due to either surgical or other penetrating traumas. *C. septicum* is one of the leading causes of occult, atraumatic, gas gangrene. Infections from this species usually results from bacteremia secondary to lesions of the gastrointestinal tract. This is often seen with colonic malignancies, especially in immunocompromised patients. Several studies have postulated that *C. septicum's* tolerance to aerobic environments may decrease the efficacy of hyperbaric therapy relative to *C. perfringens* (66, 190).

# CLINICAL CONSIDERATIONS

The four forms of necrotizing clostridial disease delineated by Altemeier in 1966 still best describe the clinical picture of "gas gangrene" (1).

## Clostridial Myonecrosis with Toxicity

The clinical scenario that is classically associated with gas gangrene is characterized by diffuse and rapid spread from the initial site of involvement. Its onset is acute and follows an incubation period with an average range between four hours and three days, however, cases have been reported after incubation periods that have lasted up to six weeks (159). The first symptom observed in most cases is pain out of proportion to the extent and timing of the correlated injury. The tissue surrounding the wound swells with edema, causing the overlying skin to become tense and blanch to the touch. From this point, the toxic process accelerates rapidly as the skin surrounding the site of involvement appears light bronze within a few hours and progressively darkening as underlying tissue dies, before finally giving way to the blebs and bullae.

Barring additional wound contamination by non-clostridial organisms, patients typically do not develop fevers above 101°F, and remain normotensive despite becoming disproportionately tachycardic, between 140-160 beats per minute. When shock develops, it marks the latter stages of the disease and is a grave prognostic sign. Most patients remain oriented to person, place, and time, but can exhibit a characteristic flattening of affect and a "la belle indifference" attitude. Drainage from the wound site is usually serosanguinous with a typical "sweetish" or "mousy" odor, unless the wound is super-infected, and may contain gas bubbles, which can be observed on exam, as crepitus within the soft tissue, or demonstrated radiographically, as free air dissecting along fascial planes. Gas in the soft tissue can also be caused by an initiating injury that introduces air into a wound, or by non-clostridal organisms contaminating the wound that are associated with gas production, such as *E. coli* and anerobic *streptococci* (31). Since there is no evidence of gas in at least half of the cases diagnosed as clostridial infections, the presence of this finding is not necessary to establish the diagnosis (64). Most cases of gas gangrene will show some evidence of hemolysis on laboratory analysis, but clinically significant levels are diagnostic for bacteremia, which is a very serious complication. When there is a high index of suspicion for clostridial infections, these patients must be managed and treated appropriately to improve their chances for survival.

## Localized Clostridial Myonecrosis

This uncommon form of the disease is usually seen following non-sterile injection of drugs. The infection tends to remain localized and few, if any, toxic symptoms are manifested. Local incision and drainage with appropriate antibiotic therapy is the appropriate management for this disease, but these patients must be monitored closely to potentially manage the more aggressive, disseminated form of the disease.

## Clostridial Cellulitis without Toxicity

The involvement of invasive clostridial disease can also be limited to the subcutaneous tissue without invading the muscle, which creates a benign lesion, commonly referred to as a "gas abscess." Definitive treatment for this issue is incision and drainage, but these patients must be followed closely for the development of toxic symptoms.

## Clostridial Cellulitis with Toxicity

A small number of patients with clostridial cellulitis can present with the same clinical picture as patients with spreading, toxic clostridial myonecrosis. If the clinical scenario goes undiagnosed or untreated, the patient has a similarly grave prognosis to those diagnosed with fulminant gas gangrene, and requires equally intensive treatment.

## EFFECTS OF HYPEBARIC OXYGEN

There is extensive evidence to support the efficacy of hyperbaric oxygen in gas gangrene, based upon *in vivo* and *in vitro* studies. Demello, et al. (32) did a comparative study on an experimental gas gangrene model in dogs by comparing the outcomes of treatment with hyperbaric oxygen, antibiotics, and surgery, both individually and in combination. They found that when all three treatment modalities were used together, the mortality was significantly lower than when they were used individually or in any other combination. In related study, the Demello group also demonstrated that hyperbaric oxygen reduces the germination rate of heat-activated spores of *Clostridium perfringens* (35).

Hill and Osterhout showed a significant increase in survival of mice who were treated with HBOT versus those who were left untreated (66). Similar findings were also published by both Kelley and Pace and Nora and associates (84, 120). Van Unnik showed that alpha toxin production by clostridial organisms is inhibited by exposing the organisms to oxygen pressures of three atmospheres absolute (154). This finding was expanded upon by Hill and Osterhout, who demonstrated that high concentrations of oxygen can overcome the effects of catalase in necrotizing tissue, and by Kaye, who showed the bactericidal effects of hyperbaric oxygen on clostridial organisms (67, 83). In a similar study, Stevens found that oxygen tensions of 40 mmHg suppress clostridial growth, while oxygen tensions of 80 mmHg suppress toxin synthesis (144).

From 1961 to 1978, hyperbaric oxygen was used in the treatment of well over 1,200 cases of gas gangrene. There are 117 case reports and comments on the efficacy of hyperbaric oxygen with regards to this disease in the world literature (1-4, 6-13, 15-19, 21-23, 27-31, 34, 37-43, 45-50, 55, 56, 59, 60, 62-66, 68, 69, 71-77, 79-81, 83, 85-88, 90-97, 102-108, 116, 117, 119, 123-125, 127,128, 130, 131, 133, 135, 138, 140-144, 146-153, 156-159, 161, 165). For this series of reports, the approximate cumulative mortality rate is 25% while the approximate disease specific fatality rate is 15%. When patients received treatment within 24 hours of the presumptive diagnosis of gas gangrene, the disease specific fatality rate was reported as 5% (64).

Many cases have been reported in the world's literature since 1978, proving that HBO has been accepted among clinicians who are aware of its benefits. Despite the evidence supporting HBOT as a non-invasive adjunct to proper surgical techniques and antibiotic therapy, gas gangrene patients must continue to be managed as multi-organ, intensive care problems. Constant vigilance and prompt intervention are essential to the successful prevention and treatment of life-threatening complications.

## DIAGNOSIS OF GAS GANGRENE

The most common initial symptom in patients with gas gangrene is pain out of proportion to the extent and timing of the correlated injury at the traumatic or surgical site. Depending on the duration of infection, gas gangrene patients can present with signs of clinical toxicity (99). The presence of gas in the soft tissue can be detected on physical exam and confirmed with various imaging modalities; however, this finding is not diagnostic for clostridial myonecrosis. Microscopic evaluation of biopsy material demonstrates necrotizing or degenerating muscle tissue, clostridial organisms, and a remarkable paucity of inflammatory cells (165, 167).

While definitive diagnosis is ultimately contingent upon demonstrating large, gram positive rods, it is essential that proper treatment not be delayed in favor of diagnostic confirmation from the laboratory. Once tissue destruction from clostridial proliferation begins, the patient's outcome depends upon the time that elapses between achieving a working diagnosis and initiating appropriate surgical intervention. The decision to proceed with treatment of clostridial myonecrosis is based primarily on the patient's current clinical status, as described above and summarized in Table 1. If the patient's clinical status does not indicate a need for immediate debridement, then the results of the anaerobic culture and tissue biopsies should be considered.

In reality, the diagnosis of gas gangrene is most often made empirically during surgical exploration in patients who present with less definitive signs and symptoms that are suggestive of gas gangrene. These patients require more aggressive debridement to prevent a more serious wound complication from developing. For patients with a confirmed diagnosis of clostridial myonecrosis, the goal of debridement is to extirpate just enough viable tissue to stop the spread of the disease. Grossly necrotic tissue should always be removed, but it is important that as much viable, well-vascularized tissue be left intact to reduce both the morbidity and length of post-operative recovery that are associated with such procedures. By combining the use of early hyperbaric oxygen treatments, it is possible to limit

## TABLE 1. COMMON PRESENTING SIGNS AND SYMPTOMS IN TOXIC CLOSTRIDIAL MYONECROSIS AND CELLULITIS

| | |
|---|---|
| Pain | Low-grade fever |
| Tachycardia | Bronzing of the skin over involved area |
| Crepitus | Formation of blebs and bullae |
| Hemolysis | Obtunded sensorium |

the spread of the clostridial organisms, thereby reducing the tissue destruction associated with the infection and the treatment, and improving the patient's final outcome.

## TREATMENT STRATEGY

The following strategy emphasizes hyperbaric oxygen as an important adjunctive therapy for the treatment of clostridial myonecrosis. Since the approach for treating both gas gangrene and its complications have changed over time, this text has been updated to reflect the current standard of care, as defined by the world's literature.

## INITIAL CARE OF HIGH RISK PATIENTS

Approximately two-thirds of patients who develop gas gangrene do so post-operatively or after suffering a traumatic wound. The remaining one third of gas gangrene cases are spontaneous in origin, and arise most often in patients with chronic medical conditions that induce sub-clinical ischemia in previously healthy tissue. Patients with pre-existing diabetes mellitus or atherosclerosis are at increased risk for developing clostridial myonecrosis following "clean," but occultly contaminated, large bowel or gall bladder procedures. This same class of chronic diseases is often present in the small number of de novo clostridial infections that have been reported.

Among high-risk patients, traumatic wounds, including minor ones suffered underwater, should be considered contaminated by default and treated accordingly. These wounds should undergo wide debridement to include tissue that shows signs of compromised circulation. Special care must be taken when removing foreign material from the wound. Pulsatile irrigation should be performed, using copious quantities of sterile electrolyte solution or a non-ionic surfactant complexed with elemental iodine. Commercially available surgical-scrub solutions should not be used for irrigation because they contain anionic detergents that have been shown to decrease tissue resistance to infection. The wounds should be left open and inspected at least daily; further debridement should be performed as necessary. Delayed primary closure can be performed approximately five days after the injury in wounds showing no evidence of infection and when the wound edges have maintained adequate perfusion for a minimum of 24 hours.

The operative patient with compromised tissue perfusion presents special problems. Such patients undergoing gall bladder or large bowel surgery have the greatest risk of postoperative clostridial infection. Meticulous attention must be paid to ensure the use of both aseptic surgical technique and appropriate instrumentation.

Electrocautery should be used judiciously to avoid inducing necrosis in neighboring tissue, thereby creating new potential sites of infection. If electrocautery must be used to achieve hemostasis, the bipolar setting should be used at all times, as it produces two-thirds less necrosis to neighboring tissue when compared with monopolar. Suture ligation should be used to control bleeding in vessels larger than 2 mm in diameter. Tissue should be approximated with minimal tension sutures and closed in layers to avoid unnecessarily compromising perfusion.

During the post-operative period, wound inspections and dressing changes must be performed daily, but the actual schedule can vary according to the rate of wound healing. Consultation with a wound care specialist may be indicated in the immediate post-operative period or to manage more complicated cases, such as non-healing wounds. The presence of significant edema surrounding the incision, non-serous drainage from the wound, or complaints of increasing pain at the operative site are all signs concerning for an emerging wound infection and demand immediate evaluation by the surgical team.

## INITIAL SURGICAL INTERVENTION

Aside from minimal debridement, few surgical procedures are required to make the initial diagnosis. This is not the case, however, for patients with extremity involvement, where thorough fasciotomies must be performed to ensure complete decompression of all anatomic compartments. While there are numerous adjunctive therapies for this disease, rapid diagnosis followed by surgical debridement, including thorough, yet conservative, fasciotomies when indicated, remains the standard-of-care for the treatment of clostridial myonecrosis. Adherence to these principles helps preserve tissue, prevents complications, improves post-operative function, and increases overall survival (176, 177).

One of the more common characteristics of clostridial infections is massive edema, which can compromise local tissue perfusion, thereby making any therapeutic procedure attempted significantly less effective. Without adequate circulation, neither high levels of oxygen nor antibiotics can be delivered to the infected area. By maintaining the hypoxic milieu, the clostridial organisms and their toxins are allowed to proliferate and eventually become intravascularly disseminated, which can result in shock. This makes both the planning and management of patients requiring surgical intervention significantly more challenging.

If the patient shows signs of being in fulminant shock, general anesthesia should be avoided in favor of local or regional blocks. A central venous line and at least one other intravenous line should be introduced by either the catheter or cut-down techniques. Particular care should be taken to keep the end of the central venous line from entering the right atrium. Patients with gas gangrene can easily develop myocardial irritability, and an uncontrollable arrhythmia can be induced by placing a catheter into the right atrium. An arterial line should be placed and secured with a heparin lock to facilitate repeated determinations of arterial blood gases for patients who are either suffering from severe trauma and are in particular danger of developing acute respiratory distress syndrome (ARDS) or are suspected of having underlying pulmonary disease.

## ANTIBIOTIC THERAPY

Based upon studies of *in vitro* susceptibility, Penicillin G remains the first-line therapy for antibiotic treatment of clostridial infections. The standard regimen for this medication is a total dose of 10 to 20 million units per day administered intravenously for two weeks. Several other antibiotics, including clindamycin, tetracycline, chloramphenicol, metronidazole, and some cephalosporins, are effective *in vitro* against both *C. perfringens* and other clostridial species (176, 177). In patients with known penicillin allergy, chloramphenicol and metronidazole can potentially be used as alternatives. When the pathology shows mixed infections, specifically with gram-negative bacilli, initial treatment should include aminoglycosides, new generation cephalosporins or choramphenicol.

One animal study showed a survival benefit in a treatment group receiving a regimen of both clindamycin and penicillin when compared to treating with penicillin alone. In this same study, another treatment group had an increase in mortality rates while receiving penicillin and metronidazole simultaneously (179). Studies also indicate that when used alone, clindamycin may have greater efficacy than penicillin in experimental models (178, 179). In experimental models of gas gangrene, clindamycin and penicillin have been shown to be rapidly bactericidal, while clincamyin has the added benefit suppressing alpha toxin production. This difference may account for clindamycin's superior performance in experimental models when compared with penicillin (180). Despite this experimental increase in activity, it is important to consider the combination of clindamycin and penicillin in clinical applications, since a small but significant percentage of clostridial strains show resistance to mono-therapy with clindamycin. Tetracycline can also be used alone or in combination with penicillin for the treatment of clostridial infections, and has been recommended as an alternative to clindamycin for its ability to rapidly inhibit toxin synthesis (180, 181).

It is important to note that these regimens were designed using evidence from both pre-clinical trials and anecdotal evidence. Unfortunately, clinical trials have not yet been performed to establish the efficacy of these proposed regimens for the treatment of clostridial myonecrosis in human subjects.

## POLYVALENT GAS GANGRENE ANTITOXIN

Even though its efficacy has never been proven, polyvalent equine antitoxin has been used intravenously to treat gas gangrene. Administration of the antitoxin resulted in a significant percentage of patients demonstrating serious allergic reactions, ranging from serum sickness to anaphylactic shock. This treatment is no longer being produced for clinical applications.

## TETANUS PROPHYLAXIS

Since the wounds being evaluated are often severe and contaminated, patients with suspected or diagnosed gas gangrene are also at increased risk for tetanus infections. In these cases, an aggressive approach to tetanus prophylaxis is indicated. The regimen for tetanus prophylaxis consists of an intramuscular injection of 500 units of tetanus immune globulin (human) and 0.5 cc of tetanus toxoid injected intramuscularly at another site.

## BLOOD AND BLOOD COMPONENTS

Whole blood should be administered to replace acute blood loss, but it should only be used sparingly. Bedridden patients show remarkable improvement when their hematocrits (HCT) fall between 30-35 %, as long as their intravascular volumes are kept within normal range. Outcome analyses have demonstrated that the overall cardiac workload increases for patients whose hematocrits are maintained above the suggested range, resulting in worsened outcomes.

Whole blood should be administered through a micro-aggregate filter to prevent patients from developing ARDS. Specific blood components, such as fresh-frozen plasma or platelets, can be used to treat platelet deficiencies or coagulopathies, as needed.

## TRANSFER OF PATIENT FOR HYPERBARIC THERAPY

If a hyperbaric chamber is not available at the initial receiving hospital, arrangements must be made quickly to transfer the patient to a facility equipped with a hyperbaric chamber within 24 hours.

The physician covering the chamber at the receiving facility should be contacted to arrange for the transfer of care. Patient transport, which should involve the most expeditious method available, is often performed by air ambulance when the distance between the two facilities is greater than 100 miles.

## HYPERBARIC OXYGEN TREATMENT

The hyperbaric oxygen treatment schedule used should closely follow the protocol that was originally promulgated by Drs. Brummelkamp and Boerema (23). The depth equivalent chamber pressure used is 66 feet of sea water (3 ATA). Some facilities treat gas gangrene patients at a depth equivalent pressure of 49.5 feet of sea water (2.5 ATA), which is the minimum pressure where oxygen has been found to be effective in the treatment of gas gangrene.

The patient breathes 100% oxygen for 90 minutes per treatment, using a tight fitting aviator's mask, anesthesia mask or endotrachial tube. The cuffs of the endotrachial tubes should be inflated with normal saline solution. The 90-minute period of oxygen treatments can be divided into two 45-minute periods or three 25-minute periods with a final 15-minute period. In either case, the oxygen breathing periods should be separated by 5-minute air breaks to minimize the potential for oxygen toxicity.

Three oxygen treatments are administered and evenly spaced over the first 24 hours. For seriously ill patients, the first two treatments are given with only 2-hour surface intervals. After the first 24 hours, 2 treatments are given every 24 hours, until toxic signs and symptoms have abated. This usually requires 7 treatments, but in no case should fewer than 5 treatments be administered.

Following each treatment, the patient can be decompressed directly to the surface since the excess oxygen that they were administered prevented the uptake of excess nitrogen into their bloodstream. Unlike the patient, the attendants inside the chamber must follow a conservative decompression schedule, such as a variant of the standard U.S. Navy Oxygen Decompression Tables, to avoid developing decompression illness.

Should symptoms of central nervous system oxygen toxicity develop during any of the treatments, the patient should be taken off 100% oxygen and allowed to breathe air for 15 minutes. Following this, the oxygen schedule should be resumed at the point of interruption, but the oxygen periods should be shortened to 20 minutes and include 5-minute air breaks. The chamber pressure should also be decreased by 5 feet of sea water, but only after any convulsive diathesis has abated. If additional episodes of oxygen toxicity occur, the chamber pressure should be decreased by increments of 5 feet of sea water and the oxygen breathing periods shortened, as needed.

In no case should the pressure be decreased to less than 49.5 feet of sea water or the oxygen breathing periods shortened to less than 15 minutes. If these limits have been reached and symptoms of oxygen toxicity continue, the treatment should be terminated. Any treatments that follow should not be attempted until a surface interval of at least 8 hours has elapsed. In the event that anticonvulsive drugs are used to prevent the convulsive diathesis, there must be strict adherence to both time and depth limits, as described in the published protocols, to prevent central nervous system damage from continued oxygen administration.

## FLUIDS, ELECTROLYTES, AND pH

The patient's fluid and electrolyte status must be monitored frequently and adjusted according to maintain homeostatic conditions. It is particularly important to maintain a full intravascular volume to avoid peripheral vasoconstriction, optimize adequate circulation, and dilute and promote the elimination of both clostridial toxins and the toxic by-products of tissue breakdown. Since the pulse rate will typically be elevated by clostridial toxins, it cannot be used to evaluate the patient's fluid status. One must rely on the central venous pressure (CVP), urinary output and clinical signs, such as mucous membrane appearance and skin turgor. Adequate intravenous fluid should be given to maintain the CVP within the normal range and a urinary output of 80-100cc per hour.

In choosing the fluids for administration, the following details should be taken into consideration. The ratio of the quantity of crystalloid retained in the intravascular compartment to the quantity administered will approximate 1:4, while colloid will be retained on a 1:1 basis. Following aggressive debridement, particularly of the trunk, insensible fluid losses can increase by a factor of three or four, even exceeding this estimate in the febrile patient. Alternating 0.9% NaCl with a balanced electrolyte solution such as Lactated Ringer's will optimize electrolyte balance while minimizing the chance of iatrogenic lactic acidosis. Finally, one liter of 5% glucose should be administered with every other liter of intravenous fluid for patients who do not receive oral nutrition to prevent catabolic metabolism and to stabilize the intravascular pH.

In the seriously ill patient, blood glucose, pH, and electrolyte status should be reevaluated every two hours. Appropriate treatments should be instituted immediately to correct any deviations from normal values. Acidosis, a common issue with critically ill patients, can occur rapidly and should be treated with intravenous bicarbonate. An early blood sugar determination must be performed to identify patients with potentially undiagnosed diabetes mellitus, a co-morbidity commonly associated with gas gangrene. Even in patients with diabetes that is diagnosed and controlled, clostridial infections can precipitate diabetic ketoacidosis that must be identified and treated immediately.

Hyperkalemia is another significant issue for these patients, and can result from both tissue breakdown and hemolysis. Elevated potassium levels can be controlled by administering an enema containing sodium polystyrene sulfonate cation resin, or kayexalate. A single, 30-50 gram dose of kayexalate usually lowers the potassium level into the normal range, and has a more predictable measurable outcome in the non-diabetic patient with gas gangrene compared to glucose and insulin, which can lower the threshold for central nervous system oxygen toxicity. When treating hyperkalemia, particular care must be taken not to avoid inducing hypokalemia, especially in the digitalized patient.

## CARE OF PATIENTS BETWEEN HYPERBARIC OXYGEN TREATMENTS

Patients who are between hyperbaric oxygen treatments demand constant monitoring and frequent evaluation, both of which are best accomplished in an intensive care unit. If ventilatory assistance is required, it is extremely important to avoid treating patients with partial pressures of oxygen above ambient levels. When $FIO_2$ levels exceed 0.2 between hyperbaric oxygen treatments, patients are at increased risk for developing pulmonary oxygen toxicity. Patients should be maintained at ambient oxygen levels, unless their arterial oxygen tension falls below 65 mmHg, and the $FIO_2$ should be titrated to ensure adequate tissue oxygenation. Any changes in the patient's fluid, electrolyte, and immunologic status should also be addressed when determining the critically ill patient's oxygen demands, as these issues can significantly alter the blood pH and result in a compensatory shift of the oxygen dissociation curve.

In addition, positive end-expiratory pressure (PEEP) is frequently used to treat gas gangrene patients requiring ventilatory assistance either during or between hyperbaric oxygen treatments. This practice minimizes the chance of atelectasis secondary to a decrease in pulmonary surfactant that may result from pulmonary oxygen toxicity and/or Acute Respiratory Distress Syndrome (ARDS).

## HYPERBARIC OXYGEN TREATMENT PRIOR TO DEBRIDEMENT

Since providing hyperbaric oxygen treatments prior to surgical intervention has been shown to arrest the growth and spread of clostridial myonecrosis, it is recommended that patients receive at least two hyperbaric oxygen treatments before undergoing debridement. The benefits of this pre-operative intervention include the improvement of the patient's overall clinical status and a decrease of both the intra-operative and anesthetic risk. Administering hyperbaric oxygen therapy also establishes the line of demarcation between viable and nonviable tissue, which limits the amount of non-necrotic tissue that is mistakenly excised. After the debridement is completed, the course of hyperbaric oxygen treatments should be performed along with the routine daily wound inspections. Additional debridements may be required until there is no evidence of necrotic tissue at the wound site. When all toxic signs and symptoms have abated, one final hyperbaric oxygen treatment should be given and the patient followed closely to monitor for reemergence of the clostridial infection. In the rare event of a clostridial re-infection, hyperbaric oxygen treatments should be reinstituted.

## COMPLICATIONS

In addition to the physiological and biochemical management issues mentioned above, the following clinical issues are complications frequently experienced by patients with clostridial myonecrosis and require immediate identification and treatment.

**ARDS:** This complication is commonly seen following severe trauma, and is characterized by poor alveolar gas exchange. ARDS is caused by inflammatory injury by damage to pulmonary capillaries or alveolar epithelium, resulting in acute or sub-acute pulmonary edema. Loss of pulmonary surfactant is part of the syndrome and can be compounded by micro-emboli from blood transfusions as well as pulmonary oxygen toxicity. As a protective measure, the use of blood transfusions and supplemental oxygen should be minimized between hyperbaric oxygen treatments.

Diagnosis is based upon arterial blood gas determinations that demonstrate inadequate alveolar gas exchange; radiographic abnormalities may be minimal or absent. Treatment consists of correction of the initiating cause, adequate fluid balance, and use of positive end expiratory pressure (PEEP) ventilation or, when necessary, continuous mechanical ventilation (CMV).

**Disseminated Intravascular Coagulopathy (DIC):** This complication is the result of dysfunctional fibrinogen and platelet activity. It is often seen concomitantly with serious infections and has two primary clinical manifestations. The hemorrhagic type presents in patients as a bleeding diathesis, and is due to a decrease in circulating platelets. The thrombotic type is characterized by the formation of platelet thrombi form in small vessels, leading to significantly decreased tissue perfusion at the arteriolar and capillary level. Generally, elements of both types are present in all cases of DIC since they share a common physiological pathway involving the conversion of fibrinogen to fibrin, fibrinolysis, an increase in platelet adhesion, and thrombocytopenia.

Making the diagnosis of DIC is based upon correlating the patient's history and clinical status with laboratory analysis, including fibrinogen levels, platelet counts (below normal), and the level of fibrin-split products (a four-fold increase is diagnostic). Treatment is based on rapid correction of the underlying disorder. While there are still no controlled studies that have demonstrated an improvement in outcome by directly treating the resulting coagulopathy, heparin may be administered intravenously by infusion pump at a dose of 500 units per hour, if the underlying cause of DIC can be controlled within 48 to 72 hours of onset. After heparin has been infused for two hours procoagulant replacement can be administered safely. Two to three units of fresh frozen plasma and four to eight units of platelets will provide an adequate amount of procoagulants.

**Oliguria and Acute Renal Failure (ARF):** While not commonly seen in gas gangrene, renal impairment can occur and must be adequately managed. In many oliguric patients, the toxic process can be reversed with hyperbaric oxygen, resulting in the reestablishment of normal renal function. If oliguria progresses to acute renal failure, treatment should focus on maintaining fluid and electrolyte balance. Dialysis should be considered when the patient's fluid and electrolyte status cannot be managed conservatively. Acute renal failure is not a contraindication to initiating or continuing hyperbaric oxygen therapy.

**Myocardial Irritability:** Several clostridial exotoxins have cardiotoxic side-effects that can result in significant myocardial irritability, especially in children. Common dysrhythmias that have been seen in both adults and children include wandering atrial pacemaker, atrial tachycardia, nodal rhythms, unifocal and multifocal premature ventricular contractions, ventricular tachycardia, and ventricular fibrillation.

These patients should receive continuous cardiac monitoring during the course of their illness to rapidly identify and treat the arrhythmias, while simultaneously undergoing detoxification to prevent additional complications. Iatrogenically-induced arrythmias have been associated with the introduction of CVP catheters, but this complication can be prevented by not allowing the catheter to enter the right atrium.

The action of hyperbaric oxygen in decreasing the toxin load appears to be adequate treatment for most supranodal arrhythmias. In more severe arrhythmias or scenarios where cardiac function is significantly compromised, specific cardio-pharmacologic agents should be used without hesitation, including rapid digitalization of patients in cardiac failure.

**Deep Vein Thrombosis (DVT):** Any patient immobilized for a prolonged period of time is in danger of developing deep vein thrombosis, particularly of the lower extremities. This danger is increased in the patient who has suffered traumatic injury to the lower extremities, recently under-gone surgery, or has pre-existing inadequate lower extremity venous drainage.

Low dose heparin and low molecular weight heparin are two commonly used pharmacologic modalities for preventing deep vein thromboses. A traditional, low-dose heparin schedule consists of the subcutaneous administration of 5,000 units of heparin every 8-12 hours. Low molecular weight heparin, such as enoxaparin, is administered at a dose of 30 mg subcutaneously every 12 hours, and is shown to be much less likely to induce immune-mediated, or heparin-induced, thrombocytopenia than unfractionated heparin (182). In addition, injured extremities should be elevated to avoid complications from dependent edema and all dressings should be carefully applied to ensure that gentle, even pressure are applied from the foot to the thigh.

**Fat Embolism:** This complication can be seen following injuries involving long bone fractures. It is a particular hazard in the gas gangrene patient who is frequently moved from the intensive care unit to the hyperbaric chamber. Immobilization of the involved extremity will minimize the risk of this disorder. There is still no proven treatment for fat embolism, although corticosteroids, maintenance of adequate intravenous fluids, and PEEP are often used as adjunctive therapies.

## CONCLUSION

While proper care of traumatic and surgical wounds can lessen the incidence of gas gangrene, it has become apparent that the disease is resistant to total eradication. No longer solely a disease of combat, it is now a real and serious threat to patients who suffer injuries in an increasingly violent and high-speed civilian society.

The devastating nature of gas gangrene created a primary need for decisive, aggressive surgical intervention directed toward stopping the potentially rapid spread of an established clostridial process. Early cases could only be treated with radical amputations and mutilating flaying procedures, and despite its profound impact on a wide variety of medical and surgical issues, the advent of antibiotic therapy had very little impact on the surgical approach to treating clostridal myonecrosis. The efficacy of hyperbaric oxygen, as originally demonstrated in the Netherlands in the early 1960s, was destined to ultimately be recognized by the medical community. Despite several decades of dogmatic resistance, the medical and surgical communities have accepted the early use of hyperbaric oxygen as an effective weapon for treating this potentially fatal disease. Though still a surgical disorder, radical surgical intervention is no longer the only tool available for the successful treatment of gas gangrene. The success of hyperbaric oxygen at rapidly detoxifying patients allows surgeons to operate with far less risk while minimizing the morbidity associated with aggressive debridement.

Despite its utility in controlling the proliferation of clostridial organisms and the elaboration of their toxins, hyperbaric oxygen therapy should not be considered a definitive treatment for clostridial myonecrosis. These patients pose multi-organ, intensive care problems throughout the course of their disease that can test the abilities of the most astute physician. Only a thorough and coordinated approach to diagnosis, maintenance, monitoring, prevention and therapy, such as the one presented in this chapter, can result in successful treatment of this disease.

# REFERENCES

1. Altemeier WA. "Diagnosis, classification, and general management of gas producing infections, particularly those produced by Clostridium perfringens. Proceedings of the Third International Conference of Hyperbaric Medicine. Brown IW Jr. and Cox, BG (Eds.) National Academy of Science-National Research Council Publication 1404, Washington, D.C. 1966:481.

2. Alvis HJ. "What hyperbaric medicine has to offer the industrial physician." J Occup Med. 1967;9:304-307.

3. Alvis HJ. "Hyperbaric oxygen therapy of gas gangrene." JAMA. 1971;218:445.

4. Baffes TG and Agustsson MH. "Changing concepts in hyperbaric oxygen therapy." Dis Chest. 1966;49:83-88.

5. Bagdade JD. "Infection of diabetes, predisposing factors." Postgrad Med. 1976;59:160-164.

6. Bahr R and Koslowski L. "Hyperbaric oxygenation in gas gangrene therapy." Helv Chir Acta. 1977;44:431-438.

7. Balldin U, Hedstrum SA, Lundgren C. "Cases of gas gangrene treated with hyperbaric oyxgen." Nord Med. 1968;79:589-591.

8. Barr PO and Dunner H. "Hyperbaric oxygen therapy." Läkartidningen. 1970;67:3538-3539.

9. Bayliss GJ and Cass C. "Hyperbaric oxygen used in the treatment of gas gangrene." Med J Aust. 1967;2:991-993.

10. Beavis JP and Watt J. "Hyperbaric oxygen therapy in the treatment of gas gangrene." J R Nav Med Serv. 1970;56:26-38.

11. Bebenerd J. "The hyperbaric oxygen therapy in gas gangrene infections in gynecology." Gynaeckol Rundsch. 1969;7:235-240.

12. Belokurov Yu, Kamennyy AN, Mormytko AS, et al. "Treatment of anaerobic infection using hyperbaric oxygenation." Vestn Khir. 1970;105:137-138.

13. Bernhard WF and Filler RM. "Hyperbaric oxygenation: Current concepts." Am J Surg. 1968;115:661-668.

14. Bes JC, Deidier C, Baulieux J, et al. "Gas gangrene after rupture of the humeral artery. Temporary by-pass on the third day." Lyon Chir. 1972;68:198-199.

15. Bhargava SK and Chopdar A. "Gas gangrene panophthalmitis." Br J Ophthalmol. 1971;55:136-138.

16. Blaise G, Noel F and Lamy M. "Treatment of gas gangrene. Interest in hyperbaric oxygen therapy." Acta Anesthesiol. 1977;28:41-52.

17. Blenkarn GD. "Hyperbaric therapy: Report of its utilization at the Toronto General Hospital." Can Med Assoc J. 1970;102:951-956.

18. Boccaletti E, Nofrini U, Josi G., et al. "Hyperbaric oyxgen therapy and its clinical uses." Policlinico Prat. 1966;1157-1170.

19. Bristow JH, Kassar B, Sevel D. "Gas gangrene panophthalmitis treated with hyperbaric oyxgen." Br J Ophthalmol. 1971;55:139-142.

20. Brown PW and Kinman PB. "Gas gangrene in a metropolitan community." J Bone Jt Surg. 1974;56:1445-1451.

21. Brummelkamp WH. "Treatment of anaerobic infections with hyperbaric oxygen." Proceedings of the Third International Conference on Hyperbaric Medicine. IW Brown, Jr. and BG Cox (Eds.) National Academy of Science-National Research Council Publication 1404, Washington, DC, 1966;492.

22. Brummelkamp WH. "Treatment of infections due to anaerobic germs by inhalation of hyperbaric oxygen." Ann Chir Thorac Cardiovasc. 1966;5:607-610.

23. Brummelkamp WH, Hoogendijk J, Boerema I. "Treatment of anaerobic infections (clostridial myositis) by drenching the tissue with oxygen under high atmospheric pressure." Surgery. 1961;49:299-302.

24. Cantillo W and Rojas L. "Postabortion septicemia caused by Clostridium welchii: Report of 4 cases." Rev Colomb Obstet Ginecol. 1971;22:247-255.

25. Caplan ES and Kluge RM. "Gas gangrene." Arch Intern Med. 1976;136:788-791.

26. Charon P and Duthois S. "Fatal gas gangrene after intramuscular injection." Nouv Presse Med. 1972;1:109.

27. Colwill MR and Maudsley RH. "The management of gas gangrene with hyperbaric oxygen therapy." J Bone Joint Surg. 1968;50:732-742.

28. Cooke JN. "Hyperbaric oxygen treatment in the Royal Air Force." Proc R Soc Med. 1971;64:881-882.

29. Darke SG, King AM, Slack WK. "Gas gangrene and related infection: classification, clinical features and aetiology, management and mortality. A report of 88 cases." Br J Surg. 1977;64:104-112.

30. Davis JC, Dunn JM, Hagood CO, et al. "Hyperbaric medicine in the U.S. Air Force." JAMA. 1973;224:205-209.

31. DeHaven KE and Evarts CM. "The continuing problem of gas gangrene: A review and report of illustrative cases." J Trauma. 1971;11:983-991.

32. Demello FJ, Haglin JJ, Hitchcock CR. "Comparative study of experimental Clostridium perfringens infection in dogs treated with antibiotics, surgery, and hyperbaric oxygen." Surgery. 1973;73;936-941.

33. Demello FJ, Hashimoto T, Hitchcock CR, et al. "The effect of hyperbaric oxygen on the germination and toxin production of Clostridium perfringens spores." Proceedings of the Fourth International Congress on Hyperbaric Medicine. J Wada and T Iwa (Eds.) Tokyo, Igaku Shoin Ltd., 1970;276.

34. Desfemmes C, Metrot J, Boussignac G, et al. "Treatment of gas gangrene with hyperbaric oxygenation. Parenteral hyperalimentation, antibiotic and heparin therapy and surgery. Apropos of 17 cases." Ann Anesthesiol Fr. 1974;15:249-267.

35. Dieminger HJ and Braune M. "On the therapy of postabortal gas gangrene infection." Zentralb Gynaekol. 1967;89:484-488.

36. Dikshit SK and Mehrotra SN. "Gas gangrene of the lower limb following femoral venepuncture." J Trop Med Hyg. 1968;71:162-164.

37. Dolatkowski A. "The necessity for organizing hospital centers dispensing oxygen hyperbaric treatment." Pol Tyg Lek. 1975;30:315-317.

38. Dominiguez, AA, Garcia FA, Diaz AM. "A case of gas gangrene caused by Clostridium treated with hyperbaric oxygen." Rev Esp Anestesiol. Reanim. 1968;15:674-676.

39. Dominguez AA, De Miguel GF, Grande MM, et al. "Personal experience in the treatment of gas gangrene using hyperbaric oxygenation." Rev Esp Anestesiol Reanim. 1969;16:545-547.

40. DuCailar J, Dossa J, Kienlen J, et al. "Results of treatment of 20 gas gangrene patients with hyperbaric oxygenation." Ann Anesthesiol Fr. 1974;15:243-248.

41. Ducailar J, Lefebvre F, Roquefeuil B, et al. "Indication for hyperbaric oxygen therapy in certain anoxic and infectious conditions." Maroc Med. 1970;50:378-382.

42. Duff JH, Shibata HOUR, Vanschaik L, et al. "Hyperbaric oxygen: A review of treatment in eighty-three patients." Can Med Assoc J. 1967;97:510-515.

43. Durant CJ and Bailey AS. "Hyperbaric oxygen in the treatment of gas gangrene." Radiography. 1971;37:61-64.

44. Dykes RG. "Gas gangrene after hip nailing." Aust NZ J Surg. 1977;47:790-792.

45. Editorial. "Gas gangrene and hyperbaric oxygen." Br Med J. 1972;3:715.

46. Editorial. "Gas gangrene and hyperbaric oxygen." Br Med J. 1972;4:174-175.

47. Editorial. "Hyperbaric oxygen." Lancet. 1968;1:336-338.

48. Eraklis AJ, Filler RM, Pappas AM, et al. "Evaluation of hyperbaric oxygen as an adjunct in the treatment of anaerobic infections." Am J Surg. 1969;117:485-492.

49. Fowler DL, Evans LL, Mallow JE. "Monoplace hyperbaric oxygen therapy for gas gangrene." JAMA. 1977;238:882-883.

50. Frichs G, Klepp G, Gollman K, et al. "Hyperbaric oxygenation in the hospital, first experiences." Zentralbl Chir. 1975;100:321-331.

51. Gazzaniga AB. "Nontraumatic clostridial gas gangrene of the right arm and adenocarcinoma of the cecum: Report of a case." Dis Colon Rectum. 1967;10:298-300.

52. Gaylis H. "Gas gangrene and intramuscular injection." Br Med J. 1968;3:59-60.

53. Glenert J. "Gas gangrene in the abdominal wall following gastrectomy." Nord Med. 1966;75:623-624.

54. Greiner PM. "Clostridial infection following appendectomy." J Am Osteopath Assoc. 1973;72:909-912.

55. Gunter V. "Gas gangrene treated by hyperbaric oxygen." Nurs Times. 1969;65:526-528.

56. Hahnloser P. "Hyperbaric oxygenation." Schweiz Med Wochenschr. 1966;96:1462-1463.

57. Halpern AA, Jameson RM, Nagel DA, et al. "Nontraumatic embolic clostridial gas gangrene: Involvement of an extremity associated with endoscopy." West J Med. 1978;129:141-145.

58. Hamburger S and Zaltse H. "Early diagnosis of biliary Clostridium welchii during cholecystectomy." Harefuah. 1972;82:553-554.

59. Hart GB, Cave RH, Goodman DB, et al. "Clostridial myonecrosis: The constant menace." Milit Med. 1975;140:461-463.

60. Hart GB, O'Reilly RR, Cave RH, et al. "The treatment of clostridial myonecrosis with hyperbaric oxygen." J Trauma. 1974;14:712-715.

61. Harvey PW and Purnell GV. "Fatal case of gas gangrene associated with intramuscular injection." Br Med J. 1968;1:774-776.

62. Hedström SA. "Differential diagnosis and treatment of gas producing infections." Acta Chir Scan. 1975;141:582-589.

63. Hedström SA. "Ten cases of gas gangrene treated with hyperbaric oxygen." Nord Med. 1970;84:989.

64. Heimbach RD, Boerema I, Brummelkamp WH, Wolfe WG. "Current therapy of gas gangrene." Hyperbaric Oxygen Therapy. JC Davis and TK Hunt (Eds.) Undersea Medical Society, Inc., Bethesda, MD, 1977;153.

65. Heimbach RD, Davis JG, Davis JC, et al. "Hyperbaric Medicine in the U.S. Air Force." Aeromed Rev. 1976;6:3-22.

66. Hill GB, and Osterhout S. "Experimental effects of hyperbaric oxygen on selected clostridial species. II. In vitro studies in mice." J Infect Dis. 1972;125:26.

67. Hill GB and Osterhout S. "In vitro and in vivo effects of hyperbaric oxygen on Clostridium perfringens." Proceedings of the Third International Conference on Hyperbaric Medicine. IW Brown, Jr. and BG Cox (Eds.) National Academy of Science-National Research Council Publication 1404, Washington, DC, 1966;538.

68. Hitchcock CR and Bubrick MP. "Gas gangrene infections of the small intestine, colon and rectum." Dis Colon Rectum. 1976;19:112-119.

69. Hitchcock CR, Haglin JJ, Arnar O. "Treatment of clostridial infections with hyperbaric oxygen." Surgery. 1967;62:759-769.

70. Hitchcock CR, Demello FJ, Haglin JJ. "Gas gangrene: New approaches to an old disease." Surg Clinics N Amer. 1975;55:1403-1410.

71. Hoffman S, Katz JF, Jacobson JH. "Salvage of lower limb after gas gangrene." Bull NY Acad Med. 1971;7:40-49.

72. Holland JA, Hill GB, Wolfe WG, et al. "Experimental and clinical experience with hyperbaric oxygen in the treatment of clostridial myonecrosis." Surg. 1975;77:75-84.

73. Hommelgaard P and Kolind-Sorenson V. "Gas gangrene treated with hyperbaric oxygen." Ugeskr Laeger. 1974;136:1073-1075.

74. Howell LM. "Hyperbaric oxygen in gas gangrene." Northwest Med. 1969;68:1016-1019.

75. "Hyperbaric oxygen therapy." Med Lett Drugs Ther. 1971;13:29-32.

76. "Hyperbaric oxygen therapy." Med Lett Drugs Ther. 1978;20:51-52.

77. Irvin, TT. "Gas gangrene and hyperbaric oxygen." Br Med J. 1972;4:47.

78. Irvin TT, Donaldson AJ, Smith G. "Clostridium welchii infection in gastric surgery." Surg Gynecol Obstet. 1967;124:77-81.

79. Jackson RW and Waddell JP. "Hyperbaric oxygen in the management of clostridial myonecrosis (gas gangrene)." Clin Orthop. 1973;96:271-276.

80. Jacobsen A and Secher O. "Hyperbaric oxygenation: Clinical results and experiences in hyperbaric oxygenation in the individual pressure chamber." Ugeskr Laeger. 1967;129:822-828.

81. Johnson JT, Gillespie TE, Cole JR, et al. "Hyperbaric oxygen therapy for gas gangrene in war wounds." Am J Surg. 1969;118:839-843.

82. Kakande I. "Gas gangrene following an injection." East Afr Med J. 1977;54:434-437.

83. Kaye D. "Effect of hyperbaric oxygen on Clostridia in vitro and in vivo." Proc Soc Exp Biol Med. 1967;124:360-366.

84. Kelley HG, Jr. and Pace WG, III. "Treatment of anaerobic infections in mice with high pressure oxygen." Surg Forum. 1962;14:46.

85. Keogh AJ. "Clostridial brain abscess and hyperbaric oxygen." Postgrad Med J. 1973;49:64-66.

86. Kindwall EP. "Gas gangrene: acute medical emergency: The role of hyperbaric oxygen." Wis Med J. 1970;69:261-263.

87. Kitamoto H. "Hyperbaric oxygen therapy." Naika. 1965;16:78-80.

88. Kokame GM, Olinde HD, Krementz ET, et al. "Gas gangrene: Successful treatment with hyperbaric oxygenation." J La State Med Soc. 1967;119:193-198.

89. Kole W, Mose JR, Ratzenhofer M. "Gas gangrene caused by war injury - 28 years later fatal gas gangrene following cholecystectomy." Zentralbl Chir. 1973;98:926-931.

90. Kucher R and Riedel W. "Treatment of gas gangrene in hyperbaric oxygen chamber." Wien Klin Wochenschr. 1969;81:308-310.

91. Lacey CG, Futoran R, Morrow CP. "Clostridium perfringens infection complicating chemotherapy for choriocarcinoma." Obstet Gynecol. 1976;47:337-341.

92. Lambertsen CJ. "Oxygen in the therapy of gas gangrene." J Trauma. 1972;12:825-827.

93. Lamy M, Lejeune G, Noel FX, et al. "Gas gangrene: Importance of early diagnosis and hyperbaric oxygen therapy." Rev Med Liège. 1977;32:589-593.

94. Lamy ML and Hanquet MM. "Hyperbaric oxygen therapy in a monoplace chamber with pure oxygen. Experience in 700 clinical cases." Maroc Med. 1971;51:602-610.

95. Larcan A, Laprevote-Huelly MC, Fieve G, et al. "Gas gangrene, apropos of 24 cases. Value of combined surgical and hyperbaric oxygen therapy." Ann Chir. 1974;28:445-454.

96. Larcan A, Laprevote-Heully, Lambert H, et al. "Gas gangrene on the basis of 19 observations. Advantages of combining surgery with hyperbaric oxygen therapy." Mater Med Pol. 1974;6:116-119.

97. Long WB III, Howatson A, Gill W. "Marlex mesh in gas gangrene." J Trauma. 1976;16:948-953.

98. MacGregor KH. "Gas gangrene complicating surgery of the colon: Report of two cases." Dis Colon Rectum. 1965;8:431-436.

99. MacLennan JD. "The histotoxic clostridial infections in man." Bacteriol Rev. 1962;26:177-276.

100. Maguire WB and Langley NF. "Gas gangrene following an adrenaline-in-oil injection into the left thigh with survival." Med J Aust. 1967;1:973-975.

101. Maretie Z, ZeCaper Z Ku, Srketic M, et al. "Gas gangrene following criminal abortion." Med Klin. 1969;64:2186-2189.

102. Maudsley RH. "Proceedings: post-operative gas gangrene managed by hyperbaric oxygen." J Bone Joint Surg Br. 1975;57:251.

103. Maudsley RH and Arden GP. "Gas gangrene and hyperbaric oxygen." Br Med J. 1972;4:362.

104. McDonald DF. "Adjunctive treatment of life-threatening emergencies with oxygen under high pressure." Tex Med. 1976.

105. Meijne NG. "Hyperbaric oxygen, increased pressure and the activities in this field in Boerema's department in the period 1956-1972." Arch Chir Neerl. 1973;25:195-213.

106. Meijne NG, Mellink HM, Kox C. "The main present-day indications for clinical treatment in a hyperbaric chamber." Pneumonologie. 1973;149:173-180.

107. Monafo WW, Brentano L, Gravens DL et al. "Gas gangrene and mixed clostridial infections of muscle complicating deep thermal burns." Archives of Surgery 1966;92:212-221.

108. Monies I, Altman, Joachims HZ, et al. "Treatment of gas gangrene of the neck by hyperbaric oxygen." Harefuah. 1973;84:538-540.

109. Monies-Chass I, Joachims HZ, Altman MM. "Hyperbaric oxygen in anaerobic infection of the mediastinum." J Laryngol. 1975;89:1147-1150.

110. Morton A. "Testicular gas gangrene after hernia repair with cord division." Med J Aust. 1967;2:605-606.

111. Mukai T, Nishoika T, Uyama A. "Acute peritonsillitis followed by gas phlegomon in the neck in a diabetic." J Otolaryngol JPN. 1975;78:1177-1183.

112. Mzabi R, Himal HS, Maclean LD. "Gas gangrene of the extremity: the presenting clinical picture in perforating carcinoma of the caecum." Br J Surg. 1975;62:373-374.

113. Nahir AM, Hasmonai M, Merzbach D, et al. "Gas gangrene: Following intramuscular injection of aqueous solution." N.Y. State J Med. 1978;78:1948-1949.

114. Nahir AM, Scharf J, Merzbach D, et al. "Gas gangrene following intramuscular injection." Harefuah. 1971;81:502.

115. Nali MN. "Fatal gas gangrene after intramuscular injection; apropos of a case." Union Med Can. 1977;1400-1401.

116. Ney R, Podlesch I, Buchard A, et al. "Indications for active surgical procedures within the area. Hyperbaric oxygen therapy for gas edema. Experiences with 42 gas edema infections." Tidsskr Nor Laegeføren. 1971;91:766-771.

117. Nichols RL and Smith JW. "Gas in the wound: What does it mean?" Surg Clin North Am. 1975;55:1289-1296.

118. Nini W, Nini N, Assouad I. "A case of fatal fulminating gas gangrene complicating surgery of acute appendicitis." Chirurgie. 1970;96:174-177.

119. Nier H, Sailer R, Palomba P. "Hyperbaric oxygen treatment in gas gangrene." Dtsch Med Wochenschr. 1978;103:1958-1960.

120. Nora PF, Bransfield J, Cheslak F, et al. "H.P.O. in clostridial toxicity and strangulation obstruction." Arch Surg. 1966;93:236.

121. Patchell RD. "Clostridial myonecrosis of the postpartum uterus with radiologic diagnosis." Obstet Gynecol. 1978;51(Suppl):145-155.

122. Prabhakar MJ, Redding ME, Anagnostopoulos CE, et al."Gas gangrene complicating aortic dissection. Report of a case." Arch Surg. 1971;103:96-97.

123. Ratner GL, Nenashev AA, Svechnikova EL, et al. "Treatment of anaerobic infection by hyperbaric oxygenation." Khirurgiya. (Moscow) 1971;47:39-44.

124. Rifkind D. "The diagnosis and treatment of gas gangrene." Surg Clin N Amer. 1963;43:511-517.

125. Roding B, Groenveld PHA, Boerema I. "Ten years of experience in the treatment of gas gangrene with hyperbaric oxygen." Surg Gynecol, Obstet. 1972;134:579-585.

126. Rush JH. "Clostridial infection in total hip replacement; a report of two cases." Aust NZ J Surg. 1976;46;45-48.

127. Sailer R, Juneman A, Ghazwinian R. "Therapy of gas gangrene. Comparison of results of the standard and hyperbaric oxygen therapy." Med Klin. 1974;69:1620-1625.

128. Saltzman HA. "Hyperbaric oxygen." Med Clin North Am. 1967;51:1301-1314.

129. Schaupp KL, Jr., Pinto D, Valentine RJ. "Hyperbaric oyxgen in therapy of gas gangrene: Report of a case following induced abortion." Calif Med. 1966;105:97-101.

130. Schautz R. "Hyperbaric oxygen therapy for gas gangrene." Dtsch Med Wochenschr. 1968;93:1328-1330.

131. Schmauss AK. "Gas gangrene following intramuscular injections." Z Aertzl Fortbild. 1974;68:41-47.

132. Schmauss AK and Bahrmann E. "Gas and oedema producing infections today - still a challenge." Zentralbl Chir. 1977;102:120-129.

133. Schmauss AK, Bahrmann, Fabian W. "Gas gangrene therapy and hyperbaric oxygenation." Zentrabl Chir. 1973;98:912-925.

134. Schonfelder M. "Gas gangrene after common bile duct exploration." Zentralbl Chir. 1971;96:96-99.

135. Schraibman IG. "Gas gangrene after amputation for peripheral vascular disease." Postgrad Med J. 1968;44:551-553.

136. Schulte JH. "The use of hyperbaric oxygen in clinical medicine." J Occup Med. 1969;11:462-465.

137. Schuppisser JP. "Gas gangrene." Langenbecks Arch Chir. 1979;348:1-5.

138. Schweigel JF and Shim SS. "A comparison of the treatment of gas gangrene with and without hyperbaric oxygen." Surg Gynecol Obstet. 1973;139:969-970.

139. Skiles MS, Covert GK, Fletcher HS. "Gas-producing clostridial and nonclostridial infections." Surg Gynecol Obstet. 1978;147:65-67.

140. Slack WK. "Hyperbaric oxygen therapy in anaerobic infections." Med Times. 1978;06:15D(82)-16D(82),21D(82).

141. Slack WK. "Hyperbaric oxygen therapy in anaerobic infections: Gas gangrene." Proc R Soc Med. 1976;69:326-327.

142. Slack WK, Hanson GC, Chew HE. "Hyperbaric oxygen in the treatment of gas gangrene and clostridial infection. A report of 40 patients treated in a single-person hyperbaric oxygen chamber." Br J Surg. 1969;56:505-510.

143. Srivolocki WP, Nick WV, Pace WG. "Gas gangrene treated by isolated perfusion with hyperbaric oxygenation." Surg Forum. 1970;21:231-232.

144. Stevens D. Personal Communications.

145. Szekely O, Szanto G, Takats A. "Hyperbaric oxygen therapy in injured subjects." Injury. 1973;4:294-300.

146. Tarbiat S. "Results of combined surgical-antibiotic and hyperbaric oxygenation therapy in gas gangrene." Chirurg. 1970;41:506-511.

147. Taylor AR and Maudsley RH. "Post-operative gas gangrene managed by early hyperbaric oxygen therapy (two cases)." Proc R Soc Med. 1968;61:661.

148. Tenev K. "Hyperbaric oxygen therapy and the treatment of anaerobic infections." Khirurgiia. (Sofia) 1975;28:154-159.

149. Thunold J, Gjengsto H, Smith-Silvertsen J. "Hyperbaric oxygenation in the treatment of anaerobic gas forming infections." Tidsskr Nor Laegeføren. 1974;94:1069-1073.

150. Thurston JG. "Place of hyperbaric oxygen in intensive care." Proc R Soc Med. 1971;64:1287-1288.

151. Trippel OH, Ruggie AN, Stanley CJ, et al. "Hyperbaric oxygenation in the management of gas gangrene." Surg Clin North Am. 1967;47:17-27.

152. Tooley AH and Watt J. "Hyperbaric oxygen therapy: Review of the present position and experiences in the management of naval patients." J.R. Nav Med Serv. 1968;54:101-128.

153. Van Hook R and Vandervelde AG. "Letter: Gas gangrene after intramuscular injection of epinephrine: Report of fatal case." Ann Intern Med. 1975;83:669-670.

154. Van Unnik AJM. "Inhibition of toxin production in Clostridium perfringens in vitro by hyperbaric oxygen." Antonie von Leeuwenhoek. 1965;31:181-186.

155. Van Zyl JJ. "Gas gangrene, the modern therapeutic approach." S Afr J Surg. 1973;11:181-185.

156. Van Zyl JJW. "Discussion of hyperbaric oyxgen." Proceedings of the Third International Conference on Hyperbaric Medicine. IW Brown, Jr. and BG Cox. (Eds.) National Academy of Science-National Research Council Publication 1404, Washington, DC., 1966;552.

157. Watt J. "Surgical applications of hyperbaric oxygen therapy in the Royal Navy." Proc R Soc Med. 1971;64:877-881.

158. Wattel F, Gosselin B, Chopin C, et al. "Current aspects of gas gangrene, apropos of 47 cases collected over a 3-year period (1974-1976)." Ann Anesthesiol Fr. 1977;18:825-830.

159. Weinstein L and Barza MA. "Medical intelligence: Current concepts, gas gangrene." New Engl J Med. 1973;289:1129-1131.

160. Wernitsch W. "Technic and administration of hyperbaric oxygenation." Med Welt. 1969;49:2668-2671.

161. Williams JM. "Fractured neck of femur and subsequent gas gangrene." Proc Pap Annu Conf Calif Mosq Control Assoc. 1966;34:63-64.

162. Willis AT. Clostridia of Wound Infection. Butterworth, London: 1969.

163. Yeo CK and McNamara JJ. "Retroperitoneal rupture of duodenum with complicating gas gangrene." Arch Surg. 1973;106:856-857.

164. Zierott G, May E, Harms H. "Changes in the evaluation of therapy of gas edema through the administration of hyperbaric oxygenation. A clinical comparative study of 31 cases of gas edema." Burns. Betr Klin Khir. 1973;220:292-296.

165. Awad MM, Bryant AE, Stevens DL, Rood JI. Virulence studies on chromosomal alpha-toxin and theta toxin mutants constructed by allelic exchange provide genetic evidence for the essential role of alpha-toxin in Clostridium perfringens-mediated gas gangrene. Mol Microbiol 1995; 15:191-202.

166. Rood JI. Virulence genes of Clostridium perfringens. Annu Rev Microbiol. 1998;52:333-60.

167. Ellemor DM, Baird RN, Awad MM, Boyd RL, Rood JI, Emmins JJ. Use of genetically manipulated strains of Clostridium perfringens reveals that both alpha-toxin and theta-toxin are required for vascular leukostasis to occur in experimental gas gangrene. Infect Immun. 1999 Sep;67(9):4902-7.

168. Stevens DL, Tweten RK, Awad MM, Rood JI, Bryant AE. Clostridial gas gangrene: evidence that alpha and theta toxins differentially modulate the immune response and induce acute tissue necrosis. J Infect Dis. 1997 Jul;176(1):189-95.

169. Williamson, ED, Titball, RW. A genetically engineered vaccine against the alpha-toxin of Clostridium perfringens protects mice against experimental gas gangrene. Vaccine 1993; 11:1253.

170. Stevens, DL, Titball, RW, Jepson, M, et al. Immunization with the C-Domain of alpha -Toxin prevents lethal infection, localizes tissue injury, and promotes host response to challenge with Clostridium perfringens. J Infect Dis 2004; 190:767.

171. Bryant, AE, Chen, RY, Nagata, Y, et al. Clostridial gas gangrene. I. Cellular and molecular mechanisms of microvascular dysfunction induced by exotoxins of Clostridium perfringens. J Infect Dis 2000; 182:799-807.

172. Bryant, AE, Chen, RY, Nagata, Y, et al. Clostridial gas gangrene. II. Phospholipase C-induced activation of platelet gpIIbIIIa mediates vascular occlusion and myonecrosis in Clostridium perfringens gas gangrene. J Infect Dis 2000; 182:808-815.

173. Whatley, RE, Zimmerman, GA, Stevens, DL, et al. The regulation of platelet activating factor production in endothelial cells — The role of calcium and protein kinase C. J Biol Chem 1989; 264:6325.

174. Stevens, DL, Troyer, BE, Merrick, DT, et al. Lethal effects and cardiovascular effects of purified alpha- and theta-toxins from Clostridium perfringens. J Infect Dis 1988; 157:272.

175. Asmuth, DA, Olson, RD, Hackett, SP, et al. Effects of Clostridium perfringens recombinant and crude phospholipase C and theta toxins on rabbit hemodynamic parameters. J Infect Dis 1995; 172:1317.

176. Gorbach, SL. Clostridium perfringens and other clostridia. In: Infectious Diseases, Gorbach, SL, Bartlett, JG, Blacklow, NR (Eds), WB Saunders, Philadelphia 1992. p.1587.

177. Lorber, B. Gas gangrene and other Clostridium-associated diseases. In: Principles and Practice of Infectious Diseases, 6th ed. Mandell, GL, Bennett, JE, Dolin, R, (Eds), Churchill Livingstone, Philadelphia, PA 2005, p.2828.

178. Stevens, DL, Maier, KA, Laine, BM, Mitten, JE. Comparison of clindamycin, rifampin, tetracycline, metronidazole, and penicillin for efficacy in prevention of experimental gas gangrene due to Clostridium perfringens. J Infect Dis 1987; 155:220.

179. Stevens, DL, Laine, BM, Mitten, JE. Comparison of single and combination antimicrobial agents for prevention of experimental gas gangrene caused by Clostridium perfringens. Antimicrob Agents Chemother 1987; 31:312.

180. Stevens, DL, Maier, KA, Mitten, JE. Effect of antibiotics on toxin production and viability of Clostridium perfringens. Antimicrob Agents Chemother 1987; 31:213.

181. Altemeier, WA, Fullen, WD. Prevention and treatment of gas gangrene. JAMA 1971; 217:806.

182. Warkentin, TE, Levine, MN, Hirsh, J, et al. Heparin-induced thrombocytopenia in patients treated with low-molecular-weight heparin or unfractionated heparin. N Engl J Med 1995; 332:1330.

183. Boenicke L, Maier M, Merger M, et al. Retroperitoneal gas gangrene after colonoscopic polypectomy without bowel perforation in an otherwise healthy individual: report of a case. Langenbecks Arch Surg. 2006 Apr;391(2):157-60. Epub 2006 Feb 8.

184. Momm F, Schafer O, Henke M. Metastatic breast cancer causing gas gangrene. J Pain Symptom Manage. 2006 May;31(5):385.

185. Chowdhury PS, Timmis SB, Marcovitz PA. Clostridium perfringens within intracardiac thrombus: a case of intracardiac gas gangrene. Circulation. 1999 Nov 16;100(20):2119.

186. Assadian O, Assadian A, Senekowitsch C, et al. Gas gangrene due to Clostridium perfringens in two injecting drug users in Vienna, Austria. Wien Klin Wochenschr. 2004 Apr 30;116 (7-8):264-7.

187. Hallagan LF, Scott JL, Horowitz BC, Feied CF. Clostridial myonecrosis resulting from subcutaneous epinephrine suspension injection. Ann Emerg Med. 1992 Apr;21(4):434-6.

188. de Virgilio C, Klein S, Chang L, et al. Clostridial bacteremia: implications for the surgeon. Am Surg. 1991 Jun;57(6):388-93.

189. Awad MM, Ellemor DM, Boyd RL, et al. Synergistic effects of alpha-toxin and perfringolysin O in Clostridium perfringens-mediated gas gangrene. Infect Immun. 2001 Dec;69(12):7904-10.

190. Stevens DL, Musher DM, Watson DA, et al. Spontaneous, nontraumatic gangrene due to Clostridium septicum. Rev Infect Dis. 1990;12 :286 –296

# SELECTED AEROBIC AND ANAEROBIC SOFT TISSUE INFECTIONS

## CHAPTER TWENTY-TWO OVERVIEW

# SELECTED AEROBIC AND ANAEROBIC SOFT TISSUE INFECTIONS

*Dirk J. Bakker*

## INTRODUCTION

Necrotizing soft tissue infections caused by aerobic, anaerobic and mixed bacterial floras are an increasing problem in surgical and medical practice. They occur with increasing frequency and seriousness, especially in immune-compromised patients.

The suppression of the immune system may be caused by underlying systemic diseases, mainly: diabetes mellitus, malignancies, vascular insufficiency and alcoholism; by the use of immunosuppressive drugs as in transplant recipients; in drug addicts, and in neutropenic patients.

These infections occur after trauma (sharp and blunt), around foreign bodies in surgical wounds, or even "spontaneously" as is seen sometimes in scrotal and penile necrotizing fasciitis (Fournier's gangrene). A large number of these infections have even been reported after a volcanic cataclysm (103) and also in children (15, 38, 65, 112, 141, 142).

Necrotizing fasciitis is also seen postoperatively e.g. after caesarean delivery in young women without risk factors (no diabetes or peripheral vascular disease) (54), after such "sterile" operations such as suction lipectomy (59, 132) and in Crohn's disease (99). As in gas gangrene every operation can be followed by necrotizing fasciitis and a high index of suspicion is necessary for the diagnosis, especially after so-called "sterile" operations.

The clinical picture can vary considerably from patient to patient. Treatment is difficult, often irrational and very often "one step behind the facts," because early recognition is difficult and etiology, bacteriology, and the clinical course are sometimes not well understood or expected to evolve in a different and more favorable way.

Considerable morbidity occurs and mortality can be very high, from 20% up to 70 or 80%. The highest mortality is found in the group of older debilitated diabetic patients with synergistic necrotizing cellulitis (127).

## HISTORY

For a proper understanding of these infections, a short historical review is necessary.

example hemolytic streptococcal gangrene) and chronic infectious skin gangrene, an example of the latter being postoperative progressive bacterial synergistic gangrene. Kingston and Seal base the conclusions in their article on the division of these infections into three different categories based on the rates of progression (from slow to rapid) (72).

Since 1926 a great variety of synergistic microorganisms both in humans and in animals have been found (for a review see Bakker, 1984) (9).

The bacteriology of these diseases has apparently changed considerably through the years. Meleney mentioned "associated organisms next to *streptococci*, concomitants, not adding to the development of the disease, in a minority of cases" (92). Wilson found *streptococci* in 58% of his patients, (141) Crosthwait in 57%, (33) Ledingham and Tehrani in 8.5% (79) and in our series we initially found *streptococci* in 13.3% of our patients (9).

When necrosis of the deep fascia was recognized as essential in hemolytic streptococcal gangrene or Meleney's ulcer in 1948 by Wilson, the disease was renamed "necrotizing fasciitis" in 1952 (141).

Giuliano et al. (53) thought that two bacteriologic types of necrotizing fasciitis could be recognized and Lamerton (78) even suggested three bacteriologic groups whose clinical pictures, however, largely overlap.

Also, many microorganisms were suggested as causing postoperative progressive bacterial synergistic gangrene throughout the years (9).

The problem is that we seldom see patients at the onset of the disease. Time elapsed since the onset and initial treatment, for example antibiotics given and possible surgical interventions, are of course very important to explain later findings, especially later bacteriological culture results. Remarkably this is never mentioned in the literature neither about necrotizing fasciitis nor about progressive bacterial gangrene. Stone and Gorbach give a very detailed description of the microbiological findings without mentioning what we stated above (128). Smith et al. wonder why normal urethral, rectal and cutaneous flora of otherwise low to moderate virulence are able to cause severe infections of this type (116). Maybe they do not. Is it possible that Meleney was right after all when he mentioned "concomitants, not adding to the development of the disease" (92). Not every microorganism that is cultured is automatically causative to the disease.

Another thing that is seldom mentioned is the location from where the cultures are taken. It can make a big difference if one takes a swab from the center of the wound or culture tissue biopsies at the spreading periphery of the disease. Brewer and Meleney had already mentioned that in their first experiments on bacterial synergy (21).

In 1883, Jean Alfred Fournier, a French venereologist, described five cases of "gangrène foudroyante de la verge," later called Fournier's gangrene. Five healthy young men (ages 24-30 years) developed penile and/or scrotal gangrene, "spontaneously or after a superficial erosion, and despite large incisions and eschar excision, mortality was 60%" (51).

Even before that time descriptions of the same clinical entity can be found in the works of Hippocrates from the 5th century BC.

He described "erysipelas, which was at its worst when it reached the private parts, the pubes and the genitals. Flesh, sinews, and bones fell away in large quantities" (62).

After Hippocrates the first description of a possible case of necrotizing fasciitis came from Baurienne in 1764 (16) in an adult, and thereafter a case in a young baby boy reported by Hebler in 1848 (57).

Also the work by the Confederate Army Surgeon Joseph Jones must be mentioned who described a variant of this disease in 1869 and 1870 that he encountered during the Civil War in the United States, which he called "hospital gangrene" (67, 108).

Extensive reviews of the literature on necrotizing soft tissue infections including Fournier's gangrene have been published by McCrea (89), Jones (68) and Stevens (117), as well as by Loudon (84), Sutherland (129), Chapnick and Abter (28), Weiss and Lavardière (138), Smith et al (116), Eke (46), Capelli-Schellpfeffer and Gerber (27) and also by Wienecke and Lobenhoffer (140). Capelli-Schellpfeffer (27) investigated the role of hyperbaric oxygen in the treatment of these infections in urology.

Meleney, 1924, found the cause of this gangrene to be "a pure invasion of hemolytic *streptococci*"(92). Fournier's gangrene could thus be considered as a special form of hemolytic *streptococcus* gangrene. In the same article Meleney described this hemolytic *streptococcus* gangrene or "Meleney's ulcer," also caused by hemolytic *streptococci* (92). This publication was based on Meleney's experience in the Imperial Hospital in Peking (Beijing).

Cullen, also in 1924, gave a description of the so-called "postoperative progressive bacterial synergistic gangrene," in a patient after an appendectomy (34).

At first a confusing variety of microorganisms was found. But in studying the spreading periphery of the lesion, both clinically and experimentally (in Guinea pigs), the interaction of a microaerophilic non-hemolytic *streptococcus* and a hemolytic *staphylococcus aureus* was found to be synergistic (21).

The confusion in the nomenclature started here, because M...

Recently a case of Fournier's gangrene was described where only Candida was cultured as the primary organism from the urine and later from perianal debrided tissues (66).

In the spring of 1994, a cluster of seven cases of invasive group A streptococcal (GAS) infections, including four cases of necrotizing fasciitis occurred in Gloucestershire (England). When the British media reported this outbreak, the stories resembled Edgar Allan Poe's horror stories at its best. Expressions like "flesh eating bacteria or virus", "galloping gangrene" and "killer bugs" were used to describe the process, and the impression was given that a whole new disease was discovered there. From the historical review given above it should be clear that this was not the case. A description of this outbreak can be found by Efstratiou et al. (45) and Monnickendam et al. (96).

Kujath and Eckmann (77) state that only a minority of necrotizing fasciitis cases is caused by *streptococci* (3 to 4 times less than cases caused by a polymicrobial flora). Podbielski et al. (106) found 10 - 18 % group A *streptococci* and 51% "other" *streptococci* in their cultures of necrotizing fasciitis. In 75 - 85% peptostreptococci were isolated (*peptostreptococci* cause a gas forming infection). Group A *streptococci* and *staphylococci* were cultured when only a monoculture was found. All other microorganisms that were found were part of a polymicrobial flora. In both articles nothing is mentioned about the time of culture in relation to the time of onset of the disease and if the patients were previously treated already. This makes it very difficult to show what the real causative microorganisms are.

A historical review of streptococcal infections with special emphasis on necrotizing fasciitis and the use of hyperbaric oxygen is given by Bakker (12).

Our conclusion is that interpretation and misinterpretation of historical facts and microbiological culture results have caused confusion and have added to the present difficulty in understanding the bacteriology, etiology and clinical findings in these soft tissue infections.

## CLASSIFICATION

An exact classification of necrotizing soft tissue infections is difficult because the distinctions between many of the clinical entities are blurred and a great variety of names have historically been given to the same clinical entity.

Classification of these infections is usually made on the basis of:

a. The assumed causative microorganism(s) (50, 53, 55, 78, 92, 107).
b. The kind of tissue involved (2, 3, 50, 79, 81, 82, 141).
c. The kind of required therapy (50).
d. The rate of progression (72).
e. The initial clinical findings (49).

Each of these classifications has its advantages and its disadvantages because they are based on only one part of the problem. It is difficult to determine the causative microorganism(s) out of the wide variety of aerobes and anaerobes that can be cultured in these infections and it can be equally difficult to diagnose the tissue primarily involved in the advanced stages of these infections when we usually see the patients.

The best therapy is almost always a combination of surgery, antibiotics and adjunctive hyperbaric oxygen.

Also, in our experience the rate of progression of these infections can change considerably from patient to patient and seems to be more dependent on the associated diseases of the patient and/or other systemic or local factors that affect the immune status, metabolism and local vascularisation than on other factors (9, 86).

Following Ledingham and Tehrani (79) we proposed the Amsterdam classification of soft tissue infections (Figure 1), based on the fact if the infections are superficial (as in progressive bacterial gangrene) or involving deeper tissues (as in necrotizing fasciitis and myositis and myonecrosis).

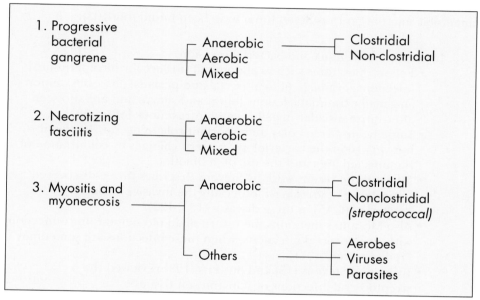

Figure 1. Amsterdam classification of soft tissue infections. In order to systematize the classification (following Ledingham and Tehrani) (28), we divided these infections into three groups: 1. Progressive bacterial gangrene, 2. Necrotizing fasciitis, and 3. Myositis and myonecrosis.

## ETIOLOGY

In these infections anaerobic microorganisms are often found in combination with aerobic Gram-negative organisms. With causes such as traumatic crush injury in the surgically or medically compromised patient, local tissue hypoxia and a decreased oxidation-reduction potential (Eh) is usually present, thus promoting the growth of anaerobic microorganisms. The vast majority of these necrotizing soft tissue infections have an endogenous anaerobic component.

Hypoxic conditions also allow the proliferation of facultative aerobic organisms since polymorphonuclear leukocytes function poorly under decreased oxygen tensions. The growth of aerobic microorganisms further lowers the Eh; more fastidious anaerobes become established and the disease process can rapidly accelerate. Clinically the most important signs of these infections are tissue necrosis, a putrid discharge, gas production, the tendency of the process to burrow through fascial planes and in many cases the absence of the classical signs of tissue inflammation (86).

The variable quantity of gas in the tissues can be used in the differential diagnosis of these infections (10, 100, 101). Carbon dioxide and water are the end products of aerobic metabolism; carbon dioxide rapidly dissolves and rarely accumulates in tissues. The major tissue gases found in mixed aerobic and anaerobic soft tissue infections are probably $H_2$ and $CH_4$, less water soluble end products of incomplete oxidation of energy sources. Nitrogen and hydrogen sulfide can also be found (101). Presence of these gases indicates a rapid bacterial multiplication at a low Eh (80, 101).

The etiology, in summary, in necrotizing soft tissue infections is multifactorial and includes local and systemic factors as well as aerobic and anaerobic microorganisms. Even fungi have been found (66, 103).

1. Local tissue trauma and bacterial invasion:
   - Follow operations such as abdominal surgery for intraperitoneal infections, drainage of ischiorectal and perianal abscesses, minor and major traumatic lesions (blunt and sharp) and are also seen after intramuscular injections and intravenous infusions.
   - Initially, *streptococci* play an important role in necrotizing fasciitis, but very soon the bacteriologic pattern changes by colonization of the infected area and the use of antibiotics.
   - Much of the recent work by Stevens describes the re-discovered importance of *streptococci*, especially the invasive Group A *streptococci* (GAS) in these diseases (121, 122).
   - Also Morantes mentions the return of an old nemesis in connection with streptococcal infections, when these infections are sometimes "rediscovered" (97).
   - Bisno and Stevens (18) and Stevens (123) reviewed the streptococcal infections of skin and soft tissues.
   - Bacterial synergism is an important mechanism in the onset of progressive bacterial gangrene but, here again, no specific bacterial combination could be found underlying the disease and the bacteriologic pattern is changing very quickly as well.

2. Local ischemia:
   - Frequently occurs in patients with diabetes mellitus, arteriosclerosis and after amputations which are necessary for diabetic and arteriosclerotic vascular insufficiency. Moreover, a relative avascularity of the fascial planes in necrotizing fasciitis can be noticed.
   - We showed that secondary gangrene of subcutaneous tissues and skin could be caused by thrombosis of the subcutaneous blood vessels (5).

3. Reduced host defense:
   - In almost all patients, serious underlying systemic diseases are present, mainly diabetes mellitus. This is reported in many series in the literature, also in necrotizing fasciitis in other locations than perianal, such as cervical. (30, 53, 78, 79, 110, 139, 139).

- Necrotizing fasciitis occurs uncommonly in the head and neck region. Chen Lin et al described an analysis of 47 cases in 12 years (83).
- However, immunologic defects specific for necrotizing soft tissue infections or specifically predisposing for these infections could not be found (11).

The importance of these different etiologic factors can vary from patient to patient and the factors are not necessarily present in every patient in the above-mentioned order.

## DIAGNOSIS

The diagnosis of these infections must primarily be made on the macroscopic appearance of the diseased area which will be described below.

The general condition of the patient, the clinical course of the disease and the bacteriologic findings, unless in a very early stage, are not decisive in this respect.

One has to realize that the classical local signs of tissue inflammation (rubor, calor, dolor, and tumor) are often absent. There are however, general signs including: evidence of fever, elevated white blood cell count and a severe systemic reaction.

Wall et al. (136) tried to develop a simple model to help distinguish necrotizing fasciitis from non-necrotizing soft tissue infections. They found that a white blood cell count (WBC) at admission above 15.4 x 10⁹/l or a serum sodium (Na) lower than 135 mmol/l were useful parameters to distinguish between both infections. However, since 70 % of their patients were IV drug users, an evaluation in other settings to prove the value of their model remains necessary (90). A high index of suspicion and careful clinical examination is always necessary.

Locally, bulla, severe pain, rapid spread and eventually gas formation can be seen. Gas forming infections can be caused by both aerobic and anaerobic soft tissue infections.

A very useful algorithm or decision-tree on gas-producing infections has been published by Nichols (101).

The initial diagnosis must be followed by immediate antibiotic and, if necessary, surgical, therapy, with adjunctive hyperbaric oxygen in selected cases (see "Therapy").

A Gram stain is taken initially but provides less information than is necessary or hoped for, because the real causative microorganisms can only be found by culturing tissue biopsies from the spreading periphery of the lesion or from the deeper tissues that are reached only when surgical debridement is performed.

An interesting publication by Ault et al. mentions a rapid streptococcal diagnostic kit, with which the authors were able to identify Group A ß-hemolytic *Streptococcus pyogenes* as the presumptive causative microorganism in cases of necrotizing fasciitis (5).

If the anatomic site of involvement is not clear, computed tomography (CT) scanning can provide this information (10) as well as sonography (97). One must, however, not lose too much time in diagnosis before surgical therapy is started.

The same goes for Magnetic Resonance Imaging (MRI). Some find this useful for an early diagnosis (41); others found the images by MRI non-specific and conclude that the preoperative diagnosis must be based on the clinical picture and the evolution of the clinical status (4).

In most patients, direct inspection or inspection of the fascia after an incision to the level of the deep fascia under local anesthesia is sufficient for determining the diagnosis; exploration and debridement under general anesthesia can follow immediately.

For a differential diagnosis on clinical signs see Table 1. In rapid spreading "closed" infections, needle aspiration and Gram stain can provide more reliable information on the microbiological cause of the infection. It is a

## TABLE 1. CLINICAL SIGNS IN DIFFERENTIAL DIAGNOSIS OF NECROTIZING SOFT TISSUE INFECTIONS

| PARAMETERS ASSESSED | PROGRESSIVE BACTERIAL GANGRENE | |
| --- | --- | --- |
| | PROGRESSIVE BACTERIAL SYNERGISTIC GANGRENE | ANAEROBIC CREPITANT OR CLOSTRIDIAL CELLULITIS |
| Incubation | 1 - 3 weeks | 1 week |
| Onset | gradual | gradual/acute |
| Systemic toxicity | (plus or minus) | (plus or minus) |
| Pain | severe | moderate |
| Exudate | none or slight serous | slight serous |
| Odor of exudate | foul | foul |
| Gas | may be present | abundant |
| Muscle | no change | no change |
| Skin | ulcer and gangrene | gangrene |
| Mortality | 5 - 15% | 5% |
| Treatment:    (5,7,33,41,64) | | |
| • Surgery | necrotomy and skin grafting | incision and drainage |
| • Antibiotics | yes (not always) | yes |
| • Adjunctive hyperbaric oxygen (HBO) | yes (compromised host and systemic toxicity) | yes (compromised host and systemic toxicity) |

well-known fact that hemolytic bacteria (for example *streptococci*), play an important role in these disease processes and do not grow in open wounds (122, 141).

## CLINICAL PICTURE AND BACTERIOLOGY

### Progressive Bacterial Gangrene

Progressive bacterial gangrene, originally described as postoperative progressive bacterial synergistic gangrene or Cullen's ulcer (34) and as chronic infectious skin gangrene (93, 94), is generally a slow advancing infectious process involving the epidermis, the dermis, the subcutaneous tissue including

## ABLE 1. CONTINUED

*(modified from LeFrock, Molavi 1982, Mader 1988)*

| NECROTIZING FASCIITIS | | MYOSITIS/MYONECROSIS |
|---|---|---|
| **STREPTOCCAL AND MIXED (FOURNIER)** | **SYNERGISTIC NECROTIZING CELLULITIS** | **NON-CLOSTRIDIAL STREPTOCOCCAL** |
| 1 - 4 days | 1 - 2 days | 1 - 4 days |
| acute | acute | acute |
| + + | + + + | + |
| moderate to severe | severe | severe |
| profuse sero-sanguinous | dishwater pus profuse | none or slight |
| foul | foul | none |
| usually not present | may be present | not present |
| viable | viable to marked change later | change later |
| cellulitis + secondary gangrene | cellulitis + secondary gangrene | minimal change |
| 35 % | 75% | 25% |
| | | |
| "fillet" procedure | "fillet" procedure | muscle removal |
| yes | yes | yes |
| yes (compromised host) | yes (compromised host) | yes (compromised host) |

lymphatic channels (14, 17) and hair follicles, but never the deep fascia (the fascial plane that envelops the muscle compartment).

Progressive bacterial gangrene includes:

- Anaerobic crepitant or Clostridial cellulitis (91).
- Ecthyma gangrenosum or gangrenous impetigo.
- Pyoderma gangrenosum (26).
- Erysipelas.
- Gangrenous or necrotizing erysipelas (105).
- Symbiotic gangrene (103).
- Phagedena geometrica (18).

***Progressive bacterial gangrene*** is directly related to skin infection. Around the site of an injury or infection, cellulitis occurs with redness, edema and a slight swelling, followed by a centrifugal necrosis of skin and subcutaneous tissues. This frequently capricious extension of necrosis is preceded by patchy, purplish discoloration of the skin. It is highly characteristic that the deep fascia, which envelops the muscle compartment, is never involved. Around the afflicted area, a 1-2 cm wide erythematous, raised border zone is present.

The speed of the extension may vary from weeks or even months to a few hours. Fresh granulation tissue with re-epithelialization may occur in the center while the centrifugal spread of necrosis still proceeds. The area is always very painful.

Bacteriologically the cause can be anaerobic, as in crepitant Clostridial cellulitis, aerobic or mixed. Bacterial synergism plays an important role, but no specific combination can be held responsible for this disease. In order to find the causative microorganisms one has to culture from the spreading periphery, preferably tissue biopsies, and not from the necrosis or the granulating center, where a great variety of concomitant microorganisms can be found that do not cause nor add to the infection.

The usual primary pathogens are group A *streptococci* (GAS) and *Staphylococcus aureus* (alone or in synergism). We found *streptococci* in 92% in needle aspirates or tissue biopsies in progressive bacterial gangrene followed by multiple other aerobic and anaerobic microorganisms such as *Bacteroides* species, *Clostridium* species and *Enterobacteriaceae*, Coliforms, *Proteus* and *Pseudomonas* (in *ecthyma gangrenosum*).

*Bacteroidaceae* as *Bacteroides fragilis* are rarely seen as a single pathogen but always as part of a mixed polymicrobial flora. The role of *Bacteroidaceae* is not a direct one in causing soft tissue infections, but it influences the immunology of the host in diminishing the interferon production and the phagocytic capacity of macrophages and polymorphonuclear neutrophil granulocytes. Clinically *Bacteroides fragilis* is often seen in combination with *Escherichia coli* (95).

***Crepitant anaerobic cellulitis*** involves Clostridial and nonclostridial cellulitis and has often been misdiagnosed as gas gangrene. In general it is a more benign disease than gas gangrene. *Clostridia* can be found in pure culture and there can be marked tissue necrosis but no involvement of the deep fascia or muscles is seen until it is in a very advanced stage. There can be abundant soft tissue gas.

In case of extensive soft tissue damage or marked vascular insufficiency of an extremity, Clostridial cellulitis can change into a true Clostridial myositis with myonecrosis.

Multiple aerobic and anaerobic organisms have been cultured including *Enterobacteriaceae*, *Clostridium* species, *Bacteroides* species and *Peptostreptococcus* species.

In our experience, in over 90% of cases of progressive bacterial gangrene there are serious underlying systemic diseases, most frequently diabetes mellitus. Malignancies and arteriosclerosis were also found, but less frequently.

## Necrotizing Fasciitis

Necrotizing fasciitis (141), originally called hemolytic streptococcal gangrene, Meleney's ulcer or acute dermal gangrene (92,93) is a progressive, generally rapid spreading, inflammatory process located in the deep fascia with secondary necrosis of subcutaneous tissues and skin.

The speed of skin involvement is directly related and proportional to the thickness of the subcutaneous tissue layer. The infection tends to spread very rapidly along the deep fascial plane.

Necrotizing fasciitis includes:

• Hospital gangrene (67).
• Suppurative fasciitis (88).
• Fournier's gangrene or disease (51).
• Synergistic necrotizing cellulitis (127).
• Hemolytic streptococcal gangrene or Meleney's ulcer (92).

Necrotizing fasciitis may start in a surgical wound, postoperatively, after a trivial injury like an insect bite, an abrasion or contusion and may even show up spontaneously, in children. (15, 38, 79, 92, 93, 142).

Usually there is a sudden onset of pain and swelling at the site of or at a certain distance from the injury with a nonspecific redness, swelling and edema. Initially the area may be very painful but later becomes numb and anesthetic. During the next hours and/or days the redness rapidly spreads, the margins fade out into the normal skin but are not raised or very sharply outlined as seen in erysipelas.

These signs and symptoms are already secondary to the most pathognomonic feature, the fascial and subcutaneous necrosis. This necrosis manifests itself as an extensive undermining of the skin and subcutis. If there is an opening in the skin, probes or gloved fingers can be passed under the skin and subcutis. In case of intact skin, the only way for diagnosis is incision into the deep fascia. This can be done at the bedside under local anesthesia.

Once the incision is made, the yellowish-green necrotic fascia becomes visible and after removal of this fascia, healthy, red, normal, bleeding muscle tissue is seen.

If the fascia is left untouched, secondary involvement of the muscles with myositis and myonecrosis can be seen in a later phase. This must be prevented, if possible, by early incision and excision of all necrotic fascia ("fillet procedure").

Without treatment a dusky discoloration of the skin appears as a small purple patch with irregular and initially ill-defined margins. This may occur at a certain distance from the injury or the operative wound. Identical patches may develop in the neighborhood which ultimately fuse and form a large plaque of gangrenous skin while the diffuse redness continues to spread. As a rule the patient is seriously ill: septic with a high fever (124).

It is highly characteristic that the spread of the fascial necrosis is more extended than the visible changes of the skin. The apparently normal skin and subcutaneous tissue are loosened from the underlying necrotic fascia over a great distance from the original wound.

Skin necrosis occurs secondary to thrombosis of subcutaneous blood vessels and the whole area may become anesthetic by necrosis of nerve fibers.

In our series, the site of necrotizing fasciitis showed an equal distribution between trunk and extremities. The head and neck were less frequently involved (139).

Fournier's gangrene or Fournier's disease (51), in its original form as scrotal gangrene, is a form of necrotizing fasciitis. Careful observation shows that the process starts with necrosis of the scrotal fascia, tenderness, local edema and redness of the scrotal skin.

Very soon thereafter the skin becomes necrotic and the diagnostic "black spot" can be seen.

When the infectious process extends from the penal-scrotal region to the abdomen or upper legs, the characteristic picture of necrotizing fasciitis is seen.

The scrotal subcutaneous layer is so thin that the majority of the patients are seen when the skin is already necrotic. In women "Fournier's gangrene" is recognized less easily as necrotizing fasciitis, because of the thicker subcutaneous layer. In the literature however Fournier's gangrene in women is more and more recognized (43). Stephenson et al. describe 29 female patients with necrotizing fasciitis of the vulva. Twenty patients or 69 % were diabetic and the mortality in the diabetic patients was 78.6 % (126).

**Synergistic necrotizing cellulitis** has been described as a different clinical entity (127). Because of the wide involvement of deeper tissues (necrosis of fascia and in a later stage, but very rapidly thereafter, involvement of subcutaneous tissue and muscles as well) together with severe systemic toxicity, we consider this to be a form of necrotizing fasciitis. Mader considers this disease to be a nonclostridial myonecrosis (86).

In our opinion the disease is the same, necrotizing fasciitis, but the clinical course of the disease differs from patient to patient, dependent on general condition, the immune status, age, associated systemic diseases and the time elapsed from the beginning of the disease to the moment when the patient is first examined.

These infections are frequently located in the peri-anal region following improperly treated peri-anal and ischiorectal abscesses. About 75-80% of the mainly elderly patients have diabetes mellitus.

Diabetes mellitus, besides age, malnutrition, hypertension and intravenous drug abuse have been recognized as considerable risk factors for mortality in necrotizing fasciitis (52).

The simple fact that the patients were mainly elderly and that a high percentage of systemic sepsis was present in the series of Stone and Martin (127), may explain the unusually high mortality of 75%, compared with the mean mortality of 38.5% in a review of 15 reports including 272 patients (3) and 3% to 45 % in the large review of 1,726 patients by Eke (46).

There is confusion and uncertainty about the exact bacteriologic cause of necrotizing fasciitis. Meleney (92) described the disease as hemolytic streptococcal gangrene and considered the cause to be "a pure invasion of hemolytic *streptococci*. This bacteriologic pattern seems to have changed as described before. (9, 33, 79, 141). Wilson was the first to consider the name "hemolytic streptococcal gangrene" inappropriate because in his patients hemolytic staphylococci were frequently cultured (141).

Mader has stated that better culture techniques have demonstrated that *Streptococcus* pyogenes only occasionally causes these infections. This, however, cannot alter the fact that Meleney indeed found only *streptococci*, strongly suggesting at least an important role for this organism. Mader explains this by saying that although most infections are mixed aerobic and anaerobic, a type of necrotizing fasciitis caused solely by *Streptococcus pyogenes* has been reported (86).

Careful bacteriologic techniques have shown anaerobes and aerobes: *Peptostreptococcus* species, *Bacteroides* species, *Fusobacterium* species together with *Streptococcus pyogenes*, *Staphylococcus aureus*, *Klebsiella pneumoniae*, *Pseudomonas aeruginosa*, *Enterobacteriaceae* and even fungi (14, 30, 47, 53, 66, 78, 79, 80, 143).

Also Clostridia have been described in 90% of cases where Fournier's disease was accompanied by myositis. Again from the description it is not clear if gas gangrene was involved. The same authors describe a large variety of microorganisms which, apparently, they all consider causal (134). Even a very rare case of necrotizing fasciitis after blunt trauma caused by a penicillin-resistant *Streptococcus pneumoniae* is reported (13).

It is, however, still very difficult to distinguish the real causative microorganisms from the concomitants.

Giuliano described two bacteriologic types of necrotizing fasciitis (53) and Lamerton even suggested three different groups (78). We could not confirm their findings in our patients (11).

A very important observation that is not mentioned in any publication is the time the organisms are cultured in relation to the time of onset of the disease and the eventual previous treatment, surgery, antibiotics, or both. We mentioned this earlier.

In our experience a pure and very early case of Fournier's gangrene, still without skin necrosis, showed *streptococci* in pure culture after needle aspiration. We found the same in other early cases of necrotizing fasciitis.

The bacteriologic pattern changes during the clinical course of the disease and seems to be more dependent on the previous use of antibiotics, the extent and frequency of debridements, the use (or non-use) of diverting colostomies, the age and immune status of the patient, and associated systemic diseases. These pattern changes make it difficult to show that the cultured bacteria can, with certainty, be declared to be causative.

Brunet et al. (125) published a study on a total of 81 patients with perineal gangrene. They advocate very systematic microbiological investigations from specific locations and repeat that after every operative debridement. They start with an antibiotic regimen directed against anaerobes, gram positive cocci and gram negative bacilli. This regimen is changed when later culture results so indicate. They stress the importance of a systematic exploration of the ischiorectal fossae.

We are convinced that for the onset of necrotizing fasciitis, *streptococci* play a very important role and that the reported changes in the bacteriologic pattern are mainly caused by other factors mentioned above.

Stevens gave a review of invasive group A streptococcal infections both clinically (119, 123, 125) and historically (120) where he also describes the ongoing research in streptococcal virulence factors; important for eventual development of new vaccines.

Recent work on streptococcal virulence factors and their possible influence on the onset of soft tissue infections can be found in Unnikrishnan et al. (133) and Norrby-Teglund et al. (102). Dele Davies and Schwarz reviewed these infections in children (38).

Stevens (124) also underlined the importance of a rapidly progressive Streptococcal Toxic Shock Syndrome that can accompany necrotizing fasciitis (strep TSS). Mortality, even with adequate therapy, is 30 – 60% of patients in 72-96 hours.

The bacteriology of synergistic necrotizing cellulitis is largely the same as in other forms of necrotizing fasciitis (86, 127).

## Non-Clostridial Myonecrosis

The most frequent and devastating anaerobic myositis and myonecrosis is Clostridial myonecrosis or gas gangrene.

We saw that some forms of synergistic necrotizing cellulitis have been categorized as nonclostridial myonecrosis (80, 86, 127) and other forms as necrotizing fasciitis.

We consider muscle involvement to be a later stage of true necrotizing fasciitis (11).

Other forms of nonclostridial myonecrosis caused by anaerobic *streptococci* (91) are found mainly in drug addicts in our patient series. Differential diagnosis between gas gangrene and streptococcal myositis can be very difficult. The muscles in streptococcal myositis have in general a more inflamed appearance than in gas gangrene. Muscle necrosis is seen later than in gas gangrene and the necrotic muscles are more greenish in color than the black muscle necrosis in gas gangrene. Also, gas production is less abundant and differently situated in streptococcal myositis. Severe systemic toxicity, however, can be the same in both diseases.

Myositis caused by aerobic microorganisms, viruses, or certain parasites are known and described but very rare and will not be discussed here (114).

# THERAPY

## Introduction

Treatment of aerobic, anaerobic and mixed necrotizing soft tissue infections is a combination of surgical debridement (timely, limited or aggressive), appropriate antibiotics, good nutritional support and optimal oxygenation of the infected tissues. In selected cases where ambient oxygen is insufficient, hyperbaric oxygen must be used.

Surgical treatment can vary in these infections from simple incision and drainage procedures to very aggressive "fillet" procedures and even amputations can become necessary.

Essential in the management is the administration of appropriate antibiotics.

The problem with this is twofold:

1. Late culture results, and
2. Treating the causative and not the concomitant microorganisms.
   My policy is to initially choose those antibiotics that cover the suspected causative pathogens (aerobic and anaerobic). Usually we start in the early stages with penicillin-G ( or clindamycin or both), metronidazole and gentamycin or tobramycin (9). Sometimes a third generation cephalosporin is indicated (86).

As early as 1952 Eagle already described the problem of treatment failure with penicillin in streptococcal infections in mice (42). Stevens repeated this phenomenon in 1988 in streptococcal myositis in a mouse model (118). Group A *streptococci* at the site of inoculation remained highly sensitive to penicillin only as long as the *streptococci* continued to grow at a rapid rate. The same was found to be true for erythromycin but not for clindamycin.

Zamboni and coworkers found penicillin therapy to be ineffective when started more than two hours after onset of a myositis in a mouse model. Although erythromycin resulted in higher survival rates, survival after clindamycin was still 70% even when treatment was started 16.5 hours after onset of the myositis (80% after 6 hours) (144). It is important to keep these data in mind when choosing a particular antibiotic treatment scheme. It seems that clindamycin is nowadays more appropriate than penicillin-G.

Hyperbaric oxygen is indicated when other measures (ambient oxygen) fail to oxygenate the infected tissues sufficiently. This must be monitored by transcutaneous or, even better, by direct intraphlegmonous and/or intramuscular $pO_2$-measurements (73, 113).

The rationale for the use of adjunctive hyperbaric oxygen and the mechanisms have been outlined extensively by Mader and Thom (85, 86, 130).

The main goals are: (a) improvement of tissue $pO_2$, necessary for normal wound healing, (b) improvement of phagocytic function by stimulating the oxygen-dependent killing mechanisms, either direct or indirect, (c) the diminishing of edema and improvement of the circulation in the affected areas, (d) stimulation of fibroblast growth, and (e) increased collagen formation. This can be roughly summarized as stimulation of the host defense and repair mechanisms.

A useful algorithm or decision tree concerning the possible use of hyperbaric oxygen in soft tissue infections has been published by Bell (17).

Because of multiple variables, clinical studies using adjunctive hyperbaric oxygen are very difficult to evaluate. The wide variety in patients makes a randomized controlled trial virtually impossible. No patient is the same or presents him or herself with the same symptoms. The variety in the bacteriological findings have been outlined sufficiently in this chapter. Almost all patients are compromised hosts. From some of the descriptions it is very difficult, if not impossible; to know which of the different clinical entities is involved. In this way it is very difficult to respond to the criticism of Tibbles and Edelsberg in their review stating that more prospective trials are necessary in order to prove the value of hyperbaric oxygen in necrotizing fasciitis (131) Maybe clinical evidence based on large numbers is sufficient to convince our adversaries. Even in gas gangrene, other gas producing infections are mixed with the true Clostridial myonecrosis. The rationale for adjunctive hyperbaric oxygen, however, is clear and based on animal studies, case reports, retrospective studies and a few prospective studies (64, 110).

Korhonen (75, 76) showed in animal experiments, in healthy volunteers and in patients with necrotizing soft tissue infections that hyperbaric oxygen raised arterial oxygen tensions seven-fold and that oxygen tensions in the vicinity of the infected area were generally higher than in healthy tissues, thus establishing a hyper-oxygenated zone around the infection. The $CO_2$ tensions rose only slightly during exposure to hyperbaric oxygen. Combining early and extensive surgery, broad spectrum antibiotics, hyperbaric oxygen and surgical intensive care gave the best results in the treatment of Fournier's disease with a mortality of 9%.

In three publications the use of honey to improve the rate of wound healing is advocated in necrotizing fasciitis (44, 46, 61).

## Progressive Bacterial Gangrene

Prognosis in progressive bacterial gangrene is generally better than in necrotizing fasciitis and is mainly determined by associated systemic diseases.

**Surgery:** Surgery can be limited to necrotomies, limited excisions in the margin of the process, the necessity of which must be judged on a day-to-day basis. Normal wound care, including temporary artificial skin substitution (for example with a polyvinyl alcohol foam) may be necessary (98). When a good granulating surface is obtained, split skin grafting can be performed. We have never been forced to more extensive excisions. If the gangrene is not responsive to the combined treatment scheme, amputation of an extremity may be necessary. Heinle et al. (58) claim superior results post grafting, with a trend to lower mortality and morbidity, by the use of 5% Mafenide Acetate Solution.

**Antibiotics:** Antibiotics should be directed to the causative and not to concomitant microorganisms. This can be very difficult because a wide variety can usually be cultured from these infections.

In one of the author's patients, a 43-year-old male with a progressive bacterial synergistic gangrene of the abdominal wall postoperatively, a flora with *E.Coli, Pseudomonas aeruginosa, Enterobacter cloacae, Enterococci, Bacteroides* species and *Acinetobacter anitratum* was cultured. The clinical picture however, professed that none of the microorganisms needed any treatment. With only local care, wound healing was uneventful.

This underlines the significance of close cooperation between the clinical bacteriologist and surgeon.

Since in 92% of the tissue biopsies taken from the margin of the process, *streptococci* were cultured followed by *staphylococci*, coliforms, *proteus*, *pseudomonas* and *clostridia*, we usually start with penicillin-G, one million IU every 3-4 hrs IV and change this regimen only when indicated by the clinical course supported by bacteriologic evidence. Because of unresponsiveness of *streptococci* depending on the stage of the process, we use more and more clindamycin (118).

**Hyperbaric oxygen:** Ledingham and Therani reported for the first time in literature that the adjunctive use of hyperbaric oxygen contributed to the arrest of the infection in four out of five of their patients (79).

Experience with hyperbaric oxygen is reported more and more in the literature. The working mechanism makes it clear, why it is useful in treating necrotic soft tissue infections.

All our patients reacted favorably when hyperbaric oxygen was added to the therapeutic regimen of surgery and antibiotics. We added hyperbaric oxygen when other treatment modalities failed. No proper prospective randomized trials are known which is a definitive disadvantage when advocating hyperbaric oxygen.

From 1978-1987, 89 patients were treated with progressive bacterial gangrene. The mortality was 5.6%. All patients had serious associated diseases, diabetes mellitus being the most frequent (74 patients or 83.1%).

Some patients had been treated for as long as 4-6 months with all known treatment modalities. Despite this, the gangrene extended progressively although slowly. At the time that amputation was considered to be unavoidable, the addition of hyperbaric oxygen stopped the progression and resulted in a clean, granulating wound suitable for grafting after approximately 3 weeks of daily treatments (14-42 days in 84 patients).

We recommend the adjunctive use of hyperbaric oxygen in progressive bacterial gangrene in cases where other treatment modalities fail, in cases with serious underlying systemic diseases and symptoms of general toxicity and in other immune-compromised patients.

## *Treatment protocol for progressive bacterial gangrene*

**Multiplace chamber:** 3 ATA 100% $O_2$, 90 minutes per treatment with appropriate airbreaks, 1-2 treatments per day. If the response is favorable, this can be diminished to 3-4 treatments per week. It is advisable to continue treatment for 10 days post grafting.

**Monoplace chamber:** In a monoplace chamber the same scheme can be used.

The question if the same results can be reached with lower oxygen pressures is difficult to answer since we do not have a clear definition of a dose of oxygen. In our experience these protocols are safe and side effects are absent or minimal. The most important thing is to establish in an oxygen challenge test that the $pO_2$ at the wound margin and/or in the wound itself is too low to expect normal wound healing; the next step is to show that this $pO_2$ can be raised by hyperbaric oxygen and not by 100 % oxygen at 1 bar. Treatment schemes with 2.4 – 2.6 ATA $O_2$ report the same results.

**Anaerobic Clostridial cellulitis,** sometimes misdiagnosed as gas gangrene, is a more benign disease than gas gangrene. *Clostridia* can be found in pure culture and there can be marked tissue necrosis. The deep fascia and the muscles however are not affected. With extensive tissue damage and/or in a seriously compromised host, a true Clostridial myositis with myonecrosis can arise.

**Surgical treatment** can be limited to incision and drainage followed by excision of the necrotic tissue.

**Antibiotics:** Penicillin-G, 8-12 million IU per day IV.

**Hyperbaric oxygen:** Adjunctive hyperbaric oxygen is recommended in immunocompromised patients and in patients with systemic toxicity. In these patients the "gas gangrene" scheme is used.

- 1st day: 3 times of 90 min. each at 3 ATA 100% $O_2$ in a multiplace
          or 2.5-2.8 ATA 100% $O_2$ in a monoplace chamber.
- 2nd day: 2 times.
- 3rd day: 2 times.

From the fourth day on, continue with one treatment per day until the wound starts granulating. Maximal treatment time is 10 days. We than found normal oxygen tissue tensions for wound healing when breathing normal air at sea level. This is the sign that hyperbaric treatment can be discontinued.

## Necrotizing Fasciitis

**Surgery:** Primary and aggressive surgical debridement is the cornerstone in the management of this disease.

Early and extensive incision of skin and subcutaneous tissue wide into healthy tissue, followed by excision of all necrotic fascia and nonviable skin and subcutaneous tissue is necessary. This has to be repeated as often as necessary. Within the first 24 hours repeated inspection of the whole infected area under general anesthesia is obligatory, with excision of further necrotized fascia, if present.

These progressive necrotizing surgical infections need a unified approach as soon as possible. It is of no use trying to determine the type of infection first by culturing the infected tissue because every delay in the start of treatment causes a significant higher mortality (32, 35, 37, 47, 52, 60, 70, 135).

In most of our patients with a necrotizing fasciitis of the peniscrotal and perianal area we performed a diverting colostomy.

The extent of fascial necrosis can easily be determined by blunt finger dissection over the deep fascial plane through the incision and by direct inspection. Viable skin flaps need not be excised and can be saved. If no further fascial necrosis is seen, the process can be considered arrested. Usually, at least in our experience, from 1-5 debridements are necessary with a mean of 3 (in 40 patients between 1985 and 1990).

A systematic exploration of the ischiorectal fossa in every case of a perianal soft tissue infection is very important (25).

**Antibiotics:** Antibiotic treatment has an important place in the combined management of necrotizing fasciitis, although second to surgery. Recommendations of drugs have changed with the development of new antibiotics and the risk of resistance. Colonization and selection of microorganisms by a former therapeutic or prophylactic regimen plays an important role (for example: antibiotic prophylaxis in large bowel surgery or treatment of a perianal abscess).

If at the time of clinical diagnosis a polymicrobial flora is present, one has to be very careful not to treat a concomitant agent instead of the causative microorganisms.

The present, confusing, bacteriologic findings in soft tissue infections are in part caused by the unnecessary, misdirected use of antibiotics.

*Streptococci* have been identified as a major pathogen in these diseases. Kaul et al. gave a recent review on the incidence of necrotizing fasciitis in Ontario, Canada (71) as did Smith et al. (116) and Corman et al. (32); the largest review, on 1726 cases, is published by Eke (46). Five cases in trauma patients were reported by Schwarz et al. (112).

The drug of choice is penicillin-G, 8-10 million IU/24 hours IV, with clindamycin more and more as the alternative. The other pathogens can be treated by metronidazole (anaerobes) and/or third generation *cephalosporins* (anaerobes, *Enterobacteriaceae*) (49).

Bacteroides fragilis can be treated with clindamycin or metronidazole (or covered by a third generation *cephalosporin*).

A useful scheme for the initial choice of antibiotics is given by Mader (86).

**Hyperbaric oxygen:** Clinical reports indicate an adjunctive role for hyperbaric oxygen in necrotizing fasciitis. Although no large controlled randomized series have been published so far, hyperbaric oxygen provides a valuable adjunct in the overall treatment management (27, 37, 63, 104). An interesting discussion on the value of adjunctive hyperbaric oxygen can be found in the Deutsche Medizinische Wochenschrift by Bock et al. and Kujath et al. (19, 77). Kujath (77) underestimates the advantages and greatly exaggerate the disadvantages of hyperbaric oxygen in necrotizing fasciitis. A useful discussion follows in a later issue of the same journal (40). (See "Discussion" in the reference list).

The overall mortality figures in this disease range from 20-75%.

1. Only Ledingham reported poor results with hyperbaric oxygen (overall mortality 8/12 = 67%, in the hyperbaric oxygen group 8/9 = 89%). However, his initial surgical management is suspect and was probably not extensive enough. Adjunctive hyperbaric oxygen cannot be successful if surgery is inappropriate (79).
2. Riegels-Nielsen reported 5 patients with a mortality of 1/5 = 20%. All five patients had necrotizing fasciitis of the external genitals and the lower abdominal wall and were treated with aggressive surgery, appropriate antibiotics and adjunctive hyperbaric oxygen (109).
3. We treated 27 patients before 1985 with necrotizing fasciitis, including 7 patients with Fournier's disease. Mortality was 5/27 = 18%. In another 40 patients (1985-1990) mortality was 5/40 = 12.5%.

Patients were treated with a combination of surgery, antibiotics and hyperbaric oxygen (9).

4. Eltorai et al. reported no mortalities in 9 patients in which hyperbaric oxygen was added to the standard therapy (48).

5. Mader reported on a retrospective evaluation of 33 patients, of which 22 had involvement of the scrotum and perianal region. Of the 22, mortality in the hyperbaric oxygen group was 25% compared with a mortality of 67% in the non-hyperbaric oxygen group. All patients were seriously compromised hosts and 14 had diabetes mellitus (86).

6. Zamboni et al. treated 6 patients with 1 late death due to complications of pneumonia (143).

7. Riseman et al. reported on 29 patients with necrotizing fasciitis treated between 1980 and 1988.

   Group I (n=12) received standard therapy and in group II (n=17) hyperbaric oxygen was added. Although group II patients were more seriously ill at admission, the mortality in this group was significantly lower (23%) than in group I patients (66%).

   Their conclusion was that the addition of hyperbaric oxygen to the surgical and antimicrobial treatment of necrotizing fasciitis significantly reduced mortality and wound morbidity (number of necessary debridements). In their view, hyperbaric oxygen should be used routinely in the treatment of necrotizing fasciitis. Following their results they conclude that withholding hyperbaric oxygen to patients when it is available will cause unnecessary deaths and is thus unethical (110).

8. Brown et al. reported on a retrospective review of the efficacy of hyperbaric oxygen. They looked only at truncal necrotizing fasciitis and identified 54 patients (30 in the HBO group and 24 without HBO). There was a trend to better survival in the HBO treated group but without statistical significance (23).

9. Shupak et al. in a retrospective study of 37 patients over a rather long period, from 1984 - 1993 also did not find statistical difference between treatment with and without hyperbaric oxygen (115).

10. Hirn presented 11 patients treated with HBO in a clinical and experimental study and found a mortality of 1 patient (9%). He advocates HBO as an adjunct in the overall treatment of necrotizing soft tissue infections (63).

11. Korhonen et al. in a retrospective study of 33 patients with Fournier's gangrene, found a mortality of 3 patients or 9%. They found that adjunctive hyperbaric oxygen reduced systemic toxicity, prevented extension of the necrotizing infection and increased demarcation, thereby improving the overall outcome (74).

12. Hollabaugh et al. reported 7% mortality in a group of patients with Fournier's gangrene when treated with adjunctive hyperbaric oxygen (n=14). In the group without hyperbaric oxygen the mortality was 42% (n=12). This difference was statistically significant. A total of 38% of their patients had diabetes mellitus; 35% had alcohol abuses.

Hyperbaric oxygen was given to patients solely on the basis of institution availability. Although the number of patients is still limited there is a good statistical paragraph concerning survival chances with and without hyperbaric oxygen (64).

Also Clark and Moon (29) underline the importance of adjunctive hyperbaric oxygen in the treatment of life-threatening soft-tissue infection. Dahm et al. (36) found that the extent of the infection as measured by the BSA (Body Surface Area) involved was a highly statistical significant independent predictor of outcome and that Fournier's gangrene with an extension of 5% BSA or greater appeared to be an indication for adjunctive hyperbaric oxygen. Their results in 50 patients did not however, reach statistical significance.

Compromised hosts with necrotizing fasciitis have extreme morbidity and mortality. From these reports it is clear that adjunctive hyperbaric oxygen in these patients is a very valuable therapeutic tool.

### Treatment protocol for necrotizing fasciitis

Proper, early, and aggressive surgical debridements remain the cornerstone of the treatment. These are surgical diseases that can only be treated with appropriate surgery first (6, 20, 35 and many others). Hyperbaric oxygen cannot compensate for bad surgery. However, the best results can only be obtained with a combination of surgery, antibiotics and hyperbaric oxygen. The same conclusion was reached at a Consensus Conference in 2000 by the French Society of Dermatology, however without the use of hyperbaric oxygen which was still considered controversial (6, 20, and 35). Mathieu (87), answering, stated that the controversy on the use of hyperbaric oxygen as a treatment for necrotizing fasciitis is more caused by the difficulty to dispose of a hyperbaric equipment that is suited for the treatment of critical patients than by doubt on its real efficiency.

**HBO Treatment scheme (necrotizing fasciitis):** After the first surgical debridement, 3 treatment sessions are given in the first 24 hours.

- In a multiplace chamber: 3 ATA, 100% $O_2$ for 90 minutes per session. Appropriate air breaks are given as necessary.
- In a monoplace chamber the same scheme can be used.

After the first day continue treatment twice daily and if the improvement of the patient permits this, once daily until granulation is obtained (10-15 treatments in total).

## Non-Clostridial Myonecrosis

**Synergistic necrotizing cellulitis:** The name "cellulitis" suggests progressive bacterial gangrene, but the disease is categorized by some as myonecrosis while, in fact, it is a necrotizing fasciitis.

This clearly demonstrates the difficulty of classification of this disease in its advanced stages when literally every kind of tissue is involved.

The therapy is the same as described under necrotizing fasciitis, but because more tissue is involved and the infection is especially fulminant, mortality reaches 75% without hyperbaric oxygen (127).

This is not so much the result of the necrotizing fasciitis itself, but of the extremely serious immune compromise of the patients, secondary to age, renal failure, arteriosclerosis, diabetes mellitus, malignancies, deficient nutrition, etc. These factors determine the danger and the rapid spread of this soft tissue infection.

In light of the above and the grim prognosis of this disease, it is only logical to give adjunctive hyperbaric oxygen where possible.

### Treatment protocol for non-clostridial myonecrosis

Again, hyperbaric oxygen has to be adjunctive to appropriate antibiotics (clindamycin or penicillin) and surgical incision and drainage, followed by excision of necrotic muscle.

Prognosis worsens progressively when muscle tissue is involved. Aggressive surgery, appropriate antibiotics and adjunctive hyperbaric oxygen following the "gas gangrene protocol."

- 1st day: 3 times of 90 min. each at 3 ATA 100% $O_2$ in a multiplace or a monoplace chamber (appropriate air-breaks as mentioned before).
- 2nd day: 2 times
- 3rd day: 2 times.

Because the myositis started in most of our patients as a "closed" disease (after drug injection in addicts), there is an early need for decompressing fasciotomy and hyperbaric oxygen.

**Anaerobic streptococcal myositis and myonecrosis:** This infection is rare. The author has seen only 7 patients since 1978. The mortality was 2/7 = 28.6%. The disease can be very fulminant, mimicking clostridial myonecrosis. Because we have demonstrated hypoxia through intramuscular $pO_2$ monitoring (73), we recommend the use of adjunctive hyperbaric oxygen. In cases of fulminant disease, systemic toxicity and a compromised host, the gas gangrene protocol may be used.

Recent reviews of invasive streptococcal disease including streptococcal myositis is given by Stevens. The incidence, reading his report, is clearly much higher than in our experience (122, 125).

Adams et al. (1) described 19 cases from the literature and added 2 of their own cases. In all cases the infection was caused by group A ß-hemolytic *streptococci*. Despite aggressive surgical and medical treatment, 18 out of 21 patients (85.7 %) died.

Demey et al. reported another 2 cases from Belgium (39).

Zamboni et al. found in a mouse myositis model using *streptococcus pyogenes* that HBO alone did not decrease mortality or bacterial proliferation in vivo significantly, but the combined treatment of penicillin with HBO exerts at least additive effects in both decreasing bacterial counts *in vivo* and increasing survival in this model (144).

# REFERENCES

1. Adams EM, Gudmundsson S, Yocum DE, Haselby RC et al. "Streptococcal myositis." Arch Int Med. 1985:145;1020-1023.

2. Ahrenholz DH. "Necrotizing soft tissue infections." Surg Clin North Am. 1988;68:199-214.

3. Ahrenholz DH. "Surgical spectrum. Clinical skin and soft tissue infection." Physicians World Communications (Monograph). West Point, Pa. Merck, Sharpe and Dohme. 1988;16-24.

4. Arslan A, Jerome CP, Borthne A. Necrotizing fasciitis: unreliable MRI findings in the preoperative diagnosis. Eur J Radiol. 2000;36(3);139-143.

5. Ault MJ, Geiderman J, Sokolov R. "Rapid identification of Group A *Streptococcus* as the cause of Necrotizing Fasciitis." Ann Emerg Med. 1996:28(2);227-230.

6. Baier VP, Imdahl A. Nekrotisierende Fasciitis. Hier hilft nur radikales Debridement. MMW-Fortschr Med. 2001:143(15);332-333.

7. Bakker DJ. "De hyperbare zuurstofbehandeling van acuut huidgangreen (necrotiserende fasciitis en progressief bacterieel gangreen)." Ned Tijdschr Geneeskd. 1980;124:2164-2170.

8. Bakker DJ. "The treatment of acute dermal gangrene with hyperbaric oxygen." Proc VIIth Int Congr Hyperbaric Medicine. Moscow, Publishing Office, Nauka:1983;238-240 (Russian).

9. Bakker DJ. "The use of hyperbaric oxygen in the treatment of certain infectious diseases especially gas gangrene and acute dermal gangrene." Drukkerij Veenman BV. Wageningen. University of Amsterdam. 1984;74-90.

10. Bakker DJ. Ibid, 42-44.

11. Bakker DJ, Kox C. "Classification and therapy of necrotizing soft tissue infections: The role of surgery, antibiotics and hyperbaric oxygen." Current Problems in General Surgery. 1988;5(4):489-500.

12. Bakker DJ. "Streptococcal infections and hyperbaric oxygen." In M Gennser (ed) "Diving and hyperbaric medicine." Proc XXIV Ann Meeting of the EUBS. Stockholm Aug 12-15. 1998. FOA report: FOA-B-98-00342-721-SE; p 140-145. Print Elanders-Gotab, Stockholm, Sweden.

13. Ballon-Landa GR, Gherardi G, Beall B et al. Necrotizing fasciitis due to penicillin-resistant *Streptococcus pneumoniae*: Case report and review of the literature. J Infect. 2001:(42);272-290.

14. Bartlett JG. "Necrotizing soft tissue infections." Nichols RL, Hyslop NE, Bartlett JG (Eds.) Decision Making in Surgical Sepsis. Decker, Philadelphia 1991;62-63.

15. Barton LL, Jeck DT. "Necrotizing Fasciitis in Children. Report of two cases and a review of the literature." Arch Pediatr Adolesc Med. 1996:150;105-108.

16. Beaurienne M. "Observation sur une plaie du scrotum." J de Med Chir Pharm 1764(20);251-256.

17. Bell WH. "Use of hyperbaric oxygen in anaerobic soft-tissue infection." Nichols RL, Hyslop NE, Bartlett JG (Eds.) Decision Making in Surgical Sepsis. Decker, Philadelphia. 1991;78-81.

18. Bisno AL, Stevens DL. "Streptococcal infections of skin and soft tissues." New Eng J Med. 1996:334(4);240-245.

19. Bock KH, Lampl L, Frey G. "Diagnose und Therapie der nekrotisierende Fasziitis. Hyperbare Oxygenation als ergänzende Therapieform." Deutsche Med Wochenschr. 1996:121(4);116-117.

20. Brandt MM, Corpron CA, Wahl WL. Necrotizing soft tissue infections: A surgical disease. Am Surg. 2000:66(10);967-970.

21. Brewer GE, Meleney FL. "Progressive gangrenous infection of the skin and subcutaneous tissues, following operation for acute perforative appendicitis." Ann Surg. 1926;84:438-450.

22. Brocq L. "Nouvelle contribution à l'étude du phagedenisme geometrique." Ann Dermatol Syph (Paris). 1916/1917;6:1-39.

23. Brown DR, Davis NL, Lepawsky M, Cunningham J, Kortbeek J. "A multicenter review of the treatment of major truncal necrotizing infections with and without hyperbaric oxygen therapy." Am J Surg. 1994:167;485-489.

24. Brun-Buisson C. Stratégie de prise en charge des fasciites nécrosantes. Conference de consensus. Texte des experts: quatrième question. Ann Dermatol Venereol. 2001:128;394-403.

25. Brunet C, Consentino B, Barthelemy A et al. Gangrènes périnéales: nouvelle approche bactériologique. Résultats du traitement médicochirurgical (81 cas). Ann Chir. 2000:125;420-427.

26. Brunsting LA, Goeckerman WH and O'Leary PA. "Pyoderma gangrenosum (Ecthyma). Clinical and experimental observations in five cases." Arch Dermatol Syph (Paris). 1930;22:655-680.

27. Capelli-Schellpfeffer M, Gerber GS. The use of hyperbaric oxygen in urology. J Urol. 1999:162;647-654.

28. Chapnick EK, Abter EI. "Necrotizing soft-tissue infections." Inf Dis Clin N Am. 1996:10(4);835-855.

29. Clark LA, Moon RE. "Hyperbaric Oxygen in the Treatment of Life-Threatening Soft-Tissue Infections." Resp Care Clin N Am. 1999:5(2);203-219.

30. Clayton MD, Fowler JE Jr., Sharifi R, Pearl RK. "Causes, presentation and survival of fifty-seven patients with necrotizing fasciitis of the male genitalia." Surg Gynecol Obstet. 1990;170:49-55.

31. Conférence de consensus de la Société Française de Dermatologie. Erysipèle et fasciite nécrosante: prise en charge. Text court. Ann Med Int. 2000:151(4);465-470.

32. Corman JM, Moody JA, Aronson WJ. "Fournier's gangrene in a modern surgical setting: improved survival with aggressive management." BJU Int. 1999:84;85-88.

33. Crosthwait RW Jr, Crosthwait RW and Jordan GL. "Necrotizing fasciitis." J Trauma. 1964;4:149-157.

34. Cullen TS. "A progressively enlarging ulcer of abdominal wall involving the skin and fat, following drainage of an abdominal abscess apparently of appendiceal origin." Surg Gynecol Obstet. 1924;38:579-582.

35. Cunningham JD, Silver L, Rudikoff D. Necrotizing fasciitis: A plea for early diagnosis and treatment. Mount Sinai J Med. 2001:68 (4&5);253-261.

36. Dahm P, Roland FH, Vaslef SN et al. Outcome analysis in patients with primary Necrotizing Fasciitis of the male genitalia. Urol. 2000:56(1);31-35.

37. Dellinger EP. "Severe necrotizing soft tissue infections. Multiple disease entities requiring a common approach." JAMA. 1981:246(15);1717-1721.

38. Dele Davies H, Schwartz B. Invasive Group A Streptococcal Infections in Children. In: Advances in Pediatric Infectious Diseases. 1999:vol 14, Ch 6; 129-145. Mosby, Inc.

39. Demey HE, Goovaerts GC, Pattyn SR, Bossaert LL. "Streptococcal myositis. A report of two cases." Acta Clin Belgica. 1991:46 (2);82-88.

40. Diskussion: Schmidt H, Welslau W, Hencke J, Siekmann U, Scharfe U, Tirpitz D, Kujath P, Eckmann C. "Die nekrotisierende Fasziitis und schwere Weichteilinfektionen durch Gruppe-A-Streptokokken." Dt Artztebl. 1998:95(39);A-2395-2401.

41. Drake DB, Woods JA, Bill TJ et al. Magnetic Resonance Imaging in the early diagnosis of group A ß Streptococcal Necrotizing Fasciitis: A case report. J Em Med. 1998:16(3);4403-407.

42. Eagle H. "Experimental approach to the problem of treatment failure with penicillin. I. Group A streptococcal infection in mice." Amer J Med. 1952;13;389-399.

43. Ecker KW, Derouet H, Omlor G, Mast GJ. "Die Fournier'sche Gangrän." Chirurg. 1993:64;558-62.

44. Efem SEE. "Recent advances in the management of Fournier's gangrene: Preliminary observations." Surg. 1993:113;200-204.

45. Efstratiou A, George RC, Tanna A et al. "Characterisation of Group A *streptococci* from necrotizing fasciitis cases in Gloucestershire, United Kingdom." Adv Exp Med Biol. 1997:418:91-93.

46. Eke N. "Fournier's Gangrene: A review of 1,726 cases". Br J Surg. 2000:87;718-728.

47. Elliott D, Kufera JA, Myers RAM. The microbiology of necrotizing soft tissue infections. Am J Surg. 2000:179(5);361-366.

48. Eltorai IM, Hart GB, Strauss MB, Montroy R, Juler GL. "The role of hyperbaric oxygen in the management of Fournier's gangrene." Int Surg. 1986;71:53.

49. Fildes J, Bannon MP, Barrett J. "Soft tissue infections after trauma." Surg Clin North Am. 1991;71:371-384.

50. Finegold SM, Bartlett JC, Chow AW, et al. "Management of anaerobic infections." Ann Intern Med. 1975;83:375-389.

51. Fournier A. "Gangrène foudroyante de la verge." Semaine Medicale. 1883;3:345-347; 1884;4:69-70.

52. Francis KR, Lamaute HR, Davis JM et al. Implications of risk factors in necrotizing fasciitis. Am Surg. 1993;59(5):304-308.

53. Giuliano A, Lewis F Jr, Hadley K, Blaisdell FW. "Bacteriology of necrotizing fasciitis." Am J Surg. 1977;134:52-57.

54. Goepfert AR, Guinn DA, Andrews WW, Hauth JC. "Necrotizing fasciitis after Cesarean delivery." Obst Gynec. 1997:89(3);409-412.

55. Gorbach SL, Bartlett JG, Nichols RL. Manual of Surgical Infections, Ch 9, Skin and Soft Tissue Infections. Brown, Boston 1984.

56. Green RJ, Dafoe DC, Raffin TA. "Necrotizing fasciitis." Chest. 1996:110(1); 219-229.

57. Hebler. "Brand des Hodensackes und vollständiger Wiederersatz." Med Zeitung. 1848:41;188.

58. Heinle EC, Dougherty WR, Garner WL, Reilly DA. The use of 5% Mafenide Acetate Solution in the postgraft treatment of necrotizing fasciitis. J Burn Care Rehab. 2001:22;35-40.

59. Heitmann C, Czermak C, Germann G. Rapidly fatal necrotizing fasciitis after aesthetic liposuction. Aesth Plast Surg. 2000:24;344-347.

60. Heitmann C, Pelzer M, Bickert B et al. Chirurgisches Konzept und Ergebnisse bei nekrotisierender Fasciitis. Chirurg. 2001:72;168-173.

61. Hejase MJ, Simonin JE, Bihrle R, Coogan CL. "Genital Fournier's gangrene: Experience with 38 patients." Urology. 1996:47(5);734-739.

62. Hippocrates. Hippocratic writings. Ed GER Lloyd. Epidemics Book I: Publ Penguin Classics. Middlesex England, 108-109, transl 1983. Idem: Book III: 121-122.

63. Hirn M. "Hyperbaric oxygen in the treatment of gas gangrene and perineal necrotizing fasciitis. A clinical and experimental study." Academic Dissertation. Eur J Surg (Acta Chir). 1993:suppl 570.

64. Hollabaugh RS, Dmochowski RR, Hickerson WL, Cox CE. "Fournier's gangrene: Therapeutic impact of hyperbaric oxygen." Plast Reconstr Surg. 1998:101(1);94-100.

65. Hsieh T, Samson LM, Jabbour M, Osmond MH. Necrotizing fasciitis in children in eastern Ontario: a case-control study. CMAJ. 2000:163(4);393-396.

66. Johnin K, Nakatoh M, Kadowaki T et al. Fournier's gangrene caused by candida species as the primary organism. Urol. 2000:56(1);153.

67. Jones J. "Investigations upon the nature, causes and treatment of hospital gangrene as it prevailed in the Confederate armies 1861-1865, New York." U.S. Sanitary Commission. Surgical Memoirs of the War of Rebellion. 1871.

68. Jones RB, Hirschmann JV, Brown GS, Tremann JA. "Fournier's syndrome: necrotizing soft tissue infection of the male genitalia." J Urol. 1979:122;279-282.

69. Käch K, Kossman T, Trentz O. "Nekrotisierende Weichteilinfekte." Unfallchirurg. 1993:96;181-191.

70. Kaiser RE, Cerra FB. "Progressive necrotizing surgical infections-A unified approach." J Trauma. 1981:21(5);349-353.

71. Kaul R, McGeer A, Low DE et al. "Population-based surveillance for group A streptococcal necrotizing fasciitis: Clinical features, prognostic indicators and microbiologic analysis of seventy-seven cases." Am J Med. 1997:103;18-24.

72. Kingston D, Seal DV. "Current hypotheses on synergistic microbial gangrene." Br J Surg. 1990;77:260-264.

73. Kley AJ vd, Bakker DJ, Lubbers MJ, Henny CP. Skeletal muscle $pO_2$ in anaerobic soft tissue infections during hyperbaric oxygen therapy. Adv Exp Med Biol. 1992:317;125-129.

74. Korhonen K, Hirn M, Niinikoski J. Hyperbaric oxygen in the treatment of Fournier's gangrene. Eur J Surg. 1998;164(4):251-255.

75. Korhonen K. Hyperbaric oxygen therapy in acute necrotizing infections. Ann Chir Gyn. 2000:suppl 214;7-36.

76. Korhonen K, Kuttila K, Niinikoski J. Tissue gas tensions in patients with necrotizing fasciitis and healthy controls during treatment with hyperbaric oxygen: A clinical study. Eur J Surg. 2000:166;530-534.

77. Kujath PE, Eckmann C. "Die nekrotisierende Fasziitis und schwere Weichteilinfektio-nen durch Gruppe-A-Streptokokken. Diagnose, Therapie und Prognose." Dt Artztebl. 1998:95(8);A-408-413.

78. Lamerton AJ. "Fournier's gangrene: non-clostridial gas gangrene of the perineum and diabetes mellitus." J R Soc Med. 1986;79:212-215.

79. Ledingham IM, Tehrani MA. "Diagnosis, clinical course and treatment of acute dermal gangrene." Br J Surg. 1975;62:364-372.

80. Lefrock JL, Molavi A. "Necrotizing skin and subcutaneous infections." J Antimicrob Chemother 9 (Suppl A). 1982;183-192.

81. Lewis RT. "Necrotizing soft tissue infections." Meakins JL (Ed.) Surgical Infection in Critical Care Medicine, Ed 20. London, Churchill Livingstone. 1985;153-171.

82. Lewis RT. "Soft tissue infection." Wilmore DW, Brennan MF, Harken AH, et al. (Eds). Care of the Surgical Patient, Ed 21. New York, Scientific American. 1989;1-15.

83. Lin C, Yeh FL, Lin JT et al. Necrotizing fasciitis of the head and neck: An analysis of 47 cases. Pals Reconstr Surg. 2001:107(7):1684-1693.

84. Loudon I. "Necrotizing fasciitis, hospital gangrene, and phagedena." Lancet. 1994:344;1416-1419.

85. Mader JT, Adams KR, Sutton TE. "Infectious diseases: Pathophysiology and mechanisms of hyperbaric oxygen." J Hyp Med. 1987;2:133-140.

86. Mader J. "Mixed anaerobic and aerobic soft tissue infections." Davis JC, Hunt TK, (Eds.) Problem Wounds: The Role of Oxygen. New York: Elsevier. 1988;153-172.

87. Mathieu D. Place de l'oxygénotherapie hyperbare dans le traitement des fasciites nécrosantes. Conférence de consensus de la Société Française de Dermatologie. Ann Dermatol Venereol. 2001:128;411-418.

88. McCafferty EL, Lyons C. "Suppurative fasciitis as the essential feature of hemolytic *streptococcus* gangrene." Surgery. 1948:24:438-442.

89. McCrea LE. "Fulminating gangrene of the penis." Clinics. 1945:4(3);796-829.

90. McGreer AJ. Commentary on Wall et al. A two factor model helped to rule out early stage necrotizing fasciitis. Evidence Based Med. 2001:6;96.

91. McLennan JD. "The histotoxic clostridial infections of man." Bact Rev. 1962;26:177-276.

92. Meleney FL. "Hemolytic *streptococcus* gangrene." Arch Surg. 1924;9:317-364.

93. Meleney FL. "A differential diagnosis between certain types of infectious gangrene of the skin, with particular reference to hemolytic *streptococcus* gangrene and bacterial synergistic gangrene." Surg Gynecol Obstet. 1933;56:847.

94. Meleney FL. "Bacterial synergism in disease process, with confirmation of the synergistic bacterial etiology of a certain type of progressive gangrene of the abdominal wall." Ann Surg. 1933;94:961-981.

95. Modai J. "Empiric therapy of severe infections in adults." Am J Med. 88 1990; (Suppl 4A):12S-17S.

96. Monnickendam MA, McEvoy MB, Blake WA et al. "Necrotizing fasciitis associated with invasive group A streptococcal infections in England and Wales." Adv Exp Med Biol. 1997:418;87-89.

97. Morantes MC, Lipsky BA. "Flesh-eating bacteria: Return of an old nemesis". Int J Dermat. 1995:34(7);461-463.

98. Mutschler W, Bakker DJ. "Temporärer Hautersatz (temporary skin replacement)." Z für Allg. med. 1088;64(24):714-720.

99. Neuber M, Rieger H, Brüwer M et al. Fulminante Fasciitis necroticans bei Morbus Crohn-assoziiertem Verlauf. Chirurg. 2000:71;1277-1280.

100. Nichols RL, Smith JW. "Gas in the wound: What does it mean?" Surg Clin North Am. 1975;55:1289-1296.

101. Nichols RL. "Gas-producing infections." Nichols RL, Hyslop NE, Bartlett JG, (Eds.) Decision Making in Surgical Sepsis. Decker, Philadelphia. 1991;60-61.

102. Norrby-Teglund A, Thulin P, Gan BS et al. Evidence for superantigen involvement in severe group A streptococcal tissue infections. J Infect Dis. 2001:184;853-860.

103. Patino JF, Castro D, Valencia A, Morales P. "Necrotizing soft tissue lesions after a volcanic cataclysm." World J Surg. 1991;15:240-247.

104. Paty R, Smith AD. "Gangrene and Fournier's Gangrene." Urol Clin N Am. 1992:19(1);149-162.

105. Pfanner W. "Zur Kenntnis und Behandlung des nekrotisierenden Erysipels. Kriegschirurgische Mitteilungen aus dem VÜlkerkrieg 1914/1918, nr 81." Dtsch Z Chir. 1918;144:108-119.

106. Podbielski A, Rozdzinski E, Wiedeck H, Lütticken R. "Gruppe-A-Streptokokken und die nekrotisierende Fasziitis." Dt Artztebl. 1998:95(8);A-414-420.

107. Pruitt BA. "Burns and soft tissues." Polk HC Jr (Ed.) Infection in the Surgical Patient. Clinical Surgery International 4. London, Churchill Livingstone. 1982;113-131.

108. Quirk WF, Sternbach G. "Joseph Jones: Infection with flesh eating bacteria." J Em Med. 1996:14(6);747-753.

109. Riegels-Nielsen P, Hesselfeldt-Nielsen J, Bang-Jensen E, Jacobsen E. "Fournier's gangrene: Five patients treated with hyperbaric oxygen." J Urol. 1984;132:918-920.

110. Riseman JA, Zamboni WA, Curtis A, Graham DR, Konrad HR, Ross DS. "Hyperbaric oxygen therapy for necrotizing fasciitis reduces mortality and the need for debridements." Surg. 1990;108:847-850.

111. Rodloff AC, Montag TH, GÜrtz G, Harnoss B-M, Ehlers S. "Mikrobiologische Aspekte von Anaerobierinfektionen." Hau T (Ed.) Anaerobierinfektionen in der Chirurgie. Upjohn Heppenheim (Germany). 1991.

112. Schwarz N, Redl H, Grasslober H, Krebitz B. "Necrotizing soft tissue infection-An increasing problem in orthopedic trauma." Eur J Trauma. 2000:2;62-68.

113. Sheffield PJ. "Tissue oxygen measurements." Davis JC, Hunt TK, (Eds.) Problem Wounds: The Role of Oxygen. New York: Elsevier. 1988;37-44.

114. Sherris JC. "Skin and wound infection." Sherris JC (Ed.) Medical Microbiology. New York, Elsevier. 1984;555-561.

115. Shupak A, Shoshani O, Goldenberg I, Barzilai A, Moskuna R, Bursztein S. "Necrotizing fasciitis: An indication for hyperbaric oxygen therapy?" Surgery. 1995:118(5);873-878.

116. Smith GL, Bunker CB, Dinneen MD. "Fournier's gangrene." Brit J Urol. 1998:81;347- 355.

117. Stevens BJ, Lathrop JC, Rice WT, Gruenberg JC. "Fournier's gangrene: Historic (1764-1978) versus contemporary (1979-1988) differences in etiology and clinical importance." Am Surg. 1993:59(5);149-154.

118. Stevens DL, Gibbons AE, Bergstrom R, Winn V. "The Eagle effect revisited: Efficacy of clindamycin, erythromycin and penicillin in the treatment of streptococcal myositis." J Inf Dis. 1988:158(1);23-28.

119. Stevens DL. "Invasive Group A *Streptococcus* infections." Clin Inf Dis. 1992; 14:2-13.

120. Stevens DL. "Invasive group A streptococcal infections: the past, the present and future." Pediatr Inf Dis J. 1994;13:561-566.

121. Stevens DL. "Streptococcal Toxic Shock Syndrome: Spectrum of disease, pathogenesis and new concepts in treatment." Em Inf Dis. 1995;1(3);69-78.

122. Stevens DL. Review: "Invasive Group A Streptococcal Disease." Infec Agents and Dis. 1996:5;157-166.

123. Stevens DL. "The Flesh-Eating Bacterium: What's next?" J Infect Dis. 1999;179(Suppl 2):S366-374.

124. Stevens DL. "Streptococcal Toxic Shock Syndrome associated with necrotizing fasciitis." Ann Rev Med. 2000:51;271-288.

125. Stevens DL. "Invasive streptococcal infections." J Infect Chemother. 2001:7;69-80.

126. Stephenson H, Dotters DJ, Katz V, Droegemueller W. "Necrotizing fasciitis of the vulva." Am J Obstet Gynecol. 1992:166(5);1324-1327.

127. Stone HH, Martin JG,Jr. "Synergistic necrotizing cellulitis." Ann Surg. 1992;175:702-711.

128. Stone DR, Gorbach SL. "Necrotizing fasciitis. The changing spectrum." Inf Dis Dermat. Dermat Clin. 1997:15(2);213-220.

129. Sutherland ME, Meyer AA. "Necrotizing soft-tissue infections." Surg Clin N Am. 1994;74(3);591-607.

130. Thom SR. "Hyperbaric oxygen therapy in septicemia." J Hyp Med. 1987;2(3):141-146.

131. Tibbles PM, Edelsberg JS. Hyperbaric oxygen therapy. N Eng J Med. 1996:334(25);1642-1648.

132. Umeda T, Ohara H, Hayashi O et al. Toxic shock syndrome after suction lipectomy. Plast Reconstr Surg. 2000:106(1);204-207. Discussion by Mladick RA 208-209.

133. Unnikrishnan M, Cohen J, Sriskandan S. Complementation of a speA negative *Streptococcus pyogenes* with speA: effects on virulence and production of streptococcal pyrogenic exotoxin A. Microb Pathogen. 2001:31;109-114.

134. Vick R, Carson CC. Fournier's Disease. Urol Clin N Am 1999:26(4);841-851.

135. Voros D, Pissiotis C, Georgantas D et al. "Role of early and extensive surgery in the treatment of severe necrotizing soft tissue infections." Br J Surg. 1993:80;1190-1191.

136. Wall DB, Klein SR, Black S, Virgilio de C. A simple model to help distinguish necrotizing fasciitis from no necrotizing soft tissue infection. J Am Coll Surg. 2000:191(3);227-231.

137. Webb R, Berg E. "Symbiotic gangrene due to Pseudomonas pyocyanea and E. coli." Austr NZ J Surg. 1966;36:159-160.

138. Weiss KA, Lavardière M. Group A *streptococcus* invasive infections: A review." Can J Surg. 1997:40(1);18-25.

139. Whitesides L, Cotto-Cumba C, Myers RAM. Cervical necrotizing fasciitis of odontogenic origin: A case report and review of 12 cases. J Or Max Surg. 2000:58(2);144-151.

140. Wienecke H, Lobenhoffer P. Nekrotisierende Weichteilinfektionen. Chirurg. 2001:72;320-337.

141. Wilson B. "Necrotizing fasciitis." Am Surgeon. 1952;18:426-431.

142. Wilson DH, Haltalin KC. "Acute necrotizing fasciitis in childhood." Am J Dis Child. 1973;125:591-595.

143. Zamboni WA, Riseman JA, Kucan JO. "Management of Fournier's gangrene and the role of hyperbaric oxygen." J Hyp Med. 1990;5(3):177-186.

144. Zamboni WA, Mazolewski PJ, Erdmann D et al. "Evaluation of Penicillin and Hyperbaric Oxygen in the treatment of streptococcal myositis." Ann Plast Surg. 1997:39(2);131-136.

CHAPTER 23

# HYPERBARIC OXYGEN IN INTRACRANIAL ABSCESS

## CHAPTER TWENTY-THREE OVERVIEW

# HYPERBARIC OXYGEN IN INTRACRANIAL ABSCESS

*Lorenz A. Lampl, Guenter Frey*

## INTRODUCTION

Based upon considerations similar to the rationale for the use of HBO in gas gangrene as well as management of necrotizing soft tissue infections, the treatment of intracranial abscess with adjunctive HBO was approved by the Undersea and Hyperbaric Medical Society in 1994 (10) followed by the ECHM in its last Consensus Conference in 2003.

The first review of the bacteriologic and pathophysiologic rationale for HBO treatment of intracranial abscesses was published in the *Journal of Hyperbaric Medicine* in 1989 (27). However, at that time as well as today, data from animal series were scarce and the number of case reports available was small.

Inasmuch as the clinical course, diagnosis, and treatment of subdural or epidural empyemas have similarities, these are included along with cerebral abscesses. All of these disorders are discussed under the term "intracranial abscesses."

As a consequence of the nature of intracranial abscess, double-blind studies of HBO's therapeutic effectiveness in humans are not to be expected. For this reason, collecting as many case reports as possible was of first priority in the past. Today, in 2006, case series from five hyperbaric centers are available internationally involving 87 patients. So, the comparison between adjuvant HBO therapy and standard management in those patients has become possible.

## MORBIDITY/MORTALITY

Intracranial abscesses account for only three to five admissions per year at a large medical center (15). Thus, the incidence is roughly in the same range or a little higher than that of gas gangrene and necrotizing soft-tissue infections.

However, the overall mortality in numerous series from various countries averages 19.2% over 25 years (see Table 1). In spite of a significantly reduced death rate in recent years to around 13%, at present (26), mortality still remains unacceptably high. Sequelae such as epileptic disorders are frequently reported in the survivors.

## TABLE 1. MORTALITY RATES FROM INTRACRANIAL ABSCESSES DURING DIFFERENT STUDY PERIODS

**a: 1981 - 1986**

| Author | yr. of. publ. | Country of Origin | No. Px | Px died | Mortality | [Ref.] |
|---|---|---|---|---|---|---|
| Yang | 1981 | PR China | 400 | 91 | 23 % | [59] |
| Alderson | 1981 | Great Britain | 90 | 9 | 10 % | [1] |
| Dohrmann | 1982 | Australia | 28 | 10 | 36 % | [9] |
| Britt | 1983 | USA | 14 | 5 | 36 % | [5] |
| Cowie | 1983 | Great Britain | 89 | 24 | 27 % | [8] |
| Harris | 1985 | USA | 15 | 3 | 20 % | [15] |
| | | | **636** | **142** | **22,3 %** | |

**b: 1987 - 1993**

| Author | yr. of publ. | Country of Origin | No. Px | Px died | Mortality | [Ref.] |
|---|---|---|---|---|---|---|
| Ferriero | 1987 | USA | 17 | 1 | 6 % | [11] |
| Pattisapu | 1987 | USA | 8 | 0 | 0 % | [43] |
| Miller | 1988 | Great Britain | 100 | 20 | 20 % | [34] |
| Schliamser | 1988 | Sweden | 54 | 17 | 31 % | [47] |
| Basit | 1989 | Saudi-Arabia | 21 | 5 | 24 % | [3] |
| Szuwart | 1989 | Germany | 38 | 10 | 26 % | [56] |
| Witzmann | 1989 | Austria | 38 | 7 | 18 % | [58] |
| Pathak | 1990 | India | 41 | 10 | 24 % | [42] |
| Kratimenos | 1991 | Great Britain | 14 | 2 | 14 % | [23] |
| McIntyre | 1991 | Australia | 14 | 3 | 21 % | [33] |
| Bagdatoglu | 1992 | Turkey | 78 | 16 | 20 % | [2] |
| Seydoux | 1992 | Switzerland | 39 | 5 | 13 % | [49] |
| Bok | 1993 | South-Africa | 21 | 5 | 24 % | [4] |
| Stapleton | 1993 | Great Britain | 11 | 3 | 27 % | [51] |
| Yang | 1993 | PR China | 140 | 11 | 8 % | [60] |
| | | | **634** | **115** | **18,1 %** | |

**c: 1995 - 2005**

| Author | yr. of publ. | Country of Origin | No. Px | Px died | Mortality | [Ref.] |
|---|---|---|---|---|---|---|
| Sharma | 1995 | India | 38 | 12 | 32 % | [50] |
| Takada | 1998 | Japan | 13 | 0 | 0,0 % | [57] |
| Stephanov | 1999 | Switzerland | 17 | 2 | 11,8 % | [52] |
| Mamatova | 2000 | Uzbekistan | 13 | 1 | 7,6 % | [30] |
| Liliang | 2001 | Taiwan | 15 | 4 | 26,7 % | [28] |
| Marchiori | 2003 | Italy | 20 | 1 | 5 % | [31] |
| Jansson | 2004 | Sweden | 66 | 3 | 4,5 % | [19] |
| Ozkaya | 2005 | Turkey | 25 | 4 | 16 % | [41] |
| | | | **207** | **27** | **13,0 %** | |

# RATIONALES FOR HBO

In 1983, we had favorable results in an anecdotal case in which HBO was initiated as a last-ditch attempt to save a young mother's life (25). A thorough literature research then led to a better understanding of HBO's potential usefulness in the treatment of intracranial abscess. Our group was able to combine this with clinical experience in a series of 22 own patients treated to date as well as with the data of four other hyperbaric centers.

## Bacteriology

Over the past 30 years, knowledge of the bacteriology of intracranial abscess has become better-defined in the literature. Anaerobes account for up to 90% of the bacteria isolated from intracranial foci. This, of course, depends on the culturing technique used.

Nevertheless, the predominance of anaerobic organisms in intracranial abscesses is well documented in the world literature (1, 5, 6, 9, 20, 26, 59).

The fact that, in the past, several studies (e.g., Ref. 59) found a high percentage of sterile cultures may be deceptive. One explanation is that anaerobic culturing either had not been done, or that it had not been done correctly.

Brook, in the *Journal of Neurosurgery* (6), reports the differential bacteriologic findings in 19 children with intracranial abscesses. In 63.2%, anaerobes were cultured exclusively; in 26.3%, both aerobes and anaerobes were found; only 10.5% of the cultures proved purely aerobic. No difference was seen in the predominance of the anaerobic organisms responsible for both brain abscess and subdural empyema. Typically, several microorganisms were found simultaneously.

These results coincide with our own. See Table 2. In 22 consecutive, non-selected patients, 35 organisms were identified. In 16 patients, cultures were purely anaerobic, including microaerophilic *streptococci*. In five patients *staphylococci* were found, combined with *enterobacter*, microaerophilic *streptococci*, and *fusobacteria*, respectively. In one septic patient with a small subdural empyema treated without surgery, only *peptostreptococci* were harvested from a blood culture, suggesting them to be the empyema's underlying cause. In a five-year-old boy, *Clostridium perfringens* was cultured from the cerebro-spinal fluid, after a penetrating skull injury; probably due to antibiotic therapy, cultures from the cerebral abscess, which emerged some days later, were sterile. See Table 3.

Most astonishing to us is the fact that anaerobes were the predominant organisms in three patients with rhinogenic intracranial abscesses when only aerobes were cultivated from the inflamed nasal sinuses, the infection's source. We do not fully understand this selection phenomenon yet. (For case reports, see Ref. 27).

The bacteriologic results quoted above are mostly from patients with endogenous intracranial abscesses. No data have been found in the literature to indicate whether the same is true in exogenous abscesses following penetrating head injuries.

The therapeutic effect of HBO on anaerobic and miscellaneous flora is well known and has been widely documented for many years (14, 16, 40, 45, 48).

## TABLE 2. BACTERIAL ISOLATES

| | | |
|---|---|---|
| **STRICTLY ANAEROBIC** | | |
| Peptostreptococci | 7 | |
| Bacteroides spp. | 4 | |
| Fusobacteria | 2 | |
| Clostr. perfringens | 1 | 53% |
| Veillonella | 1 | |
| Streptococci (anaerobic) | 4 | |
| Actinomyces spp. | 1 | |
| **INTERMEDIATE** | | |
| Streptococci (microaerophilic) | 9 | 31% |
| Enterobacter | 1 | |
| **AEROBIC** | | |
| Staphylococci spp. | 5 | 16% |

Dr. Lampl's own patient series, n=22. In 16 patients exclusively anaerobic/microaerophilic pathogens, in 10 patients more than one germ isolated.

### Perifocal Cerebral Edema

The expansive growth of an intracranial abscess and the formation of its perifocal edema may result in either secondary lesions to surrounding brain tissue or, at worst, may lead to a life-threatening increase in intracranial pressure (ICP). The beneficial influence of HBO on increased ICP has been documented for more than 40 years (35-39, 44, 53, 54).

HBO acts directly on autoregulated small blood vessels. Elevated arterial oxygen tension results in a vasoconstriction leading to a decrease in cerebral blood flow; consequently this leads to a reduction of the intracranial vascular volume. In turn, this results in the reduction of ICP. When compared with commonly applied normobaric hypocapnic hyperventilation, HBO additionally guarantees sufficient oxygen delivery to potentially hypoxic brain areas (48) and its vasoconstrictive effects are additive to those of hyperventilation. This mechanism may be of major importance in the prevention or treatment of secondary brain damage (13, 17, 18).

The therapeutic impact of these physiologic effects of HBO is expected to be even more pronounced in cases of perifocal brain swelling due to intracranial abscess. HBO acts specifically against anaerobic microorganisms as the predominant cause of intracranial abscess and the consequent brain swelling. Therefore, HBO's influence on the edema, and on elevated ICP, should tend to be curative, secondary to its attack on the underlying bacteriology. It is not just a reversible symptomatic effect, as seen with other agents used to lower intracranial pressure.

At present, there is only one anecdotal case report describing the favorable influence of adjunctive HBO on a critically elevated ICP (25) in an intracranial abscess patient.

## TABLE 3. DATA AND DIAGNOSIS, UNDERLYING DISORDERS AND BACTERIOLOGICAL FINDINGS (SEE TABLE 2)

| NO. | AGE | SEX | DIAGNOSIS | UNDERLYING DISORDER | BACTERIAL ISOLATE |
|---|---|---|---|---|---|
| 1 | 31 | f | multiple abscesses left hemisphere | septic tonsillectomy | Bacteroides fragilis peptostreptococci |
| 2 | 22 | m | epidural empyema | pansinusitis | Fusobacteria, streptococci (microaerophilic) |
| 3 | 34 | m | parietal abscess | pulmonary angioma | Bacteroides fragilis, peptostreptococci, streptococci (microaerophilic) |
| 4 | 13 | m | frontal abscess | sinusitis frontalis | streptococci (microaerophilic) |
| 5 | 15 | f | frontal abscess | pansinusitis | peptostreptococci |
| 6 | 26 | m | frontal abscess | sinusitis frontalis | Veillonella parv., Bacteroides spp. |
| 7 | 47 | m | parietal abscess | apical ostitis tooth 3/5 | peptostreptococci |
| 8 | 36 | m | frontal abscess | ? ? ? | Staph. epidermidis |
| 9 | 27 | m | subdural empyema | sinusitis maxillaris | peptostreptococci (blood culture) |
| 10 | 42 | f | frontal abscess | progressive osteomyelitis | Enterobacter, Staph. aureus |
| 11 | 48 | m | multiple abscesses left hemisphere | sinusitis frontalis | Staph. epidermidis, streptococci (microaerophilic) |
| 12 | 52 | m | frontal abscess | sinusitis maxillaris ? | streptococci (anaerobic) |
| 13 | 21 | m | multiple abscesses right hemisphere | pansinusitis | streptococci (microaerophilic) |
| 14 | 5 | m | frontal abscess | penetrating injury | Clostr. perfringens |
| 15 | 45 | m | subdural empyema | pansinusitis | —— |
| 16 | 47 | f | subdural empyema | osteomyelitis femur (?) | Fusobacteria, Staph. Sp. |
| 17 | 17 | m | epi-/subdural empyema | open skull base fracture | Staph. epidermidis streptococci (anaerobic) streptococci (microaerophilic) |
| 18 | 57 | f | subdural empyema | mastoiditis | streptococci (microaerophilic) |
| 19 | 22 | m | subdural empyema | pansinusitis | Bacteroides sp. peptostreptococci |
| 20 | 4 | m | multiple abscesses both hemispheres | pulmonary abscess | streptococci (anaerobic) streptococci (microaerophilic) |
| 21 | 19 | m | multiple abscesses | sinusitis maxillaris | Streptococci (microaerophilic) |
| 22 | 40 | m | parietal abscess | unknown | peptostreptococci Actinomyces spp. streptococci (anaerobic) |

*22 unselected patients with intracranial abscesses (own cases).*

## Enhanced Host Defense

The effects of HBO in enhancing leukocyte-mediated, host-defense mechanisms are well known to the hyperbaric community. Therefore, they need not be described in detail here.

Nevertheless, potentiation of leukocyte microbial killing seems to be of twofold importance:

1. As the predominant defense mechanism at the abscess site.
2. As an adjunct in cases of concomitant osteomyelitis.

## Concomitant Osteomyelitis of the Skull

Rhinogenic as well as otogenic intracranial abscesses are frequently combined with more or less pronounced osteomyelitic processes involving the skull's bony structure. HBO is a powerful adjuvant to surgery and antibiotics in infections of this kind. Despite its potency, however, as in other infectious diseases, it remains an adjunctive treatment.

## Other Effects

At the present time, the influence of HBO on the abscess membrane has not been assessed, nor has its influence on the extent of glial scar tissue formation been investigated in an animal model. Thus, it remains unclear whether there may be additional benefits in this regard.

Since, frequently, there is either only a slight inflammatory reaction of the meninges, or none at all in the case of intracranial abscess, achieving effective antibiotic treatment may easily pose major problems in terms of antibiotic penetration. For this reason, studies showing a reversible opening of the blood-brain-barrier by HBO, leading to an improved penetration of antibiotics through non-inflamed meninges (7), must be considered promising. Additionally, improved tissue oxygenation due to HBO is able to potentiate the antimicrobial effects of antibiotics such as aminoglykosides.

## AN EXEMPLARY CASE REPORT

**History:** Presentig the non-specific history of a flu for a few days, a 4-year old boy was admitted to the pediatric university hospital because of progressive vigilance disturbances.

**Diagnose:** Multiple cerebral abscesses predominatly in the left hemisphere (Figures 1 and 2).

**Source:** Pulmonary abscess right lower lobe (Figure 3). Bacteriology: Streptococci (anaerobic / microaerophilic).

**Course:** Neurosurgery limited to drainage ($\rightarrow$) of the most space-occupying abscess, only (Figure 4). Repeated fine-needle aspirations of all abscess formations within stereotactic reach over the following days. Comprehensive intensive care including controlled ventilation and adequate antibiosis completed by immediate HBO therapy.

Because of open lung surgery after 6 days (lobectomy of the right lower lobe) and a favourable neurological course seen at that time, already, limitation of HBO to 6 sessions alltogether before thoracotomy (Figure 5, before HBO sessions 6, mind the thoracic abscess drainage).

**Outcome:** With no neurological deficit remaining, the boy was put to school at the age of six according to national regulations.

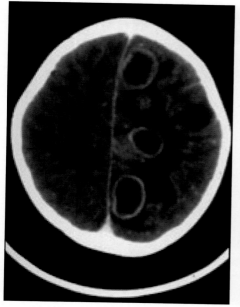

Figure 1.

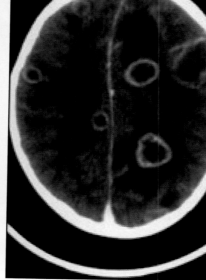

Figure 2.

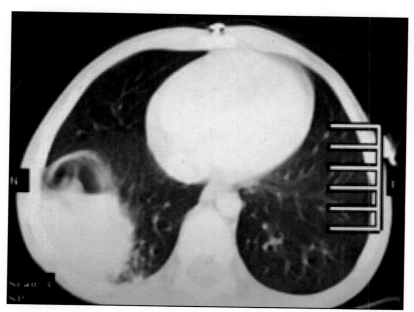

Figure 3.

Figures 1 thru 5.  A 4-year old boy with multiple brain abscesses of pulmonary origin (for details see text).

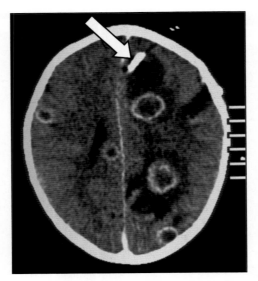

*Figure 4.*

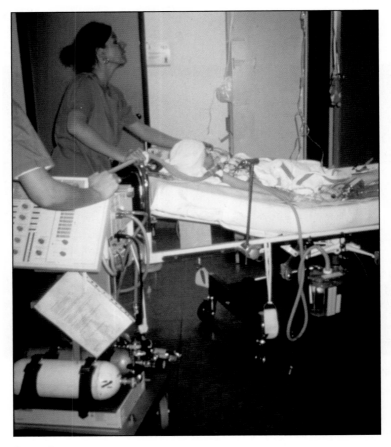

*Figure 5.*

# INTERNATIONAL CASE SERIES TREATED BY ADJUNCTIVE HBO

To date (December 2006), we have data of 22 consecutive and unrelated patients with intracranial abscess treated with adjunctive HBO at our facility from 1983 to 2006. See Table 3. In all our patients, HBO was started when at least one of the following criteria was met:

- Anaerobic or mixed pathogens.
- Multiple abscesses.
- Abscess in a deep or dominant location.

When the infection was life threatening, treatment was twice daily; otherwise there was one treatment per day at 2.5 ATA, except for patient 1 (see Table 3) who was treated at 2.8 ATA. The duration of each treatment was between 60 and 90 minutes.

Time will tell whether 2.5 ATA is the optimal pressure for this disorder; therefore, the ultimate protocol is open to discussion. However, in the entire series of 22 patients managed with 312 hyperbaric treatments, no signs of cerebral oxygen toxicity were observed, nor were other adverse effects of pressurization seen. In our opinion, when choosing the appropriate treatment pressure, treatment of the infection should be considered primary, before concerns about possible side effects.

The number of HBO sessions varied from 4 to 30, and averaged 14.2 in our patients. Usually, the number of HBO treatments depended on the patient's response, which included neurosurgical evaluation, as well as radiological findings from repeated head scans. In two cases, patient cooperation proved to be a major problem, probably secondary to psychic derangements attendant to their disease. In these cases fewer treatments than desired were given.

The mortality observed with our patients was 0,0% with a complete recovery in 73%, 77% were able to resume their former occupational work and life. See Table 4.

The favorable results that we have seen in our own patients could be confirmed by other investigators. See Figure 6. Especially, this is true for the patients treated by Mathieu, France (32, 32a): His inclusion criterion was deterioration of the patient´s neurological condition, due to lack of response to standard therapy, what, undoubtedly, means poor prognosis. Only one out of ten was lost. The same is true for a series from Graz, Austria (55): These investigators achieved a zero percent mortality in their 18 patients, beginning in the seventies at a time, when, in the international literature, the mortality of intracranial abscess patients still was up to 36%. See Table 1. The unpublished data from Kemmer, Germany (21) do fit together completely with these results as do the oberservations of Kindwall and Whelan, USA (22) and quite a number of single anecdotal case reports.

So, at present (winter 2006), data from five series enrolling 87 patients, in whom adjunctive HBO was used as a component of intracranial abscess management during the years from 1976 to 2006, are available (mortality 3,4%). See Figure 6. During the corresponding time span, from 1981 to 2005, 29 studies enrolling 1,477 patients treated conventionally with an averaging mortality of 19,2% were found in the literature. See Table 1.

## TABLE 4. NUMBER OF HBO SESSIONS AND OUTCOME IN 22 PATIENTS WITH INTRACRANIAL ABSCESSES

| NO. | AGE | SEX | HBOs | OUTCOME | |
|-----|-----|-----|------|---------|---|
| 1 | 31 | f | 14 | slightly disabled | * |
| 2 | 22 | m | 4 | complete recovery | * |
| 3 | 34 | m | 10 | severely disabled (lost follow-up) | |
| 4 | 13 | m | 16 | complete recovery | * |
| 5 | 15 | f | 10 | complete recovery | * |
| 6 | 26 | m | 10 | complete recovery | * |
| 7 | 47 | m | 6 | brachio-facial hemiparesis (in recovery, lost follow-up) | |
| 8 | 36 | m | 27 | complete recovery | * |
| 9 | 27 | m | 7 | moderate motor-dysphasia, minimal brachial hemiparesis (in recovery, lost follow-up) | |
| 10 | 42 | f | 19 | complete recovery | * |
| 11 | 48 | m | 12 | complete recovery | * |
| 12 | 52 | m | 13 | complete recovery | * |
| 13 | 21 | m | 12 | complete recovery | * |
| 14 | 5 | m | 17 | complete recovery | * |
| 15 | 45 | m | 22 | complete recovery | * |
| 16 | 47 | f | 16 | persistent aphasia | |
| 17 | 17 | m | 20 | complete recovery | * |
| 18 | 57 | f | 7 | complete recovery | * |
| 19 | 22 | m | 20 | complete recovery | * |
| 20 | 4 | m | 6 | complete recovery | * |
| 21 | 19 | m | 14 | complete recovery | * |
| 22 | 40 | m | 30** | still in therapy | |

\* Patient has returned to his / her former occupational work or school.
\*\* With kind support by BG-Unfallklinik Murnau, Germany.

Taking mortality as the criterion, and applying the one-sample test for binomial proportion (normal theory method), the results are significantly superior (p < 0.01) when HBO is applied as an adjuvant component to the standard therapeutic principles of intracranial abscess management (24). See Figure 7.

## CURRENT THERAPY AND INDICATIONS FOR ADJUVANT HBO

As with other life-threatening conditions such as gas gangrene, it is mandatory to apply HBO in intracranial abscess only in combination with currently accepted standard procedures or as a complement to them (12, 20). Above all, treatment must include appropriate neurosurgical management

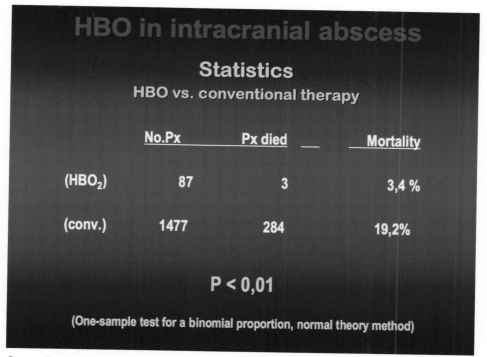

## HBO in intracranial abscess

### series available

| Author | Year | Country of origin | No. Px | Px died | Mortality |
|--------|------|-------------------|--------|---------|-----------|
| Mathieu | 2006 | France | 10 | 1 | 10,0 % |
| Kemmer, Schaan | 2006 | Germany | 29 | 2 | 6,9 % |
| Sutter | 1996 | Austria | 18 | 0 | 0,0 % |
| Kindwall, Whelan | 2001 | USA | 8 | 0 | 0,0 % |
| Lampl, Frey | 2006 | Germany | 22 | 0 | 0,0 % |
| | | | 87 | 3 | 3,4 % |

HBO-patient series compiled with assistance of the UHMS;

time span 1974 - 2006

Figure 6. Intracranial abscess patients treated by adjuvant HBO2-therapy; international series available in 2006.

## HBO in intracranial abscess

### Statistics
#### HBO vs. conventional therapy

| | No.Px | Px died | Mortality |
|--------|-------|---------|-----------|
| (HBO$_2$) | 87 | 3 | 3,4 % |
| (conv.) | 1477 | 284 | 19,2% |

### P < 0,01

(One-sample test for a binomial proportion, normal theory method)

Figure 7. Mortality rates in intracranial abscess patients; comparing adjuvant HBO2 with conventional treatment protocols.

(e.g., fine-needle aspiration, drainage or resection, depending on the individual situation) and the administration of adequate antibiotics, as well as steroids.

The benefit of steroid medication in intracranial abscess management is a controversial topic in the international literature (12). The influence of steroids on the perifocal edema in intracranial abscess may prove beneficial, but the impairment of host defense in infectious disorders must be seriously considered.

In this context, HBO certainly is a beneficial therapeutic component with proven antibiotic as well as edema-reducing efficacy. Its use is approved in the following conditions (10):

- Anaerobic or mixed pathogens.
- Multiple abscesses.
- Abscess in a deep or dominant location.
- Compromised host.
- In situations where surgery is contraindicated or where the patient is a poor surgical risk.
- No response, or further deterioration, in spite of standard surgical care (e.g., 1 - 2 fine needle aspirations) and antibiotic treatment.

The early administration of HBO seems to be of utmost importance. To delay the onset of HBO, or to start it as a last-ditch attempt when everything else has failed, will obscure the true potential benefit and may also cause avoidable brain damage.

Since the infectious component of the intracranial abscess has to be considered primary, we recommend a treatment pressure of 2.5 ATA, one or two sessions a day, depending on the clinical status of the patient. The number of HBO treatments given has to be assessed on a individual basis, in accordance with the patient's clinical response, as well as the radiologic findings.

As the mortality and long-term sequelae of intracranial abscess are substantial, HBO treatment is warranted, even in the absence of rigid double-blind studies. The number of treatments required is relatively small, and the costs of hyperbaric treatment are trivial in comparison to the total costs of managing these critically-ill patients.

In view of the high morbidity and mortality of cerebral abscess, and the fact that HBO is relatively noninvasive and carries an extremely low complication rate, the risk-benefit ratio is not arguable. The full benefit of an HBO-based protocol is expected to become even more significant once study criteria, such as epileptic sequelae and parameters such as the ability to return to work are properly documented in addition to the surveillance of the mortality rates.

# REFERENCES

1. Alderson D, Strong AJ, Ingham HR, Selkon JB (1981): Fifteen-year review of the mortality of brain abscesses. Neurosurgery 8: 1-6.

2. Bagdatoglu H, Ildan F, Cetinalp E et al (1992): The clinical presentation of intracranial abscesses. A study of seventy-eight cases. J Neurosurg Sci 36: 139-143.

3. Basit AS, Ravi B, Banerji AK, Tandon PN (1989): Multiple pyogenic brain abscesses: an analysis of 21 patients. J Neurol Neurosurg Psychiatry 52: 591-594.

4. Bok AP, Peter JC (1993): Subdural empyema: burr holes or craniotomy? A retrospective computerized tomography era analysis of treatment in 90 cases. J Neurosurg 78: 574-578.

5. Britt RH, Enzmann DR (1983): Clinical stages of human brain abscesses on serial CT scans after contrast infusion. Computerized tomographic, neuropathological, and clinical correlations. J Neurosurg 59: 972-989.

6. Brook I (1981) Bacteriology of intracranial abscess in children. J Neurosurg 54: 484-488.

7. Chambi IP, Ceverha MD, Hart GB, Strauss MB (1984): Effect of hyperbaric oxygen in the permeability of the blood-brain-barrier (Abstract only). Eighth International Congress on Hyperbaric Medicine, Long Beach CA.

8. Cowie R, Williams B (1983): Late seizures and morbidity after subdural empyema. J Neurosurg 58: 569-573.

9. Dohrmann PJ, Elrick WL (1982): Observations on brain abscesses. Review of 28 cases. Med J Austr 2: 81-83.

10. Feldmeier JJ, (Ed.) (2003): The Hyperbaric Oxygen Therapy Committee Report. Kensington, MD: Undersea and Hyperbaric Medical Society.

11. Ferriero DM, Derechin M, Edwards MS, Berg BO (1987): Outcome of brain abscess treatment in children: reduced morbidity with neuro-imaging. Pediatr Neurol 3: 148-152.

12. Garvey G (1983): Current concepts of bacterial infections of the central nervous system. J Neurosurg 59: 735-744.

13. Gött U, Holbach KH (1969): Hyperbare Sauerstofftherapie bei neuro-chirurgischen Patienten. Anaesthesist 18: 139-145.

14. Gottlieb SF (1977): Oxygen under pressure and microorganisms. In: Davis JC, Hunt TK (eds): Hyperbaric Oxygen Therapy. Undersea Medical Society, Bethesda MD, pp 79-99.

15. Harris LF, McCubbin DA, Triplett jr. JN, Haws FP (1985): Brain abscess: recent experience at a community hospital. South Med J 78: 704-707.

16. Heimbach RD, Boerema I, Brummelkamp WH et al (1977): Current therapy of gas gangrene. In: Davis JC, Hunt TK (eds.): Hyperbaric Oxygen Therapy. Undersea Medical Society, Bethesda MD, pp 153-176.

17. Holbach KH, Wassmann K, Kolberg T (1974): Verbesserte Reversibilität des traumatischen Mittelhirn-Syndroms bei Anwendung der Hyperbaren Oxygenation. Acta Neurochir 30: 247-256.

18. Holbach KH, Wassmann K, Hohelüchter KL, Jain KK (1977): Differentiation between reversible and irreversible post-stroke changes in brain tissue: its relevance for cerebrovascular surgery. Surg Neurol 7: 325-331.

19. Jansson AK, Enblad P, Sjoelin J (2004): Efficacy and Safety of Cefotaxime in Combination with Metronidazole for Empirical Treatment of Brain Abscess in Clinical Practice: A Retrospecitve Study of 66 Consecutive Cases. Eur J Clin Microbiol & Inf Dis 23: 7 - 14.

20. Kaplan K (1985): Brain abscess. Med Clin N Am 69: 345-360.

21. Kemmer A, BG-Unfallkinik Murnau, Germany (2006): Personal communication.

22. Kindwall EP (2001): Personal communication.

23. Kratimenos G, Crockard HA (1991): Multiple brain abscess: a review of fourteen cases. Br J Neurosurg 5: 153-161.

24. Lampl LA (2003): Intracranial abscess management: Are the results of adjunctive HBO therapy superior to conventional treatment? In: Cramer FS, Sheffield PJ (eds.): Proceedings of the Fourteenth International Congress on Hyperbaric Medicine. Best Publishing Company, Flagstaff, AZ, 2003: 120 - 124.

25. Lampl L, Frey G, Miltner FO, Wörner U (1987): Multiple anaerobic brain abscesses - life saving HBO therapy, integrated with comprehensive intensive care. In: Kindwall EP (ed.) Proceedings of the Eighth International Congress on Hyperbaric Medicine. Best Publishing, San Pedro CA, pp107-111.

26. Lampl LA, Frey G (2006): Intra-cranial abscess: In: Mathieu D (Ed): Handbook on Hyperbaric Medicine. Springer, Dordrecht, NL: pp 291-304.

27. Lampl L, Frey G, Dietze T, Trauschel M (1989): Hyperbaric oxygen in intracranial abscesses. J Hyperbaric Med 4(3): 111 - 126.

28. Liliang PC, Lin YC, Su TM et al. (2001): Klebsiella Brain Abscess in Adults. Infection 29 : 81 - 86.

29. Mader JT (1988): Bacterial osteomyelitis: adjunctive hyperbaric oxygen therapy. In: Bakker DJ, Schmutz J (eds.) Hyperbaric Medicine Proceedings. Foundation for Hyperbaric Medicine, Basel, pp 65-70.

30. Mamatova TS, Rasulova AK (2000): Otogenic cerebellar abscesses. Vestn Otorinolaringol 4: 47 – 50.

31. Marchiori C, Tonon E, Boscolo Rizzo P et al. (2003): Hirnabszesse nach extrakraniellen Infektionen im Kopf-Hals-Bereich. HNO 51: 813 – 822.

32. Mathieu D, Wattel F, Neviere R, Bocquillon N (1999): Intracranial infections and hyperbaric oxygen therapy: A five year experience (Abstract). Undersea and Hyperbaric Medicine 26 (Suppl.): 67.

32a. Mathieu D (2006) : Personal communication.

33. McIntyre PB, Lavercombe PS, Kemp RJ, McCormack JG (1991): Subdural and epidural empyema: diagnostic and therapeutic problems. Med J Aust 154: 653-657.

34. Miller ES, Dias PS, Uttley D (1988): CT scanning in the management of intracranial abscess: A review of 100 cases. Br J Neurosurg 2: 439-446.

35. Miller JD, Fitch W, Ledingham IM (1970): The effect of hyperbaric oxygen on experimentally increased intracranial pressure. J Neurosurg 33: 287-296.

36. Miller JD, Ledingham IM (1971): Reduction of increased intra-cranial pressure - comparison between hyperbaric oxygen and hyperventilation. Arch Neurol 24: 210-216.

37. Mogami RA, Hayakawa T, Kanai N (1969): Clinical application of hyperbaric oxygenation in the treatment of acute cerebral damage. J Neurosurg 31: 636-643.

38. Moody RA, Mead CO, Ruamsuke S (1970): Therapeutic value of oxygen at normal and hyperbaric pressure in experimental head injury. J Neurosurg 32: 51-54.

39. Ohta H, Yasui N, Kitami K (1987): Intracranial pressure and hyperbaric oxygen. In: Kindwall EP (ed.): Proceedings of the Eighth International Congress on Hyperbaric Medicine. Best Publishing, San Pedro CA, pp 68-72.

40. Ollodart RM (1966): Effects of HBO on aerobic microorganisms (abstract only). In: Brown IW, Cox BG (eds.): Proceedings of the Third International Congress on Hyperbaric Medicine. Duke University, Durham NC, Publ No 1404, pp 565-57.1

41. Ozkaya S, Bezircioglu H, Sucu HK, Ozdemir I (2005): Combined approach for otogenic brain abscess. Neurologia medico-chirurgica 45: 82 – 85.

42. Pathak A, Sharma BS, Mathuriya SN et al (1990): Controversies in the management of subdural empyema. A study of 41 cases with review of the literature. Acta Neurochir 102: 25-32.

43. Pattisapu JV, Perent AD (1987): Subdural empyemas in children. Pediatr Neurosci 13: 251-254.

44. Peirce II EC, Jacobson II JH (1977): Cerebral Edema. In: Davis JC, Hunt TK (eds.): Hyperbaric Oxygen Therapy. Undersea Medical Society, Bethesda MD, pp 287-301.

45. Petrovsky BV, Tsatsanidi K, Bogomolova N et al (1987): Treatment of peritonitis caused by non-spore-forming anaerobic bacteria. In: Kindwall EP (ed.): Proceedings of the Eighth International Congress on Hyperbaric Medicine. Best Publishing, San Pedro CA, pp 100-106.

46. Rockswold GL, Ford SE, Anderson DC, Bergmann TA, Sherman RE(1992): Results of a prospective randomized trial for treatment of severely brain-injured patients with hyperbaric oxygen. J Neurosurg 76: 929-934.

47. Schliamser SE, Baeckmann K, Norrby SR (1988): Intracranial abscess in adults: an analysis of 54 consecutive cases. Scand J Infect Dis 20: 1-9.

48. Schreiner A, Tonjun S, Digranes A (1974): Hyperbaric Oxygen therapy in Bacteroides infections. Acta Chir Scand 140: 73-76.

49. Seydoux C, Francioli P (1992): Bacterial brain abscesses: factors influencing mortality and sequelae. Clin Infect Dis 15: 394-401.

50. Sharma BS, Khosla VK, Kak VK et al. (1995): Multiple pyogenic brain abscesses. Acta Neurochir 133: 36 - 43.

51. Stapleton SR, Bell BA, Uttley D (1993): Stereotactic aspiration of brain abscesses: is this the treatment of choice? Acta Neurochir 121: 15-19.

52. Stephanov S (1999): Brain abscesses from neglected open head injuries: experience with 17 cases over 20 years. Swiss Surg 5: 288 - 292.

53. Sukoff MH, Hollin SA, Espinosa OE, Jacobson II JH (1968): The protective effect of hyperbaric oxygenation in experimental cerebral edema. J Neurosurg 29: 236-241.

54. Sukoff MH, Ragatz RE (1982): Hyperbaric oxygen for the treatment of acute cerebral edema. Neurosurgery 10: 29-38.

55. Sutter B, Legat JA, Smolle-Juettner FM (1996): Brain Abscess before and after HBO. Twelfth Proceedings Sc Soc Physiol. Styria.

56. Szuwart U, Brandt M, Bennefeld H, Tewes G (1989): Hirnabszess und subdurales Empyem aus bakteriologischer Sicht. Zentralbl Chir 114: 534-544.

57. Takada Y, Ohno K, Wakimoto H, Hirakawa K (1998): Treatment of intracranial abscess in the era of neuroimaging: an analysis of 13 consecutive cases. J Med Dent Sci 45: 69 – 76.

58. Witzmann A, Beran H, Boehm-Jurkovic H et al (1989): Der Hirnabszess. Prognostische Faktoren. Dtsch Med Wochenschr 114: 85-90.

59. Yang SY (1981): Brain abscess: a review of 400 cases. J Neurosurg 55: 794-799.

60. Yang SY, Zhao CS (1993): Review of 140 patients with brain abscess. Surg Neurol 39: 290 - 296.

CHAPTER 24

# Sternal Wound Infections, Dehiscence, and Sternal Osteomyelitis: the Role of Hyperbaric Oxygen Therapy

## CHAPTER TWENTY-FOUR OVERVIEW

# Sternal Wound Infections, Dehiscence, and Sternal Osteomyelitis: the Role of Hyperbaric Oxygen Therapy

*Max F. Riddick*

## INTRODUCTION

Infections of the sternum occurring in otherwise healthy persons are extremely rare. When it occurs, depressed immune states, illicit drug usage with unclean needles, or trauma will usually be involved to establish direct or blood borne inoculation of the causative organism (4, 18). Presentation in these cases is similar in all respects to osteomyelitis elsewhere, and successful management is expected using incision, drainage, and intravenous antibiotics.

Infections of surgical sternal wounds are both more common and present greater difficulties in management. The incidence of postoperative infection is reported between 0.5 and 5% internationally and averages 1% in clean primary operations. These potentially devastating infections have been reported in all age groups, from neonatal through geriatric (11, 24, 25, 35). The sternotomy, management of infection and dehiscence, and the role of hyperbaric oxygen therapy in that management, will be the topic of this chapter.

## STERNOTOMY

According to the Society of Thoracic Surgeons, sternotomy was performed 32,730 times in the United States in 1960. By 1996, the number of procedures had increased to 222,610. The average length of stay dropped from 12.36 to 8.72 days over the same time. Worldwide, midline sternotomy is the approach of choice for access to the mediastinum and its contents.

The procedure was first proposed during the eighteenth century. However, the sternotomy for myocardial revascularization, valve replacement, or other reconstructive cardiovascular procedures was reported by Julian et al., in 1957 (14) and became popular during the 1970s.

The technique involves incising the skin, subcutaneous tissues, and periosteum in the midline, then dividing the sternum and manubrium with a power saw. Mechanical retractors are utilized to widely expose the mediastinal structures. Hemostasis is obtained by electrocautery in soft tissues, and/or by packing exposed bone with bone wax or thrombin-soaked gelfoam. In cases of myocardial revascularization, vein grafts taken from legs or arms, and/or one or both internal mammary (internal thoracic) arteries may be utilized. Circumferential wires at multiple sites are twisted to provide relatively rigid closure and fixation of sternum and manubrium. Soft tissues are sutured by layer. Skin is closed by subcuticular suture or staples (29, 40).

The advantages of this approach are multiple. Wide, relatively easy, and rapid access to the heart, great vessels, and other mediastinal structures is afforded. Once healed, the same approach may be utilized safely should access again be needed. The rigid closure allows more rapid mobilization and recovery of the patient, and is less painful than thoracotomy. The pleural cavity is rarely entered; therefore, pulmonary function is usually not affected in the long term, nor is pleural drainage commonly required. Both right and left internal thoracic (internal mammary) arteries are accessible for myocardial revascularization. Finally, this wound is expected to heal in a very high percentage (95 to 99 %) of cases, even when one or more coexisting conditions associated with dehiscence or infection is present (2).

There are real and potential disadvantages to this approach, however. Ischemia of the sternum and surrounding tissue may be induced by utilization of one or more of the internal mammary arteries. Wire fixation may fail due to breakage or cut-out. Concomitant host or technical factors may significantly increase risk of dehiscence or infection. It is a tribute to the skill of the operating surgeons, the nursing care rendered to these patients, and the overall resiliency of the human organism, that these devastating complications occur so rarely. However, when they do occur, the implications are profound.

Mortality in noninfected cases averages 5% or less, but infection may increase mortality to 15%. In addition, mortality in the first year following operation complicated by infection rises to 25% (14, 20).

Morbidity is also significantly increased. Lengths of stay average more than two and one-half times those of non-infected cases. Utilization of intensive care, intravenous antibiotics, additional surgical procedures, and readmission are also increased.

Frequently, costs to the facility and to the patient will be far in excess of reimbursement during the period of illness. Readmission because of recurrence of active infection also drives the cost for provider and recipient above the likely reimbursement.

# STERNAL WOUND INFECTION, DEHISCENCE, AND OSTEOMYELITIS

These wound complications may appear early, that is, within fourteen days of surgery and/or during the original hospitalization. Or they may present late, more than fourteen days following surgery, and generally after the patient has left the hospital. Early infections typically behave as other wound infections with fever, redness, wound breakdown or drainage, and leukocytosis. Positive culture is usually obtained from drainage, aspirate, or blood. Late infections demonstrate fewer systemic signs; pain or crepitus is common due to instability of the unhealed sternum. Minimal drainage and redness may be present (40). Definitive culture may be more difficult to obtain, as superficial skin flora may inoculate the open wound and obscure the true infectious organism(s). Deep and/or tissue culture may be required to properly identify the causative agent. Undoubtedly, a percentage of these wounds break down due to nonhealing of the ischemic, hypoxic sternum, and only become secondarily infected.

Etiologic agents cultured from sternal wounds are varied. Among aerobic species, *Staphylococcus aureus* predominates, while other *Staphylococci, Streptococci, Enterobacter, Escherichia, Klebsiella, Proteus, Serratia,* and *Pseudomonas* species have been reported in order of frequency. *Peptostreptococci, Clostridia, Bacteriodes,* and *Propionibacter* species predominate in microaerophilic or anaerobic cultures. Polymicrobial infections occur, and when present, are associated with a significantly worsened prognosis (6, 20).

Several factors are reported to increase the risk of infection or dehiscence.

Procedural factors occurring during or immediately after surgery include: less than rigid fixation, off midline sternotomy, unclosed or unfilled "dead" space, inadequate or failed drainage, length of the procedure, number of transfused units of blood or blood products, and mobilization of one or both internal mammary (internal thoracic) arteries (5, 9, 10, 16, 20, 23, 25, 31, 32, 34).

Host factors include diabetes: obesity, macromastia, previous mastectomy, radiation or burn-damaged tissue, episodes of reduced cardiac output or hypotension in the immediate postoperative period, and chronic obstructive pulmonary disease, especially when associated with postoperative coughing. Experienced surgeons have found that one of the most common causes of sternal wound disruption is chronic lung disease, especially that associated with hyperexpanded lungs. The increase in the size of the accessory muscles used in taking each breath adds to the stress on the sternal wound. Chronic and repetitive coughing increases risk of wire breakage, or cut-through of the bone by the wire fixation. There is also evidence that some of the multiple organism infections may well arise from chronically infected bronchiectatic and/or emphysematous lungs. Of all these factors, the most significant by far are diabetes, obesity, chronic obstructive pulmonary disease, and utilization of one or both internal mammary arteries. Presence of one or more of these four factors is associated with an increased risk of dehiscence and/or infection up to 5.5% (1, 5, 6, 14, 19, 20, 24, 25, 29, 32, 34).

# HISTORICAL AND CURRENT TREATMENT TECHNIQUES

Following popularization of median sternotomy for cardiac surgery, reports of infection and dehiscence began to appear in the world's literature (14).

The treatment of this significant complication has evolved through several stages. Initially, incision, debridement, and delayed or secondary closure were utilized. However, successful outcome was uncommon and associated with prolonged treatment and hospitalization. Incision, drainage, debridement, coupled with ingress-egress irrigation using antimicrobial agents, was an improvement, but failure rates were still unacceptable (12, 33, 36).

A major advance in the management of median sternotomy wound infections came with the development of myocutaneous flaps. Procedures include pectoralis major and rectus abdominus muscle flaps, myocutaneous combination flaps, and omental flaps. Treatment of choice will depend on the condition of the wound, previous surgery, and other factors. Vascularized flaps have significantly reduced both the mortality and morbidity of sternal-wound problems. However, even with this improvement, multiple operative procedures (including the final skin graft) are required (15).

Even in the best of series, mortality during the initial hospitalization for sternal infection and dehiscence averages 14%, and rises to 25% in the first year following infection (13, 20, 21, 22, 23, 26, 28, 30, 40).

## THE ROLE OF HYPERBARIC OXYGEN THERAPY IN CASES OF STERNAL WOUND INFECTION AND DEHISCENCE

The sternal wound is, by its nature, ischemic and hypoxic. Dehiscence may occur due to nonhealing, especially of the sternum. When infection is added, the host is hard pressed to mobilize defenses and mount the healing cascade necessary for successful outcome.

For wound healing to proceed to a satisfactory conclusion, salvage of marginal tissue, reversal of local hypoxia, improvement of host defenses, healing processes, and perfusion are necessary. Adequate debridement, muscle or omental coverage, and appropriate antimicrobial therapy certainly provide at least some of those needs, and must be utilized early, and at appropriately timed intervals, in the overall care of the patient with this devastating complication.

Hyperbaric oxygen therapy is a very valuable adjunct to the care of these wounds, involving several well-documented mechanisms. Marginally perfused tissue, especially at the advancing edge of necrosis or infection, may be salvaged due to the reversal of local hypoxia. Edema, a significant factor in local hypoxia, has been shown to be reduced by hemodynamic alterations, and prevented by ATP preservation, and subsequent endothelial gap closure. Leukocyte and platelet adherence to capillary walls, with resultant sludging and thrombus formation and further decreased perfusion, is reduced or prevented.

Host defense mechanisms, such as the "oxidative burst" necessary for leukocyte killing of phagocytized bacteria, fibroblastic proliferation and subsequent fibroblast elaboration of collagen precursors, and cross-linkage to form the collagen matrix necessary for neovascularization are enhanced or allowed to proceed, when local hypoxia is reversed by hyperbaric oxygen administration.

Alteration of the local wound environment, from hypoxia and acidosis, more toward normoxia and a more neutral pH is less conducive to bacterial proliferation, and certain species are inhibited, either directly, or in their toxin production, by oxygen levels reached in clinical application of hyperbaric oxygen.

The transport of certain antibiotics across the cell membrane of microorganisms is dependent on a sufficient partial pressure of oxygen, which may be reached in the infected environment only with hyperbaric oxygen therapy.

## COMPARATIVE EVALUATION OF HYPERBARIC OXYGEN THERAPY IN CASES OF STERNAL WOUND INFECTION AND DEHISCENCE

Our initial experience was reported for a group of patients studied from June 1985 to June 1987. Twenty-six patients presented at Florida Hospital, Orlando, Florida, with sternal wound breakdown and/or infection. These included both acute infections (presenting during the hospital stay), and chronic or delayed infections (presenting after the initial stay, and requiring readmission).

Members of the same surgical group operated all patients for coronary artery bypass, and technique did not vary during the time of the study. Wound care for infected cases consisted of incision and drainage, followed by formal debridement (repeated as needed), local packing until adequately granulated, then closure by secondary suture, or myocutaneous pectoralis flap, if necessary. Wound care and treatment was augmented by culture, and sensitivity determined antibiotics, with or without hyperbaric oxygen therapy.

When hyperbaric oxygen therapy was utilized, it was by monoplace chamber, at 2.0 ATA for 90 minutes twice daily for three days, then daily thereafter. A second twice-daily course was utilized following grafting in selected cases. Therapy was discontinued when the wounds were closed and stable, usually on the tenth day following final closure.

These were studied retrospectively and analyzed as follows:

### Acute Infections and Dehiscence

#### *Group 1:*

Seven patients, presenting during initial admission, who were not treated with adjunctive hyperbaric oxygen therapy.

**Age:** Ranged from 34 to 72 and averaged 63 years.

**Sex:** There were six males and one female.

**Risk factors:** Three of the seven had transfer of internal mammary arteries and one of the seven was diabetic. None had combined internal mammary transfer and diabetes.

#### *Group 2:*

Seven patients, presenting during the initial admission, who were treated with adjunctive hyperbaric oxygen therapy.

**Age:** Ranged from 59 to 76 and averaged 69 years.

**Sex**: There were six males and one female.

**Risk Factors:** Three of seven had internal mammary (internal thoracic) artery transfers and one of the seven had diabetes alone. Three of seven had both risk factors.

## Delayed Infections or Dehiscence

### Group 3:

Five patients presenting with delayed infections, not treated with adjunctive hyperbaric oxygen therapy.

**Age**: Ranged from 46 and 64 and averaged 52 years.

**Sex:** All were male.

**Risk Factors:** Two had internal mammary (internal thoracic) artery transfers and one was diabetic. None had both.

### Group 4:

Eight patients presenting with delayed infections, treated with adjunctive hyperbaric oxygen therapy.

**Age:** Ranged from 50 to 76 and averaged 62 years.

**Sex:** Seven were male and one was female.

**Risk Factors:** Three had internal mammary (internal thoracic) transfers and four were diabetic. Two had both risk factors.

Data from patients with both acute and delayed infections are summarized in Tables 1 and 2. Time from initial surgery (sternotomy) to recognized infection (S-Ri), number of days from recognized infection to the initial formal debridement (Ri-De), number of days from recognized infection to closure of the wound (Ri-Ci), number of days from recognized infection to discharge (Ri-Dc), number of operative procedures (Proc.), number of days of intravenous antibiotics (Ab-Days), total inpatient hospital days (Hosp-Days), and number of readmissions (Re-Adm) were compared between the two acute-infected groups, and the two delayed-infected groups.

Comparison of Groups 1 and 2 produced the following information: Age was not significantly different and sex was predominantly male. Risk factors were higher in the treated group. Initial surgery to recognized infection was comparable. Recognized infection to initial formal debridement was prolonged in the nontreated group, averaging 20 days, as opposed to three days in the treated group. This was apparently due to less extensive infection in the untreated group, leading to a less aggressive debridement. Recognized infection to closure was much less in the treated group, averaging 29 days as compared to 69 days in the untreated group. In addition, two of seven in the untreated group did not close during the study. (One was hospitalized 176 days, was discharged and readmitted to another hospital, treated with hyperbaric oxygen and subsequently closed, the other was not closed when lost to follow-up one year after the end of the study.)

Recognized infection to discharge was also much less in the treated group, averaging 45 days, as compared to 72 days in the untreated group. Operative procedures were the same in both groups.

Days of intravenous antibiotics were much less in the treated group, averaging 49 days, as compared to 68 days in nontreated patients.

Total days of hospitalization averaged 63 in the treated group, and 84 in the nontreated group.

No readmissions were required in the treated group, while three occurred in the untreated group.

## TABLE 1. ACUTE INFECTIONS AND DEHISCENCES

|  | GROUP 1 (n=7) NON-HBO | | GROUP 2 (n=7) HBO | |
|---|---|---|---|---|
|  | Days Av. | Days Range | Average | Range |
| S-Ri | 12 | (4-180) | 14 | (8-22) |
| Ri-De | 20 | (1-60) | 3 | (91-8) |
| Ri-Cl | 69 | (21- *) | 20 | (19-51) |
| Re-Dc | 72 | (33-176) | 45 | (930-67) |
| Proc. | 4 | (2-10) | 4 | (3-6) |
| Ab-Days | 68 | (32-186) | 49 | (0-77) |
| Hosp-days | 84 | (32-186) | 63 | (50-91) |
| Re-Adm | 3 Patients | | 0 Patients | |

## TABLE 2. DELAYED INFECTIONS AND DEHISCENCES

|  | GROUP 3 (n=5) NON-HBO | | GROUP 4 (n=8) HBO | |
|---|---|---|---|---|
|  | Days | Days Av. | Range Av. | Range |
| S-Ri | 112 | (944-210) | 61 | (14-262) |
| Ri-De | 14 | (1-42) | 4 | (1-16) |
| Ri-Cl | NA | (21- *) | 22 | (14- *) |
| Ri-Dc | 96 | (30-250) | 46 | (25-85) |
| Proc. | 3 | (3-4) | 3 | (2-5) |
| Ab-Days | 32 | (11-44) | 35 | (12-64) |
| Hosp-days | 41 | (26-48) | 44 | (30-73) |
| Re-Adm | 4 Patients | | 2 Patients | |

**KEY TO TABLES 1 and 2:**

| | |
|---|---|
| * | = Not closed during the time of the study |
| S-Ri | = Surgery to recognized infection |
| Ri-De | = Recognized infection to debridement |
| Ri-Cl | = Recognized infection to closure |
| Re-Dc | = Recognized infection to discharge |
| Proc. | = Procedures (surgical) |
| Ab-days | = Antibiotic days |
| Hosp-days | = Hospital inpatient days |
| Re-Adm | = Number of patients readmitted during the time of the study |

This comparison indicates that hyperbaric oxygen therapy used adjunctively in acute infections and dehiscences reduced hospital stay, morbidity, and usage of antibiotics, while resulting in improved outcome.

Comparison of groups 3 and 4—delayed infections and dehiscences— was more difficult. However, some differences should be noted.

Patients who were not treated with hyperbaric oxygen therapy were significantly younger, their time from initial surgery to recognized infection was more prolonged, and careful review of their records indicated less severe infection.

The risk factors were much higher in the treated group. Time to closure of the wound was less in the treated group. However, two in the untreated group, and one in the treated group, did not close during the time of the study, and are not known to have closed up to one year after the study.

Days of intravenous antibiotics were comparable, and total hospital days were slightly higher in the treated group.

Readmission for recurrence of infection, or for further procedures, was increased in the nontreated group.

In these groups, the decrease of time to closure and discharge, once the infection was recognized, and the reduction of readmission, would indicate that hyperbaric oxygen therapy was a significant and valuable adjunct in the care of these patients.

The number of patients in each of these groups was small, and care must be taken in drawing conclusions from the direct comparison of the groups. However, the trends of each group lead us to believe that until proven otherwise, hyperbaric oxygen therapy should be considered a valuable and, perhaps, indispensable adjunct in treatment of these difficult wounds.

The very large decrease in length of stay, utilization of resources, and readmissions in the groups treated with hyperbaric oxygen therapy would indicate that, especially in the patients for whom the hospital is at risk for non-cost-based reimbursement, hyperbaric oxygen therapy should be considered extremely important, if not mandatory.

We have also studied a second group of patients, presenting from 1995 though 1997. By 1995, however, in our institution, hyperbaric therapy was considered state-of-the-art treatment for patients with severe infections. As a result, we could identify only three groups.

Surgical teams, technique, and procedure were the same for all groups. Wound care was the same as the group studied in 1985. Hyperbaric therapy was administered adjunctively by multiplace chamber at 2.4 ATA, or by monoplace chamber at 2.0 ATA. Therapy sessions were ninety minutes and the same protocols were followed as in 1985.

## Group A

Eight patients presented with minor infections or dehiscences. All had wounds that were incidental to their underlying medical problems, and none required hyperbaric therapy. Six healed with only minor intervention, but one required two readmissions for persistent infection, and was subsequently treated successfully with hyperbaric oxygen therapy. One required four readmissions, and was not healed at the end of the study.

**Age**: Range from 44 to 74 and averaged 60.
**Sex:** Three males, five females.
**Risk Factors**: Seven were diabetic, seven obese, three had COPD,
and all had IMA transfer.

## Group B

Eleven patients presented with acute infections (within 14 days of
sternotomy). All were treated aggressively with antibiotics,
debridement, and secondary closure, usually by myocutaneous flap.
All received hyperbaric oxygen therapy adjunctively.
**Age:** Ranged from 44 to 72 and averaged 63.
**Sex**: Seven males, four females.
**Risk factors:** six were diabetic, three obese, three had COPD, and
eight had IMA transfers.

## Group C

Twelve patients presented with delayed infections. Their treatment
protocols were the same as GROUP B.
**Age**: Ranged from 46 to 84 and averaged 68.
**Sex**: Five males, seven females.
**Risk Factors**: Ten were diabetic, five obese, one had COPD, and ten
had IMA transfers.

Data from these groups is summarized in Tables A, B, and C.

Risk factors were very similar in all groups. By far the most significant
risk factor in all groups was diabetes and IMA transfer.

Outcomes tracked the acuteness and severity of illness. Of interest was
the fact that none of the patients treated with hyperbaric oxygen therapy
required readmission, while two of those not treated required multiple
readmissions. One healed only after treatment with hyperbaric oxygen, and
one, which was not treated, never healed during the course of the study. This
complication, occurring in 25% of those with "minimal or incidental"
infection, underscores the significant risk that even innocuous-appearing
wounds may have major implications in morbidity. We believe that sternal
wounds, especially those that do not respond promptly to traditional forms of
treatment, should be considered for hyperbaric oxygen therapy when
available.

## COST IMPLICATIONS, UTILIZATION OVERVIEW, AND QUALITY ASSURANCE

Diagnosis-related group 106, (Coronary Artery Bypass) allows a
maximum of 11.7 days of hospital stay; the nationwide average for
uncomplicated cases is 8.2 days. Under most circumstances, a modest profit
will be realized by the hospital. However, when even a minor complication
occurs, and especially when a sternal wound becomes infected, dehisces, or
requires readmission, a significant loss of revenue will occur. The cost to the
hospital of such complicated cases has been reported to be up to two and one-
half times the uncomplicated cases.

Hyperbaric oxygen is costly. However, when the total savings of
hospital days, ancillary service utilization, and further readmission is

## TABLE A. MINOR INFECTIONS OR DEHISCENCES; NO HBO GIVEN

| Initials | age | sex | diab | ob | copd | sm | IMA | S-Ri | Ri-Db | Db-Cl | Cl-Dc | ABDys | HPDys | ICUDys | PCUDys | HBODys | HBO-Cl | ReAdm | Procds |
|---|---|---|---|---|---|---|---|---|---|---|---|---|---|---|---|---|---|---|---|
| EA | 67 | M | + | - | + | — | + | 15 | 2 | 0 | 3 | 4 | 4 | 0 | 0 | 0 | 0 | 0 | 1 |
| BC | 66 | F | + | + | - | - | + | 20 | 1 | 0 | 4 | 8 | 8 | 1 | 4 | 0 | 0 | 0 | 1 |
| MB | 74 | F | + | + | - | - | + | 8 | 0 | 0 | 7 | 7 | 8 | 0 | 0 | 0 | 0 | 0 | 1 |
| MW | 44 | F | + | + | - | - | + | 26 | 4 | 5 | 13 | 21 | 21 | 11 | 3 | 0 | 0 | 0 | 2 |
| UB | 74 | F | - | + | + | - | + | 42 | 2 | not | not | 13 | 55 | 40 | 5 | 0 | 0 | 4 | 5 * |
| LA | 67 | F | + | + | - | - | + | na-rr | 5 | 13 | 13 | 27 | 27 | 24 | 0 | 0 | 0 | 2 | 2 ** |
| DB | 44 | M | + | + | + | + | + | 9 | 2 | 5 | 10 | 11 | 11 | 10 | 0 | 0 | 0 | 0 | 0 |
| CJ | 44 | M | + | + | - | - | + | 2 | none | none | 7 | 7 | 9 | 3 | 0 | 0 | 0 | 0 | 0 ‡ |
| average | 60 | 3M | 7 | 7 | 3 | 1 | 8 | 17 | 2.3 | 7.6 | 8.1 | 12.3 | 21.6 | 11.1 | 1.5 | 0 | 0 | 0.75 | 1.5 |
| mean | 59 | 5F | | | | | | 22 | 3 | 6.5 | 8 | 15.5 | 29.5 | 20 | 2.5 | 0 | 0 | 2 | 2.5 |

* Note: never closed.  **Note: readmitted for HBO.  ‡Note: closed without surgery or HBO.

## TABLE B. PATIENTS WITH ACUTE INFECTIONS; ALL GIVEN ADJUNCTIVE HBO

| Initials | age | sex | diab | ob | copd | sm | IMA | S-Ri | Ri-Db | Db-Cl | Cl-Dc | ABDys | HPDys | ICUDys | PCUDys | HBODys | HBO-Cl | ReAdm | Procds |
|---|---|---|---|---|---|---|---|---|---|---|---|---|---|---|---|---|---|---|---|
| MW | 61 | F | + | + | - | - | + | 8 | 1 | 13 | 7 | 18 | 31 | 4 | 16 | 11 | 5 | 0 | 4 |
| JMc | 72 | M | + | - | + | - | ? | 10 | 10 | 25 | 26 | 19 | 30 | 0 | 7 | 18 | 9 | 0 | 1 * |
| SS | 63 | M | + | + | - | - | + | 5 | 3 | 3 | 10 | 0 | 8 | 0 | 4 | 4 | NA | 0 | 1 ** |
| CJJ | 71 | F | ? | ? | ? | - | + | 8 | 0 | 0 | 13 | 13 | 21 | 3 | 3 | 9 | 8 | 0 | 1 |
| DB2nds | 44 | M | + | + | + | + | + | | | | 5 | 11 | 11 | 0 | 0 | 7 | 6 | 0 | 1 |
| DD | 52 | M | - | - | - | + | - | 11 | 2 | 14 | 7 | 23 | 23 | 1 | 0 | 4 | 13 | 0 | 4 |
| CT | 72 | F | - | - | - | - | + | 7 | 2 | 15 | 8 | 24 | 31 | 1 | 0 | 12 | 6 | 0 | 2 |
| FV | 67 | M | - | - | - | - | + | 11 | 2 | 13 | 8 | 23 | 23 | 3 | 20 | 17 | 11 | 0 | 2 |
| FM | 63 | M | - | - | - | - | + | 6 | 6 | 9 | 9 | 23 | 30 | 2 | 13 | 11 | 5 | 0 | 2 |
| JW | 61 | M | - | - | - | + | + | 7 | 12 | 14 | 9 | 25 | 25 | 0 | 0 | 17 | 10 | 0 | 2 |
| JC | 64 | F | 0 | - | - | - | + | 13 | 2 | 12 | 10 | 21 | 21 | 1 | 14 | 9 | 9 | 0 | 3 |
| average | 63 | 7M | 6 | 3 | 3 | 3 | 9 | 8 | 4.4 | 13 | 10.1 | 18.1 | 23.1 | 2.3 | 7.7 | 10.8 | 8.2 | 0 | 2.2 |
| mean | | 4F | | | | | | 9 | 6.5 | 14 | 15.5 | 18 | 19.5 | 5.5 | 10 | 11 | 9 | 0 | 2.5 |

* Note: Closed prior to HBO Dehisc from brkn wire. No infect.  **Note: No debride. HBO for delayed healing.

## TABLE C. PATIENTS WITH DELAYED INFECTIONS; ALL GIVEN HBO

| Initials | age | sex | diab | ob | copd | sm | IMA | S-Ri | Ri-Db | Db-Cl | Cl-Dc | ABDys | HPDys | ICUDys | PCUDys | HBODys | HBO-Cl | ReAdm | Procds |
|---|---|---|---|---|---|---|---|---|---|---|---|---|---|---|---|---|---|---|---|
| EA | 69 | F | + | + | + | - | + | 17 | 0 | 39 | 22 | 62 | 86 | 9 | 2 | 27 | 37 | 0 | 4 |
| Emc | 81 | M | - | - | - | - | ? | 16 | 0 | 15 | 24 | 20 | 20 | 5 | 16 | 19 | 10 | 0 | 2 |
| RD | 59 | M | + | - | - | + | + | 57 | 30 | 43 | 49 | 18 | 18 | 0 | 0 | 14 | 14 | 0 | 3 |
| MP | 68 | F | + | + | - | - | + | 18 | 1 | 15 | 28 | 28 | 49 | 8 | 29 | 21 | 12 | 0 | 2 |
| MG | 81 | F | + | - | - | - | - | 24m | 2 | 25 | 5 | 31 | 31 | 17 | 10 | 10 | 11 | 0 | 3 |
| HH | 46 | M | + | + | - | - | + | 17 | 1 | 43 | 9 | 52 | 52 | 0 | 0 | 45 | 12 | 0 | 3 |
| JF | 55 | F | + | + | - | - | + | 30 | 20 | same | 7 | 7 | 7 | 0 | 0 | 6 | NA | 0 | 1 |
| DP | 60 | M | + | - | - | - | + | 16 | 2 | same | 7 | 7 | 7 | 7 | 0 | 19 | 12 | 0 | 1 |
| BT | 84 | F | + | - | - | - | + | 10y | 2 | 27 | 6 | 37 | 33 | 5 | 5 | 6 | 24 | 0 | 2 * |
| EM | 82 | F | + | - | - | - | + | 20 | 1 | 12 | 27 | 17 | 12 | 0 | 0 | 30 | 9 | 0 | 3 |
| SH | 58 | F | - | + | - | - | + | 17 | 4 | 8 | 9 | 17 | 17 | 4 | 12 | 10 | 10 | 0 | 2 |
| AR | 77 | F | + | - | - | - | + | 21 | 2 | 14 | 12 | 25 | 25 | 0 | 3 | 8 | 5 | 0 | 5 |
| average | 68 | 5M | 10 | 5 | 1 | 1 | 10 | 23 | 5.4 | 20.1 | 17.1 | 26.8 | 29.8 | 4.6 | 6.4 | 17.9 | 13 | 0 | 2.5 |
| mean | | 7F | | | | | | 37 | 15.5 | 25.5 | 27.5 | 34.5 | 46.5 | 85 | 14.5 | 25.5 | 21 | 0 | 3 |

* Note: HBO dced early.

## KEY TO TABLES A, B, and C:

| | | |
|---|---|---|
| Diab | = | Diabetic |
| Ob | = | Obese |
| Copd | = | Chronic Obstructive Pulmonary Disease |
| Sm | = | Smoker |
| IMA | = | Internal Mammary Artery used to perfuse myocardium |
| S-Ri | = | Time from initial surgery to recognized infection |
| Ri-Db | = | Number of days from recognized infection to initial formal debridement |
| Db-Cl | = | Debridement to closure |
| Cl-Dc | = | Closure to discharge |
| ABDys | = | Number of days on intravenous antibiotics |
| HpDys | = | Total number of inpatient hospital days |
| ICUDys | = | Total number of days in the ICU |
| PCUdys | = | Total days in the progressive care unit |
| HBODys | = | Total number of days HBO was given |
| HBO-Cl | = | Number of days from beginning HBO to closure |
| REAdm | = | Number of patients readmitted during the time of the study |
| Procds | = | Total number of surgical procedures |

considered, savings are possible; certainly outcomes are significantly better. See Table 3.

Utilization review should be considered as in any nonhealing wound, and decisions about continuing therapy after ten treatment days must be based on the clinical factors of progress toward healing; local wound conditions, persistence of ischemia and hypoxia in the surrounding tissues, and the general health and well-being of the patient.

Quality issues must be addressed by scrupulous attention to documentation, and the determination of benefit versus risk to the patient. Careful consideration of the special needs of these patients, some of whom are extremely ill, is mandatory. It must be assured that the intensive care provided them elsewhere in the hospital is continued in the hyperbaric unit.

## Assumptions:

1. The cost of a hospital day is the average cost in Florida (Source: Florida Hospital Cost Containment Board).
2. Hospital days are average of acutely infected patients.
3. Antibiotic costs include costs of IV fluids, set-ups, and assumes four doses/day of relatively low cost drugs.
4. HBO costs should be lower in most institutions.
5. NONE of these figures represent patient charges, but are approximations of cost of the hospital to provide them.

True cost analysis and cost savings will vary from institution to institution, and will depend on multiple factors related to severity of illness and intensity services required. Most of these patients are seriously ill, and require high intensity of services. It should be noted that no hospital caring for them,

## TABLE 3. ANALYSIS OF POTENTIAL COST SAVING: NON-HBO AND HBO

| Cost Center | | | |
|---|---|---|---|
| **Length of Stay:** | Non-HBO | 84 @ $777/day | $65,268.00 |
| | HBO | 63 @ $750/day | $47,250.00 |
| | Saving | | $18,018.00 |
| **Pharmacy as** | | | |
| **Days of ABT:** | Non-HBO: | 68 @ $200/day | $13,600.00 |
| | HBO: | 49 @ $200/day | $9,800.00 |
| | Saving | | $3,800.00 |
| **HBO Unit:** | Non-HBO | 0 @ $300/day | $00.00 |
| | HBO: | 42 @ $300/day | $12,600.00 |
| | Saving | | -$12,600.00 |
| | **Total Saving per case:** | | **$9,218.00** |

with or without hyperbaric services, should expect to realize a profit under Diagnosis Related Group reimbursement. The emphasis is on loss limitation.

It is noted that most centers that perform large numbers of sternotomies do not utilize hyperbaric oxygen therapy. In addition, a recent poll of the more active Hyperbaric Therapy Centers revealed that most are rarely called on to treat a sternal wound.

The most recent comprehensive review by a major institution treating large numbers of sternal wounds (186 over eight years), without hyperbaric oxygen therapy, reported 18.8 % flap closure complication rate and 6.5% recurrence rate (14).

In view of the better outcomes we have reported, we believe hyperbaric oxygen therapy should be considered and offered in both acute and delayed presentation of sternal wound infection and dehiscence.

## SPECIAL CONSIDERATIONS WHEN USING HYPERBARIC OXYGEN THERAPY FOR STERNAL WOUND INFECTIONS

### Known Effects to HBO in Health and Disease States

Exposure to hyperbaric oxygen results in decreased heart rate (apparently through increased vagal tone), and decreased cardiac output and stroke volume in healthy volunteers. Systemic vascular resistance and blood pressure are elevated. Cardiac work is unchanged. Coronary blood flow is reduced, but the hyperoxia achieved is sufficient to overcome any potential adverse effect of this reduction (27, 38, 41).

The effect of hyperbaric oxygen exposure in patients suffering myocardial infarction produces increased mean arterial pressure, and systemic vascular resistance as expected. Heart rate may be minimally affected, usually slowing slightly. Stroke volume, cardiac output, and circulating lactate are reduced. Cardiac work is usually unchanged. During air breaks and at the end of treatment, systemic resistance rapidly returns to pretreatment levels and cardiac output increases. The effect of increasing afterload during hyperoxia is due to vasoconstriction. Following return to normoxia, there is increased preload with the concomitant need to increase cardiac output. This results in two theoretical periods during which marginal hearts could fail if they were incapable of tolerating the increased systemic vascular resistance during treatment, and/or managing the increased load with increased output following treatment (3, 7, 37). In practical experience, only in rare cases, complicated by low ejection fractions and relative fluid overload, has decompensation been reported following hyperbaric therapy.

In cardiac muscle, increased tissue oxygen levels last approximately five minutes after ending exposure to hyperbaric oxygen (17). By inference, this time may be considered as "golden" and indicates the time available to achieve reperfusion in the event of major arrhythmia, asystole, or respiratory failure during treatment. Despite this potential advantage, patients who suffer cardiorespiratory events while in the hyperbaric unit should be treated as they would elsewhere in the institution, with BCLS and/or ACLS protocols.

In sepsis, hyperbaric oxygen has been shown to increase cardiac output and decrease pulmonary vascular resistance, both during and after treatment. During exposure, stroke volume and mean arterial pressure increase, while pulmonary wedge pressure decreases. These revert to pretreatment levels rapidly following return to air or ambient pressure respiration. In contrast to the nonseptic patient, heart rate and systemic vascular resistance may not change with hyperbaric oxygen exposure (8).

## HBO Effects on Common Cardioactive and Vasoactive Drugs and Therapies

Oxygen itself is a potent cardioactive and vasoactive drug. Reduction of hypoxia is known to suppress arrhythmias, by reduction of the irritability of hypoxic loci. Under hyperoxic conditions, heart rate is reduced (due to vagal tone effect), and cardiac output is reduced. There is intense systemic and pulmonary vasoconstriction, both venous and arterial, in nonischemic tissue. Finally, there are significant changes in afterload and preload, depending on the stage of exposure to oxygen (3, 7, 37, 39).

Hyperoxia is known to increase the effect of Angiotensin I and II. In theory, it may also effect the actions of other vasoactive and cardioactive drugs synergistically or antagonistically, although this has not proved to be a problem clinically. The effect of drugs commonly utilized in Advanced Cardiac Life Support have not been shown experimentally or clinically to be altered by hyperbaric hyperoxia. This includes the cardiotropic and/or vasoactive effect of epinephrine, the arrhythmia blocking effect of lidocaine, procainamide, and bretylium, the parasympathetic blocking effect of atropine, and the varied effects of dopamine in low (1-2 mic./kg/min), medium (2-10 mic./kg/min), or high (>10 mic./kg/min) dosages. The antihypertensive effects of nifedipine (Procardia®), sodium nitroprusside (Nipride®), and reserpine are also not altered by oxygen administered at up to three atmospheres. Furosemide (Lasix®) and digitalis preparations have been utilized without obvious alteration of effect in our center at Florida Hospital.

Cardioversion and defibrillation may be performed in the multiplace chamber, provided proper passthrough and electrodes are available so that spark and fire risk can be addressed. These modalities are incompatible with the oxygen atmosphere of monoplace chambers; patients must be decompressed and removed from the chamber before instituting synchronized cardioversion or defibrillating countershock.

Internal cardiac pacemakers are unaffected by the hyperbaric environment. However, existing commercial external pacers are not compatible with increased pressure. External pacing has been established in the chamber by connecting the external leads to a hermetically-sealed internal pacer (19).

## Pre-Treatment Evaluation of the Sternal Wound: Infected, Dehisced, or At Risk

Review of the following information may be helpful in determining the need for, possible benefit of, and risks of hyperbaric oxygen therapy in these critically ill, frequently unstable patients.

1. Presence of known risk factors, as outlined earlier.
2. Preoperative evaluations including cardiac catheterization, echo, ECG, rhythm monitoring and pulmonary function studies with special attention to:

      a. Ejection Fraction: Values of less than 40% should be approached with extra concern and care. Values of 30% or less may be considered a relative contraindication to hyperbaric therapy, especially when fluid overload is present.

      b. Pulmonary Function: Values indicative of chronic obstructive pulmonary disease indicating that a low oxygen level is the stimulus to breathe.

  3. Operative Report

      a. Vessels or valves involved.

      b. Whether a pulmonary cavity was entered.

      c. Placement and type of drains.

      d. Whether one or both mammary arteries were utilized.

      e. Difficulties during bypass or when going off the pump, and whether cardiac assist device was required.

      f. Method and success of hemostasis.

      g. Technique of closure.

These may be important in recognizing risk factors that indicate the etiology of the failed wound. Some may also be important in avoidance of complications during therapy.

  4. Post-operative Course

      a. Periods of hypoxia or hypotension.

      b. Significant blood loss and replacement.

      c. Prolonged and/or forceful coughing.

      d. Cardiac-assist device required.

      e. Cardioactive or vasoactive drugs required.

      f. Re-operation required.

      g. Length of time before sternal wound problem became apparent.

      h. Nature of any interventions that have been done since the wound problem became apparent.

      i. Nutritional assessment and maintenance.

Once again, this information may be valuable in determining whether to offer hyperbaric therapy, and what possible difficulties may be encountered in administering it.

## Sternal Wound Pre-Treatment Patient Evaluation

These patients may be quite ill, on multiple medications, have various invasive lines in place, and be under continuous hemodynamic and electrical monitoring. The pretreatment evaluation should be by a checklist and should include at least the following:

  1. Current monitoring devices, their requirements for continued monitoring during therapy, and their recent accuracy and condition.

  2. Current and recent monitored ECG, rhythm, Swan-Ganz, and/or arterial gas values should be reviewed. Of particular importance are systemic and pulmonary artery pressures and the presence of arrhythmias.

  3. Presence of drains, their condition, what space they are draining, and the volume of drainage during the proceeding time period.

  4. Number, nature, and condition of invasive lines, including arterial

and intravenous lines. Nature and volume of planned intravenous fluid, and/or feeding needed during therapy.

5. Current respiratory status, including current arterial blood gas levels, if appropriate. The need for respiratory support, including presence or need for endotrachial or tracheostomy intubation should be noted. The type of respiratory support necessary may likewise be crucial to the patient's maintenance of adequate exchange.

6. Review and listing of all current drugs, their dosage, route, rate, and time of administration. Special attention must be paid to inotropic, chronotropic, and arrhythmia-suppressive cardiac drugs. Pressor agents, dopamine and dobutamine (Dobutrex®) in particular, must also be given extra attention.

7. Intake and output during the preceding twenty-four hours, and any "carry over" positive fluid balance.

8. Most recent (and certainly within 24 hours) electrolyte and acid/base balance evaluation. While normal range values of all are important, potassium abnormalities are of such concern that postponement of treatment must be considered.

9. If diabetic, glucose levels before and, as necessary, during treatment should be determined and adjusted. In the diabetic, blood glucose levels decrease markedly during HBO treatment.

10. Assessment of anxiety, level of consciousness, and pain control.

11. Special positioning requirements and/or comfort requirements.

12. Current status of wound, evaluation, and wound management, if appropriate.

## Sternal Wound Equipment

The hyperbaric unit should be equipped to provide the same level of care as the floor or I.C.U. from which the patient arrives. Please refer to the chapter by Weaver entitled "Management of Critically Ill Patients" for specifics of the required equipment for critical care in the monoplace chamber.

## Personnel Skill Level

Our experience is that the expertise of both registered nurses and respiratory therapists is needed in caring for the more seriously-ill patients. They should be trained and experienced at the critical-care level, as well as in hyperbaric therapy.

## Sternal Wound Patient Care: a Philosophical Approach

While many of these patients will not present any greater difficulty in treatment than other patients with problem wounds, several significant exceptions may apply.

Medication administration and timing is much more critical in this patient population. Continuous monitoring and rapid response to changes in hemodynamics, rhythm, and respiratory status is mandatory.

Information exchange with the caregiver in the setting from which the patient is coming, and to which they may be going, must be clear and in keeping with the standard utilized to transfer a patient within the institution from unit to unit. In most facilities, a critical-care provider or provider team will accompany the very sick patients to the hyperbaric unit and give an oral report, as well as the patient's record to the receiving team. In turn, when the patient is sent back to the unit from which he or she came, the hyperbaric unit team will give an oral summary report to the team, as well as the record covering the time the patient was in the hyperbaric unit.

Preferably, the hyperbaric unit providing care for these patients should be located in relative proximity, and within easy access to the units where these patients are currently receiving care. Hyperbaric oxygen therapy of seriously-ill patients should not be attempted in isolated or outpatient centers and only in the presence of, or immediate availability of medical and support personnel who are capable of responding to sudden deterioration of the patient's condition.

Finally, it is essential to foster and nurture the team concept in the unit providing care for these patients. A competent, secure, and well-trained team that truly enjoys their work will find caring for these demanding patients challenging and fulfilling. Every effort should be made administratively to develop and maintain such teams in units that will offer care to the sternal wound patient.

## PRACTICAL POINTS IN AVOIDING POTENTIAL PITFALLS

1. In a small subset of patients who have low ejection fractions ($<40$) and who have become fluid overloaded, rapid development of pulmonary edema and/or right heart failure has been observed. This usually occurs within 45 minutes of the end of treatment. This complication may be avoided by careful pretreatment evaluation.

2. Special attention should be paid to drains of the pericardium. Should anything interfere with this drainage, signs of cardiac tamponade will develop, and may be initially overlooked or mistaken for other cardiac problems.

3. In patients whose mean arterial pressure is being maintained by dopamine or Dobutrex® drips, interruption of these drips, even for the short time that some pumps maybe inoperative during compression, may result in significant alterations of blood pressure. Care must be taken to assure continued administration of these agents in the face of changes in pressure.

4. Remember that standard respirators available for HBO use may not be able to maintain adequate respiratory exchange in all patients; one must be prepared to alter respirators or abort treatment in those patients whose exchange cannot be maintained adequately.

## CONCLUSION

Hyperbaric oxygen therapy should be effective for the conditions associated with the infected, failing, or failed sternal wound. Extensive practical experience has confirmed its safety and benefit. As a result, its utilization may be expected to produce savings in time, money, morbidity, and mortality when used as an adjunct to well-planned and executed treatment plans for this very serious complication of cardiac surgery. There are real and potential problems in caring for those patients who are unstable; but with adequate equipment, training, and support, these may be minimized, and the modality can be offered with a very acceptable risk/benefit ratio.

At the present time, adjunctive hyperbaric oxygen therapy is recommended for all patients with acute and delayed sternal wound breakdowns and/or infections at Florida Hospital Medical Center, unless their condition is such that the risk of treatment outweighs the potential benefits of the therapy.

## ACKNOWLEDGMENTS

I wish to give special thanks to Kerry Swartz, M.D. (Cardiology), Meredith Scott, M.D. (Cardiovascular Surgery), Barry Boyd, M.D. (Plastic Surgery), and Mark Walters, CHT., (Wound Care and HBO Unit Manager) for their invaluable insight, advice, experience, and review of the portions of this chapter covering their areas of expertise. In addition, the support and assistance of the physicians and staff of the Wound Care and Hyperbaric Medicine Unit of Florida Hospital, Orlando, Florida is deeply appreciated.

## REFERENCES

1. Arnold P and Pairolero P. "Surgical management of the radiated chest wall." Plastic and Reconstructive Surgery. 1986;77:605-612.

2. Arnold M. "The surgical anatomy of sternal blood supply." Journal of Thoracic and Cardiov Surg. 1972;64:415-426.

3. Ashfield R, Gavey C. "Severe acute myocardial infarction treated with hyperbaric oxygen, a report on forty patients." Postgrad Med Journ. 1969;45:648-654.

4. Boll K and Jurik A. "Sternal osteomyelitis in drug addicts." J of Bone and Joint Surg. 1990;72B, No. 2:328-329.

5. Bray P, Mahoney J, Anastakis D, and Yao J. ìSternotomy infections: sternal salvage and the importance of sternal stability.î Canadian Journal of Surgery. 1996;39:297-301.

6. Breyer R, Mill S, Hudspeth A, Johnson F, Cordell A. "A prospective study of sternal wound complications." Annals of Thor Surg. 1984;37:412-416.

7. Brook I. "Microbiology of the post-thoracotomy sternal wound infection" J of Clin Microbiol. 1989;27:806-807.

8. Cameron A, Hutton I, Kenmure A, Murdoch W. "Haemodynamic and metabolic effects of hyperbaric oxygen in myocardial infarction" Lancet. 1966;2:833-837.

9. Deepika K, Myers R, Crowley R. "Cardiovascular effects of hyperbaric oxygen in septic patients." Undersea Biomed Res 9. (1-Supplement). 1982;167.

10. Grossi E, Culliford A, Krieger K, Kloth D, Press R, Baumann F, Spencer F. "A survey of 77 major infectious complications of median sternotomy. A review of 7,949 consecutive operative procedures." Annals of Thoracic Surgery. 1985;40:214-223.

11. Grmoljez P, Barner H. "Bilateral internal mammary artery mobilization and sternal healing." Angiology. 1978;9:272-274.

12. Gualt D, Huddleston C, Jones B. "Infected sternotomy wounds." Europ J Cardio-Thorac Surg. 1990;4:48-50.

13. Jeevanandam V, Smith C, Rose E, Malm J, Hugo N. "Single-stage management of sternal wound infections." J Thorac and Cardiovasc Surg. 1990;99:256-263.

14. Jones G, Jurkiewicz M, et al. ìManagement of the infected median sternotomy wound with muscle flaps.î Annals of Surgery. 1997;225:766-778.

15. Josa M, Khuri S, Braunwask N, VanCisin M, Spencer M, Evans D, Barsamian E. "Delayed sternal closure." J of Thorac and Cardiovasc Surg. 1986;91:598-603.

16. Julian O, Lopez-Belio M, Dye W, Javid H, Grove W. "The median sternal incision in intracardiac surgery with extracorporean circulation, a general evaluation of its use in heart surgery." Surgery. 1953;42:753-761.

17. Jurkiewicz M, Bostwick J, Hester R, et al. "Infected median sternotomy wounds: Success of treatment by muscle flaps." Annals of Surg. 1980;191:738-744.

18. Kalush S, Cherukuri R, Teller P, Watson C, Murphey B, Shaheen S. "Bilateral mammary artery bypass and sternal dehiscence: A favorable outcome." Am Surgeon. 1990;2:487-493.

19. Kawamura M, Kinsaku S, Bunsaku S, Hitoshi K, Shigeo K, Shinichiro K, Yutaka O. "Protective effect of hyperbaric oxygen for temporary ischaemic myocardium. Macroscopic and histologic data." Cardiovasc Res. 1976;10:599-604.

20. Kelly C and Chetty M. "Primary sternal osteomyelitis." Thorax. 1985;40:872-873.

21. Kratz J, Blackburn J, Leman R, Crawford F. "Cardiac pacing under hyperbaric conditions." Am Thorac Surg. 1983;36:66-68.

22. Loop F, Bruce W, Cosgrove D, Mahfood S, McHenry M, Goormastic M, Steward R, Golding L, Taylor P. "Sternal wound complications after isolated coronary bypass grafting: Early and late mortality, morbidity, and cost of care." Annals of Thorac Surg. 1990;49:179-189.

23. Lovich S, Iverson L, Young J, Ennix C, Harrell J, Echer R, Lau G, Joseph P, May I. "Omental pedical grafting in the treatment of postcardiotomy sternotomy infections." Arch of Surg. 1988;124;1192-1194.

24. Martin R. "The management of infected median sternotomy wounds." Annals of Plast Surg. 1989;22;243-251.

25. Miller J and Nahai F. "Repair of the dehisced median sternotomy incision." Surg Clinics of N Am. 1989;69:1091-1102.

26. McDonald W, Brame M, Sharp C, Eggerstedt J. "Risk factors for median sternotomy dehiscence in cardiac surgery." So Med J. 1989;82;1361-1364.

27. Ottino G, DePaulis R, Pansini S, Rocca G, Tallone M, Comoglio C, Costa P, Orzan F, Morea M. "Major sternal wound infection after open heart surgery: A multivariant analysis of risk factors in 2,579 consecutive operative procedures." Annals of Thoracic Surgery." 1987;44:173-179.

28. Pairolero P and Arnold P. "Management of recalcitrant median sternotomy wounds." J Thorac and Cardiovasc Surg. 1989;88:357-364.

29. Pizarello J, Clark J, Lambertsen C, and Gelfand R. "Human circulatory responses to prolonged hyperbaric hyperoxia in predictive studies V." In: Proc. of the 9th Int. Symp. on Underwater and Hyperbaric Physiology. A.A. Bove, A.J. Bachrach and L.J. Greenbaum, Jr., (Eds.) Bethesda MD, Undersea and Hyperbaric Medicine Society, 1987; pp. 763-772.

30. Prevosti L, Subramainian V, Rothaus K, Dineen P. "A comparison of open and closed methods in the initial treatment of sternal wound infections." J of Cardiovasc Surg. 1990;30:757-763i.

31. Scott M. Personal communication. 1991.

32. Scully H, Leclerc Y, Martin R, Tong C, Goldman B, Weisel R, Mickelborough L, Baird R. "Comparison between antibiotic irrigation and mobilization of pectoral muscle flaps in treatment of deep sternal infections." J of Thorac and Cardiovasc Surg. 1985;90:523-531.

33. Seyfer A, Shriver C, Miller T, Graeber G. "Sternal blood flow after median sternotomy and mobilization of internal mammary arteries." Surg. 1988;104:899-904.

34. Shafir R, Weiss J, Herman O, Cohen N, Stern D, Igra Y. "Faulty sternotomy and complications after median sternotomy." J of Thorac and Cardiovasc Surg. 1988;96;310-313.

35. Shumacher H, Mandelbaum I. "Continuous antibiotic irrigation in the treatment of infection." Archives of Surg. 1963;86:384.

36. Stradtman J and Ballenger M. "Nursing implications in sternal and mediastinal infections after open heart surgery." Focus on Crit Care. 1989;16:178-183.

37. Terranova W and Crawford F. "Treatment of median sternotomy wound infection and sternal necrosis in an infant." J of Thorac Surg. 1989;48:122-123.

38. Thurer R, Bognolo D, Vargas A, et al. "The management of mediastinal infection following cardiac surgery: An experience utilizing continuous irrigation with povidine-iodine." J of Thorac Surg. 1989;68:962-968.

39. Thurston J, Greenwood T, Bending M, Conner H and Curwen MP. "A controlled investigation into the effects of hyperbaric oxygen on mortality following myocardial infarction." The Quarterly Journal of Medicine. 1973;(42)168:751-770.

40. Villanucci S, DiMarzio G, School M, Priovine C, d'Adamo C, Settimi F. "Cardiovascular changes induced by hyperbaric oxygen therapy." Proc of the Europ Undersea Biomed Soc. Amsterdam, 1990;247.

41. Visona A, Lusiani L, Rusca F, Barbiero D, Ursini F, Antonio P. "Therapeutic, hemodynamic, and metabolic effects of hyperbaric oxygenation in peripheral vascular disease." Angiology. 1988;40:994-1000.

42. Weber L and Peters R. "Delayed chest wall complications of median sternotomy." So Med J. 1986;79:723-727.

43. Williams B, Roding B, Winters P, Worthington G. "Hyperbaric oxygenation, influence on coronary blood flow and oxygen delivery to the myocardium." Archives of Surg. 1969;758-763.

# THE ROLE OF HYPERBARIC OXYGEN IN THE MANAGEMENT OF CHRONIC REFRACTORY OSTEOMYELITIS

## CHAPTER TWENTY-FIVE OVERVIEW

# THE ROLE OF HYPERBARIC OXYGEN IN THE MANAGEMENT OF CHRONIC REFRACTORY OSTEOMYELITIS

*Michael B. Strauss, Stuart S. Miller*

## INTRODUCTION

Chronic refractory osteomyelitis (CROM) is an infection of bone that involves both its cortical and medullary components which has persisted or recurred after appropriate management (Figure 1). With this fundamental definition, three presentations of chronic refractory osteomyelitis in the appendicular skeleton become apparent: 1) CROM in the compromised host, 2) CROM associated with a non-healing fracture, that is to say, the septic non-union and 3) CROM of the diffuse sclerosing type. Since hyperbaric oxygen (HBO) was first used as an adjunct for the management of chronic refractory

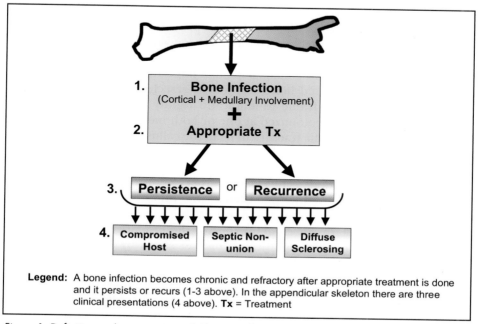

Legend: A bone infection becomes chronic and refractory after appropriate treatment is done and it persists or recurs (1-3 above). In the appendicular skeleton there are three clinical presentations (4 above). **Tx** = Treatment

*Figure 1. Definition and presentations of Chronic Refractory Osteomyelitis.*

*The contemporary use of hyperbaric oxygen for chronic refractory osteomyelitis is paradoxical. Only rarely, in contrast to the past, is hyperbaric oxygen used for this problem in long bones. However, hyperbaric oxygen now is used more than ever because of refractory bone infections in the feet. Especially in the diabetic, compromised host group.*

osteomyelits, its utilization and role has changed dramatically. Contemporary utilization of HBO for chronic refractory osteomyelitis is much different than when its benefits were first reported over 40 years ago (1, 2). The reasons are twofold: First, initially the benefits of HBO were largely thought to be due to the direct effects of HBO on the micro-organisms causing the infection; today the benefits are ascribed to its effect on host factors such as angiogenesis and neutrophil oxidative killing. Second, whereas in the past HBO was used almost exclusively for the long bones of the extremities and the jaw, today the majority of the use of HBO for chronic refractory osteomyelitis is in the small bones of the foot in patients, especially diabetics, with compromised host factors.

Since the indications for HBO were delineated by the Undersea [and Hyperbaric] Medical Society in 1977, chronic refractory osteomyelitis has been an approved use for this modality. Regardless of the change in focus, as described above, chronic refractory osteomyelitis remains an important indication for HBO. The reason HBO is rarely used for chronic refractory osteomyelitis of the long bones of the appendicular skeleton is threefold: First the incidence of this problem has decreased due to improved open fracture management, use of organism specific antibiotics, performing primary amputations for mangled extremities and staging dead space management of exposed and/or infected bone with use of antibiotic-laden bone cement. Second, the use of microvascular free flaps to provide both early coverage and augmented perfusion to the fracture site has been very effective in converting open fractures to "closed" types (3, 4, 5). Third, the Illizarov technique has added a new dimension to the management of infected, un-united fractures. In this technique, the diseased bone segment is resected after placement of a special external fixation frame to align and rigidly stabilize the extremity. Next, healthy bone is osteotomized at one or both metaphyseal levels. Rather than allowing the iatrogenic fracture to heal, the callus forming at the fracture site(s) is stretched out until the bone is lengthened enough to obliterate the segment that was resected.

As effective as these techniques are, there are predictable complication rates including non-union, persistence of infection and lower limb amputation. The complications are due to tissue hypoxia at the injury site, compromised host status or combinations of these. Mader and Cierney get credit for appreciating the significance of host status by incorporating this

*Hyperbaric oxygen (as well as other management interventions) is not always indicated for patients with chronic refractory osteomyelitis. In fact, major limb amputation or minimal interventions may be the better choices for some patients.*

important consideration in their classification of osteomyelitis (Table 1) (6). Not only does this classification consider the host-function, but by doing so it provides guidelines for when hyperbaric oxygen should be considered in the management, as will be further discussed in the management section (7, 8). We have generated a more contemporary approach to quantifying host-function by using a 0-to10 scoring system, with ten being best, based on five assessments each graded from 2 (best)-to-0 (worst) (Table 2). Judgment is required for making management decisions for patients with CROM. Hyperbaric oxygen and surgery may not always be the best decision when the severity of the problem and the patient's functional status are considered. The mating of the host score with the different presentations of chronic refractory osteomyelitis aid in deciding whether to recommend salvage of the limb, major limb amputation or the withholding of treatment interventions for the patient (Figure 2).

## PATHOPHYSIOLOGY

The factor that makes chronic refractory osteomyelitis difficult to eradicate is the impaired vascularity at the site of infection (9, 10). The

## TABLE 1. THE CIERNEY AND MADER STAGING SYSTEM OF OSTEOMYELITIS

**Anatomic Type**

Stage 1 – Medullary osteomyelitis

Stage 2 – Superficial [infected bone surface] osteomyelitis

Stage 3 – Localized [infected sequestrum] osteomyelitis

Stage 4– Diffuse [sclerosis] osteomyelitis

**Physiological Class**

A Host -   Normal host

B Host -   Systemic compromise ($B_S$)

Local  compromise ($B_L$)

Systemic & local compromise ($B_{SL}$)

C Host -   Treatment worse than the disease

**Systemic or local factors that affect immune surveillance, metabolism and local vascularity**

| Systemic ($B_S$) | Local ($B_L$) |
|---|---|
| Diabetes mellitus | Major vessel compromise |
| Renal, hepatic failure | Small and medium vessel disease |
| Malnutrition | Extensive scarring |
| Chronic hypoxia | Arteritis |
| Immunosuppression | Radiation fibrosis |
| Malignancy | Chronic lymphedema |
| Immune deficiency | Venous stasis |
| Extremes of age | Neuropathy |
| Tobacco abuse [2 packs per day] | |

## TABLE 2. QUANTIFYING HOST FUNCTION

| Assessment | 2- Points | 1 Point | 0-Points |
|---|---|---|---|
| | Use half points if mixed or intermediate between 2 grades | | |
| Age | < 40 | 40-60 | >60 |
| Ambulation | Community | Household | None |
| | Subtract ½ point if aids are used | | |
| CV/Renal (Which ever gives the lower score) | Normal | Impaired | Decompensated |
| Smoke/Steroid (Which ever gives the lower score) | None | Past | Current |
| Neurological Deficits | None | Some | Severe |

**Interpretation:** 8-10 points = Healthy host
4-7 points = Impaired host
0-3 points = Decompensated host

*Impaired blood supply to the site of infection is the factor that makes osteomyelitis refractory.*

consequences are threefold: 1) hypoxia, 2) development of an impermeable, avascular barrier between intact, healthy tissues and the focus of infection in the bone (i.e. the interface) and 3) necrotic bone (Figure 3). These interfere with the body's responses for dealing with the infection as well the delivery of antibiotics to the septic focus. Causes of hypoxia are usually a combination of systemic and local factors impairing perfusion.

The majority of factors Cierney and Mader consider in the compromised host group (B Host) are conditions, both systemic and local, that interfere with blood supply to the infection site (6, 11, 12). Without adequate blood supply, the environment around the infection site becomes hypoxic. This thwarts the host's responses for dealing with infection such as neutrophil oxidative killing of bacteria and angiogenesis as needed to deliver white blood cells, antibodies, and substrates (13).

Oxygen tensions in the tissue fluids need to be in the 30 to 40 mmHg range in order for neutrophils to generative superoxides and peroxides during the oxidative burst required for bacteria killing and for fibroblasts to

*Neutrophils lose their ability to kill bacteria by oxidative mechanisms when juxta-infection tissue fluid oxygen tensions fall below 30 mmHg to 40 mmHg.*

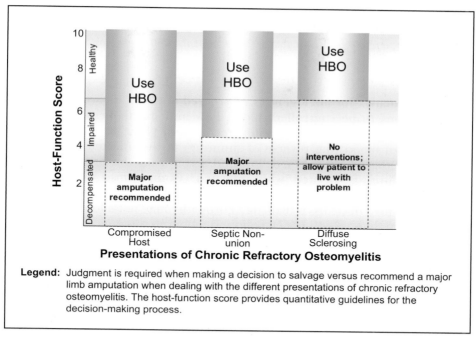

Legend: Judgment is required when making a decision to salvage versus recommend a major limb amputation when dealing with the different presentations of chronic refractory osteomyelitis. The host-function score provides quantitative guidelines for the decision-making process.

Figure 2. Host-function as a criterion in deciding whether to use hyperbaric oxygen for the different presentations of Chronic Refractory Osteomyelitis.

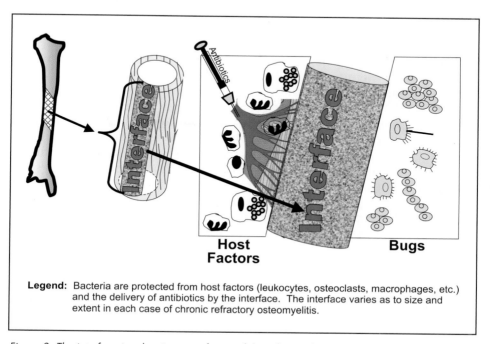

Legend: Bacteria are protected from host factors (leukocytes, osteoclasts, macrophages, etc.) and the delivery of antibiotics by the interface. The interface varies as to size and extent in each case of chronic refractory osteomyelitis.

Figure 3. The interface is a barrier to perfusion of the infection focus and a major consideration in osteomyelitis becoming refractory.

*The interface compounds the hypoxia problem at the infection focus and further protects the microorganisms causing the bone infection from host factors and antibiotics.*

elaborate a matrix for angiogenesis to proceed (14-16). For wounds to heal and infections to be controlled, blood flow and metabolic activity at the infection site must increase an estimated 20-fold (17). Vasodilatation and channeling of blood (the reverse of shunting) to the infected area are the mechanisms that increase blood flow and account for the rubor, calor and tumor (swelling) associated with infection. Compromise of an already impaired circulation at the infection site because of calcified vessels and auto sympathectomy effects from diabetic neuropathy may not allow perfusion to increase enough to meet the metabolic and mobilizations demands needed to manage the infection. Diabetes mellitus is probably the leading co-morbidity associated with this latter cause of refractory osteomyelitis and one for which hyperbaric oxygen is often used as a management adjunct. Another cause of hypoxia at the infection site is the premature thickening of the capillary basement membrane, a frequent consequence of diabetes (18). The thickened basement membrane becomes a diffusion barrier for oxygen from the capillary to the tissue fluids. A hypoxic environment also renders some antibiotics such as aminoglycosides and amphotericin ineffective since they require active transport by bacteria, an oxygen dependent process, across their cell walls (19).

The significance of the interface cannot be overemphasized. The interface is the body's response to the inflammatory reaction infected bone initiates. The response begins with edema, continues with leukocyte and fibroblast infiltration and ends with the formation of scar tissue. Each stage compounds the hypoxia problem mentioned above. Other items that may be associated with the interface include, dead bone (sequestra), cartilage, fluid collections including pus, and foreign materials such as bone cement, shrapnel and orthopaedic hardware. Edema increases the diffusion distance that oxygen molecules must traverse through tissue fluids from capillaries to target cells. It decreases by the square root of the oxygen tension of the tissue fluid adjacent to the capillary and is only 1/20th as great as the diffusion ability of carbon dioxide through tissue fluids (20, 21). The mobilization stage of leukocytes has the potential to resolve the infection. However, if the environment is hypoxic (as discussed above), these cells fail to function properly and may act as a relative barrier through abscess formation. In the presence of hypoxia, metaplasia of tissues generate fibrotic material and cicatrix. This makes the interface essentially an impermeable barrier. From one perspective the interface serves the purpose of isolating chronically infected bone from adjacent healthy tissues. From another it is counter

*The interface, as a host response, is paradoxical. It keeps the infected focus from extending to healthy host tissues. Conversely, it acts as a barrier for leukocytes, other host factors and antibiotics to get to the site of infection.*

productive, because it prevents host responses and antibiotics from getting to the site and resolving the infection. Necrotic bone is the third pathophysiological feature of refractory osteomyelitis and it too is a consequence of impaired vascularity. Necrotic bone, by definition, is avascular. When small in amount and not infected, the body can deal with it effectively by remodeling. The remodeling process is a normal, on-going physiological function of bone. Osteoclasts remodel, create vascular ingress channels and remove dead bone while osteoblasts lay down new bone. Osteoclasts are about 100 times more active than osteoblasts (22). This differential in activity explains why stress fractures occur. Bone resorption as a response to stress and a precursor to ultimate strengthening of the bone occurs 100 times faster than the formation of new bone. Another corollary of the intensified metabolic activity of osteoclasts is its oxygen requirements. In the hypoxic environment the osteoclast stops functioning. Remodeling and removal of dead bone is halted. When bone is infected, as well as dead, and the environment around the osteoclast is hypoxic, this host "debridement" mechanism ceases to function. The consequence is refractory osteomyelitis.

There are several reasons bone loses its vascularity and becomes necrotic. Traumatic disruption of blood vessels associated with fractures and crush injuries is an obvious cause (See Chapter on Traumatic Ischemias in this text). Both non-traumatic intrinsic and extrinsic causes lead to avascularity of bone. When edema, confirmed by magnetic resonance imaging, occurs in bone, it may increase the intra-osseous pressure. If the tensions are higher than the capillary perfusion pressure, the bone is rendered avascular. This mechanism is analogous to the pathophysiology of the skeletal muscle-compartment syndrome. External pressure from pus and edema formation in tightly compacted areas such as tissues adjacent to joint capsules, neurovascular compartments and tendon sheaths may also exceed the capillary filling pressure and render more distal tissues ischemic. This problem is likely to be compounded by flow that is already impeded by peripheral artery disease, hypoxia secondary to impaired oxygen diffusion through thickened capillary basement membranes and anatomical considerations where perfusion to the target tissue is an end artery or single bone perforating vessel. This latter consideration is undoubtedly the cause of refractory osteomyelitis of distal tufts of toes and metatarsal heads as so often seen in diabetic feet with sepsis adjacent to these areas.

## JUSTIFICATION FOR HYPERBARIC OXYGEN: LAB AND ANIMAL STUDIES

There have been many in vitro and in vivo studies, which have been designed to quantify and define the value of HBO in refractory osteomyelitis. The oxygen tension in osteomyelitic bone is low, rarely exceeding 25 mmHg of oxygen (10). Using animal models, Hunt et al., Kivisaari et al., and Mader et al., have shown that the oxygen tension in normal, as well as infected, tissue is increased with HBO (14, 23, 24). Values ranging from 30 mmHg to as high as 1200 mmHg have been measured in infected tissue under HBO conditions. Esterhai, et al. compared the infected tibia of a rabbit to an uninfected tibia in the same animal and demonstrated the ability of HBO to elevate the oxygen tension in osteomyelitic bone (25). Under ambient conditions, the oxygen tension in the uninfected tibia was 32 mmHg, while the oxygen tension in the infected tibia was only 17 mmHg. By treating the rabbit with 100% oxygen at two atmospheres absolute (ATA), the oxygen tension in both tibias rose to over 190 mmHg. In the Mader, et al. studies, a standard rabbit model, with diffuse *Staphylococcus aureus* osteomyelitis of the tibia was used. The animals were treated at two ATA with 100% oxygen for 2 hours daily, five times per week, for a total of 20 treatments. With the assistance of a mass spectrometer, oxygen tensions were measured in normal and infected tibias, before and during HBO treatment. It was shown that HBO increased the oxygen tensions in both the normal and osteomyelitic bone (24, 26). Under ambient conditions, the oxygen tension in the osteomyelitic bone was 23 mmHg, while in normal bone the oxygen tension was 45 mmHg. HBO increased the oxygen tension to 104 mmHg in osteomyelitic bone and 322 mmHg in normal bone. In both the Esterhai and Mader studies, the low tensions in infected bone are probably secondary to hypoperfusion and inflammation. Hypoperfusion is the direct effect of increased intramedullary pressure in the bone. Increased pressure results when purulent material and other debris fill the Haversian system and medullary canal (27).

The body's first cellular defense mechanism is the polymorphonuclear leukocyte (PMN). The PMN is primarily responsible for fighting bacterial infections. Mandell's work showed that phagocytic killing of aerobes is diminished under low oxygen tensions (28). Since a majority of aerobic organisms can also function as facultative anaerobes, hypoxic tissue is especially at risk for infection. Using a *Staphylococcus aureus* model, Mader showed a proportional relationship between oxygen tensions and phagocytic killing ability (24). At the oxygen tension found in osteomyelitic bone, 23 mmHg, there was a reduced capacity of phagocytes to kill bacteria, as compared to their bactericidal ability at normal bone oxygen tensions of 45 mmHg. Increasing the oxygen tension to 109 mmHg, the oxygen tension found in osteomyelitic bone under HBO conditions, further augmented the ability of the phagocytes to kill bacteria. Mader also showed that increasing the oxygen tension to 150 mmHg generated killing of the greatest number of *S. aureus* (24). Using normal bone oxygen tensions of 45 mmHg as a baseline, it has been shown that HBO produces increased killing by the PMN's, over ambient oxygen conditions. Hamblen also found that HBO did not reduce the initial infection rate of experimentally introduced osteomyelitis in the rabbit tibia model, however, it caused a significant increase in the healing of the established infection. Also, it was noted that part of the benefit of hyperbaric oxygen is to increase the rate of breakdown of sclerotic bone and dense scar tissue with an associated stimulus to normal repair by osteogenesis. Furthermore, Hamben's study did not detect a difference in outcomes when the animals were treated with 2 ATA vs. 3 ATA (29). The Mader study showed improved treatment of experimental *S. aureus* osteomyelitis with the adjunctive use of HBO, probably as the result of enhanced oxygen-dependent killing mechanisms. A similar result is probable with the oxygen-dependent killing mechanisms of PMNs against other organisms. This conclusion is supported by work, which shows that *Staphylococcus epidermidis, Pseudomonas aeruginosa, Escherichia coli,* as well as *S. aureus* are inefficiently killed by phagocytes while under hypoxic conditions as compared to their activity under hyperbaric oxygen tensions (>100 mmHg) (13, 30, 31).

Superoxide dismutase and catalase are among the enzymatic mechanisms used by aerobic bacteria to degrade toxic oxygen radicals (32). Anaerobic and many microaerophilic organisms lack the ability to produce these enzymes (33). Therefore, anaerobic organisms are rendered sensitive to oxygen radicals developed both intracellularlly and extracellularly during HBO therapy. As a result, increased oxygen tension is lethal to fastidious anaerobic organisms and to some microaerophilic organisms, but not aerobes (34). Using a mouse model for intrahepatic liver abscesses induced with *Bacteroides fragilis* and *Fusobacterium sp.*, Hill showed a reduction in abscess size and number in those animals receiving adjunctive HBO (35).

Another mechanism by which HBO may assist in the treatment of osteomyelitis is in the promotion of fibroblastic activity. Fibroblasts cannot synthesize collagen or migrate to the affected area when oxygen tensions are less than 20 mmHg. Elevating oxygen tensions to levels greater than 200 mmHg allows a return to normal function (15, 16). Therefore, increasing oxygen tensions with HBO therapy is a means of assisting return of fibroblastic activity to normal. The fibroblast is then able to produce collagen, which forms a protective matrix. Following their differentiation from fibroblast-like mesenchymal cells, osteoblasts lay down a layer of immature course fibrillar bone. This immature bone is then replaced by mature lamellar bone that is functionally reconstructed by resorption and deposited by osteoclasts and osteoblasts (36).

Bone healing is an important aspect in post-surgical management of refractory osteomyelitis and in the repair of bony destruction due to this infection. A number of researchers have studied the effects of HBO therapy on bone healing in animal models. Coulson, et al., found that the fractured femurs of rats treated for two hours per day at three ATA of oxygen showed greater breaking strength at two weeks post-fracture than atmospheric controls (37). Barth, et al., also demonstrated the beneficial effects of HBO therapy on bone healing by showing that the metaphyseal defects in the cortices of rat femurs were healed by primary ossification when rats were treated with once-a-day HBO treatments, for 90 minutes at two ATA (38). This group of rats also appeared to have accelerated bone repair and vessel ingrowth, compared to controls. However, in the same study, Barth found that if the HBO treatment regimen was given twice daily, the defects healed through enchondral ossification; the bone repair rate and vessel ingrowth were retarded, and the osteoclastic activity was upregulated.

This oxygenation of tissues beyond a once daily treatment, for 90-120 minutes at two to three ATA with 100% oxygen, and its effect upon bone healing has also been previously evaluated by a number of other laboratories. Wray and Rogers found that when the duration of the hyperbaric treatment was increased to six hours per day at three ATA of oxygen, the breaking strength was reduced (39). In another study, Goldhaber demonstrated that sustained hyperoxygen environments (95% $O_2$ and 5% $CO_2$) lasting for periods of up to 12 days, resulted in marked *in vitro* bone resorption due to altered distribution and increased activity of osteoclasts (40). Yablon, et al., also studied the effect of hyperbaric oxygen treatment at three ATA, twice daily on femur fractures in male rats. However, this study exposed the rats to HBO therapy for only 60 minutes per treatment. At this lower treatment time, the HBO treated animals showed the formation of more cartilage in the fracture callus, a greater conversion of this cartilage to bone, and a greater amount of new bone than controls (41). All of these studies demonstrate that bone repair is hindered when hyperbaric oxygen treatment goes beyond the optimal range: 90-120 minutes HBO treatment at two to three ATA of 100% oxygen, once daily. Oxygenation below this level (such as occurs in infected bone) will result in slow bone healing due to inhibition of fibroblast, osteoclast, osteoblast, and macrophage activity (43). When oxygen levels are raised beyond optimal levels for a sustained period, fibroblast activity is highly upregulated, resulting in a thick collagenous deposition (38). Also, many *in vitro* studies have demonstrated an upregulated osteoclast activity due to long exposures to oxygen radicals (including hydrogen peroxide) associated with hyperoxygen growth conditions (40, 42, 43). The end result of sustained hyperoxygenation is the development of a repair process that is rich in collagen and structurally weak. Therefore, maximal bone healing was achieved when HBO treatment is provided within the optimal range: once daily treatments for 90-120 minutes at two to three ATA with 100% oxygen.

The effect of HBO therapy provided during concomitant antibiotic therapy has also been studied. The aminoglycoside class of antibiotics had been the mainstay in the treatment of Gram-negative aerobic infections for many years. The class includes such drugs as gentamycin, tobramycin, amikacin, etc. An important therapeutic limitation, however, is their inability to penetrate pus and their decreased activity under low oxygen tensions (11, 44). Other antibiotics, including vancomycin, quinolones, trimethoprim/sulfamethoxazole and nitrofurantoin have also been shown to be far less active in a hypoxic environment (45). Such conditions are readily found in ischemic tissues and in normal bone. It has been theorized that HBO therapy may be beneficial in potentiating the bactericidal effects of these antibiotics. Verklin, et al. demonstrated that HBO helps certain antibiotics enter bacteria, especially in hypoxic environments (19). Mader has shown that with HBO therapy, the bactericidal activity of the aminoglycoside class of antibiotics is enhanced (24, 46). Using *Pseudomonas aeruginosa*, they demonstrated that the bactericidal activity of tobramycin was improved when oxygen tensions were elevated above hypoxic levels. The Mader study was done by comparing tobramycin under anaerobic, aerobic and simulated HBO conditions (24). The effectiveness of HBO in augmenting tobramycin activity against *Pseudomonas aeruginosa* was evaluated using a rabbit model. When Mader compared tobramycin alone, HBO alone, and the two combined, he demonstrated that adjunctive HBO enhanced eradication of the *Ps. Aeruginosa* from infected bone (46). Trimethoprim/sulfamethoxazole and nitrofurantoin have also been shown to augment antibacterial activity in enhanced oxygen environments

*The consensus of the animal and lab data is that HBO is a useful adjunct for the management of osteomyelitis. These studies consistently demonstrated improved outcomes when HBO was used in conjunction with antibiotic therapy.*

(47). Mendel, et al. used a rat model for osteomyelitis due to *Staphylococcus aureus* to compare the results of treatment with HBO, cefazolin, a combination of both, or no treatment. It was demonstrated that HBO alone compared to no treatment reduced the number of colony-forming units (CFU) in tibial bone. Antibiotic therapy alone demonstrated further reduction in the number of CFU's in tibial bone. However, changes were most marked using a 4-week combination therapy consisting of HBO and the antibiotic agent (48).

Mendel, et al. followed this study up by evaluating the synergy of HBO and a local antibiotic carrier for experimental osteomyelitis due to *S. aureus* in rats. This study demonstrated a significant reduction in CFUs in the tibial bone in either the HBO alone group or the local antibiotic carrier group. However, a synergistic effect was noted when HBO was used in combination with local antibiotic therapy. The CFU reduction was most marked in this group and, in fact, 82% of the animals had undetectable organisms in the processed bone suspension (49).

These studies demonstrate that hyperbaric oxygen increases the oxygen tension in infected tissue, including bone. While hyperbaric oxygen has a direct effect on strict anaerobic organisms through the production of toxic radicals, it has no bactericidal effect on aerobic organisms. In fact, hyperbaric conditions induce aerobic organisms to produce increased concentrations of superoxide dismutase, an oxygen–radical detoxifying enzyme. However, hyperbaric oxygenation does increase the oxygen tension in infected tissue, thereby promoting the oxygen-dependent intracellular killing mechanisms by the polymorphonuclear leukocyte. Hyperbaric oxygen also augments the bactericidal activity of the aminoglycosides, cefazolin, certain sulfonamides and likely has similar effects on other antibiotics. There is also a synergistic effect in reducing the number of organisms when combining HBO with both local and intravenous antibiotic therapy. Finally, hyperbaric oxygen provides adequate oxygen for fibroblastic activity, leading to angiogenesis and wound healing in hypoxic tissues.

## JUSTIFICATION FOR HYPERBARIC OXYGEN: CLINICAL EXPERIENCES

The first report that hyperbaric oxygen (HBO) was useful in refractory osteomyelitis was published by Slack in 1965. He reported good results with using this modality in five patients (1). A year later, Perrins reported a 71 percent arrest rate of refractory osteomyelitis cases when HBO was used as an adjunct in the management after surgery and antibiotics failed (2). Subsequently, additional reports attesting to the benefits of HBO in managing refractory osteomyelitis of long bones have appeared (Table 3) (50-53). Most are reports dealing with the use of HBO as an adjunct to surgery and antibiotics of long bones after previous failures with these latter two interventions. In total, over 200 cases are tallied. Arrest rates with the adjunctive use of HBO ranged from 61 to 89 percent. In those reports where the infection was not arrested, there was almost 100 percent unanimity in observations that the patient's infections were improved. Often, follow-ups were not mentioned or were of relative short durations, for example from 12 to 53 months (54). It is noteworthy that there have been no new published

## TABLE 3. SUMMARY OF REPORTS USING HYPERBARIC OXYGEN FOR CHRONIC REFRACTORY OSTEOMYELITIS

| Name [ref] Year | Patients | Outcomes Arrested (%)/Improved (%) | Comments/ Study Type |
|---|---|---|---|
| Slack [1] 1965 | 5 | Improved 5 (100%) | Prospective |
| Perrins [2] 1966 | 24 | 17 (71%)/ 4 (16.7%) | Previous failures with surgery & antibiotics |
| Depenbusch [50] 1972 | 50 | 35 (70%)/15 (30%) | SAA |
| Bingham [72] 1977 | 70* | 43 (61%) Arrested | SAA; Variety of sites; excludes osteomyelitis of the mandible; ~100% improved |
| Morrey [53] 1979 | 40 | 34(85%) Arrested | SAA; symptoms > 1 month |
| Davis [52] 1986 | 38 | 34 (89%) Arrested | SAA |
| Esterhai [55] 1987 | 14 | 11(78.6%) Arrested | Prospective study; all failures refused surgery—see text |

KEY: * 36 patients (51% included from Depenbusch's study, excluded mandibular osteomyelitis; SAA = Same as above, i.e. failures with surgery and antibiotic treatments

series using hyperbaric oxygen treatment for osteomyelitis of long bones for almost 20 years. This is attributed to the shift of treatment interventions to the use of muscle flaps and/or use of Illizarov principles for managing chronic refractory osteomyelitis (see introduction).

In 1980, an extensive review of refractory osteomyelits that considered both non-hyperbaric and hyperbaric managed reports was published (54). The non-hyperbaric reports which included over thirty publications were typically prospective series of outcomes with surgical techniques utilized by the primary author of each article. The hyperbaric oxygen experiences in the review consisted of 17 reports. Many were on-going series by the same authors. The majority of reports dealt with osteomyelitis of the mandible. Many of the outcomes were reported as "favorable," "effective," "successful," etc. When actual numbers were provided (percentages), the range was little different from those reported in the non-HBO management reports.

Esterhai, et al. reported on a retrospective study, of sorts, that on initial inspection undermines the benefit of hyperbaric oxygen (55). After studying a group of 14 patients who received HBO with a 78.6 percent arrest rate (3 of 14 patients failed), the authors retrospectively reviewed a similar number of patients who did not receive HBO. A 93 percent arrest rate (1 of 14 patients failed) was reported. An analysis of the failures disclosed that all occurred in patients who refused surgical management; three in the HBO limb and one in the control limb. Several questions arise as to the validity of this study including the question of whether the control group with a 90 percent arrest rate even met the definition of refractory osteomyelitis. Furthermore, the durability of results where only based on the initial arrest of the infection. In a subsequent publication from the same institution, a 62 percent arrest rate in a group of patients who did not receive HBO in their management was reported (56). How this latter outcome differs from the control group in the HBO study fuels further suspicion about the validity of their HBO experiences.

In the 1980s, Barr began displaying his experiences using HBO treatments for "seemingly impossible" to heal diabetic foot wounds (57). Incredible improvements occurred in wounds that where not differentiated as to the presence or absence of osteomyelitis. From the literature it is known that osteomyelitis is present in at least 70 percent of diabetic foot wounds where bone is exposed and/or can be probed at the base of a tract wound (58, 59). This kindled a new direction for hyperbaric medicine; its use in the management of the diabetic foot wound. In hyperbaric medical centers treatment of the diabetic foot wound has become one of the predominant indications. Criteria for using hyperbaric oxygen in this group of patients are no measurable signs of healing after a thirty day period using standard wound care, antibiotic and surgical intervention with either the presence of

> *Dr. Barr should be credited for his almost single-handed perseverance in demonstrating the usefulness of hyperbaric oxygen in the management of seemingly incurable, limb threatening diabetic foot infections/osteomyelitis.*

## TABLE 4. BENEFITS OF HYPERBARIC OXYGEN IN THE MANAGEMENT OF DIABETIC FOOT WOUNDS WITH (PRESUMPTIVE) CHRONIC REFRACTORY OSTEOMYELITIS (61, 62)

|  | Wound Healing | | Amputations | |
|---|---|---|---|---|
|  | HBO | Controls | HBO | Controls |
| Subjects | 535 | 534 | 560 | 507 |
| Healed | 453 | 256 | 98 | 235 |
| Percent | 85 | 48 | 18 | 46 |

COMMENTS: Data based on 12 reports including two randomized control trials. Complete data cited in the references listed above. Wounds not specified as to whether osteomyelitis was present or not. However, in as much as osteomyelitis is a qualifying criterion for using hyperbaric oxygen in diabetic foot wounds, the assumption is made that osteomyelitis was a component in the majority of cases.

osteomyelitis or deep abscess (60). Chronic refractory osteomyelitis is undoubtedly present in almost all of those patients where the infection persists after debridement surgery and use of antibiotics. Further discussion of this indication is found in the problem wound management chapter, but from the first author's own review, healing is almost doubled and amputations more than halved versus control groups where HBO was not used (Table 4) (61, 62).

## EVALUATION

Evaluation of chronic refractory osteomyelitis (CROM) starts with confirmation of the diagnosis and establishment of a bacteriological etiology (Figure 4). The diagnosis is confirmed by the history, examination, and imaging studies. The history provides essential information as to whether or not the problem meets the definition of CROM as given before, the type of presentation (i.e. compromised host, septic non-union or diffuse sclerosing osteomyelitis), the presence of co-morbidities, the patient's functional status (Table 2) and the patient's goals (Table 5) with respect to the bone infection problem. The latter two considerations are essential when considering the three options for management of CROM, namely salvage of the extremity, lower limb amputation or living with a chronic, stable non-healing wound. The functional status of the patient and his/her aspirations are crucial when making decisions whether to invest resources and time to arrest the infection or to proceed directly to a major limb amputation.

> The "CROM Triad" (1. Persistent wound, 2. Bone deformity and 3. Tracking to bone) is invariably present in chronic refractory osteomyelitis. The triad virtually confirms the diagnosis.

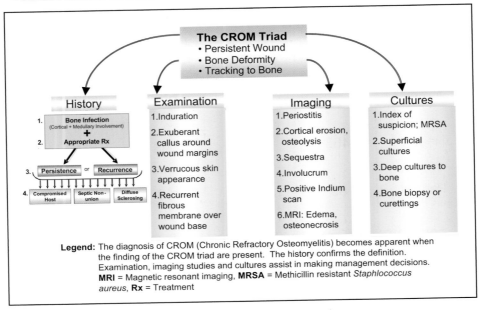

*Figure 4. Confirming the Diagnosis of Chronic Refractory Osteomyelitis.*

## TABLE 5. QUANTIFYING PATIENT'S GOALS

| Assessment | 2- Points | 1 Point | 0-Points |
|---|---|---|---|
| | Use half points if mixed or intermediate between 2 grades | | |
| Motivation | Full | Some | None |
| Comprehension | | | |
| Compliance<br>(Diabetes management, weight, skin care, etc.) | | | |
| Family/Care Giver Support | | | |
| Activities of Daily Living | | | |

**Interpretations:**

**4 or more points:**  Patient (and/or care givers) demonstrate sufficient aspirations for carrying through with wound care instructions and prevention of new wounds in the future

**Less than 4 points:**  Aspirations insufficient to justify limb salvage

The examination helps to confirm the diagnosis, define the extent of the infection and plan the strategies for managing CROM. Anytime a chronic wound persists over a deformity with exposed bone at the base, osteomyelitis is the diagnosis until proven otherwise. Osteomyelitis of the toe is invariably present when the triad of a digit wound tracking to bone, induration and fusiform swelling are present. A toe with the latter finding has been referred to as a "sausage" toe (63). Other clinical findings highly suggestive of CROM include: 1) Induration, a tense, erythematous swelling, 2) Exuberant callus formation especially with adjacent maceration of the marginal tissues and 3) A verrucous, mammilated appearance of the hyperplastic skin around the wound. The recurrent formation of a well-defined fibrinous membrane or fibrinous granulation tissue over the wound base, even after repetitive debridements, is a "soft" sign of underlying bone infection. The quantity and character of the exudate in the wound base is an unreliable sign of underlying osteomyelitis.

Imaging studies are helpful in confirming the diagnosis of osteomyelitis. Signs of osteomyelitis on plain x-rays include the triad of cortical erosion, periostial new bone formation and bone resorption. Other findings that may be observed include sequestra, involucrums and cloacae. The absence of plain x-ray confirmation of osteomyelits does not rule out this diagnosis. If the infected bone is avascular and/or exists in a hypoxic environment, the above findings which reflect host responses for dealing with the problem will not be observed. Nuclear medicine imaging is a useful adjunct in this latter situation (64). Bone scans (Technetium pyrophosphate) reflect bone metabolic activity and hence can be positive in a variety of conditions including trauma, infection, metabolic disorders (gout), arthridities and neuropathic (Charcot) osteoarthropathy. When "cold," that is no activity is observed, the bone is avascular. This does not rule out infection as explained above. To add specificity to the evaluation, a concomitant white blood cell labeled (Indium) scan will differentiate infected bone from the other conditions which may "light-up" the Technetium scan. The LeuckoScan® (anti-granulocyte Fab fragment antibody) nuclear medicine study is another scan that is reported to add specificity to the interpretation of osteomyelitis (65). Magnetic resonance imaging is the most sensitive imaging study for diagnosing osteomyelitis with greater than 90 percent positive findings (66). Unfortunately, the studies tend to be over read with specificities in the 50 percent range due to positive findings being based on bone edema. However, the magnetic resonance study is unparalleled in its ability to diagnosis necrotic bone (osteonecrosis), soft tissue fluid collections such as abscesses, septic arthritis, infected bursa, tract wounds, osteitis (cortical bone involvement) and tenosynovitis.

The need for an accurate bacteriological diagnosis from the bone causing CROM is controversial. If the infection is severe enough to cause sepsis, blood cultures and sensitivities are sufficient for antibiotic selection. If the infection is of the chronic indolent type, superficial or sinus tract cultures may be obscured by secondary contaminants. If organisms other than *Staphylococcus* are cultured, there is a 60 percent chance they represent a contamination (67). Generally, tract or wound base cultures supplemented with judgment are sufficient to initiate appropriate antibiotic therapy. Methicillin Resistant *Staphylococcus aureus* (MRSA)* is so commonly observed in the compromised host that appropriate antibiotics to deal with this pathogen are invariably indicated in the absence of actual culture and sensitivity results from bone. For example, 15% to 74% of community acquired purulent skin and soft tissue infections in patients without other intercurrent problems culture MRSA (68). In our experience, approximately 30% of patients presenting to our medical facility with *Staphylococcus* wound infections are positive for MRSA. In those with previous hospitalizations or transferring from assisted care living facilities, the frequency of MRSA infections is doubled. When the response to antibiotics is not as anticipated and/or the bacteriological diagnosis remains in doubt, bone cultures should be obtained (69). This can be done with needle biopsy preferably under computer tomography control, samples of bone debrided from the wound base, or in the operating room associated with surgical debridement and/or resection of the infected bone. The results from these techniques may be challenged if the patient is already on antibiotics. In the presence of avascular bone (osteonecrosis), it is unlikely that antibiotics will have much effect on the organisms residing in the bone. Consequently, the culture and sensitivity

*The terms Methicillin resistant Staphylococcus aureus and Oxacillin resistant Staphlococcus aureus (ORSA) can be used interchangeably. For all practical purposes the terminologies are identical. Perhaps ORSA is the more precise term since antibiotic sensitivity testing is done with Oxacillin rather than with Methicillin.*

results are expected to reflect accurately the bacterial flora of the bone. If the bone is perfused, cessation of antibiotics for 24 hours before the biopsy or the planned surgical procedure may improve the accuracy of the bacterial diagnosis. However, with the clinical presence of osteomyelitis, antibiotic management is indicated even if the bone cultures show no growth. Consequently the use and selection of antibiotics for CROM must be tempered with clinical judgment.

## MANAGEMENT

Once osteomyelitis meets the criteria of chronic refractory, that is the infection persists or recurs after treatment, three presentations become obvious, namely: 1) Refractory osteomyelitis in a compromised host, 2) Septic non-union fracture and 3) Diffuse sclerosing osteomyelitis (Figure 1) (70). Each has features that require special considerations for management and different protocols for using hyperbaric oxygen. This approach supplements and is more encompassing than the two anatomic types (namely localized osteomyelitis in the compromised host and diffuse osteomyelitis) that Mader et al. proposed for using HBO in osteomyelitis (Table 1) (7). In order to make appropriate management decisions, information about host-function and patient goals with respect to the management of CROM and avoidance of a lower limb amputation must be considered (Tables 2 and 5).

Of the three presentations of CROM (that is the compromised host, septic non-union and diffuse sclerosing types), the major indication for using HBO is in the compromised host. In our experiences over 90 percent of the use of HBO for CROM is for this presentation type. It is characterized by three features, namely: 1) Wound Hypoxia, 2) Mixed flora frequently with aerobes and anaerobes and 3) Impaired ability by the host to develop an inflammatory response. Treatment requires a five-fold strategic approach

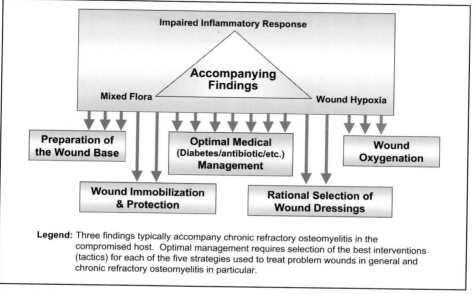

Legend: Three findings typically accompany chronic refractory osteomyelitis in the compromised host. Optimal management requires selection of the best interventions (tactics) for each of the five strategies used to treat problem wounds in general and chronic refractory osteomyelitis in particular.

*Figure 5. Management of Chronic Refractory Osteomyelitis in the Compromised Host.*

including: 1) Management of the wound base, 2) Immobilization and protection, 3) Optimizing medical interventions 4) Proper selection of dressing materials and 5) Augmentation of wound oxygenation (Figure 5). The host-function and goal-aspiration scores offer justification for using the strategic approach versus proceeding directly to a major lower limb amputation (Tables 2 and 5). If the host is decompensated and the goal-aspirations score is low, the better choice is a lower limb amputation. Salvage of the limb, in such situations, is unlikely to affect the patient's level of function.

Once, the evaluation is completed (see previous section), surgical management is usually required for preparation of the wound base strategy. The reason for this is that there is a high probability the infected bone is necrotic and without removal, the infection will burgeon as soon as the course of antibiotics has been completed. If a significant deformity is present, the wound and bone infection will inevitably recur as soon as activity is resumed even with the selection of appropriate foot wear. Surgical management may require debridement/ostectomy, partial/complete ray resection or partial foot amputation. Usually, what needs to be done surgically becomes apparent after examination and imaging studies are completed. Often time's surgery to prepare the wound base can be done in the clinic or on the ward versus being done in the operating room. Nonetheless, resourcefulness is required in order to remove the infected bone and generate flaps that will cover the wound, but still preserve a structurally stable and functionally sound foot.

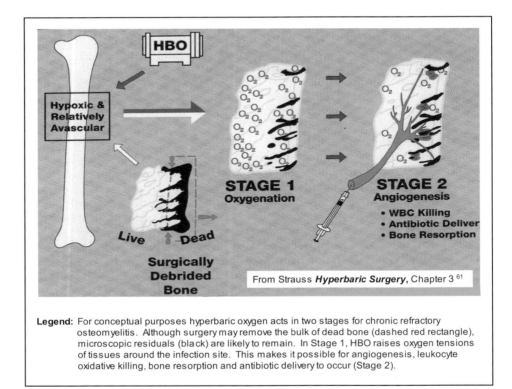

**Legend:** For conceptual purposes hyperbaric oxygen acts in two stages for chronic refractory osteomyelitis. Although surgery may remove the bulk of dead bone (dashed red rectangle), microscopic residuals (black) are likely to remain. In Stage 1, HBO raises oxygen tensions of tissues around the infection site. This makes it possible for angiogenesis, leukocyte oxidative killing, bone resorption and antibiotic delivery to occur (Stage 2).

*Figure 6. The Role of Hyperbaric Oxygen for the Management of Refractory Osteomyelitis.*

*For wound healing, infection control, and post-operative flap survival oxygen requirements may need to increase 20-fold or more for successful healing as compared to steady-state oxygen requirements for non-critical tissues (17). Inability to meet these demands result in wound healing failures. When these requirements are partially met, the wound may initially fail, slough or dehisce, but then go on to eventual healing, especially when HBO is used in the peri-operative period.*

If the soft tissue margins are of questionable viability and/or not clinically free of infection, the operative site should be left open with healing by secondary intention or later return to the operating room for delayed closure. Antibiotic selection and duration should be done in conjunction with an infectious disease consultant. If there are reasonable expectations that the bone infection has been eradicated with surgery, post-operative antibiotics should be continued for an additional two weeks after wound closure to assure that the soft tissues adjacent to the infected bone are sterilized. When concerns exist that residual infection is present in bone, antibiotics should be continued for a minimum of six to eight weeks after wound closure and consideration should be given for the long term (six months or more) of suppressive antibiotics.

For the compromised host presentation of CROM, the adjunctive use of HBO is indicated especially if the host-function and goal-aspiration scores justify attempts to eradicate the infection and salvage the limb. The effects of hyperbaric oxygen are well defined and are especially applicable to CROM in the compromised host (Figure 6). Wound hypoxia is a predominant concern in this group of patients. Without augmentation of tissue oxygenation levels, wound healing and infection control will be stymied. For the reasons discussed in the justification sections, HBO predictably improves wound oxygenation. Juxta-wound transcutaneous oxygen measurements in room air and during hyperbaric oxygen exposures predict, with nearly a 90 percent accuracy, which wounds will heal with HBO (71). Although treatment protocols need to be individualized, the recommended approach is to give this group of patients 10 to 14 HBO treatments to initiate angiogenesis and other host mechanisms before debridement surgery. After surgery, an additional 7 to 14 treatments are recommended to optimize healing of the flaps and potentiate host mechanisms during the very crucial (and oxygen-dependent) immediate post-operative period. Our experiences indicate that over 90 percent of patients with CROM who are compromised hosts will avoid lower limb amputation when HBO is used as an adjunct to surgical and antibiotic management in those patients who meet function and motivation criteria to preserve the limb.

Hyperbaric oxygen is indicated for septic non-unions when other treatment measures such as debridements and courses of antibiotics have failed and there is justification to preserve the limb as supported by host-function and goal-aspiration scores (Tables 2 and 5). Two considerations are fundamental before initiating a salvage attempt with adjunctive HBO: First, there is the potential for useful function if healing is achieved and second, intractable pain is not present. Hyperbaric oxygen will only be successful in conjunction with appropriate orthopaedic interventions such as debridement, stabilization, bone grafting and soft tissue management as well as the use of appropriate antibiotics. The recommended HBO treatment protocol for this presentation of CROM includes two weeks of daily pre-operative treatments followed by 20 to 40 post-operative sessions. This more extensive course of HBO treatments (as compared to the protocol for CROM in the compromised host) is needed in order to enhance the more slowly responding host factors, especially those associated with bone formation and remodeling. In about one third of our patients we have observed stress fractures with resumption of walking activity after healing and eradication of infection. This is attributed to the effect of the well-oxygenated environment for stimulation of the osteoclast and the resultant zealous remodeling of bone. Our limited experiences in patients with septic non-unions reveal almost 100 percent fracture healing rates when HBO is used in conjunction with appropriate orthopaedic and antibiotic management even after initial failures with these latter two interventions alone.

Diffuse sclerosing osteomyelitis is the third presentation of bone infections for which hyperbaric oxygen may be indicated. In this presentation, the bone infection involves the diaphysis and is usually extensive, poorly demarcated (in contrast to the discrete appearance of a sequestrum), and refractory to antibiotic treatment. Surgical management can be challenging since eradication of the infection by this means may compromise the structural integrity of the bone so much that useful function is unlikely. Conversely, residual infection at the margins of the debridement, which is likely to occur unless segmental resection of the diffuse, sclerosed infected bone is accomplished, allows the infection to persist and consequently be labeled refractory. As mentioned in the introduction, dead space management with antibiotic impregnated bone cement beads, use of microvascular free flaps and Illizarov healing principles have been a great asset in managing this type of refractory osteomyelitis.

When these measures fail or the extent of the infection is too widespread for the above interventions to be utilized, hyperbaric oxygen treatments should be considered especially if the patient's host-function and goal-scores merit salvaging the extremity. Saucerization (the debridement technique of creating a saucer-shaped defect in the skin and soft tissue level

*Rarely the situation occurs where the patient is too ill (this corresponds to the Cierney-Mader type C host) or is unwilling to comply with the requirements needed for post-operative management and convalescence of their diffuse, sclerosing bone infection problem. Typically these patients present with one or more chronically infected, draining sinus tracts. In these situations a course of hyperbaric oxygen plus antibiotics should be considered. A minimum of 21 hyperbaric oxygen treatments is recommended for this alternative protocol for managing diffuse, sclerosing osteomyelitis.*

*Drainage has been observed to stop and/or markedly decrease with this approach. The patient should be informed to anticipate future recurrences of drainage and if severe enough, consider additional courses of hyperbaric oxygen and antibiotics when this occurs.*

followed by generating a trough in the cortical bone to the medullary canal) is helpful in debulking the amount of infected bone. Although this technique is not likely to remove all the infected bone, when it is done in conjunction with hyperbaric oxygen treatments, host responses to the infection plus additional antibiotic therapy are often sufficient to eradicate the infection. Once the wound base has granulated, healing by secondary intention or coverage with a flap can be done. If the wound base is observed to have residual foci of avascular and/or infected bone, the patient can be returned to the operating room for second stage debridement of these foci. Hyperbaric oxygen treatment protocols for this presentation of refractory osteomyelitis are similar to those for the septic non-union. However, post-operative hyperbaric oxygen treatments are usually continued until a total of 60 treatments have been completed.

Osteomyelitis of sites other than the appendicular skeleton such as the mandible, skull and sternum are discussed in other chapters of this text. For osteomyelitis of the spine and pelvis the adjunctive use of hyperbaric oxygen is indicated if the infections meet the definition of refractory osteomyelitis. Because of the predominantly cancellous type of bone in these sites, arrest of the infection can usually be achieved with antibiotics and hyperbaric oxygen without major debridement surgery. Imaging studies and bone biopsies under CT (computer tomography) guidance should be done in order to verify the diagnosis, appreciate the extent of the infection and optimize the selection of antibiotics. Hyperbaric oxygen treatments should be given for a two to four-week period for optimizing host responses for dealing with the infection.

## REIMBURSEMENT CONSIDERATIONS

Reimbursement for the use of hyperbaric oxygen as an adjunct in the management of chronic refractory osteomyelitis (CROM) is currently authorized by the Department of Health and Human Services (DHHS), Centers for Medicare and Medicaid Services (CMS) and is covered by most third party insurance carriers. In order to justify the use of hyperbaric oxygen therapy in osteomyelitis, documentation that the condition is chronic and refractory is generally expected prior to initiation of HBO. Although CMS does not provide a specific definition for the words chronic and refractory as it relates to osteomyelitis, it is assumed that the initial acute osteomyelitis has been treated appropriately. In the event that the osteomyelitis remains or recurs despite appropriate therapy, a diagnosis of chronic refractory osteomyelitis is accurate.

Since indications on the use of hyperbaric oxygen for various conditions were first formulated by the Undersea and Hyperbaric Medical Society (UHMS), refractory osteomyelitis has been included in the Hyperbaric Oxygen Therapy Committee Report as an approved indication. The U.S. Food and Drug Administration (FDA) uses the UHMS HBO Committee Report as a primary source document when inquiries are made regarding the use of hyperbaric oxygen therapy.

The International Classification of Diseases, Clinical Modification (ICD-9-CM) code for the diagnosis of chronic osteomyelitis, unresponsive to conventional medical and surgical management is currently 730.1. A fifth digit is required as a designator of location of the infection. For example, 730.16 specifies CROM of the lower leg while 730.17 specifies CROM of the ankle and foot and 730.19 indicates CROM at multiple sites. Physician supervision of hyperbaric oxygen treatment for CROM is reimbursed by CMS and third party insurers with appropriate documentation. According to the UHMS Committee Report, utilization review is recommended after 40 HBO treatments for this condition, if additional HBO treatments are indicated. Please be aware that these codes and this reimbursement information is subject to change as new directives are promulgated.

## CONCLUSIONS

The role of hyperbaric oxygen treatments in the management of chronic refractory osteomyelitis becomes objective when the definition of this problem and the three clinical presentations as provided in this chapter are employed. During almost 30 years of experience using hyperbaric oxygen therapy as an adjunct to manage refractory osteomyelitis, the following salient observations about the usefulness of this modality are summarized below:

1. **Pre-treatment with HBO improves the environment around the CROM site:** This is the rationale for recommending two weeks of HBO before surgery and starting antibiotics, especially in the septic nonunion and diffuse sclerosing CROM presentations. Effects observed include a) decreased wound edema, induration and drainage; b) improved quality of the skin around the wound and c) better demarcation of infected from non-infected tissues.

2. **Hyperbaric oxygen helps demarcate live from dead, infected bone:** This is attributed to the angiogenesis and osteoclast stimulation effects of HBO. Observations in the operating room support the assumption that the vascularity of the tissues adjacent to the interface and dead bone are preferentially affected by pre-operative HBO treatments, with little changed in the avascular infection site itself. This assists in establishing viable, infection-free margins at the time of the debridement.

3. **Hyperbaric oxygen preferentially stimulates the osteoclast:** The osteoclast, a highly oxygen dependent derivative of the macrophage, generates acids and alkaline phosphatases to resorb bone. Its metabolic activity is 100 times greater than the osteoblast, the bone formation cell, at least with respect to bone resorption (by the osteoclast) and bone formation (by the osteoblast) (22). Osteoclast function is thwarted in a hypoxic environment. Strong evidence to support the osteoclast's role in bone resorption after HBO treatments is twofold: First, new onset x-ray evidence of bone resorption in the small bones of the feet and second, high incidences of stress fractures when patients resume ambulation after CROM has been arrested in long bones.

4. **Optimal protocols using HBO must be followed to achieve successful outcomes:** Protocols must be individualized to the clinical presentation, that is, compromised host, septic non-union or diffuse sclerosing type of CROM (Table 6). For the latter two presentations, pre-surgical, pre-antibiotic HBO treatments are given, usually during a two week period, to improve the vascularity and to reduce

## TABLE 6. HYPERBARIC OXYGEN PROTOCOLS FOR THE THREE PRESENTATIONS OF CHRONIC REFRACTORY OSTEOMYELITIS

| Presentation (and findings) | Recommended HBO Txs | | Total HBO Txs* | Comments |
|---|---|---|---|---|
| | Pre-op | Post-op | | |
| **Compromised Hosts**<br>1. Wound hypoxia<br>2. Mixed flora<br>3. Impaired host responses | 0-14 | 7-14 | 28 | If infection is eradicated, HBO is stopped<br>HBO Txs may need to be extended, if flaps are threatened |
| **Septic Non-union**<br>1. Chronic infection<br>2. Instability<br>3. Avascular interface | 14-21 | 14-28 | 50 | Surgeries may be staged; first debridement + stabilization; then bone grafting + closure |
| **Diffuse Sclerosing**<br>1. Diffuse distribution<br>2. Poor demarcation<br>3. Extensive involvement | 14-21 | 21-40 | 60 | Extended HBO Txs needed to maximize bone resorption and angiogenesis effects |

**COMMENTS:** HBO treatments are usually for 90 to 120 minute durations at 2.0 to 2.4 atmospheres absolute pressure once a day if an outpatient and twice a day if an inpatient. **HBO** = Hyperbaric oxygen, **Op** = Operation (surgery), **Txs** = Treatments, **\*TXs** = Maximum number of HBO treatments

edema in the infection site. After this, surgical debridement, fracture stabilization, if indicated and initiation of antibiotics is done. Re-debridements may be required if granulation tissue formation fails to cover the exposed bone after the initial debridement. Once the infection is arrested and the wounds are covered/closed in septic non-unions and diffuse sclerosing CROM, organism specific antibiotics should be continued for a minimum of six additional weeks. Usually two additional weeks of HBO treatments, up to a total of 60, are given after the last debridement in these two presentations to enhance host factor removal of the remaining vestiges of dead, infected bone.

5. **The duration of CROM does not have an adverse effect on the outcomes:** When HBO is used as an adjunct to both surgery and antibiotic therapy, the outcomes appear to be independent of the duration of the problem. This observation takes exception to a previous report where arrest rates decreased from 80 percent to 50 percent if CROM was present for longer than two years (72). When the protocols previously described are followed, outcomes appear to be independent of the duration the bone infection has existed.

6. **Advanced age is not a cause for poorer outcomes when HBO is used for the management of CROM:** Advancing age is recognized as a negative predictor for good outcomes especially in trauma and fracture management (73). If the bone infection meets the definition of CROM and the decision is made to avoid amputation based on the

patient's host-function and goal-scores, outcomes appear to be independent of age especially in the compromised host presentations. Hyperbaric oxygen has been reported to act as a signaling device to stimulate fibroblast activity and reconcile the effects that advancing age has on slowing fibroblast doubling times (74, 75).

7. **Outcomes with HBO are equally good whether the bone infection is caused by synergistic and/or mixed aerobic and anaerobic organisms:** This contrasts to a previous report where failures were observed in over 60 percent of the patients who had bone infections culturing synergistic bacteria (76).

8. **Once CROM has been arrested using HBO, the results are durable:** This observation is ascribed to the "jump start" effects HBO has on host factors and the continuation of these effects after surgery and antibiotics have been completed. For the compromised host with arrested CROM, strategies to prevent new or recurrent infections must be followed (77). A seemingly negative effect that supports the observation that the effects of HBO continue even after treatments have been completed is the delayed appearance of stress fractures after CROM is arrested in septic non-union and diffuse sclerotic presentations.

9. **If the decision is made to arrest CROM, management may require using interventions what were done before, but were unsuccessful in the absence of HBO:** The protocols for the managing the three presentations of CROM must be followed. Antibiotics should be selected based on bone cultures from the debridement surgery regardless of what had been cultured before. The extent of debridements must be based on clinical findings and imaging studies regardless of previous surgeries. Hyperbaric oxygen needs to be given according to the described protocols.

10. **Not every case of CROM will be arrested with the adjunctive use of HBO:** Failures, that is the need for lower limb amputations have occurred in several, somewhat predictable, circumstances including: a) Methicillin resistant *Staphlococcus aureus* infections in a subset of diabetics, b) Patients with collagen vascular diseases, especially those requiring steroids and/or other immunosuppressors, c) New onset vascular occlusive events, d) Intractable pain, e) Residual structural problems of the arrested infection site that prevent useful function and f) Insufficient patient compliance to follow the required treatment protocols.

How does hyperbaric oxygen measure up as an Evidenced Based Indication for chronic refractory osteomyelitis? Since it is used as an adjunct to surgery and antibiotics and is used when these managements fail, perhaps it needs to be judged differently than a primary treatment modality. Nonetheless, when the American Heart Association 1999 Guidelines are used, HBO meets the criteria of a Class-II indication (78). That is, it is probably useful and effective with a favorable risk/benefit ratio. The absence of a randomized control trial keeps HBO from being classified at a higher level for CROM.

It is apparent that factors other than the criteria used for Evidence Based Indications need to be considered when making decisions about selecting treatment interventions. This is certainly true for the use of HBO in CROM. Five assessments for making a decision on a treatment selection should be used (Table 7) (79). To quantify this approach, each assessment is graded on a 0-to-2 point scale with two points indicating overwhelming information to support the decision to use the treatment intervention, one point to indicate that the information is consistent with the selection and zero points if there is no information, no benefit or possible harm if the treatment is used. By adding-up the points of each of the five assessments, a 0-to-10 score (with 10 being best) is determined. If the total is five or greater, a rational basis for using the treatment is established. For the use of HBO in CROM the score is 6 (Table 7), thereby qualifying it as a rational indication for this condition.

In summary, hyperbaric oxygen has a defined role in the management of chronic refractory osteomyelitis. Laboratory studies and clinical experiences confirm its benefit in this condition. Chronic refractory can be precisely defined. Since there are three predominant presentations, HBO treatment protocols and other interventions need be selected based on the type of presentation. The patient's functional status and goals (which can be quantified; Tables 2 and 5) always need to be factored into the decision whether to try to arrest the infection or recommend a limb amputation.

## TABLE 7. A RATIONAL APPROACH FOR SELECTING HBO TREATMENT FOR CHRONIC REFRACTORY OSTEOMYELITIS

| Assessments | Criteria for Grading (Use half points if mixed or intermediate between 2 grades) | Grades for CROM | Interpretation |
|---|---|---|---|
| Experiences with the intervention based on observations and reports | 2 Points = Overwhelming information to support the intervention | Exp's = 1 | A total of 5 points or more quantifies the intervention as rational based |
| Mechanisms as supported by lab studies | | Mech's = 2 | |
| Published reports | 1 Point = Information is consistent with the intervention | Rept's = 1½ | |
| No other treatments available and/or failures with previous treatments | | No Txs = 1½ | |
| Randomized control trials and/or head-to-head studies | 0 Points = No information, no benefit or possible harm with the intervention | RCT's = 0 ___ 6 | |

COMMENTS: Based on a rational approach for selecting a treatment intervention for chronic refractory osteomyelitis, hyperbaric oxygen qualifies with a grade of 6 points.
CROM = Chronic refractory osteomyelitis, Exp's = Experiences,
Mech's = Mechanisms, Rept's = Reports, No Txs = No treatments,
RCT's = Randomized control trials

Evidenced based and rational criteria are available to support the decision-making process for using HBO in CROM.

## ACKNOWLEDGMENTS

No review on the use of hyperbaric oxygen therapy in the treatment of chronic osteomyelitis would be complete without the acknowledgement of the work of the late Jon T. Mader, MD. We are especially appreciative to Dr. Mader for the information he presented in the osteomyelitis chapter on *in vitro* and *in vivo* studies in the second edition of this text. We have included information from this section in our chapter.

# REFERENCES

1. Slack WK, Thomas DA, Perrins DJD. Hyperbaric Oxygenation in Chronic Osteomyelitis. Lancet 1965;1:1093-1094.

2. Perrins, DJD, Maudsley RH, Colwill MW, et al. OHP in the management of chronic osteomyelitis. In, Proceedings of the Third International Conference on Hyperbaric Medicine (Brown IW, Cox BG, eds.) Washington, DC, National Academy of Sciences, National Research Council 1966, pp 578-584.

3. Mathes SJ. The muscle flap for management of osteomyelitis. N Engl J Med 1985;306:294.

4. Fitzgerald RH Jr., Ruttle PE, Arnold PG, et al. Local muscle flaps in the treatment of chronic osteomyelitis. J Bone Joint Surg 1985;67A:175.

5. Weiland AJ, Moore JR, Daniel RK. The efficacy of free-tissue transfer in the treatment of osteomyelitis. J Bone Joint Surg 1984;66A:181-193.

6. Cierny G, Mader JT. Adult chronic osteomyelitis. Orthopedics 1984;7:1557-1564.

7. Mader J, Shirtliff M, Calhoun J. The use of hyperbaric oxygen in the treatment of osteomyelitis. In: Kindwall EP, Whelan HT, eds. Hyperbaric Medicine Practice, Second Edition, Flagstaff, AZ Best Publishing Co., 1999;603-639.

8. Mader J. Osteomyelitis (Refractory) In: Hampson NB, ed, Hyperbaric Oxygen Therapy: 1999 Committee Report, Kensington, MD Undersea and Hyperbaric Medical Society 1999;47-50.

9. Waldvogel FA, Medoff G, Swartz MN. Osteomyelitis: A review of clinical features, therapeutic considerations, and unusual aspects. N Engl J Med 1970;282:198-206,260-266,316-322.

10. Niinikoski J. Oxygen Tensions in Healing Bone. Surg Gynecol Obstet 1972;134:746-750.

11. Cierny G. Classification and treatment of adult osteomyelitis. CM Evarts (Ed.) Surgery of the Musculoskeletal System. New York: Churchill Livingston Inc. 1990;4337-4379.

12. Cierny G, Mader JT, Pennick JJ. A clinical staging system of adult osteomyelitis. Contemporary Orthop 1985;10:17-37.

13. Hohn DC, MacKay RD, Halliday B, et al. The effect of oxygen tension on the microbial function of leukocytes in wounds and in vitro. Surg Forum 1976;27:18-20.

14. Hunt TK, Niinikoski J, Zederfelt BH, et al. Oxygen in wound healing enhancement; cellular effects of oxygen. JC Davis and TK Hunt, (Eds.) Hyperbaric Oxygen Therapy. Bethesda, MD: Undersea Medical Society, Inc. 1977;111-112.

15. Hunt TK, Pai MP. The effect of varying ambient oxygen tensions on wound metabolism and collagen synthesis. Surg Gynecol Obstet 1972;135:756-758.

16. Hunt TK, Zederfeldt B. Goldstick TK. Oxygen and healing. Am J Surg 1969;118:521-525.

17. Strauss MB. Diabetic Foot and Leg Wounds. Principles, Management and Prevention. Primary Care Reports 2001;7(22):187-197.

18. Hansen RO, Lundback K. The basement membrane morphology in diabetes mellitus. In: Ellenberg M, Rifkin H. eds. Diabetes Mellitus: theory and practice. New York: McGraw Hill, 1970:178-209.

19. Verklin RN, Mandell GL. Alteration of effectiveness of antibiotics by anaerobiosis. J Lab Clin Med 1977;89:65-71.

20. Peirce EC II. Pathophysiology, apparatus, and methods, including the special techniques of hypothermia and hyperbaric oxygen. Extracorporeal Circulation for Open Heart Surgery. 1969, Charles C. Thomas, Springfield, IL, 84-88.

21. Textbook of Medical Physiology. 10th ed. Guyton AC, Hall JE, eds. 2000, Philadelphia, PA WB Saunders. 2000:144-194.

22. Johnson LC. Kinetics of osteoarthritis. Lab Invest 1959:Nov-Dec;8:1223-41.

23. Kivisaari J, Niinikoski J. Effects of hyperbaric oxygenation and prolonged hypoxia on the healing of open wounds. Acta Chirurgica Scandinavica 1975;141:14-19.

24. Mader JT, Brown GL, Guckian JC, et al. A mechanism for the amelioration by hyperbaric oxygen of experimental staphylococcal osteomyelitis in rabbits. J Infect Dis 1980;142:915-922.

25. Esterhai JL, JR., et al. Effect of hyperbaric oxygen exposure on oxygen tension within the medullary canal in the rabbit tibial osteomyelitis model. J Orthop Res 1986;4(3):330-6.

26. Mader JT, Guckian JC, Glass DL, et al. Therapy with hyperbaric oxygen of experimental osteomyelitis due to Staphylococcus aureus in rabbits. J Infect Dis 1978;138:312-318.

27. Turek SL (Ed.) Osteomyelitis Orthopedics: Principles and their Applications. Philadelphia: JB Lippincott Co., 1984;258-282.

28. Mandell Gl. Bactericidal activity of aerobic and anaerobic polymorphonuclear neutrophils. Infec Immunity 1974;9:337-341.

29. Hamblen DL Hyperbaric Oxygenation: Its Effect on Experimental Staphylococcal Osteomyelitis in Rats. J Bone Joint Surg 1968;50:1129-1141.

30. McRipley RJ, Sbarra AJ. Role of the phagocyte in host-parasite interactions. XI. Relationship between stimulated oxidative metabolism and hydrogen peroxide formation and intracellular killing. J Bacteriol 1967;94:1417-1424.

31. Selvaraj RJ, Sbarra AJ. Relationship of glycolytic and oxidative metablolism to particle entry and destruction in phagocytosing cells. Nature 1966;211:1272-1276.

32. Gregory EM, Fridovich I. Induction of superoxide dismutatse by molecular oxygen. Baceriol 1973;114:543-548.

33. McCord JM, Keele BB, Fridovich I. An enzyme based theory of obligate anaerobiasis: The physiologic function of superoxide dismutase. Proc Nat Acad Sci 1971;68:1024-1027.

34. Brown GL, Thompson PD, Mader JT, et al. Effects of hyperbaric oxygen upon Staphylococcus aureus, Pseudomonas aeruginosa, and Candida albicans. Aviat Space Environ Med 1973;50:717-720.

35. Hill GB. Hyperbaric oxygen exposure for intrahepatic abscesses produced in mice by nonspore-forming anaerobic bacteria. Antimicrob Agents Chemother 1976;9:312-317.

36. Mainous EG. Osteogenisis enhancement utilizing hyperbaric oxygen therapy. HBO Review 1982;3(3):181-185.

37. Coulson DB, Ferguson AB Jr., Diehl RC Jr. Effect of hyperbaric oxygen on healing fracture of the rat. Surg Forum 1966;17:449-450.

38. Barth E, Sullivan T, Berg E. Animal model for evaluating bone repair with and without adjunctive hyperbaric oxygen therapy (HBO): Comparing dose schedules. J Inves Surg 1990;3:387-392.

39. Wray JB, Rogers LS. Effect of hyperbaric oxygenation upon fracture healing in the rat. J Surg Res 1968;8(8):373-378.

40. Goldhaber P. The effect of hyperoxia on bone resorption in tissue culture. AMA Archives Path 1958;66:635-641.

41. Yablon IG, Cruess RL. The effect of hyperbaric oxygen on fracture healing in rats. J Trauma 1968;8(2):186-202.

42. Fraser JH, Helfrich MH, Wallace HM, Ralston SH. Hydrogen peroxide, but not superoxide, stimulates bone resorption in mouse calvarieae. Bone 1996;19(3):223-226.

43. Hall TJ, Chambers TJ. Molecular aspects of osteoclast function. Inflamm Res 1996;45(1):1-9.

44. Sheffield PJ. Tissue oxygen measurement with respect to soft-tissue wound healing with normobaric and hyperbaric oxygen. HBO Rev 1985;6:18-46.

45. Park MK, Meyers RA, Marzella L. Oxygen tensions and infections: modulation of microbial growth, activity of antibiotics, and immunological responses. Clin Infect Dis 1992;14:720-740.

46. Mader JT, Adams KR, Couch LA, et al. Potentiation of tobramycin by hyperbaric oxygen in experimental Pseudomonas aeruginosa osteomyelitis. Presented at the 27th Interscience Conference on Antimicrobial Agents and Chemotherapy, New York 1987.

47. Park MK, Muhvich KH, Myers RA, Marzella L, et al. Effects of hyperbaric oxygen in infectious diseases: Basic mechanisms. In: Kindwall EP, ed. Hyperbaric Medicine Practice, Flagstaff, AZ: Best Publishing Co. 1994;Ch 9:141-164.

48. Mendel V, Reichert B, Simanowski H-J, et al. Therapy with hyperbaric oxygen and cefazolin for experimental osteomyelitis due to Staphylococcus aureus in rats. Undersea and Hyper Med Society 1999;26(3):169-174.

49. Mendel V, Simanowski H-J, Scholz H CH. Synergy of HBO and local antibiotic carrier for experimental osteomyelitis due to Staphylococcus aureus in rats. Undersea and Hyper Med Society 2004;31(4):407-416.

50. Depenbusch FL, Thompson RE, Hart GB. Use of hyperbaric oxygen in the treatment of refractory osteomyelitis: A preliminary report. J Trauma 1972;12:807-812.

51. Bingham EL, Mullen JE, Winans RG, Hart GB. The treatment of refractory osteomyelitis with hyperbaric oxygen: A progress report. In: Trapp WG, Banister EW, Davison ED, Trapp PA, eds. Proceedings of the Fifth International Conference on Hyperbaric Medicine. Burnaby, Canada: Fraser University, 1973:264-269.

52. Davis JC, Heckman JD, DeLee JC, Buckwold FJ. Chronic non-hematogenous osteomyelitis treated with adjuvant hyperbaric oxygen. J Bone Jt Surg 1986;68A:1210-1217.

53. Morrey BF, Dunn JM, Heimbach RD, Davis JC. Hyperbaric oxygen in chronic osteomyelitis. Clin Orthop 1979;144:121-127.

54. Strauss MB. Chronic refractory osteomyelitis: Review and role of hyperbaric oxygen. HBO Review 1980;1:231-255.

55. Esterhai JH, Pisarello J, Brighton CT, Heppenstall RB, et al. Adjunctive hyperbaric oxygen therapy in the treatment of chronic refractory osteomyelitis. J Trauma 1987;27:763-768.

56. MacGregor RR, Grziani AL, Esterhai JL. Oral ciprofloxacin for osteomyelitis. Orthopedics 1990;13:55-60.

57. Barr PO, Perrins DJD. Prolonged use of hyperbaric oxygen (HBO) in indolent ulcers of the leg. Proceedings of the Eighth International Congress on Hyperbaric Medicine. Long Beach, California: Best Publishing Co. August 20-22, 1984;217-222.

58. Newman LG, J Waller, et al. Unsuspected osteomyelitis in diabetic foot ulcers: Diagnosis and monitoring by leukocyte scanning with Indium in 111 oxyquinoline. J Am Med Assoc 1991;266(9):1246-125.

59. Lipman, BT, BD Collier, et al. Detection of osteomyelitis in the neuropathic foot; nuclear medicine, MRI and conventional radiography, Clin Nucl Med 1998;23:77-82.

60. Medicare Coverage Issues Manual. Department of Health and Human Services (DHHS). Centers for Medicare and Medicaid Services (CMS) Transmittal AB-02-183, Appendix 35-10. December 27, 2002.

61. Strauss MB. Hyperbaric Oxygen as an Adjunct to Surgical Management of the Problem Wound. In: Bakker DJ, Cramer FS, eds. Hyperbaric Surgery, Perioperative, Flagstaff, AZ Best Publishing Co., 2002;383-396.

62. Strauss MB. Hyperbaric Oxygen as an intervention for managing wound hypoxia: Its role and usefulness in diabetic foot wounds. Foot Ankle Int 2005;26:15-18.

63. Rajbhandari SM, Sutton M, Davies C, Tesfaye S, et al. "Sausage toe": a reliable sign of underlying osteomyelitis. Diabet Med 2000;17:74-7.

64. Poirier, JY, E Garin, et al. Diagnosis of osteomyelitis in the diabetic foot with a 99mTC-HMPAQ leukocyte scintigraphy combined with a 99m Tc-MDP bone scintigraphy, Diabetes Metab 2002;28:485-490.

65. Rubello D, Casara D, Maran A, Avogaro A, et al. Role of anti-granulocyte Fab fragment antibody scintigraphy (LeukoScan) in evaluating bone infection: acquisition protocol, interpretation criteria and clinical results. Nucl Med Commun 2004;25:39-47.

66. Ledermann HP, Schweitzer ME, Morrison WB. Nonenhancing tissue on MR imaging of pedal infection: characterization of necrotic tissue and associated limitations for diagnosis of osteomyelitis and abscess. AJR Am J Roentgenol 2002;178:215-22.

67. Mackowiak PA, Jones SR, Smith JW. Diagnostic Value of Sinus-tract Cultures in Chronic Osteomyelitis. J Am Med Assoc 1978;239:2772-2775.

68. Moran GJ, Krishnadasan A, Gorwitz, R, Fosheim G, et al. Methicillin-Resistant S. aureus Infections among Patients in the Emergency Department. New Engl J of Med 2006;355:666-674.

69. Khatri G, Wagner DK, Sohnle PG. Effect of bone biopsy in guiding antimicrobial therapy for osteomyelitis complicating open wounds, Am J Med Sci 2001;321:367-371.

70. Strauss MB. Refractory Osteomyelitis. J Hyperbaric Med 1987;2(3):147-159.

71. Strauss MB, Bryant BJ, Hart GB. Transcutaneous Oxygen Measurements Under Hyperbaric Oxygen Conditions as a Predictor for Healing of Problem Wounds. Foot Ankle Int 2002 Oct;23;(10):933-937.

72. Bingham, EL, Hart GB. Hyperbaric oxygen treatment of refractory osteomyelitis, Postgrad Med 1977;61:70-76.

73. Johansen K, Daines M, Howey T, Helfet D, et al. Objective criteria accurately predict amputation following lower extremity trauma. J Trauma 1990;30:568-573.

74. Renstra WR, Buras JA, Svoboda KS. Hyperbaric oxygen increases human dermal fibroblast proliferation, growth factor receptor number and in vitro wound closure. Undersea Hyperb Med 1998; 25(Suppl):53(#164).

75. Saulis AS, Davidson JD, Mustoe TA, Moford JE. Hyperbaric oxygen modulators PDGF receptor B expression and ERK ½ activation in human dermal fibroblasts in vitro. Plastic Surgery Research Council, 45th Annual Meeting, Seattle, WA. 200:143.

76. Hall BB, Fitzgerald RH Jr., Rosenblatt JE. Anaerobic osteomyelitis. J Bone Joint Surg 1983;65(A):30-35.

77. Strauss MB. Diabetic foot problems: keys to effective, aggressive prevention. Consultant. 2001;31(13):1693-1705.

78. Handbook of Emergency Cardiovascular Care for Health Care Providers. Hazinski ME, Cummins RD, eds. American Heart Association 1999;p.3.

79. Strauss MB. Evidence review of HBO for crush injury, compartment syndrome and other traumatic ischemia. Undersea and Hyperbaric Medicine 2001;28(Suppl):35-36.

# NOTES

CHAPTER 26

# HYPERBARIC OXYGEN IN THE MANAGEMENT OF THE DIABETIC FOOT ULCER

## CHAPTER TWENTY-SIX OVERVIEW

# Hyperbaric Oxygen in the Management of the Diabetic Foot Ulcer

*Jeffrey A. Niezgoda, Luis A. Matos*

## INTRODUCTION

### The Problem

Diabetes mellitus is a major health problem affecting approximately 6.3% (18.2 million) of the U.S. population (26). A recent report released by the Yale Schools of Public Health and Medicine in conjunction with the Institute for Alternative Futures reveals that if the healthcare system in the United States continues to fail in adequately preventing and treating diabetes; by the year 2025 the number of people dying and suffering from diabetes and its complications will roughly triple (42). According to this study diabetes is one of only two major causes of death in the U.S. that continues to increase while other major causes of death are declining. These data are directly linked to the obesity epidemic. The study found that if the system remains unchanged by the year 2025:

- Diabetes-associated deaths will nearly triple from 213,062 in 2000 to 622,000.
- Amputations due to complications of diabetic foot disease will triple from current yearly numbers of 82,000 to 239,000.
- The U. S. will nearly triple its spending on costs associated with diabetes to $351 billion.
- The numbers of people living with diabetes will more than double to 50 million.

One of the most morbid complications of diabetes is foot disease ulceration and infection. It has been reported that of the total diabetic population requiring hospitalization, 20% are admitted for foot problems, and 30% have evidence of peripheral vascular disease (31). Diabetic patients account for in excess of 82,000 nontraumatic amputations in this country, and their hospitalization averages from 4 to 12 weeks (20). The economic impact of diabetic-foot complications is enormous. Direct medical costs are estimated to exceed $92 billion, while the indirect costs (disability, work loss, premature mortality) add an additional $40 billion (41). The costs reported for a partial foot amputation are $45,000 while a below knee amputation is estimated to exceed $65,000, not including rehabilitation and prosthesis.

### Diabetes Mellitus and Compromised Wound Healing

Diabetes mellitus constitutes a significant risk factor for impaired wound healing (7). Diabetes mellitus adversely affects wound healing through two principal mechanisms:

**Atherosclerosis:** severe, accelerated, infrapopliteal arterial occlusive lesions are more frequent in diabetics (5, 54). This pattern leads to severe chronic pedal ischemia resulting in impaired wound healing and lowered resistance to infection.

**Defective cellular and humoral immunity:** there is decreased phagocytosis, and a decrease in chemotaxis affecting the immunologic component of the inflammatory process. Lymphocytic function is also abnormal (18, 39, 53).

The relative insulin deficiency seen in many diabetics depresses the early phase of the inflammatory response and inhibits cellular proliferation. The synergistic effect of ischemia and impaired immune response is illustrated by Cruse's prospective study of over 23,000 patients (9). He showed that diabetic patients had a 10.7% incidence of infection in clean surgical wounds, compared to 1.8% in nondiabetics.

## REVIEW OF THE PATHOLOGIC PROCESS IN THE DIABETIC FOOT

A variety of synergistic factors predispose diabetics to the development of foot wounds, which can become secondarily infected. The peripheral neuropathy associated with diabetes leads to hypoesthesia which allows the unperceived development of traumatic foot ulcers due to trauma, friction or pressure. In addition, diminished pedal pain perception allows development of severe infection before the patient becomes aware of it. Diabetic peripheral neuropathy also involves motor nerves to the intrinsic musculature of the foot. The progressive denervation of these muscles allows deformation of the foot and results in abnormal weight bearing with increased stress over the metatarsal heads. Eventually, ulceration can develop that can become secondarily infected. Even without the development of infection, these "neurotrophic" ulcerations are difficult to heal because of continued weight bearing.

The accelerated atherosclerosis of infrainguinal arteries observed in diabetics can produce significant, asymptomatic ischemia of the foot. Many diabetic patients do not develop classic intermittent claudication or rest pain, and yet suffer severe pedal ischemia. When ulceration develops in the foot, ischemia can result in a nonhealing wound. Ischemia can also potentiate pedal infection. As an independent factor, pedal ischemia, when it reaches critical levels (ankle systolic blood pressure less than 40 mmHg, toe pressure less than 30 mmHg) (55), can result in spontaneous skin breakdown and nonhealing ulceration. Although diabetics with atherosclerosis can present with the common patterns of segmental arterial occlusion (aorto-iliac, femoro-popliteal), it is the typical tibial arterial occlusive lesion in diabetics that produces the most severe pedal ischemia (59).

It is important to note that although a characteristic microvascular angiopathic lesion (thickening of the basement membrane) has been described in the foot of diabetics (17), it is not this lesion that produces ischemia leading to ulceration. It is the macrovascular, typically tibial arterial occlusive lesion, which leads to critical ischemia (33). For this reason, most diabetics who present with nonhealing ulcerations or severe pedal infection in the presence of ischemia mandate arterial vascular interrogation and lower extremity revascularization if possible.

The hallmark of diabetic foot infection is its polymicrobial nature. Recent studies have shown that anaerobic organisms (*B. fragilis and Peptococcus*) are the most common bacteria found in deep wounds (34, 56), when adequate samples are appropriately cultured. Gram positive bacteria, such as S. *aureus*, and Gram negative coliforms remain important pathogens in infected diabetic wounds. Antibacterial resistant organisms, such as MRSA, have become a significant concern and are oftentimes the offending organism in diabetic foot infections. Infection potentiates pedal ischemia by increasing tissue demand for oxygen, while tissue blood flow is decreased due to the extrinsic compression of vessels by edema formation, potentially resulting in microvascular thrombosis. When infection extends to the deep plantar space, osteomyelitis is a frequent finding.

In a recent study, Pecoraro et al. (49) evaluated 80 consecutive diabetic men who required an initial lower extremity amputation in an effort to determine pathways leading to limb amputation. The sequence of minor trauma, cutaneous ulceration, and wound healing failure was the common pathway in 73% of the cases. However, gangrene (40%) and infection (41%) were the most frequent final components that led to the amputation. Subsequently, Pecoraro et al. (48) prospectively studied 46 consecutive outpatient diabetics presenting with full thickness lower extremity ulcers and concluded that adequate periwound cutaneous perfusion is the critical physiologic determinant for healing the diabetic ulcer. A 39-fold increased risk of healing failure was present when the TcPO$_2$ value was less than 20 mmHg.

The unique environment created by coexisting ischemia, neuropathy, and infection, is the factor most frequently leading to diabetic foot infections. It is the tissue destructive effect of uncontrolled, deeply-penetrating infection that culminates in limb loss.

## EVALUATION OF THE DIABETIC FOOT ULCER

Evaluation of the patient with the diabetic foot ulcer must begin with a complete history and head to toe physical examination. The history can provide valuable insight into the mechanism of injury or onset of the ulcer, prior complications and infections, and subjective findings suggesting the presence underlying peripheral arterial occlusive disease or neuropathy. A detailed history can also begin to formulate the management plan by identifying prior wound care strategies, diagnostic testing and therapeutic interventions. The physical must begin with a careful vascular and neurological examination to identify contributing global or systemic compromising factors (6). A focused examination of the ulcer should indentify the appearance (necrotic or granular), the depth and involvement of underlying tissues and structures, the presence of sinus tracts or abscess formation, and describe the odor, drainage and quality of the tissue surrounding the ulcer.

## Peripheral Neuropathy Assessment

A simple, reliable method to evaluate sensory perception in the diabetic foot is the use of the Semmes-Weinstein monofilament. The 5.07 monofilament is usually pressed against the skin of the plantar surface of the foot or pertinent area to the point of buckling. The inability to detect the monofilament indicates loss of protective sensation and risk for development of a pressure ulcer (32).

## Radiologic and Laboratory Testing

Radiographic examination should be performed on all patients with nonhealing diabetic foot ulcers. Routine x-rays are often initially negative due to relative osteopenia in the neurotrophic foot; however, x-rays still have clinical utility because they may demonstrate foreign bodies, fractures associated with a Charcot foot, or gas in the tissue. A repeat x-ray 2 to 4 weeks later may demonstrate the bony erosion of osteomyelitis or periosteal new bone formation associated with healing. A wound that probes to bone is almost universally considered *de facto* evidence of osteomyelitis and prompt referral to surgical specialists is critically important (19). A bone scan under these circumstances to "diagnose" osteomyelitis is almost always an unnecessary expense. Routine bone scans are expensive and only helpful if positive, but are often negative. MRI evaluation may have greater diagnostic accuracy as well as provide the additional benefit of detecting underlying abscess or necrotizing soft tissue infection.

All diabetic ulcers should be cultured. Whenever possible, it is essential that deep-tissue biopsy be used, as superficial swab cultures do not accurately reflect the organisms causing invasive infection (56). Anaerobic cultures should also be obtained in all diabetic patients.

Diabetic control is important for all diabetic patients, but it is critical in those diabetics with foot ulcers. The extent to which diabetes is controlled is assessed by measuring the levels of blood glucose and glycosylated hemoglobin (HbA1c). A measure of long-term glycemic control in people with diabetes, HbA1c is produced by the non-enzymatic glycosylation of hemoglobin at a rate proportional to the prevailing glucose concentration. The level of HbA1c depends upon the red cell lifespan and the prevailing blood glucose concentration. Providing the red cell lifespan is normal, HbA1c measures the mean blood glucose concentration over the preceding 60 days, i.e. the half-life of the red cell lifespan. Recommended levels of blood glucose and HbA1c are as follows: Type 1 diabetes 7.0 – 7.5% and Type 2 diabetes < 6.5% (1).

## Noninvasive Arterial Studies

The most reliable noninvasive indicator of global pedal perfusion is the determination of ankle-brachial index (ABI) (64). This examination is performed using a blood pressure cuff at the ankle inflated to a pressure that obliterates the Doppler signals normally audible in the posterior tibial artery behind the medial malleolus and in the dorsalis pedis artery. The return of the Doppler signal with deflation of the cuff marks the systolic blood pressure. To determine the ABI, the systolic blood pressure in both arms is measured and the higher of the two is used as the denominator in a ratio with the greatest measured pedal pressure (9). Caution must be exercised in the interpretation of this measurement in patients with diabetes or chronic renal failure. These patients may have varying degrees of medial arterial sclerosis (calcification), which may render arteries partially or totally incompressible, thereby falsely elevating the ABI.

In patients with incompressible tibial arteries, alternate means of assessing pedal perfusion must be used. The most commonly used methods are the determination of digital (toe) arterial blood pressures and plethysmographic assessment of arterial pulse volume waveforms (24). Although both of these methods give an indication of global pedal perfusion, they do not assess cutaneous circulation. This concept is important because healing of cutaneous lesions is ultimately dependent not upon total pedal perfusion, but upon local cutaneous circulation.

The most reliable methods of assessing the cutaneous circulation presently available are transcutaneous measurements of oxygen tension ($TcPO_2$) (22) and cutaneous laser Doppler velocimetry (23). From a practical viewpoint, these methods are best reserved for those patients in whom the methods of global circulatory assessment predict borderline healing potential or when there is slower than expected wound healing, despite tests showing adequate global pedal perfusion. Assessment with transcutaneous oximetry is an absolute requirement for any patients with diabetic foot ulcers when hyperbaric oxygen treatment is planned.

## Transcutaneous Oximetry

Transcutaneous oximetry is a simple, reliable noninvasive diagnostic technique that provides an objective assessment of local tissue perfusion and oxygenation. It can be used for serial assessment of the soft tissue envelope surrounding the problem wound. Uses of transcutaneous oximetry in the evaluation of the diabetic ulcer include the assessment of healing potential, selection of amputation level, and patient selection for HBO therapy (57, 58, 70). Accurate prediction of wound healing potential is essential to avoid the increased morbidity and mortality rates that accompany ischemic breakdown of failed debridement, amputation, and revascularization (36).

The transcutaneous oxygen pressure ($TcPO_2$) monitor has a Clark polarographic electrode that has been modified to include a heating element and a thermistor. The heating element should be preset at 450°C to allow maximum oxygen diffusion to the skin surface from the dermocapillaries (60). With the patient in the supine position, a skin area near the wound is selected for evaluation. This area should not overlie bone, ischemic lesions, inflammation or superficial veins. A second electrode is placed on the skin of the chest, as a control. The areas selected should be cleaned with an alcohol pad and shaved, if necessary, followed by stripping of the superficial layers of dead skin with adhesive tape. A self-adhesive ring, filled with contact solution, is used to attach the electrodes to the prepared skin areas. Serial determinations of $TcPO_2$ are made at 10, 20, and 30 minutes while the patient is breathing room air. Measurements can also be obtained while the patient is breathing 100% oxygen at 1 ATA and at 2.0-2.5 ATA. Recent comprehensive reviews of the use of tissue oxygen monitoring have been published (37, 61).

Several recent studies have shown that $TcPO_2$ is a reliable indicator to determine healing potential of problem wounds, to select amputation level, to evaluate the results of revascularization procedures, and to assess the severity and progression of peripheral vascular disease. In a study published in 1982, Franzek and colleagues determined $TcPO_2$ in 35 patients who underwent amputation of the lower extremities at various levels (30). Twenty-six patients achieved primary healing with a mean $TcPO_2$ of 36.5 mmHg ($\pm$ 17.5). In six patients who failed to heal, $TcPO_2$ levels were less than 3 mmHg. The same year, Burgess (12) measured $TcPO_2$ in 37 patients who required below knee amputation due to peripheral vascular disease. In this series, 30 patients achieved primary healing while 7 patients did not. The $TcPO_2$ values were significantly different between the two groups ($p < 0.001$). The mean $TcPO_2$ in the group with a primarily healed amputation was 42 mmHg ($\pm$ 11), but only 16 mmHg ($\pm$ 15) in those with failed amputations. Failures were due to wound dehiscence or necrosis. This study also showed a correlation between $TcPO_2$ measurements made below the knee and the healing of amputation performed at that level. Patients with $TcPO_2$ values of 40 mmHg or greater experienced no delay in healing their amputation site.

Dowd and associates (13) determined $TcPO_2$ in 161 normal volunteers and compared these values with 62 patients with peripheral vascular disease. In the normal volunteers, the $TcPO_2$ measurements on the dorsum of the foot showed a mean of 70 mmHg ($\pm$ 9), with a range of 45 to 95 mmHg. Similar values were obtained 10 cm above and below the knee, and on the chest wall. No significant differences were found with age. They also recorded $TcPO_2$ values at the site of the amputation in 24 patients. All patients with $TcPO_2$ greater than 40 mmHg healed, but those with values less than 40 mmHg did not. A group of 15 patients with intermittent claudication was found to have a mean $TcPO_2$ on the dorsum of the foot of 52 mmHg (range 26 to 72 mmHg). A group of 14 patients with ischemic skin changes had a mean $TcPO_2$ of 33 mmHg (range 16 to 49 mmHg), and a group of 33 patients with gangrene had a mean $TcPO_2$ of 10 mmHg (range 0 to 38 mmHg). A transcutaneous oxygen pressure gradient was present from the proximal to the distal part of the lower extremity in patients with peripheral vascular disease. This gradient was not observed in the normal volunteers. The authors showed that $TcPO_2$ reflected the severity of ischemia and was a more accurate guide to skin viability than clinical assessment.

In 1985 Harward et al. (42) undertook a blinded prospective study of 101 patients in whom 119 amputations (23 AK (Above Knee), 57 BK (Below Knee), 39 forefoot) were performed. The authors concluded that the initial $TcPO_2$ value, coupled with the response to 100% oxygen inhalation was an excellent predictor of healing potential. They introduced the concept of 100% oxygen inhalation, to enhance specificity of the measurement. In this study, the $TcPO_2$ values were obtained breathing air and following 10 minutes of breathing 100% oxygen. The authors concluded that $TcPO_2$ values greater than 10 mmHg on air, or an increase of more than 10 mmHg after oxygen inhalation, were excellent predictors of healed amputation. These values are significantly lower than those obtained in other studies. The reason for this discrepancy is unclear. In a retrospective analysis, the same group uncovered provocative information. In 50% of the patients who underwent an AK or BK amputation at their institution, the $TcPO_2$ values predicted healing at the next distal level of amputation. They concluded that clinical criteria alone were not reliable indicators to allow maximum tissue preservation.

In 1987, Hauser (22) prospectively assessed 159 wounds in 113 high risk patients with diabetes mellitus and peripheral vascular disease. In this study, the regional perfusion index (RPI = wound $TcPO_2$/chest $TcPO_2$) was compared to the leg-to-brachial blood pressure index (ABI). Surgical wound management in these high-risk patients consisted of 93 local debridements and 66 amputations. When the Regional Perfusion Index (RPI) was greater than 0.8 (n=30), all wounds healed. When the ratio was between 0.61 and 0.8 (n=34), 94% healed. With values between 0.4 and 0.6 (n=38), 58% healed. With RPIs between 0.2 and 0.4 (n=30), 7% healed. When the RPI value was less than 0.4, primary wound healing was achieved in only 3% (n=64). Of all surgical procedures performed, 46% failed, resulting in further vascular intervention, more proximal amputation, or death. When the RPI values were greater than 0.4, the wound failure rate was only 13%. The author proposed that the use of RPI would have dramatically reduced the rate of wound failure. A further finding of this study was that RPI predicted healing in patients requiring either debridement or amputation, while ABI did not. Although ABI was predictive of healing only in patients requiring debridement, it proved to be a less sensitive indicator than RPI.

Similarly, Oishi et al. (44) found $TcPO_2$ measurement to be a more accurate predictor of a healed amputation than segmental blood pressures or cutaneous temperatures. Lalka et al. (27) concluded that $TcPO_2$ measurements were a more reliable indicator of preoperative limb ischemia and of the outcome of revascularization, than the ankle-brachial index (ABI). Osmundson et al. (45) found that RPI was a better indicator of the results of revascularization, than was ABI, in patients with incompressible arteries.

In a recent prospective study, Ballard et al. (2) evaluated the use of $TcPO_2$ measurements in the management of 55 patients with diabetic foot problems. An absolute transmetatarsal $TcPO_2$ value of 30 mmHg was chosen to select a treatment option. The conservative treatment group (n=36, $TcPO_2$ > 30 mmHg) had a mean $TcPO_2$ of 50 mmHg at the transmetatarsal level, and 86% achieved a successful outcome with conservative treatment (i.e., minor foot amputations, debridement, local wound care). In the operative treatment group (n=24, $TcPO_2$ < 30 mmHg) the initial mean $TcPO_2$ was 11 mmHg. After revascularization, 83% (n=20/24) of the limbs had a $TcPO_2$ > 30 mmHg with a mean of 42 mmHg and achieved complete resolution of the foot problem. They concluded that transcutaneous oximetry can prospectively determine severity of foot ischemia and that it can be used to select appropriate treatment for patients with foot threatening problems. A $TcPO_2$ > 30 mmHg had a 90% accuracy in predicting diabetic foot salvage in this study. Bunt et al. (11) have validated the utility of $TcPO_2$ determination as an accurate predictor of therapy in limb salvage.

$TcPO_2$ was used by Sheffield et al. (60) to confirm local hypoxia and the increase in oxygen tension in response to hyperbaric oxygen treatment. In general, wounds in lower extremities with $TcPO_2$ values below 30 mmHg have a low probability of healing, while values higher than 40 mmHg usually predict a successful outcome. RPI values greater than 0.6 predict successful wound healing, while values less than 0.4 predict an unsuccessful outcome. The predictive value of TcPO$_2$ measurements may be enhanced by the use of 100% O$_2$ inhalation at sea level during measurement (an "oxygen challenge"), and by using an oxygen challenge at 2.5 ATA.

A recent retrospective data analysis of 1,144 patients with diabetic foot ulcer by Fife et al. (15) confirmed the reliability of TcPO$_2$ in predicting outcomes of diabetics who underwent hyperbaric oxygen therapy for lower extremity wounds. They reported that breathing oxygen at sea level was unreliable for predicting failure, but 68% reliable for predicting success after hyperbaric oxygen therapy. TcPO$_2$ measured in chamber provided the best single discriminator between success and failure of hyperbaric oxygen therapy using a cutoff score of 200 mmHg. The reliability of in-chamber TcPO$_2$ as an isolated measure was 74% with a positive predictive value of 58%. They also suggested that better predictive results can be obtained by combining information about sea-level air and in-chamber oxygen. A sea-level air TcPO$_2$ < 15 mmHg combined with an in-chamber TcPO$_2$ < 400 mmHg predicts failure of hyperbaric oxygen therapy with a reliability of 75.8% and a positive predictive value of 73.3%.

At the European Consensus Conference on the use of HBO in treatment of the diabetic foot held in 1998, there was compelling evidence to show that TcPO$_2$ measurements made at 2.5 ATA were highly sensitive, as well as predictive, in defining prognosis and properly selecting patients who would benefit from HBO treatment (37).

For the last three decades, the Doppler derived ankle-brachial systolic blood pressure index (ABI) has been the standard noninvasive method for the evaluation of the ischemic lower extremity and of the results of revascularization. However, the studies cited show that TcPO$_2$ measurement is a better predictor of wound healing, appropriate amputation site selection, and that it can provide accurate and reliable information regarding tissue viability in the ischemic diabetic foot. Determination of RPI allows the surgeon to maximize tissue conservation by predicting the most distal amputation level that will heal. If TcPO$_2$ values adjacent to the wound site are less than 40 mmHg and the Regional Perfusion Index (RPI) is less than 0.6, especially in the presence of infection, hyperbaric oxygen therapy should be considered to decrease the high probability of wound failure. The TcPO$_2$ measurement will help the hyperbaric medicine physician determine if HBO therapy is indicated, by demonstrating wound hypoxia and a favorable response to hyperbaric oxygen treatment.

## CLASSIFICATION OF DIABETIC FOOT LESIONS

A variety of classifications have been proposed for the accurate description of the diabetic foot (16, 48). The one in most widespread use is that proposed by Wagner (70). See Table 1. This system categorizes diabetic foot lesions by depth of tissue involvement, presence and extent of infection, and presence of gangrene. This scheme allows the use of a systematic management protocol for diabetic foot lesions. Its principal drawback, however, is its failure to include the severity of ischemia as an additional complicating factor in diabetic foot wounds.

## TABLE 1. WAGNER'S CLASSIFICATION OF THE DIABETIC FOOT

**Grade 0:** The skin is intact. There is no open lesion. There may be bony deformities, Charcot joint changes, and partial amputations such as toe, ray, or transmetatarsal.

**Grade 1:** There is a superficial ulcer without penetration to deep layers.

**Grade 2:** The ulcer is deeper and reaches tendon, bone or joint capsule.

**Grade 3:** Deeper tissues are involved and there is osteomyelitis, plantar space abscess or tendonitis usually with extension along the midfoot compartments of tendon sheaths. Operative debridement is mandatory.

**Grade 4:** There is gangrene of some portion of the toe, toes, and/or forefoot. The gangrene may be wet or dry, infected or noninfected, but in general, surgical ablation of a portion of the toe or foot is indicated.

**Grade 5:** Gangrene involves the whole foot or enough of the foot that no local procedures are possible and amputation must be carried out, at least, at the below the knee level.

## MANAGEMENT OF DIABETIC FOOT LESIONS

The successful management of diabetic foot lesions depends upon accurate recognition of the principal etiologic factors (i.e., ischemia, infection) involved. Additional risk factors predictive of impaired wound healing must also be identified.

If the initial assessment of the patient reveals evidence of generalized or specific compromising factors, these should be addressed and rectified to the greatest extent possible. Nutritional deficits and poor diabetic control must be corrected. Patients with evidence of poor tissue perfusion or ischemia need aggressive vascular evaluation and intervention. In addition to revascularization, a variety of adjunctive procedures may be required to achieve wound healing. Initial debridement of necrotic tissue and limited nonstandard amputations are accomplished at the time of revascularization or shortly thereafter (68). All patients with diabetic foot ulcers require offloading. A variety of orthotic and pressure redistribution devices are available.

In a prospective, controlled, clinical trial by Mueller et al. (40), 40 diabetic patients with Wagner's grade I and II lesions were randomized to treatment by total contact casting (TCC) or traditional wound management (TWM). In the TCC group (n=21), 19 healed in 42 ± 29 days, while 6 of 19 healed in 65 ± 29 days in the TWM group. This study demonstrated that TCC is effective in the management of neuropathic ulcers. If TCC is used to successfully heal the ulcer, the provision of a custom pedorthic device later may be just as important in preventing its recurrence (28). In another prospective study, Patel et al. (47) investigated the effects of metatarsal head resection (MTH) on plantar pressure distribution and ulcer healing in 16 diabetic patients with refractory neuropathic ulcers. In this study, all patients achieved complete ulcer healing within eight weeks, and the mean plantar pressure following resection was significantly reduced, irrespective of the site (p = 0.002). The use of locally applied growth factors is a recent development that may prove beneficial (25, 62).

A daily wound management program is critical to promote wound healing. Aggressive and meticulous wound care is one of the most effective means to preserve marginally perfused tissue and to control wound infection. This approach includes:

- Wound cleansing: aseptic cleansing of the wound with non-cytotoxic solutions such as hypochlorous acid 300-400AFC (Vashe), or normal saline (51).
- The following cytotoxic agents are detrimental to tissue repair, and should rarely be used: 1% povidone iodine solution, 3% hydrogen peroxide U.S.P., and 0.5% sodium hypochlorite (Dakin's solution).
- Sharp debridement is performed, as required, to remove all necrotic and devitalized tissue.
- Appropriate topical and moisture retentive dressings (e.g., enzymatic and antimicrobial agents, with foam, hydrocolloid, alginate, or collagen).
- Aggressive management of wound bioburden.
- Frequent education about proper foot care.

As mentioned previsously, patients with diabetic foot ulcers are at high risk for local and invasive soft tissue infection. All chronic wounds are colonized with bacterial organisms. One of the goals of wound management is to prevent critical colonization, as this increases the risk of skin, soft tissue and bony infection. Without fastidious attention to managing wound bioburden, the successful management of foot ulcers is impossible. Use of topical antimicrobial agents to decrease ulcer bioburden should be considered in patients showing evidence of critical colonization (localized erythema and warmth, increased drainage, odor, increased pain) or in those patients showing flattened wound healing trajectories or deterioration.

Progression of critical colonization oftentimes results in serious skin and soft tissue infection. Because of the polymicrobial nature of diabetic foot infections, presumptive intravenous antibiotic therapy must provide broad spectrum coverage. Some commonly used regimens includes either Timentin (ticarcillin and clavulanic acid), Unasyn (ampicillin and sulbactam), Zosyn (piperacillin and tazobactam), Primaxin (imipenem and cilastin), Zyvox (linezolid), Vancomycin and Invanz (ertrapenem). Combination therapy often includes clindamycin in addition to the previously mentioned antibiotics. Parenteral antibiotic therapy should be continued as long as signs of local or systemic soft-tissue infection persist. If osteomyelitis is present, long-term antibiotic coverage may be indicated, in addition to operative debridement. Frequently, the presence of invasive infection will result in difficult-to-manage hyperglycemia. However, vigorous attempts at strict glycemic control should continue.

In summary, the frequency of wound care is dictated by the severity and extent of the soft tissue injury and the degree of infection. Appropriate cleansing, debridement, and dressing techniques effectively remove non-viable tissue, reduce bacterial load, and therefore, optimize the wound healing environment. In addition to the wound care efforts directed at the ulcer, aggressive offloading, maximization of arterial flow, and optimization of the patient's nutritional status and diabetic control compliment the daily wound care regimen.

## RATIONALE FOR THE USE OF HBOT FOR THE DFU

It is well established that local-tissue hypoxia and infection are two of the primary defects underlying compromised healing in the diabetic foot ulcer (DFU). Hyperbaric oxygen therapy specifically treats both of these underlying factors. The use of hyperbaric oxygen as an adjunct is based on a rational physiologic basis, favorable *in vitro* studies, and animal research that has elucidated mechanisms of action in aerobic and anaerobic infections and wound healing (4, 29, 35, 52). These effects are corroborated by extensive clinical experience (11, 12, 50).

Hyperbaric oxygen therapy provides a significant increase in tissue oxygenation in the hypoperfused, infected wound. This elevation in oxygen tension in the hypoxic wound induces powerful positive changes in the wound-repair process. Hyperbaric oxygen therapy promotes wound healing by directly enhancing fibroblast replication, collagen synthesis, and the process of neovascularization in ischemic tissue. By providing molecular oxygen at the cellular level, it also significantly increases leukocyte bactericidal activity. The increase in tissue oxygenation, which leads to the increased formation of oxygen radicals within the leukocyte, is bactericidal or bacteriostatic to anaerobic organisms, and it may be as effective as specific antibiotic therapy, providing an added effect.

The Centers for Medicare & Medicaid Services (CMS) recently approved the use of HBOT for the management of the diabetic foot ulcer. Strict criteria have been established. The patient must have diabetes (Type I or Type II) and a lower extremity wound (Wagner Grade III or higher) due to diabetic disease. The wound must have failed standard wound care as demonstrated by no measurable signs of healing for 30 days (decrease in volume or size, decrease in exudate or decrease in necrotic tissue). Standard therapy must include assessment of vascular status, optimization of nutrition/glucose control, debridement, moist dressings, off loading and treatment of infection. Once these criteria have been satisfied and HBOT initiated, the wound must be re-evaluated every 30 days during HBOT course. Continued HBOT will not be covered if there are no measurable signs of healing during the 30-day period.

### Clinical Literature

Although there is an extensive literature describing the surgical management of the diabetic foot, it is difficult to adequately compare different approaches to therapy. The principal obstacles to interpretation of most studies are the influence of the bias introduced by "clinical judgment" and the lack of objective documentation of the severity of complicating local and systemic factors. Recently, a protocol for the management of diabetic foot wounds has been tested in a prospective, randomized fashion (14).

In 1982 (38), a retrospective report of 70 patients with nonhealing wounds treated with adjuvant hyperbaric oxygen therapy suggested a beneficial effects for this modality. This report included diabetic patients with soft-tissue infection, underlying osteomyelitis, failed skin grafts, and nonhealing amputation sites. In this series, 60% of the patients healed or showed significant improvement despite the presence of ischemia, infection or neuropathic changes.

In a prospective controlled study, Baroni et al. (3) studied the effect of HBOT on the management of grade 3 and 4 diabetic foot lesions. The groups were matched for lesion size, subfascial involvement, and duration and severity of diabetes. All patients were hospitalized, underwent daily debridement, and were maintained under strict metabolic control. The study (HBO) group consisted of 18 patients, of whom 16 healed and two underwent amputation. In the control group (n=10) 1 patient healed, five showed no change, and four underwent amputations (p = 0.001). A retrospective review in the same center revealed an amputation rate of 40%, between 1979 and 1981. Once HBO therapy became available, the amputation rate dropped dramatically to 11%. Baroni concluded that HBOT was effective in the treatment of grade 3 and 4 diabetic foot lesions as evidenced by a higher healing rate and a drastic decrease in amputation rate.

In a large clinical series of 168 patients with grade 3 and 4 diabetic foot lesions, Davis (10) reported a 70% success rate with a combined management protocol consisting of daily debridement, specific antibiotic therapy, aggressive wound care, metabolic control, and daily HBOT for 30-60 days. Most treatment failures were seen in older patients with significant occlusive vascular disease and absent pedal pulses. Oriani and colleagues (46) reported on the effect of HBO for the treatment of grade IV diabetic foot lesions. In this series, the HBO group consisted of 62 patients while the matched control group had 18. There was no significant difference in age, severity or duration of diabetes, or its complications. All patients were hospitalized and underwent daily debridement, strict metabolic control and specific antibiotic therapy. In the HBO group, 96% of the patients healed, while 4% underwent amputation. In the control group, 66% achieved primary healing, and 33% required amputation (p < 0.001).

In addition, Wattel et al. (71), evaluated the role of transcutaneous oximetry in predicting outcome in a prospective series of 59 consecutive patients with diabetic foot lesions treated with HBO therapy. In this study, the patients received an average of $29 \pm 19$ treatment sessions at 2.5 ATA, 100% $O_2$ for 90 minutes, twice daily. The benefit of HBO therapy was shown in this study with a healing rate of 87% and an amputation rate of 13%. More importantly, the outcome was predicted by $TcPO_2$ measurements in the hyperbaric chamber. The healed group attained a chamber $TcPO_2$ of $786 \pm 258$ mmHg as compared to $323 \pm 214$ mmHg for the amputation group (P < 0.005). In this study, a minimum value of 450 mmHg was shown to correlate with a successful outcome. In another large retrospective series of patients with diabetic foot lesions, Stone et al. (63) showed that the HBO-treated group (n=87) had a higher limb salvage rate (73% vs. 53%) than the non-treated group (n=382). These studies strongly suggest that HBO therapy should be an integral part of the treatment regimen of the diabetic foot to minimize lower extremity amputations and that TcPO$_2$ measurements may be of significant value in predicting outcome.

More recently, in a prospective, randomized study, Faglia et al. (14) evaluated the effectiveness of HBOT in decreasing major lower-extremity amputations in diabetic patients with Wagner's grade II, III, and IV lesions. All patients were evaluated and treated following a comprehensive protocol including aggressive surgical debridement, culture specific antibiotics, appropriate revascularization, strict metabolic control of diabetes, daily wound care, and prevention of mechanical stress. The HBO group consisted of 35 patients with the following Wagner's classification lesions: grade IV (n=22), grade III (n=9), and grade II (n=4). The control group consisted of 33 patients with grade IV (n=20), grade III (n=8), and grade II (n=5). The transcutaneous oxygen measurements on the dorsum of the foot for the HBO group were 23.25 ± 10.6 mmHg, as compared to 21.29 ± 10.7 mmHg in the control group. There were no significant differences in the clinical characteristics of the groups, including presence of infection, sensory motor neuropathy, or severity of peripheral vascular disease. The treated group underwent an average of 38 ± 8 sessions at 2.5 ATA on 100% O$_2$ for 90 minutes. The average chamber TcPO$_2$ value was 493 ± 152 mmHg.

In this trial, a significant difference in major amputation rates was observed between the two groups. The HBO group underwent 3 major amputations (8.6%, 1 AK, 2 BK) with 11 (33.3%, 4 AK, 7BK) major amputations in the control group (p = 0.016). Furthermore, the foot TcPO$_2$ values were significantly higher in the HBO treated group 37 ± 16.1 mmHg, than in the control group (26 ± 13.5 mmHg), at the time of discharge (p = 0.0002). The results obtained in this landmark randomized trial clearly document and define the effectiveness of HBO therapy, in addition to a comprehensive protocol, in decreasing major amputations in the diabetic with a compromised foot. Moreover, the transcutaneous oximetry data provides objective documentation of improved tissue oxygenation post HBO treatment.

## Guidelines for Patient Management

Currently, transcutaneous oximetry is the best method available to evaluate the severity of tissue hypoxia, to assess wound healing potential, to select amputation level, to facilitate proper patient selection for hyperbaric oxygen therapy, and to monitor progress during therapy.

Clearly, low TcPO$_2$ values reflect tissue ischemia. However, a transcutaneous oximetry threshold value that unfailingly predicts wound healing outcome in an individual patient has not been established, because of the multifactorial nature of the healing process. It is important to recognize the limitations of this non-invasive diagnostic modality, such as the inability to apply the electrode to the wound surface, or to the digits, and that the values obtained from the periwound sites may be affected by skin thickness, the presence of edema, or of infection. Presently, plantar surface values are unreliable, and should not be used, as they may often give paradoxical readings.

Hyperbaric oxygen therapy will not accelerate tissue repair in wounds with normal oxygen tensions and will only do so effectively in diabetic ulcers in which oxygen tension can be elevated to therapeutic levels. It is essential in clinical practice, before HBOT can be considered to demonstrate the presence of critical tissue ischemia and its correction with hyperbaric oxygen therapy.

Clinical pearls in documenting critical ischemia:

- During the initial evaluation, at least one transcutaneous oximetry value adjacent to the wound/amputation site must be less than 40 mmHg at sea level breathing air. If all values are greater than 40 mmHg, tissue hypoxia is not a significant etiologic factor and hyperbaric oxygen therapy is unlikely to benefit the patient, in the absence of infection.
- A representative initial transcutaneous oximetry measurement of less than 40 mmHg must be shown to increase to more than 100 mmHg in the diabetic patient while breathing 100% oxygen at sea level; failing that, at least 200 mmHg at a pressure of 2.0-2.5 ATA. If values do not reach a level of 200 mmHg at pressure in the chamber, it is extremely unlikely that hyperbaric oxygen therapy will benefit the patient (37).
- Repeated transcutaneous oximetry measurements must be obtained at least at weekly intervals during the first 14 treatments. Repeat measurements are made with the patient breathing air at the surface at least 12 hours after the previous HBO treatment. If there is no significant rise seen during the first 14 treatments, in the absence of infection, further HBO is discontinued. There is often a "latent period" during the first two weeks of HBO treatment where periwound edema and infection may decrease, but where little evidence of granulation tissue is seen in the wound. This often prompts surgeons to become discouraged with HBO treatment and to proceed with amputation. The $TcPO_2$, however, will be seen to rise during this period in those patients who will eventually respond to HBO, and the surgeon must be made aware of the results of repeated measurement.
- When a patient's wound fails to improve, despite hyperbaric oxygen therapy and adequate medical or surgical management, and if transcutaneous oximetry values, while breathing air at sea level prior to the daily hyperbaric oxygen treatment, fail to increase compared to baseline values, hyperbaric oxygen therapy should be discontinued.
- If a wound rapidly deteriorates, transcutaneous oximetry should be performed as soon as possible, to assess the severity of ischemia. A decrease in transcutaneous oximetry measurements may indicate arterial occlusion, a failed vascular reconstruction, or a compartment syndrome.
- Once a wound develops a healthy granulation base without evidence of infection, transcutaneous oximetry should be performed to determine if tissue hypoxia persists. When transcutaneous oximetry

measurements adjacent to the wound reach 40 mmHg, hyperbaric oxygen therapy should be discontinued and the patient should be followed, continuing proper wound care, as necessary, even if the wound has not healed (37). At TcPO$_2$ values of 40 mmHg or greater, the patient is said to be "host competent" as far as tissue oxygenation is concerned, and should heal on his/her own with good wound care or grafting. In most cases, this usually occurs between 20-30 treatments.

Even before hyperbaric oxygen therapy is considered, in the absence of infection, it is vital that the patient receive a complete vascular work-up and that all possibilities for angioplasty or surgical correction of the ischemia be exhausted. Patients with evidence of critical ischemia and diabetic foot ulcers should be aggressively revascularized, unless a contraindication exists. The procedure employed is dependent upon the results of noninvasive studies of lower-extremity arterial circulation and the arteriographic findings. As a general principle, proximal (aorto-iliac-superficial femoral) lesions are treated first. If inadequate revascularization of the foot results, as evidenced by poor healing and abnormal noninvasive arterial studies, then infra-popliteal revascularization is performed.

It has been shown that using modern revascularization techniques and an aggressive approach to limb salvage, more than 90% of patients who present with ischemic foot ulceration can be revascularized. To achieve these results, a multidisciplinary approach is necessary. The interventionalist must produce diagnostic arteriograms of the lower extremity that show complete arterial anatomy, including detailed arteriograms into the foot. Expertise in the performance of endovascular intervention and revascularization of the extremity involved is mandatory (68).

The vascular surgical team involved must be expert in all phases of lower extremity revascularization. In addition to the standard procedures for lower extremity revascularization (aorto-iliac and femoral-popliteal reconstructions), the vascular surgeons will need to employ techniques of tibial and pedal revascularization which will, at times, require alternate inflow sites (66, 69), and unusual approaches to arteries (43). Presently, it is clear that the best results for infra-inguinal revascularization, especially for tibial bypasses, are achieved when autogenous vein graft is employed (67). Whether results are better when a specific vein is used (greater saphenous, lesser saphenous, cephalic or combinations) (21) or when a specific method of greater saphenous vein preparation is employed (in situ, reversed, or translocated) is not definitively established (65). The specific method of vein usage and the type of vein used, is dictated by the team's experience, the availability of vein, and specific clinical circumstance.

Frequently, the eventual closure of the diabetic foot ulcer will require one or a variety of methods, such as split-thickness skin grafting, local rotation of full thickness toe flaps, or microvascular reconstruction with myocutaneous free flaps (8). Hyperbaric oxygen therapy can be essential at all stages of wound healing, especially when the foot remains compromised despite maximum revascularization. However, there is no role for topical oxygen in the treatment of diabetic foot lesions (30).

Adjunctive hyperbaric oxygen therapy in the compromised diabetic foot is only indicated for Wagner Grade 3-5 ulcers that do not respond to the standard management, which is defined as and includes optimization of vascular status, nutrition, and glucose control, debridement, moist dressings, off loading and treatment of infection. These patients can only be treated with HBOT after they have failed standard wound care as demonstrated by no measurable signs of healing for 30 days (decrease in volume or size, decrease in exudate or decrease in necrotic tissue). In many instances, these wounds remain hypoxic following revascularization, and infection remains limb-threatening despite culture-specific antibiotic therapy. In this setting, HBOT can oftentimes increase wound oxygen tension, enhanced host antibacterial mechanisms, and promotion of the wound healing process.

The hyperbaric oxygen treatments are performed at 2.0 to 2.5 ATA, with a range of 90 to 120 minutes of oxygen breathing. The frequency of treatments is dictated by the severity of the disease process. In the presence of limb-threatening infection after debridement or compromised surgical flaps following amputation, twice-daily treatments are recommended to control the infectious process and to prevent wound dehiscence. This stage is critical, since the development of wound dehiscence with infection in a compromised diabetic foot usually leads to a more proximal amputation. Once the infection recedes, as shown by the presence of early granulation tissue and the absence of tissue necrosis, purulent drainage or erythema, the patient may be placed on a once-daily treatment schedule. For closed amputations, HBOT can be decreased to once-daily when the suture line appears clean and dry, without evidence of dehiscence, necrotic or dusky edges, or infection.

In open ulcers, the decision to stop HBOT can be based on the appearance of the wound base soft tissue. A healthy granulation bed and the presence of advancing epithelial wound margins are indicative that the treatment may be discontinued safely. For most patients this usually occurs between 20 and 30 treatments. In addition, transcutaneous oxygen values greater than 40 mmHg at the periwound sites indicate adequate tissue neovascularization. In the absence of significant infection, hyperbaric oxygen therapy can be discontinued, and the patient may be managed with appropriate wound care once $TcPO_2$ values rise above 40 mmHg. In larger wounds, placement of a skin graft or a flap procedure may be required to achieve wound closure. If there is concern about graft or flap viability, a short course of HBO therapy (5-10 treatments) should be started as soon as possible post-operatively.

The objective in treating patients with complicated or compromised diabetic foot ulcers is to minimize tissue loss, resulting in a healed, functional foot. This is accomplished by developing a soft tissue environment in which local debridement or a minor amputation can be successfully performed, thus obviating the need for major amputation or extensive reconstructive procedures.

## SUMMARY

In all patients with compromised wound healing, the cornerstone of therapy is the identification and correction of the underlying etiologic and risk factors that inhibit the wound healing process. The most common etiologic factors in nonhealing diabetic foot ulcers are infection and ischemia. Diabetic patients account for the vast majority of non-traumatic amputations in this country. After eliciting a careful history and performing a detailed physical examination, pertinent laboratory data are obtained. The foot lesion is then graded using Wagner's classification. The use of noninvasive vascular studies and transcutaneous oximetry are essential to determine the degree of ischemia in the lower extremity. The use of transcutaneous oximetry in problem-wound evaluation allows assessment of healing potential, determination of amputation level, and patient selection for HBO therapy. HBO therapy is utilized for those diabetic patients with Wagner Grade 3 or higher ulcers that have failed 30 days of standard wound care which includes revascularization, antibiotic therapy, debridement, offloading, glycemic control, and aggressive wound management. Special consideration should be afforded to patients who require reconstructive surgical procedures. This approach will prevent major amputations and will result in a healed functional foot. The importance of an aggressive multidisciplinary approach to optimize the treatment of diabetic foot disease cannot be overemphasized. Hyperbaric oxygen therapy is an extremely useful adjunctive therapy in the management of patients with compromised and complicated diabetic foot ulcers.

## REFERENCES

1. American Diabetes Association http://www.diabetes.org.

2. Ballard JL, Eke CC, Bunt, TJ, Killen JD. A prospective evaluation of transcutaneous oxygen measurements in the management of diabetic foot problems. J. Vasc. Surg. 1995: 485-492.

3. Baroni G, Porro T, Faglia E, et al. "Hyperbaric oxygen in diabetic gangrene treatment." Diabetes Care. 1987;10(1):81-86.

4. Bassett BE, Bennett PB. Introduction to the Physical and Physiological Bases of Hyperbaric Therapy. JC Davis and TK Hunt (Eds.) Bethesda, MD: Undersea Medical Society, Inc., 1977;11-24.

5. Bendick PJ, Glover JL, Kuebler TW, et al. "Progression of atherosclerosis in diabetics." Surgery. 1983;93(6):834-838.

6. Calligaro KD, Veith FJ. "Proper technique of lower extremity pulse examination." Contemp Surg. 1992;40:49-51.

7. Carrico TJ, Mehrhof AI, Cohen IK. "Biology of wound healing." Surg Clinics of North America. 1984;64(4):721-733.

8. Colen LB. "Limb salvage in the patient with severe peripheral vascular disease: The role of microsurgical free-tissue transfer." Plast Reconstr Surg. 1987;79:389-395.

9. Cruse PJE, Foord R. "A prospective study of 23,649 surgical wounds." Arch Surg. 1973;107:206-210.

10. Davis JC. "The use of adjuvant hyperbaric oxygen in treatment of the diabetic foot." Clinics in Podiatric Medicine and Surgery. 1987;4(2):429-437.

11. Davis JC. "Enhancement of healing." Hyperbaric Oxygen Therapy: A Critical Review. E Camporesi and AC Barker, (Eds.) Bethesda, MD: Undersea and Hyperbaric Medical Society, Inc.; 1991;127-140.

12. Davis JC, Buckley CJ, Barr PO. "Compromised soft tissue wounds: Correction of wound hypoxia." Problem Wounds: The Role of Oxygen. JC Davis and TK Hunt, (Eds.) New York: Elsevier, 1988;143-152.

13. Dowd GSE, Linge K, Bentley G. "Measurement of transcutaneous oxygen pressure in normal and ischemic skin." J Bone Joint Surg. 1983;65B(1):79-83.

14. Faglia Ezio et al. Adjunctive Systemic Hyperbaric Oxygen Therapy in treatment of severe prevalently ischemic diabetic foot ulcer. Diabetes Care 1996 19(12) 1338-1343.

15. Fife CE, Buyukcakir C, Otto GH, Sheffield PJ, Warriner RA, Love TL, Mader J. The predictive value of transcutaneous oxygen tension measurement in diabetic lower extremity ulcers treated with hyperbaric oxygen therapy: a retrospective analysis of 1,144 patients. Wound Repair Regen. 2002 Jul-Aug;10(4):198-207.

16. Fylling CP. "A comprehensive wound management protocol including topical growth factors." Wounds. 1989;1(1):79-86.

17. Goldenburg SG, Alex M, Joschi RA, et al. "Non-atheromatous peripheral disease of the lower extremity in diabetes mellitus." Diabetes. 1959;8:261-273.

18. Goodson WH III, Hunt TK. "Wound healing and the diabetic patient." Surg Gynecol Obst. 1979;149:600-608.

19. Grayson LM, Gibbons GW, Balosh K, Levine E, Karchmer AW. Probing to bone in infected pedal ulcers. JAMA 1995: 273(9) 721-723.

20. Harrelson JM. "Management of the diabetic foot." Orthopedic Clinics of North America. 1989; 20(4):605-619.

21. Harris RW, Andros G, Dulawa LB, et al. "Successful long-term limb salvage using cephalic vein bypass graft." Ann Surg. 1984;200:785-792.

22. Hauser CJ. "Tissue salvage by mapping of skin surface transcutaneous oxygen tension index." Arch Surg. 1987;122:1128-1130.

23. Karanfilian RG, Lynch TG, Zirut VT, et al. "The value of laser Doppler velocimetry and transcutaneous oxygen tension determination in predicting healing of ischemic forefoot ulcerations and amputations in diabetic and nondiabetic patients." J Vasc Surg. 1986;4(5):511-516.

24. Kempczinski R. "Segmental volume plethysmography: The pulse volume recorder." Practical Noninvasive Vascular Diagnosis, 2nd Ed. RF Kempczinski and JST Yao, (Eds.) Chicago: Year Book Medical Publishers, Inc., 1987;140-153.

25. Knighton DR, Ciresi K, Fiegel VD, et al. "Stimulation of repair in chronic, nonhealing, cutaneous ulcers using platelet-derived wound healing formula." Surg Gynecol Obstet. 1990; 170:56-60.

26. Kozak GP and Rowbotham JL. "Diabetic foot disease: A major problem." Management of Diabetic Foot Problems. GP Kozak, CS Hoar, JL Rowbotham, et al., (Eds.) Philadelphia, PA: W.B. Saunders Company, 1984;1-8.

27. Lalka SG, Malone JM, Anderson GG, et al. "Transcutaneous oxygen and carbon dioxide pressure monitoring to determine severity of limb ischemia and to predict surgical outcome." J Vasc Surg. 1988;7(4):507-514.

28. Landsman AS, Meaney DF, Cargill II RS, Macarak EJ and Thiebault LE, "High Strain Rate Tissue deformation: A theory on the mechanical etiology of diabetic foot ulcerations." 1995, J. Am. Podiatric Med. Ass. 85(10):519-527.

29. LaVan FB, Hunt TK. "Oxygen and wound healing." Clinics in Plastic Surg. 1990;17(3):463-472.

30. Leslie C, Sapico FL, Ginunas VJ, et al. "Randomized controlled trial of topical hyperbaric oxygen for treatment of diabetic foot ulcers." Diabetes Care. 1988;11(2):111-115.

31. Levin ME. Preface. The Diabetic Foot. ME Levin and LW O'Neal, (Eds.) St. Louis, MO: CV Mosby, 4th Ed., 1988;ix-x.

32. Levine ME. Pathogenesis and management of diabetic foot lesions. The Diabetic Foot, Mosby, 1993: 17-60.

33. LoGerfo FW, Coffman JD. "Vascular and microvascular disease of the foot in diabetics. Implications for foot care." NEJM. 1984;31(25):1615-1619.

34. Louie TJ, Bartless JG, Tally FP, et al. "Aerobic and anaerobic bacteria in diabetic foot ulcers." Annals of Internal Med. 1976;85:461-463.

35. Mader JT, (Ed.,) Hyperbaric Oxygen Therapy : A Committee Report. Bethesda, MD, 1989;37-44.

36. Malone JM. Complications of Lower Extremity Amputation. WS Moore and JM Malone, (Eds.) Philadelphia, PA: Harcourt, Brace, Jovanovich, Inc. 1989;208-214.

37. Mathieu D and Wattel, FE, (Eds.) "Proceedings of the ECHM Consensus Conference on Hyperbaric Oxygen in the Treatment of Foot Lesions in Diabetic Patients" 1998, University Press, Lille, France.

38. Matos LA. "Preliminary report of the use of hyperbarics as adjunctive therapy in diabetics with chronic non-healing wounds." HBO Review. 1983;4(2):88-89.

39. Morain WD and Colen LB. "Wound healing in diabetes mellitus." Clinics in Plastic Surg. 1990;17(3):493-501.

40. Mueller MJ, Diamond JE, Sinacore DR. Total contact casting in treatment of diabetic plantar ulcers. Diabetes Care 1989 12(6): 384-388.

41. The National Institute of Diabetes and Digestive and Kidney Diseases http://www2.niddk.nih.gov.

42. New Yale Schools of Public Health and Medicine Report: Diabetes Epidemic. Business Wire, Nov 9, 2005.

43. NuÒez AA, Veith FJ, Collier P, et al. "Direct approaches to the distal portions of the deep femoral artery for limb salvage bypasses." J Vasc Surg. 1988;8:576-581.

44. Oishi CS, Fronek A, Golbranson FL. "The role of non-invasive vascular studies in determining levels of amputation." J Bone Joint Surg. 1988;70A(10:1520-1530.

45. O'Neal LW. "Debridement and amputation." The Diabetic Foot. ME Levin and LW O'Neal, (Eds.) St. Louis, MO: C.V. Mosby, 4th Ed., 1988;237-248.

46. Oriani G, Meazza D, Favales F, et al. "Hyperbaric oxygen therapy in diabetic gangrene." J of Hyperbaric Med. 1990;5(3):171-175.

47. Patel GV, Wieman JJ. Effects of metatarsal head resection for diabetic foot ulcers on the dynamic plantar pressure distribution. A.J. of Surg. 1994, 167: 297-301.

48. Pecoraro RE, Reiber GE. "Classification of wounds in diabetic amputees." Wounds. 1990;2(2):65-73.

49. Pecoraro RE, Reiber GE, Burgess EM. Pathways to diabetic limb amputation. Diabetes Care 1990 13(5) 513-521.

50. Perrins DJD and Davis JC. Enhancement of Healing in Soft Tissue Wounds. JC Davis and TK Hunt, (Eds.) Bethesda, MD: Undersea Medical Society, Inc., 1977;229-248.

51. Puricore http://www.puricore.com/developing_wound.aspx.

52. Rabkin JM and Hunt TK. "Infection and oxygen." Problem Wounds: The Role of Oxygen. JC Davis and TK Hunt, (Eds.) New York: Elsevier, 1988;1-16.

53. Robson MC, Stenburg BD, Heggers JP. "Wound healing alterations caused by infection." Clinics in Plastic Surgery. 1990;17(3):485-492.

54. Ruderman NB and Haudenschild CC. "Diabetes as an atherogenic factor: Progress in cardiovascular disease." Diabetes. 1984;26:373-412.

55. Rutherford RB, Flanagan DP, Gupta SK, et al. "Suggested standards for reports dealing with lower extremity ischemia." J Vasc Surg. 1986;4:80-94.

56. Sapico FL, Witte JL, Canawati HN, et al. "The infected foot of the diabetic patient: Quantitative microbiology and analysis of clinical features." Reviews of Infectious Diseases. 1984;6(1):S171-S176.

57. Seltzer MH, Bastidas JA, Cooper DM, et al. "Instant nutritional assessment." J Parent. and Ent. Nutr. 1979;3:157-159.

58. Seltzer MH, Fletcher HS, Slocum BA, et al. "Instant nutritional assessment in the intensive care unit." J Parent. and Ent. Nutri. 1981;5:70-72.

59. Selvin E, Wattanakit K, Steffes MW. HbA1c and Peripheral Arterial Disease in Diabetes: The Atherosclerosis Risk in Communities study. Diabetes Care 29:877-882, 2006.

60. Sheffield PJ. "Tissue oxygen measurements." Problem Wounds: The Role of Oxygen. JC Davis and TK Hunt, (Eds.) New York: Elsevier, 1988;17-51.

61. Sheffield, PJ. "Measuring tissue oxygen tension: a review." Undersea & Hyperbaric Medicine, 1998; 25:179-188.

62. Steed DL, and the Diabetic Ulcer Study Group. "Clinical evaluation of recombinant human platelet-derived growth factor for the treatment of lower extremity diabetic ulcers". J. Vasc. Surg. 1995; 21:71-81.

63. Stone JA, Scott R, Brill LR, Levine BD. The role of hyperbaric oxygen in the treatment of diabetic foot wounds. Diabetes 1995; 44 (Suppl-1)71A.

64. Strandness DE Jr, Schultz RD, Sumner DS, et al. "Ultrasonic flow detection. A useful tool in the evaluation of peripheral vascular disease." Am J Surg. 1967;113:311-320.

65. Taylor LM Jr, Phinney ES, Porter JM. "Present status of reversed vein bypass for lower extremity revascularization." J Vasc Surg. 1986;3:288-297.

66. Veith FJ, Ascer E, Gupta SK, et al. "Tibiotibial vein bypass graft: A new operation for limb salvage." J Vasc Surg. 1985;2:552-557.

67. Veith FJ, Gupta SK, Ascer E, et al. "Six-year prospective multicenter randomized comparison of autologous saphenous vein and expanded polytetrafluoroethylene grafts in infra-inguinal arterial reconstructions." J Vasc Surg. 1986;3:104-114.

68. Veith FJ, Gupta SK, Samson RH, et al. "Progress in limb salvage by reconstructive arterial surgery combined with new or improved adjunctive procedures." Ann Surg. 1981;194:386-401.

69. Veith FJ, Gupta SK, Samson RH, et al. "Superficial femoral and popliteal arteries as inflow sites for distal bypasses." Surgery. 1981;90:980-990.

70. Wagner FW. "The dysvascular foot: A system for diagnosis and treatment." Foot and Ankle. 1981;2(2):64-121.

71. Wattel FE, Mathieu DM, Fossati P, Nevierre RR, Caget JM. Hyperbaric Oxygen in the treatment of diabetic foot lesions. J. Hyperbaric Med 1991: 6 263-268.

# NOTES

CHAPTER 27

# MICROCIRCULATION AND ISCHEMIA-REPERFUSION: BASIC MECHANISMS OF HYPERBARIC OXYGEN

## CHAPTER TWENTY-SEVEN OVERVIEW

# MICROCIRCULATION AND ISCHEMIA-REPERFUSION: BASIC MECHANISMS OF HYPERBARIC OXYGEN

*Richard C. Baynosa, William A. Zamboni*

## ISCHEMIA-REPERFUSION INJURY

Patients with high-energy trauma, extremity compartment syndromes, amputated body parts, or failing flaps all experience varying degrees of tissue ischemia. Despite emergent clinical efforts that successfully restore perfusion in these situations, subsequent microcirculatory failure and tissue necrosis may still ensue (Figure 1). Prolonged periods of ischemia

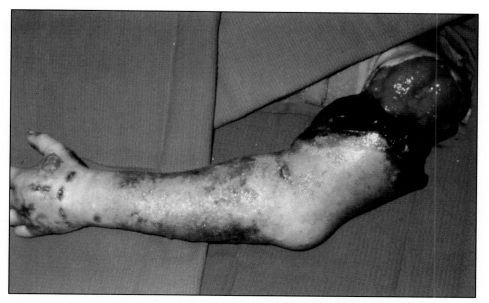

Figure 1. A 10-year old boy sustained a traumatic amputation of the upper extremity from a farm accident that was replanted after 12 hours of ischemia. The above photograph shows the extremity three days after replantation. Although the arterial and venous anastomosis remained patent and the skin perfused, all of the muscle died as a result of reperfusion injury, necessitating revision amputation.

followed by reperfusion can actually lead to accelerated microcirculatory injury and ultimate cell death in many tissues. This phenomenon is known as ischemia-reperfusion (I-R) injury and has been linked to the generation of oxygen-derived free radicals in combination with a dramatic increase in neutrophil adhesion to post-capillary venules during reperfusion. This injury can be severe in extremity traumatic ischemias due to the large muscle mass. Skeletal muscle is very sensitive to ischemia and shows progressive necrosis and loss of function as the ischemic insult is increased. Ischemia-reperfusion injury therefore becomes a significant limiting factor in the successful outcome of the surgical treatment of ischemic skeletal muscle, especially in cases of major limb replantation. Although various tissues have different tolerance levels to ischemia, the final common pathway that results in I-R injury is likely similar. This chapter focuses on the biochemical and microcirculatory mechanisms of I-R injury in addition to the effects of hyperbaric oxygen (HBO), particularly in skin and skeletal muscle.

## PATHOPHYSIOLOGY

### Free Radicals

The biochemistry of I-R injury has been studied extensively and revolves around the production of oxygen-derived free radicals (1, 26). These oxyradicals are highly unstable molecules with an unpaired electron in the outer shell. They are extremely toxic to all biological substances, causing cell death by lipid peroxidation and propagation of more free-radicals. Due to the difficulty in isolating oxyradicals, many investigators have turned to the use of free radical scavengers in animal models of ischemia-reperfusion. Several studies have shown that administration of various free radical scavengers improves survival and function in skin and skeletal muscle subjected to I-R (9, 13, 18, 19, 27). These studies provide indirect evidence that oxyradicals play a central role in the tissue destructive events that occur from I-R injury. The oxyradicals most often implicated in I-R (superoxide and hydroxyl free radicals) come from two important sources: xanthine oxidase and neutrophils (26).

The neutrophil has gained significant attention for its role in I-R injury. Neutrophils are capable of liberating large quantities of extracellular superoxide, which is formed by an enzyme in the cell membrane, NADPH oxidase (Figure 2). Superoxide can then dismutate to hydrogen peroxide, which reacts with ferritin to produce the highly toxic hydroxyl radical. Neutrophilic $H_2O_2$ can also generate the potent oxidant hypochlorous acid (HOCl) via myeloperoxidase enzymes released from azurophilic granules. HOCl may play an additional role in the activation of proteases (elastase, collagenase and gelatinase) released by neutrophils. There is growing evidence that free radical production by activated neutrophils may be more important than XO in producing the tissue-destructive events associated with I-R, particularly in skeletal muscle (14, 22, 39).

### Microcirculation

The proliferation of free radical research has provided a better understanding of the biochemistry of I-R injury. Investigators have more

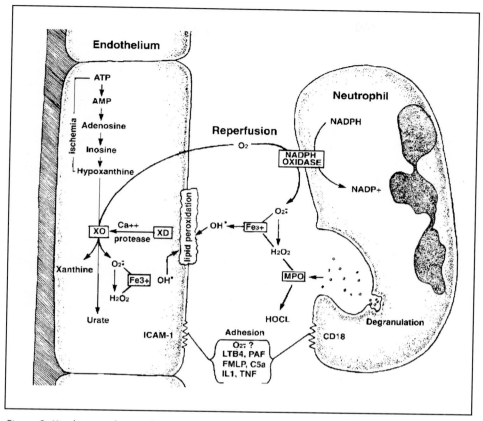

*Figure 2. Xanthine oxidase and neutrophil oxygen free radical generating systems associated with I-R injury (adapted from Inauen) (14).*

recently begun to study the microcirculatory morphology of reperfusion injury including dynamic changes in the microvessels, and the activity of the circulating cellular elements, in particular the leukocytes.

Zamboni et al. (39), using an *in vivo* rat gracilis skeletal muscle preparation, has investigated the effects of I-R on the microcirculation. Quantitative observations of the microcirculation during reperfusion in this study have provided us some insight into the morphology of I-R injury. Following four hours of global ischemia in this model, a significant increase in the number of neutrophils sticking to the endothelium of post capillary venules was noted minutes after the initiation of reperfusion that was not seen in nonischemic control preparations (Figure 3). This increase in neutrophil adhesion was maintained throughout a 3-hour reperfusion observation period. As reperfusion progressed, the venule walls became ill defined from adherent marginating and extravasating leukocytes. Disruption of the endothelial basement membrane adjacent to adherent neutrophils was noted on electron microscopy (Figure 4). These observations suggest that neutrophil adhesion and subsequent release of free radicals is an important early event leading to endothelial damage and microcirculatory failure associated with I-R injury.

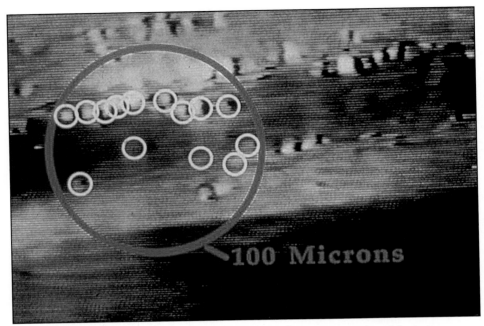

Figure 3. Leukocytes adherent to the endothelium of an ischemic microvenule at 15 minutes reperfusion (700x) were easily identified by their characteristic size and whitish color (39).

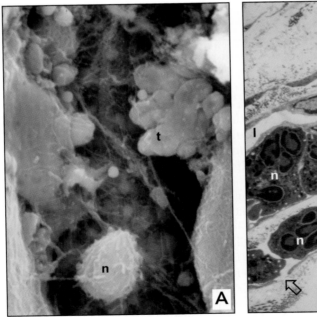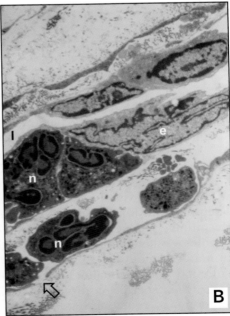

Figure 4A – 4B.
A. Scanning EM (4,500K) showing the lumen of an ischemic venule at 2 hours reperfusion. Note the neutrophil (n) and adjacent thrombus like particulate matter (t) attached to the endothelium.
B. Transmission EM (4,500K) of a similar venule. Note the neutrophils (n) invading the endothelium with disruption of the basement membrane (arrow) e – endothelial cell, l – lumen (39).

Multiple studies have also implicated increased neutrophil-endothelial adhesion as an important pathway in the development of I-R injury (12, 25, 31). Additional support of this mechanism is provided by other skeletal muscle microcirculation studies (11, 20) as well as several experiments which have demonstrated improved tissue survival by altering the number and adherence properties of neutrophils (2, 16, 29, 35). The mechanism of I-R induced neutrophil-endothelial adhesion in skeletal muscle is now known to involve the neutrophil CD18 (beta-2-integrin) adhesion molecule which binds the endothelial ICAM-1 receptor (41, 46). These studies examining this adhesion molecule demonstrated that the neutrophil CD18 adhesion molecule was upregulated by I-R injury and necessary for the initiation of neutrophil-endothelial adhesion. Subsequent confocal microscopy studies have shown that there is not only an upregulation of the CD18 adhesion molecule, but also a morphological change leading to polarization of the CD18 adhesion molecules on the neutrophil surface leading to an increased avidity of neutrophil adhesion to its associated endothelial ICAM-1 receptor (24). This polarization phenomenon in this study has been termed "capping" of the CD18 adhesion molecules on the neutrophil.

Evaluation of the vasoreactivity and flow characteristics of microarterioles is pertinent to the understanding of I-R injury. Feng, et al. (10) measured the venous washout of vasoactive prostaglandins during reperfusion in a rat hind limb ischemia model. He found a significant increase in thromboxane B2 (the stable metabolite of vasoconstricting thromboxane A2) relative to vasodilating prostaglandin E2 in limbs that went on to complete microcirculatory failure. A decrease in venous outflow, in the absence of arteriole thrombosis, was also noted. It was hypothesized from these findings that the impending no-reflow state associated with I-R injury may reflect a global "agonal" vasoconstriction in the microcirculation. Observations of 101 microarterioles in our rat gracilis skeletal muscle preparation have confirmed this hypothesis (39). Measurement of arteriole diameters during reperfusion after 4 hours global ischemia demonstrated an initial reactive vasodilation that was followed at 1 hour by a progressive and severe vasoconstriction. It was interesting that only arterioles in close proximity to venules showed this vasoconstriction, suggesting that the local environment created by the leukocyte-damaged venule is responsible for the arteriole response. Lew et al. (17) have shown that experimental exposure of the microarteriolar vascular smooth muscle to water soluble vasoactive substances produces a much greater response than luminal endothelial exposure. It is possible that the neutrophil damaged venular endothelium results in the release and interstitial diffusion of a vasoactive substance, which causes vasoconstriction in adjacent arterioles. The vasoactive substance causing the I-R induced vasoconstriction in skeletal muscle microarterioles is unknown at this time. Possibilities include thromboxane, serotonin, leukotrienes and impaired endothelial derived relaxing factor, which is now known to be nitric oxide (8, 28, 36, 42).

It is clear from these observations that neutrophil endothelial adherence and microarteriolar vasoconstriction are important morphological events leading to the microcirculatory failure associated with I-R injury. The fact that vasoconstriction occurs in the subset of arterioles adjacent to leukocyte-damaged venules may explain the "heterogeneity" of I-R injury which results in patchy muscle necrosis. This pattern of injury is seen clinically more often than "global" microcirculatory failure and complete necrosis.

# HYPERBARIC OXYGEN

## Basic Studies

The controversy surrounding the use of hyperbaric oxygen for I-R injury has been resolved by numerous studies looking at a variety of different tissues and organs. Initial concern was based on the theory that HBO therapy would exacerbate I-R injury by adding extra oxygen to the system, and increasing free radical production (3, 6). This hypothesis was tested in a rat ischemic axial skin flap experiment in which the authors expected to see decreased flap survival with HBO treatment (37). Instead, the administration of HBO during reperfusion significantly improved skin flap survival following 8 hours of global ischemia. This beneficial effect on I-R injury was also noted in a follow-up study in which laser Doppler analysis during reperfusion showed increased microvascular blood flow in ischemic skin flaps treated with HBO (38). These unexpected findings corroborate the results of Kaelin et al. (15) in which HBO treatment during reperfusion significantly improved free skin flap survival in rats following microvascular reattachment with ischemia times up to 24 hours. Experiments have also shown that hyperbaric oxygen is beneficial after a secondary ischemic insult by significantly reducing necrosis in both skin flaps and skeletal muscle (43, 44). It can be concluded from these animal studies that HBO therapy does not exacerbate, but rather counteracts the ill effects of I-R injury resulting in increased microvascular perfusion and improved skin-flap survival.

Although the skin-flap studies are interesting, the effect of HBO on I-R injury of skeletal muscle has more important clinical significance, especially with regard to limb replantation and the traumatic ischemias. HBO therapy has been shown experimentally to reduce skeletal muscle edema and necrosis in rat hind limb tourniquet ischemia (21) and dog hind limb compartment syndrome models (30). One hypothesis for this beneficial effect is hyperoxia-induced vasoconstriction, which theoretically decreases edema by reducing capillary pressure. Although hyperoxia-induced vasoconstriction may be marked in cerebral arterioles (4, 7), reducing blood flow 40%, the effect on limb blood flow reduction is minimal (4, 5) (12 to 18.9%), making vasoconstriction unlikely as the primary mechanism for reducing skeletal muscle edema. In order to further delineate additional mechanisms, Zamboni et al. (39) studied the effect of HBO on the microcirculatory morphology of I-R in rat gracilis muscle, specifically evaluating leukocyte endothelial adherence and vasoactivity by measurement of microarteriole diameters. The most striking observation during reperfusion in this study was the significant reduction of leukocytes adherent to venular endothelium in preparations treated with HBO during and immediately following 4 hours of ischemia (Figure 5). The vein walls in these treatment groups remained clear and well defined throughout the 3-hour reperfusion observation period. HBO initiated 1 hour after reperfusion also significantly reduced leukocyte adherence, but not as

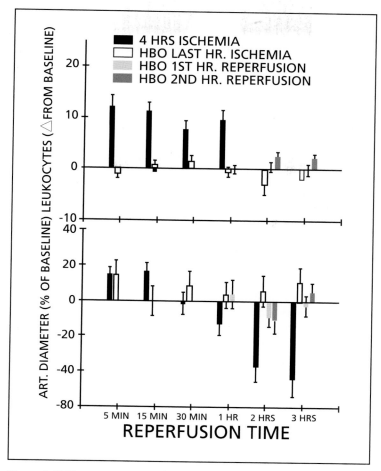

Figure 5. HBO treatment up to 1 hour reperfusion significantly reduced the number of leukocytes sticking to the endothelium (above) and inhibited the progressive vasoconstriction in arterioles adjacent to venules (below) compared to reperfused ischemic nontreated vessels (39).

effectively. The progressive arteriolar vasoconstriction seen in untreated reperfused vessels was also inhibited by HBO therapy administered during and up to 1 hour following ischemia (Figure 5). HBO administered to nonischemic muscle had no effect on subsequent leukocyte adherence or arteriolar diameters. These results demonstrate that any vasoconstriction in microarterioles occurring during HBO exposure does not persist beyond the treatment. Although HBO therapy initiated 1 hour after reperfusion prevented ischemic arteriolar vasoconstriction, deterioration of the microcirculation preparation after 3 hours obviated the addition of delayed HBO treatment groups. It is likely that the timing of HBO therapy in relation to I-R injury is important in producing a beneficial response.

The beneficial effects of HBO on ischemic tissue are systemic and not local (37). The systemic mechanism by which HBO decreases neutrophil adherence during reperfusion is not yet known but ongoing research provides optimism that this mechanism will soon be elucidated. A direct action of HBO at the neutrophil-endothelial interface is one possibility. Kaelin (15) found a significant increase in the activity of the free radical scavenger superoxide dismutase (SOD) in rats with ischemic skin flaps treated by HBO. If superoxide is playing a direct or indirect role in neutrophil endothelial adhesion, then increased SOD activity may decrease this adherence. Thom (32) studied lipid peroxidation *in vitro* and demonstrated that hyperoxia alters the free radical pathway in favor of hydroperoxyl radical formation. These quenching radicals react with lipid radicals to form nonradical products. This termination reaction antagonizes and significantly reduces lipid peroxidation. This stabilizing effect may reduce endothelial activation upon reperfusion resulting in decreased neutrophil adherence. Although we initially considered the possibility of HBO promoting preferential sequestration of neutrophils in the lungs, it is now known that this does not occur in response to skeletal muscle I-R injury (45).

Thom (33) studied an animal model of brain reperfusion injury to show that conversion of xanthine dehydrogenase (XD) to the free radical-forming XO was responsible for lipid peroxidation. More recently, Thom examined the effect of HBO exposure to human neutrophils and noted an inhibition of the CD18 (beta-2-integrin) function that prevented neutrophil adherence while having no effect on the cell surface expression of the adhesion molecules (34). This observed HBO-mediated inhibition of neutrophil CD18 function would prevent adherence/activation and release of proteases known to stimulate XD to XO conversion. It is interesting that the brain biochemical I-R studies by Thom, as well as the skeletal muscle microcirculation morphology studies done in our laboratory, appear to substantiate a final common pathway in which HBO is inhibiting neutrophil adherence and the deleterious cascade of events that follow reperfusion. It is apparent that the endothelial-neutrophil interaction associated with I-R is complex and multiple studies have recently focused on the effects of HBO on cellular adhesion molecules (CAMs) in attenuating the I-R induced neutrophil adhesion.

Experiments in a rat skeletal muscle model corroborate the observation that CD18 cell surface expression is not altered by HBO exposure (46, 49). There is recent evidence that the mechanism by which HBO inhibits neutrophil adhesion involves a qualitative change in the CD18 adhesion molecule through cellular alterations in cyclic GMP (34, 46-48). Preliminary work employing harvested neutrophils from an *in vivo* rat skeletal muscle model using confocal microscopy has suggested that the qualitative change in these CAMs may be secondary to a change in the polarization of the CD18 molecules on the neutrophil surface (23). This essentially would indicate a reversal of the neutrophil "capping" previously seen using confocal microscopy after I-R injury (24).

In addition to the scientific work centering on the effect of HBO on the neutrophil, some investigators have focused on the changes encountered by endothelial cells exposed to HBO after I-R injury. Activation of endothelial cells due to ischemia and subsequent reperfusion triggers the expression of CAMs such as E-selectin and ICAM-1 through transcription and translation (50, 51). *In vitro* studies using both bovine and human endothelial cells by

Buras et al. confirmed that mock ischemia with hypoxia and hypoglycemia was capable of inducing increased expression of ICAM-1. These investigators further showed that treatment of the endothelial cells with HBO for 90 minutes at 2.5 ATA decreased the expression of ICAM-1 with a reduction of PMN binding to the endothelial surface (52). These findings were further corroborated by *in vivo* studies in a rodent skeletal muscle flap model which also demonstrated that HBO was able to reduce ICAM-1 expression, reduce neutrophil adhesion, and improve overall flap survival (49).

Nitric oxide (NO) has been implicated as an important regulator of several aspects of I-R injury including vascular tone and neutrophil adhesion (53). Research involving the role of NO in the beneficial effects of HBO has shed further light on the possible basic mechanisms of HBO's protective effects. Studies in a rat model revealed that the decreased neutrophil adhesion provided by HBO treatment was reversed when the experimental rats were treated with the NO-blocker L-NAME (47). These investigators also suggested that the NO upregulation induced by HBO may inhibit neutrophil CD18 (beta-2-integrin) function by inhibiting membrane-associated cyclic GMP synthesis (47). More recent studies have quantitatively documented an increase in nitric oxide in the cerebral cortex and abdominal aorta of rats exposed to HBO (54, 55). While these studies implicate the neuronal-derived form of nitric oxide synthase (NOS) as the source of increased NO, they focus on the cerebral tissue and the peri-aortic area and not the microcirculation. It is likely that different organs and tissues may be influenced by other forms of NOS, particularly the endothelial-derived form (eNOS) that is associated with the endothelial cells of the microcirculation. Indeed, preliminary work in our laboratory has demonstrated a time-dependent effect of HBO on eNOS activity as well as transcription and translation in examining both the microcirculation as well as the systemic circulation (56-58). These studies suggest that after HBO treatment for I-R injury there is an early increase in eNOS activity locally followed by a late phase (24 hours of reperfusion) increase in eNOS transcription and translation in the systemic circulation (56-58). In addition, other preliminary studies have implicated vascular endothelial growth factor (VEGF) as a possible regulating factor by demonstrating an increase in VEGF transcription in the skeletal muscle subjected to I-R injury (56). Moreover, the decrease in neutrophil adherence seen in our rat muscle flap model with HBO was reversed after pretreatment of the rodents with a functional VEGF monoclonal antibody (59).

The biochemical and microcirculation studies of HBO and I-R injury are important from a mechanistic point of view and should be continued. Studies evaluating the ultimate function in skeletal muscle subjected to I-R injury may be more important and clinically relevant. Surgical restoration of blood flow following a traumatic crush injury or amputation may result in a viable extremity, but if a significant portion of the muscle dies from I-R injury, then fibrosis will occur and function will be compromised.

## Clinical Applications

The primary treatment for traumatic extremity injury with arterial compromise is surgical restoration of blood flow. Fracture fixation, arterial repair, fasciotomy to prevent compartment syndrome, and replantation in selected cases, are necessary interventions for limb salvage. Hyperbaric oxygen is an important adjunctive treatment, especially if the tissue is at risk for reperfusion injury. The skeletal muscle is particularly at risk due to its sensitivity to ischemia. The degree of muscle damage from I-R injury is proportional to the ischemic interval, especially in cases of warm ischemia. Some degree of permanent damage to the muscle can be expected when ischemia times exceed four to six hours.

It is important to understand that the majority of microcirculatory damage from ischemia occurs during the first six to seven hours of reperfusion (60). Therefore, early recognition and treatment become critical. We are currently using HBO to treat most patients with revascularized or replanted extremities, and ischemia times greater than six hours. We are also treating patients who experience the occasional free muscle flap vascular thrombosis requiring re-exploration and anastomotic revision in which a secondary ischemic interval has occurred. These patients are taken directly from the recovery room and, often from the operating room, to the hyperbaric medical unit for treatment. The traumatic ischemia protocol outlined in the Hyperbaric Oxygen Therapy Committee Report is followed. We have treated patients with ischemia times up to 14 hours (Figures 6 and 7) and have noted excellent muscle survival and a remarkable reduction in soft tissue edema.

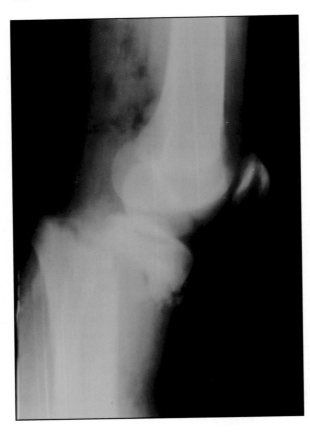

Figure 6. A teenage cheerleader involved in a 3-wheeler accident sustained a severe proximal tibia fracture (left) resulting in popliteal artery disruption. Due to extenuating circumstances, a 14-hour warm ischemia time elapsed before successful revascularization with a vein graft was accomplished. A primary amputation was considered but instead lower leg fasciotomies were performed and she was treated immediately with HBO using the traumatic ischemia protocol.

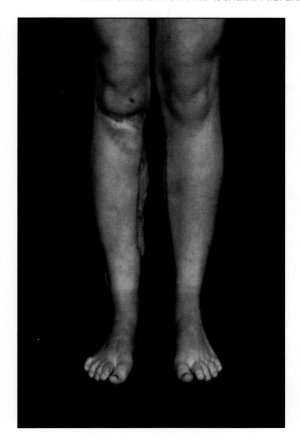

*Figure 7. The teenage cheerleader obtained 100% survival of the muscle and regained normal function of her leg (one year post-op).*

Since most of these patients are still drowsy post anesthesia, they are unable to cooperate with ear clearing techniques, and frequently develop hemotympanum (61). We are currently placing myringotomy tubes prophylactically in most patients entering the traumatic ischemia protocol, especially in the elderly age group. The HBO treatments are otherwise well tolerated by patients, and give us a readily available tool to help ameliorate the ill effects of I-R injury. Although our results have been good, we recognize that this information is anecdotal. A recent systematic review by Garcia-Covarrubias et al. regarding the use of HBO in the management of crush injury and traumatic ischemia located eight retrospective, uncontrolled studies or case series lacking a standardized methodology and one prospective controlled randomized trial with some design limitations (62). Their analysis determined that eight of the nine studies showed a beneficial effect with only one major complication. They concluded that adjunctive HBO is not likely to be harmful and could be beneficial if administered early (62). Definitive proof of the potential benefit of HBO on I-R injury will require a well-controlled, prospective, randomized clinical trial.

## SUMMARY

Acute HBO therapy does not exacerbate I-R injury. Rather, a large body of experimental evidence is accumulating from animal skin flap studies, quantitative skeletal muscle microcirculation observations, and biochemical experiments that demonstrate that HBO treatment antagonizes I-R injury. The microvascular preservation afforded by HBO (Figure 8) appears to play a central role in treating skeletal muscle I-R injury that may accompany extremity crush injury, compartment syndrome, major limb replantation/revascularization, and acutely failing flaps.

The application of HBO may eventually extrapolate to other tissues subjected to I-R injury including brain, intestine, kidney and heart. Indeed, several recent basic science studies in rodents have demonstrated a protective role for HBO in renal, intestinal, and cardiac ischemia reperfusion as well as I-R injury related to hemorrhagic and embolic stroke (63-67). The progress made in recent years has been significant but there is still a need for further quality basic-science research, as well as well-controlled prospective clinical studies to fully understand, and further define the effectiveness of HBO in the treatment of I-R injury.

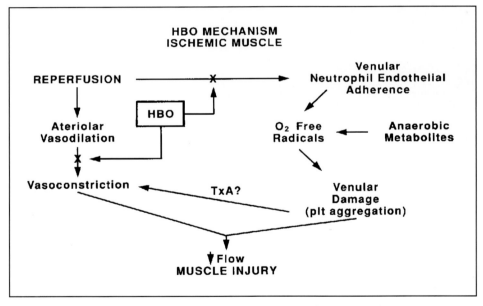

*Figure 8. Reperfusion cascade leading to skeletal muscle injury after prolonged ischemia. HBO treatment protects the microcirculation by blocking neutrophil endothelial adherence and inhibiting subsequent arteriolar vasoconstriction (39).*

## REFERENCES

1. Angel MF, Ramasastry SS, Swartz WM, et al. "Free radicals: Basic concepts concerning their chemistry, pathophysiology, and relevance to plastic surgery." Plast Reconstr Surg. 1987;79:990.

2. Belkin M, LaMorte WL, Wright JG, Hobson RW. "The role of leukocytes in the pathophysiology of skeletal muscle ischemic injury." J Vasc Surg. 1989;10:14.

3. Benke PJ. "Jessica in the well: Ischemia and reperfusion injury." JAMA. 1988;259:1326.

4. Bergofsky EH, Bertun P. "Response of regional circulations to hyperoxia." J Appl Physiol. 1966;21:567.

5. Bird AD, Telfer ABM. "Effect of hyperbaric oxygen on limb circulation." Lancet. 1965;1:355.

6. Davis JC. "Jessica in the well. Ischemia and reperfusion injury." JAMA. 1988;259:3558.

7. Dollery CT, Hill DW, Mailer CM, Ramelho PS. "High oxygen pressure and the retinal blood vessels." Lancet. 1964;ii:291.

8. Eidt JF, Ashton J, Golino P, et al. "Thromboxane A2 and serotonin mediate coronary blood flow reductions in unsedated dogs." Am J Physiol. 1989;257:H873.

9. Feller AM, Roth AC, Russell RC, et al. "Experimental evaluation of oxygen free radical scavengers in prevention of reperfusion injury to skeletal muscle." Ann Plast Surg. 1989;22:321.

10. Feng LJ, Berger BE, Lysz TW, Shaw WW. "Vasoactive prostaglandins in the impending no-reflow state: Evidence for a primary disturbance in microvascular tone." Plast Reconstr Surg. 1988;81:755.

11. Goldberg M, Serafin D, Klitzman B. "Quantification of neutrophil adhesion to skeletal muscle venules following ischemia-reperfusion." J Reconstr Micro. 1990;6:267.

12. Granger DN, Benoit JN, Suzuki M, Grisham MB. "Leukocyte adherence to venular endothelium during ischemia-reperfusion." Am J Physiol. 1989;257:G683.

13. Im JM, Manson PN, Bulkley GB, Hoopes JE. "Effects of superoxide dismutase and allopurinol on the survival of acute island skin flaps." Ann Surg. 1985;201:357.

14. Inauen W, Suzuki M, Granger DN. "Mechanisms of cellular injury: potential source of oxygen free radicals in ischemia/reperfusion." Microcirculation, Endothelium and Lymphatics. 1989;5:143.

15. Kaelin CM, Im MJ, Myers RAM, et al. "The effects of hyperbaric oxygen on free flaps in rats." Arch Surg. 1990;125:607.

16. Lee C, Kerrigan CL, Picard-Ami LA. "Cyclophosphamide induced neutropenia: effect on postischemic skin flap survival." Plast Reconstr Surg. 1992;89:1092.

17. Lew MJ, Rivers RJ, Duling BR. "Arteriolar smooth muscle responses are modulated by an intramural diffusion barrier." Am J Physiol. 1989;257:H10.

18. Manson PN, Anthenelli RM, Im MJ, et al. "The role of oxygen-free radicals in ischemic tissue injury in island skin flaps." Ann Surg. 1983;198:87.

19. Marzella L, Jesudass RR, Manson PN, et al. "Functional and structural evaluation of the vasculature of skin flaps after ischemia and reperfusion." Plast Reconstr Surg. 1988;81:742.

20. Messina LM. "*In vivo* assessment of acute microvascular injury after reperfusion of ischemic tibialis anterior muscle of the hamster." J Surg Res. 1990;48:615.

21. Nylander G, Lewis D, Nordstr_m H, Larsson J. "Reduction of postischemic edema with hyperbaric oxygen." Plast Reconstr Surg. 1985;76:596.

22. Pang CY. "Ischemia-induced reperfusion injury in muscle flaps: pathogenesis and major source of free radicals." J Reconstr Micro. 1990;6:77.

23. Jones S, Wang WZ, Nataraj C, Stephenson LL, Khiabani KT, Zamboni WA. "HBO inhibits IR-induced neutrophil CD18 polarization by a nitric oxide mechanism." Unders Hyperb Med. 2002; 35: 75 (suppl).

24. Khiabani KT, Stephenson LL, Gabriel A, Nataraj C, Wang WZ, Zamboni WA. "A quantitative method for determining polarization of neutrophil adhesion molecules associated with ischemia reperfusion." Plast Reconstr Surg. 2004; 114:1846-1850.

25. Roth AC, Russell AC, Suchy H, Kalita S. "The increased neutrophil adherence seen following ischemia in skeletal muscle is not superoxide dependent." FASEB J. 1990;4:A267.

26. Russell RC, Roth AC, Kucan JO, Zook EG. "Reperfusion injury and oxygen free radicals. A review." J Reconstr Micro. 1989;5:79.

27. Sagi A, Ferder M, Levens D, Strauch B. "Improved survival of island flaps after prolonged ischemia by perfusion with superoxide dismutase." Plast Reconstr Surg. 1986;77:639.

28. Schumacher WA, Heran CL, Allen GT, Ogletree ML. "Leukotrienes cause mesenteric vasoconstriction and hemoconcentration in rats without activating thromboxane receptors." Prostaglandins. 1989;38:335.

29. Simpson PJ, Todd RF, Mickelson JK, et al. "Sustained limitation of myocardial reperfusion injury by a monoclonal antibody that inhibits leukocyte adhesion." Circulation. 1990;81:226.

30. Strauss MB, Hargens AR, Gershuni DH, et al. "Reduction of skeletal muscle necrosis using intermittent hyperbaric oxygen in a model compartment syndrome." J Bone Joint Surg. 1983;65-A:656.

31. Suzuki M, Inauen W, Kvietys PR, et al. "Superoxide mediates reperfusion-induced leukocyte-endothelial cell interactions." Am J Physiol. 1989;257:H1740.

32. Thom SR, Elbukin ME. "Oxygen dependent antagonism of lipid peroxidation." Free Radical Biology and Medicine. 1991;10:413.

33. Thom SR. "Xanthine dehydrogenase conversion to oxidase and lipid peroxidation in brain after CO poisoning." J of Applied Physiology. 1992;73:1584.

34. Thom SR, Mendiguren I, Hardy K, Bolotin T, Fisher D, Nebolon M, Kilpatrick L. "Inhibition of human neutrophil beta2-integrin-dependent adherence by hyperbaric O2." Am J Physiol. 1997; 272: C770-777.

35. Vedder NB, Fouty BW, Winn RK, et al. "Role of neutrophils in generalized reperfusion injury associated with resuscitation from shock." Surgery. 1989;106:509.

36. Warren JB, Maltby NH, MacCormack D, Barnes PJ. "Pulmonary endothelium-derived relaxing factor is impaired in hypoxia." Clinical Science. 1989;77:671.

37. Zamboni WA, Roth AC, Russell RC, Nemiroff PM, Cassas L, Smoot EC. "The effect of acute hyperbaric oxygen therapy on axial pattern skin flap survival when administered during and after total ischemia." J Reconstr Micro. 1989;5:343.

38. Zamboni WA, Roth AC, Russell RC, Smoot EC. "Effect of hyperbaric oxygen on reperfusion of ischemic axial skin flaps: a laser doppler analysis." Ann Plast Surg. 1992;28:339.

39. Zamboni WA, Roth AC, Russell RC, Graham B, Suchy H, Kucan JO. "Morphological analysis of the microcirculation during reperfusion of ischemic skeletal muscle and the effect of hyperbaric oxygen." Plast Reconstr Surg. 1993;91:1110-1123.

40. Zamboni WA, Roth AC, Bergman BA, Russell RC, Stephenson LL, Suchy H. "Experimental evaluation of oxygen in the treatment of ischemic skeletal muscle." Undersea Biomedical Research. (Abstract). 1992;19(Suppl):78.

41. Zamboni WA, Stephenson LL, Roth AC, Suchy H, Russell RC. "Ischemia-reperfusion injury in skeletal muscle: CE18 dependent neutrophil-endothelial adhesion and arteriolar vasoconstriction." Plast Reconstr Surg 1997;99:2002-2007.

42. Billiar TR. "Nitric oxide: Novel biology with clinical relevance." Ann Surg 1995;221:339-349.

43. Stevens DM, Weiss DD, Koller, WA, Bianchi DA. "Survival of normothermic microvascular flaps after prolonged secondary ischemia: Effects of hyperbaric oxygen." Otolaryngol Head Neck Surg 1996;115:360-364.

44. Wong HP, Zamboni WA, Stephenson LL. "Effect of hyperbaric oxygen on skeletal muscle necrosis following primary and secondary ischemia in a rat model." Surgical Forum 1996;XLVII:705-707.

45. Zamboni WA, Wong HP, Stephenson LL. "Effect of hyperbaric oxygen on neutrophil concentration and pulmonary sequestration in ischemia-reperfusion injury." Arch Surg 1996;131:756-760.

46. Larson JL, Stephenson LL, Zamboni WA. "The effects of HBO treatment on PMN expression of CD18 in a rat model of ischemia reperfusion (IR)." Undersea Hyperbar Med. 1998;25.

47. Banick PD, Chen Q, Xu YA, Thom SR. "Nitric oxide inhibits neutrophil beta 2 integrin function by inhibiting membrane-associated cyclic GMP synthesis." J Cell Physiol 1997;172:12-24.

48. Chen Q, Banick PD, Thom SR. "Functional inhibition of rat polymorphonuclear leukocyte beta2 integrins by hyperbaric oxygen is associated with impaired cGMP synthesis." J Pharmacol Exp Therapeutics. 1996; 276: 929-933.

49. Hong JP, Kwon H, Chung YK, et al. "The effect of hyperbaric oxygen on ischemia-reperfusion injury: An experimental study in a rat musculocutaneous flap." Ann Plast Surg. 2003; 51: 478-487.

50. Buras JA. "Basic mechanisms of hyperbaric oxygen in the treatment of ischemia-reperfusion injury." Int Anesthesiol Clin. 2000; 38: 91-109.

51. Buras JA, Reenstra WR. "Endothelial-neutrophil interactions during ischemia and reperfusion injury: basic mechanisms of hyperbaric oxygen." Neurol Res. 2007; 29: 127-131.

52. Buras JA, Stahl GL, Svoboda KK, Reenstra WR. "Hyperbaric oxygen downregulates ICAM-1 expression induced by hypoxia and hypoglycemia: The role of NOS." Am J Physiol Cell Physiol. 2000; 278: C292-C302.

53. Lefer AM, Lefer DJ. "The role of nitric oxide and cell adhesion molecules on the microcirculation in ischaemia-reperfusion." Cardiovasc Res. 1996; 32: 743-751.

54. Thom SR, Bhopale V, Fisher D, Manevich Y, Huang PL, Buerk DG. "Stimulation of nitric oxide synthase in cerebral cortex due to elevated partial pressures of oxygen: an oxidative stress response." J Neurobiol. 2002; 51: 85-100.

55. Thom SR, Fisher D, Zhang J, Bhopale VM, Ohnishi ST, Kotake Y, Ohnishi T, Buerk DG. "Stimulation of perivascular nitric oxide synthesis by oxygen." Am J Physiol Heart Circ Physiol. 2003; 284: H1230-H1239.

56. Baynosa RC, Khiabani KT, Stephenson LL, Fang XH, Wang WZ, Zamboni WA. "The effect of hyperbaric oxygen on nitric oxide synthase and vascular endothelial growth factor expression in ischemia-reperfusion injury." J Amer Coll Surg. 2004; 199: S65 (suppl).

57. Baynosa RC, Naig AL, Murphy PS, Hansen B, Fang XH, Stephenson LL, Khiabani KT, Wang WZ, Zamboni WA. "The effect of hyperbaric oxygen on NOS activity and transcription in ischemia reperfusion injury." J Amer Coll Surg. 2005; 200: S57-S58 (suppl).

58. Baynosa RC, Graves AK, Fang XH, Stephenson LL, Khiabani KT, Wang WZ, Zamboni WA. "The effect of hyperbaric oxygen on eNOS protein expression in ischemia reperfusion injury." Plast Reconstr Surg. 2007; 120: 73 (suppl).

59. Ellis CM, Hansen BK, Baynosa RC, Stephenson LL, Khiabani KT, Wang WZ, Zamboni WA. "Hyperbaric oxygen decreases neutrophil adherence in ischemia reperfusion by a VEGF-dependent mechanism." J Amer Coll Surg. 2005; 200: S57 (suppl).

60. Olivas TP Saylor, TF, Wong, HP, Stephenson, LL, Zamboni, WA. "The Timing of Microcirculatory Injury from Ischemia Reperfusion". Plast Reconstr Surg. 2001; 107: 785-788.

61. Presswood G, Zamboni WA, Stephenson LL, Santos PM. "Effect of artificial airway on ear complications from hyperbaric oxygen." Laryngoscope 1994;104:1383-1384.

62. Garcia-Covarrubias L, McSwain NE, Van Meter K, Bell RM. "Adjuvant hyperbaric oxygen therapy in the management of crush injury and traumatic ischemia: and evidence-based approach." Amer Surg. 2005; 71: 144-150.

63. Gurer A, Ozdogan M, Gomceli I, Demirag A, Gulbahar O, Arikok T, Kulacoglu H, Dundar K, Ozlem N. "Hyperbaric oxygenation attenuates renal ischemia-reperfusion injury in rats." Transplant Proc. 2006; 38: 3337-3340.

64. Bertoletto PR, Fagundes DJ, De Jesus Simoes M, Oshima CT, De Souza Montero EF, Simoes RS, Fagundes AT. "Effects of hyperbaric oxygen therapy on the rat intestinal mucosa apoptosis caused by ischemia-reperfusion injury." Microsurgery. 2007; 27: 224-227.

65. Cabigas BP, Su J, Hutchins W, Shi Y, Schaefer RB, Recinos RF, Nilakantan V, Kindwall E, Niezgoda JA, Baker JE. "Hyperoxic and hyperbaric-induced cardioprotection: role of nitric oxide synthase 3." Cardiovasc Res. 2006; 72: 143-151.

66. Qin Z, Karabiyikoglu M, Hua Y, Silbergleit R, He Y, Keep RF, Xi G. "Hyperbaric oxygen-induced attenuation of hemorrhagic transformation after experimental focal transient cerebral ischemia." Stroke. 2007; 38: 1362-1367.

67. Henninger N, Kuppers-Tiedt L, Sicard KM, Gunther A, Schneider D, Schwab, S. "Neuroprotective effect of hyperbaric oxygen therapy monitored by MR-imaging after embolic stroke in rats." Exp Neurol. 2006; 201: 316-323.

# NOTES

CHAPTER **28**

# THE ROLE OF HYPERBARIC OXYGEN IN CRUSH INJURY, SKELETAL MUSCLE-COMPARTMENT SYNDROME, AND OTHER ACUTE TRAUMATIC ISCHEMIAS

## CHAPTER TWENTY-EIGHT OVERVIEW

# THE ROLE OF HYPERBARIC OXYGEN IN CRUSH INJURY, SKELETAL MUSCLE-COMPARTMENT SYNDROME, AND OTHER ACUTE TRAUMATIC ISCHEMIAS

*Michael B. Strauss, Stuart S. Miller*

## INTRODUCTION

Hyperbaric oxygen (HBO) has been used as adjunct for the management of crush injury and compartment syndrome since its mechanisms and indications were first delineated in 1977 (1, 2). Several other conditions including frostbite, thermal burns, threatened flaps/grafts and compromised replantations have similar pathophysiology and hence can be classified along with crush injury and compartment syndrome as acute traumatic peripheral ischemias, henceforth referred to as traumatic ischemias. In addition to all having trauma (physical, thermal, surgical) as a cause, three unifying factors are present in these conditions, namely: 1) Tissue hypoxia, 2) Edema and 3) A gradient of injury (Figure 1). Tissue hypoxia and edema lead to self-perpetuation, a "vicious circle" of the injury, and cause tissue damage of and beyond that sustained from the original trauma. The primary role of HBO for these conditions is to counteract tissue hypoxia and edema in order to prevent progression of tissue damage. This chapter will give primary attention to crush injury and compartment syndrome. Information on burns and threatened flaps are presented in other chapters in this text.

## PATHOPHYSIOLOGY OF TRAUMATIC ISCHEMIAS

It is essential that an adequate blood supply be maintained to traumatized tissues, in order for them to survive, heal and recover function. Ischemia is the major cause of tissue hypoxia in the traumatic ischemias. It may arise from injury to large, potentially surgically reparable blood vessels, blood vessels too small to be repaired surgically or both. Local hypoxia occurs because of a direct result of trauma to blood vessels or an indirect consequence

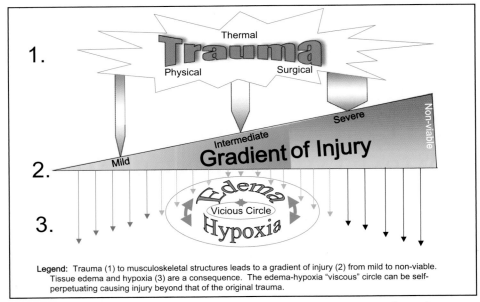

Figure 1. Factors that unify the acute traumatic peripheral ischemias (traumatic Ischemias).

of the injury. In the latter, decreased flow in the microcirculation occurs as a consequence of extravasation from the damaged blood vessels (with or without vascular collapse from the external pressure of the tissue fluid), stasis, vasoconstriction, thrombosis, or a combination of these processes (Figure 2). The consequence of the above causes of ischemia is hypoxia. Without the availability of sufficient oxygen, tissues are unable to meet their metabolic needs. During the early phase of healing and infection control, the metabolic needs of tissues increase by a factor of 20 or more (3).

Without increased blood flow, these new metabolic demands will not be met. The likelihood of non-healing wounds, non-functional tissues, necrosis, infections or combinations of these, increase in direct proportion to the amount of the ischemic insult.

Edema also contributes to tissue hypoxia. It arises either from extravasation of intravascular fluid (vasogenic causes) or leakage of intracellular fluid to the extracellar spaces (cytogenic causes). Vasogenic edema occurs after direct trauma to blood and lymphatic vessels, increased tissue-perfusion pressure, decreased venous outflow, and decreased intravascular oncotic pressure, all of which can be associated with trauma. Hypoxia is an important

*It is interesting to note that the importance of a blood supply is mentioned in the Bible, for it is stated that "...the life of all flesh [is] the blood thereof." (Leviticus 17:14)*

*During the initial phase of wound healing and infection control, the metabolic demands and blood flow requirements need to increase 20-fold or more.*

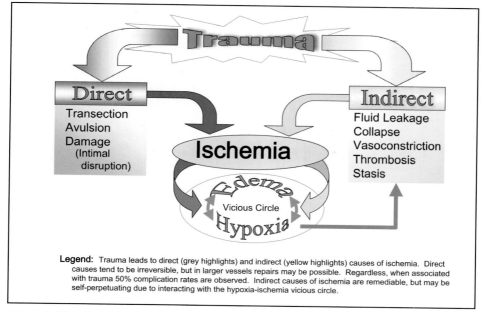

*Figure 2. Blood vessel injury types as causes of ischemia and their consequences in traumatic ischemias.*

contributor to cytogenic edema since maintenance of intracellular fluid balance is an oxygen dependent mechanism (4, 5). Edema has detrimental effects on wound healing and infection control. It increases the diffusion distance of oxygen, which is essential for cell metabolic function, through the tissue fluids from capillaries to cells (Figures 3A, 3B and 3C). Oxygen has limited diffusability through tissue fluids and falls off rapidly as the distance increases. This contrasts sharply to carbon dioxide, a waste product of cellular metabolism, which has 20 times the diffusability through tissue fluids as oxygen (6). The diffusion distance of oxygen through tissue fluid is proportional to the square root of the oxygen content in the capillary (7). Consequently, oxygen diffusion through tissue fluids is decreased by an exponential factor as edema increases the distance from the capillary to the cell.

A second harmful effect of edema is collapse of the microcirculation. This occurs as interstitial fluid pressure around the capillaries increases with accumulation of edema. This is a problem that occurs in closed spaces such as skeletal muscles enclosed in fascia, the intracranial compartment, nerve tunnels, the peritoneum (abdominal compartment syndrome) and perhaps visceral organs that are covered with well defined serosal membranes. Once the interstitial fluid pressure exceeds the capillary perfusion pressure in the closed

*Oxygen diffusability through tissue fluids is 1/20th that of carbon dioxide and decreases in an exponential fashion as the diffusion distance from the capillary to the cell increases. Consequently, edema can severely interfere with tissue oxygenation. It can be somewhat mitigated by increasing the oxygen tensions in the plasma, for example, with hyperbaric oxygen.*

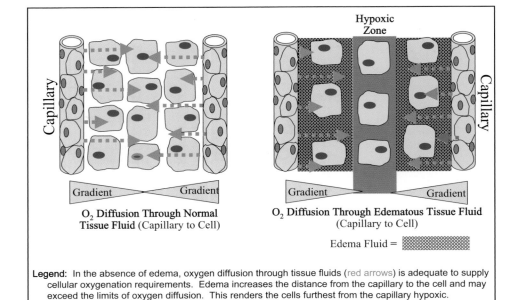

Legend: In the absence of edema, oxygen diffusion through tissue fluids (red arrows) is adequate to supply cellular oxygenation requirements. Edema increases the distance from the capillary to the cell and may exceed the limits of oxygen diffusion. This renders the cells furthest from the capillary hypoxic.

*Figure 3A. Edema as a contributor to cellular hypoxia.*

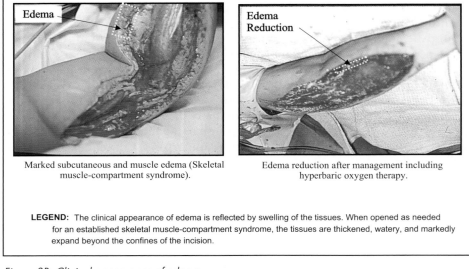

Marked subcutaneous and muscle edema (Skeletal muscle-compartment syndrome).

Edema reduction after management including hyperbaric oxygen therapy.

LEGEND: The clinical appearance of edema is reflected by swelling of the tissues. When opened as needed for an established skeletal muscle-compartment syndrome, the tissues are thickened, watery, and markedly expand beyond the confines of the incision.

*Figure 3B. Clinical appearance of edema.*

space, the capillary bed collapses, flow in the microcirculation ceases and the oxygen supply to the cell is disrupted. This is the pathophysiology that defines the skeletal muscle-compartment syndrome as well as compartment syndromes in other closed spaces.

The third unifying factor in traumatic ischemias, after hypoxia and edema, is a gradient of injury severity. At the margins of the injury site, minimal or no tissue damage occurs. At the site of maximal injury, tissues may

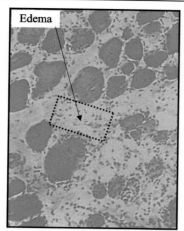

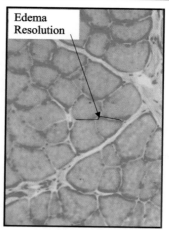

Skeletal muscle with edema separating the muscle fibers. (Dog model skeletal muscle-compartment syndrome without hyperbaric oxygen treatments.)

Edema resolution with normal appearance of muscle. (After hyperbaric oxygen treatments.)

**Legend:** Edema increases the distance between cells (for example muscle fibers as demonstrated in the figure on the left) and between capillaries and cells. This interferes with oxygen availability to cells.

*Figure 3C. Microscopic appearance of edema.*

be so severely damaged that they are rendered non-viable. In between these two zones, a continuum of injury occurs from minimal damage, with the tissues still able to carry out their functions, to barely viable and totally non-functional. Obviously, the severity of injury and the extent of the continuum of damage varies from injury to injury. This complicates the comparisons of benefits of treatment interventions and outcome measurements. Grading systems are used to measure the severity of injury in traumatic ischemias. They are attempts to establish identifiable, but arbitrary points along a gradient of injury (Figure 4). Several of the acute traumatic ischemias have established grading systems; in others the severity of injury is often described as mild, moderate or severe, even though other terms may more precisely define the seriousness of the injury. The efficacy of management interventions are based on comparisons of outcomes from injuries that have similar grades, although the grade for each injury reflects only a single point, or perhaps a zone, on the gradient of injury.

Another consideration of injury from traumatic ischemias is that they tend to be self-perpetuating due to factors of hypoxia and edema; each contributing to worsening of the other factor (Figure 1) (8, 9). As edema

*The variety of presentations of traumatic ischemias essentially makes each one different. Rather than thinking of each as conforming to a specific classification in the particular grading system, it is better to consider the injury as a point on a continuum of responses from the damage. Generally the most severely damaged tissue is used to classify the injury, but size and location are also important considerations for making management decisions and comparing outcomes.*

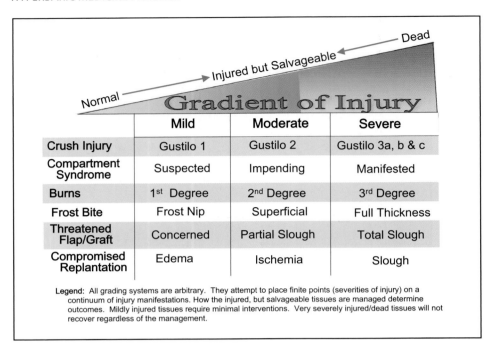

| | Mild | Moderate | Severe |
|---|---|---|---|
| **Crush Injury** | Gustilo 1 | Gustilo 2 | Gustilo 3a, b & c |
| **Compartment Syndrome** | Suspected | Impending | Manifested |
| **Burns** | 1st Degree | 2nd Degree | 3rd Degree |
| **Frost Bite** | Frost Nip | Superficial | Full Thickness |
| **Threatened Flap/Graft** | Concerned | Partial Slough | Total Slough |
| **Compromised Replantation** | Edema | Ischemia | Slough |

**Legend:** All grading systems are arbitrary. They attempt to place finite points (severities of injury) on a continuum of injury manifestations. How the injured, but salvageable tissues are managed determine outcomes. Mildly injured tissues require minimal interventions. Very severely injured/dead tissues will not recover regardless of the management.

*Figure 4. Grading systems for traumatic ischemias.*

worsens, oxygen diffusion distances increase and cellular hypoxia worsens. Hypoxia interferes with the cell's ability to maintain its intracellular fluid content, which further contributes to edema. In addition, vasodilatation of the intact blood supply proximal to the injury, a reflex response, increases perfusion to the injury site. Damage to the microcirculation makes this increased flow counterproductive with more bleeding and leakage of fluid into the interstitial spaces.

These self-perpetuating activities may cause further tissue injury after the initial traumatic event has passed. Often the full extent of the injury is not appreciated until irreversible damage has occurred and it is too late to modify the course.

Tissue destruction in traumatic ischemias results from primary or secondary causes (Figure 5). Primary destruction of tissues arises from the transfer of energy to tissues in amounts that exceed the tissues ability to absorb the energy and/or irreversible interruption of blood supply to the tissues. Each tissue has an ischemic interval that represents the time from the interruption of its blood supply until irreversible injury occurs. For the brain, it may be four minutes or less. The ischemia time for muscle is in the six hour

*The propensity for self-perpetuation (the vicious circle) is almost a universal finding in the traumatic ischemias. Management interventions are invariably directed at preventing or lessening the amount of injury from self-perpetuation of the injury. Self-perpetuation of the injury is a significant cause of secondary tissue losses and/or amputation (Figure 5).*

range. Secondary destruction of tissues is a consequence of the body's attempts to manage the injury, the inability of host reparative and infection controlling functions to respond adequately or combinations of the two. The reperfusion injury that occurs after transient periods of ischemia is also a cause of secondary tissue destruction (10, 11). During the time of frank ischemia, the non-perfused tissue temporarily acts as if it is in a state of suspended animation. During reperfusion, reactive oxygen species are generated by neutrophils that attach to the post-capillary venule endothelium in the reperfused tissue. The reactive oxygen species, in turn, cause vasoconstriction of the precapillary arterioles resulting in the "no-reflow" phenomenon and the ultimate death of the involved tissues. In addition, toxic oxygen radicals initiate lipid peroxidation of cell membranes and react with endothelial generated nitric oxide to form perioxynitrite, an extremely destructive radical (12, 13).

Stasis in microcirculation is another cause of secondary tissue loss in traumatic ischemias (Figure 6). It interferes with the delivery of oxygen and nutrients to tissues. Causes include, impaired inflow, restricted outflow, direct vessel injury and/or rheological problems arising from peripheral arterial insufficiency, venous stasis disease, diabetic microangiopathy, vasculitis, thrombophilia and hypofibrinolysis syndromes. Another cause of stasis in microcirculation is the loss of the normal deformability function of the red blood cell. The red blood cell with a 7.5 micrometer diameter must deform (elongate) to pass through the 5 micrometer diameter capillary. As red blood cells age, they lose their ability to deform and ordinarily at about 120 days are removed from the blood stream by the reticuloendothelial system and their products recycled. Hypoxia and sepsis are known to interfere with red blood

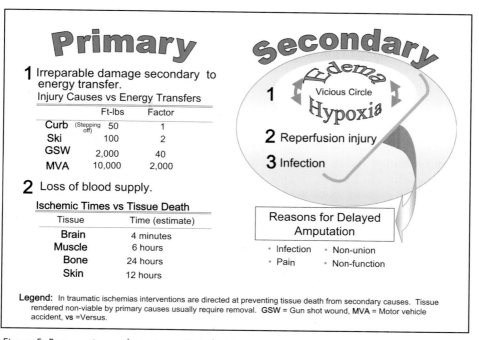

Figure 5. Reasons tissues die in traumatic ischemias.

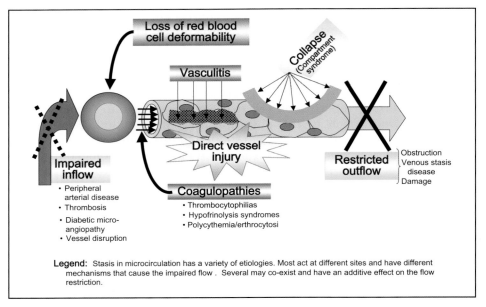

Figure 6. Causes of stasis in microcirculation.

cell deformability, both of which can be associated with traumatic ischemias and stasis in microcirculation and further contribute to tissue injury and destruction (14, 15).

Infection, impaired wound healing, and wound contractures are additional secondary problems that occur in traumatic ischemias (Figure 7). Bacteria grow without restraint in damaged tissues that have impaired blood supplies (16, 17). With the interruption of blood supply, antibiotic delivery to the site of infection is halted. In addition, as tissue oxygen levels decrease, the neutrophil's ability to kill bacteria by oxidative mechanism is impaired. These cells require tissue oxygen tensions in the 30 mmHg to 40 mmHg range in order to kill bacteria (16, 18, 19). For similar reasons, wounds will not heal unless there are equally high oxygen tension for fibroblasts to migrate to the injury site, multiply and produce a collagen matrix that is needed for angiogenesis and wound repair (20, 21). If tissues die from anoxia or infection, they are replaced by scar tissue, a replacement tissue that forms under low oxygen tensions and/or as an attempt by the body to isolate the infection site from the adjacent healthy tissues. As scar tissue matures it shortens and leads to deformities and contractures, which are sometimes observed as the endpoint responses of traumatic ischemias.

*Adequate oxygen tensions are essential for all aspects of healing from the time of the initial injury, during the control of the bioburden, through the inflammatory, reparative, and remodeling stages of repair and for the rehabilitation and restoration of function. Although tissues may not die in hypoxic environments, they become nonfunctional. With restoration of adequate oxygen tensions, function returns. This is fundamental to the management of traumatic ischemias.*

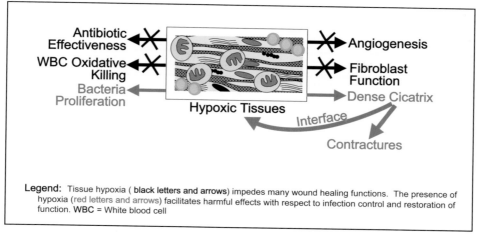

Legend: Tissue hypoxia ( **black letters and arrows**) impedes many wound healing functions. The presence of hypoxia (red letters and arrows) facilitates harmful effects with respect to infection control and restoration of function. WBC = White blood cell

*Figure 7. Hypoxia and its harmful effects on wound healing, bioburden control, and restoration of function.*

## MECHANISMS OF HYPERBARIC OXYGEN APPLICABLE TO TRAUMATIC ISCHEMIAS

Hyperbaric oxygen is a logical adjunct for the management of traumatic ischemias. It has both primary and secondary effects (Table 1). The primary and most important effect of hyperbaric oxygen is hyperoxygenation of blood and other tissues. Oxygen physically dissolves in plasma and equilibrates in tissue fluids in direct proportion to the partial pressure of oxygen in the breathing gas. This supplements the oxygen-carrying mechanisms of the red blood cell. The breathing of pure oxygen at 2.4 atmospheres absolute pressure provides sufficient physically dissolved oxygen in plasma to meet tissue oxygen requirements (22, 23). This effect is an important consideration when stasis of cellular elements restricts red blood cell flow through microcirculation. Plasma will continue to stream through microcirculation and deliver the physically dissolved oxygen it contains to tissues (Figure 8). With hyperoxygenation of the plasma, dissolved oxygen in the plasma is no more flow limited than any of its other physically dissolved components. Hyperbaric oxygen may also help improve flow through microcirculation by enhancement of the red blood cell deformability mechanism (24). Nemiroff demonstrated the synergistic effects of pentoxifylline, a medication that improves red blood cell deformability, and hyperbaric oxygen on skin flap survival (25).

Vasoconstriction is a secondary effect of hyperoxygenation that targets blood vessels. An approximately 20 percent reduction in blood flow in

*Boerema, et al. of the Netherlands published a milestone paper in 1960 reporting survival of piglets under hyperbaric oxygen conditions after removal of their red blood cells. This proved that hyperoxygenated plasma could meet short-term tissue oxygen requirements (23). For this seminal work Boerema is regarded as the "father" figure of hyperbaric medicine.*

# TABLE 1. EFFECTS OF HYPERBARIC OXYGEN USEFUL FOR TRAUMATIC ISCHEMIAS

| TYPE | MECHANISM | EFFECTS | CHARACTERISTICS |
|---|---|---|---|
| Primary<br><br>Maintain tissue viability | Hyperoxygenation | • 10-fold ↑ tissue & plasma $O_2$<br><br>• 25% ↑ blood $O_2$ content<br><br>• 3-fold ↑ in $O_2$ diffusion through tissue fluids | 1) Immediate onset<br>2) Transient effect<br>3) Proportional to inhaled $O_2$ partial pressure<br>4) Dependent on plasma transport |
| Secondary<br>(To hyper-oxygenation)<br><br>Facilitate healing & durable effects | 1) Vasoconstriction<br>2) Host Factors<br> • Fibroblast function<br><br> • Neutrophil activity<br><br> • Osteoclast and osteoblast effects<br>3) Microbial actions<br><br>4) Perturbation of reperfusion injury<br><br>5) RBC deformability | 20% ↓ in blood flow<br><br>Migration, proliferation & secretory activity<br><br>Oxidative killing of bacteria<br><br>Bone remodeling; removal of dead bone<br>Decrease bioburden & its effects<br><br>Interference with WBC adhesion to endothelium<br><br>$O_2$ exchange through capillary | Edema reduction<br><br>Wound healing & matrix for angiogenesis<br><br>Formation of superoxides & peroxides<br><br>Removal 100 times faster than formation<br>Stasis, killing, ↓ toxin formation & antibiotic synergy<br>Interrupts "no reflow" phenomenon after reperfusion<br>7.5u wide RBC passage through the 5u capillary |

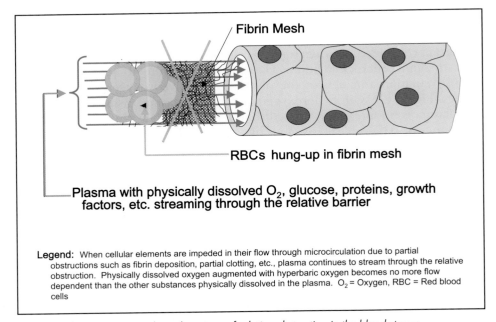

Fibrin Mesh

RBCs hung-up in fibrin mesh

Plasma with physically dissolved $O_2$, glucose, proteins, growth factors, etc. streaming through the relative barrier

**Legend:** When cellular elements are impeded in their flow through microcirculation due to partial obstructions such as fibrin deposition, partial clotting, etc., plasma continues to stream through the relative obstruction. Physically dissolved oxygen augmented with hyperbaric oxygen becomes no more flow dependent than the other substances physically dissolved in the plasma. $O_2$ = Oxygen, RBC = Red blood cells

*Figure 8. Plasma streaming through regions of relative obstruction in the blood stream.*

*Vasoconstriction of blood vessels in diabetics and patients with other causes of peripheral arterial disease probably do not occur to any significant degree in these conditions. This is due to calcification with non-compressibility of their peripheral blood vessels and auto-sympathectomy effects.*

normal vasculature and corresponding reduction in edema is observed from this effect (26-32). Filtration of plasma and/or extravasation of intravascular fluid from blood vessels is reduced secondary to decreased flow (Figure 9). The increased oxygen content of the blood flow secondary to hyperoxygenation of the plasma more than compensates for the decreased flow associated with vasoconstriction (26). The net effects are maintenance of oxygen delivery in the presence of decreased flow and edema reduction. A secondary effect of edema reduction is improved flow in the microcirculation as edema decreases and results in decreased pressure around these blood vessels.

A third mechanism of hyperbaric oxygen and another secondary effect of hyperoxygenation for traumatic ischemias is its ability to provide a sufficiently oxygenated environment so host factors for wound healing and infection control function adequately (Figure 7). As mentioned before, these required oxygen tensions are in the 30 mmHg to 40 mmHg range (16, 19, 21, 33). It appears that intermittent exposures of oxygen to achieve or exceed the above oxygen tensions, as accomplished through two or three times a day hyperbaric oxygen treatments, are sufficient to meet tissue oxygen requirements for host function. Although these effects may not be important

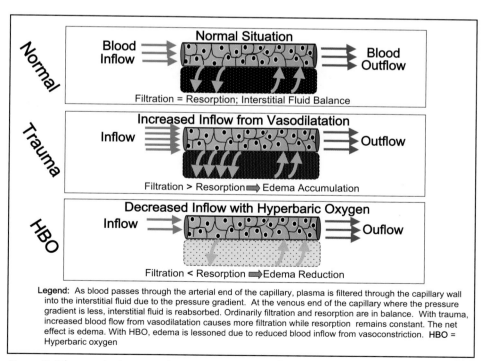

Figure 9. Edema reduction secondary to vasoconstriction from hyperbaric oxygen.

*For host factors such as fibroblast, neutrophils, and osteoclasts/osteoblasts to function, 30 to 40 mmHg oxygen tensions are required in the tissue fluids. Transient elevations of oxygen tension as achieved with intermittent hyperbaric oxygen (rather than continuous tensions above these levels) appear sufficient for functional activities in these cell types.*

for the survival of tissues immediately after the injury, their function becomes increasingly important as time progresses since they are ultimately responsible for wound healing and prevention of secondary complications, such as infection.

Finally, hyperbaric oxygen protects tissues from the harmful effects of reactive oxygen species (Figure 10) (12, 34, 35). Several mechanisms support this effect, including: First, hyperbaric oxygen antagonizes lipid peroxidation of cell membranes from toxic oxygen radicals that interact with the lipids in the membrane (13). Second, hyperbaric oxygen interferes with the sequestration of neutrophils on post-capillary venules and consequently perturbs the initiation of the reperfusion injury (36). This effect results from hyperbaric oxygen interfering with the CD-11 Beta2 integrin mechanism that involves the adherence of neutrophils to the endothelium of the post-capillary venule (12). There appears to be a window of opportunity for using hyperbaric oxygen for this purpose from one hour before until several hours after the ischemic insult (35-37). Third, hyperbaric oxygen provides sufficient oxygen to the reperfused tissues so they can generate scavengers to detoxify the reactive oxygen species (35, 38).

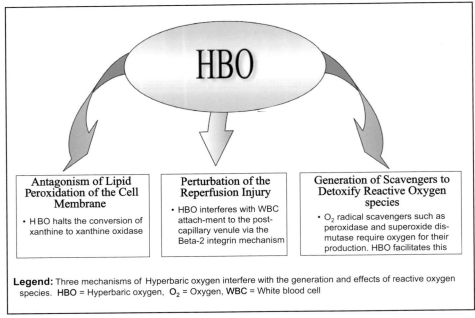

**Legend:** Three mechanisms of Hyperbaric oxygen interfere with the generation and effects of reactive oxygen species. HBO = Hyperbaric oxygen, $O_2$ = Oxygen, WBC = White blood cell

*Figure 10. Roles of hyperbaric oxygen in mitigating the harmful effects of the reperfusion injury.*

*Although hyperbaric oxygen is a possible source for the generation of reactive oxygen species, this appears to be of no clinical significance as observed in safely treating hundreds of thousands of patients with this modality. Additionally, the mechanisms that protect tissues from the harmful effects of reactive oxygen species are becoming increasingly well defined.*

## CLINICAL EXPERIENCES WITH HYPERBARIC OXYGEN FOR TRAUMATIC ISCHEMIAS

The complexity and diversity of these injuries makes interpretations of published reports using hyperbaric oxygen difficult. The first successful use of hyperbaric oxygen for a traumatic ischemia was reported in 1961, when it helped in the salvage of a foot after a near-avulsion (39). In 1964, Perrins reported that the survival of threatened flaps was improved by a three-fold factor when hyperbaric oxygen was used (40). Subsequently, two literature reviews have been published (8, 41). The first review was reported in 1981 and consisted of all the published reports on crush-type injuries and use of hyperbaric oxygen to that date (8). Over 700 case reports were identified (42-54). The cases were separated as to either being published in English (63 patients or 13 percent of the series) or Russian (634 cases or 87 percent of the series). The preponderance of patients from the Russian reports was a strong indication of their interest in using hyperbaric oxygen for traumatic ischemias, as would be expected to arise from battlefield injuries. Outcomes were almost invariably described in subjective terms such as useful, improved, beneficial, effective, etc. The most noteworthy observation from this review was that the outcomes for traumatic ischemias improved as the frequency of treatments increased; for example, 59 percent good responses with one hyperbaric treatment a day, 80 percent complete or partial recovery with three treatments a day and 100 percent salvage with six treatments a day (47, 51, 53). In the second review published in 2005, eight reports met the criteria to be included in an evidenced-based approach (41, 54-62). Seven of the eight reports were case series, with one of them being a retrospective study and the others prospective series. It is not surprising that only one of the citations in the 1981 review had enough statistical data to be included in the evidentiary review (54). One randomized control trial (discussed next) was included in the review (60).

In 1996, Bouachour, et al. reported the benefits of hyperbaric oxygen for open fracture-crush injury (Table 2) (60). His study was a randomized, double-blinded, placebo-controlled clinical trial. Thirty-six patients were randomized into two groups of 18 each. Indicated orthopedic and surgical management was provided for one arm of the study and similar management plus adjunctive use of hyperbaric oxygen in the other. Complete healing

*The 1981 review of the effects of hyperbaric oxygen for traumatic ischemias suggest that favorable outcomes improved in direct proportion to the frequency of treatments.*

occurred in 94 percent (17 of 18 patients) in the hyperbaric group as compared to 59 percent (10 of 18 patients; p = < 0.01) in the controls. Additional surgical procedures were required in six percent (1 of 18 patients) of the hyperbaric oxygen group as compared to 33 percent (6 of 18 patients; p = < 0.05) in the controls. Finally, healing in patients over 40 years of age was significantly improved in the hyperbaric oxygen group with this occurring in 7 of 8 patients (88 percent) versus 3 of 10 patients (30 percent; p = < 0.05) in the control group. The authors also demonstrated the need for adequate oxygenation for healing of open fracture-crush injuries. Transcutaneous oxygen measurements of both the injured and contralateral legs were recorded. This information allowed the authors to generate an index [that is, $P_{tc}O_{2(injured\ leg)}/P_{tc}O_{2(un-injured\ leg)}$]. In all fractures that healed the indices were 0.9 or greater with the differences being statistically significant. All patients who received hyperbaric oxygen had ratios greater than 0.9.

In 1999 Matos, et al. published an abstract that was included in the evidentiary review (62). His study is useful in that it allows comparisons of outcomes in more or less a head-to-head fashion with those reported in the orthopedic literature where hyperbaric oxygen was not used (Table 2). Twenty-three patients with open fracture-crush injuries were managed with orthopedic interventions plus adjunctive hyperbaric oxygen treatments. Fractures were subdivided into those where enough soft tissue remained after debridement and stabilization of the fracture to cover all bone tissue (Gustilo type III-A open fracture, crush injury) and those where exposed bone

## TABLE 2. CRUSH INJURY, OPEN FRACTURE STUDIES ATTESTING TO THE USEFULNESS OF HYPERBARIC OXYGEN IN THEIR MANAGEMENT

| 1. Boucher, et al. Doubled Blinded Randomized Control Trial [60] | | | |
|---|---|---|---|
| Observations | HBO Limb | Control Limb | p Value |
| Patients | 18 (50%) | 18 (50%) | |
| Primary Healing | 17 (94%) | 10(56%) | < 0.01 |
| Returns to OR | 1 (6%) | 6 (33%) | < 0.05 |
| Primary Healing (Pts. > 40 years old) | 7/8(88%) | 3/10(30%) | < 0.05 |

| Observations | Matos (HBO as an adjunct to orthopaedic management) | Caudle (Orthopaedic management without HBO) |
|---|---|---|
| Study Design | Prospective | Prospective |
| Patients | 23 | 62 |
| Primary Healing | 20 (87%) | 24 (39%) |
| Unsatisfactory Outcomes* | 3 (13%, all amputations) | 38 (61%) |

Key: *Unsatisfactory Outcomes = Amputations, infections, non-unions or combinations, HBO = Hyperbaric oxygen, OR = Operating room, VS = versus

*Recommended hyperbaric oxygen treatment guidelines for traumatic ischemias vary with what is the suspected pathophysiology of the underlying condition. Treatment schedules should be altered if justified by clinical findings, such as the need to increase the frequency of treatments for threatened flaps or when additional trailing treatments are indicated. Peer review is recommended in such situations and provides collective justification for modifying hyperbaric oxygen treatment schedules.*

remained after the initial orthopedic management (Gustilo type III-B) and those where there was a concomitant vascular injury (Gustilo type III-C) (Table 3). Twenty patients (87%) had a successful outcome with preservation of the limb, while three patients (13%) required amputations. For comparison purposes a paper published in the orthopedic literature with analogous open fracture-crush injuries, for which hyperbaric oxygen was not used as an adjunct, had an amputation rate of 25 percent (13 of 62 patients) and other unsatisfactory results in 40.3 percent (25 of 62 patients) giving an overall complication rate of 62.8 percent (Table 2) (63).

Hyperbaric oxygen treatment schedules for traumatic ischemias vary according to the desired effects being sought from this modality (Table 4). Almost all hyperbaric oxygen treatments for traumatic ischemias are done at pressures of 2.0 to 2.4 atmospheres absolute for periods of 90 to 120 minutes of pure oxygen breathing. Early application of HBO, preferably within four to six hours of the injury is recommended. Treatment schedules for traumatic

## TABLE 3. THE GUSTILO CLASSIFICATION OF OPEN FRACTURE, CRUSH INJURY (65, 66, 70)

| TYPE (Gustilo) | INJURY CHARACTERISTICS | ANTICIPATED OUTCOMES IN HEALTHY HOSTS[1] |
|---|---|---|
| I | Small (<1 cm wide) puncture wound from inside to out | Usually no different from a closed fracture |
| II | Laceration with minimal deep soft tissue damage | Same as above |
| III | Crush Injuries | Depends on Sub-type |
| A | Sufficient soft tissue too close the wound | Complications[2] ~ 10% |
| B | Flaps needed for coverage | ~ 50% incidence of complications[2] |
| C | Major vascular injury | |

Note: [1]Healthy hosts are those who do not have conditions including advancing age that would be expected to interfere with healing. Host function is quantified in Table 5.

[2]Complications include infection, failed flaps, delayed/non-union, intractable pain, non-function, and amputation)

## TABLE 4. TREATMENT RECOMMENDATIONS AND PEER REVIEW (TO JUSTIFY ADDITIONAL HBO TREATMENTS) WHEN USING HYPERBARIC OXYGEN FOR TRAUMATIC ISCHEMIAS

| CONDITION | HBO TREATMENTS AND PEER REVIEW[1] | COMMENTS |
|---|---|---|
| **Primary Conditions** | | |
| Reperfusion Injury | 1 | Minimal tissue trauma; e.g. after revascularizations, free flaps and transient ischemias |
| Crush Injury, threatened flaps, compromised replantations | 8 (TID 2 days, BID 2 days and daily 2 days) | If deterioration noted when HBO treatments are decreased, resume the previous schedule |
| Compartment Syndrome | 3 (BID day 1 and a single HBO Rx day 2) | HBO is not a substitute for fasciotomy; use HBO for the impending stage of the SMCS |
| **Residual Problems and/or Complications** | | |
| Threatened flaps and grafts | 10 (BID for 5 days) | If site remains tenuous, consider daily HBO treatments an additional 5 days |
| Problem wounds/infected wounds | 21 (BID for 7 days; daily for 7 days) | See problem wounds section |
| Refractory osteomyelitis | 21 (Daily for 3 weeks) | HBO must be integrated with a combined antibiotic and surgical strategy |
| SMCS post-fasciotomy concerns | 14 (BID for 7 days) | Concerns include massive swelling, threatened flaps, unclear demarcation, neuropathy, etc. (see text) |

Note: [1]Peer review should be done if additional HBO treatments are needed after completion of the recommended treatments for the primary condition by two or more of the following: 1) HBO consulting physician, 2) Trauma/orthopaedic surgeon, 3) Plastic/reconstructive surgeon and/or 4) Primary care physician.

Abbreviations: **BID** = Twice a day, **e.g.** = for example, **etc.** = etcetera, **HBO** = Hyperbaric Oxygen, **SMCS** = Skeletal muscle-compartment syndrome, **TID** = Three times a day

ischemias should be tailored to mitigate the suspected pathophysiology. For example, three or more treatments in a 24-hour period for critical ischemias, twice a day for threatened flaps and oxygenation of the environment so host factors can function, and daily for infections and/or remodeling/resorption of calcified tissues. For the isolated reperfusion injury, for example after a prolonged tourniquet time, revascularization and/or thrombectomy of an extremity that otherwise has sustained minimal physical trauma, a single HBO treatment, based on animal studies and limited clinical observations appears to be adequate (12, 35-37).

When hyperbaric oxygen is used as an adjunct for the management of traumatic ischemias, three distinct levels of tissue involvement/injury must be appreciated when considering its benefits and harmful effects (Figure 11) (9). Normal and non-involved tissues adjacent to and/or remote from the injury tolerate hyperbaric oxygen treatments without apparent untoward effects when accepted treatment protocols as mentioned above are used (64). Remote and seemingly non-involved tissues undoubtedly contribute to the healing process by providing adequate perfusion and oxygenation to the injured

*The tissues in the gradient of injury are the target sites for appreciating the benefits of hyperbaric oxygen, although non-injured tissues as well as irreparably damaged tissues may be benefited. Effects appreciated from hyperbaric oxygen for the injured but salvageable tissues are four-fold: preservation of tissue viability, prevention of infection, promotion of healing, and restoration of function.*

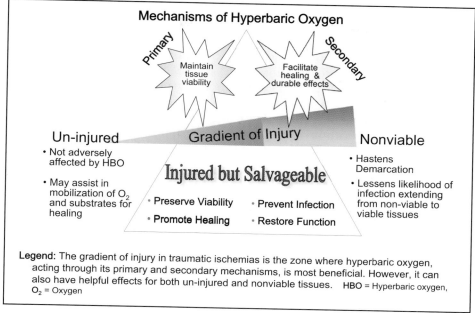

*Figure 11. Effects of hyprebaric oxygen on the three levels of tissue involvement in traumatic ischemias.*

tissues as well as mobilizing precursors for wound healing and infection control. Systemic vasoconstriction from hyperbaric oxygen does not adversely affect these activities since hyperoxygenation of plasma more than compensates for the decreased perfusion due to vasoconstriction (26). The tissues in the gradient of injury are the target area for hyperbaric oxygen treatments.

Four major goals are sought for this level of involvement:

1) Preservation of tissue viability,
2) Prevention of infection, especially during the critical post-injury hypoxic phase,
3) Promotion of healing processes, and
4) Restoration of function during the recovery and convalescent phases.

The third level of involvement concerns non-viable tissue. Although hyperbaric oxygen will not revitalize dead tissue, it hastens demarcation between the non-viable and the adjacent live tissue. As a corollary to this, it helps prevent extension of infection from the very vulnerable margins of the necrotic tissues to the adjacent severely injured tissues.

## CRUSH INJURY: SPECIAL CONSIDERATIONS AND MANAGEMENT

Crush injuries are traumatic ischemias that cause such severe damage to tissues from the energy transfer that tissue survival is in question (9). Crush injuries arise primarily from motor vehicle accidents, high velocity gun shot wounds, falls and the dropping of heavy objects onto a body part. Invariably, two or more types of tissues are injured severely enough that they are at risk of not surviving. Associated with these findings are the two other components of the traumatic ischemia triad, namely the gradient of injury and the self-perpetuating edema, hypoxia vicious circle. Gustilo's classification of open fractures is widely used for judging the severity of open fracture-crush injury (Table 3). Type III fractures meet the criteria of crush injury (65). In sub-type III-B,C open fracture-crush injury, those with insufficient soft tissue to cover bone after debridement is done and concomitant major blood vessel injury respectively, complication rates approach 50 percent, even with optimal management (66). Complications include non-union, infection, amputation or a combination of these. The Mangled Extremity Severity Score (MESS) provides a guideline to select which injured extremities, after limb threatening trauma, should undergo primary amputation (67).

These classification systems provide objective guidelines when making decisions whether hyperbaric oxygen should be used as an adjunct for managing crush injuries. It appears that most trauma surgeons classify crush injuries on an analogue scale as mild, moderate or severe based on their clinical experiences and only intuitively factor in the host status for making decisions regarding management. Naturally, hyperbaric oxygen would be indicated for the serious injuries. Regardless, the overall health and function status of the patient should always be factored into the decision-making process. This can be done objectively by using a five assessment, ten-point scoring system to determine the host status (Table 5). When the host score is integrated with the Gustilo classification, which is the most widely used open fracture-crush injury classification system, objective indications for using hyperbaric oxygen in crush injuries are apparent (Table 6). The MESS system, a third classification for crush injuries of the extremity, can also be used for similar purposes (68). For the healthy host, hyperbaric oxygen is advised for all Gustilo type III-B and C open fracture-crush injuries. In the impaired host, hyperbaric oxygen is recommended for lower Gustilo grades (Table 6). Failure to take into consideration impaired and decompensated host status when dealing with traumatic ischemias will likely increase the morbidity associated with these conditions. Indirect evidence to support this comment with respect to using hyperbaric oxygen as adjunct to managing crush injuries is two-fold: First, Renstra, et al. showed *in vitro* that the doubling times of fibroblasts from older aged subjects was reduced by approximately 50 percent (which approached the doubling times of fibroblasts from newborns) when cultured with intermittent hyperbaric oxygen exposures (69). Second, Bouachour, et al. observed that in the subgroup of patients over 40 years of age with open fracture-crush injuries, the outcomes were statistically significantly better in the hyperbaric oxygen treatment arm (60).

Management of crush injuries include direct interventions that involve surgery such as debridement, management of damaged vessels, stabilization of bony elements and repair of soft tissues. The other component of crush injury care is management of its indirect effects. The mechanisms of hyperbaric oxygen such as hyperoxygenation, increased oxygen delivery in low-flow states, perturbation of the reperfusion injury, and reduction of edema help to manage the indirect effects of the crush injury. Other considerations for

## TABLE 5. A USER FRIENDLY FIVE ASSESSMENT, 0-TO-10 POINT SCORE TO QUANTIFY HOST FUNCTION (75)

| Assessment \ Grade | 2-Points | 1-Point | 0-Points | Interpretation |
|---|---|---|---|---|
| | Use ½ points if findings are mixed or intermediate between 2 points | | | |
| Age | <40 | 40-60 | >60 | |
| | Subtract ½ point if DM or CVD Present | | | **Healthy Host** 8-to-10 points |
| Ambulation | Community | Household | None | |
| | Subtract ½ point if walking aids used | | | **Impaired, but Compensated Host** 4-to-7 points |
| Cardiac/Renal Status (Which ever gives the lower score) | OK | Impaired | Decompensated /End-stage | |
| Smoking/Steroid Use (Which ever gives the lower score) | None | Past | Current | **Decompensated Host** 0-to-3 points |
| Neurological Impairment | None | Some | Severe | |

Key:   CVD = Collagen vascular disease, DM = Diabetes mellitus

Note:   To determine Host-Function score add-up the points for each assessment; score interpretations are provided on the right.

## TABLE 6. THE PATIENT'S HOST STATUS AS A GUIDE FOR USING HBO IN OPEN FRACTURE, CRUSH INJURIES (65, 66, 75)

| Gustilo Type[1] | Host Status[1] | | |
|---|---|---|---|
| | Healthy | Impaired | Decompensated |
| I   Small (<1 cm wide) puncture wound typically from inside to out | | | Yes |
| II  Laceration with minimal deep soft tissue damage | | Yes | Yes |
| III ◄————Crush Injuries ————————————► | | | |
| A Sufficient soft tissue to close the wound primarily or secondarily | | Yes | Yes |
| B Flaps needed for coverage | Yes | Yes | Yes[2] |
| C Major blood vessel injury | Yes | Yes | Yes[2] |

Notes:  [1]Refer to Tables 4 and 5; Gustilo classification and the Host-Function Score respectively.

[2]Consider primary amputation in decompensated hosts with Grade III-B and C open fracture, crush injuries; Hyperbaric oxygen may be needed to help with primary healing of the amputation flaps.

cm = Centimeter, HBO = Hyperbaric oxygen, vs = Versus

managing the indirect effects of the crush injury include adequate fluid and blood replacement to optimize perfusion, prophylactic antibiotics to prevent infection, venous stasis disease prophylaxsis, and measures to improve flow in microcirculation. For this latter consideration, agents such as anti-platelet adhesion medications, red blood cell deformability agents, anticoagulants, and/or low molecular weight Dextran are used.

Hyperbaric treatments for Gustilo type III-B and C open fracture-crush injury should be started as soon as possible. After emergency surgical care is completed, hyperbaric treatments should commence immediately since the greatest needs for adequate wound oxygenation to ensure primary healing and prevention of infection is during the inflammatory phase of wound healing. If surgical interventions are delayed more than a few hours, a hyperbaric oxygen treatment should be given while awaiting transfer to the operating room. Once hyperbaric oxygen treatments are started for crush injuries, they should be continued three times a day for one to two days, then twice daily for two days and daily for the next couple of days. By that time, the ischemic tissues should have stabilized with restoration of blood flow in the microcirculation and reduction of edema. If the flaps are threatened, hyperbaric oxygen treatments should be continued on a twice per day schedule until the flaps appear stable, which may take up to two weeks to achieve the angiogenesis effect. Finally, if refractory osteomyelitis develops as a complication of the injury, 40 to 60 hyperbaric oxygen treatments may be required.

Experiences with hyperbaric oxygen as discussed previously show that when this modality is used as an adjunct for managing severe open fracture-crush injury complication rates are in the 20 percent range (8, 41). This is a sizable improvement from the 50 percent rates reported when hyperbaric oxygen was not used (63, 65, 66). The additional expenses associated with hyperbaric oxygen treatments would be expected to be far less than the costs of managing the 50 percent complication rates reported with Gustilo type III-B and C open fracture-crush injury (63, 65, 66, 70). In 1977, Brighton estimated that in the United States, $140,000 was the average cost per patient required to resolve the 100,000 open fracture-crush injuries that failed to heal primarily each year (71). Today, the costs would be ten or more times higher. Even with new technologies, the complication rates are predictable for the most severe open fracture-crush injuries (63, 65, 66, 70). Because of the large number of these injuries that occur in the United States each year, a reduction in complications and the morbidity associated with them could have substantial impact on health care costs and far outweigh the additional expenses associated with hyperbaric oxygen treatments. Mackay, et al. reported that lower limb amputations after failed revascularizations generated medical costs approaching $50,000 when hospitalization, surgery, prosthesis, and rehabilitation costs are considered (72). Not to be dismissed are the intangible

*Hyperbaric oxygen should be started as soon as possible after the "Big Bang." Immediately after the time of injury, the oxygen demands are the greatest and paradoxically the oxygen availability likely to be the lowest of any time in the healing process.*

benefits that primary healing and avoidance of amputations have on the patient's mental outlook, ability to function independently and return to gainful employment (73).

## COMPARTMENT SYNDROME: SPECIAL CONSIDERATIONS AND MANAGEMENT

A skeletal muscle-compartment syndrome occurs when swelling of injured skeletal muscle increases the interstitial fluid within the myofascial compartment above the capillary perfusion pressure. Ischemic injury to the muscle occurs due to blood flow interruption at the microcirculation level. Edema and tissue hypoxia are the important pathophysiological components of skeletal-muscle compartment syndrome. While direct trauma to muscle is probably the most frequent cause, other etiologies include: 1) Prolonged ischemia time from thromboses, 2) Arterial injuries, 3) Prolonged tourniquet times, 4) Venous occlusion or interruption of outflow secondary to injury, 5) External compression from devices such as bandages, casts or pneumatic compression suits, 6) Bleeding into the compartment , 7) Intravenous fluid or medication infiltration into the compartment, 8) Snake bite, 9) "Crush" Syndrome (prolonged compression of an extremity secondary to comatose posturing, that is to say i.e. lying on a limb) and 10) Disproportionate muscle swelling within the myofascial compartment secondary to unusually intense physical activity. Self-perpetuation from hypoxia and edema is an important pathophysiological feature of the skeletal muscle-compartment syndrome. This is the reason most skeletal muscle-compartment syndromes do not manifest themselves until after a lag phase; that is the time from injury to the time serious symptoms appear. The lag phase may range from a few minutes, especially with bleeding into the compartment, to several days after the inciting cause.

The skeletal muscle-compartment syndrome, like the open fracture-crush injury, represents a continuum of severities that can be divided into suspected, impending and established stages (Figure 12a and b). In the suspected stage, the compartment syndrome is not actually present, but the severity of the injury or the circumstances (for example, prolonged ischemia time) raise suspicions that a compartment syndrome could develop. In this stage hyperbaric oxygen is not recommended, but frequent neurocirculatory checks of the injured extremity are required in order to recognize the earliest possible progression to the impending stage.

If the edema-hypoxia cycle perpetuates itself, the condition may evolve into the impending stage. In this stage findings include: 1) Increasing pain, 2) Hypesthesia/paresthesia, 3) Muscle weakness, 4) Discomfort with passive stretch, 5) Tenseness in the compartment or combinations of these. If

*Most skeletal muscle-compartment syndromes do not manifest themselves until after a lag phase. The exception is frank bleeding into the compartment. The lag phase is the time interval from the injury to the time symptoms and signs of a compartment syndrome occur. The lag phase exemplifies the self-perpetuation hypoxia-edema process.*

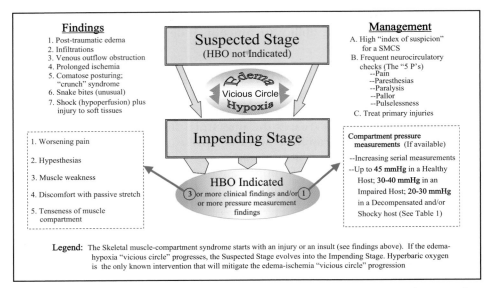

Figure 12A. Progression of the skeletal muscle-compartment syndrome from suspected to impending stages and the indication for hyperbaric oxygen (HBO).

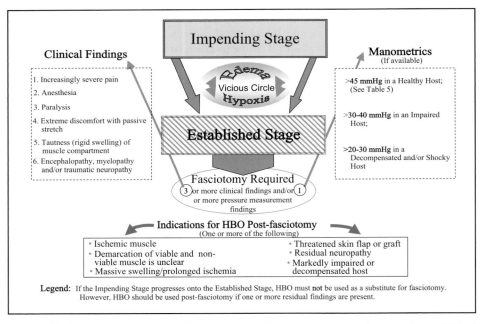

Figure 12B. Fasciotomy is required with progression of the compartment syndrome to the established stage.

any of these signs exist, compartment pressure measurements should be made. If the compartment pressures and clinical findings are such that fasciotomy is not required at that time, hyperbaric oxygen treatments should be started to prevent progression from the impending stage to the established stage. If pressure testing is not available and the compartment syndrome is not in the established stage, three or more of the above clinical findings provide sufficient indications to initiate hyperbaric oxygen treatments (Figure 12a). A second indication for hyperbaric oxygen in the impending stage, if pressure testing is available, is the finding of increasing pressures with repeated measurements. As in open fracture-crush injuries, the host score needs to be considered when making decisions to use hyperbaric oxygen for the impending stage of the compartment syndrome (Table 5).

In the established stage of the skeletal muscle-compartment syndrome signs and/or pressure measurements confirm the diagnosis and dictate that immediate fasciotomy be done (Figure 12b). Hyperbaric oxygen must not be used as a reason to defer surgery in the above situation. However, after fasciotomy hyperbaric oxygen should be used as an adjunct to wound management if significant residual problems remain such as ischemic muscle, threatened flaps, unclear demarcation between viable and non-viable muscle, residual neuropathy, marked swelling, prolonged (more than 6 hours) ischemia time and/or significant host impairment as quantified by the host score (Table 5).

Measurements of interstitial fluid pressure within the compartment provide objectivity for assessment of the skeletal muscle-compartment syndrome. Surgical decompression of the myofascial compartment is recommended when pressure measurements exceed the capillary perfusion pressure (74). If the initial pressure measurements are in the intermediate range, that is not elevated enough to justify surgical decompression, three permutations arise: 1) The pressures may decline, 2) The pressures may plateau or 3) The pressures may rise to a point where surgical decompression is required. Except for the use of hyperbaric oxygen, no interventions are available to interrupt the progression of the skeletal muscle-compartment syndrome during the impending stage (lag phase). If serial measurements of compartment fluid pressures are done at timed intervals in the patient with a suspected skeletal muscle-compartment syndrome, the time of critical pressure elevation may be missed. This is due to the fact that initial pressure increases occur gradually until the compliance of the compartment is exceeded (that is, the compartment is filled to capacity with edema fluid without a significant rise in intracompartmental pressures). After that point, additional edema formation in the compartment causes rapid elevations in pressure.

Several problems complicate the evaluation and management of the skeletal muscle-compartment syndrome. First, when compartment pressure measurements alone are used to provide an objective indication for fasciotomy, there is no agreement in the published reports as to what pressure should be used (75). Furthermore, hypotension is the only host factor

---

*If the compartment syndrome becomes "full blown" that is, progresses to the established stage, immediate fasciotomy is required. Hyperbaric oxygen should not be used as a substitute for fasciotomy when surgery is indicated. If significant residual problems remain after the fasciotomy, then hyperbaric oxygen should be used as an adjunct to wound, flap and/or recovery management.*

considered in the manometric interpretation reports. It is integrated into four of seven reports, but without unanimity in opinion as to what degree is considered significant (76-82). Second, as suggested above, hypotension lowers the threshold pressure for the skeletal muscle-compartment syndrome because it decreases capillary perfusion pressure. Consequently, the criteria for surgical decompression of the compartment based on interstitial fluid pressures alone may not be valid in the presence of shock. Third, if neuropathy develops as a consequence of the skeletal muscle-compartment syndrome, recovery of function only occurs in a small percentage of cases (76, 83). Finally, once the compartment has been surgically decompressed, it is not always apparent which tissues will survive since a gradient of injury exists as in the other traumatic ischemias.

Hyperbaric oxygen is a logical intervention for the skeletal muscle-compartment syndrome (Figures 9, 10, and 11).

The primary pathophysiology of this condition, hypoxia and edema, are corrected by the hyperoxygenation and edema reduction mechanisms of hyperbaric oxygen. This information was conclusively confirmed by skeletal muscle-compartment syndrome studies in animal experiments (30-32, 84, 85). Enhanced recovery of muscle function has been demonstrated in a rabbit skeletal muscle-compartment syndrome model with hyperbaric oxygen (86). Clinical experiences using hyperbaric oxygen for the skeletal muscle-compartment syndrome are consistent with what would have been predicted from knowing the mechanisms of hyperbaric oxygen, the pathophysiology of skeletal muscle-compartment syndrome and the laboratory studies (58, 87, 88).

When hyperbaric oxygen was initiated during the lag phase (impending stage) of the skeletal muscle-compartment syndrome, no compartment syndromes progressed to the established stage and required surgical decompression (58). When hyperbaric oxygen was started after surgical decompression had been done because of significant residual problems it sped the reduction of edema and prevented further loss of tissue and function. This facilitated wound closure, survival of threatened flaps and grafts and restoration of function. A cost-benefit review showed that when hyperbaric oxygen was started during the lag phase and aborted progression to the need for fasciotomy, the total expenses generated (hospitalization, hyperbaric oxygen treatments, medicines and surgeries) were one-quarter of those in patients whose compartment syndromes had progressed to the degree that surgical decompression was required and then subsequently received hyperbaric oxygen treatments to manage the residual problems (89).

*Why is hyperbaric oxygen not used more frequently and as a "standard of practice" for the impending stage of the skeletal muscle-compartment syndrome? The question is especially pertinent since the mechanisms of hyperbaric oxygen have been demonstrated conclusively in well-designed laboratory studies to interrupt its pathophysiology. Additionally, no other interventions are known to be effective for this stage of the skeletal muscle-compartment syndrome. Some responses to this dilemma are offered in the conclusion of this chapter.*

# THE ROLE OF HYPERBARIC OXYGEN IN OTHER TRAUMATIC ISCHEMIAS

The mechanisms of hyperbaric oxygen useful for crush injury and compartment syndrome also have applications for other traumatic ischemias such as burns, frostbite, threatened flaps and grafts and compromised replantations. Burns demonstrate a gradient of injury; first, second or third degree severity (Figure 4). The mechanism of injury from burns is thermal rather than mechanical as in open fracture-crush injury. Since hypoxia and edema are also important components of the pathophysiology, they meet the criteria of a traumatic ischemia. Components of a traumatic ischemia are also observed in threatened flaps and grafts. Hypoxia is the predominant finding, but other characteristics of traumatic ischemias such as edema and a gradient of injury are important features. In contrast to other traumatic ischemias, there is usually less actual physical injury to the threatened flaps and grafts site than in crush injuries and burns. The underlying problems are predominantly ischemia and edema from mobilizing the flap during surgery or a wound base with insufficient vascularity to support the flap or skin graft. The exception to this, of course, is the severe open fracture-crush injury where physical trauma to the flap is an important consideration in defining the seriousness of the crush injury. As in the other traumatic ischemias, the primary indications for hyperbaric oxygen in threatened flaps and grafts are to improve oxygen availability to areas where perfusion is compromised and to reduce edema. Comprehensive discussions of burns and threatened flaps and grafts are found in other chapters of this text. The following discussion supplements information about frostbite and threatened replantations.

The pathophysiology of frostbite is similar that of the other traumatic ischemias, but the etiology is that of cold injury to the tissues. Problems arise in frostbite injuries during re-warming with stasis in the microcirculation, rouleau formation of red blood cells and other consequences of reperfusion. During re-warming oxygen demands are at their greatest point, yet the ability to deliver oxygen to the injured tissues is most compromised. The role of hyperbaric oxygen in this condition is obvious, but unfortunately few clinical studies are available (90). The ideal time to initiate hyperbaric oxygen for frostbite is during the re-warming period. After the re-warming is accomplished, hyperbaric oxygen treatments should be done twice a day for edema reduction, supporting injured but salvageable tissues, aiding in demarcation between viable and irreversibly damaged tissues and lessening the chances of infection. Other adjuncts to improve perfusion, such as low molecular weight Dextran, application of nitroglycerin patches proximal to the threatened tissue, sympathetic blocks, optimization of intravascular fluid volume, maintenance of cardiac function, and use of anti-platelet, anti-agglutination medications should be considered (91). In addition, recombinant tissue plasminogin activator (r-tPA) has shown benefits in reducing injury from frostbite when it was given during the re-warming period (92).

Due to rouleau formation and vasospasm, perfusion to the microcirculation can be severely compromised. This additionally qualifies frostbite as an acute peripheral arterial insufficiency condition, which is discussed more extensively in other parts of this text.

Threatened replantations demonstrate the same pathophysiology as other traumatic ischemias. Hyperbaric oxygen has been used as an adjunct for managing this problem (55, 61, 93, 94). Typically the pathophysiology of the threatened replantation is a combination of the findings found in open fracture-crush injury and the threatened flap. Edema reduction appears to be the major benefit of hyperbaric oxygen for the threatened replantation (93). This is because post replantation arterial repairs are usually sufficient to meet the reimplant's perfusion needs while vein repairs are more tenuous. The consequence is congestion and swelling due to insufficient venous outflow. Medicinal leech therapy supplemented with hyperbaric oxygen treatments for its edema reducing mechanism is an effective combination for dealing with this threatened replantation problem. If arterial inflow is insufficient and/or the microcirculation has been compromised by the injury causing the amputation, the hyperoxygenation effect of hyperbaric oxygen will be useful for this component of the problem, also. Finally, if the ischemia time is prolonged, as is usually the situation with replantations, hyperbaric oxygen should be used for its perturbation of the reperfusion injury (95).

## CONCLUSIONS

It is obvious that hyperbaric oxygen is grossly under utilized as an adjunct for the management of traumatic ischemias. As mentioned before, the specific mechanisms of hyperbaric oxygen mitigate the pathophysiology of these conditions. The laboratory and clinical information demonstrating the benefits of hyperbaric oxygen for traumatic ischemias are as substantial as any evidence used to justify adjunctive interventions for other medical or surgical conditions. The relevant question is, why is hyperbaric oxygen not included in all traumatologists' algorithms for managing open fracture-crush injuries and other traumatic ischemia? The answers are several-fold:

- First, traumatologists are either unaware or appear to ignore the science of hyperbaric oxygen therapy and the evidenced-based information that supports its use in traumatic ischemias.
- Second, complications and wound healing failures are expected with the severest degrees of the traumatic ischemias. Unfortunately, there appears to be a general acceptance of these outcomes as meeting the "standards of practice," without any consideration for improving the outcomes with the adjunctive use of hyperbaric oxygen.
- Third, hyperbaric oxygen is too often not utilized as an adjunct to initial primary surgical and medical management of traumatic ischemias. Hyperbaric oxygen tends to be considered only after complications arise rather than as a proactive primary intervention to prevent predictable problems.
- Fourth, because hyperbaric oxygen chambers are not universally available at trauma centers, their lack of immediate availability is used as a reason to defer transfer or not consider hyperbaric oxygen treatments at all. However, transfers for other emergencies are done frequently from medical facilities where a higher level of care is unavailable at that institution. For example, life and limb threatening conditions such as limb replantations, neurosurgical emergencies, severe burns, arterial gas embolism, decompression sickness, gas

gangrene, and carbon monoxide poisoning are transferred to facilities that can provide the level of care required for these problems. Is it not ironical that these latter four conditions are often transferred specifically for primary or adjunctive hyperbaric oxygen therapy? Should not the same standards be used to reduce predictable complications with the use of hyperbaric oxygen for the most serious types of traumatic ischemias?

• Finally, there seems to be reluctance for hyperbaric medicine facilities themselves to encourage the use of hyperbaric oxygen for traumatic ischemias. This is a two-part problem. First, the complexity of managing patients with traumatic ischemias, often with associated complex medical problems, is problematic for hyperbaric medical facilities that do not regularly treat critical care patients. Second, because of Diagnosis-Related Group (DRG) payments, third party payer contracts, or the patient being uninsured, reimbursements for hyperbaric oxygen treatments for traumatic ischemia may be extremely limited or non-existent.

How does hyperbaric oxygen measure up as an evidenced-based indication for open fracture-crush injury and skeletal muscle-compartment syndrome? Since it is used as an adjunct to surgery and medical management, perhaps hyperbaric oxygen therapy needs to be judged differently than how a primary treatment modality is judged. Nonetheless, when the American Heart Association 1999 Guidelines are used, hyperbaric oxygen meets the criteria of a Class-I-b indication for crush injury and a Class II indication for compartment syndrome (96). For open fracture-crush injury, a favorable randomized controlled trial exists (Class-I-b indication) and for the skeletal muscle-compartment syndrome, it is probably useful and effective with a favorable risk/benefit ratio (Class II indication). The absence of a randomized control trial for the skeletal muscle-compartment syndrome is the reason hyperbaric oxygen is not classified at a higher evidence-based indication level for this condition.

It is apparent that factors other than the criteria used for evidence-based indications need to be considered when making decisions about selecting treatment interventions. This is true for using hyperbaric oxygen for open fracture-crush injury, skeletal muscle-compartment syndrome, and other traumatic ischemias, as it is for selecting management interventions for any other medical and surgical condition. We recommend that five assessments be used to justify the use of hyperbaric oxygen therapy for open fracture-crush injury, skeletal muscle-compartment syndrome and other traumatic ischemias (Table 7) (97, 98). To quantify this approach, each assessment is graded on a 0 to 2 point score, with two points indicating overwhelming information to support the assessment, one point to indicate that the information is consistent with the assessment and zero points if there is no information, no benefit or possible harm for the assessment. By adding-up the points of each of the five assessments, a 0 to 10 score (with 10 being best) is determined. If the total is six or greater, we feel a rational-based, evidence appropriate indication exists for using the treatment. When using this guide, open fracture-crush injury scores a 7 and compartment syndrome scores a 6; thereby qualifying each as a rational based, evidence appropriate indication for using hyperbaric oxygen (Table 7).

## TABLE 7. RATIONAL-BASED, EVIDENCE-APPROPRIATE (RBEA) EVALUATION TO GUIDE DECISION MAKING FOR SELECTING TREATMENT INTERVENTIONS (97, 98)

| ASSESSMENT | Scoring Criteria[1,2] (For justifying the intervention) | RBEA EVALUATION FOR USING HBO | |
|---|---|---|---|
| | | Crush Injury | Compartment Syndrome |
| 1. Treating physician's experiences based on judgement & outcomes | **2 Points** (Overwhelming evidence) | 1 | 1 |
| 2. **Mechanisms & lab studies** of the intervention appropriate for the pathophysiology of the condition | | 2 | 2 |
| 3. Literature reports | **1 Point** (Evidence is consistent) | 1 1/2 | 1 |
| 4. No other treatments available (Failures with interventions or poor outcomes with usual management) | | 1 | 2[3] |
| 5. Randomized control trials and/or head-to-head studies (2 or more reports). | **0 Points** (No information, no benefit or possible harm) | 1 1/2 | 0 |
| | | 7 Points | 6 Points |

Notes: [1]Use half points if the information is between two of the scoring criteria.

[2]Six or more points qualifies the intervention as a rational-based, evidence-appropriate indication.

[3]Especially true regarding the impending stage of the skeletal muscle-compartment syndrome.

Since indications on the use of hyperbaric oxygen for various conditions were first formulated by the Undersea and Hyperbaric Medical Society (UHMS), crush injury, compartment syndromes and other acute ischemias have been included in the *Hyperbaric Oxygen Therapy Committee Report* as approved indications (1, 99). The U.S. Food and Drug Administration (FDA) uses the UHMS HBO Committee Report as a primary source document when inquiries are made regarding the use of hyperbaric oxygen therapy. Reimbursement for the use of hyperbaric oxygen as an adjunct in the management of acute traumatic peripheral ischemia and open fracture-crush injuries is currently authorized by the Department of Health and Human Services (DHHS), Centers for Medicare and Medicaid Services (CMS) and is covered by most third party insurance carriers (100). In order to justify the use of hyperbaric oxygen therapy in these conditions, appropriate documentation is necessary.

## SUMMARY

Hyperbaric oxygen therapy as an adjunct in the management of crush injury, skeletal muscle-compartment syndrome and other traumatic ischemias, has the scientific basis, outcome expectations and reimbursement justifications for its use. It is anticipated that as clinicians become better informed about the use of hyperbaric oxygen, demands for better outcomes increase and the availability of hyperbaric oxygen treatment facilities expand, this important therapy will assume its appropriate role in the these conditions.

# REFERENCES

1. Kindwall, EP (Ed.) Hyperbaric Oxygen Therapy Committee Report Undersea Medical Society, Bethesda, MD, 1977.

2. Hyperbaric Oxygen Therapy Davis JC, Hunt TK (Eds.) Undersea and Hyperbaric Medical Society, Bethesda, MD, 1977.

3. Strauss MB. Diabetic Foot and Leg Wounds. Principles, Management and Prevention. Primary Care Reports 2001; 7(22)187-197.

4. Christensen O. Mediation of cell volume regulation by Ca++ influx through stretch-activated channels. Nature. 1987; 330:66-68.

5. Malinoski DJ, Slater MS, Mullins RJ. Crush Injury and rhabdomyolysis. Crit Care Clin. 2004; 20:171-192.

6. Textbook of Medical Physiology 10th ed. Guyton AC, Hall JE (Eds.) Philadelphia, PA. WB Saunders; 2000:144-194.

7. Peirce EC II. Pathophysiology, apparatus, and methods, including the special techniques of hypothermia and hyperbaric oxygen. Extracorporeal Circulation for Open-Heart Surgery Charles C. Thomas, Springfield, IL. 1969;84-88.

8. Strauss MB. Role of hyperbaric oxygen therapy in acute ischemias and crush injuries – an orthopedic perspective. HBO Review. 1981; 2:87-108.

9. Strauss MB, Hart GB. Crush injury and the role of hyperbaric oxygen. Topics in Emergency Med. 1984; 6:9-24.

10. McCord JM. Oxygen derived free radicals in post-ischemic tissue injury. N Engl J Med. 1985; 312:159-163.

11. Vedder NB, Fouty BW, Winn RK, Harlan JM, et al. Role of neutrophils in generalized reperfusion injury associated with resuscitation from shock. Surgery. 1989; 106:509-516.

12. Thom SR. Functional inhibition of neutrophil B2 integrins by hyperbaric oxygen in carbon monoxide mediated brain injury. Toxicology and Applied Pharmacol. 1993; 123:248-256.

13. Thom SR. Antagonism of CO-mediated brain lipid peroxidation by hyperbaric oxygen. Toxicol Appl Pharmacol. 1990; 105:340-344.

14. Hurd TC, Dasmhapatra KS, Rush BF, Machiedo GW. Red blood cell deformability in human and experimental sepsis. Arch Surg. 1988; 123:217-220.

15. Powell RJ, Machiedo, GW, Rush, BF. Decreased red blood cell deformability and impaired oxygen utilization during human sepsis. Am Surg. 1993; 59:65-68.

16. Howe CW. Experimental studies on determinants of wound infection. Surg Gynecol Obstet. 1966; 123:507-514.

17. Tran DT, Miller SH, Buck D, Imatani J, et al. Potentiation of infection by Epinephrine. Plast Reconstr Surg. 1985; 76:933-934.

18. Hohn DC. Oxygen and leukocyte microbial killing. In: Hyperbaric Oxygen Therapy Davis JC, Hunt TK, (Eds.) Undersea Medical Society, Inc., Bethesda, MD. 1977;101-110.

19. Hunt TK, Linsey M, Grislis G, Sonne M, et al. The effect of differing ambient oxygen tensions on wound infection. Ann Surg. 1975; 181:35-39.

20. Hunt TK, Pai MP. The effect of varying ambient oxygen tensions on wound metabolism and collagen synthesis. Surg Gynecol Obstet. 1972; 135:561-567.

21. Hunt TK, Zederfeldt, Goldstick TK. Oxygen and healing. Am J Surg. 1969; 118:521-525.

22. Bassett BE, Bennett PB. Introduction to the physical and physiological bases of hyperbaric therapy. In: Hyperbaric Oxygen Therapy Davis JC, Hunt TK, (Eds.) Undersea Medical Society, Inc., Bethesda, MD. 1977;11-24.

23. Boerema I, Meijne NG, Brummelkamp WK, et al. Life without blood. A study of the influence of high atmospheric pressure and hypothermia on dilution of the blood. J Cardiovasc Surg. 1960; 1:133-146.

24. Mathieu D, Goget J, Vinkier L, Saulnier F, et al. Red blood cell deformability and hyperbaric oxygen therapy. (Abstract) HBO Review. 1985; 6:280.

25. Nemiroff PM. Synergistic effects of pentoxifylline and hyperbaric oxygen on skin flaps. Arch Otolaryngol Head Neck Surg. 1988; 114:977-981.

26. Bird AD, Telfer ABM. Effect of hyperbaric oxygen on limb circulation. Lancet. 1965; 1:355-356.

27. Meijne NG. Hyperbaric oxygen and its clinical value, with special emphasis on biochemical and cardiovascular aspects. Charles C. Thomas, Springfield, IL, 1970.

28. Nylander G, Lewis D, Lewis D, Nordstom H, et al. Reduction of post-ischemic edema with hyperbaric oxygen. Plast Reconstr Surg. 1985; 76:596-601.

29. Schraibman IG, Ledingham I McA. Hyperbaric oxygen and local vasodilation in peripheral vascular disease. Br J Surg. 1969; 56:295-299.

30. Skyhar MJ, Hargens AR, Strauss MB, Gershuni DH, et al. Hyperbaric oxygen reduces edema and necrosis of skeletal muscle in compartment syndromes associated with hemorrhagic hypotension. J Bone Joint Surg. 1986; 68A:1218-1224.

31. Strauss MB, Hargens AR, Gershuni DH, Greenberg DA, et al. Reduction of skeletal muscle necrosis using intermittent hyperbaric oxygen in a model compartment syndrome. J Bone Joint Surg. 1983; 65A:656-662.

32. Strauss MB, Hargens AR, Gershuni DH, Hart GB, et al. Delayed use of hyperbaric oxygen for treatment of a model anterior compartment syndrome. J Orthop Res. 1986; 4:108-111.

33. Grief R, Akea, et al. Supplemental perioperative oxygen to reduce the incidence of surgical-wound infection. N Eng J Med. 2000; 342(3):61-67.

34. Burt JG, Kapp JP, Smith RR. Effects of HBO on infarcts in gerbils. Surg Neurol. 1987; 28:265-268.

35. Thomas MP, Brown LA, Sponseller DR, Williamson SE, et al. Myocardial infarct size reduction by synergistic effect of hyperbaric oxygen and recombinant tissue plasminogen activator. Am Heart J. 1991; 120:791-800.

36. Zamboni WA, Roth AC, Russel RC, Nemiroff PM, et al. The effect of acute hyperbaric oxygen therapy on axial pattern skin flap survival when administered during and after total ischemia. J Reconstr Microsurg. 1989; 5:343-347.

37. Shandling AH, Ellestad MH, Hart GB, Crump R, et al. Hyperbaric oxygen and thombolysis in myocardial infarction: the "Hot MI" pilot study. Am Heart J. 1997; 134:544-50.

38. Ferrari R, Ceconi C, Cunnello S, et al. Oxygen-mediated damage during ischemia and reperfusion: role of the cellular defense against oxygen. J Mol cell Cardiol. 1985; 17:937-41.

39. Smith G, Stevens J, Griffiths JC, et al. Near-avulsion of foot treated by replacement and subsequent prolonged exposure of patients to oxygen at two atmospheres pressure. Lancet. 1961; 2:1122-1123.

40. Perrins DJ. The effect of hyperbaric oxygen on skin flaps. In: Skin Flaps Grabb WC, Myers MB, (Eds.) Boston, Little, Brown and Co., 1975;53-63.

41. Garcia-Covarrubias l, McSwain NE, Van Meter K, et al., Adjuvant hyperbaric oxygen therapy in the management of crush injury and traumatic ischemia: an evidenced-based approach, Am Surg. 2005; 71:141-151.

42. Barthelemy L, Bellet L, Michaud A, Carbon P. The value of thermography in the appreciation of the effectiveness of hyperbaric oxygen therapy in treatment of acute arteritis of the lower limbs. Bordeux Med. 1976; 9:1095-1100.

43. Davidkin NF. Experience with clinical use of hyperbaric oxygenation in traumas and their complications. Ortop Travmatol Protez. 1977; 9:33-35.

44. Gismondi, AG Micalella F, Colonna SS. Possible use of hyperbaric oxygen in the treatment of certain vascular disease. Ann Med Nav. 1978; 83:547-558.

45. Illingworth CFW, Smith G, Lawson DD, Ledingham McA I, et al. Surgical and physiological observations in an experimental pressure chamber. Br J Surg. 1961; 49:222-227.

46. Isakov YV, Atroschenko ZB, Bailik IF, Grigorjev NG, et al. Hyperbaric oxygenation in the prophylaxis of wound infection in the open trauma of the locomotor system. Bestn Khir. 1979; 123:117-121.

47. Loder RE. Hyperbaric oxygen therapy in acute trauma. Ann R Coll Surg Engl. 1979; (3):39-43.

48. Lukich VL, Filimonova MV, Bazarova VS. Changes of the gaseous exchange in hyperbaric oxygenation in patients with regional ischemia. Vrach Delo. 1979; (3):39-43.

49. Lukich VL, Fillimonova MV, Fokina TS, Novikova LL, et al. Employment of hyperbaric oxygenation in out-patients. Khirurgiia. 1976; (2):82-86.

50. Maudsley RH, Hopkinson WI, Williams KG. Vascular injury treated with high pressure oxygen in a mobile chamber. J Bone Joint Surg. 1963; 2(B):346-350.

51. Schramek A, Hashmonai M. Vascular injuries in the extremities in battle casualties. Br J Surg. 1977; 64:644-648.

52. Skurikhina LA. Therapeutic use of changed barometric pressure (barotherapy, vacuumtherapy, hyperb). Vopr Kurortol Fizioter Lech Kult. 1976; 3:83-89.

53. Slack WD, Thomas DA, DeJode LRJ. Hyperbaric oxygen in the treatment of trauma, ischemic disease of limbs, and varicose ulceration. In: Proc of the Third Int'l Conf on Hyperbaric Med. (Brown IW, Cox BG, Eds.) National Academy of Science, National Research Council, Publ 1404, Washington DC, 1966;621-624.

54. Szekely O, Szanto G, Takats A. Hyperbaric oxygen therapy in injured subjects. Injury. 1973; 4:294-300.

55. No authors. Hyperbaric oxygen therapy in replantation of severed limbs. A report of 21 cases. Chin Med J. 1975; 1:197-204.

56. Monies-Chass, I, Hashmonai M, Hoerer D, et al. Hyperbaric oxygen treatment as an adjuvant to reconstructive vascular surgery in trauma. Injury. 1977; 8:274-277.

57. Shupak A, Gozal D, Ariel A, et al. Hyperbaric oxygenation in acute peripheral posttraumatic ischemia. J Hyperbaric Med. 1987; 2:7-14.

58. Strauss MB, Hart GB. Hyperbaric oxygen and the skeletal muscle-compartment syndrome. Contemp Orthop. 1989; 18:167-174.

59. Radonic V, Baric D, Petricevic A, et al. War injuries of the crural arteries. Br J Surg. 1995; 82:777-83.

60. Bouachour G, Cronier P, Gouello JP, et al. Hyperbaric oxygen therapy in the management of crush injuries: A randomized double-blind placebo-controlled clinical trial. J Trauma. 1996; 41:333-9.

61. Kiyoshige Y. Effect of hyperbaric oxygen therapy as a monitoring technique for digital replantation survival. J Reconstr Microsurg. 1999; 15:327-30.

62. Matos LA, Hutson JJ, Bonet H, et al. HBO as an adjunct treatment for limb salvage in crush injuries of the extremities. Undersea Hyperb Med. 1999; 26(Suppl):66-7.

63. Caudle RJ, Stern, PJ. Severe open fractures of the tibia, J Bone Joint Surg. 1987; 69(Am):801-807.

64. Hart GB. Hyperbaric oxygen as clinical therapy: hoax or breakthrough. Proceedings San Diego Biomed Symposium. 1973; 12:313-320.

65. Gustilo RB, Williams DN. The use of antibiotics in the management of open fractures. Orthopedics. 1984; 7:1617-1619.

66. Gustilo RB, Mendoza RM, Williams DN. Problems in the management of type III (severe) open fractures: A new classification of type III open fractures. J Trauma. 1984; 24:742.

67. Johansen K, Daines M, Howey T Helfet D, et al. Objective criteria accurately predict amputation following lower extremity trauma. J Trauma. 1990; 30:568-573.

68. Strauss, MB. Crush injury, compartment syndrome and other acute traumatic peripheral ischemias, Hyperbaric Medicine Practice 2nd Edition, 1999, (Eds.) Kindwall E, Whelan H. Best Publishing, Flagstaff, AZ, pp753-771.

69. Renstra WR, Buras JA, Svoboda KS. Hyperbaric oxygen increases human dermal fibroblast proliferation, growth factor receptor number and in vitro wound closure. Undersea Hyperb Med. 1998; 25(Suppl):53.

70. Gustilo R. Management of Open Fractures and their Complications, 1982, WB Saunders, Philadelphia, pp202-208.

71. Brighton CT. Quoted in Hospital Tribune Vol. 4, 9 May, 1977.

72. Mackey W, McCulloughs, Conlon Tp, et al. The costs of surgery for limb threatening ischemia. Surgery. 1986; 99:26-35.

73. MacKenzie, EJ, Bosse, Pollak AN, et al. Long term persistence of disability following severe lower-limb trauma. Results of a seven-year follow-up, J Bone Joint Surg. 2005; 87(A):1801-1809.

74. Mubarak SJ, Owen CA, Hargens AR, Garetto LP, et al. Acute compartment syndromes: Diagnosis and treatment with the aid of the wick catheter. J Bone Joint Surg. 1978; 60A:1091-1095.

75. Strauss MB. Hyperbaric Oxygen For Crush Injuries and Compartment Syndromes: Surgical Considerations. In: Bakker DJ, Cramer FS, (Eds.) Hyperbaric Surgery Perioperative Care Flagstaff, AZ Best Publishing Co., 2002; 341-359.

76. Matsen FA III, Winquist RA, Krugmire RB Jr. Diagnosis and management of compartment syndrome. J Bone Joint Surg. 1980; 62(A):286-291.

77. Whitesides TE Jr., Haney TC, Morimoto K, Harada H. Tissue pressure measurements as a determinant for the need of fasciotomy. Clin Orthop Rel Res. 1975; 113:43-51.

78. Matsen FA, Mayo RA, Sheridan GW, Krugmire RB. Monitoring of intramuscular pressure. Surgery. 1976; 79:702-709.

79. Mubarak SJ, Hargens AR. Acute compartment syndromes. Surg Clin North Am. 1983; 63:539-565.

80. Heckman MM, Whitesides TE Jr., Grewe SR, et al. Histologic determination of ischemic threshold of muscle in the canine compartment syndrome model. J Orthop Trauma. 1993; 7:199-210.

81. Matava MF, Whitesides TE Jr., Seiler JG III, Hutton WC. Determination of the compartment threshold pressure of muscle ischemia in the canine model. Orthopedic Transactions. 1993-1994; 17(3):667-668.

82. McQueen MM, Christie J, Court-Brown CM. Acute compartment syndrome in tibial diaphyseal fractures. J Bone Joint Surg. 1996; 78-B:95-98.

83. Bradley El III. The anterior tibial compartment syndrome. Surg Gynecol Obstet. 1973; 136:289-297.

84. Nylander G, Nordstr H, Franzen L, et al. Effects of hyperbaric oxygen in post-ischemic muscle. Scand J Plast Reconstr Surg. 1988; 22:31-39.

85. Nylander G, Otamiri DH, Larsson J. Lipid products in post-ischemic skeletal muscle and after treatment with hyperbaric oxygen. Scand J Plast Reconstr Surg. 1989; 23:97-103.

86. Bartlett RL, Stroman RT, Nickels M, Kalns JE, et al. Rabbit model of the use of fasciotomy and hyperbaric oxygenation in the treatment of compartment syndrome. Undersea and Hyperbaric Medicine. 1998 Supplement; 25:29, #77.

87. Fitzpatrick DT, Murphy PT, Bruce M. Adjunctive treatment of compartment syndrome with hyperbaric oxygen. Mil Med. 1998; 163(8):577-579.

88. Oriani G. Acute indications of HBO therapy—final report, Handbook of Hyperbaric Medicine. 1996, (Ed.) G Oriani, et al., Springer, NY, pp 93-103.

89. Strauss MB, Hart GB. Cost-effective issues in hyperbaric oxygen therapy complicated fractures. J Hyperbaric Med .1988; 3:199-205.

90. Thom SR, Strauss BM. Frostbite: Pathophysiology, treatment and role of hyperbaric oxygen. HBO Review. 1985; 6:99-113.

91. Strauss MB, Winant DM. Contact Point. Letter to the Editor: More on frostbite. Biomechanics. 1998; V(5):9.

92. Skolnilek AA. Early data suggest clot-dissolving drug may help save frostbitten limbs from amputation. JAMA. 1992; 267(15):2008-2010.

93. Buncke HJ, Alpert BS, Johnson-Giebink R. Digital replantation. Surg Clin N Am. 1981; 61:383-394.

94. Kiyoshige Y, Tsuchida H, Watanabe Y. Color monitoring after replantations. Plast Reconstr Surg. 1996; 97:463-468.

95. Zamboni WA, Roth AC, Russell RC, et al. Morphological analysis of the microcirculation during reperfusion of ischemic skeletal muscle and the effect of hyperbaric oxygen, Plas Reconstr Surg. 1993; 91:1110-1123.

96. Handbook of Emergency Cardiovascular Care for Health Care Providers. Hazinski ME, Cummins RD (Eds.) American Heart Association. 1999; p. 3

97. Strauss MB. Evidence review of HBO for crush injury, compartment syndrome and other traumatic ischemia. Undersea and Hyperbaric Medicine. 2001; 28(Suppl):35-36.

98. Strauss MB. The Role of Hyperbaric Oxygen in the Surgical Management of Chronic Refractory Osteomyelitis. In: Bakker DJ, Cramer FS, (Eds.) Hyperbaric Surgery Perioperative Care Flagstaff, AZ Best Publishing Co., 2002; 37-62.

99. Feldmeier JJ (Ed.) Hyperbaric Oxygen 2003 Indications and Results, Hyperbaric Oxygen Therapy Committee Report, Undersea and Hyperbaric Medical Society, Kensington, MD, 2003.

100. Medicare Coverage Issues Manual. Department of Health and Human Services (DHHS). Centers for Medicare and Medicaid Services (CMS), CIM 35-10 Dec 2002, Rev. 48 Issued 03-17-06.

CHAPTER 29

# HBO AND EXCEPTIONAL BLOOD-LOSS ANEMIA

## CHAPTER TWENTY-NINE OVERVIEW

# HBO AND EXCEPTIONAL BLOOD-LOSS ANEMIA

*Bob Bartlett*

## INTRODUCTION

The skillful management of extreme blood-loss anemia requires a great deal of interpersonal, clinical, and sometimes legal coordination. The medical management of extreme anemia is clinically challenging and requires a detailed understanding of oxygen delivery - which is clearly the pervue of an oxygen-based therapy like hyperbaric medicine. With extreme anemia, hyperbaric oxygen provides a supportive bridge until the patient produces sufficient hemoglobin to meet the base physiologic requirements of oxygen delivery.

Following the publication of Boerema's famous "Life without Blood" paper, it is only natural that the medical community turns to the hyperbaric physician as the resident expert on "oxygen therapeutics" (1). This chapter will provide the reader with the necessary background to clinically manage those patients for which traditional transfusion is not an option. A successful recovery of patients with extreme anemia is possible only when the hyperbaric physician understands the appropriate physiologic triggers for beginning and ending hyperbaric therapy as well as the medical management. When the patient's condition warrants a hyperbaric consult, the hyperbaric physician, by necessity must become the managing physician as very few physicians have the skill or knowledge required to medically manage a patient in the absence of transfusion.

The original dosing of HBO by Hart and others was largely empirical and utilized a symptom based approach (2). With the development of the oxymetric pulmonary artery catheter it is now possible to continuously monitor oxygen delivery and consumption and identify deteriorating physiology and provide more timely evidenced-based treatment before organ failure and complications develop. The physiologic approach outlined in this chapter integrates the oxymetric based recommendations pioneered by Shoemaker and the Critical Care Society into an algorithmic guide to the dosing of HBO and medical management of the patient.

## DEFINITION OF EXCEPTIONAL BLOOD-LOSS ANEMIA

Exceptional blood-loss anemia occurs when the hemoglobin level has dropped to a concentration that the circulation can no longer meet the oxygen delivery requirements of life, which leads to cell damage, organ dysfunction or death. The hemoglobin level at which this occurs is extremely variable and will depend on the age and health of the patient and their capacity to compensate. Some patients may decompensate at 6 grams/dl while others may tolerate as little as 2 grams/dl. For example, Weiskoff demonstrated that acute isovolemic reduction of hemoglobin to 5 gm in conscious healthy resting human volunteers is well tolerated (3). There was no evidence of inadequate systemic oxygen transport as assessed by consumed oxygen ($VO_2$), lactate, and Holter monitoring. What is not tolerated is anemia and hypovolemia. The more anemic the patient the more attentive one must be to maintaining adequate vascular volume at all times. Lapin detailed a series of 73 patients all with hemoglobin values less than 5 gm who received orthopedic surgeries with 100% survival (4). Three of these patients had hemoglobin values less than 2 grams/dl, specifically 1.9, 1.8 and 1.4 grams/dl. The take home message should be clear - *there is extreme case to case variability in tolerance and in the clinical arena, you should "treat the patient, not the laboratory values."*

Based on the experience gained from a Bloodless Medicine and Surgery program that manages extreme anemia cases without transfusion, the source of hyperbaric referrals can be divided into two broad categories where transfusion is not an option. They are medical and religious and the religious category comprises 95% of the case consultations for hyperbaric therapy.

## Medical

Cases occasionally arise where there are cross-match difficulties and no compatible blood is readily available. Warm antibody's to cross-matched blood are particularly difficult to manage as is idiopathic autoimmune hemolytic anemia. In addition, there is the perennial blood shortages that are especially problematic for those with special cross-match requirements. For example, sickle cell patients who have received multiple transfusions often develop multiple antibodies that make cross-matching increasingly difficult. In all of these cases, HBO may be required for short term support, while special units of donor blood are located and transferred to the managing institution.

## Religious

The Jehovah's Witness Society is the most rapidly growing religious organization in the western world, with an estimated six million active members. For most healthcare providers, the Society is best known for its refusal of blood products. This abstention is based on three biblical passages that have been interpreted to forbid transfusion:

- Genesis 9:3,4: "every moving thing that liveth shall be meat for you....but the blood thereof, ye shall not eat."
- Acts 15:19-21: "for it seemed to the Holy Ghost, and to us, to lay upon you no greater burden than these necessary things; that ye abstain from meats offered to idols, and from blood..."
- Leviticus, 17:10-16: "therefore I say unto the children of Israel, ye shall eat the blood of no manner of flesh: for the life of all flesh is the blood thereof: whoever eateth it shall be cut off."

Conscious acceptance of blood products means loss of Jehovah's favor and the chance of everlasting life.

The Watchtower and Bible Tract Society still opposes the administration of whole blood and blood components, such as packed red cells, white cells, platelets, and plasma (5). Other biblical passages (Leviticus 17:13, Deuteronomy 12:15,16 and 15:23) rule out pre-operative collection and storage of autologous blood (6). The majority of Jehovah's Witnesses accept crystalloid solutions, colloid solutions, perfluorochemicals and erythropoietin. On an individual basis, some Jehovah's Witnesses find minor blood fractions acceptable, such as immunoglobulin, interferon, interleukins and albumin. Some Jehovah's Witnesses will allow cardiopulmonary bypass, dialysis, plasmaphoresis, intra-operative blood donation and intra-operative cell salvage, provided no allogeneic blood prime is used and the intravenous "circuit" from vein to reservoir and back is not broken. In this regard, acute normovolemic hemodilution has proven value for elective cases where the beginning hemoglobin mass is near normal.

The refusal of potentially life-saving blood products creates ethical and legal dilemmas. The conflict pits the respect of an individual's right to choose against the Hippocratic Oath to preserve life. Clearly, the refusal of standard therapy necessitates the use of alternative strategies.

## Ethical and Legal Considerations

In 1914 on the matter of Schloendorff v Society of New York Hospital, Justice Cordoza provided one of the most important legal opinions governing modern medical care. "Every human being of adult years and sound mind has a right to determine what shall be done with his own body; and a surgeon who performs an operation without his patient's consent commits an assault, for which he is liable in damages" (7). The concept of self-determination is well established in courts around the world and extensively supported by case law. In refusing blood products, Jehovah's Witnesses are exercising their right to independent decision-making, without external coercion. Healthcare professionals must respect and promote the choices of competent patients, even treatment refusal. "Rights are subject to compromise only when they collide with conflicting rights vested in others. The right of free exercise of religion protects more than mere beliefs. Religiously grounded actions or conduct are often beyond the authority of the state to control" - 1985 US Appellate Court Ruling (8). In a 1992 ruling it was noted, "This right of choice is not limited to decisions which others might regard as sensible. It exists whether the reasons for making the choice are rational, irrational or unknown" (9).

Traditionally, parental consent is required in order to perform medical procedures on children, including adolescents. However in emergencies or life threatening situations, this does not apply. Courts recognize that parents have rights, but have noted that these rights are not absolute and exist only to promote the welfare of children. Parental rights to raise children are qualified by a duty to ensure their health, safety, and wellbeing. "Parents may be free to become martyrs themselves. But it does not follow that they are free, in identical circumstances, to make martyrs of their children..." This principle applies whether or not the child is in imminent danger, as parents are always required to make decisions in the child's best interests. Parents cannot make decisions that may permanently harm or otherwise impair their healthy development. If treatment refusal results in a child suffering, the courts are asked to exercise their power under the doctrine of parens patriae, which allows state interference to protect a child's welfare.

Unfortunately, where the courts have been consistent regarding young children, they have been inconsistent where adolescent Jehovah's Witnesses are concerned. Traditionally, minors remain under parental jurisdiction until they reach the age of majority. Over the past century, however, legislation has altered this, allowing minors to obtain treatment for specific conditions without parental consent and, in some states, make medical treatment decisions. Although not recognized by the US Supreme Court, some states have a "mature minor" doctrine, which allows some minors to consent to medical treatment without parental consent. The Illinois Supreme Court recognized that minors have a common law right to refuse medical treatment and determining that, individual judges could determine "whether a minor is mature enough to make health care choices." The most recent case confuses the issue further as the Massachusetts Appeals court granted minors the right to determine their own medical treatment (10). Placing emphasis on the evaluation of a minor's maturity, the court directed judges to consider a minor's wishes and religious convictions and to receive the testimony of minors. At the present time only three states use the mature minor exception to consent to or refuse specific medical treatment, and the majority of adolescents rely on parental decision-making (11). In summary, one should be aware that case precedence is always evolving. For the present one should be aware of the "mature minor" concept until the age of majority is reached for the state in which the case resides.

## MEDICAL MANAGEMENT

### Erythropoietin

Under normal conditions, the circulating red cell mass is remarkably constant. However erythropoiesis is increased by hypoxia suggesting a humoral feedback mechanism. By the early 1950s several investigators had demonstrated the existence of such a humoral erythropoietic factor. This humoral factor was named erythropoietin, as it did not appear to affect white cell or platelet production. During the past 30 years the biochemistry and physiology of this hormone has been extensively studied and culminated in the genetic cloning of the erythropoietin gene in 1985 by Jacobs and Lin (12). Using recombinant DNA technology it has become possible to commercially produce recombinant human erythrpoietin (rHuEPO). Its immediate application was in the management of anemia associated with renal disease. The loss of kidney function is commonly associated with anemia and reflects the fact that erythropoietin is produced primarily by the kidney. Several other anemias have also been found to be responsive. Recombinant human erythrpoietin is also given to normal patients to increase autologous donation (13).

In the management of the acute blood loss anemia patient it serves two purposes. The first purpose is to offset any possible effects of the hyperoxia of HBO as a negative feedback signal to suppress endogenous erythropoietin production (14). The second purpose is the induction of a supranormal bone marrow response. The bone *marrow has a clear dose dependent response to erythropoietin* - the higher the dose, the better the response (15). Regardless of which commercial form of erythropoietin is used, it must be *given at or exceeding maximum doses*. With extreme anemia, there is a race against time and the high dosing is justified, given the scenario that survival is on the line. Beyond the immediate clinical urgency, there are physiologic reasons that require higher than normal doses based on the recent recognition that critically ill patients have a depressed bone marrow response to erythropoietin (16). The depression is mediated by inflammatory cytokines and altered iron metabolism that are associated with critical illness and stress. However an increased dose of erythropoietin will restore red cell production (17). The optimal dose of erythropoietin is still unclear, especially when treating critically ill patients with life-threatening acute blood loss. One high dose rHuEPO regimen is to provide 600 IU kg every other day (18).

Besides stimulating erythropoiesis, rHuEPO appears to provide cellular protection against hypoxic and ischemic injury in different tissues (19). Accumulating evidence indicates that erythropoietin is a cellular survival factor in neurons and can cross the blood–brain barrier (20). Erythropoietin can provide cellular protection against apoptosis by inhibiting specific cellular protein kinase cascades and plays a specific role in repair and regeneration, including the recruitment of stem cells into the region of damage (21). Erythropoietin may be a novel therapeutic approach to limiting myocardial injury after ischemic events and minimizing ventricular dysfunction. This protection is associated with decreased myocyte apoptosis and is supported by the absence of myocardial ischemia or dysfunction in our patient (22).

## Intravenous Iron

The demand for hemoglobin synthesis imposed by rHuEPO will exceed the capacity of the reticuloendothelial system to release iron to transferring. Goodnough and others have observed that "oral iron supplementation may be sufficient to keep pace with endogenously stimulated erythropoiesis, it may not be adequate to prevent iron-restricted erythropoiesis during rHuEPO therapy" (23). Thus, many patients may have a blunted response to epoietin because of a "functional" iron deficiency anemia. Current concepts regarding iron and in particular intravenous iron have changed considerably in recent years (24).

The accurate determination of iron status in these patients can be a challenging task, which is made more difficult by inflammation, infection, and the large number of co-morbid conditions that can affect commonly used indices of body iron stores. Despite their limitations, transferrin saturation and serum ferritin remain the cornerstones of iron status assessment. Because these values can be altered by a number of non-iron-related factors, it is necessary to go beyond these measures and draw upon additional sources of information to determine the patient's iron status. Other important factors to consider when assessing the need for iron therapy include evidence of underlying inflammatory processes that may block iron mobilization and distort the standard iron indices, the results of alternative iron indices, and the patient's recent history of iron administration. Frequently, the response to a gram of intravenous iron is a safe and effective way to determine the role of iron deficiency in the anemia of the problematic patient. The newer intravenous preparations of IV iron, such as Ferelecit, have established an effective record of safety and efficacy. At a minimum, transferrin saturation should be maintained above 20% at all times through periodic doses of intravenous iron.

## Androgens

Before the advent of epoietin, androgens were used with some success in treating the anemia associated with renal disease. A study by Ballal et al. indicates that the androgen nandrolone decanoate potentiates the effect of low dose epoeitin. One hundred mg of nandrolone was given IM once a week during a 12-week period. It appears to enhance the effect of epoietin by increasing the sensitivity of erythroid progenitor cell lines such as colony forming units (CFU- E) and burst forming units (BFU-E). The benefit of using an androgen with low dose epoeitin is clear. No androgen side effects were reported in Ballal's study. As an anabolic steroid, there may be additional benefits to this approach as detailed by others (25).

## Hemostatic Agents

The most common circumstances that precede a hyperbaric consult involve a Jehovah's Witness who has sustained recent trauma, has gastrointestinal bleeding, or had unplanned complications during surgery. All three of these may be associated with some slow, continuing blood loss. In the absence of transfusion, it is important to have a strategy to reduce ongoing blood loss or for planned surgical interventions to reduce blood loss.

Concerns regarding the safety of transfused blood have led to the development of a range of interventions to minimize blood loss during major surgery. Three useful interventions to keep in mind are fibrin glue, antifibrinolytic amino acids, and desmopressin. Fibrin glue has proven value and on a case to case basis, it may be acceptable to Jehovah's witnesses. This agent is only of value intraoperatively.

The antifibrinolytic amino acids, also known as lysine analogues include the two drugs tranexamic acid and aminocaproic acid. These agents have been widely used in cardiac surgery and orthopedic surgery to reduce blood loss and the need for transfusion. These agents prevent the breakdown of the stabilizing fibrin element of a blood clot; hence the term "antifibrinolytic." They exert their antifibrinolytic effect through the reversible blockade of lysine binding sites on plasminogen molecules and prevent the conversion to plasmin, which is responsible for splitting fibrin. This blockade ensures that nature's bandage, the blood clot, remains in place. This results in significant reduction in postoperative "oozing". A common concern has been the possible development of deep venous thrombosis. Meta-analyses have consistently documented that short term use of these medications is not associated with thromboembolic events. In short, they stabilize existing blood clots, but do not contribute to the formation of new blood clots.

Desmopressin (1-desamino-8-D-arginine vasopressin or DDAVP) improves the bleeding time and provides surgical hemostasis for many patients with von Willebrand disease, mild hemophilia, primary or acquired platelet disorders, and uremia. Recent observations indicate that this treatment shortens the bleeding time in normal patients as well. Desmopressin is a synthetic vasopressin analogue that lacks vasopressor activity. It apparently shortens bleeding time by inducing the release of factor VII and possibly has an effect on vessel walls that increases platelet adhesion. In a double-blind, prospective randomized trial of intraoperative DDAVP to reduce blood loss during cardiac surgery in hemostatically normal patients, the drug significantly reduced blood loss; 1,300 ml in the treatment group vs 2,200 ml in the placebo group (26). The recommended dose is 0.3 ug/kg IV over 20 minutes (27).

## Hypothermia

Induction of mild hypothermia to a core temperature of 34°C (93.2°F) causes a significant reduction in oxygen consumption. This technique has been widely used in cardiovascular surgery to reduce the oxygen requirements during cardiopulmonary bypass. For every 1°C decrease in temperature, oxygen consumption will decrease approximately 6%. Thus at 34°C there is an 18% reduction in oxygen requirements (28).

There is a great deal of clinical experience detailing the use of therapeutic hypothermia for cardiac surgery and there is accumulating evidence that mild hypothermia may improve outcomes for hemorrhagic shock. In a clinically relevant, large animal model with trauma and intensive care, mild hypothermia improve survival after hemorrhagic shock (29). Because muscle shivering increases oxygen consumption 50% to 70%, it is imperative that the patient is paralyzed before inducing hypothermia and maintained until the hypothermia is completed. If surgery is anticipated or there is ongoing blood loss, hypothermia may be associated with increased bleeding (30).

With hypothermia, the oxyhemoglobin curve shifts to the left. In other words, there is an increased affinity for oxygen. There has been a concern that this increase in hemoglobin's affinity for oxygen would adversely affect $DO_2$, however, there is no *in vivo* evidence linking the P50 change (affinity) to impaired oxygen extraction. One theory suggests there may also be a proportional increase in the affinity of tissues for oxygen, thus preventing any diffusion imbalance between hemoglobin and tissue affinities (31).

Other possibilities could account for normal oxygen delivery despite a left shift in the oxyhemoglobin dissociation curve. These include a change in the Krogh oxygen diffusion coefficient or possibly the minimum tissue $PO_2$ required for aerobic metabolism may be lower in hypothermia. Finally, an increase in capillary transit time with hypothermia, would allow the erythrocytes more time to release their $O_2$ during their passage through the capillary beds.

Oxygen solubility in plasma increases as blood temperature decreases (32). There is a reported 10% increase in dissolved oxygen when the plasma is cooled to 30°C. With a normal Hb level, the increase plasma $O_2$ solubility is of minor importance, but at the extremely low levels of Hb that is encountered in the acute blood loss patient the relative contribution of dissolved oxygen becomes increasing important even under normobaric conditions. For example a patient with a hematocrit of 5% will transport 50% of the oxygen by hemoglobin and 50% by plasma at a temperature of 30 degrees with a 10% AV extraction (99 to 89% sat) and a $PvO_2$ of 40 mmHg.

Blood viscosity increases with hypothermia. For patients with a normal hematocrit, the viscosity is 23% higher at 30°C than at 37°C. For the acute blood loss patient these changes are considerably less because of the extreme "dilution" of the blood. Viscosity changes may be partially offset by the use of pentoxiphylline, a theobromine that increases erythrocyte deformability and reduces resistance to flow in capillaries (33). Use of this drug improves oxygen extraction and reduces the critical $DO_2$ value of hypothermic dogs. There is accumulating evidence that pentoxyfilline may have other benefits. Several experimental studies have demonstrated improved outcomes from hemorrhagic shock by reducing white cell activation and pro-inflammatory mediators (34).

## HYPERBARIC OXYGEN THERAPY

### Historical Perspective

Based on Henry's law, the amount of oxygen dissolved in plasma is quite small (0.003 ml/mmHg). However, at 3 atmospheres absolute (ATA), the arterial $pO_2$ is in excess of 2,000 mmHg, which will dissolve 6.3 volumes percent of oxygen in the plasma. At this pressure the oxygen content of plasma will meet the body's resting requirement of 6 volumes percent. These mathematical considerations were put to a physiological test by Boerema using pigs. In a study entitled "Life without Blood," he exchanged the pig's whole blood with an acellular perfusate - lowering the pig's hemoglobin to 0.4 grams/dl while they were inside of a hyperbaric chamber (1). Despite the near absence of red cells, the pigs survived without complications. Based on Boerema's classic study, Ammonic was the first to demonstrate that HBO would also support humans at an extremely low hematocrit. Further use of HBO by Hart et al. extended the clinical experience greatly and established HBO's role in the management of acute blood loss anemia (35).

### Experimental Evidence

It is not surprising that HBO can be used to augment oxygen delivery in the setting of anemia. But can HBO still be effective when the patient is hypovolemic or has significant vasoconstriction? The answer appears to be yes. Several shock models indicate that HBO provides significant protection against irreversible shock. In a hemorrhagic canine shock model employed by Doi et al., the animal's blood pressure was lowered to 30 mmHg by removal of blood through the femoral artery into a reservoir bottle (36). This pressure was maintained for 90 minutes. A control group breathed air during the 90 minutes while the experimental group received HBO at 2 ATA. At the end of the 90 minutes, their blood was reinfused. In the control group oxygen consumption was decreased to 2 ml/kg/min. An oxygen debt subsequently accrued during the hypotensive period. In the hyperbaric group, the decrease in oxygen consumption was negligible as was the change in lactate. In the control group, all animals with an oxygen debt in excess of 140 ml/kg died.

Similar findings were reported by Attar, utilizing a comparable hemorrhagic shock model. Animals were held at a mean arterial pressure of 30 mmHg for 2 1/2 hours. During that time the control group breathed air and the experimental group received HBO at 3 ATA. At the end of the 2 1/2 hr period only 17% of the control animals were alive in contrast to 74% of the HBO group (37, 38).

In a canine model of controlled hypotension of (40 mmHg for 2 hours), Elliot investigated survival rates for animals on room air, 100% $O_2$, 100% $O_2$ by ventilator, and HBO at 3 ATA. Mortality rates were 90% in the control, 50% in those receiving normobaric oxygen with or without a ventilator, and 27% for those given HBO (39).

The understanding of hemorrhagic shock as a cytokine trigger has grown considerably in recent years. Many shock induced cytokines are responsible, in part, for the evolution of organ failure hours to days later. HBO has established benefit as an aid to recovery from reperfusion mediated injury. Yamashita recently reported on the effect of hyperbaric oxygen treatment on cytokine induction after hemorrhage in a rat model. The HBO treatment group had a significant reduction in TNF-α, IL-6 as well as mortality compared to the room air controls. It would appear that the benefits of hyperbaric oxygen are far more substantial than the simple notion of oxygen as a metabolite (40).

## Clinical Experience

Typically HBO is employed in those instances where the patient has religious convictions that prescribe the use of blood or blood products. In rare instances it may be required to temporarily support a patient when there are blood shortages, cross-match problems or warm antibody hemolytic anemia. Hart summarized a series of 26 patients with severe anemia who were managed with HBO between 1970 and 1987. Clinical management consisted of replacing lost volume with dextran and later with hetastarch, generous doses of hematenics (vitamins B, C and iron) and intermittently wrapping of the lower extremities with ace bandages. The particular details of the patient treatment profiles were not published; however, the average survivor required HBO for 10 days. No instances of pulmonary or CNS oxygen toxicity occurred.

Concern is sometimes raised that HBO might blunt the erythropoietic response to anemia. This should not be a concern for two reasons. First, these patients should already be on high doses of erythropoietin, in which case endogenous production is not a factor. Second, Wright demonstrated that HBO facilitates a more rapid recovery from hemorrhage, independent of any exogenous erythropoietin. In their rabbit blood loss model involving 30% loss of hemoglobin they found a faster recovery with the HBO-treated group reaching the baseline level of hemoglobin in 11 days as opposed to 14 days for the control group (p < 0.001) (41).

Historically HBO was administered according to Hart's criteria: 1) systolic blood pressure below 90 mmHg or patients requiring vasopressors, 2) disorientation or coma, 3) ischemic ECG changes or 4) ischemic gut (1). However, these criteria have a number of limitations. Ischemic diarrhea is often a pre-terminal event where HBO may be "too little, too late." ECG changes in the form of flipped T waves can be caused by a variety of factors. Disorientation often times cannot be assessed because paralysis, sedation, and mechanical ventilation is continued post-operatively to reduce unnecessary oxygen consumption and finally, current concepts of shock no longer endorse a blood-pressure-based definition.

## A PHYSIOLOGICAL APPROACH

### Goal-Directed Oxymetric Monitoring

On an individual basis, the tolerance for anemia is quite variable. For this reason the decision to transfuse should not be based solely on the hemoglobin concentration. The current concept in transfusion medicine is to treat "the physiology, not the lab" (42). Where HBO is involved, a clear understanding of physiologic principles is required as a basis for determining the frequency and duration of therapy. Central to this understanding is an appreciation for the total amount of oxygen delivered and consumed. To utilize an oxygen based therapy without measuring the substance in question, oxygen, would be a step backward into simple empirical practice. In the same way that modern hyperbaric programs explore wounds with transcutaneous oxygen probes to determine whether hypoxia is a problem, we may not intelligently approach cases of extreme anemia utilizing whole body oxymetrics.

In the past it was difficult to measure oxygen delivery and consumption, but it was easy to measure blood pressure. This was unfortunate for the understanding of circulatory function. "Blood pressure cuffs have had a fatal influence on clinical practice because blood pressure and blood flow are not equivalent. Organs respond to blood flow, and hence, oxygen delivery, not blood pressure" (43). In a large series of carefully monitored, critically ill, postoperative patients, over 50,000 values of the five most commonly measured variables were evaluated: mean arterial pressure, heart rate, central venous pressure, pulmonary artery wedge pressure and cardiac output. These values were restored to normal in 76% of non-survivors who, nevertheless, still died. Thus traditional indicators do not have a clear relationship to outcome. They are useful descriptors of end-stage circulatory failure, but are neither sensitive nor accurate as an *early warning* of circulatory impairment (44, 45).

Shock is more appropriately characterized as a state in which oxygen delivery ($DO_2$) is inadequate. For this reason, responsible use of hyperbaric oxygen therapy requires an understanding of oxygen dynamics. Whether the etiology is anemia, hypovolemia, cardiogenic, respiratory, septic, or toxic, the net effect is the same; tissue hypoxia, a cumulative oxygen debt, and the cessation of oxidative metabolism. Failure to provide adequate amounts of oxygen will result in cellular injury owing to the loss of electrochemical gradients. When a critical mass of cells in an organ is injured, organ function is impaired, and an inflammatory process follows. Through the release of inflammatory mediators, cellular oxygen and substrate delivery suffer further, leading to the multiorgan failure syndrome. Early identification of failing physiology permits a more timely use of oxygen therapeutics.

A recent meta-analysis showed significant benefit when pulmonary artery catheter data is used to guide therapy during the intraoperative and immediate postoperative period (46). Goal-directed therapy is ineffective in the late stages of oxygen debt after the onset of organ failure. No amount of extra oxygen will restore irreversible oxygen debt, failed organs, or dead cells. In the late stage of acute illness after organ failure has occurred, aggressive therapy directed to improve oxygen delivery is generally futile. *The goal of oxymetric monitoring is to detect significant physiologic change before it becomes clinically obvious.* The ability to monitor delivered and consumed oxygen, permits a more timely intervention. Early intervention prevents tissue ischemia and secondary organ dysfunction.

## Tissue Oxygen Debt in the Surgical Setting

Postoperative multi-organ failure is a major problem associated with circulatory insufficiency. Because of the vital interdependence of organs, the failure of one organ almost invariably sets the stage for failure of other organs. When metabolic processes are limited by insufficient oxygen over prolonged periods, multiple organ failure ensues. First described by Baue, this condition has been regarded as a common ICU syndrome associated with postoperative death (47, 48).

Shoemaker advanced the concept that a tissue oxygen debt is reflected by inadequate oxygen consumption ($VO_2$) in the intraoperative and immediate postoperative periods (49). Oxygen debt is a common determinant of multisystem organ failure and death (50). Earlier work by other investigators calculated the cumulative $VO_2$ deficit in dogs subjected to hemorrhagic shock (51). When the oxygen debt was less than 100 ml/kg there was no mortality. When the calculated $VO_2$ deficit increased to 120 ml/kg the mortality increased to 50% and when the $VO_2$ deficit was greater than 140 ml/kg, mortality was greater than 95%. Shoemaker observed that the cumulative oxygen deficit averaged 33 $L/m^2$ in patients who died, 27 $L/m^2$ in survivors with one or more organ failures, and 8 $L/m^2$ in survivors who had no shock related complications. In addition the temporal pattern of the $VO_2$ deficit was important. The duration of the oxygen deficit averaged 35 hours for nonsurvivors, 24 hours for survivors with organ failure and 8 hours for survivors without any complications. All of these patients had normal preoperative hemodynamic values and did not have any existing handicaps such as trauma, sepsis, cirrhosis, or major cardiovascular problems.

For the past 25 years intensivists has been studying the hemodynamic and oxygen transport responses to operative trauma (52). Increased cardiac index, oxygen delivery, and oxygen consumption characterized the physiologic status of surviving high risk patients. Relatively normal $DO_2$ and $VO_2$ values were associated with nonsurvivors who developed an early oxygen debt followed by progressive organ failure and death. The oxygen transport differences were sufficiently large and consistent to be used to predict outcome. An outcome predictor based on CI, $DO_2$, and $VO_2$ values was tested prospectively on a series of high risk postoperative patients and found to be correct in 94% of the patient. It was most accurate in the first 24 hours (53). It was concluded that the "supranormal" values of $DO_2$ and $VO_2$ were necessary compensatory responses for survival (54). It seemed clear that the use of normal values as therapeutic goals in an abnormal situation (e.g. recovery from operative trauma) may not be appropriate. Compensatory increases in $DO_2$ and $VO_2$ are needed to quickly correct intraoperative oxygen debt, overcome impaired peripheral perfusion, and meet the increased metabolic demands or recovery from operative trauma.

## Understanding Oxygen Delivery ($DO_2$) and Consumption ($VO_2$) Relationships

To properly manage a patient with significant blood loss anemia physicians must understand the principle factors governing oxygen delivery ($DO_2$) and consumption ($VO_2$). The adequacy of tissue oxygenation depends upon the volume of oxygen delivered to the tissues and the volume consumed. This supply/demand balance is determined by five factors that are readily measured and a sixth that cannot be measured. The five measured factors are hemoglobin concentration, the affinity of hemoglobin for oxygen (P50), the percentage of arterial hemoglobin saturated with oxygen ($SaO_2$), oxygen consumption ($VO_2$) and the cardiac output (CO). The sixth factor is the distribution of perfusion. If oxygen delivery is reduced by a partial loss in any of the five measurable factors, compensations will occur among the others.

Under normal conditions oxygen delivery or availability greatly exceeds oxygen consumption. For this reason oxygen consumption is considered to be supply independent. In other words increasing the delivery of oxygen does not cause an increase in consumption. A change in delivery only results in a reciprocal change in oxygen extraction from blood. Increasing delivery results in less oxygen being extracted per unit volume. Conversely, decreasing oxygen delivery produces a higher oxygen extraction ratio. In a case where oxygen delivery is greatly reduced, there exists for tissue a critical oxygen delivery value after which the oxygen extraction ratio cannot increase enough to meet oxygen consumption. At this point, oxygen consumption becomes "supply dependent." When this occurs, oxygen consumption varies directly with the delivery of oxygen. When oxygen consumption is supply dependent, anaerobic metabolism begins, oxygen debt accrues, and the patient is now in the first stage of shock (55, 56)

The relationship between $DO_2$ and $VO_2$ has been the subject of numerous studies. As previously mentioned, under normal conditions there is an abundant oxygen supply and $VO_2$ is a function of metabolic rate, not oxygen supply. As the supply of oxygen is reduced, there is a compensatory increase in the oxygen extraction ratio and $VO_2$ is unchanged. However, this extraction reserve can be exhausted when there are severe reductions in $DO_2$. At this point $VO_2$ becomes completely dependent on oxygen delivery and will directly fluctuate with the changes in $DO_2$. This state of affairs is pathologic and referred to as supply dependent oxygen consumption. The $DO_2$ value at which this occurs is termed the "critical $DO_2$" ($DO_2$crit). Below the critical $DO_2$, the tissues begin to consume energy stores in the form of phoshpocreatine, eventually turning to anaerobic glycolysis with lactate production. When perfusion is appropriately regulated and the oxygen requirements are met, $VO_2$ is maximal ($VO_2$ max). Basal $VO_2$ is approximately 2 ml/kg/min. and is typically constant when the $DO_2$ is in the range of 7-9 ml/kg/min (57, 58).

# Understanding Mixed Venous Blood Gas Analysis - $SvO_2$

Mixed venous blood gas analysis is the cornerstone for assessing the adequacy of global oxygen transport. So long as the patient maintains appropriate capillary regulation, $SvO_2$ will serve as a global index of oxygen supply/demand balance. Because a decrease in $SvO_2$ may indicate inadequate oxygen transport, continuous monitoring is desirable. It will not identify the precise cause, but will bring to attention any change in supply and demand. The mixed venous saturation is a flow weighted average of the oxygen extraction for all tissues. Some tissues such as skin, resting muscle, or kidneys extract less oxygen than other tissues such as the heart. The magnitude of the effect of oxygen extraction by any organ on $SvO_2$ is proportional to the blood flow to that organ so that low-consumption/high-flow organs, such as the kidneys have a greater effect on $SvO_2$ than do high consumption organs like the heart.

Normally, venous oxygen saturation is maintained within a narrow range. Decreases in $SvO_2$ occur frequently in patients with cardiopulmonary complications. The changes in $SvO_2$ often precede changes in blood pressure. The decrease may correlate with the magnitude of cardiopulmonary impairment and decreases in $SvO_2$ that do not improve with therapy are associated with a poor prognosis. Severe venous hypoxemia has been associated with lactic acidosis and a high mortality. In 20 patients with severe cardiac or pulmonary disease or both, mixed venous $pO_2$ ($PvO_2$) correlated better with both hyperlactemia and survival than did cardiac output or arterial $pO_2$ ($PaO_2$). A $PvO_2$ below 28 mmHg was usually associated with death in this study (59).

Swan measured $PvO_2$ during cardiopulmonary bypass and found a close correlation to increases in lactic acid (60). They concluded that maintaining patient levels above 35 mmHg will ensure adequate tissue oxygenation and prevent lactic acidosis. Conversely, if the $PvO_2$ drifts below 30 mmHg, lactic acidemia will develop. In dogs, the lactate production threshold for $PvO_2$ was 27 mmHg whether caused by arterial hypoxemia, low cardiac output, or a combination of these variables. These observations suggest that when vasoregulation is intact there is a threshold value, or critical $PvO_2$ of about 28 mmHg, below which anaerobic metabolism is usually manifest as an increase in blood lactate. Despite a general lack of knowledge regarding the precise relationships between $PvO_2$ levels and the adequacy of tissue oxygenation, there exists a strong interdependence.

These observations suggest that oxygen requirements are being met when $PvO_2$ is above 28 mmHg. However, metabolic compromise may occur at higher perfusion levels even when the $PvO_2$ is more than 28 mmHg. For example, lactate production by isolated tissues (muscle) might be compensated for with increased lactate consumption by heart, kidney, and liver. The threshold value of 28 mmHg marks an oxymetric level where lactate production is no longer compensated for by the liver. In other words, tissue hypoxia may occur at higher $PvO_2$ levels; however the lactate production is typically compensated for by increased liver consumption (61).

The microcirculatory physiology of extreme anemia is uniquely different (62, 63). Traditionally it was thought that mixed venous oxygen saturation values would be similar during hypoxic hypoxia and anemic hypoxia. Using a pig model to duplicate conditions of hypoxic hypoxia and anemic hypoxia, van der Hoeven followed $SvO_2$, oxygen delivery, oxygen extraction, and determined critical values based on lactate and oxygen consumption (64). In comparison with hypoxic hypoxia, critical values of $SvO_2$ are higher in anemic hypoxia (26% vs. 55%), indicating that oxygen unloading from blood to tissues is impaired in anemic hypoxia. Because the red blood cell velocity is increased and the red blood cell residence time is reduced during isovolemic hemodilution, a decrease in precapillary oxygen release and in diffusional oxygen transfer to other microvessels is thought to account for a higher critical $SvO_2$ value. These characteristics in oxygen transport and capillary hemodynamics should be taken into consideration when $SvO_2$ is used in clinical critical care.

## Microcirculatory Regulation

Early investigators evaluating $DO_2$, $VO_2$, or $SVO_2$ patterns in general ICU populations reported conflicting clinical outcomes. It was hoped that a relationship as fundamental as $DO_2$ and $VO_2$ would produce a set of universal parameters that would transcend any particular disease state. With the passage of time it became apparent that more meaningful relationships could be found when critically ill patients are divided into the following five categories: (1) posttraumatic and/or postoperative, (2) cardiogenic, (3) septic (4) cirrhotic and (5) adult respiratory distress syndrome (ARDS). This division reflects the observation that some diseases produce tissue hypoxia by limiting the ability to extract sufficient oxygen despite an adequate cardiac output with normal arterial oxygen content. Specifically patients with sepsis, cirrhosis, and adult respiratory distress syndrome have reduced extraction capacity, which reflects disordered microcirculatory regulation (65, 66).

Although $SvO_2$ is an indicator of the supply/demand balance for perfused tissues, its value as a threshold marker for anaerobic metabolism depends on appropriate vasoregulation. When vasoregulation is impaired due to multiorgan failure, sepsis, etc, the utility of $SVO_2$ as a guide to therapy is greatly diminished. However, *oxygen extraction relationships appear to remain intact for the critically ill post-hemorrhage or postoperative patients.* This is a key concept as 90% of exceptional blood loss cases will either be the result of trauma-related blood loss or surgical-related blood loss.

## Lactate Levels

Beyond pulmonary artery catheter data other measures of tissue perfusion should be considered as a guide to the frequency and duration of HBO therapy. In patients with poor tissue oxygenation, cells increase anaerobic metabolism and lactate levels rise. The clinician may, therefore, monitor serial lactate levels in patients with normal hepatic function as measures of global perfusion. Waxman et al. followed sequential perioperative lactate levels in 12 high risk surgical patients (67). There was a marked increase in lactate values intraoperatively. This increase did not correspond to decreases in either mean arterial pressure or cardiac output, but did correlate with $VO_2$. Postoperatively, lactate levels remained elevated, and this elevation correlated with the intraoperative oxygen deficit. Rashkin, et al. had similar findings in 44 critically ill patients with and without adult respiratory distress syndrome (68). Blood lactate was used as an indicator of tissue hypoxia independent of cardiac output. Survival was good (55%) and blood lactate was near normal for those with oxygen delivery greater than 8 ml/kg/min. Below this level, survival was poor (14%) and blood lactate markedly increased (69). In a series of surgical ICU patients, lactate levels > 10 mmole/L were associated with 100% mortality, levels between 5 and 10 mmole/L with 75% mortality, and 36% mortality for levels between 2.5 and 5 mmole/L (70). A notable finding was the lack of an anion gap. More than half of the patient had no anion gap. This underscores the importance of directly measuring lactate levels. In summary, lactate levels can cross validate to oxymetric measurements and strengthen the clinical determination of clinical stability and physiologic adaptation for a given level of hemoglobin.

The physiologic concepts relevant to circulatory failure from blood loss can be summarized as follows: (1) among the metabolic substances transported by the circulatory system, oxygen has the highest extraction ratio and is the most flow dependent, (2) the general adequacy of circulation system can be evaluated by the mass movement of oxygen in terms of the $DO_2$; (3) the $VO_2$ reflects the sum of all oxidative metabolism; thus $DO_2$ and $VO_2$ provide the best measure of the functional adequacy of both circulation and metabolism; (4) the pattern of oxygen transport ($DO_2$ and $VO_2$) correlates with survival or death. The hyperbaric implications of the foregoing should be clear - if the postoperative survival goals for $DO_2/VO_2$ cannot be reached using conventional therapies HBO should be added to the regimen. Other factors to weigh into the decision process would include ischemic ECG changes as an indicator of isolated cardiac failure and lactate levels. These general considerations of oxygen dynamics can serve as a guide to the intelligent and timely use of hyperbaric oxygen or oxygen therapeutics.

## TREATMENT PROTOCOL

### Bioavailability of Oxygen

If the goal of hyperbaric oxygen therapy is to physiologically repay the oxygen debt, it is reasonable to ask what is the pressure and duration required. All hyperbaric medicine classes teach the common concept of arterial oxygen pressures at different A; e.g. at 1 ATA the $pO_2$ is 760 mmHg and at 3 ATA it is more than 2,000 mmHg. However, rarely do we consider the concept of bioavailability. This concept transcends simple gas pressures and answers the question of oxygen delivery to the tissues.

For example, if a patient with a hemoglobin of 2 gm/dl, has accumulated an oxygen debt of 20 liters over the past 12 hours, do we actually repay that debt with a single HBO treatment at 2 ATA for 60 minutes? The answer to the question requires a consideration of bioavailability or more precisely, oxygen delivery. Assume in this example a normal cardiac output of 6 liters/min. For simplicity, we will ignore the contribution of the hemoglobin that is present as it is typically 100% saturated under room air conditions. Using Henry's law, we can calculate the volume of oxygen delivered by plasma alone. The solubility of oxygen in plasma is 0.003 ml/dl/mmHg or 0.03 ml/liter/mmHg. Under hyperbaric conditions at 2 ATA of pure oxygen, we would achieve a plasma-mediated delivery of 16.4 liters of oxygen. Using this simple model, we would fall short of our goal of 20 liters. If the treatment were extended to 90 minutes, we would deliver 24.6 liters. If we extended the duration to 120 minutes, we could deliver as much as 32.8 liters of oxygen.

## Treatment Schedule

There have been no experimental dosing studies of HBO to examine the variables of pressure (2 verses 2.5 ATA), time (60 verses 90 verses 120 minutes), and frequency. Based on what is known about tissue oxygen half lives, the generating of energy stores, shock-mediated reperfusion injury with up-regulated white cell activity and the clinical reports that have been published to date, an approximate starting point can be offered. It should always be subject to change based on the physiologic data that is available e.g. ECG changes, lactate levels, oxygen consumption, and oxygen debt. (See Figure 1 Algorithm.)

If significant lactate elevation is present, ST segment depression or T wave changes, the first treatment should begin at 3 ATA for 30 minutes followed by a 5-minute air break and a reduction of pressure to 2 ATA for an additional 90 minutes with 5-minute air breaks being given every 30 minutes. (See Figure 2 ) This HBO protocol is very similar to the protocol advanced by Weaver for the management of carbon monoxide (71).

The obvious initial benefit of 3 ATA is to quickly load the tissues with oxygen. This pressure may offer additional benefits by limiting the pathophysiology of shock mediated white cell adhesion and cytokine production. Current concepts of circulatory shock detail the adverse effects of white cell activation and cytokine production. Much of the physiology of shock is similar to a reperfusion injury as both are triggered by circulatory failure followed by restoration. HBO's ability to limit white cell activation is more pronounced at higher pressures such as 3 ATA, and is probably achieved in as little as 30 minutes. The HBO mechanisms for reperfusion injury attenuation are cited elsewhere in this textbook.

Following the first treatment, repeat measurements of delivered and consumed oxygen, mixed venous saturation, and lactate. Continued presence of lactate with a high oxygen extraction ratio ($SvO_2$ of 50%) indicate a continuing oxygen debt and promptly repeat treatments of 60-90 minute duration with 5-minute air breaks given every 30 minutes, followed by one hour surface intervals. Air breaks are given to reduce the risk of pulmonary oxygen toxicity. It is important that the oxygen administration in between treatments is administered by a venti-mask at the lowest $FIO_2$ required for 100% saturation of hemoglobin. It is well recognized that pulmonary oxygen toxicity will develop if the lungs are continuously exposed to an $FIO_2 > 60\%$.

The HBO treatment intensity can be relaxed if the post-treatment lactate levels have fallen and the $SvO_2$ has increased. The interval between treatments is now governed by obtaining the lactate level and $SvO_2$ just prior to the next treatment. If the values are acceptable, this suggests that the treatment intervals could be lengthened further. The minimum treatment frequency is b.i.d.

## OXYGEN THERAPEUTICS - A NEW ERA OF MEDICINE

The quest for blood substitutes has spanned half a century. Some of the established limitations to the use of banked blood include the following: (1) a limited shelf life of 42 days, (2) the time-consuming process of cross-matching

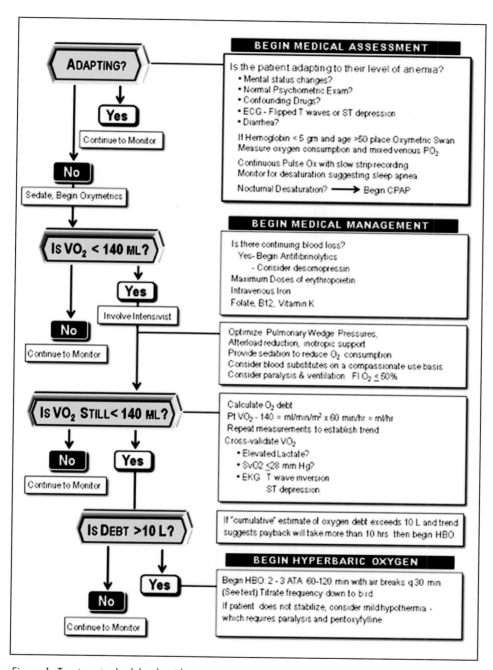

*Figure 1. Treatment schedule algorithm.*

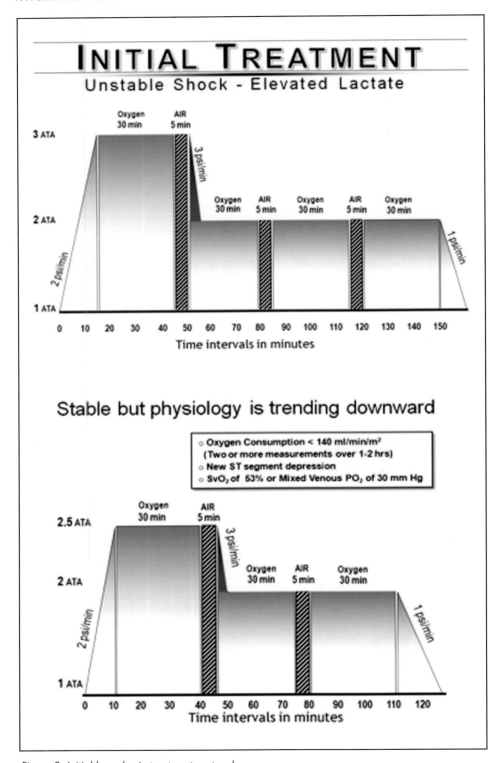

Figure 2. Initial hyperbaric treatment protocol.

(3) the risk of viral and bacterial transmission and (5) the limited oxygen transport capacity of banked blood during the initial hours following transfusion.

Additional concerns surrounding transfusion encompass the known transmissible diseases as well as the yet-to-be-discovered diseases. Transfusion science has been humbled sufficiently in recent history, to regard blood as an "ever-present vector" for disease transmission. In addition, the case for immune suppression is well established. The clinical significance of this suppression has been verified with increased infection rates and tumor recurrence. There is now evidence that links transfusion to multiorgan failure syndrome in the setting of trauma resuscitation (72). Many of these adverse side effects have been linked to the presence of residual leukocytes, which has prompted blood banks to switch to leukodepletion, adding additional expense. Although leukodepletion appears to offer benefits, there is growing evidence that it will not completely eliminate transfusion mediated immune depression, bone marrow depression or the multiorgan failure syndrome (73, 74).

With each passing decade, the need for a solution with gas transporting properties similar to blood has increased. The ideal blood substitute should not require cross-matching or refrigeration, which would permit ease of use in prehospital care. More importantly, it should also have a long shelf life and be disease free. Although the term "blood substitutes" has been popularized in the literature, it is a technical misnomer given the variety of functions carried out by this "liquid organ" blood. With oxygen delivery as the singular goal of these man-made solutions, a more appropriate term is red cell substitutes or the more generic term "oxygen therapeutics." Oxygen therapeutics offer features not found in natural red cells. The most important feature may be their ability to penetrate into compromised capillary beds that exhibit the phenomenon of plasma streaming.

There are currently four broad categories of oxygen therapeutics to consider. The hemoglobin-based oxygen carriers are chemically modified derivatives of hemoglobin or recombinant DNA derivatives of hemoglobin. Presently, the base hemoglobin is either human or bovine. The second category is the use of perflourocarbons which have a high solubility coefficient for oxygen. The third category employs the use of synthetic allosteric modifiers to shift the oxyhemoglobin dissociation curve to the right, which produces a greater release of oxygen in the capillary beds. The fourth category is hyperbaric oxygen, which makes use of the natural gas laws to dissolve large volumes of oxygen in plasma.

## The Hemoglobin-Based Oxygen Carriers

### Physiological challenges
In the 1930s and 1940s it was learned that removal of the red cell membrane eliminated the antigenicity associated with blood types and eliminates the need for cross-matching. Such "stroma free" hemoglobin also had a relatively long shelf life. Experiments with lactated Ringer's solution containing hemoglobin demonstrated that animals could undergo a complete exchange transfusion. However several significant problems are associated

with the use of simple hemoglobin solutions. These include a very high affinity for oxygen, high oncotic pressures, methemoglobin formation, renal and neurotoxicity and short intravascular half-lives. To produce a viable carrier these problems needed to be addressed through some form of chemical modification of hemoglobin.

### Oxygen affinity

Red cells are more than membrane envelopes for hemoglobin. The cytosol of the red cell is designed to protect and regulate hemoglobin. The high intracellular concentrations of adenosine triphosphate and 2,3-diphosphoglycerate decrease the oxygen affinity of hemoglobin. Typically the P50 for hemoglobin inside a red cell is ~26 mmHg. The $P_{50}$ represents the oxygen pressure at which 50% of the hemoglobin is carrying oxygen. In contrast, the P50 for hemoglobin outside of the red cell is ~12 mmHg. In the absence of intracellular ATP and 2,3 DPG "stroma free hemoglobin" exhibits a very high affinity for oxygen that interferes with "appropriate" oxygen release within the tissue beds. Several different strategies have been used to readjust the affinity of extracellular hemoglobin. One method is to chemically bind organic phosphate to serve the function of 2,3-diphosphoglycerate and adenosine triphosphate. The most common approach is to cross-link the dimers into tetramers.

### Oncotic properties

The presence of the red cell membrane maintains an osmotic balance between the high concentration of hemoglobin inside and the plasma outside. In the absence of the red cell membrane, a solution of free hemoglobin exerts a significant oncotic force. Fortunately stroma free hemoglobin is commonly cross-linked and polymerized to improve intravascular retention. This has the added advantage of lowering the oncotic pressure by reducing the overall number of molecules. Current solutions consist of a mix of 2-, 3-, and 4- hemoglobin molecule polymers. Solutions of cross-linked tetramers must be diluted to reduce the oncotic pressure and therefore have a lower concentration than an equivalent volume of blood. These solutions generally have a lower viscosity than blood, which is thought to be a desirable trade off.

### Half-life

Within the red cell, hemoglobin normally exists as a tetramer composed of 2 beta units complexed with 2 alpha units. Following membrane lysis, hemoglobin rapidly dissociates from the tetrameric form into smaller alpha-beta dimers and monomers that are readily filtered by the kidney. The intravascular half-life of these lower molecular weight subunits is 2-4 hours. Increasing the molecular size by polymerizing the subunits prolongs the half-life. They appear to saturate the endothelial system early and then follow a zero-order pattern of clearance, which ranges from 12-24 hours.

The "effective" half-life of stroma-free hemoglobin is also a function of heme oxidation from the ferrous ($Fe^{2+}$) to the ferric ($Fe^{3+}$) which is methemoglobin (MetHb). This oxidized form of hemoglobin does not transport oxygen. Red cells contain MetHb reductase that reduces MetHb back to hemoglobin; however, this enzyme is lost with the removal of the red cell membrane. At the time of infusion, the MetHb content of hemoglobin based oxygen carriers is ~5% and increases rapidly in the circulation (75, 76). If this were not cleared by the reticuloendothelial system it would become a problem. Clinically, it has not been determined whether there is a maximum cumulative dosing that would overload the reticuloendothelial system.

### Hypertension and smooth muscle effects

One of the formidable problems associated with hemoglobin-based oxygen carriers is vasoconstriction and hypertension. Several mechanisms have been considered (77). The predominant mechanism is most likely the result of heme-mediated absorption of nitric oxide (NO), also known as endothelial-derived relaxing factor (EDRF), which relaxes vascular smooth muscle and lowers blood pressure (78). When hemoglobin is enclosed within the red cell membrane, there is a controlled absorption and dissemination of NO that may actually facilitate the delivery of oxygen by producing local vasodilatation (79). When hemoglobin is deprived of a regulatory membrane, it becomes an unregulated scavenger of NO, resulting in hypertension.

In human trials with hemoglobin based oxygen carriers, gastrointestinal side effects are common. The symptoms include generalized pain, heart burn, dysphagia, nausea, vomiting, and diarrhea; although they rarely require treatment. These symptoms are believed to be related to NO binding, causing gastrointestinal smooth muscle contraction (80).

Initially the vasoconstrictive effect of hemoglobin-based oxygen carriers was attributed to the binding of intravascular NO. Later investigations revealed that much of the hypertensive effect was due to scavenging of NO in the extravascular space by small nonpolymerized 64 kilodalton tetramers, which easily diffuse out of the blood vessels. The production of polymerized hemoglobin requires several steps designed to provide a pure, fully polymerized, end product. Nonetheless, some small nonpolymerized hemoglobin tetramers are found in the final product. The hemoglobin-based carriers that have the lowest number of tetramers are also associated with the least amount of extravasation and hypertension.

Working on the theory that vasoconstriction is solely a result of NO binding by hemoglobin, Baxter Healthcare developed a recombinant form of hemoglobin with almost no affinity for NO. Although there was a significant reduction in hypertension, it was not eliminated. This study and others suggested that mechanisms other than NO regulation were at play (81).

Today the hypertensive effect of oxygen therapeutics is also attributed to delivering excess $O_2$ to terminal arterioles, thus triggering vasoconstriction (82). Intaglietta developed a method for the measurement of $PO_2$ in the microcirculation and showed that it drops continuously as blood passes from systemic vessels into progressively smaller vessels until it reaches tissue capillaries, after which $PO_2$ rises again (83). This observation confirms the concept that significant amounts of oxygen exit the circulation from pre-capillary vessels. Within this zone of circulation the pre-capillary arterioles exert a regulatory role that is believed to be governed in part by $PO_2$ (84, 85). This form of control is referred to as the autoregulation theory of blood flow. Facilitation of $O_2$ diffusion by $O_2$ carriers (hemoglobin, myoglobin) was demonstrated many years ago by Scholander (86). Since that time, other investigators have showed that cell-free hemoglobin augments both the uptake and release of $O_2$.

### Free radicals

Heme and free iron, can contribute to the generation of oxygen free radicals in tissue. The ferrous iron ($Fe^{2+}$) center frequently loses an electron to $O_2$, resulting in superoxide ($O_2$-) and the ferric ($Fe^{3+}$) iron state of MetHb. Normally, if this is occurring within the red cell membrane, the superoxide radical is neutralized by MetHb reductase present in the cytosol of the red cell. In the absence of MetHb reductase, $O_2$- can react with NO to produce peroxynitrite (ONOO-), which readily decays to yield hydroxyl radicals (OH-) that are highly reactive and denature proteins. In addition this process consumes NO and exacerbates vasoconstriction. Additional protection is provided by superoxide dismutase and catalase, which are present in the cytosol and convert superoxide into hydrogen peroxide, which in turn is converted into water and oxygen.

## Types of Hemoglobin-Based Oxygen Carriers

**Human hemoglobin** – Human hemoglobin solutions have the advantage of being derived from a naturally occurring product that has been extensively studied. The primary disadvantage relates to limitations in the availability of outdated red blood cells. Currently, only 5% to 15% of the 14 million units of blood donated in the United States each year are discarded.

**Bovine hemoglobin** – Animal hemoglobin as a substrate is potentially inexpensive and widely available. Bovine derived hemoglobin has a P50 of 30 mmHg, which is remarkably close to that of human red cells (P50 of 26.5 mmHg) (87). In addition there is a more pronounced Bohr effect (the rightward shift in the $O_2$ dissociation curve in the presence of $CO_2$) of bovine hemoglobin, providing for better $O_2$ unloading in an acidic environment. In its natural state, the concentration of chloride ions in solution controls the $O_2$ dissociation curve of bovine hemoglobin. Thus, bovine hemoglobin does not shift to the left (increasing its $O_2$ affinity) with a drop in pH to the degree that human hemoglobin does. There remains a level of uncertainty regarding animal pathogens (e.g. bovine spongiform encephalitis) that may require purification. If bovine hemoglobin was used as the substrate, a herd of about 150,000 cows could generate enough hemoglobin to make the equivalent of 6 million units per year.

**Recombinant hemoglobin** – Utilizing recombinant DNA technology, the human gene for hemoglobin has been inserted into the DNA of *Escherichia coli* bacteria, which in turn produce the final hemoglobin protein (88). Recombinant hemoglobin has as its primary limitations the costs of the technical facilities required to produce the enormous volumes of bacterial culture, and the need for stringent purification methods. The obvious potential benefit of recombinant hemoglobin is the product source, theoretically devoid of the microbiologic contamination of human or animal sources. Furthermore, genetic control over the product source allows for future adjustments or improvements to the current generation of products to be simply written into the code. Indeed, since the initial creation of genetically recombinant hemoglobin 1.1 (rHb1.1) a new form rHb 2.0 has been created by Somatogen, Inc. (Boulder CO) (89). The first generation rHb had an NO scavenging rate similar to that of native human hemoglobin and produced the undesirable side effects of inappropriate vasoconstriction. A second-generation hemoglobin rHb 2.0 has an NO scavenging rate 20 to 30 fold lower than that of rHb1.1 (90). Like rHb 1.1, rHb2.0 is expressed in *E. coli* and the alpha chains are fused to prevent dissociation. Amino acid substitutions were made in the distal heme pocket by site-directed mutagenesis to reduce the rate of NO scavenging. Recombinant Hemoglobin 2.0 is also polyethylene glycol-polymerized and is formulated at a concentration of 100 g/l in a gluconated electrolyte solution. At this hemoglobin concentration, rHb 2.0 has a viscosity of 2.3 cP, a colloid osmotic pressure of 62 Torr and a P50 of 34 Torr.

**Encapsulated hemoglobin** – Liposome-encapsulated (HbV) hemoglobin is created from stroma-free hemoglobin that is then emulsed or encapsulated within double phospholipid membranes coated with polyethylene glycol (91). The encapsulation of hemoglobin prolongs the circulation time in the organism and prevents direct contact of hemoglobin with the endothelial lining, thus suppressing vasoconstriction due to NO scavenging, which has been attributed to chemically modified hemoglobin. Another major advantage of the HbV is that oxygen affinity may easily be adapted to the needs of the tissue by supplementing the appropriate amount of coencapsulated allosteric effector (pyridoxal 5'-phosphate). The size of the vesicles averages 250 nm. The oxygen carrying capacity of a typical solution is 9 ml $O_2$/100ml (Blood is ~ 20 ml $O_2$/100ml) with an oncotic pressure that is about twice that of blood. HbVs have not been produced on a scale that would permit human testing, but small animal studies indicate that it is well tolerated. Encapsulated hemoglobin, also known as hemoglobin vesicles, has been associated with stimulation of the reticuloendothelium system. Experiments in rats show that repeated dosing with HbVs doubles the weight of the liver and spleen and; therefore, are still restricted to preclinical work (92).

**Arenocola hemoglobin** – The discovery of this hemoglobin occurred just recently. This hemoglobin is found in a common marine worm, Arenicola marina, and does not appear to be associated with any of the complications associated with vertebrate derived hemoglobin when administered to mice (93). The molecule's large size and natural cross-linking make it an ideal oxygen carrier with limited extravasation. According to biologist Franck Zal of the Université Pierre et Marie Curie in Paris, "We don't have to modify anything, only collect it and purify it" (94). At the present time, this hemoglobin is undergoing further animal evaluation.

## Allosteric Modifiers

Allostery is a branch of biochemistry, which focuses on influencing protein activity by changing protein conformation by other molecules or proteins. The oxygen dissociation curve for hemoglobin demonstrates such allosteric phenomenon in the presence of 2,3 diphosphoglucose. Oxygen affinity will decrease in physiologic conditions characterized by oxygen deprivation; however, this compensatory change takes several days to occur.

The use of an intravenous "synthetic allosteric modifier" that could instantly reduce hemoglobin's affinity for oxygen would increase delivery – especially if the patient were to breathe supplemental oxygen to ensure complete "oxygen loading" of the red cells.

## Perfluorocarbons

Fluorocarbons are carbon fluorine compounds characterized by a high gas-dissolving capacity ($O_2$ and $CO_2$), low viscosity, and chemical and biological inertness. The $O_2$ transport characteristics of modified hemoglobin solutions and fluorocarbon emulsions are fundamentally different. Hemoglobin-based oxygen carriers exhibit a sigmoid $O_2$ dissociation curve similar to blood. In contrast, the fluorocarbon emulsions are characterized by a linear relationship between $O_2$ partial pressure and $O_2$ content. The content of $O_2$ in arterial plasma is directly proportional to the partial pressure of $O_2$ in the lungs. Consequently, supplemental oxygen must be provided to maintain relatively high arterial $O_2$ partial pressures that are necessary to maximize the $O_2$ transport capacity of fluorocarbon emulsions. Despite these fundamental differences, the efficiency of both groups of artificial $O_2$ carriers has been demonstrated experimentally and clinically.

The only blood substitute that was approved in the United States was a perfluorocarbon, Fluosol 20. This first generation product, which is no longer available, may soon be replaced by a second-generation version known as perflubron (*Oxygent*), produced by Alliance Pharmaceuticals. This newer formulation is easier to handle, has few side effects, and dissolves more oxygen per unit volume. It is administered as an emulsion containing particles with a diameter of approximately 0.2 microns and is eliminated unchanged by the lungs.

The amount of oxygen dissolved into the perflourocarbon is linearly related to the $PaO_2$. Intravascular perflourocarbon solutions loaded with oxygen at a Pa $O_2$ of 200 mmHg can deliver 5 vol% of oxygen per dL of perflourocarbon. Because perflourocarbons release 80% of their carried oxygen it can deliver approximately four times the oxygen that would be delivered by the same volume of hemoglobin. Giving 120 ml of *Oxygent* to a 70 kg patient is equivalent to 500 ml transfusion of whole blood. (See Figure 3.)

This graph depicts the oxygen performance curves for hemoglobin transport vs perflourocarbon transport. Hemoglobin transport relies on ac chemical binding of $O_2$ whereas perflourocarbons (*Oxygent*) physically dissolve $O_2$. This results in a number of important distinctions:

1. $O_2$ loading and unloading is approximately twice as rapid with *Oxygent* as with hemoglobin.

2. Only about 20-30% of the $O_2$ carried by hemoglobin is actually extracted (delivered) to the tissues and consumed; extraction of dissolved $O_2$ from *Oxygent* is generally greater than 90%.

3. Each hemoglobin molecule has a fixed capacity to carry a maximum of four $O_2$ molecules; in contrast, the $O_2$-carrying capacity of *Oxygent* can be maximized by increasing the concentration of $O_2$ inspired by the patient.

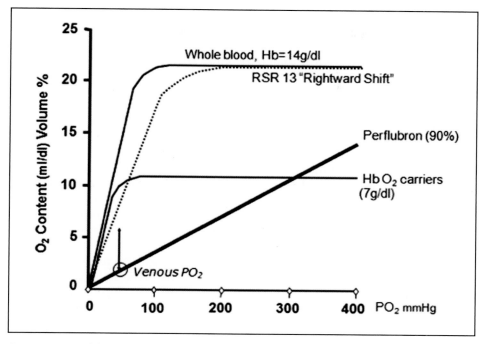

Figure 3. Hemoglobin-based vs. Oxygent-based transport and delivery of $O_2$.

4. Because the $O_2$ carried by *Oxygent* is in a dissolved state, *Oxygent* increases the partial pressure of oxygen within the blood vessels, providing an additional driving gradient that facilitates diffusion of $O_2$ into the tissues.

## PRODUCTS CURRENTLY UNDER CLINICAL INVESTIGATION

### Hemoglobin-Based Oxygen Carriers

The first studies demonstrating the *in vivo* ability of hemoglobin solutions to transport $O_2$ in mammals was reported in 1933 (95). From these early investigations they proceeded to use lysed RBC solutions in 14 patients, documenting the ability of free hemoglobin's ability to transport oxygen and reporting its nephrotoxic side effect (96). In the 1960s the US military started a formalized research program to develop a stroma-free hemoglobin under the belief that the red cell membrane was responsible for many of the side-effects of lysed RBC solutions. By the late 1970s it was determined that highly purified hemoglobin still had side effects that were attributed to the dissociation of the hemoglobin tetramer into dimers and monomers. In the 1980s private industry pioneered a variety of cross linking methods to stabilize and polymerize hemoglobin. There are currently three companies with chemically modified hemoglobin based carriers that have completed phase III studies: Northfield Laboratories product *PolyHeme®*, which is a glutaraldehyde cross-linked human hemoglobin; Hemosol's product

*Hemolink* (o-raffinose polymerized hemoglobin) and Biopure's product *Hemopure,* which is a glutaraldehyde cross-linked bovine hemoglobin. Biopure has received U.S. approval for its veterinary product *Oxyglobin* and South African approval for it human product *Hemopure.*

### Polyheme® – Northfield laboratories

*PolyHeme* is now in phase III (efficacy) trials and appears to lack the vasopressor effect of some of the other blood substitutes. Northfield completed the first randomized clinical trial comparing *PolyHeme* with blood in trauma patients (97). Forty-four patients with severe injury (mean injury severity score of 21) were randomized to receive red cells or up to 6 units of *PolyHeme.* The *PolyHeme* group experienced no adverse events and reduced the initial use of allogenic blood. While there were no differences in circulating hemoglobin levels, the mean number of allogenic red cell transfusions within the first 24 hours was only 7.8 units in the *PolyHeme* group, while controls received 10.4 units (P < 0.05).

Favorable outcomes were found in a recent prospective cohort study comparing the 30-day mortality of trauma patients given *PolyHeme* versus a historical control of 300 patients who abstained from blood due to religious grounds. One hundred and seventy one patients received rapid infusion of 1 to 20 units of *PolyHeme* as the initial management for trauma and urgent surgery. Forty of the patients had nadir red cell hemoglobin ≤ 3 gm/dl. Thirty-day mortality was 25% compared with 64% in the control group.

Beyond the reduction in allogenic blood use, a secondary benefit may be the risk reduction for multi-organ failure syndrome, which appears to be partially linked to allogenic blood transfusions. It is now clear that a number of mediators present in stored packed red blood cells have the potential to contribute to multiple organ failure through priming of circulating neutrophils. *PolyHeme* is devoid of such natural priming agents and should attenuate neutrophil priming during resuscitation. In a prospective study of trauma patients resuscitated with either *PolyHeme* or packed red blood cells, no leukocyte priming occurred when *PolyHeme* was used.

Northfield recently completed pivotal Phase III study designed to evaluate the safety and efficacy of *PolyHeme* when used to treat patients in hemorrhagic shock following traumatic injuries (*www.clinicaltrials.gov*). This was the first U.S. trial of a hemoglobin-based oxygen-carrying resuscitative fluid in which treatment began in the prehospital setting. Thirty-two Level 1 trauma centers throughout the U.S participated in the trial. Enrollment in the trial was 720 patients. Treatment began at the scene of injury, continued in the ambulance during transport, and for up to 12 hours post-injury or 6 units in the hospital. The trial is designed to evaluate *PolyHeme* compared to the current standard of care, namely salt water in the ambulance followed in the hospital by donated blood, when needed. The primary endpoint is survival at 30 days. The final analysis has not been published at this time.

### Hemolink® – Hemosol Inc.

The o-raffinose cross-linked human hemoglobin is prepared from outdated human red blood cells obtained from the Canadian Red Cross Blood Transfusion Service. The cells are washed to remove plasma proteins and lysed by gentle osmotic shock. The crude hemoglobin is separated from red cell ghosts by filtration and then pasteurized for 10 hrs at 62°C. The pasteurized hemoglobin is purified by a combination of anion and cation exchange chromatography that yields a preparation of hemoglobin $A_0$ which is > 99% pure. *Hemolink* is prepared by reacting purified deoxygenated hemoglobin $A_0$ with o-raffinose to covalently link the alpha-beta dimmers. The chemically modified, cross-linked hemoglobin is mixed with lactated Ringer's solution to give a final concentration of 10 g/dL. The product is then frozen and stored at -80°C.

Hemolink was evaluated in a Phase III clinical trial in Canada and the United Kingdom. This trial involved 299 patients undergoing coronary artery bypass grafting in conjunction with autologous normovolemic hemodilution. The *Hemolink* group had a higher rate of complete transfusion avoidance (83%) and fewer units of blood transfused. There was no difference in the adverse events profile between the two groups. However, Hemosol recently suspended enrollment of patients into its HLK 213 trial of *Hemolink* for coronary artery bypass graft patients due to an imbalance in the number of myocardial infarctions occurring in the *Hemolink* group. The matter is currently under review.

### *Hemopure® – Biopure Inc.*

*Hemopure* is ultrapurified, glutaraldehyde-polymerized, bovine hemoglobin in a balanced electrolyte solution. It has a lower oxygen affinity than human hemoglobin (p50 = 38 mmHg compared with 26 mmHg for human hemoglobin) which facilitates the unloading of oxygen. It also has a markedly reduced viscosity of 1.3 cP (similar to crystalloid solutions and about one-third that of blood). *Hemopure* does not require refrigeration and is stable at room temperature for 2 years. *Hemopure* has been in 22 clinical trials involving more than 800 subjects and completed Phase III studies in both Europe and the United States where it has been shown to reduce transfusion requirements in 35-40% of patients (99). The New England Journal of Medicine featured a dramatic case report of a patient with a hemolytic anemia who was supported for several days with *Hemopure* and ultimately recovered from her hemolytic process (100). *Hemopure* has been approved in South Africa for the treatment of adult surgical patients who are acutely anemic and for the purpose of eliminating, delaying or reducing the need for allogenic (donated) red blood cells. Biopure intends to submit an FDA protocol for a Phase 2 randomized trial in 2008 for the treatment of autoimmune hemolytic anemia and other forms of hemolytic anemia, including alloantibody anemia, but excluding sickle cell anemia. The company has already submitted an application to the British government in 2007 for the elective use of *Hemopure* in orthopedic case.

## The Next Generation of Hemoglobin-Based Oxygen Therapeutics

Capitalizing on past experience, developers are engineering the next generation of oxygen therapeutics (101). To offset the problems of nitric oxide binding a new form of human recombinant hemoglobin has been developed that has less affinity for nitric oxide. This new tetrameric recombinant hemoglobin does not cause vasoconstriction when infused into animals. However, there was a change in the oxygen release characteristics (lower P50) that was corrected through further genetic changes, which replaced the distal histidine with glutamine resulting in a normal oxygen release curve.

Superoxide dismutase and catalase are normal constituents of red cells where they convert superoxide into hydrogen peroxide that is, in turn, converted into water and oxygen. This activity may be especially important in the presence of reperfusion injuries with damaged tissue such as stroke, heart attacks and resuscitation from hemorrhagic shock. Steps are underway to cross link superoxide dismutase and catalase enzymes to polymerized hemoglobin (102).

Small hemoglobin-filled spheres are created using biodegradable polymers such as polylactides or polyglycolides, which are commonly used in absorbable sutures (103). These capsules would have the long half-life and limited NO scavenging advantages of liposome encapsulated hemoglobin without reticuloendothelial system engorgement. The diameter of these "artificial cells" range from 80 to 200 nm, which is quite small compared to a red cell diameter of 7,500 nm. Polylactide is first degraded into lactic acid and then into water and carbon dioxide. For a 500-mL suspension, the total lactic acid produced is 83 mEq. This is only a small fraction of the normal human lactic acid production (1,000–1,400 mEq day).

Winslow has advanced a new paradigm for the design characteristics of second generation products. It was originally believed that a low viscosity (1 cP) was desirable; however the new paradigm espouses a viscosity closer to blood (4 cP) to preserve normal sheer forces (104). The osmotic pressure should be higher to maintain vascular volume. Oxygen affinity should also be higher than normal hemoglobin. This characteristic is based on the concept that vasoconstriction is mediated in part by high precapillary $pO_2$ values. This occurs through premature release of oxygen or increased diffusion of oxygen. Because of their small size, these agents easily move into the extravascular space where they facilitate the diffusion of oxygen from the bloodstream.

Sangart Inc (San Diego, CA) has formulated a new hemoglobin derivative based on the new paradigm (105). This product (*MP4*) is formulated by taking the basic hemoglobin tetramer and attaching six molecules of polyethylene glycol to produce a larger molecule that does not easily move into the extravascular space. *MP4* has been shown to be free of vasoconstriction in the hamster microcirculation (106). In a phase I trial in Sweden there were none of the customary side effects of hypertension and gastrointestinal distress. The second novel characteristic of *MP4* is its high $O_2$ affinity – a P50 of 7 mmHg. Research with this product in hamster shock model has shown that it is very effective in oxygenating hypoxic tissue as a result of this high $O_2$ affinity.

Researchers at the University of Maryland recently reported their experience with their new hemoglobin derivative called zero-linked hemoglobin. This product is created by a direct coupling of hemoglobin molecules and produces a very large polymer that is easily purified to eliminate any of the smaller extravasation prone polymers. Other useful attributes include a high $O_2$ affinity, which is believed to be more desirable, and a slightly negative charge, which reduces movement across the basement membrane. In animal models, zero-linked hemoglobin lacks any vasoconstrictive effect (107).

Rather than creating large polymers, Researchers at Wasada University, have selected a large natural protein, albumin, and linked heme groups to it. Albumin does not extravasate and this new preparation does not scavenge NO (108, 109). This novel approach has yet to reach a clinical trial stage.

SynZyme Technologies (Irvine, CA) is developing a second-generation blood substitute called *HemoZyme*. *HemoZyme* consists of a hemoglobin carrier and a caged nitric oxide complex that remains in blood vessels, delivers oxygen to tissues, and catalytically removes reactive oxygen and reactive nitrogen species. Termed "polymerized polynitroxyl hemoglobin," it contains caged nitric oxide, which is a stable free radical referred to as nitroxide. In the bloodstream, free nitric oxide combines with reactive oxygen species to form peroxynitrate, a toxic radical. However caged nitric oxide breaks down peroxynitrate into a nontoxic specie. Still in the early phase of development, SynZyme states that *HemoZyme* can treat ischemia and post-reperfusion phenomena and has significant advantages over other HBOCs. These include dilation of blood vessels, antioxidant and anti-inflammatory properties.

Distinct from the physical and chemical properties of the HBOCs, it is important to recognize that a patient's underlying illness and clinical condition may also influence the physiologic responses to any of these agents.

HemoBioTech's product, *HemoTech*, was designed to diminish the toxic intrinsic effects of hemoglobin and help eliminate the pathological reactions associated with hemorrhagic shock (110). Beyond oxygen transport, *HemoTech* has additional pharmacological activities that eliminate blood vessel constriction, improve the release of oxygen, and produce an anti-oxidant and anti-inflammatory effect. *HemoTech* reacts pure bovine hemoglobin with o-adenosine 5'-triphosphate (o-ATP), o-adenosine, and reduced glutathione (GSH) to produce intra and intermolecular linkage resulting in a large molecule with high purity, a favorable surface charge, and antioxidant properties that are bestowed by the presence of glutathione.

Since its initial development, *HemoTech* has been tested in different *in vitro* and *in vivo* models including pre-clinical studies conducted at the Research Toxicology Centre S.p.A. (Rome, Italy) and a human clinical trial (111). The results of these studies are favorable, indicating that this novel red cell substitute has vasodilation activity; reduces the vasoconstriction that follows hemorrhage; prolongs intravascular persistence; functions as a physiological oxygen carrier; and produces no adverse nephrotoxic, neurotoxic, oxidative, or inflammatory reactions.

## *Oxygent – Alliance Pharmaceutical*

Perfluorocarbons are lipophilic solutions that have a high solubility for all gases, including oxygen and carbon dioxide. In 1965 the world saw a dramatic demonstration of rats submerged in this liquid, yet still alive. (Leland Clark) Equilibrated with 100% oxygen at the surface, the rats were able to breathe in this liquid and meet their metabolic requirements for oxygen and carbon dioxide transport. In 1968, a perflourocarbons micro emulsion was used to perform a complete exchange transfusion in a rat, which survived, breathing 100% oxygen, with a hematocrit of zero. This experiment established the practical viability of pursuing the clinical application of these agents.

The first generation perflurocarbon (*Fluosol*) had poor oxygen-carrying characteristics and had to be stored frozen. Despite FDA approval for use with angioplasty in 1989, its production was terminated in 1994. A second-generation perflurocarbon emulsion, perfluorooctylbromide developed by Alliance Pharmaceuticals, San Diego, CA is called *Oxygent*, and contains 45% perflubron (C8F17) by volume. This flourocarbon is emulsified with lecithin, has a viscosity of 4.0 cP (about 30% thicker than blood) and is stable at room temperature for 6 years.

When the inspired atmosphere contains 90% to 100% oxygen, this solution releases about 10 mL of oxygen per 100 mL or about twice that of normal blood. No serious adverse events have been reported with the use of *Oxygent*. A 10-24% reduction in platelet account does occur on the second day after infusion, but no bleeding abnormalities have been noted. *Oxygent* elimination occurs first through the reticuloendothelial system which is followed by pulmonary excretion of the perflourocarbon. The emulsion is typically cleared within 24 hours.

An international, multicenter phase III transfusion avoidance study in noncardiac elective surgical patients was recently completed (112). This study enrolled 492 patients with expected blood loss of 20 to 70 mL/kg. Control patients were transfused at a hemoglobin of 8 gm/dL, or at predefined physiologic triggers. Perflourocarbon patients underwent hemodilution to a hemoglobin of 8 gm/dL, and then received perflourocarbon and were given transfusions at a hemoglobin of 5.5 gm/dL, or at the same physiologic triggers as control patients. The perflourocarbon patients required significantly less allogeneic blood. In the patient population specifically targeted by this study protocol (i.e., surgical procedures with an anticipated blood loss > 20 mL/kg), *Oxygent* treatment resulted in a highly significant (p < 0.001) reduction and avoidance of blood transfusion, which translated into an overall sparing of allogeneic units compared to the control group. Safety assessments, performed quarterly during the conduct of the study by an independent data safety monitoring board, indicated that *Oxygent* was well tolerated.

### RSR13 – Allos Therapeutics

In the 1980s two antilipidemic drugs, clofibrate and benzofibrate demonstrated an allosteric effect on the oxyhemoglobin dissociation curve by shifting it to the right (113, 114). Such a shift means there is a decreased affinity for oxygen resulting in a greater release or desaturation of oxygen in the tissue beds. This effect was an *in vitro* phenomenon and is extinguished by albumin when used *in vivo*. Nontheless the concept of creating an allosteric agent was born. Allos therapeutics, has committed considerable efforts toward the development of a compound known as *RSR13*, which decreases hemoglobin's affinity for oxygen. This effect is dose-related, and current dosing regimens result in approximately a 10-mmHg shift in the p50 Although the right shift of the oxyhemoglobin provides for an increase release of oxygen to the tissues, it also means that there is a corresponding decrease in the uptake of oxygen in the lungs. This can be compensated for by providing supplemental oxygen to ensure complete saturation of hemoglobin. At the present time this agent is being evaluated as a radiation sensitizer for hypoxic tumors. Hypoxic tumors are notoriously radio-resistant. By providing a more complete release of oxygen within the tumor, the $pO_2$ elevates rendering the tumor more susceptible to radiation.

Using electron paramagnetic resonance to directly measure cortical $pO_2$, Miyake examined whether *RSR13* would improve brain tissue $pO_2$ following hemorrhagic shock in rats. After a 30-minute shock period, resuscitation was performed by infusion with Ringer lactate plus *RSR13* or saline. Following hemorrhage, brain $pO_2$ decreased by 14 mmHg in both groups. Following crystalloid resuscitation brain $pO_2$ remained depressed in the control group, but returned to the pre-hemorrhage values in the *RSR13* treated rats. *RSR13* immediately increased and maintained the $pO_2$ while controls had a very gradual return to pre-hemorrhage values. There was no difference in the blood pressure or heart rate between groups. Whar et al. recently evaluated the safety and dosing schedules in surgical patients. A shift of 10 mmHg was achieved at 75mg/kg. There were no adverse events and further studies are planned to more fully evaluate *RSR13* for the management of acute blood loss anemia.

Myocardial and cerebral hypoxia in the setting of cardiopulmonary bypass surgery is another potential application for allosteric modulation. *RSR13* improves myocardial oxidative metabolism and contractile function in models of myocardial ischemia. In cardiopulmonary bypass patients, *RSR13* improved pO2 and reduced neuronal cell death following cerebral ischemia (116, 117). Allosteric modification of the oxyhemoglobin dissociation curve by *RSR13* represents a unique therapeutic strategy. Tables 1 and 2 summarize the status of major oxygen therapeutics

## POTENTIAL APPLICATIONS

The short half-life, side effects and expense of oxygen therapeutics preclude the indiscriminate use of these agents based simply on a hemoglobin level. In recent years it has become clear that the singular use of a hemoglobin level is overly simplistic and does not accurately predict whether the patient is compensating for the anemic state.

FDA licensure of oxygen therapeutics requires demonstrated safety and efficacy. Safety and the concept of adverse events is easily defined. However, the definition of efficacy is quite nebulous given the lack of consensus on a transfusion trigger, especially when co-morbid problems exist. The efficacy endpoints may include transfusion avoidance, mortality and organ perfusion. Because the FDA has focused more so on transfusion avoidance, manufacturers have designed trails with that index as a primary outcome variable. Although the oxygen therapeutics will make their greatest contribution in the management of trauma patients, the majority of the clinical studies have been performed in the more controlled setting of elective surgery.

Accordingly, the first area of licensure will probably be for transfusion avoidance during elective orthopedic or cardiovascular surgery. However,

## TABLE 1. CHARACTERISTICS OF MAJOR OXYGEN THERAPEUTICS

| CHARAC- TERISTIC | BANKED BLOOD | HBOC* | PFC | ALLOSTERICS | HBO |
|---|---|---|---|---|---|
| Shelf life | 42 days | 3 years | 2 years | Years | Unlimited |
| Storage Temperature | Refrigeration | Room Temp | Refrigeration | Room Temp | Room Temp |
| Size | 7 micron | 0.007 micron | 0.2 micron | NA | NA |
| Cross-matching | Required | Not Required | Not Required | Not Required | Not Required |
| Risks | Disease transmission, Immune depression, Transfusion reactions, RBC Storage Defects | NO scavenging | Mild decrease in platelet count | None apparent | Oxygen toxicity |

*Hemoglobin-Based Oxygen Carrier
**NA Not Applicable

## TABLE 2. STATUS OF MAJOR OXYGEN THERAPEUTICS

| COMPANY | PRODUCT | TYPE | STATUS |
|---|---|---|---|
| Northfield | Polyheme® | Human | Phase III Elective Surgery / Trauma Resuscitation |
| Biopure | Hemopure® | Bovine | Phase III:* Approved in S Africa Elective Surgery |
| Hemosol | Hemolink® | Human | Phase III Elective Surgery |
| Alliance | Perflubron (Oxygent) | Perflurocarbon | Phase III Elective Surgery |
| Allos | RSR13 | Allosteric Modulator | Phase II |
| NA | Oxygen | Hyperbaric | Approved |

*FDA Application filed October 2004. Approved for clinical use in South Africa granted 2001.

once a product is clinically available it will most likely be used in a variety of off-label scenarios. Several different applications could be considered.

**Trauma** – The popularization of the "golden hour" of trauma management underscores the importance of rapidly restoring oxygen transport. The ability to provide these agents at the scene would be invaluable.

In addition, there could be a substantial saving of banked blood when these agents are given during the initial resuscitation (118). It is far more desirable to have a patient "bleeding" oxygen therapeutics as opposed to red cells. This would conserve the use of banked blood for transfusion after bleeding has been controlled. As noted earlier, other potential benefits for the use of oxygen therapeutics in trauma include possible reduction in multiorgan failure syndrome and the elimination of red cell storage defects; thereby, insuring an immediate improvement in oxygen delivery (119, 120).

**Remote Settings** – The long shelf life of these agents would be of immediate value in first aid stations that provide care in locations that are in remote settings. A second "delayed care" scenario would be disaster relief where neither bank blood or definitive care are readily available. The elimination of cross-matching further contributes to the practical aspects of having these agents readily available to buy time for patient transport.

**Elective Surgery** – To completely avoid allogenic blood use in this setting will require several different strategies. The first would be to conserve the patient's red blood cell mass by using an enhanced form of acute normovolemic hemodilution (ANH) (121). At the present time, ANH is limited by the amount of blood that can be safely withdrawn into a holding reservoir (122). If large amounts are withdrawn the patient is at risk for accruing a significant introperative oxygen debt, myocardial infaction or stroke (123). However if the hemodilutional agent is an oxygen therapeutic, substantially more blood can be withdrawn without the risk of hypoxia related events (124). In essence these agents will afford the patient an "oxygen bridge" to carry them through the operative bleeding, after which their red cells can be safely returned (125-127). Because oxygen therapeutics have a short half-life (< 24 hours), multiple administrations will be required for 5 to 7 days if ANH is not performed or is inadequate. During this time the use of recombinant erythropoietin will accelerate the endogenous replacement of red cells. Ideally, rHuEPO would be initiated prior to surgery to compensate for the reticulocytosis production time. (See the chapter by Clark entitled "Oxygen Toxicity.")

**Acute Vascular Occlusions** – The small particle size and reduced viscosity of these agents offer therapeutic promise to enhance both direct and collateral oxygen delivery following acute obstructions such as myocardial infarctions, strokes, and failing flaps (128-130). Several favorable reports have been published that substantiate this area to be worthy of further investigation.

**Sickle Cell Anemia** – Sickle cell anemia is well known for the sickling phenomenon that may occur whenever the tissue $pO_2$ drops. As the cells sickle, they cause obstruction, which could be compensated for by oxygen carriers smaller than red cells. A number of reports have detailed the use of hemoglobin based substitutes in the management of painful crisis, aplastic crisis, and acute chest syndrome (131). All of the investigators believed there was a beneficial effect. Clearly further work needs to be done in this area.

**Radiation Sensitizer** – The relationship of radiation and oxygen is an important determinate of successful tumor kill (132). It is well recognized that hypoxic tumors are notoriously resistant to radiation. Some of the earliest applications of hyperbaric therapy were directed toward tumor oxygenation. Although there was limited success there has been a resurgence of interest in recent years for HBO and brain tumors. The use of oxygen therapeutics is technically easier to administer and has also shown promise as a radiation sensitizer.

**Septic Shock** – Although the mechanisms of septic shock are complex, recent work has focused on the unregulated production of NO by an endotoxin-inducible form of nitric oxide synthase. This observation has led investigators to speculate on the utility of using NO scavenging attributes of hemoglobin based oxygen carriers in a therapeutic capacity. Unlike synthetic NO synthetase inhibitors, hemoglobin-based oxygen carriers are capable of down-regulating NO concentrations while maintaining physiological levels of this important messenger. Curacyte (Durham, NC) has employed this strategy using its PHP product. Pyridoxalated Hemoglobin Polyoxyethylene (PHP) is a natural human hemoglobin that is chemically modified in order to preserve its physiological functions and to deliver them to locations affected by inflammation. Curacyte has just completed a Phase IIc study in patients suffering from distributive shock. Although promising, the application of HBOC in septic shock is still largely theoretical.

## SUMMARY

The development of oxygen therapeutics parallels man's quest for flight. It took less than 100 years from the achievement of the first flight to lunar landing. In a similar fashion it was only 100 years from Karl Landsteiner's description of blood types, which made transfusion possible, to the commercial release of the first "blood substitute," *Hemopure*, in South Africa. Because the four classes of oxygen therapeutics have different delivery mechanisms and side-effect profiles, each can be expected to have its own unique clinical applications as the characteristics of the individually designed products are better understood. Increasing volunteer-blood-donor shortages, coupled with increasing blood-transfusion needs, as well as an expanding list of pathogens and adverse effects continue to fuel the demand for further development of these products.

The skillful management of extreme anemia requires a vertical understanding of oxygen physiology from the bone marrow production of red cells to the bedside coordination of care. Because hyperbaric oxygen therapy is based on oxygen physiology, it follows that the hyperbaric physician would serve as one of the resident experts on oxygen-based therapies that will soon involve more than the manipulation of pressure alone.

# REFERENCES

1. Boerema I, Meijne NG, Brummelkamp WH, et al.: Life without blood. J Cardiovasc Surg 1960; 182:133-146.

2. Hart G: Exceptional blood loss anemia: Treatment with hyperbaric oxygen therapy. JAMA 74;228:1028-1029.

3. Weiskopf RB, et al. Human cardiovascular and metabolic response to acute, severe isovolemic anemia. JAMA Jan 21, 1998 Vol 279 : 217-21.

4. Lapin R, Major Surgery in Jehovah's Witnesses. (1980), 2(9) Contemporary Orthopaedics 647-654.

5. Watchtower and Bible Tract Society. Blood as medicine. The Watchtower 2004;15 June:21–7.

6. Online Bible: New World Translation of the Holy Scriptures. www.watchtower.org.bible/index.htm.

7. Schloendorff v Society of New York Hospital 105 NE 92, 93 (NY 1914).

8. 20 In re Brown 478 So2d 1033 (MS 1985)].

9. Re T (An Adult) (Consent to Medical Treatment) [1992] 2 Fam 458, 460.

10. In re Rena 705 N.E. 2d 1155 (Mass. 1999).

11. Dwyer JG. The Children we Abandon: Religious Exemption to Child Welfare and Education Laws as Denials of Equal Protection to Children of Religious Objectors. North Carolina L. Rev 1996;74:1321.

12. Jacobs K, Shoemaker C, Rudersdorf R, et al. Isolation and characterization of genomic and cDNA clones of human erthropoietin. Nature 1985; 313: 806-810.

13. Jaspan D. Erythropoietic therapy: cost efficiency and reimbursement. Am J Health Syst Pharm. 2007 Aug 15;64(16 Suppl 11):S19-29.

14. Rosen AL, et al.: Erythropoietic response to acute anemia. Crit Care Med 1990;18(3):298.

15. Eschbach JW, et al.: Correction of the anemia of end-stage renal disease with recombinant human erythropoietin. NEJM 1987 Jan 8;316(2):73.

16. Rogiers P, Zhang H, Leeman M, et al. Erythropoietin response is blunted in critically ill patients. Intensive Care Med. 1997 Feb;23(2):159-62.

17. Krafte-Jacobs B. Anemia of critical illness and erythropoietin deficiency. Intensive Care Med. 1997 Feb;23(2):137-8.

18. Schalte G, Janz H, Busse J, et al. Life-threatening postoperative blood loss in a Jehovah's Witness, treated with high-dose erythropoietin. Br J Anaesth 2005; 94: 442–4.

19. Siren AL, Fratteli M, Brines M, et al. Erythropoietin prevents neuronal apoptosis after cerebral ischemia and metabolic stress. Proc Natl Acad Sci USA 2001; 98: 4044–9.

20. Digicaylioglou M, Lipton SA. Erythropoietin mediated neuroprotection involves cross talk between Jak and NF-kappaB signal cascades. Nature 2001; 412: 641–7.

21. Ehrenreich H, Hasselblatt M, Dembowski C, et al. Erythropoietin therapy for acute stroke is both safe and beneficial. Mol Med 2002; 8: 495–505.

22. Parsa CJ, Matsumoto A, Kim J, et al. A novel effect of erythropoietin in the infarcted heart. J Clin Invest 2003; 112: 999–1007.

23. Goodnough LT. The role of iron in erythropoiesis in the absence and presence of erythropoietin therapy. Nephrol Dial Transplant. 2002;17 Suppl 5:14-18.

24. Auerbach M, Coyne D, Ballard H. Intravenous iron: From anathema to standard of care. Am J Hematol. 2008; Jan 29:1-9.

25. Navarro JF, Mora C, Macía M, et al. Randomized prospective comparison between erythropoietin and androgens in CAPD patients. Kidney Int. 2002 Apr;61(4):1537-44.

26. Salzman EW, et al.: Treatment with desmopressin acetate to reduce blood loss after cardiac surgery. NEJM 1986 May;314(22):1402.

27. Stone DJ, DiFazio CA. DDAVP to reduce blood loss in Jehovah's Witnesses (letter). Anesthesiology 1988 Dec;69(6):1028.

28. Hegnauer AH, Schriber WJ, Haterius I, et al.: Cardiovascular response of the dog to immersion. Am J Physiology, 1950; 455-465.

29. Wu X, Kochanek PM, Cochran K, Nozari A, Mild hypothermia improves survival after prolonged, traumatic hemorrhagic shock in pigs. J Trauma. 2005;59:291-9.

30. Rajagopalan S, Mascha E, Na J The effects of mild perioperative hypothermia on blood loss and transfusion requirement. Anesthesiology, 2008 Jan;108(1): 71-7.

31. Longmuir IS: The effect of hypothermia on the affinity of tissues for oxygen. Life Sci 1962;1:297-300.

32. Hedley-Whyte J, Laver MB: O2 Solubility in blood and temperature correction factors for pO2 . J Appl Physiol 1964:19(5); 901-906.

33. Hershenson MB, Schena JA, Loyano PA et al.: Effect of pentoxiphylline on oxygen transport during hypothermia. J Applied Physiol 1989: 66; 96-101.

34. Deree J, de Campos T, Shenvi E, Hypertonic saline and pentoxifylline attenuates gut injury after hemorrhagic shock: the kinder, gentler resuscitation. J Trauma 2007 Apr;62(4):818-27.

35. Hart GB: Hyperbaric oxygen in exceptional acute blood-loss anemia. J Hyperbaric Med 1987;2(4):205-210.

36. Doi Y, Onji Y: Oxygen deficit in haemorrhagic shock under hyperbaric oxygen. Pro 4th Int Congress on Hyperbaric Med 1969 Sept; Japan, p181.

37. Attar S, Esmond WG, Cowley RA: Hyperbaric oxygenation in vascular collapse. J Thor and Cardio Surg 1962; 44(6): 759.

38. Attar S, Esmond WG, Blair E, et al.: Experimental aspects of the use of hyperbaric oxygen in hemorrhagic shock. The American Surgeon 1964; 30: 243-246.

39. Elliott DP, Paton BC: Effect of 100% oxygen at one and three atmospheres on dogs subjected to hemorrhagic hypotension. Surgery 1965; 57: 401-408.

40. Yamashita, M., Yamashita, M. Hyperbaric oxygen treatment attenuates cytokine induction after massive hemorrhage. Am. J. Physiol. 2000;278: 811-816.

41. Wright JK, Ehler W, McGlasson DL, Thomson W. Facilitation of Recovery from Acute Blood Loss with Hyperbaric Oxygen. Arch Surg. 2002;137:850-853.

42. Spahn DR. Perioperative Transfusion Triggers for Red Blood Cells. Vox Sang. 2000;78 Suppl 2:163-6.

43. Shoemaker WC, Kram HB: Effects of crystalloids and colloids on hemodynamics, oxygen transport, and outcome in high-risk surgical patients. In: Debates in General Surgery, Simmons RL, Udekwu AO (Eds). Chicago, Year Book Medical Publishers. 1990, pp263-302.

44. Schwartz S, Frantz A, Shoemaker WC: Sequential hemodynamic and oxygen transport responses in hypovolemia, anemia, and hypoxia. Am J Physiol 1981;241(6):864-71.

45. Cone JB: Monitoring of tissue oxygenation, in Snyder JV, Pinsky JR (eds): Oxygen Transport in the Critically Ill. ISBN 0-8151-7903-0; Chicago, Year Book Medical Publishers 1987, pp 164-176.

46. Kern JW, Shoemaker WC. Meta-analysis of hemodynamic optimization in high-risk patients. Crit Care Med. 2002 Aug;30(8):1686-92.

47. Baue AE: Multiple, progressive or sequential system fauilure: A syndrome of the 1970's. Arch Surg 1975; 110:779.

48. Baue AE, Chaudry IH: Prevention of multiple systems failure. Surg Clin North Am 1980; 60(5): 1167-78.

49. Shoemaker WC, Appel PL, Kram HB: Tissue oxygen debt as a determinant of lethal and nonlethal postoperative organ failure. Crit Care Med 1988; 16: 1117-20.

50. Shoemaker WC, Appel PL, Kram HB: Tissue oxygen debt as a determinant of lethal and nonlethal postoperative organ failure. Crit Care Med 1988; 16: 1117-20.

51. Crowell JW, Smithe EE: Oxygen deficit and irreversible hemorrhagic shock. Am J Physiol 1964; 106: 313.

52. Shoemaker WC, Czer L, Chang P, et al.: Cardiorespiratory monitoring in postoperative patients: I Prediction of outcome and severity of illness. Crit Care Med 1979; 7:237.

53. Shoemaker WC, Appel PL, Kram HB: Measurement of tissue perfusion by oxygen transport patterns in experimental shock and high risk surgical patients. Intensive Care Med 1990; 16: S135.

54. Shoemaker WC, Appel PL, Kram HB, et al.: Oxygen transport measurements to evaluate tissue perfusion and titrate therapy: dobutamine and dopamine effects. Crit Care Med 1991; 19(5):672-88.

55. Schumacker PT, Cain SM: The concept of a critical oxygen delivery. Intensive Care Med 1987;13:223-29.

56. Reinhart K, Hannemann L, Kuss B: Optimal oxygen delivery in critically ill patients. Inten Care Med 1990;16(Suppl 2):S149-S155.

57. Shibutani K, Komatsu T, Kubal K, Sanchala V, Kumar V, Bizzarri DV: Critical level of oxygen delivery in anesthetized man. Crit Care Med 1983;11:640-43.

58. Buran MJ: Oxygen consumption, in Snyder JV, Pinsky JR (eds): Oxygen Transport in the Critically Ill. ISBN 0-8151-7903-0; Chicago, Year Book Medical Publishers 1987, pp 16-23.

59. Kasnitz P, Druger GL, Yorra F, el al: Mixed venous oxygen tension and hyperlactatemia. JAMA 1976;236:570.

60. Swan H, Sanchez M, Tyndall M, Koch C: Quality control of perfusion: monitoring venous blood oxygen tension to prevent hypoxic acidosis. J Thorac Cardiovasc Surg 1990 May;99(5):868-72.

61. Cain SM: Assessment of Tissue Oxygenation. Crit Care Med 1986 Jul;2(3):537.

62. Trouwborst A, Tenbrinck R, van Woerkens ECSM: Blood gas analysis of mixed venous blood during normoxic acute isovolemic hemodilution in pigs. Anesth Analg 1990; 70: 523-529.

63. Kuo L, Pittman RN: Effect of hemodilution on oxygen transport in arteriolar networks of hamster striated muscle. Am J Physiol 1988; 254:H331-H339.

64. Van der Hoeven MAHBM, Maertzdorf WJ, Blanco CE. Relationship between mixed venous oxygen saturation and markers of tissue oxygenation in progressive hypoxic hypoxia and in isovolemic anemic hypoxia in 8- to 12-day-old piglets. Crit Care Med 1999; 27:1885-1892.

65. Weg JG: Oxygen transport in adult respiratory distress syndrome and other acute circulatory problems: relationship of oxygen delivery and oxygen consumption. Crit Care Med 1991;19(5):650-7.

66. Dantzker DR, Foresman B, Gutierrez G: Oxygen supply and utilization relationships. Am Rev Respir Dis 1991; 143:675.

67. Waxman K, Nolan LS, Shoemaker WC: Sequential perioperative lactate determination: Physiological and clinical implications. Crit Care Med 1982;10:96.

68. Rashkin MC, Bosken C, Baughman RP: Oxygen delivery in critically III patients: Relationship go blood lactate and survival. Chest 1985; 87(5): 580-583.

69. Komatsu T, Shibutani K, Okamoto K, et al.: Critical level of oxygen delivery after cardiopulmonary bypass. Crit Care Med 1987; 15:194.

70. Iberti TJ, Leibowitz AB, Papadakos PJ, Fischer EP: Low sensitivity of the anion gap as a screen to detect hyperlactatemia in critically ill patients. Crit Care Med 1990 Mar;18(3):275-7.

71. Weaver LK, Hopkins RO, Chan KJ, et al. Hyperbaric oxygen for acute carbon monoxide poisoning. N Engl J Med. 2002 Oct 3;347(14):1057-67.

72. Moore FA, Moore EE: Evolving concepts in the pathogenesis of postinjury multiple organ failure. Surg Clin North Am 1995;75:257-277.

73. Zallen G; Moore EE; Ciesla DJ; Stored red blood cells selectively activate human neutrophils to release IL-8 and secretory PLA2. Shock - 2000 Jan; 13(1): 29-33.

74. Ghio M, Contini P, Mazzei C, et al. In vitro immunosuppressive activity of soluble HLA class I and Fas ligand molecules:do they play a role in autologous blood transfusion? Transfusion 2001; 41: 988-996.

75. Gould SA, Moore EE, Moore FA, et al.: Clinical utility of human polymerized hemoglobin as a blood substitute after acute trauma and urgent surgery. J Trauma 1997;43:325-332.

76. Phillips WT, Lemen L, Goins B, et al.: Use of oxygen-15 to measure oxygen-carrying capacity of blood substitutes in vivo. Am J Physiol 1997;272:H2492-H2499.

77. Gulati A, Sharma AC, Singh G: Role of endothelin in the cardiovascular effects of diaspirin crosslinked and stroma reduced hemoglobin. Crit Care Med 1996;24:137-147.

78. Hindman BJ, Dexter F, Cutkomp J, et al.: Diaspirin-crosslinked hemoglobin does not increase brain oxygen consumption during hypothermic cardiopulmonary bypass in rabbits. Anesthesiology 1995;83:1302-1311.

79. Jia L, Bonaventura J, Stamler JS, et al.: S-nitrosohemoglobin: A dynamic activity of blood involved in vascular control. Nature 1996;380:221-226.

80. Gould SA, Moss GS: Clinical development of human polymerized hemoglobin as a blood substitute. World J Surg 1996;20:1200-1207.

81. Matheson B, Razynaka A, Kwansa H, Bucci E: Vascular response to infusions of a nonextravasating hemoglobin polymer. J Appl Physiol 2002, 93:1479–1486.

82. Winslow RM. Alternative Oxygen Therapeutics: Products, Status of Clinical Trials, and Future Prospects. Current Hematology Reports 2003, 2:503–510.

83. M. Intaglietta, P. Johnson and R. Winslow, Microvascular and tissue oxygen distribution. Cardiovasc. Res. 32 (1996), pp. 632¯643.

84. Homer L, Weathersby P, Kiesow L. Oxygen gradients between red blood cells in the microcirculation. Microvascular Res 1981; 22: 308–23.

85. Biro G, Anderson P, Curtis S, Cain S. Stroma-free hemoglobin: its presence in plasma does not improve oxygen supply to the resting hindlimb vascular bed of hemodiluted dogs. Can J Physiol Pharmacol 1991; 69:1656.

86. Scholander P. Oxygen transport through hemoglobin solutions. Science 1960; 131: 585–90.

87. Vlahakes GJ, Lee R, Jacobs EE Jr, et al.: Hemodynamic effects and oxygen transport properties of a new blood substitute in a model of massive blood replacement. J Thorac Cardiovasc Surg 1990;100:379-388.

88. Looker, D, Abbott-Brown D, Cozart P, Durfee S, Hoffman S, Mathews AJ, Miller-Roehrich J, Shoemaker S, Trimble S, Fermi G, Komiyama NH, Nagai K, and Stetler GL. A human recombinant haemoglobin designed for use as a blood substitute. Nature 356: 258-260, 1992.

89. Resta TC, Walker BR, Eichinger MR, Doyle MP. Rate of NO scavenging alters effects of recombinant hemoglobin solutions on pulmonary vasoreactivity J Appl Physiol 2002; 93: 1327-1336.

90. Resta TC, Walker BR, Eichinger MR, Doyle MP. Rate of NO scavenging alters effects of recombinant hemoglobin solutions on pulmonary vasoreactivity J Appl Physiol 2002; 93: 1327-1336.

91. Sakai H, Tsai A, Rohlfs R, et al.: Microvascular responses to hemodilution with Hb vesicles as red blood cell substitutes: influence of O2 affinity. Am J Physiol 1999, 276:H553–H562.

92. Sakai H, Horinouchi H, Tomiyama K, Ikeda E, Takeoka S, Kobayashi K, Tsuchida E Hemoglobin-vesicles as oxygen carriers: influence on phagocytic activity and histopathological changes in reticuloendothelial system. Am J Pathol. 2001 Sep;159(3):1079-88.

93. Nature News Service 4 June 2003 / Macmillan Magazines. Blood substitute from worms shows promise Haemoglobin from sea creature could replace red cells. Hannah Hoag.

94. Zal, F., Lallier, F.. & Toulmond, A. Utilisation comme substitut sanguin d'une hémoglobine extracellulaire de poids moléculaire élevé. French Patent No. 00 07031, granted August 2, 2002.

95. Amberson WR, Mulder AG, Steggerda FR, et al. Mammalian life without red blood corpuscles. Science 1933;78:106-7.

96. Amberson WR, Jennings JJ, Rhode CM. Clinical experience with hemoglobin-saline solutions. J Appl Physiol 1949;1:469-89.

97. Gould SA, Moore EE, Hoyt DB, et al. The first randomized trial of human polymerized hemoglobin as a blood substitute in acute trauma and emergent surgery. J Am Coll Surg. 1998;187:113-20.

98. Gould SA, Moore EE, Hoyt DB, et al. The life-sustaining capacity of human polymerized hemoglobin when red cells might be unavailable. Journal of the American College of Surgeons 2002:195; 445-452.

99. Sprung J, Kindscher JD, Wahr JA, et al. The use of bovine hemoglobin glutamer-250 (Hemopure) in surgical patients: results of a multicenter, randomized, single-blinded trial. Anesth Analg. 2002 Apr;94(4):799-808.

100. Mullon J, Giacoppe G, Clagett C, et al. Brief Report: Transfusions of Polymerized Bovine Hemoglobin in a Patient with Severe Autoimmune Hemolytic Anemia. The New England Journal of Medicine. 2000;342:1638-1643.

101. Chang TMS Future generations of red blood cell substitutes. J Intern Med 2003;253:527-535.

102. Powanda DD, Chang TM. Cross-linked polyhemoglobin-superoxide dismutase-catalase supplies oxygen without causing blood-brain barrier disruption or brain edema in a rat model of transient global brain ischemia-reperfusion. Artif Cells Blood Substit Immobil Biotechnol 2002;30:23-37.

103. Chang TM: Modified hemoglobin-based blood substitutes: cross-linked, recombinant and encapsulated hemoglobin. Vox Sang 1998, 74:233–241.

104. Winslow RM. Alternative oxygen therapeutics: products, status of clinical trials, and future prospects. Curr Hematol Rep. 2003;6:503-10.

105. Tsai AG, Vandegriff KD, Intaglietta M, et al. Targeted $O_2$ delivery by low-P50 hemoglobin: a new basis for $O_2$ therapeutics. Am J Physiol Heart Circ Physiol 2003;285: H1411–H1419.

106. Wettstein R, Tsai A, Erni D, et al.: Resuscitation with polyethylene glycol-modified human hemoglobin improves microcirculatory blood flow and tissue oxygenation after hemorrhagic shock in awake hamsters. Crit Care Med 2003, 31:1824–1830.

107. Matheson B, Razynaka A, Kwansa H, Bucci E: Vascular response to infusions of a nonextravasating hemoglobin polymer. J Appl Physiol 2002, 93:1479–1486.

108. Huang Y, Komatsu T, Nakagawa A, Tsuchida E, Kobayashi S Compatibility in vitro of albumin-heme ($O_2$ carrier) with blood cell components. J Biomed Mater Res. 2003 Aug 1;66A(2):292-7.

109. Zunszain PA, Ghuman J, Komatsu T, Tsuchida E, Curry S. Crystal structural analysis of human serum albumin complexed with hemin and fatty acid. BMC Struct Biol. 2003 Jul 7;3(1):6. Epub 2003 Jul 07.

110. Simoni J, Simoni G, Wesson DE, Griswold JA, Feola M.A novel hemoglobin-adenosine-glutathione based blood substitute: evaluation of its effects on human blood ex vivo. ASAIO J. 2000 Nov-Dec;46(6):679-92.

111. Feola M, Simoni J, Angelillo R, et al. Clinical trial of a hemoglobin based blood substitute in patients with sickle cell anemia. Surg Gynecol Obstet 1992;174:379-86.

112. Spahn DR, Waschke KF, Standl T, et al. Use of perflubron emulsion to decrease allogeneic blood transfusion in high-blood-loss non-cardiac surgery: Results of an European phase 3 study. Anesthesiology 2002;97:1338-49.

113. Perutz MF, Poyart C. Bezafibrate lowers oxygen affinity of haemoglobin. Lancet 1983;2(8355):881-2.

114. Poyart C, Marden MC, Kister J. Bezafibrate derivatives as potent effectors of hemoglobin. Methods Enzymol 1994;232:496-513.

115. Wahr JA, Gerber M, Venitz J, et al. Allosteric modification of oxygen delivery by hemoglobin. Anesth Analg 2001;92:615-20.

116. Miyake M, Grinberg OY, Hou H, Steffen RP, Elkadi H, Swartz HM. The effect of RSR13, a synthetic allosteric modifier of hemoglobin, on brain tissue $pO_2$ (measured by EPR oximetry) following severe hemorrhagic shock in rats Adv Exp Med Biol. 2003;530:319-29.

117. Grinberg OY, Miyake M, Hou H, Steffen RP, Swartz HM. The dose-dependent effect of RSR13, a synthetic allosteric modifier of hemoglobin, on physiological parameters and brain tissue oxygenation in rats. Adv Exp Med Biol. 2003;530:287-96.

118. Knudson MM, Lee S, Erickson V, Morabito D, et al. Tissue oxygen monitoring during hemorrhagic shock and resuscitation: a comparison of lactated Ringer's solution, hypertonic saline dextran, and HBOC-201. J Trauma. 2003 Feb;54(2):242-52.

119. Moore EE. Blood substitutes: the future is now. J Am College of Surgeons 2003;196: 1-17.

120. Standl T, Freitag M, Burmeister MA, et al. Hemoglobin-based oxygen carrier HBOC-201 provides higher and faster increase in oxygen tension in skeletal muscle of anemic dogs than do stored red blood cells.J Vasc Surg. 2003 Apr;37(4):859-65.

121. Spahn DR, van Brempt R, Theilmeier G, Reibold JP, et al. Perflubron emulsion delays blood transfusions in orthopedic surgery. European Perflubron Emulsion Study Group.Anesthesiology. 1999 Nov;91(5):1195-208.

122. Levy JH, Goodnough LT, Greilich P, et al. Polymerized bovine hemoglobin solution as a replacement for allogeneic red blood cell transfusion after cardiac surgery: results of a randomized, double-blind trial. J Thorac Cardiovasc Surg 2002;124:35-42.

123. Hill SE, Gottschalk LI, Grichnik K. Safety and preliminary efficacy of hemoglobin raffimer for patients undergoing coronary artery bypass surgery. J Cardiothorac Vasc Anesth. 2002 Dec;16(6):695-702.

124. Hill SE, Leone BJ, Faithfull NS, et al. Perflubron emulsion (AF0144) augments harvesting of autologous blood: a phase II study in cardiac surgery.J Cardiothorac Vasc Anesth. 2002 Oct;16(5):555-60.

125. Krieter H, Hagen G, Waschke KF, et al.: Isovolemic hemodilution with a bovine hemoglobin-based oxygen carrier: Effects on hemodynamics and oxygen transport in comparison with a nonoxygen-carrying volume substitute. J Cardiothorac Vasc Anesth 1997;11:3-9.

126. Schubert A, Przybelski RJ, Eidt JF, et al. Diaspirin-Crosslinked Hemoglobin Reduces Blood Transfusion in Noncardiac Surgery: A Multicenter, Randomized, Controlled, Double-Blinded TrialAnesth Analg 2003 97: 323-332.

127. Levy JH The use of haemoglobin glutamer-250 (HBOC-201) as an oxygen bridge in patients with acute anaemia associated with surgical blood loss. Expert Opin Biol Ther 2003;3:509-17.

128. Niquille M, Touzet M, Leblanc I, Baron JF. Reversal of intraoperative myocardial ischemia with a hemoglobin-based oxygen carrier. Anesthesiology 2000;92:882-5.

129. Saxena R, Wijnhoud AD, Carton H, et al. Controlled safety study of a hemoglobin-based oxygen carrier, DCLHb, in acute ischemic stroke. Stroke 1999;30:993-6.

130. Claudio C, Schramm S, Wettstein R, et al. Improved oxygenation in ischemic hamster flap tissue is correlated with increasing hemodilution with Hb vesicles and their O2 affinity. Am J Physiol Heart Circ Physiol 2003; 285: H1140–H1147.

131. Lanzkron S, Moliterno AR, Norris EJ. Polymerized human Hb use in acute chest syndrome: a case report. Transfusion. 2002 Nov;42(11):1422-7.

132. Teicher BA, Schwartz GN, Alvarez Sotomayor E, et al. Oxygenation of tumors by a hemoglobin solution. J Cancer Res Clin Oncol 1993;120:85-90.

CHAPTER 30

# HYPERBARIC OXYGEN IN SKIN GRAFTS AND FLAPS

## CHAPTER THIRTY OVERVIEW

# HYPERBARIC OXYGEN IN SKIN GRAFTS AND FLAPS

*Paul M. Nemiroff*

## SKIN GRAFTS AND FLAPS

### Rationale

Hyperbaric oxygen therapy is not necessary nor recommended for the support of normal, uncompromised skin grafts or flaps. However, following preoperative or postoperative irradiation or in other cases where there is decreased microcirculation or hypoxia, HBO has been shown to be extremely useful in preservation of these tissues. HBO can help maximize the viability of the compromised tissue, thereby reducing the need for regrafting or repeat flap procedures.

With respect to HBO's specific effect on flap survival, several mechanisms have been demonstrated. Reinisch (71, 72) has suggested that skin flap failure is secondary to the development of arteriovenous shunts in the distal portion of the flap. This results in a reduced flow to the critical nutrient capillary network. The vasoconstrictive properties of HBO may act to close the shunts selectively in non-ischemic areas and thereby allow greater blood flow to the nutrient capillary circulation in ischemic tissue.

Compromised tissues are frequently hypoxic, with oxygen tensions frequently below 15 mmHg (77). Tissue oxygen tensions of 30 to 40 mmHg are necessary for the synthesis of fibroblasts and subsequent development of a collagen matrix for capillary budding in avascular areas (27, 29, 37, 65, 80, 81, 87). Hyperbaric oxygen can deliver these levels of oxygen, thereby stimulating fibroblasts and enhancing collagen synthesis (76, 78). Being a facultative anaerobe, the fibroblast is thought to be stimulated by both intermittent hypoxia (the lactate stimulus) and hyperoxia (28, 37, 52). By restoring abnormally low tissue oxygen tension values to physiologic levels, HBO has been shown to support the otherwise hypoxic tissue until adequate circulation is reestablished (9) and promote capillary proliferation (26, 34, 48, 54, 58).

Thus, the ability of HBO to hyperoxygenate tissues, stimulate fibroblasts, and enhance collagen synthesis and neovascularity, as well as possibly close off arteriovenous shunts, are all mechanisms that contribute to improved skin flap survival.

A plethora of work has shown the efficacy of HBO on enhancement of flap and graft survival in a variety of experimental and clinical situations. A review of relevant animal and human studies is presented below.

## Animal Studies

Champion and colleagues, using a rabbit model pedicle flap, were able to obtain complete 100% survival of HBO treated flaps in rabbits at 2 ATA for 2 hours twice a day for 5 days, whereas all control flaps had significant areas of necrosis to greater than 40%. The increase in flap survival was noted with elevation of alveolar as well as skin surface oxygen levels. The authors concluded that this increase in oxygen levels under HBO supports hypoxic tissue until adequate circulation can recur (9). Similarly, work by McFarlane and Wermuth concluded that "HBO has been of definite value in preventing necrosis in a pedicle flap in the rat and also limited the extent of necrosis in a free composite graft." In addition, the authors noted that their particular design was a severe test of treatment and attests to the value of HBO in preventing necrosis (44).

In a study of healing tissues of full thickness and partial thickness wounds in rats, Shulman and Kron found that HBO lowered the healing time significantly. Further, the combination of repeated skin grafting and HBO reduced the healing time of partial thickness wounds to one half of that of nontreated controls. The authors conclude that the combined effect of grafting and HBO has "...the startling effect of a reduction in healing time of 50%, thus seemingly improving on nature itself" (79). Also, noted in the above study was the fact that no attempt at sterilizing was made in performing surgeries. Superficial contamination did occur in all animals, but infection was entirely absent in the groups treated with HBO. Mader has demonstrated that HBO significantly enhances leukocyte bacterial killing ability at tissue oxygen pressures up to 150 mmHg both in *vitro* and with an *in vivo* osteomyelitis model (46, 47).

Wald et al. found that HBO for two hours (four times a day) at 2.4 ATA produced a 22% increase in survival of skin flaps (84).

Niinikoski found a 51% improvement in length of the viable portion of tubed skin flaps in rats treated with HBO (2.5 ATA for two hours twice daily for two days) compared to air-breathing controls (64). The author suggested that the enhanced diffusion of oxygen into the area of disturbed circulation was the mechanism for improvement in tissue viability.

Gruber et al. showed that in skin flaps in rats, HBO at 3 ATA raised mean tissue tensions to 600 mmHg, whereas 100% oxygen at sea level did not raise mean flap $pO_2$ (23).

Arturson and Khanna in an experimental study on standard dorsal skin flaps in rats designed to give a predictable and constant degree of necrosis, revealed that HBO treatment had a significant improvement in flap survival over untreated controls (p<0.05) (1). Other flap enhancing agents were studied, and in some cases also enhanced flap survival. However, the best results were found in rats treated with hyperbaric oxygen. The authors note that all therapies had a marginal effect on survival of flaps when circulation to the area had ceased completely. This is expected, since any modality will be unable to revitalize tissue which is already "dead."

Jurell and Kaijser using a cranially based pedicle flap in rats showed that rats treated with HBO had significantly longer flaps, than controls (p < 0.001) (33). With 24 hours of intermittent treatment with HBO at 2 ATA, the surviving area was approximately twice that of the control group. Even when the start of hyperbaric treatment was delayed for 24 hours after surgery, there was still a significantly greater survival area of HBO treated flaps when compared with controls (p < 0.01) (33). The increase in surviving area was less, however, than if the HBO therapy was begun immediately after surgery. This emphasizes the importance of initiating HBO therapy as soon as a problem is suspected. This finding has been noted by others. If a significant delay in HBO treatment occurs, the beneficial results will be diminished (see Nemiroff 1985) (60).

Greenwood and Gilchrist demonstrated the effectiveness of HBO in reducing the extent of ischemic necrosis of skin flaps created in previously irradiated rats. All animals in the study were given 2,600 rads. At six months post exposure, a rectangular pedicle was created on the back of each animal. Half the animals were treated with HBO (at 2.0 ATA for 14 days) and half were treated with air. Mean flap necrosis was significantly greater (p < 0.05) in the control (air) group (21).

Kivisaari and Niinikoski in a study on rats showed that HBO at 2 ATA had no effect on the healing rate of open wounds in which circulation was left intact (i.e., "non-compromised" wounds). When the wound edges were devascularized, however, HBO enhanced wound closure rate significantly over control groups, thus counteracting the delay caused by disturbed blood supply in "compromised" wounds (36).

Related to the area of compromised grafts is a study by Calderwood, who studied the effect of HBO on transplantation of epiphysical growth cartilage in the rabbit. In the group of rabbits given HBO, approximately half of the transplants were regarded as successful when examined histologically six weeks after operation, versus only 28% in the group not treated with HBO (8).

Although not directly related to skin flap survival, a study by Jacobs, et al. on the histocompatibility of grafts and graft rejection, indicated that repeated daily exposure of mice to HBO significantly prolonged skin allograft survival (32).

Related to the area of wound healing and flap survival is the area of wound epithelialization of wounds after thermal injury. An example of this is a controlled study of Korn et al., who showed faster epithelialization of second degree burn wounds in guinea pigs treated with adjunctive HBO at 2 ATA. The authors noted earlier return of capillary patency in the HBO treated group (39).

Also, Winter and Perrins conducted studies with pigs and shallow wounds and found that intermittent treatments with HBO at 2 ATA resulted in 80% epidermal coverage versus 49% in controls (87).

Some of the work demonstrating that HBO enhances wound healing, grafts, and flaps by way of enhancement of capillary proliferation has been demonstrated by a number of researchers, and will be discussed later (26, 34, 48, 54, 58).

Tan et al., studied the effect of HBO and air under pressure on skin survival in acute 8 x 8 cm neurovascular island flaps in rats (82). Skin flaps treated with 8% hyperbaric oxygen (equivalent to room air at standard pressure) exhibited no improvement in skin survival. Skin flaps treated with hyperbaric air (21% oxygen) and hyperbaric 100% oxygen exhibited significant increases in survival. The extended treatments used with HBO resulted in no mortality, but in significant beneficial effects on flap survival. The authors cite other studies that emphasize tissue oxygen tension of pedicle flaps is lower than that of normal skin, and the fact that tissue oxygen tension can be raised by hyperbaric 100% oxygen, but not by 100% oxygen at standard pressures. Pedicle flaps treated with just 100% oxygen at ambient pressure exhibit no improvement in survival.

A controlled, randomized study of the effects of HBO and irradiation on experimental skin flaps has been performed by Nemiroff et al. (59). One hundred eighty-five Sprague-Dawley rats weighing between 195 and 275 grams were randomly assigned to one of 15 conditions, including all possible ordering effects of HBO, radiation and flap elevation, as well as controls which included flap elevation only, radiation only, and HBO groups. Cranially based skin flaps measuring 3 x 9 cm were elevated on the dorsum. The surviving length, in centimeters, was evaluated seven days after the operation using a fluorescein dye technique. Rats receiving HBO were subjected to four consecutive two-hour treatments of 100% oxygen at 2.5 ATA, with half-hour intervals of room air breathing. Depending on the treatment condition, HBO was given either 48 hours or 24 hours before flap elevation, or within four hours or 48 hours after flap elevation. Rats receiving radiation (cobalt 60) received a single dose of 1,000 rads to the dorsum using the Theratron 780 cobalt unit. Pre- and post-treatment weights were measured on all rats. Additionally, flaps from each of the 15 groups were removed (at random) and placed in 10% formalin for histopathologic analysis at a later date.

Results showed that all groups receiving HBO within four hours after flap elevation had significantly greater flap survival length ($p < 0.05$), with as much as a 22% increase in the surviving flap. Additionally, HBO given 48 hours prior to flap elevation significantly improved flap survival over that of controls ($p < 0.05$), whereas HBO given 24 hours prior to flap elevation resulted in no significant differences from controls. Immediate effects of radiation either pre- or post-flap elevation in conjunction with, or without HBO, appeared to have no significant effect on flap survival. However, rats receiving radiation, regardless of other factors, gained significantly less weight than did controls ($p < 0.001$) (60).

The authors note that HBO needs to be initiated as soon after the operation as possible. In this case, the flaps were designed to "fail." In clinical practice, a surgeon obviously does not design or plan a flap to fail. The implication here is that HBO in a clinical situation needs to be started as soon as a problem is detected - during or after surgery. As shown in Nemiroff's work, waiting 48 hours prior to initiation of HBO did not improve flap survival. This has been noted in other experimental studies as well as clinical studies (7, 33, 67-70). Thus, to be maximally effective, HBO treatment should be started as soon as there is any doubt as to the viability of the flap. Flap viability can be assessed by clinical judgement as well as a variety of other techniques (e.g., fluorescein dye, laser Doppler flow) (45). The important fact to appreciate is that once circulation has ceased completely, HBO will have a marginal effect. Further, if a surgeon cuts the principal vessel in an axial flap (e.g., the thoracoacromial artery in a pectoralis myocutaneous flap), then HBO will be of no value in saving the flap. HBO cannot "resurrect" dead tissue.

Further work by Nemiroff and Lungu revealed some of the mechanisms whereby HBO enhanced flap survival (58). Flaps from a previous study (60) were randomly chosen and placed in 10% formalin. A longitudinal strip (1 x 9 cm) was harvested from each flap. Sections 1 mm thick were routinely processed and stained with hematoxylin-eosin. At a standard power, and with the aid of an ocular micrometer, a middle segment from each flap of 3 to 6 cm was analyzed for number and size of vessels.

Results of the previous study (1985) showed that all groups receiving HBO within four hours after flap elevation had significantly greater flap survival length (p < 0.05). In the 1987 study, the absolute number of blood vessels in the microvasculature was significantly greater for all of these HBO groups when compared with that in controls (p < 0.01). The mean surface area of vessels of these "flap-HBO" groups was significantly greater than in controls in all but one group (p < 0.01).

The authors conclude that starting hyperbaric oxygen significantly enhanced flap survival, by increasing and/or maintaining the number and possibly the size of vessels within the microvasculature. To be most efficacious, HBO must be administered as soon after surgery as possible (i.e. as soon after a problem is suspected).

These findings are consistent with those documented by other researchers who have shown that HBO can enhance healing and flap survival by affecting angiogenesis (26, 48, 52, 54).

Manson, who used histochemical staining of the ATPs (Adenosine 5'-Triphosphate) to visualize small blood vessels, clearly demonstrated that capillaries grew almost three times further distally in pedicle flaps of guinea pigs that were treated with HBO, compared to age-matched controls (48).

Rubin et al. studied the effects of HBO in composite skin grafts in rabbit ears (73). Experimental animals received 100% $O_2$ at 2 ATA twice daily for 21 treatments. Grafts in HBO animals demonstrated significantly greater survival than grafts in control animals.

Recently, two additional controlled animal studies using entirely different flap models (random and axial) have clearly shown that HBO can significantly enhance flap survival (61, 88).

Nemiroff's 1988 study investigated the effects of pentoxifylline and hyperbaric oxygen (HBO) on experimental skin flaps in rats under four conditions (62). Sixty animals were randomly divided into one of four groups; (1) a control group (2) A pentoxifylline treated group (3) an HBO-treated group, and (4) a pentoxifylline-plus-HBO-treated group (Pentoxifylline is a rheologic agent which enhances capillary circulation by increasing the flexibility of red blood cells). Cranially based skin flaps were elevated on the dorsum. The surviving length was evaluated with fluorescein dye seven days after the operation. Rats that were treated with pentoxifylline received 20 mg/kg intraperitoneally at 24, 12, and 1 hour(s) before flap elevation and every 12 hours after the operation for seven days. Rats that were treated with HBO received a total of 14 two-hour treatments of 2.5 absolute atmospheres in divided doses. Results indicated that the surviving length of flaps in the pentoxifylline- or HBO treated groups were significantly longer than those in the control group, but were not significantly different from each other. Animals treated with both pentoxifylline and HBO had significantly greater flap survival than animals in any of the other three groups (p < 0.001). This reflected a 30% to 39% improvement over animals treated with pentoxifylline alone or animals treated with HBO alone, and an 86% improvement over control animals. Mechanisms of action of this apparent synergistic effect on flap survival were discussed.

Zamboni et al. examined the effect of hyperbaric oxygen on axial pattern flap survival in male Wistar rats when administered during and immediately following prolonged total flap ischemia (88). Eighty-one 3 x 6 cm rectangular epigastric skin flaps were elevated, and the inferior epigastric pedicle of each flap occluded for eight hours. The animals were divided into a control and three experimental groups: Control (n=27) - 8 hours flap ischemia, no HBO; group 1 (n=21) - HBO therapy (100% $O_2$ - three 1.75 hour dives at 2.5 ATA) during the ischemia; Group 2 (n=21) - HBO therapy (two 1.75 hour dives) following the ischemia; Group 3 (n=12) - HBO treatment during ischemia but with the flap contained in a metal-coated mylar bag to prevent oxygen diffusion. The percentage of flap necrosis was calculated on postoperative day six.

Mean flap necrosis for controls was 28% (± 21 SD) while HBO treatment during ischemia or during reperfusion significantly reduced this necrosis to 9% (± 11) and 12% (± 14) respectively (p < 0.01). The percentage of necrosis for Group 3, with the local effect of HBO on the flap blocked by the diffusion barrier, was 5% (± 7), also significantly better than the controls (p < 0.0005) but no different than the other two HBO groups. Hyperbaric oxygen treatment significantly increased the percentage of axial pattern skin flap survival when administered during or immediately following total flap ischemia. The improved flap survival was demonstrated to be a systemic and not a local effect.

In summarizing the experimental studies, it can be noted that a variety of animal models, simulating human clinical flaps, have been investigated (43). Results of the preponderance of work in the literature clearly show the efficacy of HBO with respect to enhancement of wound healing, skin/graft and flap survival. Of import is the fact that different types of flaps were analyzed in the studies, including free skin grafts, pedicle flaps, random flaps, irradiated wounds/flaps, composite grafts as well as axial pattern flaps. Although the blood supplies are very different in these flaps, a key factor to flap necrosis is tissue hypoxia. The results indicate that viability of flaps can be enhanced with HBO by a reduction of the hypoxic insult. Other mechanisms of action whereby HBO enhances flap survival are discussed elsewhere.

## Clinical Studies

Perrins demonstrated the value of adjunctive HBO in skin grafts (67-70). This was first shown in some case studies in 1966 and then later in a controlled clinical trial in 1967. In the latter study, he showed that significant improvement occurred in patients receiving HBO. Forty-eight patients were studied, random assignment to treatment or controls were used. Half were treated with HBO and half served as controls. Complete survival of grafts occurred in 64% of the treated groups as opposed to only 17% of the controls (p < 0.01).

Results of this study clearly showed that "whole-body exposure to HBO" significantly enhanced healing. Similar positive results in the clinical situation have been described by Monies-Chass et al. (55). In general, these cases represented failures of other available methods, after which HBO was undertaken.

Greenwood and Gilchrist examined the effect of HBO and wound healing in post irradiated "compromised wounds" in laryngectomy patients (20). The authors conclude that healing was significantly improved by hyperbaric oxygen therapy. As mentioned previously, controlled animal studies by these same researchers (21) on irradiated flaps revealed significantly better results in HBO-treated animals (p < 0.05). They also comment on the fact that randomized clinical trials are not practical or feasible. Welsh and Matos (1980) also discuss the benefits of HBO on improving skin flap survival (85). Other favorable case reports were noted by Barr et al. (5, 6). Bowersox et al., in a review of 105 patients with ischemic skin flaps or grafts (where 90% of the graft patients had risk factors that were considered to be poor prognostic indicators of graft or flap survival) found that 89% of threatened flaps and 91% of threatened skin grafts were salvaged (7). Thus, there was an average failure rate of approximately 10%. Compare this with other studies where failure rates with some complications can reach 67% in compromised tissues (24).

Kim et al. reported that in digits severed distally to the distal interphalangeal joint, HBO was essential to survival to the digits. He reported a 76% survival rate (35).

Bao also reported on the benefit of using HBO to improve survival of reimplanted severed limbs (2).

Neubauer et al. discussed the use of HBO as a useful adjunct in the successful reanastomosis of the severed ear (63).

Hyperbaric oxygen also has been shown to improve the survival of ischemic skin flaps of the face and to be an adjunct in periorbital reconstruction (16).

Related to wound healing in compromised tissues is a study by Hart et al. (25). In a randomized double blind study of 191 burn patients, the researchers showed that HBO decreases healing time, morbidity and mortality significantly.

Controlled animal studies on compromised burn wounds have shown similar positive results (22, 39, 66).

Baroni and colleagues examined the benefits of HBO in compromised diabetic lesions of the foot (4). Success in the HBO group of patients was significantly better than nonhyperbaric oxygen treated control patients (p < 0.001). All other variables between groups were reported to be essentially equal. In practical terms, the authors state that HBO treatment drastically reduced the incidence of leg amputations.

Related to the area of compromised wounds is the effect of hyperbaric oxygen in the treatment of radiation injuries. The work by Marx and associates (49-52) as well as others (17, 40, 83, 86) has shown the tremendous benefits of adjunctive HBO in "tissue deficient" and compromised wounds associated with bone necrosis. In addition to its therapeutic effectiveness against osteoradionecrosis (ORN), HBO has been proven useful in the treatment of soft tissue radiation-induced necrosis (10,

14, 15, 41). Farmer and associates demonstrated the usefulness of HBO in the management of radiation-induced injury to the larynx, nose, and floor of the mouth (14). Recently, Ferguson reported that HBO was used successfully to treat seven of eight patients with laryngeal radionecrosis. The authors concluded that HBO therapy was a useful adjunct in the management of laryngeal radionecrosis (15).

HBO therapy produces sufficient oxygen partial pressures in poorly perfused tissues to allow fibroblastic activity and collagen production, which creates a matrix for capillary budding and neovascularization. The daily elevation of oxygen tension in hypoxic bone and soft tissue results in the ingrowth of functioning capillaries, fibroblastic proliferation, collagen synthesis, and capillary angiogenesis. By these mechanisms, HBO has been reported to improve reconstructive attempts in the maxillofacial area (16, 52).

A recent paper reported successful treatment of osteoradionecrosis of the temporal bone in a 10-year-old child with rhabdomyosarcoma of the infratemporal fossa. This child had suffered with 6 years of otorrhea, which was refractory to other forms of therapy, prior to adjunctive HBO treatments (41).

Thus, there are a number of articles in the literature which demonstrate the usefulness of HBO on compromised flaps in the clinical situation. The preponderance of evidence from controlled animal studies also clearly shows the salutary effects of HBO on flap survival. Of course the controversy regarding the relative value of various animal models for flap experiments continues (13, 30). However, Hurn (30) has shown that by using a standardized flap design and method of evaluation, as well as sufficient sample sizes, rodent flaps can provide useful information relating to methods to enhance skin flap survival in the clinical situation.

Also, the issue of "double-blind controlled, randomized studies" on human flaps arises. Besides being virtually impossible to establish meaningful "double-blind" studies in these highly variable wounds and flaps, it would appear unethical to withhold HBO treatment from a patient in light of the findings of controlled, randomized "blinded" animal studies, as well as the clinical studies that have been performed.

Although numerous alternative methods have been tried to augment skin flaps, few have been routinely successful in animal or human settings.

Many methods of augmenting skin flaps have been reported (12), including cooling (38), the use of gravity (31, 57), raising systemic blood pressure (57), transforming rheological characteristics of blood (dextran) (18, 19), application of vasodilators (phenoxybenzamine, alpha-adrenergic blockers (3), histamine (11), a beta-adrenergic receptor, isoxsuprine (75), and increased humidity (74). However, all methods other than a "delay" technique, or HBO, have usually been unsuccessful. Of course, "delay techniques" are of no value once a flap has already been raised and inserted into its recipient bed. Further, delayed flaps are even less tolerant of ischemia than fresh flaps (56). Also, McFarlane et al. (42) found no difference in the survival of either delayed or fresh flaps.

From a practical point of view, many flap techniques do not permit the use of a "delay." Of course, when a delay technique is used, it results in a second or third surgery (with additional costs in re-hospitalization, surgical fees, etc.). Further, "delayed flaps" are known to be sub-optimal when the recipient sites are "compromised" (e.g., by previous radiation, trauma, etc.). On the contrary, the animal evidence and clinical work on using HBO have shown that it can enhance flap survival in compromised wounds, grafts, and flaps in a multitude of situations.

In closing, it should be emphasized that HBO is not necessary nor recommended for the support of normal, uncompromised skin grafts or skin flaps. However, following preoperative or postoperative irradiation or in other cases of compromised flaps, HBO can be a useful and even critical adjunct to other medical and surgical therapies. For the head and neck surgeon, for example, the problems of skin slough and tissue necrosis in compromised wounds and flaps with its resulting increase in various complications (e.g., infections, fistulas, carotid "blow-outs", etc.) is very serious. For example, Habel has noted a post-irradiation surgical complication rate of 67% (24). Besides the increased morbidity and mortality, the costs of longer hospitalizations, re-hospitalizations, repeat surgical interventions, etc. are tremendous. The fact that adjunctive HBO can reduce these costs has been presented in the previous pages. If one takes a hypothetical example, the savings become obvious. For example, if one compares the cost of the one "lost flap" on a patient (say for example a pectoralis major flap covering a hypopharyngeal fistula), one can quickly compare the increased costs of additional surgery (which may still not work), increased hospitalization stay, increased morbidity, etc. In conservative terms with a failed flap of this sort, the cost will be an additional $5,000-$10,000 in surgical and assistant's fees alone, as well as at least $15,000-$20,000 of increased hospitalization fees (assuming for example, two weeks additional time in the hospital including ICU care).

Compare this with the cost of 10-20 hyperbaric treatments needed to "save the flap" (e.g., at $300/treatment = $3,000-$6,000 versus $20,000-$30,000 if the flap fails.

In a more formal analysis, the report of Marx et al. on the prevention of one of the complications of post-irradiation extractions (i.e., osteoradionecrosis) shows the economic savings using HBO (53). In a randomized prospective clinical study, the HBO group had significantly less incidence of postoperative complication relating to osteoradionecrosis (5.4%) versus nontreated patients (29.9%). The potential cost savings per patient (in the HBO group) was estimated at $60,000.

## General Recommendations

Treatments are given at a pressure of 2.0 to 2.5 ATA and range from 90 to 120 minutes (depending on type of HBO facility available, patient status, etc.). Initial treatment should be twice daily. Once the graft or flap appears more viable and stable, once-daily treatments may suffice.

Peer review is required after 20 treatments when preparing a recipient site for a flap or graft and following 20 treatments after a flap or graft has been placed into its recipient site.

## REFERENCES

1. Arturson GG, Khanna NN. "The effects of hyperbaric dimethyl sulfoxide and complamin on survival of experimental skin flaps." Scan J Plast Reconst Surg. 1970;4:8-10.

2. Bao JYS. "HBO therapy in reimplantation of severed limbs: A report of 34 cases." In: (E.P. Kindwall, Ed.) Proceedings of the 8th International Congress on Hyperbaric Medicine. Flagstaff, AZ, Best Publishers. 1984;182-186.

3. Barisoni DM and Veall N. "Effects of thymoxamine circulation in skin flaps and in denervated skin." Lancet. 1969;1:400-401.

4. Baroni G, Porro T, Faglia E, Pizzi G, et.al. "Hyperbaric oxygen in diabetic gangrene treatment." Diabetes Care. 1987;10(1):81-86.

5. Barr PO, Enfors W, Erickssen G. "Hyperbaric oxygen therapy in dermatology." Br J Dermatology. 1972;86:631-635.

6. Barr PO, Liljedahl SO, Nylén B, "Enfarenheter av hyperbar O2 inom rekonstruktiv kirurgi." Nord Med. 1969;82:1223.

7. Bowersox JC, Strauss MB, Hart GB. "Clinical experiences with hyperbaric oxygen therapy in the salvage of ischemic skin flaps and grafts." J of HBO. 1986;1:141-149.

8. Calderwood JW. "The effect of hyperbaric oxygen in the transplantation of epiphyseal growth cartilage in the rabbit." J Bone Joint Surg. 1974;56B:735-759.

9. Champion WM, McSherry CK, Goulian D Jr. "Effect of hyperbaric oxygen on survival of pedicled skin flaps." J Surg Res. 1967;7:583-586.

10. Davis JC, Dunn JM, Gates GA, et al. "Hyperbaric oxygen: A new adjunct in the management of radiation necrosis." Arch Otolaryngol. 1979;105:58-61.

11. DeHaan C and Stark RB. "Changes in efferent circulation of tubed pedicles and in the transplantability of large composite grafts produced by histamine ionophoresis." Plast and Reconstr Surg. 1961;28:577.

12. Donegan JO. "The assessment and enhancement of skin flap viability." Head and Neck Surg. 1980;2:470-475.

13. Donovan WE. "Experimental models in skin flap removal research." Skin Flaps. WC Grabb and MB Myers (Eds). Boston: Little Brown and Co., Inc., 1975;11-20.

14. Farmer JC Jr, Shelton DL, Angelillo JD, et al. "Treatment of radiation-induced tissue injury by hyperbaric oxygen." Ann Otol Rhinol Laryngol. 1978;87:707-715.

15. Ferguson BJ, Hudson WR, Farmer JC Jr. "Hyperbaric oxygen therapy for laryngeal radionecrosis." Ann Otol Rhinol Laryngol. 1987;96:1-6.

16. Gonnering RS, Kindwall EP, Goldmann RW. "Adjunct hyperbaric oxygen therapy in periorbital reconstruction." Arch Opthalmol. 1986;104:439-443.

17. Goode RL and Linehan JW. "The fluorescein test in post-irradiation surgery." Arch Otolaryng. 1970;91:526-528.

18. Goulian D Jr. "The use of bromphenol blue in the assay of rheomacrodex effects on flap viability." Plast and Reconstr Surg. 1967;39:227.

19. Grabb WC and O'Neal RM. "The effect of low molecular weight dextran on the survival of experimental skin flaps." Plast and Reconstr Surg. 1966;37:406.

20. Greenwood TW, Gilchrist AG. "Hyperbaric oxygen and wound healing in post-irradiation head and neck surgery." Br J Surg. 1973;60:394-397.

21. Greenwood TW, Gilchrist AG. "The effect of HBO on wound healing following ionizing radiation." In: Trapp WC, et al.(Eds.) Proc of the Fifth Int'l Congress on Hyperbaric Med. Vol.1. Burnaby, Canada: Simon Frazier Univ. 1973; pp 253-263.

22. Gruber RP, Brinkley FB, Amato JJ, Mendelson JA. "Hyperbaric oxygen and pedicle flaps, skin grafts, and burns." Plast Reconstr Surg. 1970;45:24-30.

23. Gruber RP, Heitkamp DH, Lawrence JB. "Skin permeability to oxygen and hyperbaric oxygen." Arch Surg. 1970;101:69-70.

24. Habel DW. "Surgical complications in irradiated patients." Arch Oto. 1967;82:382-386.

25. Hart GB, O'Reilly RR, Broussard ND, Cave RH, Goodman DB, Yanda RL. "Treatment of burns with hyperbaric oxygen." Surg Gyn Obst. 1974;139:693-696.

26. Hartwig J, Kohnlein HE, Scherer D. "The influence of hyperbaric oxygen therapy and Dextran 40 on the endangered survival of skin-pedicle flaps." (German) Chirurg. 1973;44(10):452-456.

27. Hunt TK and Pai MP. "The effect of varying ambient oxygen tensions on wound metabolism and collagen synthesis." Surg Gyn Obstet. 1972;135:561-567.

28. Hunt TK, Van Winkle W. "Fundamentals of wound management in surgery." Wound Healing Normal Repair. New York: Appleton-Century-Crofts, 1976.

29. Hunt TK, Zederfeldt BH, Goldstick TK. "Oxygen and healing." Am J Surg. 1969;118:521-525.

30. Hurn IL, Fischer JC, Arganese T, et al. "Standardization of the dorsal rat flap model." Ann Plast Surg. 1984;2:210-213.

31. Hynes W. "The 'blue flap' - a method of treatment." Brit J Plast Surg. 1950;4:166.

32. Jacobs BB, Thuning CA, Sacksteder MR, Warren J. "Extended skin allograft survival in mice during prolonged exposure to hyperbaric oxygen." Transplantation. 1979;28:70-72.

33. Jurell G, Kaijser L. "The influence of varying pressure and duration of treatment with hyperbaric oxygen on the survival of skin flaps. An experimental study." Scand J Plast Reconstr Surg. 1973;7:25-28.

34. Ketchum III, SA, Thomas AN, Hall AD. "Angiographic studies of the effects of hyperbaric oxygen on burn wound revascularization."In: (J Wada and T Iwa Eds.) Proc of the Fourth Int'l Congress on Hyperbaric Med. Baltimore, Williams and Wilkins. 1970;388-394.

35. Kim SS, Kim D, Kim W, Baek S. "Treatment of amputated digit distal to DIP joint." Plast Surg Forum. 1987;10:241.

36. Kivisaari J and Niinikoski J. "Effects of hyperbaric oxygen and prolonged hypoxia on the healing of open wounds." Acta Chir Scand. 1975;141:14-19.

37. Knighton TR, Silver IA, Hunt TK. "Regulation of wound healing angiogenesis: Effect of oxygen gradient and inspired oxygen concentration." Surgery. 1981;90:262-269.

38. Körlof B and Ugland O. "Flaps and flap necrosis." Acta Chir Scand. 1966;131:408-412.

39. Korn HN, Wheeler ES, Miller TA. "Effect of hyperbaric oxygen on second degree burn wound healing." Arch Surg. 1977;122:732-737.

40. Kraut RA. "Prophylactic hyperbaric oxygen to avoid osteoradionecrosis when extractions follow radiation therapy." Clin Rev Dent. 1985;7:17-20.

41. Kveton JF. "Surgical management of osteoradionecrosis of the temporal bone." Otolaryngol Head Neck Surg. 1988;98:231-234.

42. McFarlane RM, Heazy FC, Rodin A, et al. "A study of the delay phenomenon in experimental pedicle flaps." Plast Reconst Surg. 1965;35:245-265.

43. McFarlane RM, DeYoung G, Henry RH. "The design of a pedicle flap to study necrosis and its prevention." Plast Reconst Surg. 1965;35:177-182.

44. McFarlane RM, Wermuth RE. "The use of hyperbaric oxygen to prevent necrosis in experimental pedicle flaps and composite skin grafts." Plast Reconstr Surg. 1966;37:422-430.

45. McGraw JB, Myers B, Skanklin KD. "The value of fluorescein in predicting viability of arterialized flaps." Plast Reconst Surg. 1977;60:710-719.

46. Mader JT. "Phagocytic killing and hyperbaric oxygen. Antibacterial mechanisms." HBO Rev. 1981;2:37-49.

47. Mader JT, Brown GL, Guckian JC, et al. "A mechanism for amelioration by HBO of experimental staphylococcal osteomyelitis in rabbits." J Infect Dis. 1980;142:915-922.

48. Manson PN, IM MJ, Myers RA, Hoopes JE. "Improved capillaries by hyperbaric oxygen in skin flaps." Surg Forum. 1980;31:564-566.

49. Marx RE. "Osteoradionecrosis of the jaws: Review update." HBO Rev. 1984;5:78-126.

50. Marx RE. "Osteoradionecrosis. Part I. A new concept in its pathophysiology." J Oral Maxillofac Surg. 1983;41:283-288.

51. Marx RE. "Osteoradionecrosis. Part II. A new concept in its treatment." J Oral Maxillofac Surg. 1983;41:351-357.

52. Marx RE, Ames JR. "The use of hyperbaric oxygen therapy in bony reconstruction of the irradiated and tissue deficient patient." J Oral Maxillofac Surg. 1982;40:412-420.

53. Marx RE, Johnson RP, Kline SN. "Prevention of osteoradionecrosis: A randomized prospective clinical trial of hyperbaric oxygen versus penicillin." J Am Dent Assoc. 1985;111:49-54.

54. Meltzer T, Myers B. "The effect of hyperbaric oxygen on the bursting strength and rate of vascularization of skin wounds in rats." Amer Surgeon. 1986;52:659-662.

55. Monies-Chass I, Hashmonai M. "Hyperbaric oxygen treatment as an adjunct to reconstructive vascular surgery in trauma." Injury. 1977;8:274-277.

56. Myers MB and Cherry G. "Mechanisms of the delay phenomenon." Plast Reconstr Surg. 1969;44:52-57.

57. Myers MB and Cherry G. "Enhancement of survival in devascularized pedicles by the use of phenoxybenzamine." Plast and Reconst Surg. 1968;41:254-260.

58. Nemiroff PM and Lungu AP. "The influence of hyperbaric oxygen and irradiation on vascularity in skin flaps: A controlled study." Surg Forum. 1987;38:565-567.

59. Nemiroff PM, et al. "HBO and irradiation on experimental skin flaps in rats." Surg. Forum. 1984;35:549-550.

60. Nemiroff PM, Merwin GE, Brant T, Cassissi NJ. "Effects of hyperbaric oxygen and irradiation on experimental flaps in rats." Otolaryngol Head Neck Surg. 1985;93:485-491.

61. Nemiroff PM, Ryback LP. "Applications of hyperbaric oxygen for the otolaryngologist-head and neck surgeon." Am J Otolaryng. 1988;9:52-57.

62. Nemiroff PM. "Synergistic effects of pentoxifylline and hyperbaric oxygen on skin flaps." Arch Otolaryngol Head Neck Surg. 1988;114:977-981.

63. Neubauer RA, Pinella J, Hill K, Bright DE. "The use of hyperbaric oxygen in the successful re-anastomosis of the severed ear: three cases." Proc. of EUBS Annual Meeting XIV. Sept. 5-9, 1988.

64. Niinikoski J. "Viability of ischemic skin in hyperbaric oxygen." Acta Chir Scand. 1970;136:567-568.

65. Niinikoski J and Hunt TK. "Oxygen tension in human wounds." J Surg Res. 1972;12:77-82.

66. Nylander G, Nordström H, Eriksson E. "Effects of hyperbaric oxygen on oedema formation after a scald burn." Burns. 1980;10:193-196.

67. Perrins DJD. "Hyperbaric oxygenation of skin flaps." Br J Plast Surg. 1966;19:440.

68. Perrins DJD. "Influence of hyperbaric oxygen on the survival of split skin grafts." Lancet. 1967;1:806-871.

69. Perrins DJD. "The effect of hyperbaric oxygen on ischemic skin flaps." Skin Flaps. WC Grabb and MB Myers (Eds.) Boston: Little Brown and Co., Inc. 1975;53-63.

70. Perrins DJD, Davis JC. "Enhancement of healing in soft tissue wounds." In: JC Davis and TK Hunt (Eds.). Hyperbaric Oxygen Therapy. Bethesda, MD: Undersea Medical Society, 1977;229-248.

71. Reinisch JF: Pathophysiology of skin flap circulation." Plast Reconstr Surg. 1974;54:585.

72. Reinisch JF. "The role of arteriovenous anastomoses in skin flaps." Skin Flaps. WC Grabb and MB Myers (Eds.) Boston: Little Brown and Co., 1975;81-92.

73. Rubin JS, Marzella L, Myers RA, Suter C, Eddy H, Kleiman L. "Effects of hyperbaric oxygen on the take of composite skin grafts in rabbit ears." J Hyperbaric Med. 1988;3(2):79-88.

74. Sasaki A, Fukuda O, Soeda S. "Attempts to increase the surviving length in skin flaps by a moist environment." Plast Reconstr Surg. 1979;64:526-531.

75. Sasaki A, Harii K. "Lack of effect of Isoxsuprine on experimental random flaps in the rat." Plast Reconstr Surg. 1980;66:105-108.

76. Sheffield PJ. "Tissue oxygen measurements with respect to soft tissue wound healing with normobaric and hyperbaric oxygen." HBO Rev. 1985;6(1):18-46.

77. Sheffield PJ, Dunn JM. "Continuous monitoring of tissue oxygen tension during hyperbaric oxygen therapy." In: G Smith (Ed.) Proc of the Sixth Int'l Congress on Hyperbaric Med. Aberdeen, Scotland: Aberdeen University Press. 1977;125-129.

78. Sheffield PJ, Workman WT. "Noninvasive tissue oxygen measurements in patients administered normobaric and hyperbaric oxygen by mask." HBO Rev. 1985;6:47-63.

79. Shulman AG, Kron HL. "Influence of hyperbaric oxygen and multiple skin allografts on the healing of skin wounds." Surg. 1967;62:1051-1058.

80. Silver IA. "Oxygenation and epithelialization." In: HI Maibach and DT Rovee (Eds.) Epidermal Wound Healing. Chicago: Year Book Medical Publishers. 1972;291-305.

81. Silver IA. "The measurement of oxygen tension in healing tissues." In: H. Herz (Ed.) Progress in Respiration Research. Vol III. Basel, Switzerland: Skarger, 1969;124-125.

82. Tan CM, Im MJ, Myers RA, Hoopes JE. "Effect of hyperbaric oxygen and hyperbaric air on survival of island skin flaps." Plast Reconstr Surg. 1974;73:27-30.

83. Tobey RE, Kelly JF. "Osteoradionecrosis of the jaws." Otolaryngol Clin North Am. 1979;12:183-186.

84. Wald HI, Georgiade NG, Angelillo DDS, Saltzman HA. "Effect of intensive hyperbaric therapy on survival of experimental skin flaps in rats." Surg Forum. 1968;19:497.

85. Welsh F, Matos L. "Medical hyperbaric therapy." Ohio State Med J. 1980;76:582-585.

86. Wilcox JW, Kolodny SC. "Acceleration of healing of maxillary and mandibular osteotomies by use of hyperbaric oxygen." Oral Surg. 1976;41:423-429.

87. Winter GD, Perrins DJD. "Effects of hyperbaric oxygen treatment on epidermal regeneration." In: J Wada and T Iwa (Eds.). Proc of the Fourth Int'l Congress on Hyperbaric Med. Baltimore: Williams and Wilkins, 1970;363-368.

88. Zamboni WA, Roth AC, Russell RC, Nemiroff PM, Casa L, Smoot C. "The effect of acute hyperbaric oxygen therapy on axial pattern skin flap survival when administered during and after total ischemia." J of Reconst Microsurg. 1989;5:343-347.

CHAPTER 31

# RADIATION INJURY TO TISSUE

## CHAPTER THIRTY-ONE OVERVIEW

# RADIATION INJURY TO TISSUE

*Robert E. Marx*

## THE UNIQUE CHARACTER OF RADIATION INJURY

The effect of hyperbaric oxygen (HBO) on tissues radiated to a dose of more than 5,000 cGy (centi-Gray) is one of capillary angiogenesis and fibroplasia. This effect alone is unique in therapeutics. The mechanism by which hyperbaric oxygen accomplishes this is complex but is related to normal wound revascularization and healing. This mechanism is made possible only because of the unique pattern of tissue injury that radiation creates a pattern which does not permit the normal revascularization that occurs in other tissue injuries.

When tissue is radiated in the treatment of a malignancy, normal tissue cells are also damaged. In spite of the concerted efforts of radiation therapists to enhance tumor kill and reduce normal nontumor damage such as fractionation, hyperfractionation, supervoltage, beam collimation, etc., normal tissue is nevertheless damaged (10, 25). The nontumor cells that are in the field of radiation are heterogeneous in their type (fibroblasts, endothelium, muscle, nerve, etc.) and heterogeneous in their sensitivity to radiation. This is partially because of the inherent radiation sensitivity of different cell types. In descending order of sensitivity are tumor cells, endothelium, fibroblasts, muscle, and nerve cells. Varying effects may also be seen because radiation may either kill any cell type outright or inflict lethal damage so that it dies later. Radiation may also incapacitate a cell so that it does not produce daughter cells or collagen. The surviving cells may produce defective collagen or defective regulatory enzymes. Individual cells may totally escape damage. The result is a residual tissue which develops a progressive loss of vascularity and cellularity over time as cells live out their life span and are not replaced or fail to contribute to tissue integrity.

The progressive radiation fibrosis and capillary loss with time have been shown to be almost linear and are an inescapable aftermath of therapeutic radiation. See Figure 1 (23, 25).

It may even progress to spontaneous radionecrosis of soft tissue or bone if the radiation dose has been sufficiently high. Breakdown may also occur as a complication of surgical wounding when the tissue is required to meet the increased demands of healing.

## ANGIOGENESIS AND FIBROPLASIA IN RADIATED TISSUE

A hyperbaric chamber, per se, is not the therapeutic agent which produces angiogenesis and fibroplasia in radiated tissue. Oxygen is actually the

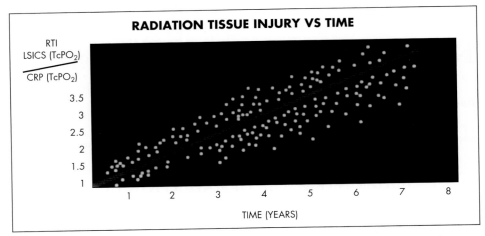

*Figure 1. Inverse of capillary density curve shows an increasing radiation tissue hypovascularity with time. It is due to the late cellular effects which stop endothelial cells, and fibroblasts in particular, from replenishing their populations and maintaining sound structures. Therefore, they lose their prime function of providing vessels for perfusion and collagen synthesis for tissue repair. The resultant tissue has been termed "Three-H" tissue (23, 25, 26). It is hypovascular, hypocellular, and hypoxic. Importantly, it will continue to become more so with time. See Figures 2 and 3.*

therapeutic drug, with the chamber serving merely as a dosing device. Oxygen at normobaric (1 ATA) pressure has been shown incapable of producing angiogenesis (see Figures 4 and 5) or fibroplasia (see Figures 6 and 7) in animal models (24).

It seems that increasing pressures to the optimum of 2.4 ATA brings the dosage of oxygen into a therapeutic range while avoiding toxicity. Thus oxygen, like any other medically useful drug, can be applied in insufficient dosage and as such may be subtherapeutic, or it can be given in too high a dose and thus produce toxic symptoms.

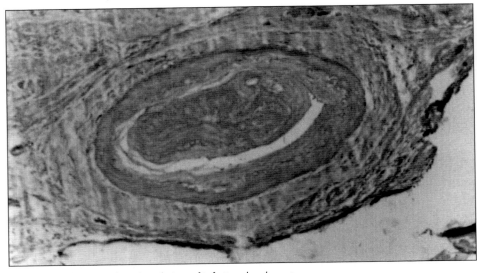

*Figure 2. Radiation-induced occlusion of inferior alveolar artery.*

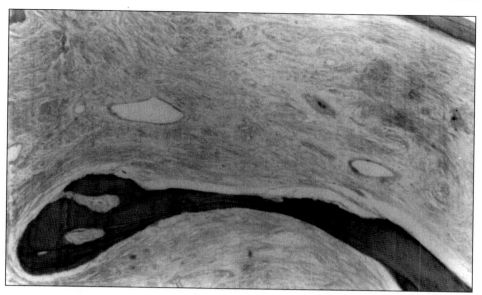

*Figure 3. Radiation-induced hypovascular-hypocellular-hypoxic tissue (Three-H Tissue).*

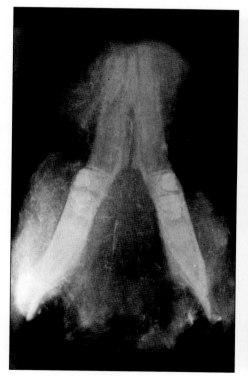

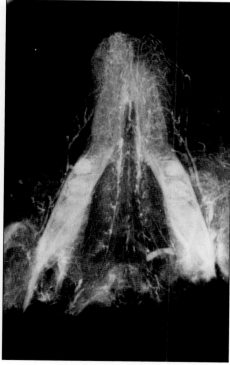

*Figure 4. Tissue angiogram of radiation induced three-H tissue in a rabbit model after 20 exposures to 1 ATA of 100% oxygen. Little angiogenesis is noted.*

*Figure 5. Tissue angiogram of radiation induced three-H tissue in same rabbit model after 20 exposures to 2.4 ATA 100% oxygen. A measured eight fold increase in vascular density is noted.*

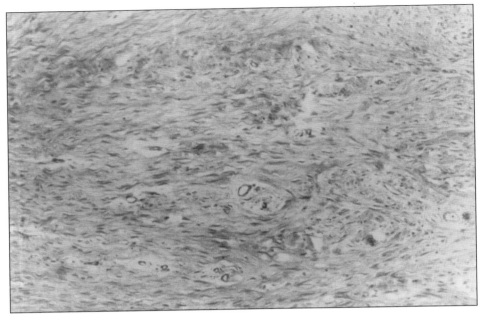

Figure 6. Tissue histology of radiation induced three-H tissue in same rabbit model after 20 exposures to 1 ATA of 100% oxygen. Marked hypovascularity within a fibrotic stroma.

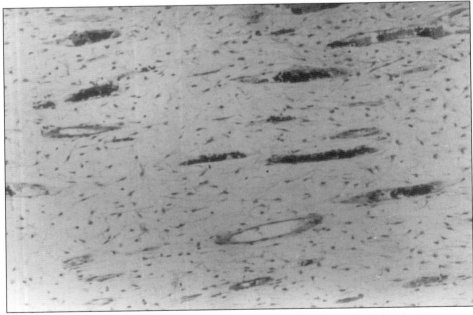

Figure 7. Tissue histology of radiation induced three-H tissue in same rabbit model after 20 exposures to 2.4 ATA of 100% oxygen. Increased vascular density, reduced fibrosis, and increased cellularity are seen.

The pressures and exposure times necessary to create angiogenesis and fibroplasia in radiated tissue have been elucidated (23, 24, 25). Initially, studies documented both angiogenesis and fibroplasia in radiated head and neck cancer patients through biopsy of human tissues before and after hyperbaric oxygen. See Figures 8 and 9 (23). Later, human transcutaneous oxygen measurements and animal studies traced the time course of this angiogenesis and fibroplasia (see Figure 10).

As seen in Figure 10, angiogenesis and fibroplasia develop in response to HBO of 2.4 ATA, 90 minutes each session, 5 days a week over a 20-session treatment course. Uncomplicated radiated tissue, after the usual dose of 6,000 to 8,000 cGy for malignant tumors, exists with a capillary density only 20% to 40% of that in nonradiated tissue (24, 26). The first response of this "Three H" tissue to HBO is known as the "lag phase" because no measurable change is seen with the crudeness of a transcutaneous oxygen monitor (26). However, histologic studies have shown capillary budding and cellular collagen synthesis. The radiated tissue's response begins with macrophage activity, fibroblastic collagen production and endothelial proliferation, which occur during the first six to eight hyperbaric oxygen exposures.

After eight hyperbaric treatments the curve in Figure 10 begins a steep upward deflection known as the "rapid rise phase" (26). This rise is caused by the proliferation of lumenized and functional capillaries, which is measured by the transcutaneous monitor as increased capillary density. Histologic evidence shows a geometric development of capillaries from the few preexisting ones. That is, one capillary buds into two, those two into four, and onward at a rate to the exponent of two. This vascular proliferation continues until twenty sessions of hyperbaric oxygen is attained, after which it levels off to between 75% and 85% of that seen in nonradiated tissue. This leveling off of angiogenic response is termed the "plateau phase."

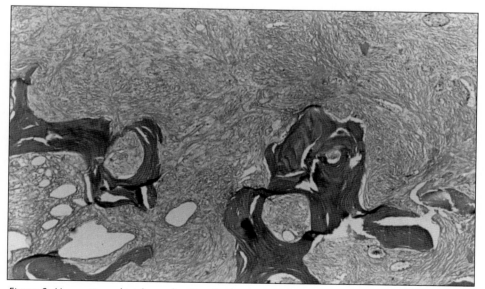

Figure 8. Human tissue histology of radiated tissue prior to hyperbaric oxygen exposures. Three-H picture is evident.

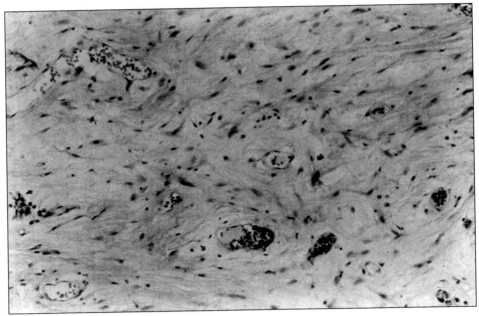

Figure 9. Human tissue histology of radiated tissue after 20 hyperbaric oxygen exposures at 2.4 ATA. Angiogenesis and fibroplasia are apparent.

The plateau phase consists of maximum revascularization where the stimulus for further angiogenesis ceases. Histologically, it is associated with an observed reduction in tissue macrophages, capillary budding, and collagen synthesis as compared to the "lag" and "rapid rise" phases. Most importantly, as illustrated in Figure 10, the angiogenic effect is maintained for at least four years. Those patients who were restudied demonstrated the same level of

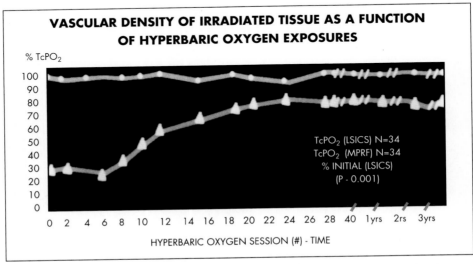

Figure 10. Graph of capillary density versus number of hyperbaric oxygen exposures showing non-radiated tissue and radiated tissue responses.

angiogenesis after four years as they had immediately after their hyperbaric oxygen treatment. Apparently, the new vessels induced by hyperbaric oxygen do not involute after cessation of HBO treatment any faster than vessels involute at the normal rate of aging.

Also observed in Figure 10 is the lack of any response in nonradiated tissue. Hyperbaric oxygen does not induce a supervascularization in nonradiated, otherwise normal tissue and therefore cannot be expected to accelerate healing in tissue which does not have a compromised wound healing potential.

## PROTOCOLS FOR HYPERBARIC OXYGEN WHEN SURGERY IS PERFORMED IN RADIATED TISSUE

From the research data illustrated in Figure 10, and from clinical experience, the most effective protocol for the application of HBO as an adjunct to healing in radiated tissue is:

1. Twenty sessions prior to surgical wounding.
2. Surgical wounding.
3. Ten sessions after surgical wounding.

A hyperbaric treatment is defined as breathing 100% oxygen for 90 minutes at 2.4 ATA.

Some chamber facilities prefer to use, or can only use, 100% oxygen at 2.0 ATA. This may be less than ideal, but is clinically acceptable if when using the reduced pressure, an increased exposure time of 120 minutes is offered. This protocol has produced clinically similar results to the 2.4 ATA protocol but has been less used. Recent animal studies by the author indicate increasing tissue response up to 3 ATA, but 3ATA is potentially too toxic to be of clinical use for multiple treatments. The 2.4 ATA protocol has been studied extensively and has been proven effective.

Similarly, some have suggested a twice-daily session of HBO to reduce the time of overall treatment, but this concept is empirical and is untested. A twice-a-day protocol is not recommended because it is both unproven and theoretically may afford insufficient time for the radiated tissue to respond with angiogenesis and fibroplasia.

## MECHANISMS OF HYPERBARIC OXYGEN INDUCED ANGIOGENESIS AND FIBROPLASIA

The mechanism by which hyperbaric oxygen achieves angiogenesis and fibroplasia in radiated tissue has been studied (26) and found to be stimulated by a similar oxygen-gradient phenomenon that Knighton, Silver and Hunt have found to be central in the angiogenesis and fibroplasia of normal wound healing (13, 15, 38). Radiated tissue does not spontaneously revascularize as do other wounded tissues because of the unique physics and pattern of tumoricidal radiation delivery. Normal wounds have a central area of tissue injury or hematoma surrounded by relatively normal tissue with normal perfusion. Therefore, the oxygen tension in the central area of the wound is extremely low (often 0 to 5 mmHg) and the adjacent tissue is normal (approximately 50 to 60 mmHg). The oxygen gradient is thus naturally steep across a short distance. Such steep oxygen gradients have been shown to be the physio-chemotactic factor attracting wound regulating macrophages to a wound. (14, 38) Steep oxygen gradients, along with the lactate, iron, and acid inherent in wounds, stimulate macrophage derived angiogenesis factor (MDAF) and macrophage derived growth factor (MDGF) which in turn promote the capillary budding and collagen synthesis of wound healing (14).

Radiated tissue does not spontaneously revascularize because the wounding pattern is so diffuse that only shallow oxygen gradients are created. Therefore, the physiochemical response which identifies an injured area as a wound does not develop, and the body, in a sense, does not recognize the radiation injury as a wound. In fact, as the late radiation effect on cells makes the tissue worse with time, the continuation and worsening of the "Three H" pattern make the natural tissue oxygen gradients even less. See Figure 1.

The diffuse pattern of radiation injury is created chiefly by the isodose concept of tumoricidal radiotherapy. That is, a tumor is conceptualized as a spheroidal mass with the greatest number of target cells in the diameter of its equator. A greater dose or boost dose is given to the tumor's center. At incremental distances from the equator, the tumor's cellular mass is less, and therefore the delivered radiation dose is less. This progressively diminishing dose from the tumor's center to the periphery of the planned radiated area creates a gradual lessening of tissue injury and therefore a gradual or shallow oxygen gradient. The divergence of the radiation beam from its source further contributes to this shallow oxygen gradient. Even with attempts at higher speed emissions (super or megavoltage) and collimated beams there is some divergence. This creates greater cellular damage at the center of the radiation port than at the periphery.

The effect of hyperbaric oxygen on the diffuse wounding pattern of radiated tissue is illustrated in Figures 11 through 15.

Studies have identified that the center of an uncomplicated radiation injured area has oxygen tensions around 5 to 10 mmHg. This value is not far above the 3 mmHg of oxygen tension at which spontaneous wound breakdown is thought to occur. Measurements taken at 1 cm increments from the center show a gradual improvement in tissue oxygen tensions until one reaches the limits of the radiated field, where the normal 55 to 60 mmHg oxygen tension is found. See Figure 11. During exposure of the patient to hyperbaric oxygen at 2.4 ATA, measurements indicate a seven to ten-fold rise at each 1 cm increment, including the nonradiated tissue outside the radiated field. Since each incremental area shows an increase in oxygen tension, the underlying shallow oxygen gradient is magnified into a steep oxygen gradient. See Figure 12. In addition, at every increment, increased oxygen is available at the cellular level. After ten exposures, when the radiated tissue is in the early portion of the rapid-rise phase, the oxygen gradients move centrally, indicating that much of the angiogenesis comes from outside of the radiated field. See Figure 13. After 18 exposures, when the radiated tissue is in the later portion of the rapid rise phase (see Figure 14), the oxygen gradient is not only seen to move more centrally but is eliminated at the outer areas. This indicates that the bulk of the angiogenesis comes from outside of the radiated field and suggests that angiogenesis in that area eliminates the oxygen gradient altogether. After 20 to 24 exposures, oxygen gradients are either eliminated or

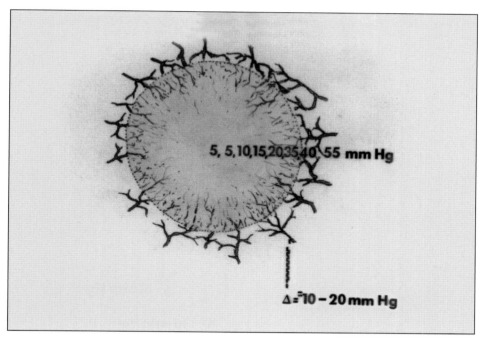

*Figure 11. Shallow oxygen tension gradients can be measured within a radiated tissue field. Such shallow oxygen gradients prevent initiation of revascularization.*

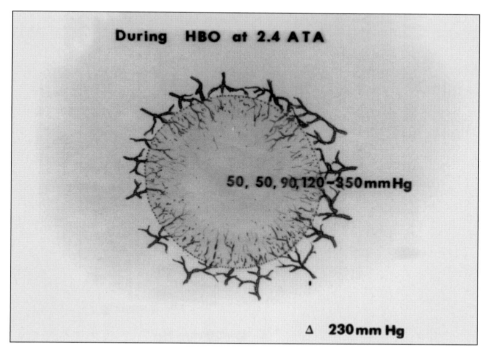

*Figure 12. Steep oxygen gradients can be measured within a radiated tissue during hyperbaric oxygen exposures. The creation of oxygen gradients in excess of 20 mmHg is theorized to initiate angiogenesis.*

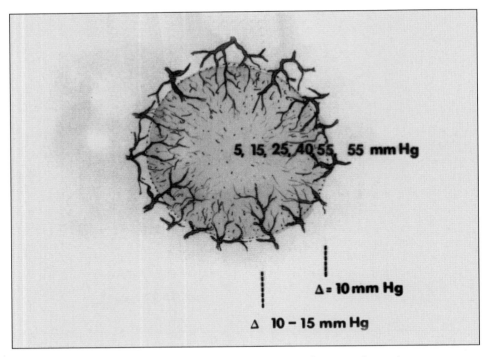

Figure 13. After 10 hyperbaric oxygen exposures, oxygen gradients are observed to move centrally indicating an angiogenesis front from the periphery and the deep wound margin.

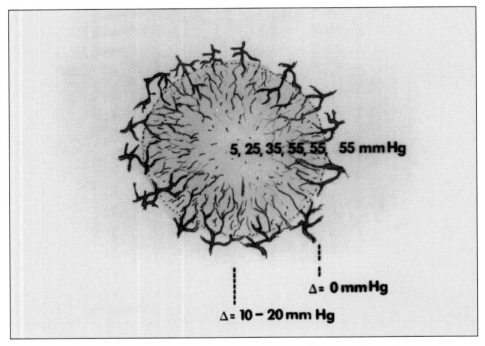

Figure 14. After 18 hyperbaric oxygen exposures, oxygen gradients are observed to continue to move centrally and are actually eliminated at the periphery.

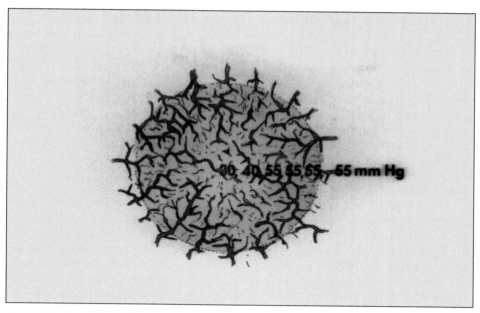

*Figure 15. After 24 hyperbaric oxygen exposures, oxygen gradients were either eliminated or reduced to a point where gradients above 20 mmHg can no longer be achieved, even under hyperbaric conditions, and thus further angiogenesis ceases.*

are so small that gradients above 20 mmHg cannot be achieved even with hyperbaric oxygen. See Figure 15. Thus, hyperbaric oxygen creates steep oxygen gradients in radiated tissues which cannot develop them naturally as do other wounds. These steep oxygen gradients then trigger the recognition of the radiated tissue as a wound and initiate the series of biochemical steps seen in normal tissue angiogenesis. The angiogenesis induced by hyperbaric oxygen remains under the same regulatory control as normal wound angiogenesis, so that when sufficient capillary perfusion develops to eliminate oxygen gradients, the biochemical messenger-response sequence shuts off and over-angiogenesis is prevented. It is important to emphasize that HBO stimulates angiogenesis to create a vascular architecture of 75% to 85% that of nonradiated tissue. This seems to hinge on the fact that angiogenesis shuts off when oxygen gradients dip below a fixed point (suggested to be 20 mmHg), not necessarily when the gradient is absolutely zero (34, 35).

This mechanism may also explain why HBO produces angiogenesis in certain other nonradiated wounds such as diabetic ulcers, crush injuries, failing flaps, etc. Compromised wounds have in common a lack of steep oxygen gradients. A notable example is the diabetic ulcer, which has a similarly diffuse, hypoxic vascular pattern due to its microangiopathy.

In nonradiated, noncompromised wounded tissue, there is already a steep oxygen gradient. HBO only adds to the steepness of the gradient which is already producing a maximal stimulus, and the capacity for further response is lost. Since oxygen gradients stimulate angiogenesis, rather than increased oxygen availability, a mere increase in oxygen availability will not enhance wound healing in normal tissue.

# CLINICAL APPLICATIONS OF HYPERBARIC OXYGEN

The protocol of 20 sessions of HBO prior to surgery and 10 sessions afterwards (the 20/10 protocol) is the one most commonly used for surgery in uncomplicated radiated tissues. A different and more directed protocol is used in more serious situations where frank soft tissue and/or osteoradionecrosis is present. Nevertheless, the 20/10 protocol has now been studied and found effective with randomized, prospective studies in at least three areas of head and neck post-radiation surgery: bone graft reconstruction, soft tissue vascular flaps, and tooth removal. Therefore, it is presently the definitive protocol whenever any elective surgery or wounding is performed within radiated tissues.

## Bony Reconstruction of the Jaws

Some of the first experiences with hyperbaric oxygen involved jaw surgery and reconstruction (17). In its early application hyperbaric oxygen was used only after surgery to oxygenate tissue and enhance healing (19). Early workers empirically applied hyperbaric oxygen in the postoperative phase because of an insufficient knowledge concerning its mechanism, time course, and the basic tissue angiogenesis response (11, 19). Results were disappointing, as one might anticipate (11, 19), until Marx and Ames focused the attention of hyperbaric oxygen on the preoperative phase (23). Since then, Marx and Johnson (25), Marx, Johnson, and Kline (27), and Marx, Ehler et al. (24), have elucidated the mechanisms and time course of angiogenesis and fibroplasia as discussed earlier.

The importance of preoperative HBO relates to the basic biology of bone graft healing. Hyperbaric oxygen has literally revolutionized facial bone reconstruction of the radiated patient because it has made outcomes predictable and functional. The patient's healing is less complicated. Prior to the regular use of the 20/10 hyperbaric oxygen protocol, mandibular reconstruction success rates were 40% to 50% (1, 16). With the use of the 20/10 hyperbaric oxygen protocol, success rates meeting six rigid criteria have been 90% to 93% (23, 26). See Tables 1 and 2.

Our group conducted a controlled, randomized, prospective study of specific hemimandibular jaw reconstructions in tissue beds radiated to greater than 6,400 cGy. With 52 patients in the hyperbaric group, as compared to 52 patients in the nonhyperbaric group, the complication rate was 9% versus 22% respectively and the percentage meeting the six rigid success criteria was 92% versus 65% respectively. See Table 1 and 2, Figures 16, 17, and 18.

The reason for increased success in the hyperbaric oxygen group relates directly to the induced angiogenesis and fibroplasia. Live bone cell transplantation into HBO treated tissue produces a greater survival of cellular elements and greater bone formation. Such grafts are known to undergo a two-phased regeneration into a functional bone ossicle. The first phase requires a vascular tissue bed to support bone cell survival and the production of osteoid and mineralized early bone. The second phase, which is a bone remodeling/maturation phase, requires a vascular and cellular tissue bed. The vascularity supports the metabolic activity of the bone-resorption, bone-apposition, bone mineralization sequence inherent in remodeling. Cellularity supplies a cell population of inducible cells which develop into endosteum and periosteum in the grafts. See Figures 19 and 20.

## TABLE 1. HEMIMANDIBULAR RECONSTRUCTION IN RADIATED TISSUES

|          | N  | COMPLICATIONS | MET (6) CRITERIA OF SUCCESS |
|----------|----|---------------|-----------------------------|
| Non-HBO  | 52 | 11(22%)       | 34 (65%)                    |
| HBO      | 52 | 5 (9%)        | 48 (92%)                    |

## TABLE 2. SIX CRITERIA TO MEASURE "SUCCESS" IN JAW RECONSTRUCTION

**RESTORATION OF:**

1) Continuity

2) Aleveolar Bone Height

3) Osseous Bulk

4) Soft Tissue Deficiencies Eliminated

5) Facial Form

6) Maintenance of Bone (18 months minimum)

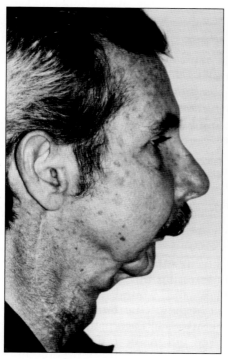

*Figure 16. Radiated cancer patient with hemimandibular defect before bone graft reconstruction supported by the 20/10 hyperbaric oxygen protocol.*

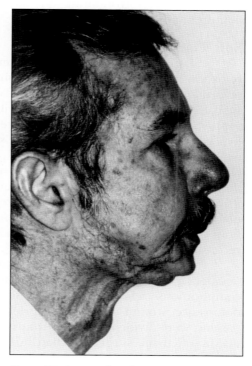

*Figure 17. Same radiated cancer patient after bone graft reconstruction supported by the 20/10 hyperbaric oxygen protocol.*

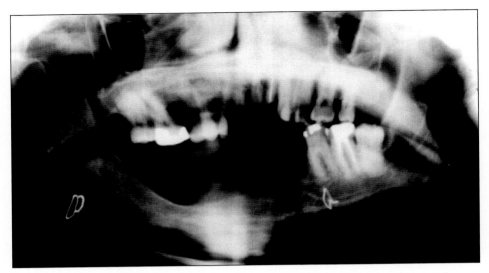

*Figure 18. Panoramic radiograph showing seven year follow-up of same patient's bone grafts, demonstrating a well consolidated graft, which has withstood functional demands.*

It is endosteum and periosteum which also make the graft long lasting and capable of withstanding the functional demands of chewing, speech, dentures and dental implants.

## Soft Tissue Flaps

Extirpative cancer surgery removes significant soft tissue, while radiation more subtly necroses and contracts soft tissue. Therefore pedicled myocutaneous or free microvascular flaps are often required to reconstruct such defects. Although these flaps will bring with them their own blood supply, they nevertheless must adhere to and heal into the hypovascular-hypocellular-hypoxic radiated tissue. Use of such flaps does not eliminate the need for the hyperbaric oxygen 20/10 protocol. Flaps which bring their own blood supply do not increase the blood supply of the radiated tissue into which they heal. If bone graft placement is required into an area of flap and radiated tissue, the flap tissue will support bone regeneration, but the radiated tissue will not. Use of the 20/10 hyperbaric oxygen protocol, however, will support bone graft healing in all previously radiated tissue and therefore make reconstruction of such patients possible.

Our department at the University of Miami has accomplished a detailed, randomized, prospective study assessing three aspects of wound complications related to soft tissue flaps and wound healing: wound dehiscence, wound infection, and delayed healing. One hundred and sixty patients were divided into two groups of eighty each. Each patient required a major soft tissue surgery or flap introduced into tissue radiated to a dose greater than 6,400 cGy. One group underwent surgery without preoperative hyperbaric oxygen. The other group underwent their indicated surgery by the same surgeons using the 20/10 hyperbaric oxygen protocol. The results are shown in Tables 3A, 3B, and 3C.

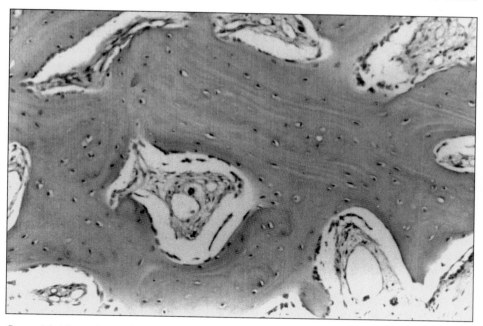

Figure 19. Mature human bone graft in radiated tissue with prominent endosteum derived from hyperbaric oxygen induced cellularity in recipient tissue.

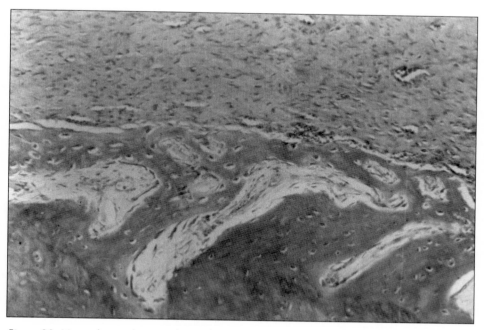

Figure 20. Mature human bone graft in radiated tissue with functioning periosteum derived from hyperbaric oxygen-induced cellularity in recipient tissue.

**Wound Dehiscence:** The control group developed a 15% incidence of minor wound dehiscence and a 33% incidence of major wound dehiscence, while the 20/10 hyperbaric group developed a 7.5% incidence of minor wound dehiscence and a 3.5% incidence of major wound dehiscence. In this study a minor wound dehiscence was defined as one which healed within three weeks with wound care and dressings. A major wound dehiscence was defined as one unhealed within three weeks and/or which required secondary surgery or hyperbaric oxygen. See Figures 21, 22, 23, and 24. The total wound dehiscence difference was 48% to 11% with a p-value of 0.001.

**Infection:** The control group developed a 7.5% incidence of minor wound infections and a 16% incidence of major wound infections. The 20/10 hyperbaric group developed a 3.5% incidence of minor wound infections and a 2.5% incidence of major wound infections. In this study a minor wound infection was defined as one which responded to culture specific antibiotics and local wound irrigations. A major wound infection required debridement surgery in addition to culture specific antibiotics and wound irrigations. See Figures 25 and 26. The total wound infection difference was 24% to 6% with a p-value of 0.005.

**Length of Hospital Stay:** Delayed wound healing was evident in many of the patients who developed a dehiscence with or without wound infection, or a wound infection alone. The totals of all cases were striking. In the control

## TABLE 3A. WOUND INFECTIONS IN RADIATED TISSUE

|         | N  | MINOR    | MAJOR    | TOTAL    |
|---------|----|----------|----------|----------|
| Non-HBO | 80 | 6 (7.5%) | 13 (16%) | 19 (24%) |
| HBO     | 80 | 3 (3.5%) | 2 (2.5%) | 5 (6%)   |

p = 0.001

## TABLE 3B. WOUND DEHISCENCE IN RADIATED TISSUE

|         | N  | MINOR     | MAJOR    | TOTAL    |
|---------|----|-----------|----------|----------|
| Non-HBO | 80 | 12 (15%)  | 26 (33%) | 38 (48%) |
| HBO     | 80 | 6 (7.5%)  | 3 (3.5%) | 9 (11%)  |

p = 0.001

## TABLE 3C. DELAYED WOUND HEALING

|         | N  | DELAYED HEALING |
|---------|----|-----------------|
| Non-HBO | 80 | 44 (55%)        |
| HBO     | 80 | 9 (11%)         |

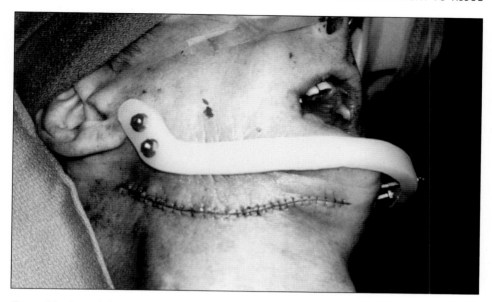

Figure 21. Wound closure of reconstruction patient who did not receive hyperbaric oxygen.

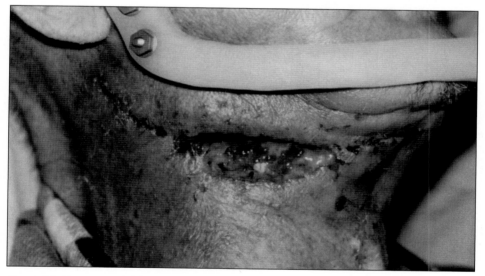

Figure 22. Major wound dehiscence in same patient required hyperbaric oxygen to heal.

group over one half of all patients (55%) experienced a wound healing delay as compared to the hyperbaric group, in which only one of every nine (11%) (p=0.005) experienced a wound healing delay. In this study, wound healing delay was defined as an increase in the in-patient hospital stay specifically to treat the radiated tissue wound. See Figures 27 and 28.

This study clearly quantitates and confirms the historical observations of many other authors who have reported such complications when surgery is performed in radiated tissues (9, 12, 18). It also quantitated the value of the 20/10 hyperbaric oxygen protocol as an adjunct prior to any surgery in

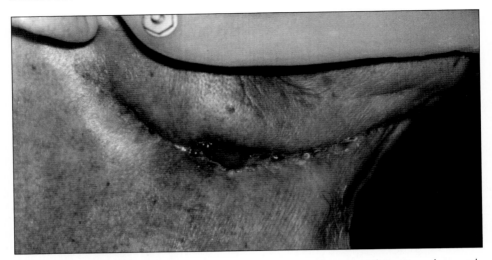

Figure 23. Same patient after 19 hyperbaric oxygen exposures shows granulating tissue base and a periphery-to-central-core direction of healing.

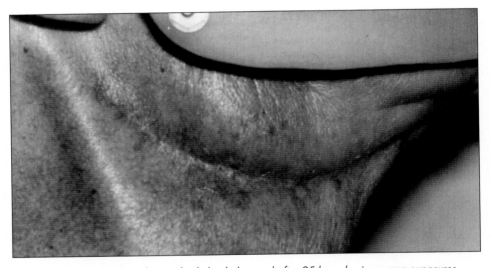

Figure 24. Same patient with completely healed wound after 25 hyperbaric oxygen exposures.

radiated tissue. What should also be evident is that use of the 20/10 hyperbaric oxygen protocol reduces the need for prolonged care and additional surgeries. It also reduces deformity, disability, and total cost of care.

## Tooth Removal

Osteoradionecrosis is the most dreaded complication of radiation therapy. The single most common precipitating event leading to osteoradionecrosis of the jaws is the post-radiation removal of teeth. Eighty-nine percent of all trauma-induced osteoradionecrosis is secondary to tooth removal. When a tooth is removed from a jaw which has previously received 6,000 cGy or more, the bone and surrounding mucosa are wounded. The

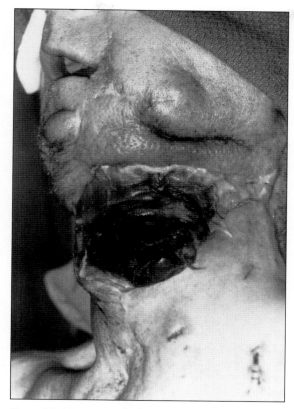

Figure 25. Major wound infection in radiated patient who did not receive hyperbaric oxygen.

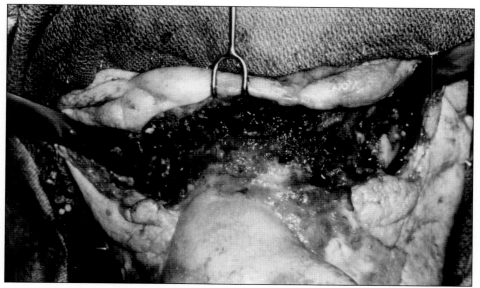

Figure 26. Major wound infection required debridement in addition to irrigation and wound care to achieve healing.

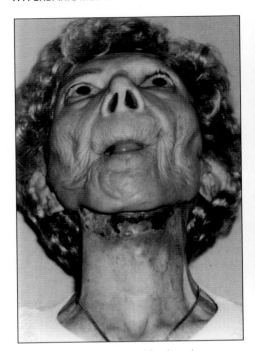

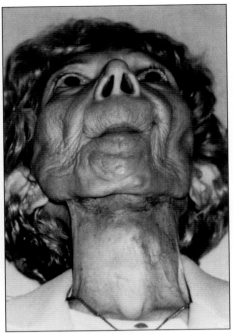

Figure 27. Delayed wound healing due to dehiscence and minor infection extending hospital stay of radiated patient who did not receive hyperbaric oxygen.

Figure 28. Completed healing of same patient without further surgery or hyperbaric oxygen, but delayed by approximately 21 days including an extension of in-patient care for 7 days.

greater the elapsed time after completion of radiotherapy, the more hypoxic and hypocellular the tissue becomes, and the less likely it is to meet the demands of healing. An open tooth socket requires a tertiary type of healing to fill a void and cope with the bacterial contamination of the oral flora. This radiated soft tissue-bone composite, which in the usual case can barely maintain its own physiologic homeostasis, often cannot repair itself post-radiation, if a breakdown occurs due to surgical wounding. Hence, it develops into osteoradionecrosis.

In 1985, Marx, Johnson, and Kline published the first randomized, prospective study dealing with the effects of HBO on radionecrosis (27). The study involved 74 patients who needed teeth removed from high-dose radiated mandibles. All patients were considered at high risk because of a minimal dose of 6,800 cGy and an average dose of over 7,200 cGy. The patients were randomized into two groups. One group of 37 underwent the indicated tooth removals using standard techniques and antibiotics, which were the recommended prophylaxis of the day. In this study, 1 million units of penicillin G were used intra-operatively, followed by 500 mg QID orally for ten days. Excluded from the study were all penicillin-allergic patients and those with other conditions affecting wound healing. The other group of 37 underwent the 20/10 hyperbaric oxygen protocol. Tooth removal using standard technique was accomplished, and no antibiotics were given at any time. All patients were followed to a single end-point to eliminate bias. At six months those with exposed, nonhealing mandibles were considered to have osteoradionecrosis. The results are shown in Table 4. See Figures 29, 30, 31, 32, 33, and 34.

The antibiotic group developed a 29.9% incidence of osteoradionecrosis versus 5.4% in the hyperbaric group (p=0.005). In addition, eight of the eleven patients who developed osteoradionecrosis in the antibiotic group required jaw resection and hyperbaric oxygen for resolution. Of the two patients in the hyperbaric oxygen group who developed osteoradionecrosis, neither required jaw resection, indicating a less severe form of necrosis. Since 1985, the 20/10 protocol has become the standard in oral and maxillofacial surgery and the dental profession. It is recommended for single and multiple tooth removals alike, as it is for any surgery in a radiated tissue (25, 27).

## Osseointegrated Dental Implants

One of the truly great advances that emerged from the orthopedic and dental professions in the 1980s was the biology of osseointegration and its use as anchorage for oral prostheses (3). Osseointegration is the remodeling of bone about an implanted metal interface without intervening soft tissue. Clinically, root-form metal cylinders become incorporated into bone

## TABLE 4. TOOTH REMOVALS IN RADIATED MANDIBLES

|  | N | # TEETH | ORN | % ORN |
|---|---|---|---|---|
| Non-HBO | 37 | 135 | 11 | (29.9%) |
| HBO | 37 | 156 | 2 | (5.4%) |
| p = 0.005 | | | | |

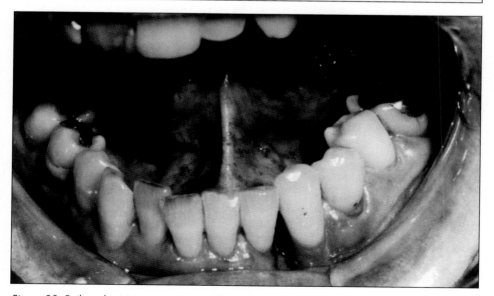

Figure 29. Failing dentition in a patient randomized to the penicillin arm of the study.

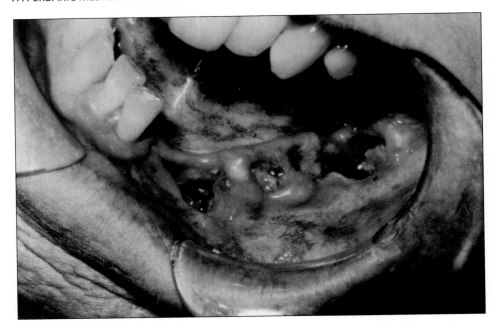

*Figure 30. Six months later all tooth removal sockets evidence exposed non-healing bone indicative of osteoradionecrosis.*

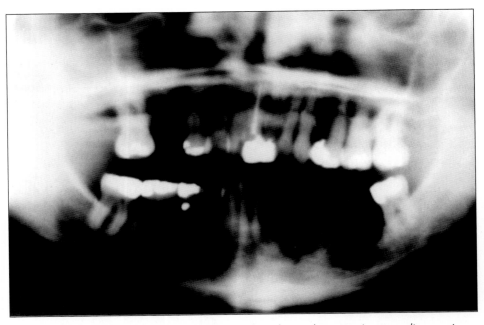

*Figure 31. Panoramic radiograph shows extensive bone loss in this patient's osteoradionecrosis that required hemimandibulectomy and hyperbaric oxygen to resolve.*

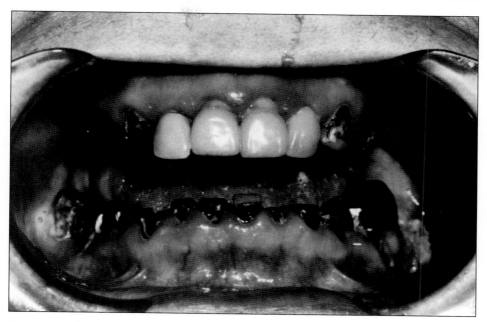

Figure 32. Failing dentition in a patient randomized to the hyperbaric oxygen arm of the study.

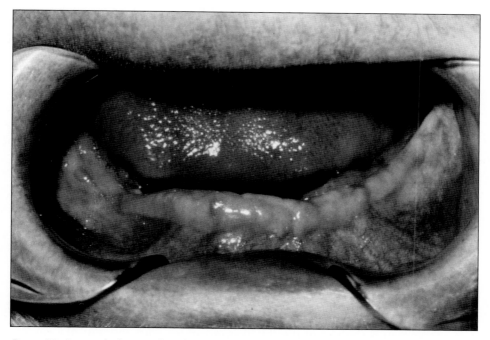

Figure 33. Six months later tooth sockets have healed and bone has remodeled so that a denture prosthesis can be made.

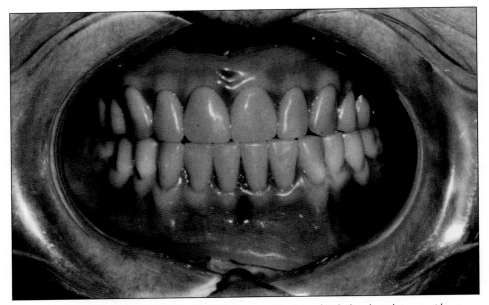

*Figure 34. Same patient functioning with a denture prosthesis on healed radiated tissue without tendency for breakdown.*

(osseointegration) and thus may serve to replace individual teeth or several teeth via bridgework. Osteointegrated prostheses offer greater stability and retention over conventional ones (4).

Head and neck cancer survivors have often undergone removal of all or part of their jaws and many of their teeth. Such missing natural tissues combine with surgical and radiation damage to impair tongue function, palatal function, and the pharyngeal phase of swallowing. The salivary glands are damaged, creating xerostomia which disables these patients greatly. In addition to the soft and hard tissue reconstructive surgery which is necessary, osseointegrated implants are needed in these patients, more so than in others. However, implant placement, which is a surgical procedure in itself, as well as the loading forces on these implants when prostheses are constructed, has been a concern. Current data indicate that hyperbaric oxygen makes it feasible to afford radiated patients the same advantage of osseointegrated implants as nonradiated patients. So far, our center has placed 79 osseointegrated fixtures in bone radiated to greater than 6,400 cGy. Sixty-four (81%) have integrated completely and have withstood a minimum of one year's loading by a prosthesis. Fifteen implants (19%) have failed to osseointegrate. Each failed during the initial six months of osseointegration. Each became mobile and was removed. None precipitated an osteoradionecrosis, and all that did integrate are continuing to be functional under loading forces. The lack of development of osteoradionecrosis and the acceptable osseointegration rate of 81% recommends the use of the 20/10 protocol for such implant placement. This is contrasted with our experience with fourteen cases where osseointegrated implants precipitated osteoradionecrosis when HBO was not used. Thus it appears that HBO has as much value post-radiation in osseointegration as it has in bone grafting and soft tissue repair.

The osseointegration rate of 81% with implants placed into radiated bone using HBO is still less than the 94% published for implants placed into nonradiated bone (3, 4, 41). This is probably due to the fact that although HBO induces an angiogenesis and fibroplasia in all radiated tissues, including bone, it does not seem to increase the osteoblast population. Since osteoblasts are the primary cells in forming and maintaining osseointegration and since radiated bone has a reduced osteoblast population (2), a lesser success rate is expected. Its greater value is in using HBO for the soft tissue healing and especially the prevention of osteoradionecrosis. See Figures 35, 36, 37, 38, 39A, and 39B.

## OSTEORADIONECROSIS

This disease has been reported in nearly every bone in the skeleton (5, 9, 26). However, it is most common in the jaws, particularly the lower jaw due to frequent radiation for oral and oropharyngeal cancers. Serial woundings from periodontal inflammation, pulpal disease, chewing trauma, and the need for oral surgical procedures also contribute to osteoradionecrosis of the jaws.

The pathophysiology of osteoradionecrosis was redefined in 1983 as a sequence beginning with (1) radiation; which produces (2) hypovascular-hypocellular-hypoxic tissue; which may undergo (3) tissue breakdown; which

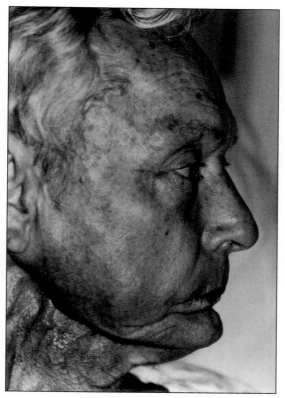

*Figure 35. Cancer patient after extirpative surgery and radiotherapy exhibiting thin radiated tissue is still a candidate for osseointegrated fixtures if the 20/10 hyperbaric oxygen protocol is used.*

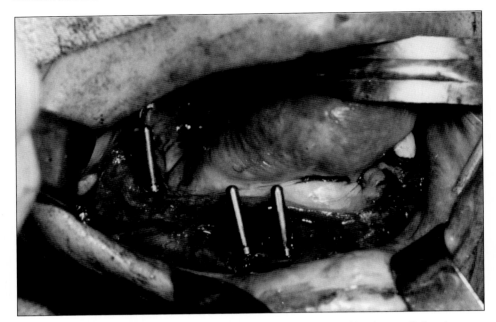

Figure 36. Osseointegrated fixtures must be placed parallel as dictated by the maxillofacial prosthodontist and accomplished with minimal reflection of vascular tissue from bone.

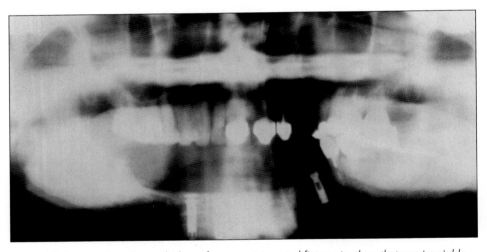

Figure 37. Panoramic radiograph shows four osseointegrated fixtures in place that require viable and vascular bone to properly integrate into the bone over a six-month period.

is an imbalance where cell death and collagen lysis exceed the homeostatic mechanisms of cell replacement and collagen synthesis. This in turn develops into (4) a non-healing wound, where the metabolic demands exceed the oxygen and vascular supply. See Table 5 (21, 22).

Prior to 1983 osteoradionecrosis was thought to be an infection of radiated bone (31, 37). However, several good studies have firmly documented osteoradionecrosis as a defect in wound healing (21, 25, 27). The

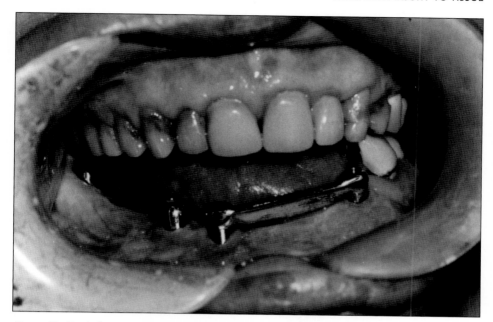

Figure 38. Healed osteointegrated fixtures act as supports for two retention bars which allow the prosthesis to snap on to it.

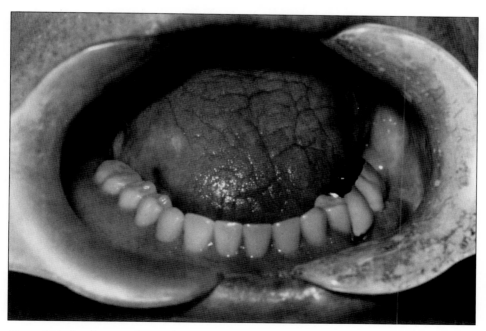

Figure 39A. Prosthesis in place with excellent arch form. Prosthesis has a lip plumper addition to support denervated lower lip.

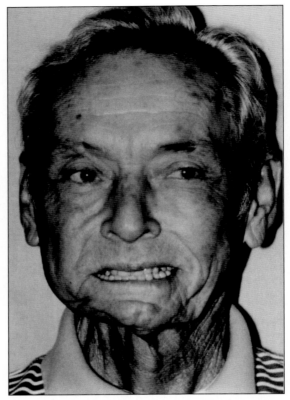

*Figure 39B. Patient demonstrating ability to bite with force on implant supported prosthesis where implants were placed into a highly radiated bone.*

importance of this concept is that antibiotics are not the main focus of therapy for osteoradionecrosis (7). Whenever bone develops osteoradionecrosis, surgical debridement is required, together with the absolute requirement of adjunctive hyperbaric oxygen.

Clinically, osteoradionecrosis of the jaws develops in three situations or as three types. See Figure 40.

The first type occurs when radiation and surgical wounding are coupled close together. The woundings become synergistic with hypoxia and the bone becomes overtly osteoradionecrotic. This happens in three very well known clinical scenarios. The most common situation is when teeth are

## TABLE 5. PATHOPHYSIOLOGY OF OSTEORADIONECROSIS

| |
|---|
| 1) Radiation |
| 2) Hypovascular-hypocellular-hypoxic tissue |
| 3) Tissue breakdown |
| 4) Non-healing wound |

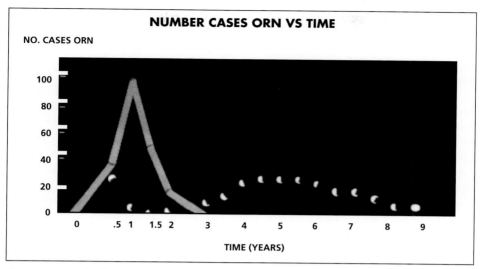

*Figure 40. Graph of 536 cases of mandibular osteoradionecrosis showing three distinct types and times of occurrence of osteoradionecrosis.*

removed in a jaw to be radiated and less than 21 days are allowed for tissue recovery and healing. Studies have shown that if 21 days or more can be afforded before radiation begins, osteoradionecrosis will rarely develop, unless the radiation dose becomes extremely high (25). Fourteen to twenty-one days have a reduced incidence of osteoradionecrosis, but breakthrough cases do develop in this period of time. Radiation that absolutely must begin within 21 days or even within 14 days to gain better tumor control is in some cases understandable, but this is done with the patient accepting a much greater risk for osteoradionecrosis. The next most common scenario is the mandibulotomy procedure, which is a transection of the mandible to gain access to what is usually a lingual or pharyngeal tumor. The reflection of the mandible's vascular periosteum and the fixation methods used in this approach, coupled with the tissue damage of post-surgical radiotherapy, often create an overt osteoradionecrosis. The third scenario is tooth extraction in the middle of a radiotherapy sequence. Teeth that develop symptoms during radiotherapy are best palliated with pulpectomies, drainage, antibiotics, analgesics, etc., rather than treated by removal (40). The supposedly trivial surgical wounding from even a single tooth removal, if coupled with ongoing radiotherapy, can cause the highest production of osteoradionecrosis. In addition, interrupting a radiotherapy sequence reduces the tumor response through repopulation of tumor cells and requires a greater total dose, thereby worsening the cancer prognosis and increasing the risk of osteoradionecrosis as well. These three developmental scenarios of osteoradionecrosis are collectively referred to as "Type I trauma induced osteoradionecrosis."

The second type of osteoradionecrosis often occurs years after radiotherapy, but most commonly within three to six years. Typically in this scenario the patient has been functioning well since radiotherapy but may develop dental caries or periodontal disease. The wounding event is most often tooth removal, but has also been biopsy, elective dental care, reconstructive surgery or irritation from dentures (40). Bone and overlying soft tissues which had been able to maintain homeostasis in the "Three-H" state undergo breakdown secondary to the effects of surgical or traumatic wounding. This "Type II trauma induced osteoradionecrosis" is the one most familiar to both clinicians and laymen.

The third type of osteoradionecrosis is not related to any external trauma or surgery but stems from the effect of radiation alone. It is associated with the higher doses of radiotherapy, neutron beam therapy, and interstitial or "implant" therapy. It may also be enhanced or accelerated by concomitant chemotherapy or hyperthermia therapy. This type of breakdown is known as "spontaneous osteoradionecrosis." It usually occurs between six months to two years after completion of radiation treatment.

Figure 41 shows the relationship of the three types of osteoradionecrosis. This graph of radiation pathology graph also demonstrates the roles of trauma, inflammation, and HBO. Clearly defined is subclinical damage or what has been referred to as tissue radiation injury. The graph also defines an arbitrary clinical threshold above which clinical damage occurs. This may present as soft tissue or bone necrosis.

The first plot shows ascending subclinical damage ending just below the clinical threshold. This point correlates with the cessation of radiotherapy. However, if excessive radiation is given, or, more commonly, surgical wounding occurs, the added damage carries over the clinical threshold into Type I (trauma induced) osteoradionecrosis (indicated by the **** line). If the first plot peaks just below the clinical threshold, (indicative of very high dose radiotherapy) but does not cross over the line into overt osteoradionecrosis, there is a recovery period of about four months. In this time period, the histologic inflammation diminishes and the clinical dermatitis and/or mucositis subsides. However, as the late effects of radiation develop, the progressively

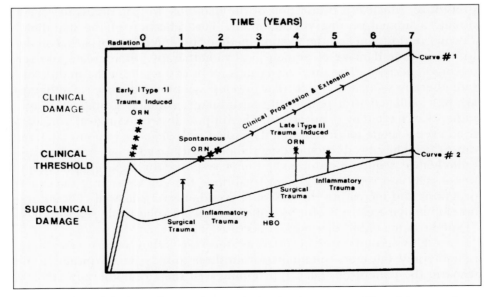

Figure 41. The radiobiology of osteoradionecrosis showing the progress of tissue injury over time.

more severe "Three-H" state in the subclinically damaged area increases. Because the initial radiation dose brought the damage level to just below the clinical threshold with only limited recovery, the late radiation damage will exceed the clinical threshold. This curve describes "spontaneous osteoradionecrosis," which will develop sometime within the patient's lifetime, usually within two years.

The usual dosage range of radiotherapy is described by the second plot, which ascends in the subclinical area but ends well below the clinical threshold. After the recovery period the progressive "Three-H" state of late radiation begins. Because the initial dose was less, the slope of the line is less and the distance it must ascend before it crosses the clinical threshold is greater. In most cases the time it will take to cross the clinical threshold is longer than the patient's life span, hence the well reported low total incidence of osteoradionecrosis, which is estimated to be 5% to 10%. However, if inflammation or surgical trauma occurs, tissue damage vertically accelerates the curve. One sees that trauma inflicted later after completion of radiotherapy has a much greater possibility of exceeding the clinical threshold. By contrast, it is also seen that hyperbaric oxygen deflects the curve vertically downward, reducing the probability of exceeding the clinical threshold. The place of hyperbaric oxygen in the development of osteoradionecrosis is also seen in Figure 42.

The slopes of the lines were derived in a study measuring before-and-after vascular densities by histologic examination and transcutaneous oxygen measurements. Not only was hyperbaric oxygen able to reduce the subclinical damage, but it reduced the rate of progression of late radiation effects.

The graph in Figure 41 shows one other noteworthy feature. During the recovery phase after radiotherapy and before the "Three-H" state develops, hyperbaric oxygen has no value. This four-month period immediately after radiotherapy has been termed the "golden period" because required surgeries can be accomplished during this time with fewer wound healing complications and without the need for hyperbaric oxygen.

## TREATMENT PROTOCOL FOR OSTEORADIONECROSIS

The treatment of frank osteoradionecrosis is different from the 20/10 protocol which is applicable to lesser radiation injuries. The osteoradionecrosis treatment is termed the 30/10 protocol because it requires a full 30 sessions prior to any surgical intervention. One reason for the additional ten treatments is that osteoradionecrosis is an advanced tissue radiation injury which has already undergone breakdown resulting in a nonhealing wound. Another reason is that the 30/10 protocol is intended to treat the radiated tissue that is not yet necrotic and which may heal and respond without surgery or with less aggressive surgery. Thus a full 30 presurgical sessions of HBO are used so that an unequivocal maximum response is obtained. The protocol becomes progressive, beginning with nonsurgical care and advancing to more aggressive debridements. The protocol, published in 1983 and developed at the United States Air Force Wilford Hall Medical Center and the University of Miami, begins by treating all patients who have had at least six months of exposed, non-healing bone with 30 HBO sessions (20). These patients begin in what is referred to as Stage I. See Figure 43.

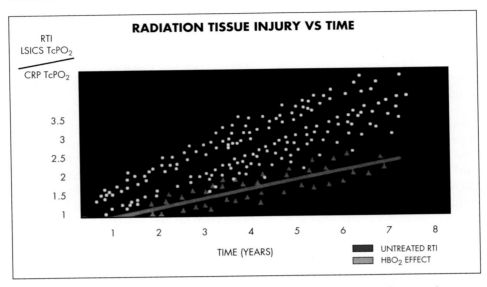

Figure 42. Graph of radiation tissue injury versus time. Two slopes are observed. One without exposure to the 20/10 hyperbaric oxygen protocol, the other after exposure to the 20/10 hyperbaric oxygen protocol.

However, if the patient initially presents with an orocutaneous fistula (see Figure 44), a pathologic fracture (Figure 45), or radiographically evident osteolysis to the inferior mandibular border, he/she is advanced directly to Stage III. See Figure 46. Any one of these clinical signs is indicative of advanced disease that requires more aggressive surgery as part of Stage III.

## Stage I

In Stage I all patients undergo an initial trial of 30 sessions of HBO. Antibiotics are often discontinued but may need to be used if there is evidence of soft tissue infection. No surgery or debridement is carried out during this time other than irrigation and removal of sequestered, mobile bone fragments. After 30 sessions, the exposed bone is examined for response. Responding tissue will show a softening of the bone, granulation tissue, and an absence of inflammation. See Figure 46. If the tissue is assessed as responding, the softened bone is removed and the patient allowed to undergo an additional 10 sessions of hyperbaric oxygen. If the wound responds with complete healing without further treatment (see Figures 47A and 47B), the patient is termed a Stage I responder. If the exposed bone shows no sign of response after 30 sessions of hyperbaric oxygen, the patient is termed as a Stage I nonresponder and is advanced to Stage II.

## Stage II

In Stage II the patient has already received 30 sessions of hyperbaric oxygen. See Figure 48. Therefore, the patient undergoes a surgical removal of exposed bone. The type of surgery accomplished in Stage II is dependent on the location of the exposed bone but in a general sense is a transoral peripheral resection. If the exposed bone is alveolar, the surgery would be an

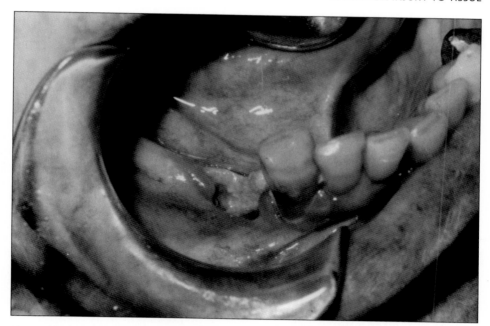

Figure 43. Stage I osteoradionecrosis is an uncomplicated, exposed, radiated bone that has failed to heal over six months.

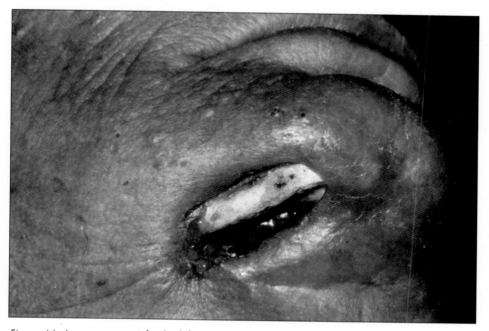

Figure 44. An orocutaneous fistula defines a patient as having Stage III osteoradionecrosis.

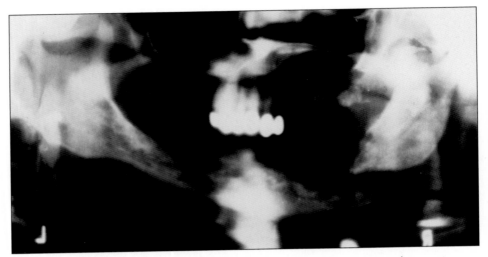

Figure 45. A pathologic fracture also defines a patient as having Stage III osteoradionecrosis.

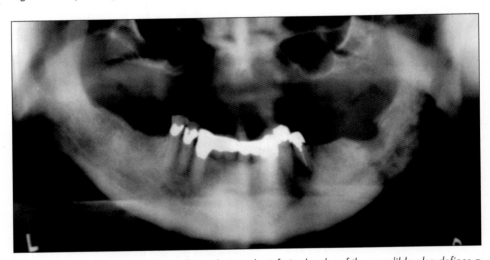

Figure 46. Radiographic evidence of osteolysis to the inferior border of the mandible also defines a patient as having Stage III osteoradionecrosis.

alveolar sequestrectomy. If the exposed bone were either the lingual or buccal cortex alone, surgery would be a cortical plate removal. All Stage II surgeries retain the inferior border and thus the continuity of the mandible. See Figure 49. The bone is removed with a saline cooled saw rather than a heat generating burr. The soft tissue is reflected minimally from the bone to preserve the blood supply to the remaining mandible. See Figure 50.

Closure is in two or three layers. After surgery the patient will complete the final 10 hyperbaric oxygen sessions. See Figure 51.

If the patient heals without further exposed bone, he or she is termed a Stage II responder. See Figure 52.

If the wound dehisces, exposing bone once again, the patient is termed a Stage II nonresponder and is advanced to Stage III.

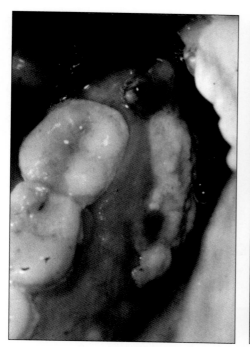

Figure 47A. Osteoradionecrosis after 30 sessions of hyperbaric oxygen showing response by bone softening, absence of inflammation, and granulation tissue.

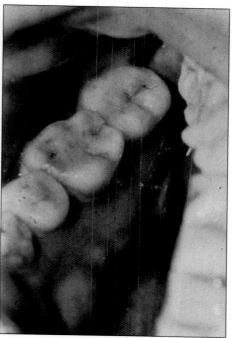

Figure 47B. Stage I responders will sequester non-viable bone and heal over the residual viable bone.

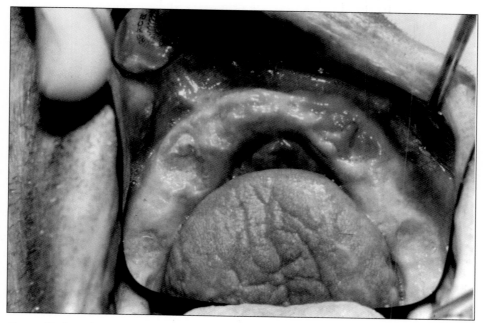

Figure 48. Stage I non-responder as evidenced by continued exposure of radiated bone is advanced to Stage II.

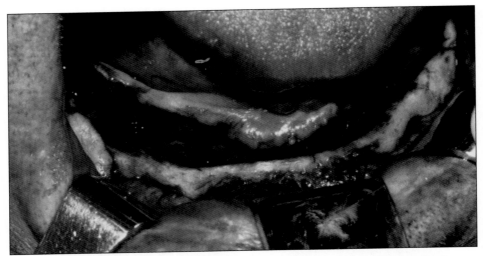

Figure 49. Stage II surgery retains jaw continuity. Here, alveolar resection back to bleeding bone margins retains the mandible's inferior border.

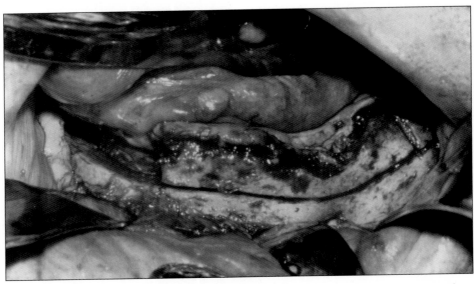

Figure 50. During Stage II surgery it is of paramount importance that the surgeon retain as much vascular tissue attachment to the remaining mandible as possible.

## Stage III

Stage III patients are those who have failed to respond in Stage I and Stage II or have been defined as such on initial presentation. Essentially this group possesses such a great quantity of nonviable bone that hyperbaric oxygen alone or combined with limited surgical debridement cannot resolve the disease. In Stage III the patient has already received 30 hyperbaric sessions. The patient will therefore undergo a transoral continuity resection of the involved portion of the mandible and an excision of any necrotic soft tissue. See Figures 53 and 54.

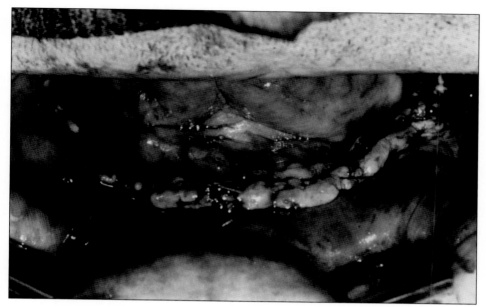

Figure 51. Stage II surgery defines a primary closure over residual viable bone by vascular soft tissue.

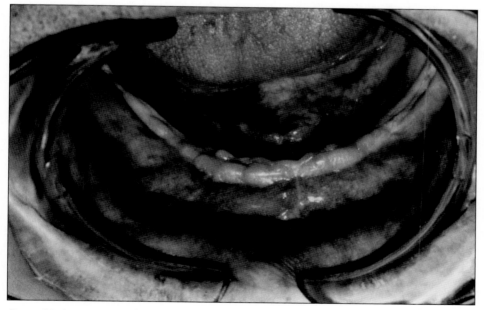

Figure 52. Stage II responders will heal over residual viable bone without further bone exposure.

The resection margins of the mandible are determined by observation at the time of surgery. Bleeding bone margins provide the best guideline as to the viability of the remaining mandibular segments. Similarly, the margins for soft tissue excision are determined by bleeding observed at the time of surgery. The two best alternatives for maintaining mandibular alignment are

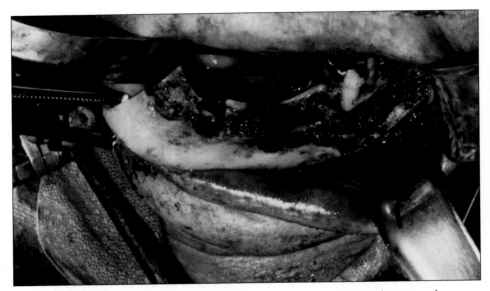

*Figure 53. Stage III surgery involves a continuity resection of the mandible and excision of any necrotic soft tissue as well.*

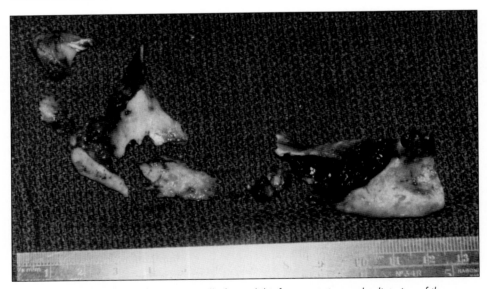

*Figure 54. Stage III osteoradionecrosis will often exhibit fragmentation and splintering of the osteoradionecrotic bone. It is important to remove all non-viable bone. Leaving small foci of non-viable bone will eventuate in wound healing complications.*

external skeletal fixation (Joe Hall-Morris Pin Fixation) (see Figure 55) or, less ideally, maxillomandibular fixation.

Rigid internal fixation bridging plates are used with caution. Frequent dehiscences and plate exposures occur when this type of fixation is used in osteoradionecrosis resections. See Figure 56.

At the time of osseous resection soft tissue loss must be assessed. If soft tissue has been excised and there is no overt infection, the soft tissue may be

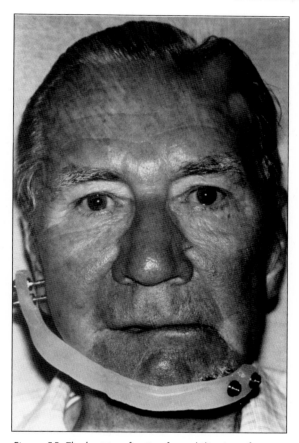

*Figure 55. The best jaw fixation for stabilization of an osteoradionecrosis-related resection remains Joe Hall-Morris type external skeletal pin fixation. This fixation allows jaw opening and other movements while keeping foreign bodies out of the radiated tissue.*

immediately reconstructed with a myocutaneous flap or a free vascular transfer. See Figures 57 and 58. The pectoralis major myocutaneous flap has proven to be one of the most predictable and useful in such defects. See Figure 59 and 60 (29).

The patient should then undergo the final 10 hyperbaric oxygen sessions to complete the 30/10 protocol.

Patients who require a Stage III approach to resolve their disease usually undergo bony reconstruction of the jaw at three months. See Figures 61, 62, and 63.

If such bone grafting or other surgery is required it can be accomplished without the need for further hyperbaric oxygen. Earlier protocols and publications indicated that a retreatment with the 20/10 protocol would be necessary (20, 22, 28). However, studies since 1986 (24, 25, 26) have shown that the angiogenesis and fibroplasia are long lasting and need not be reinforced. Indeed current clinical practice has supported the use of a single but complete protocol of hyperbaric oxygen.

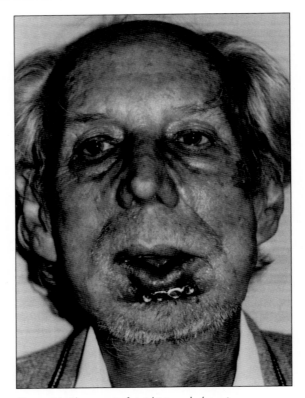

Figure 56. Placement of rigid internal plates in an osteoradionecrosis resection frequently results in mucosal or skin exposure of the plates, requiring their removal.

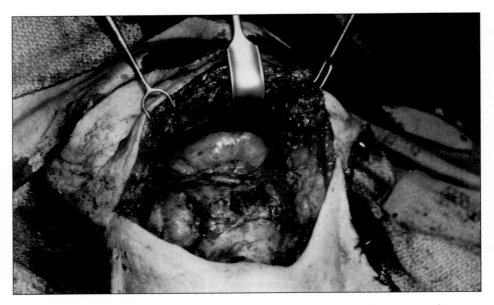

Figure 57. Since soft tissue radiation necrosis always accompanies osteoradionecrosis, soft tissue defects are often unmasked at the time of an osteoradionecrosis resection.

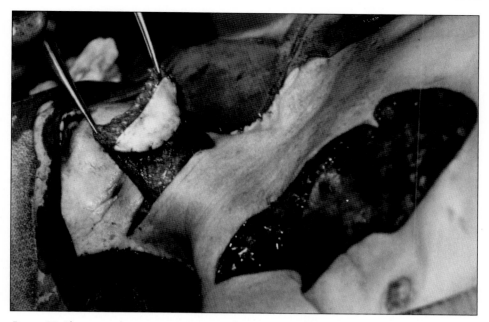

*Figure 58. The pectoralis major myocutaneous flap is the most useful, predictable, and least morbid of the available soft tissue reconstructions.*

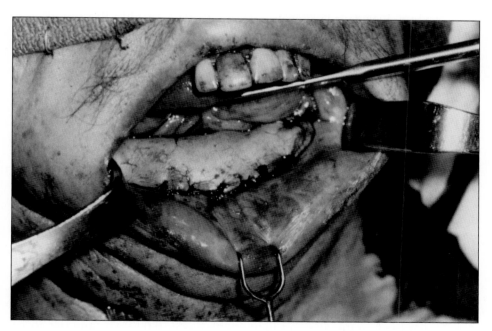

*Figure 59. Here the pectoralis major myocutaneous flap is used to resurface lost oral mucosa in the floor of the mouth and provide tissue volume for a later bone graft.*

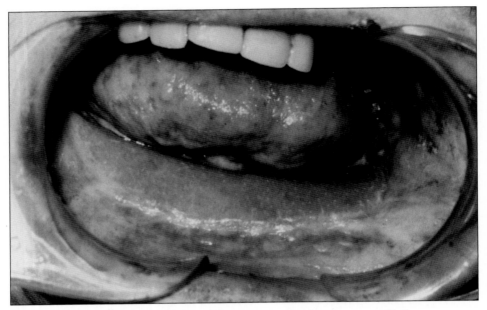

*Figure 60. Healed skin paddle in floor of mouth three months after placement will allow introduction of a bone graft into a vascular tissue bed of sufficient volume.*

These protocols have been successfully used by most institutions and private practices since 1983. They have generally proven to be effective and predictable, leading to reconstructed patients. Their value resides in the staging of the radionecrotic process, which selects those who can respond to nonsurgical or lesser surgical approaches and expeditiously prepares every patient requiring reconstructive surgery in a minimum of time (three months).

## COST ANALYSIS OF OSTEORADIONECROSIS TREATMENT

At the time of this writing, politicians, the press and the public are voicing concerns about the availability and costs of medical care. No doubt this tug-o-war will continue for decades. However, where do osteoradionecrosis and hyperbaric oxygen stand in the costliness of today's health care? Table 6 illustrates a complete review of all known cost factors of 300 patients who were treated for osteoradionecrosis and has been updated to January 1, 1992, U.S. dollars.

An overall analysis of these findings indicates that osteoradionecrosis is obviously an expensive disease once it develops, no matter how it is treated. Certainly the preventive efforts already known, such as radiotherapy dose fractioning, pre-radiation dental consultations, fluoride carriers, removing mandibular teeth in the direct radiation path if over 6,000 cGy, and the 20/10 hyperbaric oxygen protocol if surgery is anticipated, are to be encouraged and should become standards.

If one looks carefully at these data, one can see the most costly approach to osteoradionecrosis is one where hyperbaric oxygen is not used. The average yearly costs were $38,000 and the total cost was $140,000. Worse

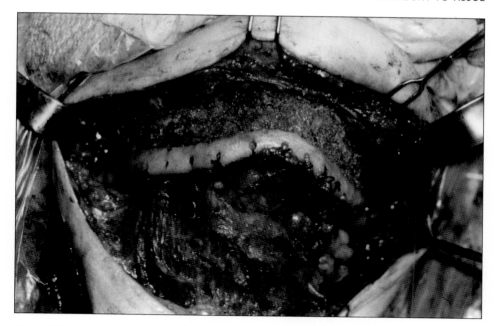

Figure 61. Bony reconstruction of a large osteoradionecrosis defect with an allogeneic mandible crib and autogenous cancellous bone.

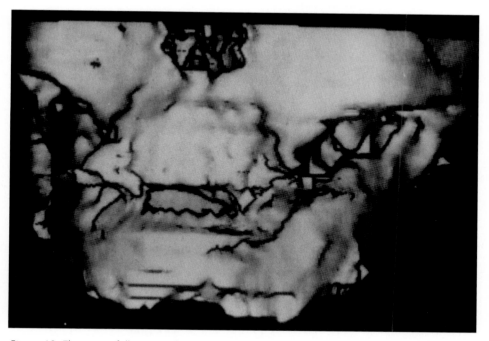

Figure 62. Three year follow-up radiograph that shows fully reconstructed mandible after an osteoradionecrosis resection.

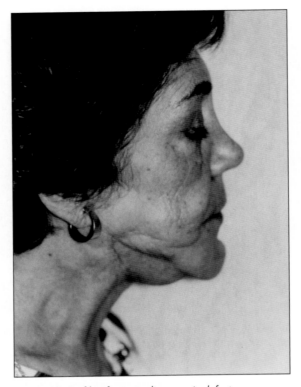

*Figure 63. Profile of osteoradionecrosis defect reconstruction shows prominent jaw projection and balanced nose-lip-chin contour.*

yet is that $140,000 dollars is a low figure because only 8% of cases were resolved. This means that 92% of patients went elsewhere for continued treatment and accrued additional costs not appearing in this table. The high costs were mainly due to hospitalizations and drugs. These patients required serial admissions, serial debridements, many office visits, and great quantities of antibiotics and analgesics. All of this added up to the enormous costs shown in Table 6. What is not shown in Table 6 is the health care provider's resources

## TABLE 6. COST ANALYSIS OF OSTEORADIONECROSIS (300 PATIENTS, JANUARY 1, 1992, U.S. DOLLARS)

| TREATMENT | # PTS. | AVG. 1 YR COST | AVG. TOTAL COST | RESOLUTION RATE |
|---|---|---|---|---|
| Non-HBO | 65 | $38,000 | $140,000 | 8% |
| HBO alone | 51 | $33,000 | $85,000 | 17% |
| WHMC-UM Protocol | 130 | $44,000 | $44,000 | 100% |
| WHMC-UM Protocol in a private practice | 54 | $42,000 | $42,000 | 100% |

which were devoted to these patients' care, the lack of productivity and absence from the work place, and the degraded quality of family life these patients endured, all of which were significant.

The next most costly approach was when hyperbaric oxygen was used without surgery. This amounted to an average yearly cost of $32,000 and an average total cost of $85,000. This approach is essentially similar to Stage I cases where HBO by itself was able to resolve the problem in only 17% of the cases. The remaining 83% were treated and retreated with several hyperbaric oxygen courses to build the high total cost of $85,000.

The main cost in this approach was the repeated hyperbaric oxygen fees followed by hospitalization and health care provider fees. This approach to osteoradionecrosis was popular in the late 1960s and 1970s before the pathophysiology of osteoradionecrosis was known and before a definitive protocol to resolve the disease was established (17, 19). Common approaches during that era called for serial hyperbaric oxygen courses every six months. Such approaches resolved the osteoradionecrosis only on rare occasions because surgical debridement of nonviable bone was not carried out. Such results are a reminder that hyperbaric oxygen cannot resurrect dead bone. Dead bone is best managed by surgical removal. It is also a reminder that the target tissue of hyperbaric oxygen is not the dead tissue but the radiation damaged tissue that is not yet dead.

The costs for patients treated with the staged protocols discussed in this chapter incurred an average yearly cost of $44,000 with a total cost of $44,000. The total cost and the yearly cost are the same because the disease is resolved rather than allowed to become chronic with ongoing costs. The $44,000 cost in this protocol is indeed expensive, but is an average of Stage I, Stage II, and Stage III responders. The costs include fees for hyperbaric oxygen, surgeons' fees, hospitalization, reconstruction fees and even prosthetic fees to replace teeth. Stage III patients were the most costly (isolated Stage III costs were $53,000) due to a greater requirement for hospitalization and surgery, but were still significantly below the costs of any other approach.

Osteoradionecrosis is documented to be an expensive entity. However, HBO, if used in a strict protocol along with surgery, has been shown to be the most effective approach. In addition to cost savings, the intangible benefits are immeasurable. By resolving a painful and debilitating disease, patients become productive once again, as they return to their families and to the workplace.

This protocol's effectiveness in both disease resolution and cost containment has also been demonstrated in a private practice setting. Table 6 shows that the same results were obtained in a private practice as was seen in a university setting, indicating the protocol's value rests with its biologic principles, rather than with the technical aspects of management.

## THE RELATIONSHIP OF HYPERBARIC OXYGEN TO ORAL CANCER

The natural concern of many has been the potential effect of increased oxygen levels on cancer which may be residual within patients or within histologically dysplastic mucosa. Patients who have had radiotherapy for head and neck cancers often harbor a treacherous prognosis. They may have residual tumor which surgery or radiation did not fully eradicate. They may also have altered mucous membrane cells from years of tobacco and alcohol use, much of which is premalignant dysplasia. They can also present with tissue breakdown and fistulae which are cancers mimicking osteoradionecrosis. They may even have radiation induced dysplasias and carcinomas. An entire array of statistics applies to this group. Some of the more important to keep in mind are the following.

Patients who have had one oral cancer and who continue to smoke have a 33% chance of developing a new primary in the foregut within five years (39). Our statistics indicate that 83% of patients who develop an oral cancer associated with smoking continue to smoke after treatment for their cancer. Squamous cell carcinoma of the oral cavity has a 50% overall five year survival rate. Ten percent of patients referred into a major medical center (The University of Miami) with a diagnosis of osteoradionecrosis have residual oral cancer along with their osteoradionecrosis. The point of all these statistics is simply that even with the best diagnostic techniques one cannot be sure these patients are tumor free. Because of this, we and several other authors have studied the relationship of cancers, particularly oral cancers, to hyperbaric oxygen.

## Animal Studies

The most common and best animal model has been that of the hamster cheek pouch using a 1, 2-9, 10 dimethyl benzanthracene (DMBA) as the carcinogen. Our first study assessed the development of dysplasia and its progression to cancer over 22 weeks as well as the growth rate of the cancers once they emerged. The animals all had the DMBA applied three times a week in a 0.5% solution in acetone. One group received daily hyperbaric oxygen at 2.4 ATA for 90 minutes each day, the other group did not receive any hyperbaric oxygen. The results are graphed in Figures 64 and 65. The graph in Figure 64 compares the hyperbaric oxygen treated group to the control group, assessing the cheek pouches of serially euthanized animals. The results indicated that surprisingly, hyperbaric oxygen actually suppressed the dysplasia and delayed the emergence of carcinomas from the dysplasia by one month. Figure 65 shows that the growth rates of tumors induced by the DMBA are equal between the hyperbaric oxygen and nonhyperbaric group (8, 26).

In a similar study, McMillan, et al. (30) also found that hyperbaric oxygen suppressed the emergence of oral cancers and suppressed dysplasias. They did observe, however, that tumors in the hyperbaric oxygen group were bigger, but they did not measure growth rates (30). In related studies, Nemiroff has shown no acceleration of the growth rate of primaries or metastases from lung tumors in mice (32, 33). In a second study we developed fully mature cheek pouch cancers in the hamsters. One group was exposed to hyperbaric oxygen, another group was injected with an oxygen radical generating system of a cross-linked enzyme of glucose oxidase and horseradish peroxidase, a third group received both, and a fourth group served as controls (6, 36). The findings indicated that oxygen radicals (superoxide, singlet oxygen, hydroxyl radical, etc.) have antineoplastic properties based on lipid peroxidation of cell membranes. It seems that tumor

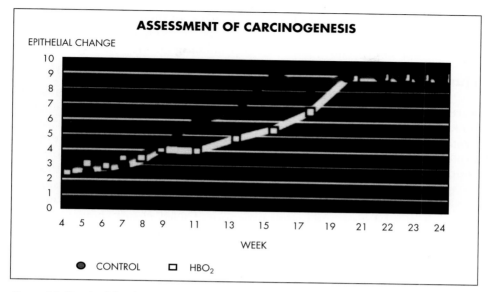

Figure 64. *Graph of developing mucosal carcinoma versus time, identifying a suppression of dysplasia and a slowing of overt carcinoma in the hyperbaric oxygen group.*

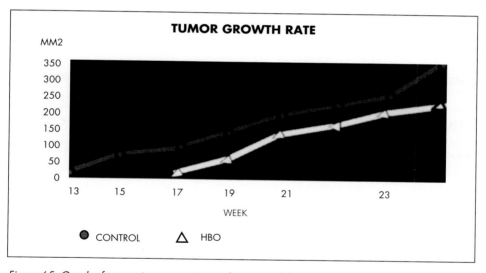

Figure 65. *Graph of tumor size versus time, indicating a delayed emergence of carcinoma in the hyperbaric oxygen group and parallel slopes identifying equal growth rates.*

cells are somewhat selectively lysed due to their inability to produce superoxide dismutase as a scavenger of oxygen radicals. These studies also indicate that oxygen radicals are more deleterious to smaller tumors and dysplasias than to larger tumors of greater mass.

Animal studies, in summary, imply some suppression of early tumor formation and no acceleration of growth or metastatic potential. However, these animal models, as good as they are, are not the equivalent of human studies. Only human studies can be looked upon as a reliable index of the potential harmful effects of clinical hyperbaric oxygen on a population of patients who have already had one foregut cancer and have been exposed to a variety of carcinogens and other cancer promoting factors.

## Human Studies

From 1985 through 1991 we have been able to follow 405 patients who were treated for oral squamous cell carcinoma by surgery and radiation therapy or radiation therapy alone. Of these patients, 245 underwent a protocol of hyperbaric oxygen for either reconstructive surgery (the 20/10 protocol) or for the treatment of osteoradionecrosis (the 30/10 protocol). The results of these findings are presented in Table 7, where the results are stratified according to the TNM classification of the Joint Commission on Cancer Staging from Stage I to Stage IV. The higher stages are indicative of more advanced disease and poorer prognosis. Table 7 clearly shows a reduced incidence of recurrence in every stage of squamous cell carcinoma in those who have been exposed to hyperbaric oxygen. The differences are small and only somewhat statistically significant. The interpretation of these results must be cautious. It may reflect a slight chemopreventative effect, as has been implied by the animal studies and in published data related to retinoids and B-carotene (11). It may instead reflect the greater radiation doses applied to those who required hyperbaric oxygen and one therefore could anticipate better tumor control. Nevertheless, it seems that a reliable interpretation shows no ability of hyperbaric oxygen, in animals or humans, to accelerate cancer or cause more to emerge from dysplastic mucosa. It remains a safe and effective modality for radiated head and neck cancer patients despite continued carcinogen exposure and the many forms of their malignancies.

## TABLE 7. FIVE-YEAR CANCER RECURRENCE OF SQUAMOUS CELL CARCINOMA

| STAGE | NON-HBO | RECURRED | HBO | RECURRED |
|---|---|---|---|---|
| I | 29 | 6 (21%) | 36 | 6 (16%) |
| II | 58 | 14 (24%) | 94 | 17 (18%) |
| III | 50 | 16 (32%) | 92 | 19 (21%) |
| IV | 23 | 9 (38%) | 23 | 6 (28%) |

## REFERENCES

1. Adamo AR, Szal RL. "Timing, results and complications of mandibular reconstructive surgery: Report of 32 cases." J Oral Surg. 1979;37:755-762.

2. Boyne PJ. "Effect of increased oxygenation on osteogenesis enhancement." In: Hyperbaric Oxygen Therapy. JC Davis and TK Hunt, (Eds). Bethesda, MD: Undersea and Hyperbaric Medical Society, 1988;205-216.

3. Brånemark PI, Adell R, Albrektsson T, Lekholm U, Lundkvist S, Röckler B. "Osseo-integrated titanium fixtures in the treatment of edentulousness." Biomaterials. 1983;4:25-28.

4. Brånemark PI, Lindström J, Hallén O, Breine U, Jeppsson PH, Öhman A. "Osseointegrated implants in the treatment of the edentulous jaw. Experience from a ten year period." Scand J Plast Reconstr Surg. (Suppl 16). 1977;1-132.

5. Bump RL, Young JM, Davis JC, et al. "Hyperbaric oxygen: Treatment of osteoradionecrosis and osteomyelitis." Med Serv Dig. 1971;26:13-18.

6. Ehler WJ, Marx RE, Kiel J, Ravelo JI, Cissik JH. "Induced regression of oral carcinoma by oxygen radical generating systems." J Hyperbaric Med. 1991;6:111-118.

7. Hahn G and Corgill DA. "Conservative treatment of radionecrosis of the mandible." Oral Surg. 1967;24:707-711.

8. Harmon FW and Marx RE. "The effect of hyperbaric oxygen on carcinogenesis and tumor growth rate." Proceedings of the 65th Annual Meeting of the Annual Meeting of the American Association of Oral and Maxillofacial Surgeons, 1983.

9. Hart GB and Mainous EG. "The treatment of radiation necrosis with hyperbaric oxygen." Cancer. 1976;37(6):2580-2586.

10. Heimbach RD. "Radiation effects on tissue." In: Problem Wounds – The Role of Oxygen. JC Davis and TK Hunt (Eds.) New York: Elsevier, 1988; Chapter 3:53-63.

11. Hong WK, Lippman SM, Itri LM, Karp DD, Lee JS, et al. "Prevention of second primary tumors with isotrelinon in a squamous cell carcinoma of the head and neck." N Engl J Med. 1990;323:795-801.

12. Joseph DL and Shumrick DL. "Risks of head and neck surgery in previously irradiated patients." Arch Otolaryngol. 1973;97:381-384.

13. Knighton DR, Hunt TK, Schenestuhl H, et al. "Oxygen tension regulates the expression of angiogenesis factor by macrophages." Science. 1983;221:1283-1289.

14. Knighton DR, Oredsson S, Banda M, et al. "Regulation of repair: Hypoxic control of macrophage mediated angiogenesis." In: Soft and Hard Tissue Repair. TK Hunt, RB Heppenstall, E. Pines, et al. (Eds.) New York: Praeger, 1984;41-49.

15. Knighton DR, Silver IA, Hunt TK. "Regulation of wound healing angiogenesis: Effect of oxygen gradients and inspired oxygen concentrations." Surgery. 1981;90:262-270.

16. Komisar A. "The functional result of mandibular reconstruction." Laryngoscope. 1990;100:364-374.

17. Mainous EG. "Hyperbaric oxygen in maxillofacial osteomyelitis, osteoradionecrosis, and osteogenesis enhancement." In: Hyperbaric Oxygen Therapy. JC Davis and TK Hunt (Eds.) Bethesda, MD: Undersea and Hyperbaric Medical Society, 1988;191-203.

18. Mainous EG and Boyne PJ. "Hyperbaric oxygen in total rehabilitation of patients with mandibular osteoradionecrosis." Int J Oral Surg. 1974;3:297-302.

19. Mainous EG, Boyne PJ, Hart GB, Terry BC. "Restoration of resected mandible by grafting with a combination of mandible homograft and autogenous iliac marrow, and post-operative treatment with hyperbaric oxygenation." Oral Surg. 1973;35:13-20.

20. Marx RE. "A new concept in the treatment of osteoradionecrosis." J Oral Maxillofacial Surg. 1983;41:351-358.

21. Marx RE. "Osteoradionecrosis: A new concept of its pathophysiology." J Oral Maxillofac Surg. 1983;48:283-289.

22. Marx RE. "Osteoradionecrosis of the jaws: Review and update." HBO Review. 1984;5:78-128.

23. Marx RE and Ames JR. "The use of hyperbaric oxygen therapy in bony reconstruction of the irradiated and tissue deficient patient." J Oral Maxillofac Surg. 1982; 40:412-419.

24. Marx RE, Ehler WJ, Tayapongsak PT, Pierce LW. "Relationship of oxygen dose to angiogenesis induction in irradiated tissue." Am J Surg. 1990;160:519-524.

25. Marx RE and Johnson RP. "Studies in the radiobiology of osteoradionecrosis and their clinical significance." Oral Surg. 1987;64:379-390.

26. Marx RE and Johnson RP. "Problem wounds in oral and maxillofacial surgery: The role of hyperbaric oxygen." In: Problem Wounds – The Role of Oxygen. JC Davis and TK Hunt (Eds.) New York: Elsevier, 1988; Chapter 4:65-123.

27. Marx RE, Johnson RP, Kline SN. "Prevention of osteoradionecrosis: A randomized prospective clinical trial of hyperbaric oyxgen versus penicillin." JADA. 1985;111:49-54.

28. Marx RE and Kline SN. "Principles and methods of osseous reconstruction." Int Adv in Surg Oncol. 1983;61:167-228.

29. Marx RE and Smith BR. "An improved technique for development of the pectoralis major myocutaneous flap." Oral Maxillofac Surg. 1990;48:1168-1180.

30. McMillan T, Calhoun KH, Nader JT, Stiernberg, Rhaaramans CM. "The effect of hyperbaric oxygen therapy on oral mucosal carcinoma." Laryngoscope. 1989;99(3):241-244.

31. Meyer I. "Infectious diseases of the jaws." J Oral Surg. 1970;28:27-33.

32. Nemiroff PM. "Effects of hyperbaric oxygen on growth and metastases on Lewis lung tumors in mice." J Hyperbaric Med. 1988;3(2):89-95.

33. Nemiroff PM. "Effects of hyperbaric oxygen on tumor metastases in mice." Clin Radiol. 1991;22:538-540.

34. Niinikoski J. "Effect of oxygen supply on wound healing and formation of experimental granulation tissue." Acta Physiol Scand Suppl. 1969;334:1-72.

35. Niinikoski J and Hunt TK. "Oxygen tensions in healing bone." Surg, Gynecol. Obstet. 1972;134:746-750.

36. Ravelo JI and Marx RE. "The effects of oxygen radicals on tumorigenesis in hamsters." Am Assoc Oral and Maxillofac Surg Scient Abstr Session. 68th Annual Meeting, Sept. 16, 1988.

37. Rubin P, Casarett GW. Clinical Radiation Pathology, Vol. II. Philadelphia, PA: W.B. Saunders, 1968;557-608.

38. Silver IA. "Cellular microenvironment in healing and non-healing wounds." In: Soft and Hard Tissue Repair. TK Hunt, Heppenstall RB, Pines E, et al. (Eds.) New York: Praeger, 1984;50-66.

39. Silverman S and Shillitoe EJ. "Etiology and predisposing factors." In: Oral Cancer. S Silverman, (Ed.) New York: American Cancer Society, Publ. 1981;6-35.

40. Strauss SE and Spatz SS. "Irradiated dentition: The dentist's responsibilities." J Prosthetic Dent. 1972;27:209-214.

41. Van Steenburghe D, Sullivan DY, et al. "A retrospective multicenter evaluation of the survival rate of osseointegrated fixtures supporting bridges in the treatment of partial edentulism." J Prosthet Dent. 1989;61:217-223.

# NOTES

CHAPTER 32

# PELVIC RADIATION NECROSIS AND RADIATION CYSTITIS

## CHAPTER THIRTY-TWO OVERVIEW

# PELVIC RADIATION NECROSIS AND RADIATION CYSTITIS

*James A. Williams Jr., Dick Clarke*

## INTRODUCTION

The efficacy of radiation therapy in the control and treatment of malignant disease is well established. The goal is to eradicate tumor with minimum possible adverse effects to adjacent tissue. In recent years, a better understanding of radiobiological principles, in conjunction with fractionated exposure protocols and high-energy radiation delivery systems, has served to reduce both the incidence and degree of iatrogenic tissue injury.

In spite of these improvements, localized radiation-induced tissue breakdown continues to occur, and may lead to complex and potentially devastating complications. While the most commonly reported form of this disease is osteoradionecrosis of the mandible (12, 27, 39, 42), radiation tissue injury has been reported in a wide variety of other bony and soft tissues (14, 19, 24, 46). This propensity for radiation-induced mandibular necrosis has been explained as secondary to the high incidence of head and neck cancers, the effectiveness of tumor control at these sites, and the presence of teeth that may subsequently require extraction (38). The long accepted and empirically-derived sequence of radiation, trauma, and infection leading to localized radiation tissue damage (41) has been replaced by a description that more accurately describes the biochemical and cellular pathology (35). Histologic analysis of tissue biopsies from a series of patients led to the identification of the post-radiation iatrogenic process as one of a progressive, obliterative endarteritis (35). This process ultimately results in a decrease in blood flow, leading to a hypovascular, hypoxic, and hypocellular tissue bed.

The treatment of local-tissue breakdown secondary to radiation therapy is a frustrating medical and surgical dilemma. Hypovascularity acts as a foundation for spontaneous or minor trauma-induced tissue breakdown. Radiation induced ulcerations can cause severe pain, requiring the use of addicting medications. Ulcerations may also involve vascular structures and result in significant bleeding, which may be life-threatening. The ulceration may represent only the "tip of the iceberg," as adjacent tissues are also hypovascular and hypoperfused. Attempts at surgical excision of the obvious lesion may lead to the development of a larger non-healing wound (25, 49). Covering external wound with skin grafts or flaps typically requires repeated procedures and, in many cases, may still prove unsuccessful (27, 37, 49).

The role of hyperbaric oxygen in the management of soft-tissue radionecrosis has evolved from clinical and laboratory studies that have addressed the pathophysiology and management of osteoradionecrosis of the mandible (14, 34-36, 40, 43). This chapter will review the effects of radiation tissue injury on pelvic structures, and present evidence for the utilization of hyperbaric oxygen therapy within the overall treatment plan.

## RADIATION TISSUE INJURY

Essentially, any tumor can be eradicated if the absorbed dose of radiation is high enough. A major limiting factor, however, is the amount of radiation that the surrounding healthy tissue can safely tolerate. The goal of radiation therapy is achieved when the tumor is completely destroyed while the surrounding tissues show minimal evidence of structural or functional injury. Improved delivery systems and a better understanding of radiobiological principles have served to reduce the incidence and degree of radiation tissue injury. However, localized radiation damage to healthy tissue continues to occur (12, 46, 23). The pathophysiologic sequence of radiation-induced tissue injury has been described by Berdjis (4) as four specific periods:

**Acute (first six months):** Organ damage accumulates. This period may be clinically silent, unless tissue-tolerance limits are exceeded.

**Subacute (second six months):** Recovery from acute damage ends. Persistence and progression of permanent residual damage is evident. Clinical changes may become apparent, depending on the degree of vascular impairment.

**Chronic (second to fifth year):** Progression of permanent residual damage occurs. The most significant problems arising during this period result from hypoperfusion because of progressive deterioration of the involved microvasculature.

**Late (after the fifth year):** Clinical conditions similar to chronic phase, but progression is slower.

The chronic and late changes can represent particularly difficult management challenges.

Radiation has been shown to produce swelling, degeneration, and necrosis of the vascular endothelium. This results in edema, fibrosis, and thickening of the vessel wall, with degeneration of the elastic and muscular coating (14). These are the characteristic changes of obliterative endarteritis, which progress as slowly after radiation exposure to produce a hypocellular, hypovascular and hypoxic tissue bed (35). Involved tissue becomes very susceptible to breakdown, either spontaneously or following minor trauma, and resistant to the processes of normal wound healing. In an area of impaired microcirculation, the increased metabolic demands of the healing wound may not be met.

Irradiated tissue, unlike other injured tissues, is largely incapable of revascularization or recovery (39). Humoral mechanisms involved in tissue repair are unable to gain access to the injured area to promote wound healing. Oxygen, in combination with the release of growth factors from tissue macrophages in otherwise hypoxic tissues, improves angiogenesis (28, 29). Oxygen permits the production of collagen and the development of a new connective tissue network. Hyperbaric doses of oxygen have been demonstrated to stimulate angiogenesis in irradiated tissue, thus increasing the vascular density supported by the new collagen matrix (40). This stimulation of neovascularization provides a mechanism for delivering oxygen to irradiated tissue and initiating re-epithelialization.

## GYNECOLOGIC RADIATION TISSUE INJURY

The genital organs are among the most common sites of cancer in women. In 1993, gynecologic cancer accounted for more than 71,000 new cancer cases and 24,000 deaths in the United States (1, 6). Major sites include the uterine corpus and cervix, vagina, and vulva. Radiation is used as an adjuvant to surgery in uterine corpus and vulvar cancer. Early stage, and small volume cervix and vaginal, cancers may be treated with radical surgical procedures. However, radiation therapy has had a long history of limited success in the treatment of high stage and larger volume malignancies of the female lower genital tract.

Two types of radiation therapy are used to treat cervical cancer; brachytherapy (intracavity and interstitial), and external-beam pelvic radiation therapy. The intracavity method permits high tumoricidal doses of radiation to be delivered directly to the cervix with minimum complications to adjacent tissue. The interstitial method, using hollow 18-gauge needles inserted into the parametrium, may increase morbidity, and long-term studies are needed to clarify these concerns. External-beam radiotherapy is indicated when tumor has extended into extrauterine pelvic soft tissue and lymph nodes. Combination intracavity and external beam radiation therapy, particularly in high doses, inevitably affects organs adjacent to the cervix. Since the beneficial effect of radiation is produced by tissue destruction, and since there is no way to restrict the radiation to the tumor cells alone, normal tissue must inevitably be injured during radiotherapy. In almost 1,000 patients treated with radiotherapy for stage I and II cervical cancer, Strockbine and colleagues (52) reported serious complications, such as radionecrosis of the vaginal wall, bladder fistula and rectal fistula in 22 patients.

Vulvar cancer is primarily a surgically-managed disease and, today, radiation is rarely used as primary treatment. The role of radiation is generally limited to treating disease in lymph nodes of the groin and pelvis, and is usually administered postoperatively. Radiation to the vulva itself is generally avoided due to the difficulty of directing the beam to this area. Also, the vulvar skin is very moist and patients develop painful, desquamating vulvitis, which often results in interruption of treatment (17).

Radiation-induced injuries following treatment for gynecologic malignancies are uncommon. Up to 10% of patients may suffer from a very superficial vaginal necrosis as an acute response to irradiation; this is generally mild and self-limiting (17). Few patients suffer late or chronic effects of irradiation months to years after completing therapy. Estimates vary, but following radical pelvic/perineal radiation, some 2-4% of patients will develop necrosis in the field of radiation (11, 48). This is a particularly debilitating condition. A painful non-healing ulceration develops, generally in the upper vagina, resulting in a continuous malodorous, serosanguinous discharge from the vagina. The necrotic wound also produces varying degrees of pain, often requiring narcotic analgesics. Many of these patients become socially isolated and in constant pain. They often require hospitalization for pain control and nutritional support, and the condition generally worsens.

The nature of radionecrotic wounds is one of progression, and these vaginal ulcers may involve surrounding organs, resulting in vesicovaginal and/or rectovaginal fistulae. Occasionally, an enterovaginal fistula may develop if a loop of small bowel is adherent to pelvic peritoneum and receives full-dose irradiation.

## TREATMENT

Traditional therapy for these necrotic wounds has involved attempts at topical wound care to enhance healing and re-epithelialization. Douches with hydrogen peroxide, antiseptic solutions, and antibiotics, have been used, as well as topical estrogen cream to stimulate the surrounding "normal" vaginal mucosal tissue. Failure to respond to this regimen is common. Using these conservative treatments methods on twelve patients with radionecrosis of the vulvar and distal vagina, Roberts and co-workers reported that it "did not result in even partial healing in any patient" (48).

Surgical treatment of radionecrotic lesions has generally been considered only after fistula development has already occurred. The first step in the management of vaginal fistulae involves diverting the urinary and/or GI tract to allow adequate debridement of necrotic tissue.

Surgical repair of vaginal fistulae is often difficult, if not impossible. Attempts at using tissue flaps to repair the defect have met with some limited success. These operations are difficult and, if unsuccessful, patients may require more radical surgery, including permanent urinary and colonic diversion.

## HYPERBARIC TREATMENT

Several early, non-randomized, and limited clinical series have reported the healing of previously refractory radionecrotic sites when hyperbaric oxygen was used. Hart and Mainous (24) discussed 69 patients who suffered radiation injury at a variety of anatomic sites. Radiation injury occurred in the pelvic area in five patients, all of whom had been treated for carcinoma of either the vagina, cervix, or uterus. While specific wound sites were not described, "all patients improved." Hart and Mainous speculated that the favorable wound-healing effects seen in full-thickness lesions, acute thermal burns, and ischemic ulcerations, when treated with hyperbaric oxygen, were suggestive of improved vascular supply. They further stated that based upon this assumption, late radiation-induced obliterative endarteritis should also benefit from hyperbaric oxygen therapy. Glassburn and Brady (22) reported 24 patients with late radiation-tissue injury who had failed to respond to conservative care. Conservative care included antibiotic agents, as infection was still thought to be a major factor in the development of radiation necrosis. Within this series, twelve patients suffered vaginal vault or perineal necrosis. This latter subset were treated at 3 ATA $O_2$ for approximately sixty minutes daily, for an average total of 23 treatments. Outcome was reported as marked improvement in eight patients, recurrent tumor in three patients, and the final patient going on to develop fistula.

In their report of radiation-induced tissue injury at various sites treated with hyperbaric oxygen, Farmer and colleagues (19) described one case of vaginal necrosis. The patient underwent "at least 40 treatments at 2.0 ATA for 120 minutes daily." Results in the vaginal case were "excellent," with complete healing and relief of pain.

## OUR CLINICAL EXPERIENCE

In 1992, we reported a clinical series of patients treated at Palmetto Richland Memorial Hospital who had developed late radiation-tissue injury, secondary to cancer control efforts (57). Hyperbaric oxygen therapy was undertaken at 2.0 ATA for 90 minutes, once daily. Four patients did not complete their prescribed course. Three of these patients were found to have recurrent disease, and the fourth patient suffered unmanageable confinement anxiety. Eleven patients had radionecrosis of the vaginal vault alone, two patients had both vaginal vault disease and rectovaginal fistula. The remaining patient was treated for necrosis of the abdominal wall. The average number of treatments was 44. Each of the eleven patients with vaginal vault necrosis alone showed marked improvement or complete resolution. Complete resolution was seen in all eleven patients within eight weeks of completing hyperbaric therapy. Minimum follow-up was nine months in this group. Both patients with rectovaginal fistulae underwent fecal diversion by loop colostomy, followed by hyperbaric oxygen with resolution of necrosis. Rectovaginal fistula repair was performed with subsequent closure of loop colostomy. Three years after surgery, there was no evidence of recurrent necrosis or fistula. The only treatment failure occurred in the one patient who developed massive necrosis of the abdominal wall, sacrum and vagina, with rectovaginal and vesicovaginal fistulae. She eventually succumbed as the necrosis, complicated by infection, continued to progress.

Since this publication, an additional 67 such patients have been referred for hyperbaric oxygen therapy. Of this number, 21 patients did not receive treatment. Reasons included patient refusal, unacceptable risk factors, cancer recurrence, and insurmountable transportation problems. Of the 46 who underwent hyperbaric oxygen therapy, 37 (80%) had significant improvement or complete healing of the area of necrosis. Of the remainder, 1 had tumor recurrence, and eight were non-compliant to the treatment course.

It is our impression that hyperbaric oxygen therapy for radiation-induced vaginal vault necrosis is a safe and effective therapy for controlling necrosis and promoting wound healing, when used in conjunction with surgical debridement, appropriate antibiotic therapy, and nutritional support. In those patients who developed fistulae, hyperbaric oxygen after fecal diversion may decrease morbidity and increase the likelihood of successful fistula repair. It is imperative that patients who are unresponsive to hyperbaric oxygen have a complete re-evaluation to rule out recurrent malignancy, as this is the greatest predictor of failure.

## TREATMENT PROTOCOLS

Our current hyperbaric treatment protocol at the University of South Carolina School of Medicine/Palmetto Richland Memorial Hospital for pelvic soft tissue radionecrosis is, as follows:

After signed informed consent:

    A. 2.5 ATA oxygen for 90 minutes, for an initial course of 20 treatments. These treatments are typically provided on a q. d. outpatient basis, but may be undertaken while patients remain hospitalized.

    B. Reassessment, in conjunction with referring specialists, after 20 treatments.

    C. Where the lesion is found to be largely resolved after 20 treatments, hold any further HBO therapy. Patients are followed by their referring physician with re-consultation if the subsequent clinical course does not result in complete resolution within 60 days.

    D. Where the lesion is found to have improved following 20 treatments, but remains significant:

        1. Ten additional treatments, at 2.5 ATA for 90 minutes each, on a q. d. basis.

    E. Reassessment after 30 treatments in conjunction with referring physician.

        1. Where significant improvement has been made during the second series of 10 treatments, hold further HBO therapy. Follow-up per referring physician.

        2. Where progress has been made, but concern remains regarding adequate healing responses, follow for another 4-6 weeks. Consider 10 additional treatments, if healing responses plateau prior to complete resolution.

    F. Where no evidence of early healing response is apparent after the initial series of 20 treatments, evaluate as follows:

        1. Reconsider diagnosis.

        2. Persistent/recurrent tumor; biopsy suspicious lesion.

        3. Persistent smoking against advice.

        4. Non-responder to hyperbaric oxygen therapy.

Any decision to exceed 40 hyperbaric treatments must be preceded by peer review.

## RADIATION CYSTITIS

    Radiation therapy for malignancies within the pelvic viscera, particularly effective in patients with carcinoma of the cervix, is not without significant morbidity. Urologic complications have been reported by a number of authors (13, 16, 30), in which the incidence of radiation cystitis has been placed at between 1% and 2.5%. Complication rates have been reported at much greater than this (31). However, apparent failure to establish pre-existing or recurrent tumor before ascribing the effects of radiation has tended to artificially elevate the incidence of urologic complications. Apparently, this is a common finding. Dean and Lylton (16) reported that 95% of patients who had developed urologic problems after receiving less than 60 gray had a tumor present.

    Bladder biopsies show a typical histology of obliterative endarteritis, with thrombi and hemorrhage of small vessels. Symptoms of radiation cystitis include urinary frequency, urgency, nocturia, and gross hematuria. Radiation cystitis is a progressive disease that will not resolve spontaneously once in an advanced stage. The mainstay of therapy for radiation cystitis has been the instillation of formalin into the defunctionalized bladder (3). This represents only a temporary cauterizing effect, is painful, and leads to further shrinkage of the bladder volume. Other palliative measures reported in the literature include bladder dilation, antibiotics, fibrinolytic drugs, and instillation of alum and silver-nitrate. Many of these procedures fail to relieve recurrent bleeding, often necessitating urinary diversion. In 1985, Weiss and colleagues (54) reported three patients who were treated with hyperbaric oxygen for persistent radiation-induced gross hematuria. Patient follow-up was 4, 11, and 14 months respectively. The hyperbaric protocol was 2.0 ATA $O_2$ for 2 hours, for a total of 60 treatments. The authors based this protocol on that which had been reported for the management of osteoradionecrosis (39).

The following year, Schoenrock and Cianci added one additional case report to the literature (51). This patient had received 61.5 Gy of external-beam radiation to the pelvis. Eleven years after completing radiotherapy, she developed radiation cystitis and was ultimately admitted, due to gross hematuria and clot retention. Her subsequent clinical course became increasingly critical, with bladder rupture, the development of a large vesicocutaneous fistula, and persistent bleeding. Because her condition had been refractory to conventional management and surgery, hyperbaric oxygen was initiated. The patient was treated at 2.0 ATA oxygen for 105 minutes, for a total of 19 exposures. This treatment course resulted in the healing of the fistula, and the patient was reported as symptom-free with no gross or microscopic hematuria for 18 months of follow-up. The authors rationalized that the same principles that apply to hyperbaric treatment of soft-tissue radionecrosis of the head, neck, abdomen, and vulva, pertained to closure of this patient's fistula. They added that "unexpectedly, at the same time, this patient also seems to have complete relief from radiation necrosis."

Weiss and Neville (55) updated their earlier report by adding five more patients. The three previous patients had remained free of symptoms of intractable hematuria for an average of 40 months. Four of the five patients added to their case series had remained improved during a follow-up period averaging 24 months. Weiss and Neville suggested that hyperbaric oxygen should be considered the treatment of choice for radiation-induced hemorrhagic cystitis, although they cautioned that a larger number of patients will need to be treated in order to reliably attribute the salutary effects of hyperbaric oxygen in these cases. A clinical series of 12 patients, who had failed all other conventional attempts at management, was reported at the 1991 Undersea and Hyperbaric Medical Society Annual Scientific Meeting (44). Having ruled out recurrent malignancy, they were treated at 2.5 ATA oxygen for 90 minutes, five to six times weekly, for an average of 20-30 treatments. With follow-up of six months to three years, outcome was reported as follows:

| | |
|---|---|
| Complete relief of symptoms | 5 |
| Marked improvement | 5 |
| Minimal improvement | 1 |
| Treatments halted due to concurrent illness | 1 |

The authors of this study recommended hyperbaric oxygen therapy as an "efficacious modality in patients who fail other forms of treatment."

Rijkmans and colleagues reported a series of ten patients (47). As before, all had failed conventional therapy, and bladder biopsies confirmed a diagnosis of late radiation tissue injury. This report was interesting in that in six of the ten patients, macroscopic hematuria stopped completely after a mean of 18 hyperbaric oxygen exposures. In the four remaining patients, macroscopic hematuria diminished significantly. However, recurrent bladder tumor was apparent in these four patients. It was significant that these malignancies could not be recognized by cystoscopy before the hyperbaric treatment course due to the presence of necrosis and bleeding. The authors concluded that hyperbaric oxygen was effective in the treatment of radiation cystitis, as it both treated hematuria and demarcated recurrent tumor. They added that "this effect of hyperbaric oxygen therapy is of special interest in patients in whom one cannot distinguish between radiation cystitis, tumor growth, necrosis and edema of catheter effect at cystoscopic examination."

Researchers from the Academic Medical Center, in Amsterdam, have prospectively studied 40 patients (5). All had been treated by one or more "standard" measures, without success. Most patients required multiple blood transfusions to control hematuria. Inclusion criteria was severe hemorrhagic radiation-induced cystitis not responding to conventional therapies. Exclusion criteria were tumor recurrence in the bladder, and significant patient-specific risks for hyperbaric oxygen exposure. Hyperbaric treatments were delivered at 3.0 ATA, with patients undergoing 20 daily sessions of 90 minutes each. At follow-up, three groups could be distinguished according to response:

> Group 1 - No hematuria (mean follow-up 29.3 months: range 3-74) - 30 pts.
> Group 2 - Occasionally slight hematuria (mean follow-up 5.1 months: range 1-13) - 7 pts.
> Group 3 - No improvement - 3 pts.

No adverse effects from HBO therapy were noted.

Random site bladder biopsy prior to HBO therapy was negative for tumor and positive for late-radiation injury in all 40 patients. Nine patients were subsequently found to have tumor recurrence after HBO. Consistent with other reports, the Amsterdam group considered that HBO therapy served to identify suspicious areas within the bladder (not revascularizing). Random pre-treatment biopsy within extensively compromised bladder is frequently hit or miss. Areas of the bladder wall that do not respond to HBO therapy should be viewed with suspicion and biopsied accordingly.

In 1996, a second group of 40 patients were reported (32). These patients were very similar to those noted above, in terms of clinical findings, previous management, and refractory nature. While the pressure and time of each treatment was similar, the average course of HBO therapy was almost doubled, at 39 treatments. Hematuria was arrested in 33 (82.5%), and reduced in 6 (6.6%). One patient ultimately required in ileal conduit. Mean follow-up was 21 months (range 3-49 months).

Distinct benefits have resulted from the utilization of hyperbaric oxygen in this disease process. In most instances, however, HBO has been provided after conventional management had proven unsatisfactory. It would appear that earlier utilization of HBO, as proposed by Weiss (55), might further reduce morbidity. Although clinical evidence for the utilization of hyperbaric oxygen is supportive, further prospective and, perhaps, crossover trials should be undertaken, in order to fully validate this therapeutic option.

## RADIATION PROCTITIS

Application of radiotherapy in the management of gynecologic and urologic malignancy involves the risk of radiation proctitis, due to the rectum's close proximity to the pelvic organs. The incidence of radiation-induced proctitis has been placed at between 1% and 5% (16, 44). Complications may occur during radiation treatment. See Table 1. Acute onset symptoms are thought to be the result of a direct effect of radiation on the mucosa of the bowel. Severe symptoms may necessitate interruption of the radiation course; however, they are generally self-limiting and reversible.

Symptoms of late radiation-induced proctitis (see Table 2) may develop months to years after completion of radiotherapy. Radiation proctitis, in this setting, may manifest as stricture, fistula, perforation, endothelial degeneration, necrosis, stenosis, rectal wall ulceration or frank hemorrhage. Clinically-significant, chronic-radiation damage results from a combination of ischemia and fibrosis secondary to an obliterative endarteritis (9). In general, treatment measures have been discouraging, and morbidity and mortality from late-radiation-induced proctitis are substantial (20). Surgical management of damaged bowel involves colostomy or resection, the latter a high risk procedure for complication (21, 50).

Conservative management of minor bleeding has involved topical rectal steroids and control of diarrhea. As late radiation proctitis is considered to be the result of vascular damage and progressive ischemia, one would not expect anti-inflammatory agents to be useful. Multiple blood transfusions may be required to correct anemia in more severe cases, and laser treatments have recently been successful in arresting hemorrhage (8, 33, 45). However, laser treatments carry the risk of perforation when applied to radiation injured tissue.

The 1986 edition of the UHMS Hyperbaric Oxygen Committee report (26) listed radiation proctitis as an investigational indication for hyperbaric oxygen therapy. The report did not clarify the precise role of

## TABLE 1. ACUTE CLINICAL PRESENTATION (2)

**RADIATION TREATMENT COMPLICATIONS:**

| Symptom |
| --- |
| Diarrhea |
| Nausea |
| Vomiting |
| Cramping Pain |

## TABLE 2. DELAYED CLINICAL PRESENTATION (2)

**RADIATION TREATMENT COMPLICATIONS:**

| Symptom | Mean Onset (mos.) |
| --- | --- |
| Diarrhea | 8 |
| Rectal Bleeding | 9 |
| Tenesmus | 5 |
| Abdominal pain | 13 |
| Constipation | 8 |

hyperbaric oxygen, and no supportive literature was provided. A single case was reported in 1991, describing the use of hyperbaric oxygen to arrest severe hemorrhagic radiation proctitis (10). The patient had received high-dose, fractionated radiation therapy (65 Gy) in conjunction with resection three years previously, for prostatic cancer. Two years later, he developed low-grade rectal bleeding. Biopsy was significant for radiation changes, in the absence of recurrent cancer. Five months later, he was admitted for severe rectal bleeding and anemia (Hb 7.0). Two laser treatments failed to arrest bleeding, and continued blood transfusions were necessary. Colostomy was considered, but HBO therapy was initiated and the surgical option held. The protocol used was 2.5 ATA for 90 minutes, b.i.d., for 41 days. Fifteen days after starting HBO, rectal bleeding progressively decreased and no further transfusions were required. A ten-month follow-up period was significant for no further bleeding. As the authors noted, this was the first case of severe hemorrhagic radiation proctitis treated with hyperbaric oxygen.

From Fremantle, Australia, Woo and colleagues retrospectively reviewed their experience involving 18 cases (56). All had changes consistent with radiation proctitis, visualized by protoscope, sigmoidoscope, or colonoscope. Symptoms were classified according to four main groups: bleeding, pain, incontinence, and diarrhea. The authors considered improvement as complete if a symptom(s) resolved entirely, partial, if improvement was sustained for three months, with subsequent relapse, or less than complete resolution. Treatments were provided at 2.0 ATA for 105 minutes each, on a 6-day a week basis. The average number of treatments was 24 (range 12-40). Overall outcome was reported as complete resolution of all symptoms in two patients (11.0%), resolution of some, but not all, symptoms in eight patients (44.4%), with the remaining eight patients experiencing no change in their symptoms. Five patients experienced transient myopia. Objectively, outcome was difficult to gauge, as few of the patients had post-treatment colonoscopy, and none consented to have the procedure just for this purpose.

An additional 14 patients have been reported by Warren and colleagues (53). Treatments varied from 2.0 to 2.36 ATA from 90 to 120 minutes, respectively, on a q.d. basis. There were nine "responders," seven of whom were fully resolved at completion of therapy. The eighth fully resolved within a few weeks of completing treatment, the remaining patient improved from daily bleeding and substantial pain, to minor bleeding and occasional minimal rectal discomfort. Five patients were classified as non-responders. In this series, the average course was 45 treatments, with the range not provided. Follow-up sigmoidoscopy was available in five responders, all of which were significant for improvement in mucosal appearance, resolution of erythema, and decreased ulceration (one case). In three non-responders, in which such follow-up was available, none showed significant improvement over baseline examination.

While these reports are retrospective in nature, they do suggest a favorable healing response in 55-64% of those who undergo HBO therapy. While this compares well with more traditional therapies, prospective trials ideally including a cross-over arm, will be necessary to more clearly define the precise role of HBO therapy.

# REFERENCES

1. Gusberg, SB, Runuwicz CD. Gynecologic Cancer, In American Cancer Society Textbook of Clinical Oncology AI Holleb, DJ Fink, GP Murphy, (Eds.), Atlanta: American Cancer Society 1991;481.

2. Anseline PF. "Radiation injury to the rectum." Annals Surgery. 1981;194(6)716-724.

3. Benham K et al. "Intravesical instillation of formalin for hemorrhagic cystitis secondary to radiation of gynaecologic malignancies." Gynaec Oncol. 1988;16:31-33.

4. Berdjis, CC. "Cell" In: Pathology of Irradiation. CC Berdjis (Ed.) 1971;18. Baltimore: Williams and Wilkins.

5. Bevers, RFM, et al. "Hyperbaric oxygen treatment for haemorrhagic radiation cystitis". Lanced;346:803-805.

6. Boring, CC et al. "Cancer statistics 1993." CA: A Cancer Journal for Clinicians. 1993;43(1):7-26.

7. Boronow, RC. "Management of radiation-induced vaginal fistulas." Am. J. Obstet. and Gynecol. 1971;110:1-8.

8. Buchi KN & Dixon JA. "Argon laser treatment of hemorrhagic radiation proctitis." Gastrointest Endoscopy. 1987;33:27-29.

9. Carr ND et al. "Microvascular studies in human radiation bowel disease." Gut. 1984;25:448-454.

10. Charneau J et al. "Severe hemorrhagic radiation proctitis advancing to gradual cessation with hyperbaric oxygen." Digestive Disease and Sciences 1991;36(3)373-375.

11. "Clinical oncology. A multidisciplinary approach." Sixth Edition, 1983;5:58-71. American Cancer Society.

12. Curi MM, Dib LL. "Osteoradionecrosis of the jaws: a retrospective study of the background factors and treatment of 104 cases". J. Oral Maxillofacial Surg. 1997;(55):540-544.

13. Cushing RM et al. "Major urologic complications following radium and x-ray therapy for carcinoma of the cervix." Am. J. Obstet. & Gynecol. 1968;107:750.

14. Davis JC et al. "Hyperbaric oxygen: A new adjunct in the management of radiation necrosis." Arch. Otol. 1979;105:58-61.

15. Davis JC. "Soft tissue radiation necrosis: The role of hyperbaric oxygen." HBO Review. 1987;2(3):153-167.

16. Dean R & Lytton B. "Urologic complications of pelvic irradiation." J. Urology. 1978;119:64-67.

17. DiSaia PG et al. Clinical Gynecologic Oncology. St. Louis: CV Mosby Co. 1993.

18. Editorial. "Radiation induced proctosigmoiditis." Lancet. 1983;1:1082-1083.

19. Farmer, JC et al. "Treatment of radiation-induced tissue injury by hyperbaric oxygen." Ann. Otol. 1978;87:707-715.

20. Fischer L. "Late progress of radiation - induced proctitis." Acta Chir Scand. 1990;156:801-805.

21. Galland RB & Spencer J. "Surgical aspects of radiation therapy to the intestine." Br. J. Surg. 1979;66:135-138.

22. Glassburn JR and Brady LW. "Treatment of necrotic wounds with hyperbaric oxygen." Proc. 6th Int. Cong. on Hyperbaric Medicine. G. Smith (Ed.) Aberdeen: Aberdeen University Press, 1977;279-285.

23. Hamberger AD, et al. "Analysis of the severe complications of irradiation of carcinoma of the cervix: whole pelvis irradiation and intracavity radium". Int. J. Radiation Oncology, Biology, Physiology 1983;9:367-371.

24. Hart, GB and Mainous EG. "The treatment of radiation necrosis with hyperbaric oxygen (OHP)." Cancer 1976;37:2580-2585.

25. Heimbach,RD. In: "Problem Wounds: The Role of Oxygen." J.C. Davis & T.K. Hunt (Eds.) 1988;3:62. New York: Elsevier Science Publishing Co., New York.

26. "Hyperbaric oxygen therapy: A committee report." JT Mader (Ed.) Undersea and Hyperbaric Medical Society, Publication Number 30CR(HBO)1989. Bethesda, Maryland: Undersea and Hyperbaric Medical Society.

27. Joseph, DL and Shumrick, DL. "Risks of head and neck surgery in previously irradiated patients." Arch. Otolaryngol. 1973;97:381-384.

28. Knighton DR et al. "Regulation of Wound Healing Angiogenesis: Effect of oxygen gradients and inspired oxygen concentrations." Surgery. 1981;90:262.

29. Knighton DR et al. "Oxygen tension regulates the expression of angiogenesis factor by macrophages." Science. 1983;221:1283.

30. Kottmeier H. "Complications following radiation therapy in carcinoma of the cervix and their treatment." Am. J. Obstet. & Gynecol. 1964;88:854.

31. Lang, EK et al. "Complications in the urinary tract related to treatment of carcinoma of the cervix." South. Med. J. 1973;66:28.

32. Lee HC, et al. "Hyperbaric oxygen therapy in hemorrhagic radiation cystitis: a report of 40 cases". Proceedings: Int. Joint Meeting on Hyperbaric and Underwater Medicine. Eds. A. Marroni, G. Oriani, F. Wattel. Milan, Italy 1996.

33. Leuchter RS et al. "Nd:YAG laser therapy of rectosigmoid bleeding due to radiation injury." Obstet Gynecology. 1982;59:655-675.

34. Mansfield MJ et al. "Hyperbaric oxygen as an adjunct in the treatment of osteoradionecrosis of the mandible." J. Oral Surg. 1981;39:585-589.

35. Marx, RE. "Osteoradionecrosis: A new concept of its pathophysiology." J. Oral Maxillofac Surg. 1983;41:283-288.

36. Marx RE. "A new concept in the treatment of osteoradionecrosis." J. Oral . 1983;41:351-357.

37. Marx RE and Kline SN. "Principles and methods of osseous reconstruction." In: International Advances in Surgical Oncology. AP Murphy (Ed.) 1983;167-228. New York: Alan R. Liss Inc.

38. Marx, RE. "Osteoradionecrosis of the jaws: Review and update." HBO Review. 1984;5:78-126.

39. Marx, RE. In: Problem Wounds: The Role of Oxygen. JC Davis and TK Hunt (Eds.). "Problem wounds in oral and maxillofacial surgery: The role of hyperbaric oxygen." New York: Elsevier Science Publishing Co. 1988;4:65-123.

40. Marx RE et al. "Relationship of oxygen dose to angiogenesis induction in the irradiated and tissue deficient patient." Am. J. Surg. 1990;160:519-524.

41. Meyer, L. "Infectious diseases of the jaws." J. Oral Surg. 1970;28:17-26.

42. Murray, CG, Herson J., Daly TE, et al. "Radiation necrosis of the mandible: A 10 year study." Part I. Factors influence the onset of necrosis. International Journal Radiation Oncology Biology Physics. 1980;6:543-548.

43. Myers RAM and Marx RE. "Use of hyperbaric oxygen in postradiation head and neck surgery." NCI Monogr. 1990;9:151-157.

44. Norkool DM et al. "Hyperbaric oxygen therapy for radiation-induced cystitis." UHMS Annual Scientific Meeting 1991. San Diego, California: Abstract #195.

45. O'Conner JJ. "Argon laser treatment of radiation proctitis." Archives Surgery. 1989;124:749.

46. Perez CA, et al. "Irradiation of carcinoma of the prostate localized in the pelvis: analysis of tumor response and prognosis". Int. J. Radiation Oncology, Biology and Physiology 1980;6:555-563.

47. Rijkmans BG et al. "Successful treatment of radiation cystitis with hyperbaric oxygen." European Urology. 1989;16:354-356.

48. Roberts WS et al. "Management of radionecrosis of the vulva and distal vagina." Am. J. Obstet. and Gynecol. 1991;164:1235-1238.

49. Samuels L, et al. "Reconstruction of radiation-induced chest wall lesions". Annals of Plastic Surgery 1993;31(5):399-405.

50. Schmitt EH & Symmonds RC. "Surgical treatment of radiation induced injuries to the intestine." Surgery, Gynecology and Obstetrics. 1981;153:896-900.

51. Schoenrock GJ & Cianci P. "Treatment of radiation cystitis with hyperbaric oxygen." Urology. 1986;27(3):271-272.

52. Strockbine MF, Hancock JE and Fletcher GH. "Complications in 831 patients with squamous cell carcinoma of the intact uterine cervix treated with 3,000 rads or more of whole pelvis radiation." Am. J. Roentgend. Radium Ther. Nucl.Med. 1970;108:293-304.

53. Warren DC, et al. "Chronic radiation proctitis treated with hyperbaric oxygen". Journal of Hyperbaric Medicine 1997;24(3):181-184.

54. Weiss JP et al. "Treatment of radiation-induced cystitis with hyperbaric oxygen." J. Urol. 1985;134:352-354.

55. Weiss JP & Neville EC. "Hyperbaric oxygen: Primary treatment of radiation-induced hemorrhagic cystitis." J. Urol. 1989;142:43-45.

56. Woo TCS, et al. "Hyperbaric oxygen treatment for radiation proctitis". Int. J. Radiation Oncology, Biology, Physiology 1997;38(3):619-622.

57. Williams JA, Clarke D, Dennis WA, et al. "The treatment of pelvic soft tissue radiation necrosis with hyperbaric oxygen." Am. J. Obstet. Gynecol.1992; 167:412-416.

# NOTES

CHAPTER 33

# ADJUNCTIVE HYPERBARIC OXYGEN THERAPY IN THE TREATMENT OF THERMAL BURNS

## CHAPTER THIRTY-THREE OVERVIEW

# Adjunctive Hyperbaric Oxygen Therapy in the Treatment of Thermal Burns

*Paul E. Cianci*

## INTRODUCTION

The use of hyperbaric oxygen therapy as an adjunct in the treatment of thermal injury remains a subject of considerable controversy. It is frequently condemned as being too dangerous and/or too expensive for routine use. A comprehensive review of the world literature fails to support these conclusions. Indeed, a significant body of data suggests it is of great benefit. Any therapy should pass scrutiny based on its merits; that is, can it favorably affect the pathology? Will it improve currently accepted results? Is it cost effective? Is it safe? In this chapter we will explore how the specific application of hyperbaric oxygen therapy in the treatment of thermal injury is related to the pathophysiology, show how it can favorably affect outcome, discuss relevant side effects or complications, and demonstrate its cost effectiveness when utilized as part of a comprehensive program of burn care.

The use of hyperbaric oxygen therapy in the treatment of thermal burns began in 1965 when Ikeda and Wada noted more rapid healing of second-degree burns in a group of coal miners being treated for carbon monoxide poisoning (52). They followed this serendipitous observation with a series of experiments that demonstrated a reduction of edema and improved healing in animal studies (27). The Japanese experience (26-28, 51, 52) stimulated interest in other countries and there followed a series of reports of uncontrolled clinical experience with favorable results (33, 49). In 1970, Gruber (18), working at the U.S. Army biophysics laboratory at the Edgewood Arsenal in Maryland, devised a series of experiments placing rats in a hyperbaric chamber breathing 100% oxygen at sea level and at 2 and 3 atmospheres, respectively. He demonstrated that the area subjacent to a third-degree burn was hypoxic when compared to normal skin and that the tissue oxygen tension could only be raised by oxygen administered at pressure (Figure 1). This important study suggested that hyperbaric oxygen therapy could have a direct effect on the pathophysiology of the burn wound.

## PATHOPHYSIOLOGY

In order to understand the rationale for therapy, it is necessary to review the physiology of the thermal injury. The burn wound is a complex and

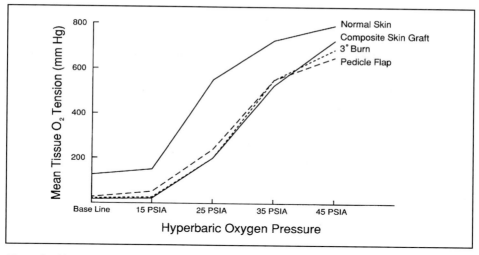

*Figure 1. Mean oxygen tension of normal skin and various hypoxic tissues as a function of hyperbaric oxygen pressure. Note: Oxygen tension rises in burned skin only with increasing pressure. (With permission.)*

dynamic injury characterized by a central zone of coagulation, surrounded by an area of stasis, and bordered by an area of erythema. The zone of coagulation or complete capillary occlusion may progress by a factor of 10 during the first 48 hours after injury. Ischemic necrosis quickly follows. Hematologic changes, including platelet microthrombi and hemo-concentration, occur in the postcapillary venules. Edema formation is rapid in the area of the injury but also develops in distant, uninjured tissue. There are also changes occurring in the distal microvasculature where red cell aggregation, white cell adhesion to venular walls, and platelet thrombo-emboli occur (7). "This progressive ischemic process, when set in motion, may extend damage dramatically during the early days after injury" (23). The ongoing tissue damage seen in thermal injury is due to the failure of surrounding tissue to supply borderline cells with oxygen and nutrients necessary to sustain viability (4). The impediment of circulation below the injury leads to desiccation of the wound as fluid cannot be supplied via the thrombosed or obstructed capillaries. Topical agents and dressings may reduce, but cannot prevent, desiccation of the burn wound and the inexorable progression to deeper layers.

## INFECTION

Susceptibility to infection is greatly increased owing to the loss of the integumentary barrier to bacterial invasion, the ideal substrate present in the burn wound, and the compromised or obstructed microvasculature which prevents humoral and cellular elements from reaching the injured tissue. Additionally, the immune system is seriously affected, demonstrating decreased levels of immunoglobulins and serious perturbations of polymorphonuclear leukocyte (PMNL) function (1, 2, 16, 51), including disorders of chemotaxis, phagocytosis, and diminished killing ability. These functions greatly increase morbidity and mortality; infection remains the leading cause of death from burns.

Regeneration cannot take place until equilibrium is reached; hence, healing is retarded. Prolongation of the healing process may lead to excessive scarring. Hypertrophic scars are seen in about 4% of cases taking 10 days to heal, in 14% of cases taking 14 days or less, in 28% of cases taking 21 days, and up to 40% of cases taking longer than 21 days to heal (13). Therapy for burns, then, is directed towards minimizing edema, preserving marginally viable tissue, protecting the microvasculature, enhancing host defenses, and providing the essential substrate necessary to sustain viability.

## EXPERIMENTAL EVIDENCE

A significant body of animal data supports the efficacy of hyperbaric oxygen in the treatment of thermal injury. Ikeda noted a reduction of edema in burned rabbits (27). Ketchum, in 1967, reported an improvement in healing time and reduced infection in an animal model (31). He later demonstrated dramatic improvement in the microvasculature of burned rats treated with hyperbaric oxygen therapy (30). In 1974, Hartwig (22) working in Germany, reported similar findings and additionally noted less inflammatory response in those animals that had been treated with hyperbaric oxygen. He suggested at that time that hyperbaric oxygen might be a useful adjunct to the technique of early debridement. Wells and Hilton (54), in a carefully designed and controlled experiment, reported a marked increase in extravasation of fluid in a series of dogs with 40% flame burns.

The effect was clearly related to oxygen and not simply increased pressure. See Figure 2. They also reported a reduction in hemoconcentration and improved cardiac output in treated dogs. Nylander, (40) in a well-accepted animal model, showed that hyperbaric oxygen therapy reduced the generalized edema associated with burn injury. See Figure 3.

Kaiser (28) showed that hyperbaric oxygen treatment resulted in shrinkage of third-degree (full thickness) injury in a rbbbit model. Untreated animals demonstrated the expected increase in wound size during the first 48 hours. Treated animals showed shrinkage of their wounds. At all times treated animal wounds remained smaller than those of controls See Figure 4.

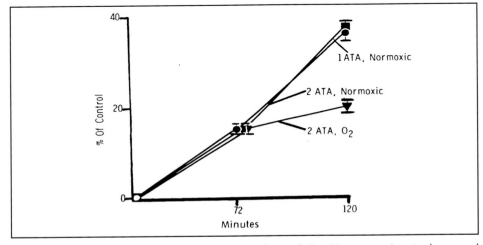

*Figure 2. Plasma volume losses after burn in untreated animals (1 ATA, normoxic), animals exposed to hyperbaric oxygen (2 ATA $O_2$) and to pressure alone (2 ATA, normoxic). (With permission.)*

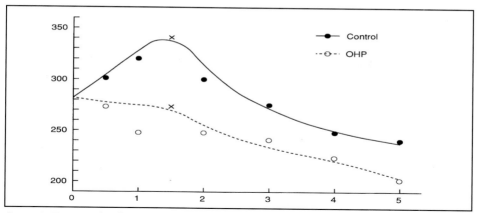

*Figure 3. Kaiser and colleagues have recently demonstrated a significant reduction of subcutaneous edema in burned animals treated with HBO. He reported progression of the burn wound in controls, while in the hyperbaric-treated animal wound size decreased (27).*

Korn and colleagues (32) in 1977 showed an early return of capillary patency in the hyperbaric-treated animals using an India ink technique. They also demonstrated survival of the dermal elements and more rapid epithelialization from these regenerative sites. He suggested the decreased desiccation of the wound they observed was a function of subjacent capillary integrity noted in the HBO-treated animals. Saunders (45) and colleagues have reported similar studies with similar results. They have also shown an improvement in collagen synthesis in HBO-treated animals. Perrins failed to show a beneficial effect in a small scald wound in a pig model treated with HBO (42). Niccole (37) in 1977 reported that HBO offered no advantage over topical agents in controlling wound bacterial counts. He proposed that HBO acted as a mild antiseptic. His data, however, supported the observation of improved healing of partial thickness injury noted by earlier investigators. Stewart (47, 48) and colleagues subjected rats to a controlled burn wound resulting in a deep partial thickness injury. See Figure 5. Both experimental groups were treated with topical agents. The hyperbaric oxygen treated

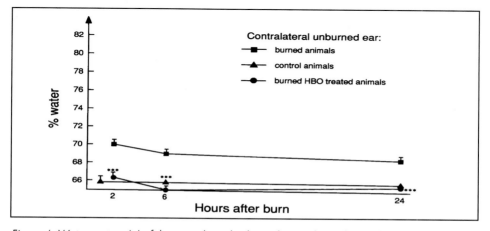

*Figure 4. Water content (+) of the contralateral unburned ear in burned animals with and without HBO treatment. (With permission.)*

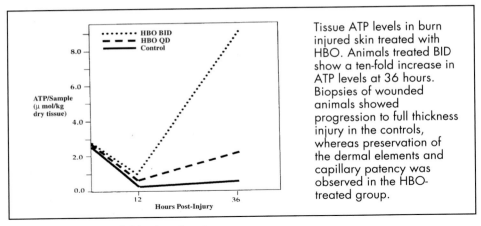

Tissue ATP levels in burn injured skin treated with HBO. Animals treated BID show a ten-fold increase in ATP levels at 36 hours. Biopsies of wounded animals showed progression to full thickness injury in the controls, whereas preservation of the dermal elements and capillary patency was observed in the HBO-treated group.

*Figure 5. Rats: Burn with Silvadene Dressing*

group showed preservation of dermal elements, no conversion of partial to full thickness injury, and preservation of adenosine triphosphate (ATP) levels; whereas, the untreated animals demonstrated marked diminution in ATP levels and conversion of partial to full thickness injury.

These studies may relate directly to the preservation of energy sources for the sodium pump. Failure of the sodium pump is felt to be a major factor in the ballooning of the endothelial cells that occurs after burn injury and subsequent massive fluid losses (3). Bleser (6), in 1973, in a very large controlled series reported reduction of burn shock and a fourfold increased survival in 30% burned animals as compared to controls. Reduction of PMNL killing ability in hypoxic tissue has been well documented by Hohn et al. (24). The ability of hyperbaric oxygen to elevate tissue oxygen tension and the enhancement of PMNL killing in an O2 enriched animal model as demonstrated by Mader (34), suggests that this may be an additional benefit of HBO. Data from Zamboni (56) suggest that hyperbaric oxygen is a potent blocker of white cell adherence to endothelial cell walls, interrupting the cascade which causes vascular damage. The mechanism is felt to be an inhibitory effect on the CD18 locus (57). Germonpre's data tends to bear out this observation and may explain the beneficial effect of hyperbaric oxygen therapy on the microcirculation previously observed (14, 22, 45, 47, 48). Shoshani reported no benefit of HBO in a rat model where all animals received standard sulfadiazine treatment. There was no improvement reported in Doppler studies of blood flow, epithelialization, or wound contraction (46). The author states that this was the first study utilizing standard burn care (topical agents). The findings are in contradistinction to Stewart's group who, in fact, utilized silvadene dressings and confirmed preservation of dermal elements by observation and biopsy (47, 48). In 1973 Bleser and Benichoux (6) reported a very large controlled series showing reduction in burn shock and a fourfold increased survival in 30% burned animals vs. controls. Hussman et al., have shown no evidence of immunosuppression in a carefully controlled animal model (25). Tenenhaus has reported reduced bacterial translocation from the gut in an animal model (50). Bacterial translocation is felt to be a major source of burn wound infection. Thus, the overwhelming evidence in a large number of controlled

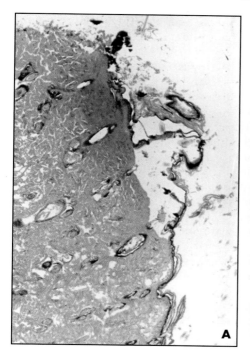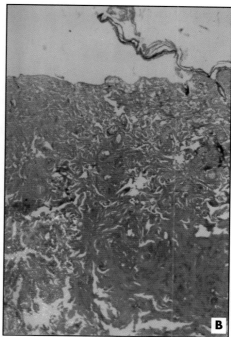

*Figure 6A – 6B. Biopsy of experimental partial thickness burns at 5 days.*
*A. HBO-treated animals show preservation of the dermal elements.*
*B. Nontreated animals show coagulation necrosis.*

animal studies suggests that hyperbaric oxygen reduces edema, prevents conversion of partial to full thickness injury, preserves the microcirculation, preserves ATP, and perhaps secondarily, the sodium pump, improves survival, and though not yet proven, may enhance PMNL killing. In a recent randomized controlled study, Bilic et al., showed a significant reduction of the post-burn edema after treatment with $HBO_2$ (p=0.009). $HBO_2$ had a beneficial effect on neoangiogenesis (p=0.009). The number of preserved regenerator, active follicles was significantly higher (p=0.009), and epithelia regeneration was more rapid in the experimental group (p=0.048). There were no significant differences for margination of leukocytes (p=0.55) or necrosis staging (p = 1.0) beneficial in the healing of burn wounds (5).

## CLINICAL EXPERIENCE

Beginning with the reports of Wada in 1965 and continuing with Ikeda (26-28, 51, 52), Lamy (33), and Tabor (49), reports of clinical series began to accumulate. In 1974 Hart (21) reported a controlled, randomized series showing a reduction of fluid requirements, faster healing, and reduced mortality when his patients were compared to controls and to U.S. National Burn Information Exchange standards. Waisbren (53), in 1982, reported a reduction in renal function, a decrease in circulating White Blood Cells (WBCs) and, an increase in positive blood cultures in a retrospective series of patients who had received hyperbaric oxygen therapy. He stated he could demonstrate neither a salutory nor deleterious effect; however, his data showed a 75% decrease in the need for grafting in the hyperbaric treated group. Grossman and colleagues (17, 18, 55) have reported a very large clinical series showing improved healing, reduced hospital stay, and reduced mortality. Merola (36) in 1978, in a randomized study, reported faster healing of partial thickness burns in 37 patients treated with HBO as compared to 37 untreated controls. Niu and his associates (39) from the Naval burn center in Taiwan, have reported a very large clinical series showing a statistically significant reduction in mortality in 266 seriously burned patients who received adjunctive hyperbaric oxygen, when compared to 609 control patients who did not receive this additional modality of therapy. Hammarlund and colleagues (20) have reported a reduction of edema and wound exudation in a carefully controlled series of human volunteers with ultraviolet irradiated blister wounds.

The author has shown a significant reduction in length of hospital stay in burns of up to 39% total body surface area (10).

Additionally, a reduction in the need for surgery, including grafting, in a series of patients with up to 80% burns, was noted when they were compared to non-HBO treated controls.

HBO-treated patients in this study experienced an average savings of $95,000 per case (8). In a series of patients with burns of up to 50% Total Body Surface Area (TBSA), averaging 28% total body surface area injury, similar results were obtained (12). In a retrospective, blinded review, this same group examined resuscitative fluid requirements in a group of severely burned patients. A 25% reduction in resuscitative fluid administration and a statistically significant reduction in maximum weight gain and percent weight gain were noted in the hyperbaric oxygen-treated group as compared to the controls (9). Maxwell and colleagues, in 1991, reported a small controlled series showing a reduction of surgery, resuscitative weight gain, intensive care days, total hospitalization time, wound sepsis, and cost of hospitalization in the hyperbaric oxygen-treated group (35). Data from our facility demonstrate continuing improvement in outcome of large burns, with a reduction of surgeries of 86% (p < 0.03) (11). Niezgoda and colleagues have demonstrated a similar reduction of wound exudate and wound size in a randomized, blinded study utilizing human volunteers with normoxic controls.

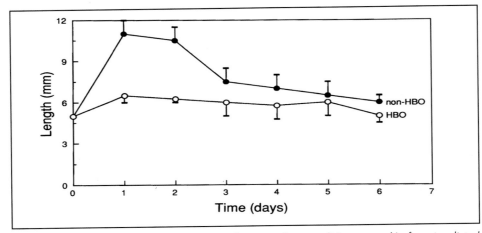

Figure 7. Maximum length (including edema adjacent to the wound) (mean ± s.d.) of u.v.-irradiated (•) and HBO-treated U.V.-irradiated (º) blister wounds as a function of time. The value on day 0 is approximately the diameter of the suction cup used to create the blister. (p<0.05)

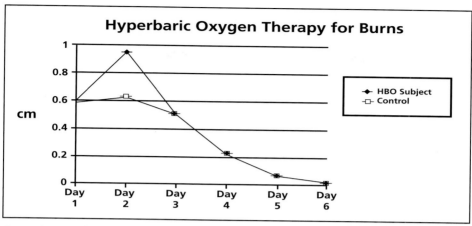

*Figure 8. Wound size measurements (cm) of ultraviolet-irradiated suction blister wounds in control group (□) and hyperbaric oxygen group (◆).*

Considerable attention has been given to the use of hyperbaric oxygen in inhalation injury. There is fear that it may cause worsening of pulmonary damage, particularly in those patients maintained on high levels of inspired $O_2$. Grim et al. (15), have studied products of lipid peroxidation in the exhaled gases in HBO-treated burn patients and found no indication of oxidative stress. Ray et al. (43), have analyzed serious burns being treated for concurrent inhalation injury, thermal injury, and adult respiratory distress syndrome. They noted no deleterious effect, even in those patients on continuous high inspired oxygen. More rapid weaning from mechanical ventilation was possible in the HBO-treated group (5.3 days vs. 26 days, $p < 0.05$). A significant saving in cost of care per case ($60,000) was effected in the HBO-treated patients ($p < 0.05$). There is presently no evidence to controvert these studies.

Brannan et al. (9), failed to show any reduction in length of stay or the number of surgical procedures in a recent study. The failure to demonstrate any reduction in surgical procedures is not surprising as both groups underwent very early and aggressive excision, thus invalidating an important study parameter. There was, however, a reduction in overall cost of care in the group treated with hyperbaric oxygen.

## SURGICAL PERSPECTIVES

Over the past 20 years, the pendulum has swung rapidly to an aggressive surgical management of the burn wound, i.e., tangential excision and early grafting of the deep second-degree, probable third-degree burns, especially to functionally important parts of the body. Hyperbaric oxygen, as adjunctive therapy, has allowed the surgeon yet another modality of treatment for these deep second-degree burns to the hands and fingers, face and ears, and other areas where the surgical technique of excision and coverage is often imprecise. These wounds, not obvious third degree, are then best treated with topical antimicrobial agents, bedside debridement, and adjunctive hyperbaric oxygen therapy, allowing the surgeon more time for healing to take place and definition of the extent and depth of injury (39). Adjunctive hyperbaric

## TABLE 1. COMPARISON OF FACTORS IN HBO AND NON-HBO GROUPS IN PATIENTS WITH 18-39% TBSA

| Variable | HBO (n=8) | Control (n=12) | |
|---|---|---|---|
| **Age** | | | |
| Average | 29.5 | 30.9 | |
| Range | 16-47 | 18-42 | p<0.57NS |
| Standard Deviation | 9.6 | 8.5 | |
| **Total Body Surface Burn (%)** | | | |
| Average | 24.0 | 25.8 | |
| Range | 20-33 | 18-39 | p<0.91NS |
| Standard Deviation | 4.3 | 7.6 | |
| **Full Thickness Injury** | | | |
| Average | 5.2 | 5.6 | |
| Range | 0-18 | 0.20 | p<0.96NS |
| Standard Deviation | 6.1 | 6.2 | |
| **Surgeries** | | | |
| Average | 1.3 | 1.7 | |
| Range | 0-2 | 0.3 | p<0.42NS |
| Standard Deviation | 0.88 | 1.2 | |
| **Days Hospitalized** | | | |
| Average | 20.8 | 33.0 | |
| Range | 16-33 | 16.58 | p<0.012* |
| Standard Deviation | 6.7 | 13.1 | |
| **Cost of Burn Care** | | | |
| Average | $44,838 | $55,650 | |
| Range | $27,600-$75,500 | $21,500 $98,700 | p,0.47NS |
| Standard Deviation | $9,200 | $11,300 | |

NS, Not Significant
*p<.012, significant (Mann-Whitney U test)

oxygen therapy has drastically reduced the healing time in the major burn injury, especially if the wounds are deep second degree (8, 10, 11, 35).

There is some theoretical benefit of hyperbaric oxygen therapy for obviously less well defined third-degree burns (29); fourth-degree burns, most commonly seen in high-voltage electrical injuries, are benefited by reduction in fascial compartmental pressures, as injured muscle swelling is lessened by preservation of aerobic glycolysis and later by a significant reduction of anaerobic infection.

Finally, reconstruction utilizing flaps and composite grafts, e.g., ear to nose grafts, has been greatly facilitated using this technique. Often the decision to use hyperbaric oxygen has been made intraoperatively as a surgeon is concerned about a compromised cutaneous or musculocutaneous flap. In many instances, the patient is prepared pre-operatively about the possibility of receiving this form of adjunctive therapy immediately after surgery.

## TABLE 2. COMPARISON OF CONTROLS AND HBO TREATED PATIENTS WITH 40-80% TBSA BURNS

| Variable | Control (n=7) | HBO (n=11) | HBO Since'87 (n=6) |
|---|---|---|---|
| **Age** | | | |
| Average | 26 | 31.3 | 35 |
| Range | 14-24 | 20-60 | 24-60 |
| **Total Body Surface Burn (%)** | | | |
| Average | 48% | 61.8% | 60% |
| Range | 40-60% | 45-80% | 40-80% |
| **Days Hospitalized** | | | |
| Average | 108 | 51.8 | 44.6 |
| Range | 47-184 | 22-95 | 22-80 |
| **Cost of Burn Care** | | | |
| Average | $391,000 | $215,000 | $200,000 |
| Range | $151,000-801,000 | $72,000-350,000 | $76,000-394,000 |
| **Surgeries** | | | |
| Average | 7.8 | 2.1 | 1.1 |
| Range | 3-12* | 0-6* | 0-6* |
| **Average HBO Tx** | | | |
| Average | 0 | 40 | 32 |
| Range | | 13-77 | 13-64 |
| **HBO Cost*** | | | |
| Average | 0 | $16,600 | $17,000 |
| Range | | $5,000-$23,000 | $5,000-$27,000 |
| **% Reduction** | | | |
| Days Hospitalized | | 53 | 86 |
| Surgeries | | 73 | 59 |
| Care cost | | 46 | 49 |

*p<0.03

## PATIENT SELECTION

Hyperbaric oxygen therapy is presently utilized to treat serious burns, i.e., greater than 20% total body surface area, partial or full thickness injury, or with involvement of the hands, face, feet or perineum. Patients with trivial burns or those not expected to survive are not accepted for therapy.

## TREATMENT PROTOCOLS

We utilize a twice-a-day regimen of 90 minutes at 2 atmospheres plus descent and ascent time. Treatments typically take 105 minutes. Treatment is rendered as soon as possible after injury, often during initial resuscitation.

## TABLE 3.

| Variable | HBO (n=6) | Control (n=6) | |
|---|---|---|---|
| **Age** | | | |
| Average | 25.7 ± 4.6 | 33.3 ± 9.8 | |
| Range | 20 - 31 | 14 - 42 | p=0.064NS |
| **Total Body Surface Burn (%)** | | | |
| Average | 61.7 ± 18.6 | 49.8 ± 8.5 | |
| Range | 40 - 80 | 40 - 60 | p=0.309NS |
| **Full Thickness Injury (%)** | | | |
| Average | 23.7 ± 21.3 | 23.5 ± 15.5 | |
| Range | 0 - 50 | 7 - 50 | p=0.818NS |
| **Surgeries** | | | |
| Average | 3.7 ± 2.6 | 8.0 ± 3.4 | |
| Range | 0 - 6 | 3 - 12 | p=0.04 |
| **Days Hospitalized** | | | |
| Average | 65.3 ± 23.4 | 111.0 ± 57.7 | |
| Range | 42 - 95 | 47 - 184 | p=0.132NS |
| **Total Cost of Burn Care** | | | |
| Average | $185,000 ± 90,500- | $292,300 ± 184,300 | |
| Range | $110,000 - 318,000 | $114,000 - 602,000 | p=0.309NS |
| **Cost of HBO\*** | $15,500 ± 10,000 | | |
| Average | $4,800 - 25,900 | | |

\*Eight percent of the total hospital bill.)
NS = Not Significant

Patients are carefully monitored during initial treatments until stable and as necessary thereafter. Children are treated for 45 minutes twice-a-day (17). In the monoplace configuration, we are now able to monitor blood pressure non-invasively using a special cuff. We attempt to treat three times in the first 24 hours and b.i.d. (twice daily) thereafter. Treatments are rendered twice during a normal workday, that is, a normal 8-10 hour period. Careful attention to fluid management is mandatory. Initial requirements of burn patients may be several liters per hour, and pumps capable of this delivery at pressure must be utilized in order to maintain appropriate fluid replacement. Patients can be maintained on ventilatory support during treatment. This is frequently the case in larger burns. Maintenance of a comfortable ambient temperature must be accomplished, and treating patients within two hours of tubbing or dressing changes is not recommended as temperature control may be difficult. Febrile patients must be closely monitored and fever controlled as $O_2$ toxicity is reported to be more common in this group. We have not observed evidence of $O_2$ toxicity in the patients we have treated.

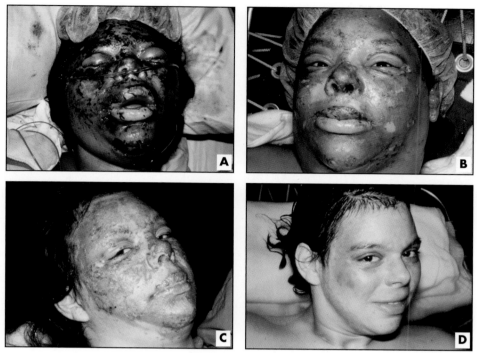

Figure 9A – 9D.
A. 23-year old white female with facial burns from flaming gasoline and tar 12 hours after injury.
B. 24 hours later (36 hours after injury) after two HBO treatments. Note resolution of edema.
C. 72 hours later (84 hours after injury) after six HBO treatments
D. Shortly before discharge.

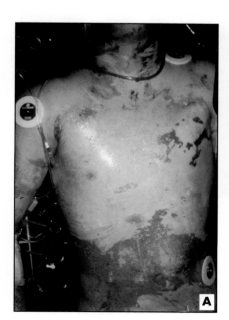

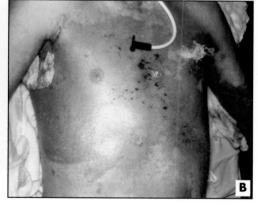

Figure 10A – 10B.
A. 19-year old white man with flame burn of chest from burning clothing estimated to be deep-partial to full-thickness burn.
B. One month later with no grafting required. Patient received adjunctive HBO therapy twice daily.

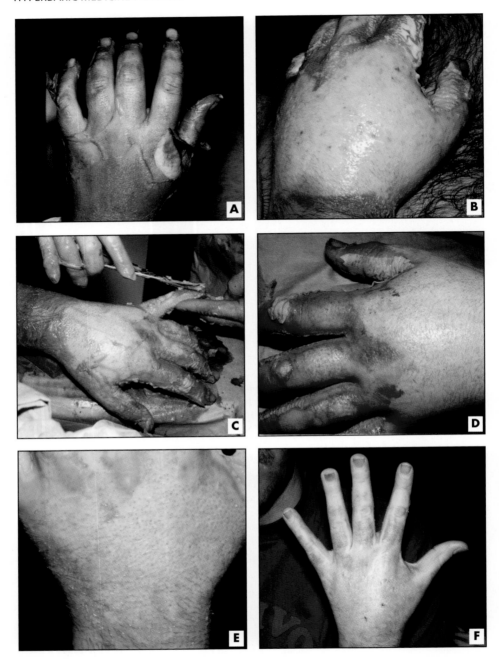

*Figure 11A – 11F.*
*A. Deep partial thickness burn of hand in 30-year old male with 60% total body surface burn and inhalation injury on admission.*
*B. 6 days later.*
*C. At surgery, light debridement.*
*D. Immediately after surgery. Note the preservation of dermal appendages.*
*E. Two weeks after admission. Note re-epithelialzation.*
*F. Appearance on discharge 25 days post-injury. Healed without grafting.*

Patients may be treated in a multiplace or monoplace hyperbaric chamber. Monoplace chamber treatment appears to be easier in terms of maintaining the patient environment, especially in head and neck burns. A multiplace chamber is obviously preferable, if available, for those patients who are hemodynamically unstable. Movement over long distances is not recommended. Patients should not be transported to a hyperbaric chamber that is not within the burn center facility. Careful attention to infection control is mandatory. In large burns of 40% TBSA or greater, treatment is rendered for 10-14 days in close consultation with the burn surgeon. Many partial thickness burns will heal without surgery during this time frame and obviate the need for grafting. Treatment beyond 30 sessions is usually utilized to ensure graft take. While there is no absolute limit to the number of hyperbaric treatments rendered, it is rare to exceed 40-50 except in very unusual circumstances.

## SIDE EFFECTS

Barotrauma to the ears is common, particularly in burns of the head and neck (44). Routine ear, nose, and throat (ENT) evaluation and early myringotomy are recommended in this subset of patients. We have established capabilities for myringotomy in our hyperbaric unit as this will often facilitate more rapid and more comfortable treatment.

In larger burn injuries, adequate fluid and electrolyte resuscitation during the first 24 hours can be problematic. Certain patients have developed hypotension shortly after exiting the chamber. We feel this represents hypovolemia that was masked during hyperbaric oxygen treatments. Careful volume replacement and assessment is mandatory prior to, during, and immediately after hyperbaric treatment. We have elected to increase fluids during ascent to compensate for any masked hypovolemia. We have not seen $O_2$ seizures or pulmonary toxicity in our patients.

## RECOMMENDATIONS

We recommend that units planning treatment of burn patients are thoroughly versed in the management of critical care patients in the hyperbaric setting, and to the peculiar problems of burn patients, prior to initiation of a therapy program. Patients with severe burns are among the most challenging encountered in medicine. The hyperbaric team must be experienced in the management of central lines, ventilators, and all aspects of critical care in the hyperbaric chamber. HBO treatment must be carefully coordinated to work around the busy schedule of the burn center. Our hyperbaric department is an extension of the burn center. Our personnel are trained in burn care and hyperbaric medicine and are an integral part in the "team approach" to burn care.

## SUMMARY

Current data show that hyperbaric oxygen therapy, when used as an adjunct in a comprehensive program of burn care, can significantly improve morbidity and mortality, reduce length of hospital stay, and lessen the need for surgery. It has been demonstrated to be safe in the hands of those thoroughly trained in rendering hyperbaric oxygen therapy in the critical care setting and with appropriate monitoring precautions. Careful patient selection and screening is mandatory.

## REFERENCES

1. Alexander JW, Meakins JL. "A physiological basis for the development of opportunistic infections in man." Annals of Surgery. 1972;176:273.

2. Alexander JW, Wilson D. "Neutrophil dysfunction and sepsis in burn injury." Surg Gynec Obstet. 1970;130:431.

3. Arturson G. "The pathophysiology of severe thermal injury." J Burn Care Rehabil. 1985;6(2):129-146.

4. Arturson G. "Pathophysiology of the burn wound." Ann Chir Gynaecol. 1980;66:178-190.

5. Bilic I, Petri NM, Bezic J, Alfirevic D, Modun D, Capkun V, Bota B. "Effects of hyperbaric oxygen therapy on experimental burn wound healing in rats: A randomized, controlled study." Undersea & Hyperbaric Medicine. 2005;32(1):1-9.

6. Bleser F, Benichoux R. "Experimental surgery: The treatment of severe burns with hyperbaric oxygen." J Chir. (Paris). 1973;106:281-290.

7. Boykin JV, Eriksson E, Pittman RN. "*In vivo* microcirculation of a scald burn and the progression of postburn ischemia." Plast and Recon Surg. 1980;66:191-198.

8. Brannen AL, Still J, Haynes M, Orlet H, Rosenblum F, Law E, Thompson WO. "A randomized prospective trial of hyperbaric oxygen in a referral burn center population." American Surgeon. 1997;63:205-208.

9. Cianci P, Lueders H, Lee H, Shapiro R, Sexton J, Williams C, Green B. "Adjunctive hyperbaric oxygen reduces the need for surgery in 40-80% burns." J Hyper Med. 1988;3:97-101.

10. Cianci P, Lueders H, Lee H, Shapiro R, Sexton J, Williams C, Green B. "Hyperbaric oxygen and burn fluid requirements: Observations in 16 patients with 40-80% TBSA burns." Undersea Biomed Research Suppl. 1988;15:14.

11. Cianci P, Lueders HW, Lee H, Shapiro RL, Sexton J, Williams C, Sato R. "Adjunctive hyperbaric oxygen therapy reduces length of hospitalization in thermal burns." J Burn Care Rehab. 1989;10:432-435.

12. Cianci P, Sato R, Green B. "Adjunctive hyperbaric oxygen reduces length of hospital stay, surgery, and the cost of care in severe burns." Undersea Biomed Research Suppl. 1991;18:108.

13. Cianci P, Williams C, Lueders H, Lee H, Shapiro R, Sexton J, Sato R. "Adjunctive hyperbaric oxygen in the treatment of thermal burns: An economic analysis." J Burn Care Rehab. 1990;11:140-143.

14. Deitch E, Wheelahan T, Rose M, Clothier J, Cotter J. "Hypertrophic burn scars: Analysis of variables." J Trauma. 1983;23:895-898.

15. Germonpre P, Reper P, Vanderkelen A. "Hyperbaric oxygen therapy and piracetam decrease the early extension of deep partial-thickness burns." Burns 1996;22(6):468-473.

16. Grim PS, Nahum A, Gottlieb L, Wilbert C, Hawe E, Sznajder J. "Lack of measurable oxidative stress during HBO therapy in burn patients." Undersea Biomed Research Suppl. 1989;16:22.

17. Grogan JB. "Altered neutrophil phagocytic function in burn patients." J Trauma. 1976;16:734.

18. Grossman AR. "Hyperbaric oxygen in the treatment of burns." Ann Plast Surg. 1978;1:163-171.

19. Grossman AR, Grossman AJ. "Update on hyperbaric oxygen and treatment of burns." HBO Review. 1982;3:51-59.

20. Gruber RP, Brinkley B, Amato JJ, Mendelson JA. "Hyperbaric oxygen and pedicle flaps, skin grafts, and burns." Plast and Recon Surg. 1970;45:24-30.

21. Hammarlund C, Svedman C, Svedman P. "Hyperbaric oxygen treatment of healthy volunteers with u.v.-irradiated blister wounds." Burns. 1991;17(4):296-301.

22. Hart GB, O'Reilly RR, Broussard ND, Cave RH, Goodman DB, Yanda RL. "Treatment of burns with hyperbaric oxygen." Surg Gynecol Obstet. 1974;139:693-696.

23. Hartwig VJ, Kirste G. "Experimentelle untersuchungen Ñber die revaskularisierung von verbrennungswunden unter hyperbarer sauerstofftherapie." Zbl Chir. 1974;99:1112-1117.

24. Heggers JP, Robson MC, Zachary LS. "Thromboxane inhibitors for the prevention of progressive dermal ischemia due to the thermal injury." J Burn Care Rehab. 1980;6:466-468.

25. Hohn DC, McKay RD, Halliday B, Hunt TK. "effect of oxygen tension on the microbicidal functiion of leukocytes in wounds and *in vitro*." Surg Forum 1976;27:18-20.

26. Hussman J, Hebebrand D, Erdmann D, Roth A, Kucan JO, Moticka J. "Lymphocyte subpopulations in spleen and blood after early wound debridement and acute/chronic treatment with hyperbaric oxygen." Hanchir Mikrochir Plast Chir 1996;28(2):103-107.

27. Ikeda K, Ajiki H, Kamiyama I, Wada J. "Clinical application of oxygen hyperbaric treatment." Geka (Japan) 1967;29:1279.

28. Ikeda K., Ajiki H, Nagao H, Karino K, Sugh S, Iwa T, Wada J. "Experimental and clinical use of hyperbaric oxygen in burns." Proceedings of the Fourth International Congress on Hyperbaric Med. J Wada and T Iwa, (Eds.) Tokyo: Igaku Shoin, Ltd., 1970;370-380.

29. Iwa T. Discussion. In: JW Brown and BG Cox, (Eds.) Proceedings of the Third International Conference on Hyperbaric Medicine. Washington, DC; National Academy of Science - National Research Council Publication No. 4, 1966;611-612.

30. Kaiser VW, Schnaidt U, Von der Lieth H. "Auswirkungen hyperbaren sauerstoffes auf die frische brandwunde." Handchir Mikrochir Plast Chir. 1989;21:158-163.

31. Ketchum SA, Thomas AN, Hall AD. "Angiographic studies of the effect of hyperbaric oxygen on burn wound revascularization." Proceedings of the Fourth International Congress on Hyperbaric Med. J Wada and T Iwa, (Eds.) Tokyo: Igaku Shoin, Ltd., 1970;388-394.

32. Ketchum SA, Zubrin JR, Thomas AN, Hall AD. "Effect of hyperbaric oxygen on small first, second and third degree burns." Surg Forum. 1967;18:65-67.

33. Korn HN, Wheeler ES, Miller TA. "Effect of hyperbaric oxygen on second-degree burn wound healing." Arch Surg. 1977;112:732-737.

34. Lamy ML, Hanquet MM. "Application opportunity for OHP in a general hospital - a two years experience with a monoplace hyperbaric oxygen chamber." Proceedings of the Fourth International Congress on Hyperbaric Med. J Wada and T Iwa, (Eds.) Tokyo: Igaku Shoin, Ltd., 1970;517-522.

35. Mader JT, Brown GL, Guckian JC, Wells CH, Reinarz JA. "A mechanism for the amelioration of hyperbaric oxygen of experimental staphylococcal osteomyelitis in rabbits." J Inf Disease. 1980;142:915-922.

36. Maxwell G, Meites H, Silverstein P. "Cost effectiveness of hyperbaric oxygen therapy in burn care." Winter Symp on Baromedicine. 1991.

37. Merola L, Piscitelli F. "Considerations on the use of HBO in the treatment of burns." Ann Med Nav. 1978;83:515-526.

38. Niccole MW, Thornton JW, Danet RT, Bartlett RH, Tavis MJ. "Hyperbaric oxygen in burn management: A controlled study." Surgery. 1977;82:727-733.

39. Niezgoda JA, Cianci P, Folden BW, Ortega RL, Slade JB, Storrow AB. "The effect of hyperbaric oxygen therapy on a burn wound model in human volunteers." Plast Reconstr Surg 1997;99(6):1620-1625.

40. Niu AKC, Yang C, Lee HC, Chen SH, Chang LP. "Burns treated with adjunctive

hyperbaric oxygen therapy: A comparative study in humans." J Hyper Med. 1987;2:75-86.

41. Nylander G, Nordström H, Eriksson E. "Effects of hyperbaric oxygen on oedema formation after a scald burn." Burns. 1984;10:193-196.

42. Ogle CK, Alexander JW, Nagy H, Wood S, Palkert D, Carey M, Ogle JD, Warden GD. "A long-term study and correlation of lymphocyte and neutrophil function in the patient with burns." J Burn Care Rehab. 1990;11(2):105-111.

43. Perrins DJD. "Failed attempt to limit tissue destruction in scalds of pig's skin with hyperbaric oxygen. Proceedings of the Fourth International Congress on Hyperbaric Med. J Wada and T Iwa, (Eds.) Tokyo: Igaku Shoin, Ltd., 1970;381-387.

44. Ray CS, Green B, Cianci P. "Hyperbaric oxygen therapy in burn patients: Cost effective adjuvant therapy (poster presentation). Undersea Biomed Res Suppl. 1991;18:77.

45. Ross JC, Cianci PE. "Barotitis media resulting from hyperbaric oxygen therapy. A retrospective study of 395 consecutive cases." Undersea Biomed Res Suppl. 1990;17:102.

46. Saunders J, Fritz E, Ko F, Bi C, Gottlieb L, Krizek T. "The effects of hyperbaric oxygen on dermal ischemia following thermal injury." Proc of Am Burn Assoc. 1989;58.

47. Shoshani O, Shupak A, Barak A, Ullman Y, Ramon Y, Lindenbaum E, Peled Y. "Hyperbaric oxygen therapy for deep second degree burns: an experimental study in the guinea pig." Brit J Plast Surg 1998;51:67-73.

48. Stewart RJ, Yamaguchi KT, Cianci PE, Knost PM, Samadani BA, Mason SW, Roshdieh BB. "Effects of hyperbaric oxygen on adenosine triphosphate in thermally injured skin." Surg Forum. 1988;39:87-90.

49. Stewart RJ, Yamaguchi KT, Cianci PE, Mason SW, Roshdieh BB, Dabbass N. "Burn wound levels of ATP after exposure to elevated levels of oxygen." Proc of the Am Burn Assoc. 1989;67.

50. Tabor CG. "Hyperbaric oxygenation in the treatment of burns of less than forty percent." Korean J Int Med. 1967.

51. Tenenhaus M, Hansbrough JF, Zapata-Sirvent R, Neumann T. "Treatment of burned mice with hyperbaric oxygen reduces mesenteric bacteria but not pulmonary neutrophil deposition." Arch Surg 1994;129(12):1338-1342.

52. Wada J, Ikeda K, Kegaya H, Ajiki H. "Oxygen hyperbaric treatment and severe burn." Jap Med J. 1966;13:2203.

53. Wada J, Ikeda T, Kamata K, Ebuoka M. "Oxygen hyperbaric treatment for carbon monoxide poisoning and severe burn in coal mine (Hokutanyubari) gas explosion." Igakunoaymi (Japan) 1965;54:68.

54. Waisbren BA, Schultz D, Collentine G, Banaszak E, Stern M. "Hyperbaric oxygen in severe burns." Burns. 1982;8:176-179.

55. Wells CH, Hilton JG. "Effects of hyperbaric oxygen on post-burn plasma extravasation." Hyperbaric Oxygen Therapy. JC Davis and TK Hunt, (Eds). Undersea Medical Society, Inc., 1977;p259-265.

56. Wiseman DH, Grossman AR. "Hyperbaric oxygen in the treatment of burns." Crit Care Clin. 1985;2:129-145.

57. Zamboni WA, Roth AC, Russell RC, Graham B, Suchy H, Kucan JO. "Morphologic analysis of the microcirculation during reperfusion of ischemic skeletal muscle and the effect of hyperbaric oxygen." Plast Reconstr Surg 1993;91(6):1110-1123.

58. Zamboni WA, Stephenson LL, Roth AC, Suchy H, Russell RC. "Ischemia-reperfusion injury in skeletal muscle: CD18 dependent neutrophil-endothelial adhesion." Undersea & Hyperbaric Medicine 1994, (Suppl to Vol 21), 53.

# SECTION III
# HYPERBARIC OXYGEN USED IN OFF-LABEL DISORDERS AND INVESTIGATIONAL AREAS

The following chapters deal with disorders that have not yet been approved by the UHMS Hyperbaric Oxygen Committee even though some have had good clinical success. Those that have shown selective value clinically include Fungal Disease, Brown Recluse Spider bite, Incomplete or Functional Ileus following surgery, Femoral Head Necrosis, Myocardial Infarction, and Hansen's Disease. The others are strictly investigational.

CHAPTER 34

# FEMORAL HEAD NECROSIS AND HYPERBARIC OXYGEN THERAPY

## CHAPTER THIRTY-FOUR OVERVIEW

# FEMORAL HEAD NECROSIS AND HYPERBARIC OXYGEN THERAPY

*Michael B. Strauss, Tomas Dvorak, Yehuda Melamed, Daniel N. Reis*

## INTRODUCTION

Non-traumatic osteonecrosis (ON) also known as avascular necrosis of bone (AVN) is a potentially disabling condition affecting mainly young adults at the prime of their lives. Historically necrosis of the head of the femur has been in the forefront of the treatment of osteonecrosis because of its frequency and its potential for serious disability. Therefore almost all published material on the use of HBO in osteonecrosis is on this subject.

The precise cause of the disease is as yet unknown. In traumatic ON the femoral head is also the commonest site following a sub-capital fracture in the elderly or a dislocation of the hip joint in a young age group. Here a disruption of the arterial blood supply is the primary cause.

The various aspects of ON are dealt with extensively in orthopedic and rheumatologic text books (1) and ongoing reviews (2, 3, 4).

## ETIOLOGY AND PATHOGENESIS

Sites particularly vulnerable to ischaemic necrosis are the femoral head, the femoral condyles, the head of the humerus, the capitulum and the proximal parts of the talus and scaphoid. These sub-articular localities lie at the most remote part of the bone's vascular tree and are enclosed by cartilage, restricting access to local blood vessels.

The sub-chondral bone is supplied by endarterioles having very little collateral circulation. The vascular sinusoids of bone have no adventitia and therefore their patency depends on the volume of fluid in, and pressure exerted by, the surrounding marrow, the whole being encased on an unyielding bony cortex. In such an enclosed compartment one element can expand only at the expense of the others. Hence lessened blood flow, bleeding, or any cause of marrow swelling can lead rapidly to a vicious cycle of ischaemia, more reactive oedema, increasing intraosseous pressure and additional ischaemia. This pathogenetic process may come about by the severance of the local arteries, venous stasis with retrograde arteriolar occlusion, intravascular thrombosis, or simply by the compression of the sinusoids and capillaries by local marrow oedema. This ischaemia leads to cell death. Eventually the dead bone, particularly when weakened by osteoclastic resorbtion, cannot withstand repeated cyclical loading resulting in collapse of the subchondral bone and the irreversible disruption of the joint surface which in turn causes a progressive osteoarthritic process (5).

In traumatic ON the aetiology is clearly the disruption of the vascular anatomy such as occurs commonly in intracapsular fracture of the neck of the femur. In non-traumatic ON the pathogenetic pathways are complex and poorly understood but lead to the same vicious circle of events. Many cases have a pathological background of steroid treatment, alcoholism, storage disease, haemoglobinopathy, dysbaric injury, or coagulation disorder (Table 1 presents a detailed list of conditions associated with avascular necrosis of bone). There remains a large group of so called idiopathic cases in which the cause is unknown.

When blood supply is totally interrupted, osteocytes begin to lose their viability within 12 hours. Histologic changes become evident 48 hours later. Soon thereafter, bone marrow edema changes may be recognized on magnetic resonance imaging. Because bone remodeling changes are slower to occur, radiologic changes do not become evident until 2 months after the injury (6).

In the initial stages of femoral head necrosis (FHN), cell death results in cytogenic edema and initiation of the inflammatory response. These are believed to be the cause of pain, which is usually the presenting symptom. Swelling in the confined space of the femoral head is thought to lead to a localized compartment syndrome (7). Later, during the remodeling, reparative process, granulation tissue grows into the injury site and dead bone is reabsorbed by osteoclasts. If the remaining mixture of necrotic bone, live bone, and granulation tissue is insufficient to provide structural integrity for the femoral head, collapse of the femoral head, loss of articular congruity, and arthritic changes occur. New bone may be formed during the reparative phase around the dead, collapsed bone, causing a sclerotic, hyperdense appearance on x-ray. Glueck reports that underlying thrombophilia or hypofibrinolysis were present in approximately 70% of the cases in their FHN series (8). Prior to this information, most presentations of FHN were thought to be idiopathic, although steroid use, trauma, alcoholism, hyperlipidemia conditions, coagulopathies and decompression sickness can all cause FHN, as well (Table 1; 9).

## MANAGEMENT

The management of FHN is an unresolved orthopedic problem. (10) The observation that multiple approaches are used for management of this problem suggests that no single approach yields uniformly good results. The outcomes from total hip arthroplasties (THA) in patients with FHN are less satisfactory than the outcomes of virtually any other group of THA patients (10). The majority of FHN patients are young, by THA criteria, and have life expectancy that makes arthroplasty revisions probable during their lifetime. The complication rates and likelihood of poor outcomes increase with each successive THA revision surgery. Consequently, any intervention that will preserve the femoral head and delay or eliminate the need for THA deserves consideration (10, 11, 12, 13). Hyperbaric oxygen (HBO) therapy has been used as an adjunct to manage FHN (Table 2).

## TABLE 1. PATHOLOGIES ASSOCIATED WITH OSTEONECROSIS (9)

| PATHOLOGY GROUP | PATHOLOGY | FREQUENCY |
|---|---|---|
| Trauma | Fractures, Dislocations, Vascular Trauma, Burns | Common; in uncommon burns |
| Idiophatic | | Common |
| Dietary or Environmental Factors | Dysbaric Conditions (Decompression Illness), Alcohol Abuse, Cigarette Smoking | Common |
| Iatrogenic | Corticosteroids, Radiation Exposure, Hemodialysis, Organ Transplantation, Cytotoxic Therapy, Laser Surgery, Hip Surgery | Common |
| Hematologic | Hemoglobinopathies (Sickle-Cell Anemia, Thalassemia), Disseminated Intravascular Coagulation, Other Coagulopathies, Polycythemia, Hemophilia | Common |
| Metabolic/ Endocrinologic | Hypercholesterolemia, Gout, Hyperparathyroidism, Pregnancy, Hemochromatosis, Hyperlipidemia, Cushing Disease, Chronic Renal Failure, Gaucher Disease, Diabetes, Obesity, Fabry Disease | Less common Common in Chronic Renal Failure |
| Neoplastic Congenital | Marrow Infiltrative Disorders, Gaucher's Disease | Less common |
| Gastrointestinal | Pancreatitis, Inflammatory Bowel Disease | Less Common |
| Infectious | Osteomyelitis, HIV, Meningococciemia | Less common |
| Vascular/ Rheumathologic/ Connective Tissue Disorders | Lupis, Polymyositis, Polymyalgia Rheumatica, Raynaud Disease, Rheumatoid Arthritis, Ankylosing Spondolytis, Siögren Syndrome, Giant Cell Arteritis, Thrombophlebitis, Fat Embolism, Ehler-Danlos Syndrome | Less common Common in SLE |
| Orthopedic Problems | Slipped Capital Femoral Epiphysis, Congenital Hip Dislocation, Hereditary Dysostosis, Legg-Calvé-Perthes Disease | Less Common Common in Legg-Calvé-Perthes Disease |

The rationale for commonly used interventions for FHN, including HBOT is summarized in Table 3.

In addition, outcomes from natural history (non-intervention) and treatment interventions are meta-analyzed in Table 4.

Since treatment differs according to the stage of the disease, staging is an essential step in the management.

## TABLE 2. FEMORAL HEAD NECROSIS OUTCOMES WITH HYPERBARIC OXYGEN THERAPY THROUGH 1997

| AUTHOR | HIPS | SURVIVAL (%) 12-24 MONTHS | SURVIVAL (%) > 24 MONTHS | COMMENT |
|---|---|---|---|---|
| Baixe[6] (1969) France | 41 | 41/41 (100) | - - - | 20 HBO (1 Hr) sessions at 2.8 ATA. Excellent pain reduction and very good functionality; moderate radiological improvement. |
| Conti[20] (1969) France | 5 | 4/5 | - - - | 10-20 (1Hr) HBO sessions at 2 ATA. Improvement in pain and function; no radiological improvement. |
| Sainty[102] (1983) France | 9 | 7/9 (78) | - - - | 10-42 (1 Hr) HBO sessions a 2.2-2.5 ATA; Pain was lessened in nearly every case. |
| Lepawski[67] (1983) Canada | 1 | - - - | 1/1 (100 0 | 19-year-old female renal transplant patient on steroids with bilateral FHN; significant reduction in pain and return to ambulation. |
| Mao[73] (1986) China | 20 | 17/20 (85) | - - - | Outcomes better on young adults with known etiologies, and on early cases. |
| Neubauer[90] (1989) USA | 1 | 1/1 (100) | - - - | 108 (1.5 Hr) HBO sessions at 2.2-2.4 ATA; excellent clinical improvement and x-ray reversal of FHN lesion size. |
| Sanchez[104] (1990) Mexico | 1 | 1/1 (100) | - - - | 60 (1.5 Hr) HBO sessions at 2-2.4 ATA; bone scan showed improved arterial blood flow to the femoral head. |
| Turanti[132] (1991) Italy | 36 | 32/36 (90) | - - - | 75 (1.25 Hr) HBO sessions at 2-2.4 ATA; 2-year follow-up 100% reduction in pain in Ficat Stages I & II. |
| Iapicca[46] (1992) Italy | 15 | - - - | 13/15 (87) | 20 (1.25 Hr) HBO sessions at 2.2 ATA; 2.5-year follow-up 100% reduction in pain in Ficat Stages I & II. |
| Iwata[49] (1993) Japan | 12 | - - - | 8/12 (67) | Clinical improvement with HBO. |
| Maronna[77] (1996) Germany | 38 | - - - | 28/38 (74) | Completew remission and/or clinical improvement in Ficat stages I & II. |
| Ramon*[98] (1997) Israel | 21 | 17/21 (81) | - - - | Follow-up results reported at 3 months 50 HBO sessions; significalnt healing of FHN using MRI criteria. |
| Lepawski**[68] (1997) Canada | 5 | 5/5 (100) | - - - | 30-40 HBO sessions with significant pain relief in all 5 hips. |
| Stein[116] (1995) israel | 4 | - - - | 4/4 (100) | 60-100  HBO Sessions; excellent results in all 4 hips. HBO reserved for Ficat Stage III hips in conjunction with pedicle bone grafting. |
| Strauss[124] (1997) USA | 6 | 2/4 (50) | 2/2 (100) | 30-40 (1.5 Hr) HBO sessions; Ficat Stage I - III. One military patient with 100 HBO treatments |

* Study not included in meta-analysis, since reporting of results did not satisfy our criteria (follow-up period was less than 12 months)
** Personal communication

* Study not included in meta-analysis since reporting of results did not satisfy our criteria (follow-up period was less than 12 months).
** Personal communication

## TABLE 3. RATIONALE FOR FHN INTERVENTIONS

| MODALITY | PRIMARY RATIONALE | SECONDARY RATIONALE | COMPLICATIONS | REFERENCES |
|---|---|---|---|---|
| Core Decompression | Relieve pressure (Compartment Syndrome) by decompression. | Allow access channel for revascularization. | Femoral neck fracture. | 3,36,84,97 |
| Osteotomy | Change weight distribution in the affected area of femoral head. | Possibly stimulate new blood suply through osteotomy healing site. | Abnnormal femoral head mechanics. | 5,26,82,129 |
| Bone Graft | Support femoral head. | Augment blood supply Decompress femoral head. | Long surgical times using micro-vascular techniques. Pain and donor site dysfunction. | 38,80,133, 136 |
| Electrical Stimulation | Stimulation of osteogenesis. | Possible stimulation of revascularization. | - - - | 2,8,117,129 |
| Pharmacological | Counteract thrombophilia & hypofibrinogenemia states. | – | Bleeding. | 31 |
| HBO | Oxygenation of ischemic bone cells. Edema reduction. | Revascularization Osteogenesis. | Possibly increased vulnerability to collapse during remodeling. | 4,12,18,34, 45,50,108, 111,123 |

## TABLE 4. SUMMARY OF OUTCOMES

| MODALITY | ANALYSIS CRITERIA | HIPS | SURVIVAL (%) < 24 MONTHS | SURVIVAL (%) > 24 MONTHS | REFERENCES |
|---|---|---|---|---|---|
| Natural History | Yes | 268 | 10/11 (91%) | 82/257 (32%) | 8,14,23,25,44,52,54,57,58, 60,65,84,86,87,93,94,100, 103,117,118,119,127,130, 131 |
| | No | 574 | 113/271 (42%) | 95/303 (331%) | |
| | **Total** | **842** | **123/282 (44%)** | **177/560 (32%)** | |
| Core Decom-pression | Yes | 1405 | 95/182 (52%) | 724/1223 (59%) | 1,3,11,18,19,27,29,41,42,43, 53,57,59,62,63,64,75,76,83, 84,97,100,103,105,109,112, 114,115,125,127,131,135 |
| | No | 101 | 16/17 (94%) | 25/84 (30%) | |
| | **Total** | **1506** | **111/199 (56%)** | **749/1307 (57%)** | |
| Bone Grafting | Yes | 415 | 16/20 (80%) | 311/395 (79%) | 7,9,11,13,17,27,30,37,38,39, 53,66,69,70,71,72,74,79,85, 89,95,101,103,107,110,113, 118,120,133,136,139,141 |
| | No | 460 | 21/21 (100%) | 290/439 (66%) | |
| | **Total** | **875** | **37/41 (90%)** | **601/834 (72%)** | |
| Osteotomy | Yes | 291 | None | 228/291 (78%) | 5,9,10,22,24,26,28,35,40,47, 48,52,55,56,61,82,92,99,103, 106,128,129,140 |
| | No | 354 | 41/48 (85%) | 223/306 (73%) | |
| | **Total** | **645** | **41/48 (85%)** | **451/597 (76%)** | |
| Electrical Stimulation | Yes | 145 | None | 108/145 (74%)* | 1,2,8,117,119 |
| | No | 22 | 19/22 (86%)** | None | |
| | **Total** | **167** | **19/22 (86%)** | **108/145 (74%)** | |
| HBO | Yes | 27 | None | 21/27 (78%) | 6,20,46,49f,67,68,73,77f,90, 98,102,104,116f,124f,132 |
| | No | 162 | 83/86 (97%) | 62/76 (82%) | |
| | **Total** | **189** | **83/86 (97%)** | **83/103 (81%)** | |

* Includes two studies with bone grafting and electrical stimulation
** Includes one studies with bone grafting and electrical stimulation
f Some patients had HBO treatments combined with other orthopaedic interventions

## Staging Avascular Necrosis of the Head of the Femur

The advent of magnetic resonance imaging (MRI) as the most sensitive diagnostic tool for the diagnosis of the earliest stages of ON has resulted in the Steinberg classification (Table 5) which includes all the MRI criteria.

## Treatment Modalities

The aim of all treatments for the early stages of the disease is to preserve the sphericity of the femoral head. Non-weight bearing for extended periods is necessary and common to all treatments. Medullary decompression, a variety of bone grafting techniques, osteotomies, and electrical stimulation have met with unpredictable success. In general the better results were achieved when treating stages I and II (2-4). More recently the administration of bisphosphonates has been shown to lesson the incidence of femoral head collapse (15-17). From stage III onwards, in which the subchondral bone is fractured, there is little hope in preventing the collapse of the head and

## TABLE 5. STEINBERG CLASSIFICATION OF FEMORAL HEAD NECROSIS (14)

| STAGE | CRITERIA |
|---|---|
| 0 | Normal or non-diagnostic X-Ray, MRI and/or Bone Scan |
| I | Pain - Normal X-Ray - abnormal MRI and/or Bone Scan<br>A – Mild        (< 15% of head)<br>B – Moderate    (15% - 30%)<br>C – Severe      (> 30%) |
| II | Sclerotic changes or cystic lesions<br>A – Mild        (< 15%)<br>B – Moderate    (15% - 30%)<br>C – Severe      (> 30%) |
| III | Subchondral fracture without flattening<br>A – Mild        (< 15% of articular surface)<br>B – Moderate    (15% - 30%)<br>C – Severe      (> 30%) |
| IV | Flattening of the femoral head<br>A – Mild        (< 15% of surface and < 2 mm depression)<br>B – Moderate    (15% - 30% of surface or 2-4 mm depression)<br>C – Severe      (> 30% of surface and > 4 mm depression) |
| V | Joint narrowing and/or acetabular involvement<br>A – Mild<br>B – Moderate<br>C – Severe |
| VI | Advanced degenerative changes |

progressive arthritic changes, leading finally to the need to perform a hip joint replacement. Therefore hyperbaric oxygen (HBO) treatment is suited only for stages I and II.

## HYPERBARIC OXYGEN AS AN INTERVENTION FOR FHN

Many interventions have been used to alter the natural history of FHN. These include surgical procedures such as core decompression, bone grafting, and osteotomy, and non-surgical procedures such as electrical stimulation, pharmacological treatment (to manage coagulopathy problems), and hyperbaric oxygen. Each intervention has a primary mechanism for altering the underlying pathophysiology of FHN; many also have secondary mechanisms. Unfortunately, undesirable side effects can be associated with treatment interventions for FHN. See Table 2.

### Rationale of HBO Treatment

The known effects of HBO treatment which creates a high concentration of dissolved oxygen in the plasma specifically counteract the above described pathogenetic pathways: HBO rapidly and powerfully reduces oedema (due to the oxygen osmotic pump (18) and vasoconstriction phenomena) and thereby reduces the intraosseous pressure bringing about an improvement in venous drainage and in the microcirculation. This improves oxygen delivery to the site of the pathology. By flooding the extracellular fluid with diffused oxygen, oxygen becomes available to the ischaemic bone cells without the need for circulating haemoglobin and without the energy normally required for the disassociation of oxygen from the haemoglobin (see the chapter entitled "The Physiologic Effects of Hyperbaric Oxygenation"). HBO stimulates angiogenesis, a process needed for the healing of ON. Furthermore osteoclast and osteoblast function is $PO_2$ dependent and is therefore stimulated by the high level of $PO_2$ (6).

Oxygen is necessary for bone viability, healing, and remodeling (19, 20, 21). Osteocytes, the "resting" bone cells, have the lowest requirement for oxygen; hence, they have the ability to tolerate traumatic ischemia for up to 12 hours (6). Osteoblasts, the bone-forming cell, have an intermediate oxygen requirement. This is reflected in an eight-fold or greater blood flow increase in healing fractures. Finally, osteoclasts, the bone-resorbing cells, have the highest oxygen requirement. Their metabolic activity may be 100 times greater than the osteocyte's (6). Bassett reported that multipotential cell precursors of fibroblastic origin form bone when exposed to increased oxygen tensions and compressive forces. However, when oxygen tensions were low, cartridge was formed (22). Studies have shown beneficial effects of HBO on mobilization of bone precursors, osteoid formation, and fracture healing (23, 24, 25, 26, 27, 28). Coulson stated that the great advantage of the early use of HBO for bone healing is that it provides "an availability of oxygen to cells with osteogenic potential at a time when hemoglobin-borne oxygen is not generally available" (29). Increased oxygen enhances bone resorption and remodeling through stimulation of the osteoclasts (30, 31, 32, 33, 34, 35, 36). Since FHN is a challenge to the body's bone repair mechanisms, HBO is a logical intervention and as said before it has the potential to specifically mitigate the pathophysiology of FHN.

To summarize the primary effects of HBO in FHN are two-fold. First, it improves oxygen tension in tissue fluids at the site of bone necrosis. This prevents further loss of ischemic bone cells that is thought to occur because of the early, diffuse, self-perpetuating effects of edema and ischemia. Second, hyperbaric oxygen-induced vasoconstriction directly decreases edema, (37, 38, 39) which allows better perfusion to the injury site as would be expected if the symptoms are due to a compartment syndrome. This may provide an explanation of why early pain relief is observed with HBO treatments. With vasoconstriction plus hyperoxygenation, blood inflow to an injury site is reduced while oxygenation and blood outflow is maintained. The secondary effect of HBO is to enhance the reparative process by providing an improved oxygen environment for osteoclastic function, angiogenesis and osteogenesis (40). A concern about using HBO for FHN is that the hyperoxic effect will preferentially stimulate osteoclastic resorption of dead bone and make the femoral head more vulnerable to collapse (33, 41, 42). In one HBO series, pain symptoms resolved after 30 treatments, but later bone collapse occurred in some patients (34). However, more recent reported series do not demonstrate this to be a problem (Table 2). Improved long-term outcomes, including radiological improvements, were observed in patients who received 100 or more HBO treatments (35).

## META-ANALYSIS: MATERIALS, METHODS, AND RESULTS

We performed a comprehensive review of articles and abstracts in which no interventions (the natural history group), or various orthopedic interventions were used for management of FHN. As mentioned previously, we also summarized all reported cases where HBO was used for managing this problem. We located over 4,200 cases of FHN, which included 189 HBO cases. In order to compare reports that used different grading systems, outcome criteria, or follow-up time periods, we established the following criteria for analysis: (43) the information was available from a published article or abstract, (44) the severity of the FHN in the publication was graded using one of the standard classification systems (Table 6).

The necrotic index, which is a summation of the arcs of bone necrosis in anterior and lateral x-ray projections, was not considered in this review, since only a few articles used these measurements. We only reviewed those cases which were classified in stages I - III. See Table 7. Most reports indicate that outcomes in stages IV and higher are poor regardless of interventions, due to collapse of the femoral head and advanced hip joint arthrosis. Patients with this degree of involvement almost always require total hip arthroplasty (45, 10, 11, 12, 13). The follow-up period was at least 12 months to allow sufficient time for negative outcomes to occur. If a report met the grading system criteria, it was included in the primary analysis; if it did not, it was analyzed in a secondary analysis of all reported cases.

Outcomes were classified as either a success or a failure. In a successful outcome, the involved hip remained functional and was essentially pain free. In a failure, the clinical outcome was unsatisfactory due to pain and loss of function, the patient was awaiting or received a total hip replacement, x-rays demonstrated radiological progression to femoral head collapse, or any combination of these. Follow-up duration was separated into short-term

## TABLE 6. FEMORAL HEAD CLASSIFICATION SYSTEMS (IMAGING CRITERIA)

| STAGE | FICAT[29] CLASSIFICATION | MARCUS[74] CLASSIFICATION | STEINBERG[118] CLASSIFICATION | USED FOR META-ANALYSIS |
|---|---|---|---|---|
| 0 | Not designated | Not designated | Normal or equivocal radiograph, bone scan, and MRI. | No |
| I | Normal or equivocal radiograph, bone scan, and MRI. | Normal or equivocal radiograph, bone scan, and MRI. | Normal radiograph, abnormal bone scan and/or MRI. | Yes |
| II | IIA: Diffuse porosis, sclerosis, or cyst IIB: Flattening or crescent sign. | Sclerotic or cystic lesions. | Abnormal radiograph showing cystic and sclerotic changes. | Yes |
| III | Broken contour of head. | Cresent sign. | Subchondral collapse producing crescent sign without flattening. | Yes |
| IV | Decreased joint space, flattened countour, collapse of head. | Step-off in outline of subchondral bone. | Flattening of femoral head without joint narrowing. | No |
| V | Not designated | Narrowing of cartilage space with degenerative changes. | Joint narrowing with or without acatabular involvement. | No |
| VI | Not designated | Not designated | Advanced degenerative changes. | No |

survival for outcomes reported for 12 to 24 months, and long-term survival for outcomes reported longer than 24 months. When data on individual patients were not available, the mean follow-up duration of the group was used for assignment into 12-24 months, or greater than 24 months categories.

### Results of the Mata-Analysis

Four thousand two hundred twenty four (4,224) case reports were included in the study. See Tables 2 and 4. Of these, 842 (20%) had no interventions and comprised the natural history group. In this control group, the long-term successful outcomes were 32%. In the orthopedic intervention group there were 3,193 (76%) cases reported. Successful outcomes were reported in 66% of the long-term cases. Finally, 189 (4%) of the reported cases were managed with hyperbaric oxygen therapy. In this group 81% of the long-term outcomes were successful. See Figure 1.

## ADDENDUM

### New studies supporting the use of HBO for FHN.

Not included in the meta-analysis is a unique study by Reis et al. (Hyperbaric oxygen therapy as a treatment for stage I avascular necrosis of the

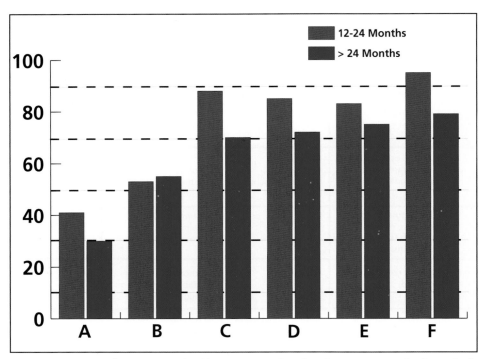

Figure 1. Percntage of success rate: A = No intervention, B = Core Decompression, C = Bone Graft, D = Electrical Stimulation, E = Osteotomy, F = Hyperbaric Oxygen.

femoral head. Journal Bone Joint Surgery 2003:85-B:375) who have reported a limited controlled clinical trial of stage I AVN (avascular necrosis) of the head of the femur treated by HBO and followed up by MRI studies (The protocol used was 100% oxygen at 2-2.4 ATA for 90 minutes daily). The follow up MRI was done after 60 sessions: a return to a normal MRI signified the cessation of HBO treatment; an MRI which still showed abnormality was an indication to continue a further 30 sessions. They report that overall, 81% of patients who received HBO therapy showed a return to normal on MRI as compared with 17% in the untreated group (47). They therefore concluded that hyperbaric oxygen is effective in the treatment of stage-I AVN of the head of the femur. Vezzani et al. (personal communication) abandoned their protocol in a controlled prospective trial of HBO in stage II AVN of the femoral head because they felt it unethical not to give HBO after finding a significant advantage in the HBO treated group.

Furthermore, in keeping with Vezzani et al.'s results, they found that stage II AVN is frequently arrested and its progression prevented by HBO therapy. During the period 1996-2004 they treated 9 cases of stage II idiopathic AVN: in 8 preservation of the sphericity of the head was achieved and 1 collapsed and required a total hip arthroplasty. Even in steroid or trauma induced disease (24 cases of grade I and II AVN), which is usually considered to have a worse prognosis, the progression was arrested in 14 cases (MRI appearance unchanged), in 4 there was an improvement (MRI showed reduction in lesion size), and in 3 the marrow oedema disappeared but the lesion remained unchanged, and 3 the head has collapsed and a hip arthroplasty was performed (Melamed and Reis unpublished material)

HBO treatment may also have a role in the prevention of post-traumatic AVN such as threatens fractures of the talus, the carpal and tarsal scaphoids, and lunate dislocations.

## ANIMAL EXPERIMENTAL STUDIES

The stimulation of bone healing and remodeling by HBO in a rabbit model FHN has been demonstrated (50). It was found that the resulting increased oxygen tension of the tissues provided the optimal settings for reparative processes. Paradoxically, rapid healing was associated with the collapse of the head (49). These results suggest that hyperoxygenation mediates relief of ischemia, and thereby enhances the fibroblastic, angioblastic, osteoblastic, and osteoclastic activities so that healing of the femoral heads is expedited. Strict non-weightbearing is critical for the preservation of the shape of the head especially during remodeling when osteoclastic activity may outstrip osteoblastic new bone formation. Collapse of the head during the remodeling process may be prevented by bisphosphonates.

## DISCUSSION

Although the number of HBO-managed subjects is small compared to the natural history and orthopedic intervention groups, a number of observations can be made. First, the meta-analysis further validates the reports that interventions do improve outcomes of FHN, when compared to the natural history of this disorder. All interventions, including HBOT, had successful outcomes double or more than those of the natural history group. Second, outcomes were similar between each intervention, regardless of whether the report met the analysis criteria or not. Even though most of the HBO patients did not meet the analysis criteria we established, we felt it reasonable to include them in this meta-analysis, since the other outcomes were similar, regardless of meeting the analysis criteria or not. Third, some of the reported follow-ups were of relatively short duration. The short term, a 12 to 24-month follow-up, is sufficient to define a treatment failure; however, there is no consensus about what time period should define a treatment success. For successful outcomes, the short time interval has little meaning, since the goal is for the involved hip to last a lifetime. Nonetheless, any intervention that delays a total hip replacement for even a short period is considered useful.

Based on our analysis, hyperbaric oxygen improves outcomes of patients with FHN, as compared to the natural history group of this disorder, and is comparable to outcomes from orthopedic interventions. Eighty-three of 86 patients (97%) treated with HBO had satisfactory short-term results, while 83 of 103 patients (81%) had satisfactory long-term results. Patients had HBO treatments combined with other orthopedic interventions. The number of combination-therapy cases reported is, nonetheless, too small to draw any meaningful conclusion about the effect of HBO when used as an adjunct to other orthopaedic interventions.

The question whether HBO facilitates bone remodeling remains to be answered, but there is an indication that this occurs from analysis of the information in Table 4 and results of the animal experiments recorded above. One study reports bone remodeling and decrease in the size of the necrotic area on radiographs in patients receiving 100 or more HBO treatments (40). It is unclear from most of the orthopedic reports whether orthopedic interventions merely prevent progression of FHN, or whether they also lead to radiologically identifiable bone healing. From an analysis of treatment mechanisms, it may be desirable to combine HBO with orthopedic interventions for optimal outcomes. The primary and secondary mechanisms of two different interventions may complement each other. For example, core decompression ameliorates the excessive pressure induced by edema and provides an access channel for granulation tissue, while HBO facilitates angiogenesis and enhances the environment for local bone remodeling responses. Both may contribute to edema reduction. Furthermore, if FHN is a progressive, on-going process, then the hyperoxygenation effect of HBO would immediately preserve the viability of those osteocytes in jeopardy of dying from the hypoxic insult, while the effects of the orthopedic intervention would be realized gradually. Similarly, bone grafting and electrical stimulation may enhance osteogenesis, while HBO would improve the milieu in which this occurs. As noted above, the reported cases using HBO in combination with other orthopedic interventions in FHN are very limited at this time.

Few side effects have been observed with HBO use. The theoretical concern about increased vulnerability of the femoral head to collapse from the enhanced osteoclast action, thought to be initiated by HBO, has not been specifically reported in the 189 case reports we analyzed. Baixe, in his HBO series, reports later bone collapse in some of his patients, even though pain symptoms uniformly resolved after 30 HBO treatments (6). Whether this represents increased vulnerability to femoral head collapse from osteoclast stimulation, or simply the expected observation of the treatment failure (as reported in all other series we reviewed), cannot be ascertained from the available data. Just as in the other interventions, the hip must, nonetheless, be protected from collapse with non-or limited weight bearing for 6 to 12 months.

Consequently, the use of bisphosphonate for depression of osteoclast may be an important adjunct to use with HBO, but interference with remodeling of necrotic bone by the osteoclast may be counterproductive.

The use of HBO in FHN needs to be considered carefully from an economic perspective. The cost of a series of HBO for FHN in the United States ranges from $12,000 to $40,000 (in Israel $8000) This expense may be greater than that for a core biopsy and drilling operative intervention: However, the long-term savings potentially realized from prevention of multiple total-hip arthoplasty operations and revisions may outweigh the initially high cost of HBO treatment. This is especially true in those patients who later develop contralateral FHN

## CONCLUSIONS

The mechanisms of HBO are directed at the underlying pathophysiology of femoral head necrosis. In the early stages, they facilitate edema reduction and oxygenation of hypoxic tissues. Later, they enhance the host's remodeling processes through stimulation of bone resorption, revascularization, and osteogenesis. Hyperbaric oxygen is beneficial in conjunction with non-weight bearing and possibily with bisphosphonates. The role of HBO is to minimize the volume of bone death, to stimulate healing and remodeling, whilst the bisphiosphonates may protect against femoral head collapse during the healing process.

We recommend HBO be considered as a primary treatment in Steinberg's (MRI stages) I and II FHN possibly in combination with the administration of bisphosphonatse to prevent femoral head collapse. It should be used as an adjunct to other orthopedic interventions in the management of pre-collapse stages of FHN in young patients, when the goal is to prevent altogether or delay total hip arthoplasty as long as possible. It also merits consideration in patients whose femoral head ischaemia may be due to vascular disease, diabetes mellitus, coagulopathies and injury. Finally, in special circumstances such as Caisson's dysbaric osteonecrosis in compressed air workers, HBO should be initiated at the first onset of symptoms.

A course of HBO treatment for FHN may be more costly than using the orthopedic interventions alone (not including THA). However, immediate economic considerations may be compensated by improved and durable results.

HBO contributes accumulated clinical and experimental evidence for a role for HBO in the treatment of early AVN together with prolonged strict non-weight bearing, and possibly the addition of bisphosphonate therapy supported by the co-authors (Reis et al.) recent study.

## REFERENCES

1. Aaron R.K. et al., The Conservative Treatment of Osteonecrosis of the Femoral Head, Clinical Orthopaedics and Related Research, 249:209-218, 1989.

2. Aaron R.K., et al., Stimulation of Experimental Endochondral Ossification by Low-Energy Pulsing Electromagnetic Fields, Journal of Bone and Min. Research 4:227-233, 1989.

3. Adam G et al., The MR Tomography of Avascular Necrosis of Bone: The Primary Findings and the Follow-up Observations after Core Decompression, Rofo. Fortschritte auf dem Gebiete der Rˆntgenstrahlen und der Neuen Bildgebenden Verfahren 163:330-334, 1995.

4. Asher M.A., et al., Hyperoxia and In-Vitro bone resorption. Clinical Orthopaedics and Related Research. 61: 48-51. 1968.

5. Atsumi T, Modified Sugioka's Osteotomy: More Than 130( Posterior Rotation for Osteonecrosis of the Femoral Head With Large Lesion, Clinical Orthopaedics and Related Research 334:98-107, 1997.

6. Baixe J.H., et al., Treatment of Osteonecrosis of the Femoral Head by Hyperbaric Oxygen, Bulletin Med. Sub. Hyp. 1:2, 1969.

7. Baksi D.P., Treatment of Osteonecrosis of the Femoral Head by Drilling and Muscle-Pedicle Bone Grafting, Journal of Bone and Joint Surgery 73B:241-245, 1991.

8. Bassett C.A.L., et al., Effects of Pulsed Electromagnetic Fields on Steinberg Ratings of Femoral Head Osteonecrosis, Clinical Orthopaedics and Related Research, 246:172-185, 1989

9. Beijneveld W.J., et al., Results of Trochanteric Rotational Osteotomy in the Treatment of Avascular Necrosis of the Femoral Head, Journal of Bone and Joint Surgery 79B(Suppl II):217, 1997.

10. Belal M.A., et al., Clinical Results of Rotational Osteotomy for Treatment of Avascular Necrosis of the Femoral Head, Archives of Orthopaedic and Trauma Surgery 115:80-84, 1996.

11. Bhatia D. et al., Long Term Results in Core Decompression of the Hip, Journal of Bone and Joint Surgery 75B(Supp 1):40, 1993.

12. Bird A.D., et al., The Effect of Oxygen at 2 Atmospheres on Reactive Hyperemia in the Human Forearm, Surg Gynecol Obstet. 124: 833-836, 1967.

13. Boettcher W.G. et al., Non-Traumatic Necrosis of the Femoral Head, Journal of Bone and Joint Surgery 52A:322-329, 1970.

14. Bradway J.K., et al., The Natural History of the Silent Hip in Bilateral Atraumatic Osteonecrosis, Journal of Arthroplasty 8:383-387, 1993.

15. Brighton C.T., Schaffzin E.A., Comparison of the Effects of Excess Vitamin A and High Oxygen Tension on In-Vitro Epiphyseal Growth. I. Morphologic Growth, Calcified Tissue Research 6:151-161, 1970.

16. Brighton C.T., Krebs A.G., Oxygen Tension of Healing Fractures in the Rabbit, Journal of Bone and Joint Surgery 54A:323-332, 1972.

17. Buckley P.D. et al., Structural Bone-Grafting for Early Atraumatic Avascular Necrosis of the Femoral Head, Journal of Bone and Joint Surgery 73A:1357-1364, 1991.

18. Camp J.F. et al., Core Decompression of the Femoral Head for Osteonecrosis, Journal of Bone and Joint Surgery 68A:1313-1319, 1986.

19. Chang M.C. et al., Core Decompression in Treating Ischemic Necrosis of the Femoral Head, Chinese Medical Journal 60:130-136, 1997.

20. Conti V.J., et al., Limits of Hyperbaric Oxygen in the Treatment of Aseptic Bone Necrosis in the Femoral Head, Bulletin Med. Sub. Hyp. 1:3-4, 1969.

21. Coulson D.B., et al., Effective Hyperbaric Oxygen on the Healing Femur of the Rat, Surgical Forum 17:449-450, 1966.

22. Courpied J.P., Trans-trochanteric Rotation Osteotomy for Femoral Head Necrosis. Long-term Results, Revue de Chirurgie OrthopÈdique et Reparatrice de l 'Appareil Moteur. 80:694-701, 1994.

23. Cruess R.L., et al., Steroid-Induced Osteonecrosis: a Review, The Canadian Journal of Surgery 24:567-571, 1981.

24. Cullen M.C., et al., The Management of Severe Avascular Necrosis Following Slipped Capital Femoral Epiphysis by Transtrochanteric Rotational Osteotomy. Results of Successful Treatment in Two Cases with Long-Term Follow-up, Iowa Orthopaedic Journal, 15:209, 1995.

25. D'Aubigne R.M., et al., Idiopathic Necrosis of the Femoral Head in Adults, Journal of Bone and Joint Surgery 47B:612-633.

26. Dean M.T., et al., Transtrochanteric Anterior Rotational Osteotomy for Avascular Necrosis of the Femoral Head: Long-Term Results, Journal of Bone and Joint Surgery 75B:597-601, 1993.

27. Dunn A.W., et al., Aseptic Necrosis of the Femoral Head: Treatment with Bone Grafts of Doubtful Value, Clinical Orthopaedics and Related Research 122:249-254, 1977.

27. Fairbank A.C., et al., Varus Osteotomy for Avascular Necrosis of the Femoral Head: Results of Long-Term Follow-up, Orthopaedic Transactions 18:176-177, 1994.

28. Fairbank A.C. et al., Long-Term Results of Core Decompression for Ischemic Necrosis of the Femoral Head, Journal of Bone and Joint Surgery 77B:42-49, 1995.

29. Ficat R.P., Idiopathic Bone Necrosis of the Femoral Head, Journal of Bone and Joint Surgery 67B:3-9, 1985.

30. Fujiwara M, et al., Vascularized Pedicled Iliac Bone Graft as a Treatment for Avascular Necrosis of the Femoral Head, Journal of Bone and Joint Surgery 79B(Suppl II):217, 1997.

31. Glueck C.J., et al., Thrombophilia and Hypofibrinolysis: Pathophysiologies of Osteonecrosis, Clinical Orthopaedics and Related Research 334:43-56, 1997.

32. Goldhaber P, The Effect of Hyperoxyia on Bone Resorption in Tissue Culture, Archives of Pathology 6:635-641, 195833.

33. Goulon M, et al., Five Cases of Suppurated Pseudoarthrosis (Osteomyelitis) Treated by Hyperbaric Oxygenation, In: Brown IW, Cox BG (eds.) Proceedings of the Third International Conference on Hyperbaric Medicine, National Academy of Sciences, National Research Council, Publication 1404, Washington, D.C., 1996, p.585.

34. Gray D.H., et al., The effects of varying oxygen tensions upon bone resorption in vitro. Journal of Bone and Joint Surgery 60B: 575-578, 1978.

35. Guenzi F, et al., Sugioka Rotational Osteotomy in Ischemic Osteonecrosis of the Femoral Head, Annali Italiani di Chirurgia, 65:583-585, 1994.

36. Gulli B., and Templeman D., Compartment Syndrome of the Lower Extremity, Orthopaedic Clinics of North America 25:677-684, 1994.

37. Harpstrite J.K. et al., Core Decompression and Autogenous Fibular Bone Grafting for Atraumatic Avascular Necrosis of the Femoral Head, Orthopaedic Transactions 18:872, 1994.

38. Hasegawa Y, et al., Vascularized Pedicle Bone-Grafting for Nontraumatic Avascular Necrosis of the Femoral Head. A 5- to 11-year follow-up, Archives of Orthopaedic and Trauma Surgery, 116:251-258, 1997.

39. Heinrich J.T. et al., The Gluteus Minimus Muscle Pedicle Graft in the Treatment of Femoral Head Avascular Necrosis, The American Journal of Orthopedics 24:615-623, 1995.

40. Helwig U, et al., Adaptation of Osteotomy in Idiopathic Femoral Head Necrosis, Zeitschrift f r Orthopadie und Ihre Grenzgebiete 133:14-18, 1995.

41. Hofmann S. et al., Bone-marrow edema syndrome and transient osteoporosis of the hip. An MRI-controlled study of treatment by core decompression, Journal of Bone and Joint Surgery 75B:210-216, 1993.

42. Holman A.J. et al., Quantitative Magnetic Resonance Imaging Predicts Clinical Outcome of Core Decompression for Osteonecrosis of the Femoral Head, Journal of Rheumatology, 22:1929-1933, 1995.

43. Hopson C.N. et al., Ischemic Necrosis of the Femoral Head, Journal of Bone and Joint Surgery 70A: 1048-1051,1988.

44. Hungerford D.S. et al., The Treatment of Ischemic Necrosis of Bone in Systemic Lupus Erythematosus, Medicine 59:143-148, 1980.

45. Hunt T.K., et al., The Effect of Varying Ambient Oxygen Tensions on Wound Metabolism and Collagen Synthesis. Surg Gynecol Obstet. 135: 561-567, 1972.

46. Iapicca M., et. al., Necrosis of the Femoral Head and HBO: A Therapeutical Approach, In: Proceedings of the Tenth International Congress on Hyperbaric Medicine, Best Publications, Flagstaff, AZ, pp.167-170, 1992.

47. Iwasada S, et al., Transtrochanteric Rotational Osteotomy for Osteonecrosis of the Femoral Head. 43 Patients Followed for at Least 3 Years, Archives of Orthopaedic and Trauma Surgery 116:447-453, 1997.

48. Iwase T, Transtrochanteric Anterior Rotational Osteotomy for Gaucher's Disease. A Case Report, Clinical Orthopaedics and Related Research 317:122-1125, 1995.

49. Iwata H., et al., Indications and Results of Vascularized Pedicle Iliac Bone Graft in Avascular Necrosis of the Femoral Head, Clinical Orthopaedics and Related Research 295:281-288, 1993.

50. Jones J.P., et al., The Effects of Hyperbaric Oxygen on Osteonecrosis, Orthopaedic Transactions 15:588-589, 1991.

51. Jones J.P. Jr., Fat Embolism, Intravascular Coagulation, and Osteonecrosis, Clinical Orthopaedics and Related Research 292:294-308, 1993.

52. Joseph B., et al., Management of Perthes Disease of Late Onset in Southern India, Journal of Bone and Joint Surgery 78B:625-630, 1996.

53. Kane S.M. et al., Vascularized Fibular Grafting Compared with Core Decompression in the Treatment of Femoral Head Osteonecrosis, Orthopedics 19:869-872, 1996.

54. Katz K. et al., The Natural History of Osteonecrosis of the Femoral Head in Children and Adolescents Who Have Gaucher Disease, Journal of Bone and Joint Surgery 78A:14-19, 1996.

55. Kerboul M, et al., The Conservative Surgical Treatment of Idiopathic Aseptic Necrosis of the Femoral Head, Journal of Bone and Joint Surgery 56B:291-296, 1974.

56. Kittredge B, et al., Intertrochanteric Rotational Osteotomy for Treatment of Avascular Necrosis of the Femoral Head: Long-Term Results, Orthopaedic Transactions 18:908, 1994.

57. Koo K.H. et al., Preventing Collapse in Early Osteonecrosis of the Femoral Head. A Randomised Clinical Trial of Core Decompression, Journal of Bone and Joint Surgery 77B-870-874, 1995.

58. Krahn T.H., et al., Long-term Follow-up of Patients with Avascular Necrosis After Treatment of Slipped Capital Femoral Epiphysis, Journal of Pediatric Orthopedics 13:154-158, 1993.

59. Kristensen K.D. et al., Core Decompression in Femoral Head Osteonecrosis, Acta Orthopaedica Scand 62:113-114, 1991.

60. Kruczynski J. et al., Long-term Clinical Assessment of the Hip Joint After Conservative Treatment of Development Dislocation Complicated by Avascular Necrosis, Chirurgia Narzadow Ruchu I Ortopedia Polska 61:53-58, 1996.

61. Langlais F, et al., Rotation Osteotomies for Osteonecrosis of the Femoral Head, Clinical Orthopaedics and Related Research 343:110-123, 1997.

62. Lausten G.S. at al., Core Decompression for Femoral Head Necrosis, Acta Orthopaedica Scand 61:507-511, 1990.

63. Learmonth I.D. et al., Core Decompression for Early Atraumatic Osteonecrosis of the Femoral Head, Journal of Bone and Joint Surgery 72B:387-390, 1990.

64. Leder K. et al., Results of Medullary Space Decompression in the Early Stage of So-Called Idiopathic Femur Head Necrosis, Zeitschrift f r Orthopadie und Ihre Grenzgebiete 131:113-119, 1993.

65. Lee C.K., et al., The "Silent Hip" of Idiopathic Ischemic Necrosis of the Femoral Head in Adults, Journal of Bone and Joint Surgery 62A:795-800, 1980.

66. Lee C.K., et al., Muscle-Pedicle Bone Graft and Cancellous Bone Graft for the 'Silent Hip' of Idiopathic Ischemic Necrosis of the Femoral Head in Adults, Clinical Orthopaedics and Related Research 158:185-194, 1981.

67. Lepawski M, et al., Avascular Osteonecrosis Ameliorated by Hyperbaric Oxygen, In: Eighth Ann Conf Clin Appl HBO, Long Beach, CA, 8-10 June 1983, p. 21.

68. Lepawski 1997- personal communication.

69. Leung P.C., Femoral Head Reconstruction and Revascularization, Clinical Orthopaedics and Related Research, 323:139-145, 1996.

70. Louie B., et al., Free Vascularized Fibular Grafting for Osteonecrosis of the Femoral Head: An Analysis of Surgical Outcome and Patient Health Status, Journal of Bone and Joint Surgery 79B(Suppl II):67, 1997.

71. Malizos K.N. et al., Osteonecrosis of the Femoral Head in Immunosuppressed Patients: Hip Salvaging with Implantation of a Vascularized Fibular Graft, Microsurgery 15:485-491, 1994.

72. Malizos K.N. et al., Osteonecrosis of the Femoral Head: Hip Salvaging with Implantation of a Vascularized Fibular Graft, Clinical Orthopaedics and Related Research 314:67-75, 1995.

73. Mao W.H., Treatment of Avascular Bone Necrosis by Hyperbaric Oxygentaion: A Report of 44 Cases, In: Fifth Chinese Conference On Hyperbaric Medicine, Fuzhou, China, 26-29 September 1986, p.27.

74. Marcus N.D. et al., The Silent Hip in Idiopathic Aseptic Necrosis: Treatment by Bone Grafting, Journal of Bone and Joint Surgery 55A:7 1351-1366, 1973.

75. Markel D. et al., Core Decompression of the Femoral Head for Osteonecrosis in Systemic Lupus Erythematosis, Orthopaedic Transactions 18:907, 1994.

76. Markel D. et al., Core Decompression for Osteonecrosis of the Femoral Head, Clinical Orthopaedics and Related Research, 323:226-233, 1996.

77. Maronna U., Idiopathische H(ftkopfnekrosen des Erwachsenen. In: Almeling M., Welslau W. (eds.) Grundlagen der hyperbaren Sauerstofftherapie, Archimedes-Verlag, Strande, 1996, pp.35-37.

78. Meijne N.G., Hyperbaric Oxygen and Its Clinical Value, with Special Emphasis on Biochemical and Cardiovascular Aspects. Charles C. Thomas, Springfield, IL 1970.

79. Meyers M.H., The Treatment of Osteonecrosis of the Hip with Fresh Osteochondral Allografts and with the Muscle Pedicle Graft Technique, Clinical Orthopaedics and Related Research 130: 202-209, 1978.

80. Meyers M.H., Osteonecrosis of the Femoral Head: Pathogenesis and Long-term Results of Treatment, Clinical Orthopaedics and Related Research 231:51-61, 1988.

81. Mont M.A., and Hungerford D.S., Non-Traumatic Avascular Necrosis of the Femoral Head, Journal of Bone and Joint Surgery 77A:459-474, 1995.

82. Mont M.A., et al., Corrective Osteotomy for Osteonecrosis of the Femoral Head: The Results of a Long-Term Follow-up Study, Journal of Bone and Joint Surgery 78A:1032, 1996.

83. Mont M.A. et al., Core Decompression for Osteonecrosis of the Femoral Head in Systemic Lupus Erythematosus, Clinical Orthopaedics and Related Research, 334:91-97, 1997.

84. Mont M.A. et al., Core Decompression for Avascular Necrosis of the Distal Femur, Clinical Orthopaedics and Related Research 334:124-130, 1997.

85. Mont M.A., et al., The Trapdoor Procedure Using Autogenous Cortical and Cancellous Bone Grafts for Osteonecrosis of the Femoral Head, Journal of Bone and Joint Surgery 80B:56-62, 1998.

86. Mulliken B.D., et al., The Prevalence and Natural History of Early Osteonecrosis of the Femoral Head, Iowa Orthopaedic Journal 14:115-119, 1994.

87. Musso E.S., et al., Results of Conservative Management of Osteonecrosis of the Femoral Head: A Retrospective Review, Clinical Orthopaedics and Related Research 207:209-215, 1984.

88. Natiella J.R., et al., The Effect of Hyperbaric Oxygenation on Bone Healing After Cryogenic Injury, In: Trapp WG, et al. (eds.), Proceedings of the Fifth International Conference on Hyperbaric Medicine, Simon Fraser University, B.C., Canada, 1974, p.270.

89. Nelson L.M., et al., Efficacy of Phemister Bone Grafting in Nontraumatic Aseptic Necrosis of the Femoral Head, Journal of Arthroplasty 8:253, 1993

90. Neubauer R.A., et al., Use of Hyperbaric Oxygen for the Treatment of Aseptic Bone Necrosis: A Case Study, Journal of Hyperbaric Medicine 4:69-76, 1989.

91. Niinikoski J., et al., Hyperbaric Oxygenation and Fracture Healing. A Biochemical Study With Rats, Acta Chir Scand.; 138: 39-44, 1972.

92. Notzli H.P., et al., Open-Reduction and Intertrochanteric Osteotomy for Osteonecrosis and Extrusion of the Femoral Head in Adolescents, Journal of Pediatric Orthopaedics 15:16-20, 1995.

93. Ohzono K., et al., Natural History of Nontraumatic Avascular Necrosis of the Femoral Head, Journal of Bone and Joint Surgery 73B:68-72, 1991.

94. Patterson R.J. et al., Idiopathic Avascular Necrosis of the Head of the Femur, Journal of Bone and Joint Surgery 46A:267-282, 1964.

95. Pavlovcic V., Vascularized Pedicular Bone Graft as Treatment for Avascular Necrosis of the Femoral Head, Journal of Bone and Joint Surgery 79B(Suppl II):217, 1997.

96. Plancher K.D, et al., Management of Osteonecrosis of the Femoral Head, Orthopaedic Clinics of North America, 28:461-477, 1997.

97. Powell E.T., Core Decompression for Early Osteonecrosis of the Hip in High Risk Patients, Clinical Orthopaedics and Related Research 335: 181-189, 1997.

98. Ramon Y. et al., Avascular Necrosis and Hyperbaric Oxygen Therapy, Presented at Sirot '97 Haifa Inter-Meeting (Societe Internationale de Recherche OrthopÈdique et de Traumatologie), Haifa, Israel, August 31-September 5, 1997.

99. Reichel H, et al., Long-Term Outcome of Dega Acetabuloplasty, Zeitschrift f r Orthopadie und Ihre Grenzgebiete 134:131-136, 1996.

100. Robinson H.J. et al., Success of Core Decompression in the Management of Early Stages of Avascular Necrosis: A Four-Year Prospective Study, Orthopaedic Transactions 16:707, 1992.

101. Rosenwasser M.P. et al., Long Term Follow-up of Thorough Debridement and Cancellous Bone Grafting of the Femoral Head for Avascular Necrosis, Clinical Orthopaedics and Related Research 306:17-27, 1994.

102. Sainty J.M., et al., The Place of Hyperbaric Oxygen Therapy in the Treatment of Aseptic Osteonecrosis of the Hip, Med Aeronaut Spat Med Sub Hyp 19:215, 1980.

103. Saito S, et al., Joint-preserving Operations for Idiopathic Avascular Necrosis of the Femoral Head: Results of Core Decompression, Grafting, and Osteotomy, Journal of Bone and Joint Surgery 70B:78-84, 1988.

104. Sanchez E.C., et al., Hyperbaric Oxygen Therapy in Avascular Necrosis of the Hip, Undersea Biomedical Research Suppl., p.58, 1990.

105. Satterwhite Y.E. et al., Clarifying the Role of Core Decompression for Osteonecrosis of the Femoral Head, Orthopaedic Transactions 16:707, 1992.

106. Scher M.A., et al., Intertrochanteric Osteotomy and Autogenous Bone-Grafting for Avascular Necrosis of the Femoral Head, Journal of Bone and Joint Surgery 75A:1119-1133, 1993.

107. Schonecker G, et al., Mid-term Follow-up in Revascularization of Avascular Necrosis of the Femoral Head With Vascularized Iliac Bone Graft, Journal of Bone and Joint Surgery 79B(Suppl II):216, 1997.

108. Schraibman et al., Hyperbaric Oxygen and Local Vasodilatation in Peripheral Vascular Disease, British Journal of Surgery, 56: 295-299, 1969.

109. Seiler J.G. et al., Core Decompression as a Treatment for Patients on Chronic Glucocorticoids with Osteonecrosis of the Femoral Head, Orthopaedic Transactions 15:823, 1991.

110. Shaffer J.W. et al., Radical Core Debridement and Vascularized Fibular Grafting for Advanced Necrosis of the Hip, Orthopaedic Transactions 15:823, 1991.

111. Shaw J.L., et al., The Effects of Varying Oxygen Concentrations on Osteogenesis and Embryonic Cartilage In Vitro, Journal of Bone and Joint Surgery 49: 73-80, 1967.

112. Shibuya T et al., Long Term Results of Core Biopsy of the Femoral Head, Orthopaedic Transactions 19:501, 1995.

113. Smith K.R. et al., Non-Traumatic Necrosis of the Femoral Head Treated with Tibial Bone-Grafting, Journal of Bone and Joint Surgery 62A:845-847, 1980.

114. Smith S.W. et al., Core Decompression of the Osteonecrotic Femoral Head, Journal of Bone and Joint Surgery 77A:674-680, 1995.

115. Solomon L, Idiopathic Necrosis of the Femoral Head: Pathogenesis and Treatment, The Canadian Journal of Surgery, 24:573-578, 1981.

116. Stein H, et al., Avascular Necrosis of the Femoral Head Treated by Decompression and Pedicle Bone Graft, Annual ARCO (Association-Research-Circulation-Osseous) Meeting and International Symposium, Vienna, Austria, October 5-7, 1995, Abstract p.28.

117. Steinberg M.E., et al., Treatment of Avascular Necrosis of the Femoral Head by a Combination of Bone Grafting, Decompression, and Electrical Stimulation, Clinical Orthopaedics and Related Research, 186:137-153, 1984.

118. Steinberg M.E., et al, The "Conservative" Management of Avascular Necrosis of the Femoral Head, In: Bone Circulation, p.334-337. Edited by Arlet, Ficat, and Hungerford. Baltimore, Williams and Wilkins, 1984.

119. Steinberg M.E., et al., Osteonecrosis of the Femoral Head: Results of Core Decompression and Grafting With and Without Electrical Stimulation, Clinical Orthopaedics and Related Research, 249: 199-208, 1989.

120. Steinberg ME, et al., Core decompression of the femoral head for avascular necrosis: indications and results, Canadian Journal of Surgery 38(Suppl I):S18-S24, 1995.

121. Stern B, et al., The Effect of Various Oxygen Tensions on the Synthesis and Degradation of Bone Collagen inTissue Culture, Proceedings of the Society for Experimental Biology and Marine, 121:869-872, 1966.

122. Strauss M.B, Hart G.B., Clinical Experiences with OHP on Fracture Healing, In: Smith (ed.), Proceedings of the Sixth International Congress on Hyperbaric Medicine, G. Aberdeen University Press, Aberdeen, Scotland, 1977, pp.329-332.

123. Strauss M.B., et al., Effect of Hyperbaric Oxygen on Bone Resorption in Rabbits. Presented at the Seventh Annual Conference on the Clinical Applications of Hyperbaric Oxygen, Anaheim, CA, June 9-11, 1982.

124. Strauss M.B., A "Meta-analysis" and Economic Appraisal of Osteonecrosis of the Femoral Head Treated with Hyperbaric Oxygen, Presented at Sirot '97 Haifa Inter-Meeting (Societe Internationale de Recherche Orthopedique et de Traumatologie), Haifa, Israel, August 31-September 5, 1997, abstract p.90.

125. Stulberg B.N. et al., Making Core Decompression Work, Clinical Orthopaedics and Related Research, 261:186-195, 1990.

126. Stulberg B.N., et al., Multimodality Approach to Osteonecrosis of the Femoral Head, Clinical Orthopaedics and Related Research, 240:181-193, 1991.

127. Stulberg B.N. et al., Osteonecrosis of the Femoral Head: A Prospective Randomized Treatment Protocol, Clinical Orthopaedics and Related Research 268:140-151, 1991.

128. Sugioka Y., Transtrochanteric Anterior Rotational Osteotomy of the Femoral Head in the Treatment of Osteonecrosis Affecting the Hip: A New Osteotomy Operation, Clinical Orthopaedics and Related Research 130:191-201, 1978.

129. Sugioka Y, et al., Transtrochanteric Anterior Rotational Osteotomy for Idiopathic and Steroid-Induced Necrosis of the Femoral Head: Indications and Long-Term Result, Clinical Orthopaedics and Related Research 277:111-120, 1992.

130. Takatori Y., et al., Avascular Necrosis of the Femoral Head: Natural History and Magnetic Resonance Imaging, Journal of Bone and Joint Surgery 75B:217-221, 1993.

131. Tooke S.M.T. et al., Results of Core Decompression for Femoral Head Osteonecrosis, Clinical Orthopaedics and Related Research, 228:99-104, 1988

132. Turanti A., et al., HBO in Treatment of Aseptic Necrosis of Femoral Head, In: 1991 International Society of Hyperbaric Medicine: V World Meeting of Hyperbaric Medicine, 1991.

133. Urbaniak J.R. et al., Treatment of Osteonecrosis of the Femoral Head with Free Vascularized Fibular Grafting. A long-term Follow-up Study of one hundred and three hips, Journal of Bone and Joint Surgery 77A:681-694, 1995.

134. Vujnovic D., The Influence of Oxygen on Fracture Healing, HBO Review, 5:10, 1984.

135. Warner J.J.P. et al., Studies of Nontraumatic Osteonecrosis: The Role of Core Decompression in the Treatment of Nontraumatic Osteonecrosis of the Femoral Head, Clinical Orthopaedics and Related Research, 225:125-127, 1987.

136. Wassenaar R.P. et al., Avascular Osteonecrosis of the Femoral Head Treated with a Vascularized Iliac Bone Graft: Preliminary Results and Follow-up with Radiography and MR Imaging, Radiographics 16:585-594, 1996.

137. Wray J.B., et al., Effect of Hyperbaric Oxygenation Upon Fracture Healing in the Rat, Journal of Trauma 8:168, 1968.

138. Yablon I.G., The effect of hyperbaric oxygen on fracture healing in rats, Journal of Trauma, 8:186-202, 1968.

139. Yoo M.C., et al., Free Vascularized Fibula Grafting for the Treatment of Osteonecrosis of the Femoral Head, Clinical Orthopaedics and Related Research 277:128-138, 1992.

140. Zimmermann A, et al., Management of Early Avascular Femur Head Necrosis by Flexion Osteotomy. 2-year Follow-up, Magyar Traumatologia Ortopedia Kezsebeszet Plasztikai Sebeszet 37:153-159, 1994.

141. Zimmermann A. et al., Management of Early Avascular Femur Head Necrosis by Implantation of a Muscle-Bone Graft, Magyar Traumatologia Ortopedia Kezsebeszet Plasztiakai Sebeszet, 37:217-222, 1994.

CHAPTER 35

# USE OF ADJUNCTIVE HYPERBARIC OXYGEN IN THE MANAGEMENT OF INVASIVE FUNGAL INFECTIONS

## CHAPTER THIRTY-FIVE OVERVIEW

# USE OF ADJUNCTIVE HYPERBARIC OXYGEN IN THE MANAGEMENT OF INVASIVE FUNGAL INFECTIONS

*Joseph C. Farmer, Diana M. Barratt,*
*Lisardo García-Covarrubias, Eric P. Kindwall*

## INTRODUCTION

The last decade witnessed changes in the epidemiology and prevalence of Invasive Fungal Infections (IFIs) (25). The incidence of these infections has risen dramatically, due in large part to the increasing size of the population at risk that includes patients with AIDS, recipients of solid organ or hematopoietic stem cell transplants, patients with hematologic malignancies, patients receiving broad-spectrum antibiotics, diabetics, and other individuals with immunosuppression (10, 11).

The management of these infections includes antifungal medications, treatment of the underlying or predisposing disease and surgical debridement. However, in spite of the advancements in new antifungal drugs, the mortality rate is approximately 40%-50% (2, 34). Hyperbaric oxygen has been advocated as an adjunct to treat IFIs mainly mucormycosis and aspergillosis. In this chapter we review the most relevant evidence including bench and clinical studies on the use of hyperbaric oxygen in invasive mycoses.

## PATHOPHYSIOLOGY AND RATIONALE FOR HYPERBARIC OXYGEN

Typically, the fungus enters the body through the respiratory tract. Local proliferation can lead to invasion of the tissues and blood vessels, resulting in hypoxia, hemorrhagic infarction, necrosis and potential hematogenous extension to distal sites (29). The hypoxic/acidotic conditions compromise antibiotic action and may promote spread of the infection (7).

Phagocytes, particularly macrophages and neutrophils, play a major role in controlling fungal infections (43). Their fungicidal activity is mediated by means of different oxygen intermediates; their killing capacity is directly proportional to available oxygen (44, 35).

Amphotericin B (AMB) remains as the mainstay of therapy for IFIs (38). Sokol-Anderson and cols. reported that under hypoxic conditions, AMB's fungicidal capacity is reduced as much as 80% compared with normoxic conditions (41).

Hyperbaric oxygenation elevates oxygen levels in severely hypoxic tissue and has an additive effect when combined with AMB (39, 24). In addition, pulmonary alveolar macrophages' fungicidal activity to *Neurospora crassa* is augmented when exposed to 100% oxygen (40).

## *IN VITRO* STUDIES

*In vitro* studies have shown a lag phase in the growth curve of *Candida albicans, Aspergillus fumigatus* and *Mucor sp.* when exposed to high partial pressures of oxygen (9, 24). Fungicidal activity was achieved using 10 ATM for 28 days (8). Furthermore, the addition of HBO in presence of AMB exhibited an additive effect on the growth of *Candida albicans* (24). Sokol-Anderson and cols. showed that hypoxia severely decreases AMB-fungicidal action. Another relevant issue mentioned by these authors was the oxidative anti-fungal mechanism of AMB. This was elegantly demonstrated by means of combining AMB with catalase and superoxide dismutase, two biological antioxidants, resulting in a significant decrease in the AMB-fungicidal activity (41).

Obviously some of the pressures and length of treatment used in the above *in vitro* studies are incompatible with human life. However they shed light in the potential application of hyperbaric oxygen in human mycoses.

## ANIMAL STUDIES

To our knowledge there are only two animal studies that have looked at the effect of hyperbaric oxygen in IFIs. The first one by Barratt and cols. (3) was a prospective randomized placebo-controlled animal trial designed to determine whether the addition of HBO (2.0 ATA/2 hours bid) to AMB improved survival function in mice with zygomycosis. Infection was induced by injection of *Rhizopus arrhizus* via the tail vein and ethmoid sinus. Prior to the inoculation, mice received intraperitoneal deferoxamine as a predisposing agent for the infection. Next, the animals were randomized as follows: HBO/AMB; Air/AMB; and No Treatment. On day 14, survivors were euthanized. Histopathology was performed on 5 brains from the No Treatment animals that died prior to day 14. Survival was as follows: HBO/AMB—42% (21/50); Air/AMB—46% (22/48); and No Treatment—31% (15/48). Histopathology revealed branching hyphae in 100% (5/5) of brains. Analysis of survival function (Wilcoxon test) did not demonstrate a significant difference between the HBO/AMB and Air/AMB groups (p = 0.72). Treatment with either HBO/AMB (p = 0.01) or Air/AMB (p = 0.067) improved survival function over No Treatment by reducing the initial death rate and increasing the survival rate. However, only HBO/AMB significantly improved survival function over No Treatment. The authors concluded that the addition of hyperbarics to Amphotericin B did not improve survival function over Amphotericin B and air.

The second study was by García-Covarrubias and cols. (18). In this study mice were administered intraperitoneal cyclophosphamide to induce immunosuppression before tail-vein injection of *Rhizopus arrhizus*. The animals received AMB in addition to HBO. Based on the lack of significant improvement using a pressure of 2 ATA (3), this study increased the pressure to 2.5 ATA. Each HBO treatment consisted of a 90-minute session. After inoculation, the animals were randomly placed in one of the following groups:

AMB plus HBO group (N=30). Three HBO treatments were administered during the first 24 hours after inoculation followed by twice daily from day 2 to day 6. Thereafter HBO was administered on a daily basis until day 14 post-inoculation, for a total of 21 HBO treatments. AMB group (N=31) received AMB only. Cages of this group were transported to the HBO room along with cages of group No. 1 to assure that both groups were exposed to the same stress, temperature and light intensity. Control group (N=22) received no treatment. Mice were monitored for 14 days and time to death was recorded. On day 14 survivors were euthanized and kidney colony forming units (CFUs) were assessed. Deaths in all groups began to occur between days 4-5 post-inoculation. All animals in the control group had died by day nine. Fifteen days after inoculation, survival rate was 40% (12/30) in the HBO-AMB group vs. 35.4% (11/31) in the AMB group. This difference in favor of the HBO-AMB group was not sufficient to achieve statistical significance. Regarding the colony counts, the HBO-AMB group showed a slightly lower number (718.5 cfu/gr) compared with the AMB group (799.9 cfu/gr). However, this difference was not significant (p = 0.92).

It is important to note that although neither of the animal studies showed a significant benefit from HBO the models do not replicate the typical clinical scenario as the infection induced in the mice was severely disseminated where a main component of the standard of care, namely surgical debridement, was lacking. Clearly a better model is needed to further assess the impact of HBO in IFIs.

## CLINICAL EXPERIENCE

Most of the clinical series on the use of HBO in IFIs deal with its application to mucormycosis. Recently a small series on aspergillosis was reported. Reports of treatment of other invasive fungi are so few as to be almost anecdotal. A few of these reports are included in this section.

### Mucormycosis

The term mucormycosis encompasses a rare group of necrotizing infections caused by fungi belonging to the order of the *Mucorales* (42). *Rhizopus* species are responsible for 70% of rhino-orbital-cerebral mucormycosis (ROCM) (45).

This infection occurs most commonly in the immunocompromised host. The typical patient profile is that of a poorly controlled diabetic with ketoacidosis. Other common comorbidities include hematologic malignancies, organ and bone marrow transplantation, end stage renal disease with concurrent deferoxamine administration, major burns, and severe trauma (12, 13).

This order of fungi has the ability to invade blood vessels with infections localizing at a variety of anatomic sites (27). In its most common forms, ROCM and pulmonary mucormycosis, inhalation is the natural route of infection. However, traumatic implantation has been described, specifically with the organism *Apophysomyces elegans* (33).

*Apophysomyces elegans* is an interesting specie as it typically infects previously healthy individuals and the mechanism of infection is traumatic. García-Covarrubias and cols. (20) reported a case of a 24-year-old previously healthy male who sustained severe craniofacial trauma secondary to a motorcycle accident. Initial management was complicated by a right forehead necrotizing infection requiring right orbital exenteration due to its poor response to antibiotics. *Apophysomyces elegans* was identified as the culprit. The patient was successfully managed with a multidisciplinary approach including liposomal Amphotericin B, surgery, hyperbaric oxygenation and granulocyte colony-stimulating factor (G-CSF). In the same article the authors reviewed 20 more cases of mucormycosis secondary to *A. elegans* confirming the fact that the majority of these individuals were previously healthy and infected by a traumatic mechanism.

Prior to 1960 ROCM was almost uniformly fatal (17). In 1980, Blitzer and cols. (6) reviewed the English language literature analyzing 179 cases. The overall mortality was 50%; a 70% survival was noted in cases reported from 1970 to 1979. This improved survival in later years was, perhaps, related to the increased use of Amphotericin B and radical surgery. However, as the authors of this review pointed out, these mortality figures are likely to be inaccurate because of the inclusion of case reports that appear to have been written only because the patient survived. Seventy percent of the survivors had significant residual defects such as blindness, cranial nerve palsies, hemiplegia, ophthalmoplegia, or significant cosmetic defects.

When cerebral extension occurs a high fatality rate persists, in spite of the use of radical surgery and Amphotericin B (1, 30, 36). Price and Stevens (37) reported a successful outcome in a case of extensive cerebral mucormycosis.

Ferguson and cols. (16) reviewed 12 patients with rhinocerebral mucormycosis treated with surgery and Amphotericin B, from 1969 to 1988. Of the six patients treated with Amphotericin B, and surgical debridement, without adjunctive HBO, prior to 1983, four died as a direct result of fungal infection. Of the six patients treated with surgery, Amphotericin B and adjunctive hyperbaric oxygen therapy, two died, with one of these exhibiting improving mucormycosis, related to a difference in the aggressiveness of the use of Amphotericin, medical therapy, or surgery.

Couch and cols. (14) reported two patients with rhinocerebral mucormycosis with brain mucor abscesses, clinical deterioration, and progression of infection, despite aggressive surgical debridement, Amphotericin therapy, and medical control of the underlying diabetic acidosis. Both patients exhibited significant clinical improvement coincident with the addition of adjunctive HBO therapy. Treatments were at 2.5 ATA for 90 minutes, six days a week. One patient received a total of 79 HBO treatments; the other received 85 such treatments. No complications of treatment were encountered and the patients remained free of disease 21 months after hospital discharge. The survival of these patients is particularly noteworthy since both had intracerebral mucor abscesses, with one having total occlusion of an internal carotid artery, complications that had formerly resulted invariably in death. One patient was reported as doing well with only residual blindness, having had to undergo debridement of an orbit. The second patients were reported as being fully alert, ambulatory, and capable of self-care, with only a short-term memory deficit.

Noting that survival is uncommon in bilateral cerebro-rhino-orbital mucormycosis, De La Paz and cols. (15) achieved eradication of the infection in a 66-year-old diabetic, using HBO combined with bilateral orbital exenteration and Amphotericin B. The patient was well one-and-a-half years later.

Melero and cols. (31) reported a 16-month remission in a diabetic patient with rhino-sinuso-orbital disease who had maintained an active infection despite two debridements and Amphotericin B. Further debridement with adjunctive HBO halted the infection.

Okhuysen and cols. (33) reported a case of a previously healthy man who presented with severe cutaneous and renal mucormycosis due to *A. elegans*. The patient was successfully treated with liposomal Amphotericin B, HBO, and interferon-gamma obviating the need for nephrectomy.

Yohai and cols. (45) reviewed 208 cases in the literature since 1970, 139 of which were presented in sufficient detail to assess factors prognostic for survival. To those were added data from six of their own patients. The histories of those 145 patients were analyzed for the following variables: 1) Underlying conditions associated with mucormycotic infections; 2) Incidents of ocular and orbital signs and symptoms; 3) Incidence of non-ocular signs and symptoms; 4) Interval from symptom onset to treatment; and 5) The pattern of sinus involvement seen on imaging studies and noted at the time of surgery. Factors related to a lower survival rate include: 1) Delayed diagnosis and treatment; 2) Hemiparesis or hemiplegia; 3) Bilateral sinus involvement; 4) Leukemia; 5) Renal disease; and 6) Treatment with deferoxamine. Facial necrosis fell just short of statistical significance, but appears clinically important. Hyperbaric oxygen was found to have a favorable effect on prognosis.

More recently a small series was reported by García-Covarrubias and cols. (19). A chart review of mucormycosis patients referred to the HBO service was performed. Also an electronic search in Medline of relevant literature was undertaken. Five mucormycosis patients referred for HBO had complete charts available. Four had craniofacial involvement and one had left upper extremity involvement. The predisposing diseases were leukemia (N=3), diabetes mellitus plus sarcoidosis (N=1), and trauma (N=1). All patients were managed with Amphotericin B, surgical debridement and HBO. Survival was 60% (3/5) three months after the diagnosis was established. The literature was scarce, but favors HBO. The authors concluded that considering the pathophysiology of mucormycosis, adjuvant HBO therapy seems reasonable. However, they acknowledge that the clinical experience is still too limited to make HBO part of the standard of care and that prospective, randomized, controlled trials will help to define the role of HBO in this devastating infection.

In the previous edition of this book Farmer and Kindwall recommended the following treatment protocol for patients with rhinocerebral mucormycosis:

1. Patients with immunocompromise who have historically-confirmed mucormycosis with tissue invasion and destruction, with or without orbital or intracranial extension, should be considered for treatment.
2. All patients should receive standard clinical care including appropriate therapy to control the underlying primary disease,

Amphotericin B, and surgical debridement. Some have suggested that only those patients, who exhibit progression of the disease in spite of adequate conventional therapy, should be considered for hyperbaric treatment. However, in many cases, the disease is rapidly progressive with extensive intracranial and orbital invasion, despite "adequate" treatment. This, plus the high morbidity and mortality of the disease, indicates that adjunctive HBO should be considered in any patient with invasive mucormycosis.

3. HBO therapy should consist of exposures to 100% oxygen for 90 minutes to two hours, at pressures from 2.0 to 2.5 atmospheres, with one to two such exposures daily. Although Mader recommended about 40 treatments to achieve eradication in the usual case (Mader JT., personal communication), up to 80 treatments have been used in the past. Determining the end point may be difficult if the patient becomes asymptomatic, as there is always the fear of stopping too soon and having the patient suffer a recurrence that may be more difficult to eradicate. Nevertheless, fungal cultures obtained from biopsy, and the clinical condition of the patient, must govern one's judgment. In any case, the patient should receive at least 40 treatments.

## Aspergillosis

Invasive Aspergillosis is now the leading cause of early death in many transplant centers and has a major impact on the management of leukemia (23, 26). This fungal organism is widespread in nature and usually does not cause disease in healthy individuals; however, it is responsible for opportunistic infections in immuno-compromised patients. Pulmonary and rhinosinusinal are the most common clinical presentations.

Oxygen levels are often decreased in the infected tissue of patients with aspergillosis, as this fungus invades blood vessels, causing obstruction, thrombosis, and hypoxia (4). This hypoxic environment results in tissue necrosis, diminishes the oxidative anti-fungal effect of Amphotericin B and impairs the oxidative killing capacity and phagocytosis of white cells (5, 35, 41).

There have been few reported cases of invasive Aspergillosis treated with hyperbaric oxygen. Recently a case of aspergillosis in the right temporomandibular joint with a history of parotid carcinoma and post-irradiation otitis was reported. Previous treatment attempts with surgery and antibiotics were unsuccessful. Radical debridement of the glenoid fossae, supplemented with Amphotericin B and adjunct HBO therapy, successfully resolved the symptoms (28).

Kindwall had success in treating a 43-year-old white male with rhinocerebral Aspergillosis following homologous bone-marrow transplant and immunosuppression. The patient initially had been suffering from non-Hodgkin's lymphoma. Maxillary and ethmoidal exenteration and Amphotericin B had failed to halt the infection. He developed complications from Amphotericin. The patient was treated 40 times at 2.4 ATA for 90 minutes. Seven years later, the patient was alive and well, and was working full-time as an electrical engineer (Kindwall E, personal communication). Price and

Stevens (37) reported treating invasive Aspergillosis with hyperbaric oxygen as a last resort, with success.

The largest experience in this area was reported by García-Covarrubias and cols. (21). A retrospective study of all the patients with histologic specimens suggestive of invasive Aspergillosis referred to a hyperbaric medicine unit located in a large county hospital was conducted. The main assessment of outcome was survival three months after initiation of HBO. The study included ten immunocompromised patients with rhino-sinusinal infection. All patients were managed with AMB, surgery and HBO. In addition, throughout the HBO course four patients received granulocyte colony-stimulating factor (G-CSF) and one patient received granulocyte infusions. The mean time between the onset of symptoms and initiation of AMB was 10.6 days whereas for HBO initiation, it was 44.1 days. HBO treatments were administered at a pressure of 2 ATA for 90 minutes. Patients received an average of 19.8 hyperbaric treatments. Complications from HBO included seizures in one patient, mild shortness of breath in two patients, and mild confinement anxiety in one patient. Six patients were alive three months after initiation of HBO therapy. The authors noted that the delay in initiating HBO seemed to indicate that it was utilized as a last resort in most of the patients.

The limited experience with HBO and invasive Aspergillosis precludes strong recommendations. Nevertheless, on the basis of the pathophysiology of invasive fungal infections and sound physiological principles of HBO, prompt initiation of HBO appears reasonable in patients with either overwhelming rhinocerebral fungal infections or host compromise.

The protocol routinely used with our patients is 10 to 20 initial treatments of 90 minutes at 2.0 to 2.5 ATA, followed by re-assessment of their condition. Patients are initially treated every 8 hours during the first day and twice a day thereafter. A five-minute air break is given every 25-min. Once the patient's condition has stabilized, once a day treatments are given until no further evidence of fungal infection is noted. Higher pressures (2.5 to 3.0 ATA) are used for necrotizing soft tissue infections such as gas gangrene and necrotizing fasciitis. However, because of the common involvement of the CNS, the treatment benefit of higher pressures for invasive fungal infections must be weighted against the risk of oxygen toxicity seizures.

## Others

### *Candidiobolus Coronato*

This extremely rare disorder is caused by another order of *Phycomycetes* family, the *Entomophthorales*. But unlike mucormycosis, the lesions caused by these organisms do not cause vascular thrombi or extensive necrosis. Nathan et al. reported the successful eradication of the disease in an otherwise healthy bulldozer operator who had the invasive rhinocerebral form, but was very intolerant to Amphotericin B (32). He had been pursuing a downhill course. He received 51 HBO treatments at 2.4 ATA for 90 minutes daily, following a partial maxillectomy, and resection of a zygomatic fungoma. This was accompanied by Amphotericin B therapy of only 5 to 10 mg per day. He received a total of 1,510 mg of the drug. Three weeks after the first surgery, re-exploration revealed no evidence of new necrosis or infection.

### Coccidioidmycosis

This disorder, also termed San Joaquin Valley fever, is usually a self-limited respiratory disease, but in the chronic form it can produce cavitation or granuloma ("coin lesion") formation. In endemic areas, people who are exposed for many years may develop the more ominous progressive form with spread to the bones, joints, viscera, skin, brain, and meninges. The fatality rate in the progressive form is 55% to 60%. Therapy is with *Amphotericin B* and *ketoconazole*. Prolonged intrathecal therapy may be necessary for meningeal involvement. Price and Stevens (28) have reported fulminant Coccidioidmycosis to respond to HBO when it has been given as "last resort."

### Pseudosallescheria Boydii

Granström and cols. (22) reported eradication of this organism in a 62-year-old *diabetic* who suffered from an ear canal and mastoid infection of the temporal bone for over two years. The CT scan was normal, but the patient developed paralysis of the 5th and 9th cranial nerves. Surgical exploration revealed the mastoid cavity to be filled with granulation tissue containing micro abscesses. A scintigram of the external bony part of the auditory canal showed increased uptake. Despite antibacterial antibiotics, the patient's condition deteriorated. Nine months following the initial surgery, a Technetium scan revealed increased uptake in the temporal bone and a CT scan confirmed involvement of the pterygoid apex. Cerebrospinal fluid (CSF) analysis indicated *blood-brain barrier* damage with *leukocytosis*. Cultures from the external canal finally yielded *P. boydii*. Oral Itraconazole (a congener of Ketoconazole) was given for one year. HBO therapy, at 2.4 ATA for 90 minutes, was then conducted daily for 60 days. Following HBO, the Technetium scan normalized, and repeated cultures were negative. An MRI scan indicated no spread of the infection in the soft tissues of the face. The CSF analysis returned to normal and the patient remained disease-free one and a half years after diagnosis.

## SUMMARY

Invasive fungal infections continue to pose a severe threat to the immunocompromised patient. Current standard of care includes control of the underlying condition, parenteral antifungal medications, and surgical debridement. Nevertheless morbidity and mortality remain high. Other treatment modalities have been incorporated to the standard of care aiming at improving the poor outcome of these patients. The role of hyperbaric oxygen as and adjuvant therapy has been investigated in the lab and clinically. Results in animal models are somewhat limited, because of the poor resemblance with the clinical picture. Case reports and small clinical series, mainly in mucormycosis and aspergillosis, suggest that HBO may be beneficial. From the current evidence we can also conclude that HBO is not likely to be harmful in this setting. A better animal model and larger clinical studies are needed to better assess the role of HBO in these devastating infections.

## REFERENCES

1. Abedi E, Sismanis A, Choi K, et al. Twenty-five years' experience treating cerebro-rhino-orbital mucormycosis. Laryngoscope. 1984; 94:1060-1062.

2. Almyroudis NG, Sutton DA, Linden P, et al. Zygomycosis in solid organ transplant recipients in a tertiary transplant center and review of the literature. Am J Transp. 2006; 6:2365-2374.

3. Barratt DM, Van Meter K, Asmar P, et al. Hyperbaric oxygen as an adjunct in zygomycosis: randomized controlled trial in a murine model. Antimicrob Agents Chemother 2001; 45;3601-3602.

4. Bennett JE. Aspergillus species. In: Principles and practice of infectious diseases. Mandell GL, Bennett JE, Dolin R (eds). New York, Churchill Livingstone. 4th Ed, 1995, pp. 2306-2311.

5. Bjerknes R, Neslein IL, Myhre K, Andersen HT. Impairment of rat polymorphonuclear neutrophilic granulocyte phagocytosis following repeated hypobaric hypoxia. Aviat Space Environ Med 1990; 61:1007-1011.

6. Blitzer A., et al. Patient survival factors in paranasal sinus mucormycosis. Laryngoscope. 1980; 90:635-648.

7. Bullen JJ, Roquers HJ, Spalding PB, et al. Natural resistance, iron and infection: a challenge for clinical medicine. J Med Microbiol. 2006 Mar; 55:251-258.

8. Caldwell J. Effects of high partial pressures of oxygen on fungi. Nature 1963; 197:772-774.

9. Cairney WJ. Developmental effects of hyperbaric oxygen on selected human pathogenic fungi in culture [Ph.D. thesis]. 1977; New York, NY: Cornell University.

10. Clark TA, Hajjeh RA. Recent trends in the epidemiology of invasive mycoses. Curr Opin Infect Dis 2002; 15:569-574.

11. Chayakulkeeree M, Ghannoum MA, Perfect JR. Zygomycosis: the re-emerging fungal infection. Eur J Clin Microbiol Infect Dis. 2006; 25:215-229.

12. Cocanour CS, Miller-Crotchett P, Reed RL II, Johnson PC, Fischer RP. Mucormycosis in trauma patients. J Trauma 1992; 32: 12-15.

13. Cooter RD, Lim IS, Ellis DH, Leitch IOW. Burn wound zygomycosis caused by Apophysomyces elegans. J Clin Microbiol 1990; 28: 2151-2153.

14. Couch L, Theilen F, Mader JT. Rhinocerebral mucormycosis with cerebral extension successfully treated with adjunctive hyperbaric oxygen therapy. Arch Otolaryngol Head Neck Surg 1988; 114:791-794.

15. De la Paz MA, Patrinely JR, Marines HM, et al. Adjunctive hyperbaric oxygen in the treatment of bilateral cerebro-rhino-orbital mucormycosis. Am J Ophthalmol 1992; 114: 208-211.

16. Ferguson BJ, Mitchell TG, Moon R, et al. Adjunctive hyperbaric oxygen for treatment of rhinocerebral mucormycosis. Rev Infect Dis 1988; 10: 551-559

17. Ferry AP. Cerebral mucormycosis (phycomycosis). Ocular findings and review of the literature. Surv Ophthalmol 1961; 6: 1-24.

18. García-Covarrubias L, Barratt DM, Bartlett R, et al. Hyperbaric oxygen and amphotericin B in the management of mucormycosis: a randomized controlled trial in the murine model. Undersea Hyperb Med 2002; 29:141.

19. García-Covarrubias L, Barratt DM, Bartlett R, et al. Treatment of Mucormycosis with adjunctive hyperbaric oxygen: five cases treated at the same institution and review of the literature. Rev Invest Clin 2004; 56:51-55.

20. García-Covarrubias L, Bartlett R, Barratt DM, et al. Rhino-orbitocerebral mucormycosis attributable to Apophysomyces elegans in an immunocompetent individual: case report and review of the literature. J Trauma 2001; 50: 353-357.

21. García-Covarrubias L, Barratt DM, Bartlett R, et al. Invasive aspergillosis treated with adjunctive hyperbaric oxygenation: a retrospective clinical series at a single institution. South Med J 2002; 95: 450-456.

22. Granström G, Hanner P, et al. "Malignant external otitis caused by Pseudoallescheria boydii treated with hyperbaric oxygen." (Abstract only) Undersea Biomedical Research 1990;17(Suppl):38.

23. Groll AH, Shah PM, Mentzel C, et al. Trends in the postmortem epidemiology of invasive fungal infections at a university hospital. J Infect 1996; 33:23-32.

24. Gudewicz TM, Mader JT, Davis CP. Combined effects of hyperbaric oxygen and antifungal agents on the growth of Candida albicans. Aviat Space Environ Med. 1987; 58:673-678.

25. Kauffman CA. Fungal Infections. Proc Am Thorac Soc. 2006; 3:35-40.

26. Latge JP. Aspergillus fumigatus and aspergillosis. Clin Microbiol Rev 1999; 12:310-350.

27. Lehrer RI, Howard DH, Sypherd PS, Edwards JE, Segal GP, Winston DJ. Mucormycosis (UCLA Conference). Ann Int Med 1980; 93: 93-108.

28. Lo WL, Chang RC, Yang AH, et al. Aspergillosis of the temporomandibular joint following irradiation of the parotid region: a case report. Int J Oral Maxillofac Surg 2003; 32: 560-562.

29. Lopes Bezerra LM, Filler SG. Interactions of Aspergillus fumigatus with endothelial cells: internalization, injury, and stimulation of tissue factor activity. Blood 2004; 103:2143-2149.

30. Maniglia AJ, Mintz DH, Novak S. Cephalic phycomycosis: A report of eight cases. Laryngoscope. 1982;92:755-760.

31. Melero M, Kaimen MI, Tiraboschi N, Botargues M, Radisic M. Adjunctive treatment with hyperbaric oxygen in a patient with rhino-sinuso-orbital mucormycosis. Medicina (B Aires) 1991; 51:53-55.

32. Nathan MD, Keller AP jr, Lerner CJ, et al. Entomophthorales infection of the maxillofacial region. Laryngoscope 1982; 92: 767-769.

33. Okhuyusen PC, Rex JH, Kapusta M, Fife C. Successful treatment of extensive post-traumatic soft-tissue and renal infections due to Apophysomyces elegans. Clin Infect Dis 1994; 19: 329-331.

34. Pagano L, Caira M, Candoni A, et al. The epidemiology of fungal infections in patients with hematologic malignancies: the SEIFEM-2004 study. Haematologica 2006; 91:1068-1075.

35. Park MK, Myers RAM, Marzella L. Oxygen tensions and infections: modulation of microbial growth, activity of antimicrobial agents, and immunologic responses. Clin Infect Dis 1992; 14:720-40.

36. Pillsbury HC and Fisher ND. Rhinocerebral mucormycosis. Arch Otolaryngol Head and Neck Surg. 1997; 103:600-604.

37. Price JC and Stevens SDL. Hyperbaric oxygen in the treatment of rhinocerebral mucormycosis. Laryngoscope. 1980; 90:737-747.

38. Shao PL, Huang LM, Hsueh PR. Invasive fungal infection-laboratory diagnosis and antifungal treatment. J Microbiol Immunol Infect. 2006; 39:178-188.

39. Shefield PJ. Measuring tissue oxygen tension: a review. Undersea Hyper Med 1998; 25: 179-188.

40. Smith RM, Mohideen P. One hour in 1 ATA oxygen enhances rat alveolar macrophage chemiluminescence and fungal cytotoxicity. Am J Physiol, 1991; 260: L457-463.

41. Sokol-Anderson ML, Brajtburg J, Medoff G. Amphotericin B-induced oxidative damage killing of candida albicans. J Infect Dis 1986; 154:76-83.

42. Sugar AM. Agents of mucormycosis and related species. In: Mandell GL, Bennett JE, Dolin R eds. Principles and practice of infectious diseases. 4th ed. New York: Churchill Livingstone, 1995, pp. 2311-2321.

43. Waldorf AR, Ruderman N, Diamond RD. Specific susceptibility to mucormycosis in murine diabetes and bronchoalveolar macrophage defense against Rhizopus. J Clin Invest. 1984; 74:150-160.

44. Washburn RG, Gallin JI, Bennett JE. Oxidative killing of Aspergillus fumigatus proceeds by parallel myeloperoxidase-dependent and –independent pathways. Infect Immun 1987; 55:2088-2092.

45. Yohai RA, Bullock JD, Aziz AA, Markert RJ. Survival factors in rhino-orbital-cerebral mucormycosis. Surv Ophthalmol 1994; 39: 3-22.

# NOTES

CHAPTER 36

# TREATMENT OF THE BROWN RECLUSE SPIDER BITE WITH HYPERBARIC OXYGEN THERAPY

## CHAPTER THIRTY-SIX OVERVIEW

# Treatment of the Brown Recluse Spider Bite with Hyperbaric Oxygen Therapy

*Ronald P. Bangasser*

*On May 3, 2007, Dr. Ronald P. Bangasser, who served as California Medical Association president passed away. Ron, a family practitioner, was always an example of what a doctor should be, operating his wound care clinic, his practice, all the while serving his patients and colleagues through his advocacy for the CMA.*

*This chapter is dedicated to Ron's contribution to hyperbaric medicine.*

## BACKGROUND

The Brown Recluse Spider (*Loxosceles reclusa*) first mentioned in the literature in 1872 by Caveness (9) has been shown to produce, by envenomation, a dermato-necrotic lesion with possible severe life-threatening systemic manifestations referred to as loxoscelism, necrotic arachnidism, and gangrenocutaneous arachnidism. Years passed until, in 1940, the etiology of what was called the "gangrenous spot of Chile" was found to be the *Loxosceles laeta*, South American cousin, by Machiarello (21). Ten more years passed before the physicians in the United States were made aware of necrotic loxoscelism through the work of Atkins et al. (3) in the American Midwest, who showed that this lesion was secondary to the necrotizing properties of the venom and not infection. Only 10% of all bites result in serious dermato-necrotic lesions (27).

## DISTRIBUTION

*Loxosceles reclusa* is the most important species in the United States, with occurrences spanning the country from New Jersey to California, and Hawaii (4, 8). It is mainly, however, an inhabitant of the South Central United States, primarily Arkansas, Missouri, Kansas, and Oklahoma.

It is usually found lurking in dark, dry, secluded places, i.e., under rocks, wood piles, and debris when outdoors, and in basements, attics, and storage areas indoors (18). This has been true in several cases where some patients report being bitten after putting on clothes that have been stored in the basement or attic. The spider is passive, in that it usually will not bite until provoked or threatened. The spider moves around at night, increasing the probability of human contact. Sixty percent of bites occur in bed. It is described as rugged; it is capable of surviving up to six months without food or water. The spider has a life span of 550 to 625 days. The incidence of bites (17) from the Brown Recluse Spider is highest in April through November. The Brown Recluse Spider is unique in many ways, especially in its physical characteristics. It ranges in length from one to 5 cm leg to leg, fawn to brown in color, with a distinctive dark-colored, violin-shaped marking located on its dorsal cephalothorax; thus it is commonly referred to as "fiddleback" by medical entomologists. The Brown Recluse Spider has only three pairs of eyes, in contrast to four pairs in most spiders. Both sexes are venomous. The legs are long and slender, imparting rapid mobility.

## VENOM/PATHOGENESIS

Most of what is known about the venom of the Brown Recluse Spider was discovered in the 1970s. In the early 1970s, the venom was shown to consist of nine different cytotoxic and inflammatory complex peptides (11). Further work by Geren et al., in 1975 and 1976 (14, 15) revealed that 99.8% of crude venom was composed of a spreading factor (such as hyaluronidase) and other enzymes. Only 0.02% of the venom consists of a skin-necrotizing factor (SNF). In the late 1970s, Finkle et al. (12) were able to identify the SNF as sphingomyelinase D. They demonstrated that the direct lytic action of RBCs was secondary to the venom without the aid of complement, or the energy systems of the cells. Phospholipases, which are lipolytic, cause microemboli that occlude capillaries, devitalize tissue, and result in indolent ulcerations in fatty sites (24).

The venom hemolysin was calcium-dependent, heat-labile (90 degrees C for 30 minutes), with an optimal pH of 7.1 (13). Rees et al. (25) contributed further scientific findings by producing antivenin raised against brown recluse spider bite venom (crude extract) in New Zealand white rabbits. His study revealed that if given within 24 hours, the specific antivenin blocked or markedly attenuated the toxic effect of the venom in the rabbit-model system. Humans appear capable of mounting an active humoral immunity to the venom; however, this has not been well studied (1). Protective immunization of humans is not yet available. Passive immunization via antivenin has yet to be produced.

## DIAGNOSIS

In most cases, the diagnosis of a Brown Recluse Spider bite is purely presumptive, and often made in retrospect by obtaining a complete bite history, and by the signs and symptoms that later develop. Even pieces of the crushed spider are enough for positive identification by experts. Berger (7) developed an immunologic test that used lymphocytes incorporating thymidine into a nucleoprotein to provide a quantitative response (2). More recently, Callahan (24) has developed an ELISA (enzyme-linked immunosorbent assay) directed against circulating venom antigen. This test requires that the blood specimen be drawn within 72 hours of the bite. Within 72 hours, there are 91% specificity and 94% sensitivity. Turn around time by FedEx or Delta Air Express is 8-16 hours. The test is sensitive to all of the *Loxosceles* species in the U.S.

The differential diagnosis of necrotic arachnoidism must include bites from snakes, ticks, scorpions, and other envenomating spiders. Other medical etiologies must be considered, such as Lyme disease, infection, focal vasculitis, foreign body, trauma, and injections of drugs and emboli.

Laboratory studies should include a CBC, PLTs, electrolytes, glucose, BUN/Cr, PT, PTT, and urinalysis. WBC may range from 20,000 to 30,000/ul, signifying the presence of systemic involvement, but often it is in the normal range. A falling hematocrit signifies hemolysis (rare), and severe DIC may follow. Hemolysis can be detected by hemoglobinuria, indicating the potential for renal problems.

## CLINICAL PRESENTATION

The clinical presentation ranges from a mild local reaction to death. The severity of clinical response is related to the amount of venom injected, the location of the bite (with areas of high fat content, such as buttocks, thighs, or abdomen being more severe) and the immune status of the patient. Many bites go unnoticed because they fail to show the characteristic changes or systemic involvement (7). Occasionally, a stinging sensation will be felt at the same time of the bite, while others will come to recognize the lesion several hours later, after the skin changes have begun. First, only redness is noted. Then in two to 12 hours, the skin will take on a dusky, mottled appearance, creating concentric rings of erythema and ischemia with a sharply demarcated border around the bite site. Over three to four days, the dusky area will gradually sink below the level of the normal skin and become progressively necrotic. The area of necrosis is often surrounded by a ring of pallor or "halo" which is in turn, surrounded by a large area of erythema. The toxic effect of the venom actually extends beyond the outer border of the lesion. Blisters are frequently present over the involved area. Initially painless, the bite rapidly becomes painful. In four to seven days, the ischemic base later results in eschar formation. The area then becomes indurated and, at 7 to 14 days, the central area becomes mummified and the eschar falls off, leaving an ulceration. This lesion heals slowly over six to eight weeks, or longer. In areas of fatty necrosis, some lesions are more extensive and have more severe scar formation (10, 29). Some continue to spread, since some patients can mount only minimal neutralizing effects against the venom. Wounds can extend to 10 cm or more.

Some patients experience systemic involvement, usually with the onset at one to two days post bite. Most common symptoms are fever, chills, headache, nausea/vomiting, malaise, diffuse pruritic morbilliform rash, and arthralgia. Further effects include thrombocytopenia, DIC, convulsions and hemolysis leading to hemoglobinemia, hemoglobinuria, renal failure, and death (14, 23). This is the result of the action of the venom and the overstimulation of inflammatory cytokines, such as Interleukin-1 Beta, and tumor necrosis factor alpha.

## TREATMENT

Dapsone is a sulfone derivative with a variety of antibacterial and antituberculosis effects currently used worldwide as a treatment for leprosy (16). Dapsone has also been found to be effective in skin disorders involving prominent polymorphonuclear infiltrates (6). It is thought that Dapsone inhibits leukocyte myeloperoxidase (6), thus decreasing the "innocent bystander" damage to surrounding tissues during acute inflammatory responses. Dapsone has several side effects, including methemoglobinemia and a dose-dependent hemolysis (19, 30). Dapsone was first used for brown spider bites by Rees and King, who have reported 31 patients treated with Dapsone, with only one patient needing skin grafting (25). Results of Dapsone-treated patients were much better than those of a cohort of patients treated with early excision of the lesion. The dosage of Dapsone, given orally, is 1-2 mg/kg/24 hour divided into two doses, up to a maximum of 100 mg b.i.d. In patients with severe envenomation, it should be started as soon as possible. The hematocrit must be followed. Dapsone can be used only after ensuring that the patient is not glucose-6-phosphate dehydrogenase (G6PD) deficient. Patients who are G6PD deficient may develop hemolysis from Dapsone, just as the *Loxosceles* venom can cause hemolysis. No antivenin is commercially available for *Loxosceles laeta* of South America.

All patients with severe disease should be monitored for hemolysis and kept well hydrated. If hemolysis is noted, the urine should be kept alkaline. Dialysis is rarely needed.

Early excision is unwise because it may be both ineffective and unnecessary. General wound care, tetanus immunization, and antibiotics, if appropriate, are given for most lesions. Debridement is necessary to remove necrotic tissue locally, and, in come cases, the wound is large enough that skin grafting later may be required. Grafting can be prevented in most cases with early hyperbaric oxygen treatment.

## CLINICAL SERIES

Hyperbaric oxygen (HBO) is a recently reported treatment for Brown Recluse Spider bites. Hyperbaric oxygen is thought to exhibit its effects through enhanced tissue oxygenation, and possibly direct inactivating effects on *Loxosceles* venom. In two different reports of clinically-diagnosed, brown spider envenomation treatment with hyperbaric oxygen, only one patient out of 48 required grafting (20). In another unpublished study of 35 patients, none of the patients required grafting, after receiving between 2 and 18 HBO treatments (5).

Treatment protocols call for the patient to be seen and diagnosed as soon as possible. If the patient presents in the first 48 hours and a strong presumptive diagnosis of a Brown Recluse Spider bite is made, the patient is treated once a day at 2.0 ATA for 120 minutes, for an average of five treatments, with a low of 2, and a high of 18 treatments. A reassessment of the brown spider bite site is made after each treatment, and additional treatments are ordered at the recommendation of the attending physician.

Some patients initially required hospitalization, depending on the severity of the wound, and the presence of systemic symptoms. The average length of a hospital stay was three days, with most patients requiring no inpatient stay, to a high of 14 days.

Medications used during hyperbaric oxygen treatments, included Valium®, or Ativan®, Actifed® or Entex®, Afrin® or Beconase® and Vitamin E.

The sizes of the dermato-necrotic lesion and surrounding erythema, along with the continuance and/or disappearance of systemic symptoms, are monitored on a daily basis. After completion of hyperbaric oxygen treatment, patients are followed as outpatients in the office.

## RESULTS

The most dramatic effect of hyperbaric oxygen therapy is the change in the color of the dermato-necrotic lesion to normal pink skin color while in the chamber. Also noted is a dramatic improvement in the diffuse morbilliform rash with which several patients have presented. By the time of the publication of the first edition of this text, Kendall (20), who contributed the chapter on the Brown Recluse Spider, had amassed a total of 90 clinically-diagnosed cases treated with HBO. All but four healed without significant scarring, or the need for surgery or skin grafting. If grafting is required, surgeons have noted anecdotally that skin grafts may have a tendency to slough for up to six months after the bite, in the absence of HBO therapy.

## DISCUSSION

The most difficult aspect of treating Brown Recluse Spider bites with hyperbaric oxygen is in establishing the diagnosis. The amount of envenomation and the time lapse between the bite and the treatment are highly variable conditions.

The first mention of hyperbaric oxygen therapy in the treatment of Brown Recluse Spider bites was by Fred J. Svendson, M.D., in October of 1986. Six cases of clinically-diagnosed Brown Recluse Spider bites were treated with hyperbaric oxygen therapy. All lesions healed promptly, without hospitalization, surgery, third-degree skin slough, or significant scarring. Svendson theorized that the necrosis of tissue in Brown Recluse Spider bites was at least partially caused by tissue hypoxia, secondary to the vasospastic and thrombotic effects of the venom. He initially felt that if the prolonged ischemia of the wound could be ameliorated, tissue necrosis could be prevented. He speculated that hyperbaric oxygen therapy might actually inactivate the necrotic venom component of the Brown Recluse Spider venom (28). Maynor et al. (22) in 1992, reported in the *Journal of Hyperbaric Medicine* on 14 patients, all of whom healed without scarring, disability, or the need for skin grafting. Bangasser et al. (5) has had experience with 35 patients with similar results.

Treatment of Brown Recluse Spider bites with hyperbaric oxygen appears to be effective at reducing scarring and complications. However, there have been no controlled animal or human studies conclusively demonstrating the efficacy of this treatment.

## REFERENCES

1. Anderson PC. "Brown Recluse Spider bites - some immunologic aspects." Illinois Med J 1978;150-153.

2. Anderson P. "What's new in loxoscelism." Mo Med 1973;70:711-718.

3. Atkins JA, Wingo CW, Sodemann WA. "Probable cause of necrotic spider bite in the Midwest." Science 1957;126:73.

4. Auer A, Hershey F. "Surgery for necrotic bites of the brown spider." Arch Surg 1974;108:612.

5. Bangasser R, Dexter J, Armijo J, Gil E, Anderson D. "Hyperbaric Oxygen treatment for the Brown Recluse Spider bite." (Unpublished)

6. Barranco V. "Dapsone - other indications." Int J Dermatol 1982;21(9):513-514.

7. Berger R. "The unremarkable Brown Recluse Spider bite." JAMA 1973;225:1109-1111.

8. Butz W. "Envenomation by the Brown Recluse Spider and related species." Clin Toxicol 1971;4:515.

9. Caveness WA. "Insect bite complicated by fever." Nashville J of Med and Surg (2nd series) 1872;10:333.

10. Dos SK, et al. "Management of Brown Recluse Spider bites. A retrospective study of case impact." Contemp Surg 1990;35(6).

11. Elgert B, Wright RP, Campbell BJ, Barrett JT. "Radiolabeling of polypeptide components of Missouri brown spider venom." Fed Proc Abstract #223 1973.

12. Finkle J, Campbell BJ, Barrett JT. "A diagnostic test for Loxosceles reclusa bites." Abstract, Annual meeting of the American Soc. of Microbiology 1973;97.

13. Forrester LJ, Barrett JT, Campbell BJ. "Red blood cells lysis induced by the venom of the Brown Recluse Spider: The role of Sphingomyelinase D." Arch Biochem Biophys 1978;187:355-365.

14. Geren CR, Chan TK, Hewell DE, Odell GV. "Isolation and characterization of toxins from Brown Recluse Spider venom (Loxosceles reclusa)." Arch Biochem Biophys 1976;174:90-99.

15. Geren CR, Chan TK, Hewell DE, Odell GV. "Partial characterization of the low molecular weight fractions of the extract of the venom apparatus of the Brown Recluse Spider and its hemolymph." Toxicon 1975;13:233-238.

16. Goodman and Gilman. The Pharmacological Basis of Therapeutics. 7th Ed. New York: McMillan Publishing Co., 1985;1212-1213.

17. Hall RD, Anderson PC. "Brown Recluse Spider bites: Can they be prevented?" Missouri Med 1981;78(5):243-247.

18. Hile JM, Gladney WJ, Lancaster JL Jr., Whitcomb WH. "Biology of the Brown Recluse Spider." Univ Ark Agr Exp Sta., Bull. 711 1966.

19. Iserson K. "Methemoglobinemia from Dapsone therapy for a suspected Brown Spider bite." J Em Med 1985;3:285-288.

20. Kendall TE, Caniglia RJ. "Hyperbaric oxygen with treatment of clinically diagnosed Brown Recluse Spider bites: A review of 48 cases." Undersea Biomed Res Suppl to Vol. 16 1989. (Abstract only)

21. Machiarello A. "Cutaneous arachnidism or gangrenous spot of Chile." Public Health Trop Med 1947;22:425.

22. Maynor ML, Abt JL, Osborne PD. "Brown Recluse Spider bite: beneficial effects of hyperbaric oxygen." J Hyperbaric Medicine 1992;7(2):89-101.

23. Novak R, Kumar M, Thopson E, Billmeier G. "Severe systemic toxicity from a spider bite in a six year old boy." J Tenn Med Assoc 1979;72:110-111.

24. Pitts RM, Callahan M, Owings E, King W. "Tough Spiders: identifying and treating their bites." Emergency Pediatrics 1992;5(4):72-74.

25. Rees R, Alternbuern D, et al. "Brown Recluse Spider bites: A comparison of early surgical excision versus Dapsone and delayed surgical excision." Ann Surg 1985;220(5):659-663.

26. Rees R, Shack RB, Withers E, Madden J, Franklin J, Lynch JB. "Management of the Brown Recluse Spider bite." Plastic and Reconstruct Surg J 1979;68(5):768-773.

27. Strain GM, Snider TG. "Hyperbaric oxygen effects on Brown Recluse Spider envenomation in rabbits." Toxicon 1991;29:989-996.

28. Svendson F. "Treatment of clinically diagnosed Brown Recluse Spider bites with HBO: A clinical observation." J Ark Med Soc 1986;83:199-204.

29. Wasserman GS, Siegel CJ. "Loxoscelism (Brown Recluse Spider Bites); A review of literature." Vet Human Tox 1977;19:256-258.

30. Wille C, Morrow J. "Case report: Dapsone hypersensitivity syndrome associated with treatment of the bite of a Brown Recluse Spider." Am J Med Sci 1988;296:270-271.

# NOTES

CHAPTER 37

# HBO in Adhesive or Incomplete Ileus Associated with Abdominal Surgery

## CHAPTER THIRTY-SEVEN OVERVIEW

# HBO in Adhesive or Incomplete Ileus Associated with Abdominal Surgery

*Hideyo Takahashi*

## BACKGROUND

Ileus is defined as an obstructive disorder of the intestinal tract which can have a neural, humoral, metabolic, inflammatory, or traumatic cause. It may have a post-surgical origin (paralytic ileus), or it may be due to any mechanical etiology such as tumor, adhesion, or intestinal strangulation (mechanical ileus). When the Japanese Society for Hyperbaric Medicine (JSHM) published the first edition of its Safety and Treatment Guidelines for HBO in 1969, only paralytic ileus was included as an indication for HBO among the intestinal disorders. The guidelines were later revised, however, as it was discovered that HBO can be useful in adhesive ileus, as well (5). Adhesive ileus is an often-refractory complication associated with abdominal, gynecologic, urologic, and even orthopedic surgery, where the abdomen is invaded to repair lumbar vascular anomalies. Extensive clinical experience suggested there was good evidence for the efficacy of HBO in its management. Although the author has always recommended the use of the multiplace chamber, many HBO units in Japan are equipped only with the monoplace unit. It was found that if the patients were not critically ill, requiring an inside tender and IV lines during treatment, monoplace treatment could also produce a favorable outcome. Thus, in Japan, ileus has become one of the most important and common indications for HBO.

## ADHESIVE ILEUS

By classical definition, ileus is divided into two groups: paralytic (adynamic) and mechanical (dynamic or hyperdynamic ileus). Adhesive ileus belongs to the mechanical group, and its incidence has been increasing over the past 10 to 15 years. Before 1986, at the Department of Hyperbaric Medicine, University Hospital of Nagoya, mechanical ileus comprised only 18% of the intestinal diagnoses treated; whereas, the other 82% were post-operative paralytic ileus. Since 1987, however, this ratio has been reversed. Between 1987 and 1995, mechanical ileus comprised 95% of the cases, with the remainder being paralytic. The reasons for this change are several. First was the development of chemical agents which can activate peristaltic movement, and many paralytic cases have become treatable with prostaglandins (Dinoprost). In addition, the progress realized in intravenous hyperalimentation made surgery possible in many elderly, high-risk patients, which would not have been previously contemplated. In recent years, it has become quite common to see radical operations for advanced visceral cancer carried out in very elderly patients which was not heretofore possible. In these cases, if the patients develop a post-operative adhesive ileus, the surgeon is reluctant to perform a repeat laparotomy to find and relieve an adhesion; in such high-risk patients, repeated surgery imposes a severe stress. Repeat surgery often creates further adhesions and leads to a vicious cycle. For this reason, it makes logical sense for a surgeon to refer his patient to the HBO Center for a non-invasive and safe treatment, if it appears to be efficacious.

Intestinal obstruction is not complete in almost all cases of adhesive ileus. Usually there is only minimal passage of small amounts of gas or stool, and the patients exhibit abdominal distention and complain of severe cramping pain. Adhesive ileus can also be defined as an incomplete ileus. Persistent gas figures in the intestine are a characteristic finding in adhesive ileus.

## HISTORICAL BACKGROUND AND RATIONALE FOR HBO IN ILEUS

The direct effect of high environmental pressure on an air-containing, closed intestinal loop was first described by Fontaine (4). He noted that the use of hyperbaric pressure made it easier to reduce an air-filled, intestinal hernia, in accordance with Boyle's Law. In 1952, Cross and Wangensteen (1) opened the gateway to the treatment of ileus using HBO. Cross described a series of elaborate experiments which demonstrated the efficacy of HBO in gas removal from the gut of dogs with artificially-created, closed-loop obstructions. He found that six hours of oxygen breathing at 2 ATA removed 45% of the gas from a closed-loop obstruction, and that 2 ATA was better than surface oxygen (2). This can be considered the direct effect of elevating the gas diffusion gradient, in accordance with Dalton's Law of partial pressures. On examining the effects of Boyle's Law per se on intestinal function, it was found that pressure alone could reduce gas volume and the luminal diameter of the affected intestinal loop. In addition, pressure alone maintained intestinal contractility, viability and peristaltic motor tone, even if the animals were breathing hyperbaric air (1, 3).

Based on these experimental results, the rationale for HBO treatment hinges on the following three physiological effects:

1) Reduction in volume of the luminal air (Boyle's Law).
2) Enhanced inert gas diffusion from the intestinal lumen into the blood (Dalton's Law).
3) Oxygenation of hypoxic intestinal tissue by HBO.

In accordance with Boyle's Law, intestinal gas is reduced in volume when the environmental pressure increases. The over-distended intestinal wall relaxes gradually resulting in reperfusion of the compromised microcirculation in the intestinal wall. HBO ameliorates the hypoxia of the intestinal tissue, which leads to preservation of intestinal viability and recovery of motility. As stated above, the large inert-gas pressure gradient between the luminal space and the blood accelerates reduction of the intestinal gas volume.

In addition, Mader has shown that HBO enhances the bactericidal activity of leukocytes, which may inhibit bacterial proliferation and the resultant production of endotoxins (7). The diaphragms, elevated by the distended gut, return to their normal position as the intestinal gas is reduced in volume and the pressure within the peritoneal cavity lessens. This results in increased venous return and improved respiratory function, which may be critical to recovery in these high-risk patients.

## PROTOCOLS FOR THE HYPERBARIC TREATMENT OF ILEUS

The protocol for the HBO treatment of ileus used at University Hospital, Nagoya is as follows:

1) If it is available, the author's personal preference is to use a multiplace chamber to facilitate care during treatment. This is particularly true if the patient has multiple IV lines, is on a ventilator, and is critically ill. In these situations, it is more convenient to have an inside tender with the patient who can more easily manage his care.

2) HBO treatment is usually administered twice a day; at 2 ATA in the morning and at 3 ATA in the afternoon. The HBO treatment duration at 2 ATA is timed for 60 minutes, beginning at the start of compression and ending at the maximum time at 2 ATA. Decompression takes an additional 20 minutes, the patient being on oxygen the entire time he is in the chamber. Thus the total chamber time is 80 minutes. Treatment at 3 ATA is timed in an identical fashion, except that 30 minutes is taken for decompression, with the total treatment time taking 90 minutes. This is to enhance the effects of Boyle's and Dalton's Laws, and is very important during the acute period.

*Editor's Note: In Japan, a loose-fitting, plastic oxygen mask is used in the multiplace chamber, resulting in a lower FIO2. If the 3 ATA-protocol described above is used with a hood or tight-fitting mask or in a monoplace chamber, it would be advisable to give one or two 5-minute air breaks to lessen the chances of oxygen toxicity. The use of 3 ATA provides additional mechanical compression of intestinal gas. Cross and Wangensteen found mechanical compression significantly effective, even breathing air (1). The reasons for using two different treatment pressures are not based on gas laws or physiology, but have to do with local time constraints for scheduling and patient preference. Dr. Takahashi feels that 3 ATA is more efficacious but it takes longer, and some patients complain that two 3 ATA treatments per day tires them too much.*

3) If for any reason HBO can only be given once a day, a treatment pressure of 3 ATA is preferred.

4) Milestones and the end point of HBO treatment are important considerations. They are:
   A) Documentation of when the first flatus and/or feces is noted.
   B) Documentation of when normalized bowel sounds are heard.
   C) Complete disappearance of intestinal gas, air-fluid levels, and dilated Kerckring's folds as seen on plain abdominal x-ray films.
5) As HBO is not the sole treatment for adhesive ileus, all other standard therapeutic measures must be fully utilized.
6) If HBO proves to be ineffective after 3 days or 6 treatments, laparotomy is urgently indicated. These patients are in considerable pain, and further temporizing imposes unacceptable risk.

## CLINICAL CASES

Two typical cases of adhesive ileus which had a successful outcome following HBO treatment are described below (6).

### Case 1: Simple Adhesive Ileus

A 42-year-old female had surgery for rectal carcinoma (Mile's Operation) combined with hysterectomy, unilateral adnexectomy, and a colostomy. Eight days following surgery she showed symptoms of adhesive ileus, which was managed with a laparotomy to relieve the adhesion. Following the second operation, her recovery progressed smoothly and she was discharged from the hospital. Four years later she complained of severe abdominal pain and gradually increasing fullness which caused her to be readmitted. At the time of her admission, her complaints were sporadic colicky pain and the absence of bowel movements. Abdominal x-rays showed massive amounts of gas and air-fluid levels in the small intestine. She was diagnosed with adhesive ileus, and a naso-gastric tube was placed, with HBO started the day after her admission.

The first HBO treatment was at 3 ATA which brought about the disappearance of her flatulence and colicky pain. Using our standard protocol, she was continued twice a day at 2 ATA in the morning and at 3 ATA in the afternoon. On the third day she was passing flatus intermittently and the air-fluid levels had almost disappeared from her roentgenogram. On the fourth hospital day, after 6 HBO treatments, the air-fluid levels had disappeared completely, the naso-gastric tube was removed and oral intake of water was started. HBO was discontinued after 7 treatments and there was no further recurrence of her ileus.

### Case 2: Adhesive Ileus

A 66-year-old male underwent gastrectomy, and extended surgery for clearing regional lymphatics following diagnosis of advanced gastric cancer. His post-operative course progressed smoothly and he was discharged without any complication.

Eight years later he began feeling ill with the frequent appearance of abdominal pain, tenesmus, nausea, and anorexia. Later his abdominal pain and nausea gradually worsened and he experienced occasional vomiting and abdominal distention.

Following an acute episode of severe, uncontrollable abdominal pain, he was returned to the University Hospital by ambulance and was immediately readmitted. The patient's abdomen was tympanitic and remarkably distended. There were no bowel sounds. A naso-gastric tube was placed immediately. The next morning a small amount of feces was passed, and on the same day the first HBO treatment was given at 3 ATA. About 10 hours after the first HBO treatment, a large amount of flatus was produced per rectum. The next day frequent flatus and a large amount of muddy stool were noted and bowel sounds became audible. What we term an ileus tube (a long, balloon-tipped tube) was advanced and HBO was continued on a twice a day basis, 2 ATA in the morning and 3 ATA in the afternoon. One week after admission, the ileus tube was removed as the ileus had completed resolved. HBO was continued, however, for a total of 30 treatments over 19 days until gas figures had completely disappeared from the small intestine.

## CUMULATIVE RESULTS

During the nine year period from 1987 to 1995, 37 cases of post-operative ileus were referred for hyperbaric treatment. Two cases (5%) were paralytic and 35 cases (95%) were adhesive. Of the 35 cases of adhesive ileus, the ileus was resolved in 24 cases (69%), but HBO was ineffective in the remaining 11 (31%).

## CONCLUSION

In mechanical ileus, HBO is particularly effective for those cases of adhesive ileus which are not accompanied by mesenteric infarction. Surgical intervention to lyse adhesions results in further adhesions in a significant number of cases. HBO is a safe and non-invasive therapeutic modality worth trying before choosing repeat laparotomy, particularly in elderly or high-risk patients.

## REFERENCES

1. Cross, FS, and Wagensteen, OH; "Effect of increased atmospheric pressures on the viability of the bowel wall and the absorption of gas in closed loop obstructions." Surg. Forum 3:111-116; 1952.

2. Cross, FS, "Effect of increased atmospheric pressure on the inhalation of 95% oxygen and helium oxygen mixtures on the viability of the bowel wall and the absorption of gas in closed loop obstructions." Surgery 36: 1001-1026, 1954.

3. Cross, FS, "Hyperoxic treatment of experimental intestinal obstruction." Dis. Of the Chest 47:374-381, 1965.

4. Fontaine, JA, "Emploi chirurgical de l'air comprimé." Un. Medic. 28:448, 1879 From Jacobson, JH Jr., Morsch JHC and Rendell-Baker L: The historical perspective of hyperbaric therapy. In: Clinical Application of Hyperbaric Oxygen (Boerema I, Brummelkamp WH and Meijne NG, Eds.) Elsevier, Amsterdam pp. 7-19, 1964.

5. Japanese Society for Hyperbaric Medicine: Safety and Treatment Guidelines for HBO. November 16, 1995.

6. Kobayashi, S. and Takahashi, H.: "Clinical results of HBO for adhesive ileus." In: Proceedings of the Twelfth International Congress on Hyperbaric Medicine, (Marroni, A., Oriani, G., and Wattel, F. Eds.) Best Publishing Company, Flagstaff, AZ pp. 400-408. 1998.

7. Mader, JT, "Phagocytic killing and hyperbaric oxygen: Antibacterial mechanisms." HBO Review 2:37-49, 1981.

CHAPTER 38

# HYPERBARIC OXYGEN FOR TRAUMATIC BRAIN INJURY

## CHAPTER THIRTY-EIGHT OVERVIEW

# Hyperbaric Oxygen for Traumatic Brain Injury

*Sarah B. Rockswold, Gaylan L. Rockswold*

## INTRODUCTION

Traumatic brain injury (TBI) is called the silent epidemic of the United States of America. Two million people suffer a TBI each year in the USA and approximately one million of them require an emergency room visit; 500,000 are hospitalized and 50,000 die. This results in direct and indirect costs of 56 billion dollars annually to our country (1). The magnitude of the problem is shown in the statement by Dr. Thomas A. Ginnarelli, a neurosurgeon specializing in TBI: "In the last 12 years, the number of deaths from head injury has exceeded all the military deaths in all the wars [up to the Vietnam War] fought by this nation since 1776." Various drug and hypothermia multi-center trials have failed to show improvement in functional outcome and mortality rates in patients suffering from TBI (2-5). In recent years, however, there has been promising animal and clinical research in the area of oxygen ($O_2$), especially hyperbaric oxygen (HBO), for the treatment of severe TBI (6-10).

The use of HBO in the treatment of TBI has been controversial. Oxygen toxicity and safety concerns have been at the forefront of this controversy. In truth, the complications from HBO have been rare and reversible in the authors' experience. Historically, HBO was seen as a mechanism to decrease cerebral blood flow (CBF) and intracranial pressure (ICP) while increasing $O_2$ availability to injured brain cells (11-13). As highly technical equipment has become available in both TBI animal and clinical studies, however, HBO appears to be working at the mitochondrial level to improve cerebral aerobic metabolism after brain injury (7, 8, 10). Clinically, HBO has been shown to decrease mortality rates and improve functional outcome in severely brain-injured patients (6, 14, 15). As research on HBO continues, the goal is to accomplish a multi-center prospective randomized clinical outcome trial by which the efficacy of HBO in the treatment of severely brain-injured patients is evaluated.

## PATHOPHYSIOLOGY OF TRAUMATIC BRAIN INJURY

Ischemia has been implicated as a major cause of secondary brain injury and death following severe brain injury (16-18). Inadequate $O_2$ supply to the traumatized brain results in the conversion of aerobic metabolism to anaerobic metabolism (19, 20). Anaerobic metabolism results in acidosis and depletion of cellular energy. As the demands for energy production are no longer met, the brain cells lose their ability to maintain ionic homeostasis. Abnormally high intracellular concentrations of calcium result (21-23). A combination of cellular acidosis and excessive concentrations of calcium activate various important intracellular proteins. This abnormal cellular environment results in the release of excitatory amino acids and in the formation of highly reactive free radicals that are extremely damaging to cell membranes (24-26). The high levels of calcium also have been shown to lead to excessive calcium being absorbed on neuronal mitochondria membranes leading to the impairment of mitochondrial respiratory chain-linked oxidative phosphorylation leading to further functional failure of aerobic metabolism (27, 28). Mitochondrial dysfunction can persist for days following the initial insult (29-32).

Paradoxically, during this early phase of injury, metabolic needs of the injured brain tissue are increased and cerebral blood flow and delivery of $O_2$ in substrate are decreased. This results in what has been termed a "flow/metabolism mismatch" (27). Oxygen delivery to brain tissue is impaired not only by decreased cerebral blood flow but by reduced $O_2$ diffusion into cells caused by vasogenic and cytotoxic edema. Studies also have shown that local brain tissue oxygen ($PtO_2$) levels are significantly correlated with ischemia and outcome (33-35). Van den Brink, et al. demonstrated the presence of early ischemia at the tissue level with reduced initial $PtO_2$ and found that low $PtO_2$ was an independent predictor of death and unfavorable outcome (34).

Many studies indicate that increased cerebrospinal fluid (CSF) lactate product is a marker for this anaerobic metabolism status caused either by a lack of $O_2$ (ischemia) and/or by damage to the mitochondria (18, 19, 33, 36, 37). A continued high level of lactate in the brain has been shown to be a poor prognostic indicator after brain injury (19, 37-39).

The time from the primary brain injury to the occurrence of irreversible cell damage resulting from ischemia and hypoxia varies considerably, depending upon the severity of the injury and the degree of hypoxia (40). Brain tissue cannot survive without adequate delivery of $O_2$, and even short periods of $O_2$ deprivation may result in the activation of pathological events that contribute to secondary cell damage. Supporting the aerobic processes of the threatened cells could possibly preserve viable, but nonfunctioning tissue.

## HISTORICAL REVIEW OF HYPERBARIC OXYGEN

### Early Studies

The first paper published measuring the effect of HBO on CBF was done by Lambertson, et al. in 1953 (41). By using the nitrous-oxide method developed by Kety and Schmidt, they found a reduction of 24% in the CBF of conscious normal volunteers breathing $O_2$ at 3.5 atmospheres absolute (ATA) compared to 1 ATA (42). However, their subjects hyperventilated at increased pressure, resulting in a fall of arterial $PCO_2$ by 5 mmHg. They concluded that the reduction in CBF was from the arterial hypocapnia.

There were no further published reports on HBO until the following decade. Early in the 1960s, there were two published articles by Illingworth, et al. and Smith, et al., who found there may be possible therapeutic value to HBO where it gave protection to an ischemic brain shown by electroencephalography (43, 44). However there was debate whether this protection was negated by the cerebral vasoconstriction found by Lambertson, et al. (41). Jacobson, et al. undertook an experiment in 1963 measuring CBF and arterial and venous blood gasses with constant arterial $PCO_2$ in non-injured dogs (45). They found a 21% reduction in CBF between dogs receiving 100% $O_2$ at 1 ATA versus 2 ATA. The venous $PO_2$ remained relatively constant while there were large increases in the arterial $PO_2$ leading to an increased arterial-venous difference of oxygen ($AVDO_2$). They felt that this increase in the $AVDO_2$ showed that there was a homeostatic mechanism that exists to maintain tissue-oxygen levels within fairly close limits and served to mitigate against the deleterious effects of HBO on the central nervous system. Also, because the arterial $PCO_2$ was held constant, they felt the decrease in CBF was a direct consequence of vasoconstriction. Tindall, et al. also studied the effect of HBO on CBF in baboons (46). He did not control arterial $PCO_2$ and found there was a drop in CBF as well as arterial $PCO_2$ during the dive. Their conclusions were similar to Lambertson, et al. (41).

During the mid 1960s, there were reports that the use of HBO may be beneficial in the treatment of cerebral ischemia (47-49). However, there was one conflicting report by Jacobsen, et al. that there were larger infarcts in the cerebrum following middle cerebral artery occlusion when HBO was used (50). Of note, the number of subjects described in all of these reports was very small.

The first study in which HBO was used to treat experimental TBI was done in 1966 by Dunn, et al. (51). The authors exposed dog brains to liquid nitrogen simulating brain contusion. The animals were divided into six groups according to pressure and $O_2$ received. The mortality for all groups receiving hyperoxia was significantly decreased (15%) in comparison to those that did not (56%). The sizes of the lesions also were reduced in the treated group, although this finding did not reach statistical significance.

In 1967, Sukoff, et al. used two methods to produce cerebral edema in dogs; psyllium seeds and the extradural balloon technique (52). Both series of dogs were divided into a HBO treated group (3 ATA for 45 minutes) and a control group. Mortality in the psyllium seed group was 27% for the HBO group and 83% for the control group. In the extradural balloon group, mortality was 50% for the HBO group and 100% for the control group. All surviving HBO treated dogs were neurologically normal. All animals were sacrificed and their brains showed gross evidence of cerebral edema. However, the HBO treated brains weighed significantly less than the control brains. They concluded that HBO has a protective effect against experimental cerebral edema and compression.

In 1968, Sukoff, et al. published another paper on the effects of HBO on experimental edema (11). This study was performed again in dogs, using the psyllium seed technique to produce a space occupying lesion. The animals were exposed at 3 ATA for 45 minutes at 8 hours intervals. The results were as follows: mortality rate for the control group was 83% compared to 27% in the HBO treated group. Cisternal CSF pressure was steadily reduced in the HBO treated group as compared to the control group which showed steady increase in ICP. They felt that the main action of HBO was at the level of the cerebral blood vessel. HBO caused cerebral vasoconstriction and decreased CBF reducing cerebral edema yet at the same time there was increased availability of $O_2$ at the cellular level. For these reasons, HBO could protect the injured brain against ischemia secondary to cerebral edema.

In 1970 a similar study was performed by Moody, et al., using an extradural balloon in dogs (53). The 95% mortality rate in the control group was reduced to 50% by treatment of the dogs with 100% $O_2$ at 2 ATA for four hours following balloon decompression. The quality of survival was good among the survivors of the treated group. They also concluded that HBO produces better tissue oxygenation during low CBF seen following this type of experimental brain injury.

The next important study on the effect of HBO on CBF was published in 1969 by Wullenberg, et al. from Dr. Holbach's group in Germany (54). This study was the first to measure CBF in severely brain-injured patients during HBO treatments. They used thermoprobes to measure the CBF. In contrast to previous published results, they found that CBF increased during the dive during increasing pressures, but once the pressure reached 2.5 ATA no further rise occurred. During the same time period, blood pressure, pH and arterial $PCO_2$ remained normal. Arterial $PO_2$ increased to 1,100 mmHg but venous $PO_2$ increased only slightly. The concentration of lactate and pyruvate decreased corresponding to the rise in arterial $PO_2$. The CBF remained slightly elevated after the dive. They concluded that HBO is indicated in cases of severe brain injury.

Mogami, et al. in 1969 was one of the first to describe the effect of HBO on ICP in severely brain-injured patients (55). Sixty-six patients in whom most (51) had traumatic brain injuries were studied. The HBO treatment was usually given at a pressure of 2 ATA for one hour, two times a day; six of these treatments, however, were given at 3 ATA for 30 minute. In total, 143 treatments were given to the 66 patients. During HBO, 33 patients (50%) showed clinical improvement during the treatment, but usually, regressions occurred after the treatments. CSF pressure was measured during treatment. The pressure was found to decrease during the beginning of treatment, stay at a low level during treatment and then rebound after treatment. The authors also found that lactate/pyruvate ratios were mildly decreased. This was the first published article that challenged that ICP decreases only from vasoconstriction. The group asserted that HBO may be affecting and stabilizing the blood brain barrier. They also felt that TBI has such heterogeneous pathophysiology that HBO may affect individuals differently.

Hayakawa, et al. in 1971 demonstrated clinical evidence that HBO treatment decreased CSF pressure (56). There were two parts to this article, a clinical and experimental portion. The clinical study measured changes in CSF pressure in 13 patients with acute cerebral damage, nine who had a TBI and four who under went craniotomy for a brain tumor. $PCO_2$ was not controlled or measured. The authors described three main patterns during HBO treatment at 2 ATA for one hour: 1) In nine patients, CSF pressure decreased at the beginning of the dive, but rose again at the end; 2) In two patients, CSF pressure fell and remained lower after the dive; and 3) In two patients, CSF pressure showed little change with the dive. In the experimental study, HBO was administered to 46 dogs at 3 ATA for one hour. Twelve of these dogs underwent extradural balloon technique to produce a brain injury. Both CBF and CSF pressure were measured. The response of the brain-injured dogs to the HBO was variable but for the most part, no or little change in CBF or CSF pressure was seen during and after HBO treatment. The authors concluded that there is considerable variation in the response of CSF pressure to HBO in patients and animals with brain injury, and like Mogami, et al., these differences needed to be studied and defined before HBO could be used in the treatment of TBI patients.

During the late 1960s and early 1970s, studies on HBO also were being done in Glasgow, Scotland. Miller, et al. published several experimental animal studies which showed HBO could reduce CBF and ICP by direct cerebral vasoconstriction in injured dogs (57). In one study, they showed that increased ICP was reduced by 23% by breathing 100% $O_2$ at normobaric pressures and 37% at 2 ATA in a HBO chamber (57). The arterial blood pressure and arterial $PCO_2$ remained constant. They felt ICP was only responsive to HBO when autoregulation was still responsive to carbon dioxide. Another study in 1971 showed that elevated ICP dropped during HBO treatment (26%), but not as much as with hyperventilation (34%) (13). However, when HBO was used in conjunction with hyperventilation, an additional 25% drop in ICP was recorded. There was no significant change in CSF lactate in the HBO group. Their conclusion was that HBO caused vasoconstriction but at the same time improved cerebral tissue oxygenation which protected the cells from damage.

The first article written by Holbach, et al. studying the effect of HBO on glucose metabolism was published in 1972 (58). The main objective of this study was to determine the limits of $O_2$ tolerance in severely brain injured patients in order to advance the use of HBO in the treatment of TBI. In this study, the effects of different HBO pressures (1 to 3 ATA ) on cerebral glucose metabolism were studied in ten patients with severe TBI. The $AVDO_2$, arterial-venous differences of glucose (AVDG), lactate (AVDL) and pyruvate were taken. The glucose oxidation quotient (GOQ), which represents cerebral glucose oxidative metabolism, was then calculated. At 1.5 ATA, a well-balanced cerebral glucose metabolism was maintained, indicated by a normal GOQ of 1.35. There was also a decrease in lactate and lactate/pyruvate ratio. However, Holbach, et al. found that exposure of HBO at 2 ATA led to a decrease in oxidative glucose metabolism shown by a significantly reduced uptake of $O_2$ in comparison to glucose as well as a rise in lactate and lactate/pyruvate levels (58). They felt the increased pressure interfered with oxidative energy formation and led to a compensatory increase of anaerobic energy production and hyperglycolysis.

By 1973 K.H. Holbach wrote, "The real indication for the hyperbaric oxygen therapy is the deficiency of oxygen in the brain tissue since brain hypoxia is an essential factor of...secondary hypoxic brain lesions" (59). He reviewed his past work, stating HBO caused a marked rise in arterial $O_2$ pressure (8-10 fold increment at 1.5 ATA and 12 fold increment at 2 ATA) while the arterial $O_2$ pressure in the jugular bulb venous flow rose only slightly resulting in a marked increase in cerebral $AVDO_2$. He also reiterated the findings of the 1972 study which showed that 1.5 ATA was the ideal pressure based on oxidative glucose metabolism. Finally, the results of a randomized trial between patients treated with 1.5 ATA versus 2.0 ATA were described.

Two hundred and sixty-seven HBO treatments were given to 102 patients: 50 patients treated with 1.5 ATA and 52 treated with 2.0 ATA. Forty-eight percent of the patients treated with 1.5 ATA had a good outcome versus 25% of the patients treated with 2.0 ATA. This improvement in functional outcome was statistically significant.

An important clinical study was published by Holbach, et al. in 1974 (14). This paper strongly suggested that HBO applied systematically may improve the outcome of patients who were severely brain-injured. The study included 99 patients with traumatic midbrain syndrome, every other one of whom was treated with HBO at 1.5 ATA for 30 minutes. Each patient received between one and seven treatments which was determined on each patient's response to the HBO. The overall mortality rate for the 49 HBO patients was 33% as compared to the control patients which was 74%. Functional outcome also was improved with 33% of the HBO patients having a good outcome compared to 6% of the control patients. Patients with cerebral contusions less than 30 years of age were particularly benefited by HBO. They felt that the increased survival and functional outcome in the HBO treated group was secondary to decreased ICP as well as improved oxidative glucose metabolism.

The final publication by Holbach, et al. was in 1977 (60) This study measured the effect of HBO at 1.5 ATA and 2 ATA on cerebral glucose metabolism in 23 TBI patients and seven anoxic brain-injured patients. Many of their previous findings on the effect of pressure on glucose metabolism were replicated in this study. They found that the injured brain would not tolerate HBO exposure at 2 ATA for 10-15 minutes, but exposure at 1.5 ATA for 35-40 minutes was well tolerated and glucose metabolism was improved. An important finding for future work was that the $AVDO_2$ values remained unchanged after the 1.5 ATA HBO treatments from baseline measurements.

Another clinical study was published by Artru, et al. in 1976 evaluating the effectiveness of HBO in the treatment of severely brain-injured patients (15). The study was a prospective trial of 60 patients randomized into an HBO treatment group and a control group. The HBO was administered at 2.5 ATA for 60 minutes. The treatment sequence was ten daily sessions, no session for four days, followed by ten more daily sessions until the patient either recovered consciousness or died. There was a time delay between injury and onset of HBO treatment averaging 4.5 days. Only 17 of the 31 patients received four daily treatments in the first week secondary to treatment interruptions. No difference in mortality at one year was seen between the two groups; however infectious complications were the primary reason for death in both groups. Functional outcome was improved at one month, in younger patients treated with HBO, who had a clinical picture of brain stem contusion. The authors felt the delay in treatment and frequent interruptions of treatment may have led to the study's poor results.

A second paper written by Artru, et al., also published in 1976, studied the effect of HBO on cerebral metabolism in severely brain-injured patients (61). Six patients were treated with HBO at 2.5 ATA, timing between dives is not known. Cerebral blood flow, $AVDO_2$, AVDG and AVDL as well as CSF parameters were measured at two hours pre-dive and two hours post-dive. The cerebral metabolic rate of oxygen ($CMRO_2$), glucose and lactate were calculated from those measurements. Pre-dive arterial and CSF lactate levels were found to be high while pre-dive CBF and $CMRO_2$ were lower than normal. They found that the $AVDO_2$ remained constant before and after the dives as had Holbach, et al. (60). The CBF was raised in patients who had low CBF values prior to the dive and was reduced in the patients who started with a high CBF. Each patient's $CMRO_2$ values followed the direction of their CBF. The effects of the HBO treatment did not last until the next pre-dive measurement and the patients reacted to each HBO treatment consistently. The spinal CSF lactate, CMRL, and CMRG did not significantly change. The authors concluded that HBO can improve CBF when there is cerebral edema or intracranial hypertension.

In 1982, Sukoff, et al. published an article studying the effect of HBO on CBF and ICP in TBI (12). Their theory was that HBO reduced ICP by decreasing CBF but concomitantly increased cerebral oxygenation leading to a decrease in cerebral ischemia. Entered into the study within six hours of injury, 50 comatose TBI patients were treated with HBO at 2 ATA for 45 minutes every eight hours for 2–4 days. The ICP was decreased in all patients in whom measurements were obtained. This reduction ranged between 4 to 21 mmHg below the pre-dive level and was sustained for two to four hours after HBO treatment was completed. Sukoff, et al. recorded only the lowest ICP value during the HBO treatment and did not report all ICP measurements recorded throughout the dive (12). There were no reports of pulmonary toxicity. They felt additional studies on the effect of HBO on ICP and cerebral metabolism were needed.

The above investigations of HBO had several weaknesses. Most of the protocols were not uniform and the number of subjects was small. Although Holbach, et al. had shown that the ideal depth was 1.5 ATA for treatment of TBI, HBO was delivered at 2–3 ATA in most of the experimental and clinical studies (14, 58-60). In the clinical trials, the severity of brain injury is not known as Glasgow Coma Scale (GCS) scoring was not used. In addition, none of the trials were truly randomized. Despite these shortcomings, positive results on the efficacy of HBO in TBI were consistently found.

In 1988, the first paper to show that HBO had a persistent effect on cerebral glucose metabolism following treatment was published by Contreras, et al. (62). The authors measured glucose utilization with the autoradiographic 2-deoxyglucose technique in rats injured by a focal parietal cortical freeze lesion. This cold lesion was felt to correspond with a focal brain contusion. Four groups of rats were used; 1) sham-lesioned group, no treatment; 2) sham-lesioned, HBO treatment; 3) cold-lesioned, no treatment; 4) cold-lesioned, HBO treatment. The HBO treatments at 2 ATA for 90 minutes were done daily for four consecutive days. Initially, glucose utilization was decreased throughout the brain, especially ipsilateral to the lesion. Glucose utilization, however, tended to be increased five days after injury in the HBO treated cold-lesioned rats as compared to the control cold-lesioned group. This improvement reached statistical significance in five of the 21 structures examined, which were the auditory cortex, the medial geniculate body, the superior olivary nucleus, the lateral geniculate body ipsilateral to the lesion and the mamillary body. An interesting finding was that HBO decreased glucose utilization in sham-lesioned rats. The authors felt that their results indicate HBO improves glucose utilization in a cold-lesion rat model, especially in the gray matter structures close to the actual lesion. Their novel finding was that the increase persisted for at least one day after termination of HBO exposure. They were unsure of the mechanism involved with this persistence, but felt further studies were indicated.

A paper which studied the effects of HBO on the blood-brain barrier was published by Mink, et al. in 1995 (63). Rabbits were subjected to cerebral ischemia by CSF compression. They were allowed to reperfuse for 30 minutes and then either treated with HBO at 2.8 ATA for 125 minutes followed by 90 minutes of 100% $FiO_2$ or with 100% $O_2$ for 215 minutes. CBF and vascular permeability were measured at the end of the reperfusion period and 90 minutes after termination of the treatments. HBO treatment statistically lowered CBF in the HBO treated group as compared with the controls. Vascular permeability also was statistically lowered by 16% in the gray matter and 20% in the white matter. Somatosensory evoked potentials (SEP) were similar between both groups. The authors concluded that HBO was promoting the blood brain barrier integrity following global cerebral ischemia in a rabbit model. CBF also was reduced and this effect was not associated with a reduction in the SEP recovery. They felt that the results suggested that if there were any detrimental effects of free radical generation with HBO treatment, they were outweighed by the beneficial effects of HBO.

An important paper investigating the mechanisms by which HBO improved ischemic tissue $O_2$ capacitance was published in 1997 by Siddiqui, et al. (64). The authors measured subcutaneous tissue $O_2$ treatment in an ischemic rabbit ear model before, during, and after HBO treatment followed by 100% $O_2$ versus those treated only with 100% $O_2$. The HBO treatment, which was at 2 ATA for 90 minutes, was performed daily for 14 treatments. The tissue responsiveness, measured by $O_2$ tissue tension, was found to increase on successive days from an ischemic baseline to well above a non-ischemic level. The authors felt that there was "a consistent and striking response to 100% oxygen (at 1 ATA) by ischemic tissue undergoing serial hyperbaric oxygen therapy." This responsiveness was not found in tissue that was treated only with 100% $O_2$ at 1 ATA. The group asserted that this tissue responsiveness represents the tissue's ability to accept and potentially utilize $O_2$ and that HBO was responsible for this change. They felt that cells in the ischemic region may see the supraphysiologic elevation of tissue $O_2$ partial pressure as a trigger that signals that enough $O_2$ is in the environment to proceed with normal healing. Subsequent exposure to 100% $O_2$ reinforces this signal and also supplies the $O_2$ needed to continue the repair. They concluded "that molecular oxygen, when delivered at high pressure, can function both as a respiratory metabolite and as a signal transducer."

## Modern Perspective on HBO Research

Rockswold, et al. published the first modern prospective randomized clinical trial on the efficacy of HBO in the treatment of severely brain-injured patients (6). All patients who were entered had suffered closed head injury with a GCS score of nine or less. The patients were entered into the study between 6 and 24 hours post-injury. One hundred and sixty-eight severely brain-injured patients were randomized into two groups; the first group receiving HBO treatments and the second serving as a control group. Eighty-four patients received HBO with 100% $O_2$ at 1.5 ATA for 60 minutes. Treatments were given every eight hours for 14 days unless the patient began following commands or became brain dead. Treatments were discontinued if the patient required a fraction of inspired oxygen ($FiO_2$) of 50% or greater to maintain an arterial $PO_2$ greater than 70 mmHg. The Glasgow Outcome Scale (GOS) was used as the primary tool for assessing outcome. Of the 168 patients, only two control patients were lost to follow-up at 12 months.

The mortality rate for the 84 HBO-treated patients was 17% and for the 82 control patients was 32% ($p < 0.05$). This improvement represents a 50% relative reduction in mortality. In addition, mortality rate was improved in specific subgroups. In the 47 patients with ICP values persistently greater than 20 mmHg, the mortality rate was 21% as opposed to 48% mortality in the 40 patients with elevated ICP who served as controls ($p < 0.02$). Functional recovery was evaluated at 12 months post injury using the GOS. Favorable outcome was defined as good recovery or moderate disability. Overall, there was no significant improvement in favorable outcome in the 84 patients treated with HBO in comparison to the 82 control patients. However, some specific subgroups did show improved favorable outcome. The 33 patients with surgically evacuated mass lesions had a 45% favorable outcome at one year as opposed to a 34% favorable outcome in the 41 patients with surgically evacuated mass lesions who served as control. This represents a 33% relative improvement. It is now thought with an appropriately increased "n," this difference would be statistically significant. Mean peak ICP was significantly reduced in HBO treated patients as opposed to controls.

Of major importance, is the fact that the 84 patients in the treatment group received a total of 1,688 HBO treatments for an average of 21 treatments. Considering the number of treatments delivered, relatively few complications occurred. They were all pulmonary in nature, manifested by an increased $FiO_2$ requirement, and frequently, chest x-ray infiltrates. In ten patients, the HBO treatments were stopped. All pulmonary changes were reversible. There were no permanent sequelae that occurred from the 1,688 HBO treatments that were delivered.

The authors concluded that this clinical outcome study showed that HBO can be administered to severely brain-injured patients safely and systematically and that mortality rates for severely brain-injured patients are reduced by about 50% with HBO treatments, particularly in patients with GCS scores of four to six, those with mass lesions, and those with increased ICP. These three factors are interrelated and without HBO treatment, the mortality rate would be highest in these groups of patients since all are indicative of poor prognosis. Thus, through reducing ICP and, most likely, improving aerobic glucose metabolism, HBO allowed these severely brain-injured patients to survive. The authors were unsure why the functional recovery overall was not improved with this treatment paradigm but hypothesized that too much $O_2$ was given to patients with less severe injuries (i.e. higher GCS score, contusion, or normal ICP). They felt that the protocol should be more individualized.

Many questions persisted about the efficacy and application of HBO in TBI following the above prospective randomized clinical study. Further investigation was needed to elucidate the potential metabolic effects of HBO on severely brain-injured patients. A prospective, clinical physiologic study, therefore, was undertaken by the same group to determine the effects of HBO on CBF, cerebral metabolism, and ICP (7).

Thirty-seven patients treated for severe TBI were entered into the study within 24 hours of admission. All patients had a GCS score eight or less and CT scan scores were ≥ II in conformance with the classification system of the Traumatic Coma Data Bank. The patients received HBO with 100% $O_2$ at 1.5 ATA for 60 minutes. The mean time from injury to initial HBO treatment was 23 hours. Treatment was administered on subsequent days for a total of five treatments. CBF using the nitrous oxide method; $AVDO_2$; $CMRO_2$; ventricular CSF lactate levels; and ICP values were obtained one hour prior to HBO and one hour and six hours post HBO. The patients were then assigned to reduced, normal, or raised categories according to the CBF classification system developed by Obrist, et al. and modified by Robertson, et al. (65, 66).

In patients in whom CBF levels were reduced before HBO, both CBF and $CMRO_2$ were raised one hour and six hours after HBO ($p = 0.001$). In patients in whom CBF levels were normal before HBO, both CBF and $CMRO_2$ levels were increased at one hour ($p < 0.05$), but not at six hours. CBF was reduced one hour and six hours after HBO ($p = 0.007$), but $CMRO_2$ was unchanged in patients who exhibited raised CBF before HBO.

Levels of CSF lactate were consistently decreased one hour and six hours after HBO, regardless of the patients' CBF category before undergoing HBO ($p = 0.011$). Pre-dive CSF lactate levels for individual HBO treatments were inversely related to the pre-dive CBF values demonstrating that in those HBO sessions in which patients began with a reduced CBF value, CSF lactate pretreatment levels were significantly greater than those seen in HBO in which patients began with normal or raised CBF ($p = 0.003$). This finding may indicate that patients with reduced pre-dive CBF were the most ischemic or had the most severe cellular dysfunction in the brain and responded to HBOT most dramatically.

Intracranial pressure was measured prior, during the HBO treatment, and until the next HBO treatment. The ICP values rose through-out the dive except for a trend for patients with elevated ICP (≥ 15 mmHg) to improve during the pressurization phase and first 15 minutes of the HBO treatment. Patients with elevated ICP also showed a consistent and highly significant decrease in their intracranial pressure from the time of the completion of the HBO treatment to six hours post-treatment ($p = 0.006$).

The results of this study indicate that HBO may have improved the ability of ischemic or damaged brain tissue to utilize the $O_2$ received in baseline $FiO_2$ for at least six hours following the HBO. This improved utilization led to improved $CMRO_2$ and decreased CSF lactate levels, which also persisted for at least six hours, indicating a shift toward aerobic metabolism. The authors hypothesized that CBF rises in response to this increased cerebral metabolism. When CBF and $CMRO_2$ are normally metabolically coupled, the ratio between them does not change. In other words, the $AVDO_2$ remains constant. This trend for HBO to normalize metabolic coupling of CBF and cerebral metabolism was most apparent in patients with reduced CBF or with ischemia as documented by high lactate levels.

The authors felt that the potentially noxious stimuli of heat and pressure in the paranasal sinuses may have overridden any benefit that HBO had on the patient's ICP during treatment. However, in patients who began their dive with a high ICP, HBO reduced their ICP (≥ 15 mmHg) for at least six hours following treatment. In this study, HBO also lowered CBF in patients who began their treatment with a raised CBF and did so without significantly reducing their $CMRO_2$. Raised CBF or hyperemia has been shown to be related to increased ICP, brain edema, and poor outcome. The authors felt that HBO may promote blood-brain barrier integrity, reducing cerebral edema and hyperemia, which in turn helped to lower elevated ICP.

## Recent Studies

A basic science article by Rogatsky et al. showed similar findings for intracranial pressure and mortality as Rockswold et al. (6, 67). Rats were subjected to a severe fluid percussion brain injury and several parameters were measured using a multiparametric assembly developed in the authors' laboratory (68). These parameters included NADH redox state, ICP, CBF, extracellular potassium, calcium, and hydrogen concentrations, which were continuously measured and downloaded electronically. Group A served as the control group and Group B received 60 minutes of HBO at 1.5 ATA beginning two hours after injury. Changes in the ICP level were analyzed every 30 minutes for eight hours after brain injury and at the end of the experiment (20 hours). Mean levels of ICP were significantly lower in the HBO group than the controls beginning four hours after the trauma. The mortality was 0% in the HBO group and 43% in the control group. The authors theorized that the diminishing ICP in the HBO group was due to the retarded development of cerebral edema caused by stabilization of the blood brain barrier.

Two separate publications, both published in 2004, showed evidence that HBO reduces necrosis area, cerebral edema, and secondary brain damage in animals following experimentally induced traumatic brain injury (69, 70). Niklas et al. showed a significant increase in brain $PtO_2$ in cold-injury-induced brain trauma rabbits treated daily with HBO for 90 minutes at 2.5 ATA for three days as compared to controls (69) Mean $PtO_2$, measured with permanently implanted Licox oxygen microprobes, was 169 mmHg during the first HBO session, 305 mmHg during the second session and 420 mmHg during the final session. The mean area of necrosis was 16.2 $mm^2$ in the HBO group and 19.9 $mm^2$ in the control group. The area of brain edema was significantly smaller in the HBO group. Mortality was 0% in the HBO group and 20% in the control group. They hypothesized that "idling neurons" in the penumbra were saved by HBO treatment by reducing cerebral edema and intracranial pressure.

In the second study, by Palzur et al., five groups of rats were subjected to dynamic cortical deformation (DCD) induced by negative pressure applied to the cortex described by Shreiber et al. (70, 71). The five groups included: 1) DCD alone; 2) DCD followed by HBO (2.8 ATA for two consecutive 45 minute treatments daily for three days); 3) DCD and post-operative hypoxia; 4) DCD and postoperative hypoxia followed by HBO 5) DCD and normobaric hyperoxia (100% $FiO_2$ for two consecutive 45 minute treatments daily for three days). All animals were sacrificed on day four and histological sections taken. Secondary brain damage was assessed by counting the number of terminal deoxynucleotidyl transferase-mediated dUTP nick end labeling (TUNEL) and caspase 3-positive cells in successive perilesional layers, each 0.5 mm thick. The HBO treated group showed a significant decrease in both the radius and severity of brain damage. The lesion surface was significantly reduced from $5.9 \pm 2.2$ mm$^2$ in non-treated animals to $2.3 \pm 0.6$ mm$^2$ in HBO treated animals. In the rats subjected to post-traumatic hypoxemia, reduction of lesion volume and severity by HBO was even more pronounced than after DCD alone. In animals treated by normobaric hyperoxia, a similar trend in the reduction of TUNEL-positive cells was demonstrated, although to a lesser extent than seen in the HBO group. The authors felt that the study demonstrated that HBO showed a definite reduction of the extent and severity of secondary brain damage.

A recent article published in 2006 by the same Israeli group showed that HBO reduced neuroinflammation and matrix metalloproteinase-9 (MMP-9) expression in rats injured with the DCD model described by Shreiber et al. (71, 72). In this study, 20 rats underwent DCD followed by HBO (2.8 ATA, two sessions of 45 minutes), ten rats underwent DCD followed by normobaric hyperoxia, and ten animals underwent DCD and served as controls. TUNEL assay was used for quantitative evaluation of cell death in the posttraumatic penumbra. Neutrophils were revealed by myeloperoxidase staining and immunohistochemical staining for MMP-9 was performed. The HBO group had a significant decrease in the number of TUNEL-positive cells and neutrophilic inflammatory infiltration as compared to the normobaric and control groups. The expression of MMP-9 also was significantly lower in the HBO group. The authors felt that HBO decreased the extent of secondary cell death and reactive neuroinflammation in this TBI model. They also felt that the decline of MMP-9 expression after HBO may contribute to the protection of brain tissue in the perilesional area. They were unclear if the decrease of apoptotic cells in the traumatic penumbra was the result of anti-apoptotic effects of HBO or the secondary consequence of the reduction of harmful inflammatory reaction.

In 2004, an important basic science article was published by Daugherty et al. studying the mechanism of action that HBO has on TBI (9). The authors produced strong supporting experimental data for Rockswold, et al. clinical observations (7). Four groups of rats were compared: 1) sham-injured, 30% FiO$_2$ for four hours; 2) sham-injured, one-hour HBO (1.5 ATA) followed by three hours of 100% FiO$_2$ at 1 ATA; 3) fluid percussion injured, 30% FiO$_2$ for four hours; 4) fluid percussion injured, one-hour HBO (1.5 ATA) followed by three hours 100% FiO$_2$ at 1 ATA. Fluid percussion injury was delivered at $2.1 \pm 0.05$ ATM to the rats (73, 74). PtO$_2$ levels were measured by a Licox probe into the cortex near the cortical hippocampal junction. This placement allowed for the measurement of brain PtO$_2$ under the injury site. *Ex vivo* measurements of global brain tissue oxygen consumption (VO$_2$) were made using the Cartesian diver microrespirometer methodology described by Levasseur, et al. (75). *Ex vivo* measurements of mitochondrial metabolic activity (redox potential) were carried out in a synaptosomal preparation to enrich for mitochondria. Mitochondrial redox potential was measured using an Alamar blue fluorescence technique (76, 77).

Brain PtO$_2$ was significantly improved in both the injured and sham-injured animals that received HBO treatment as compared to the ones receiving only 30% O$_2$. Injured animals tended to have a lower brain PtO$_2$ levels as baseline compared to the sham-injured ones. Baseline brain PtO$_2$ levels were 37.7 mmHg in injured animals receiving 30% O$_2$. This value went to approximately 103 mmHg on 100% $O_2$ at 1.0 ATA and finally to 247 mmHg on HBO at 1.5 ATA. The dramatic relative 250% increase in brain $PtO_2$ levels, when going from 100% $O_2$ at 1 ATA to 100% $O_2$ at 1.5 ATA, was not clear. Under normobaric conditions, the amount of dissolved $O_2$ in the blood is relatively small (0.3 ml/dl in air at atmospheric pressure). HBO at 1.5 ATA increases the amount of dissolved $O_2$ by tenfold (3.2 ml/dl), therefore increasing the arterial $PO_2$. One hypothesis for explaining the relatively high brain $PtO_2$ in relationship to arterial $PO_2$ is that this dissolved $O_2$ in plasma is more readily available to brain tissue than hemoglobin bound $O_2$.

The combined HBO/100% $FiO_2$ treatment paradigm described also caused a highly significant increase in global $VO_2$ in both injured and sham-injured animals when compared to control animals receiving 30% $O_2$. Brain tissue $VO_2$ is a marker for cerebral aerobic metabolism and corresponds to $CMRO_2$ values used clinically in patients. CBF and $VO_2$ are closely coupled and respond to cellular activity. Daugherty, et al. felt that the findings of increased $VO_2$ after HBO treatment strongly supports HBO improves aerobic metabolism in the injured brain (9).

Mitochondrial redox potential was significantly reduced by the fluid percussion injury when compared to sham-injured animals in both the HBO and 30% $FiO_2$ groups at the completion of one hour of treatment. However, following the one-hour HBO treatment plus three hours of 100% $O_2$ at 1 ATA, mitochondrial redox potential was reversed to near sham-injured animal levels. When the authors compared the effects of the different treatments at four hours, the injured animals that had received the HBO treatment had significantly increased mitochondrial redox potential in all areas of the brain sampled when compared to the injured animals that had received 30% $O_2$. These data indicate that mitochondrial function may be depressed after TBI, but there is a potential for mitochondrial functional recovery and that HBO can enhance this recovery.

Recent experimental evidence in the same lateral fluid percussion TBI rat model has demonstrated improved cognitive recovery, increased cerebral ATP levels, and reduced hippocampal neuronal cell loss with HBO followed by normobaric hyperoxia (10). For the cognitive recovery portion of the study, two hundred and five rats were divided into four groups 15 minutes after injury: 1) sham-injured; 2) fluid percussion injured, 30% $FiO_2$; 3) fluid percussion injured, 100% $O_2$ in the HBO chamber at 1.5 ATA for one hour and at 1 ATA for an additional three hours; 4) fluid percussion injured, 100% $O_2$ in the HBO chamber at 1 ATA for four hours. On days 11 to 15 following injury, cognitive function was assessed by the Morris Water Maze test. The results demonstrated that when compared to sham animals, all three injured groups described above had longer goal latencies. However, the combined HBO/$FiO_2$ treated group showed significantly shorter goal latency than the other two groups for all time points. By day 15, the cognitive deficit was markedly attenuated in the HBO/100% $O_2$ treated group, but not in the 100% $O_2$ treated group or control animals.

For ATP measurement, the rats in each group were given only one hour of treatment, whether it was 30% $O_2$, HBO, or normobaric hyperoxia. The combination of HBO and 100% $O_2$ was not studied. ATP was extracted from the cerebral cortex and measured using high performance liquid chromatography system. Immediately following injury, ATP levels were significantly decreased in all injured animals when compared to sham-injured animals. However, after one hour of treatment, both groups of animals that received hyperoxia had significantly elevated ATP levels when compared with the injured animals that received 30% $O_2$. In fact, the ATP levels were close to the levels of the sham-injured group.

At 21 days post injury, four rats in each group were sacrificed to assess hippocampal neuronal loss. Cranial sections throughout the hippocampus were examined with an Olympus Image System Cast Program. The HBO/100% $FiO_2$ combined group had significantly reduced injury-induced cell loss in the CA2-3 region of the hippocampus when compared to control or animals receiving normobaric hyperoxia alone. No significant differences in peroxide, peroxynitrite or free radical production between the sham-injured animals and the injured animals treated with 30% $O_2$, 100% $O_2$, or HBO at one or four hours post-treatment were found. The results of this study strongly corroborate the findings that HBO used in combination with normobaric hyperoxia enhances cellular metabolism and supports the concept that this enhancement provides a protective effect for severe TBI.

## Chronic TBI

The above scientific publications studied the actions of HBO on relatively acute TBI. There is rather scant literature about the role of HBO in chronic TBI. Although Dr. Richard Neubauer has published many studies about the use of HBO in chronic neurological disorders, there are few which focus exclusively on TBI (78, 79). In one case report, Neubauer et al. asserts that single photon emission computed tomography (SPECT) imaging, used in conjunction with HBO, is useful in identifying potentially recoverable brain tissue or "idling neurons" in cases of TBI, as well as in stroke and hypoxic encephalopathy (78, 79). SPECT imaging showed a marked defect of the right posterior temporoparietal cortex in a patient who suffered a severe TBI. After a single 60 minute HBO treatment at 1.5 ATA, there was filling of this defect. Based on these data, 188 HBO treatments were given and there was improvement in the SPECT scans as well as neuropsychological testing. In another study by Neubauer's group, 50 patients (of whom 26% had a chronic TBI) were given HBO treatments (80). The number, frequency, and depth of these HBO treatments, as well as time from insult, varied. SPECT imaging was obtained prior to initiation, midpoint, and at the conclusion of the HBO treatments. CBF statistically improved in the cortical regions of these patients, but not in the pons or cerebellum.

A study published in 2004 by Barrett et al. investigated regional CBF in chronic stable TBI patients treated with HBO (81). Five TBI patients were treated with HBO (1.5 ATA, 60 minutes) and received 120 treatments (80 treatments, five-month rest, 40 treatments). Another five TBI patients were matched for age, sex, and type of injury, and five healthy subjects served as normal controls. Both the HBO-treated and non-treated TBI patients underwent serial SPECT imaging as well as brain magnetic resonance imaging (MRI), neurologic, neuropsychometric, and exercise testing. Although an earlier abstract for the same study stated that the HBO group had permanent increases in CBF to penumbral areas and a regression to a mean CBF range, this publication states that HBO did not cause clinical or regional CBF improvements (82). There also were not significant objective changes in neurologic, neuropsychometric, exercise testing or MRIs.

## POTENTIAL MECHANISM OF ACTION OF HYPERBARIC OXYGEN

Historically, the mechanism through which HBO worked was felt to be vasoconstriction of the cerebral blood vessels which led to decreased CBF and ICP. The vasoconstriction was not felt to be deleterious because $O_2$ availability to the injured cells was greatly increased (11, 13). As experimental research continued and more evidence accumulated, however, HBO appeared to be decreasing cerebral edema and stabilizing the blood-brain barrier as well (52, 55, 63). Recent clinical studies on the effect of HBO corroborate these findings with elevated ICP being improved persistently after treatment (6, 7, 12).

HBO appears to improve aerobic metabolism in severely brain-injured patients. Following severe TBI, there is a relative energy crisis with depression of cerebral mitochondrial function. Impaired mitochondrial respiration results in a shift from aerobic to anaerobic metabolism with resultant increased lactate and reduced ATP production (29, 30). At the same time, delivery of $O_2$ to the brain tissue is reduced by both decreased local CBF as well as diminished $O_2$ diffusion secondary to cerebral edema. HBO allows the delivery of supranormal amounts of $O_2$ to the injured brain cells through increasing dissolved $O_2$ in the blood and improved CBF (7, 9). In addition, work by several investigators suggests that HBO allows the injured brain to utilize baseline amounts of $O_2$ more efficiently following treatments and has a persistent effect on the injured brain tissue (7, 9, 60-62). There is a growing amount of experimental animal evidence that this change occurs at the mitochondrial level (9, 10). The exact mechanism by which HBO may enhance mitochondrial recovery is unknown.

## SAFETY AND OXYGEN TOXICITY ISSUES

Most neurosurgeons treating severe TBI are only familiar with HBO treatment in a relatively vague way. Even amongst neurosurgeons more familiar with the technique, the idea of placing an intubated, severely brain-injured patient with multiple injuries into an HBO chamber, particularly a monoplace, seems prohibitive (83). One of the challenges in establishing HBO as an accepted therapy for severe TBI is to establish its safety as well as the efficacy of the treatment.

Fortunately, for both the TBI patient and the treating physician, the landmark investigations of Holbach, et al., established the ideal HBO treatment pressure at 1.5 ATA (58-60). This is a relatively "shallow dive" as far as HBO treatment protocols are concerned, which are typically in the 2.0 to 3.0 ATA level. The intermittent 60-minute HBO treatment administered every 8–12 hours at 1.5 ATA greatly reduces potential safety and toxicity issues.

Based on our own past and ongoing investigations, as well as that of Weaver, et al. placing severe TBI patients in either a monoplace or multiplace HBO chamber at 1.5 ATA for 60 minutes is a very low risk procedure (6, 7, 84-87). Monoplace chambers are much less expensive than multiplace chambers and can be placed in or near the intensive care unit. In fact, the monoplace chamber becomes an extension of the critical care environment. Continuous monitoring of ICP, MAP, CPP, end tidal $CO_2$, and brain tissue oxygen can be performed. In addition, central venous pressure or Swan Ganz catheter monitoring are done if needed. Careful evaluation of the patient's pulmonary status prior to HBO treatment is critical. In our work, we have regarded a baseline $FiO_2$ requirement of greater than 50% and a positive end expiration pressure (PEEP) of greater than ten to maintain adequate oxygenation as contraindications to HBO. It is essential to maintain adequate ventilation throughout the treatment. In the case of an emergency, an intubated ventilated patient can be decompressed and out of the chamber in two minutes. We routinely perform myringotomy to reduce patient stimulation during treatment, and thereby, ICP (6).

The lung is the organ most commonly damaged by hyperoxia since the $O_2$ tension in the lungs is substantially higher than in other tissues (88). The mechanism by which pulmonary injury occurs has been termed oxidative stress (89, 90). Central to this process is the release of proinflammatory cytokines by alveolar macrophages, specifically IL-8 and IL-6, and the subsequent influx of activated cells into the alveolar air space (91, 92). Measurement of these proinflammatory cytokines in bronchial alveolar lavage has been shown to be predictive of acute lung injury and pulmonary infection in exposure to super physiological concentrations of inspired $O_2$ (93). There has not been an increase in these proinflammatory cytokines in HBO treated patients compared to control patients in our current prospective randomized trial (unpublished data).

The concept of a "unit pulmonary toxic dose" (UPTD) has been developed and allows comparison of the pulmonary effects of various treatment schedules of hyperoxia (94, 95). One UPTD is equal to one minute of 100% $O_2$ at 1 ATA. Appropriate conversion factors (Kp), that is, multipliers of one minute of 100% $O_2$ at 1 ATA, allow one to quantitate the pressure (ATA) of the $O_2$ exposure. In general, it is recommended that total $O_2$ exposure in a single treatment be limited to a UPTD of 615 or less. The extreme limit of a single $O_2$ exposure is 1,425 UPTD. This dose will produce a predicted 10% decrease in vital capacity in a normal individual. A one-hour HBO treatment at 1.5 ATA is equal to 60 x 1.78 Kp or 106.8 UPDT. In our first study, one-hour treatments at 1.5 ATA were delivered every eight hours producing 320 UPDT per day (6). The 24 hours of 100% $O_2$ at 1 ATA, which was described in the recent article by Tolias, is the equivalent of 1,440 UPDTs (8). This number exceeds the extreme upper limit for a single $O_2$ exposure. Therefore, relatively speaking, a one-hour HBO treatment of 1.5 ATA delivers a low dose of $O_2$. In the clinical trial described previously in which 84 TBI patients received 1,688 HBO treatments, no permanent sequelae resulted (6). Pulmonary complications occasionally occurred (ten of 84 patients), but all were reversible.

Oxygen, especially under increased pressure, also may cause potential cerebral toxicity. Brain tissue is especially vulnerable to lipid peroxidation because of its high rate of $O_2$ consumption and high content of phospholipids. Additionally, the brain has limited natural protection against free radicals, i.e., it has limited scavenging ability, poor catalase activity, and is rich in iron, which is an initiator of radical generation in brain injury (25, 96-98). There are experimental studies demonstrating increased formation of reactive $O_2$ radicals and secondary lipid peroxidation in the brain, but the depth and duration of HBOT in theses studies are much greater than used in our clinical investigations (99-101). There is no clinical evidence for cerebral toxicity using an HBO treatment paradigm of 1.5 ATA for 60 minutes. However, to further evaluate this issue, we are monitoring ventricular CSF F2 isoprostane which is isometric to cyclo-oxygenase and is derived from prostaglandin F2 (102, 103). CSF F2 isoprostane is exclusively produced from free radical catalyzed peroxidation of arachidonic acid. It is a specific quantitative biomarker of lipid peroxidation *in vivo* in the brain. F2 isoprostane values have not been elevated in our current study (unpublished data). In addition, there have been recent experimental scientific studies which show that HBO may have a protective effect against secondary brain damage, cerebral edema and necrosis (63, 69-71).

In conclusion, HBO treatments at a depth of 1.5 ATA can be delivered to the severe TBI patient with or without multiple injuries in either a monoplace or multiplace chamber with relative safety and low risk of $O_2$ toxicity.

## PRESENT AND FUTURE DIRECTIONS

The authors are currently carrying out a prospective, randomized clinical trial for severe TBI patients designed as three-treatment comparison, i.e., HBO, normobaric hyperoxia, and control, funded by the National Institute of Neurological Disease and Stroke. HBO is delivered for 60 minutes at 1.5 ATA and normobaric hyperoxia (100% $FiO_2$) for three hours. The treatments are given every 24 hours for three days. Recent studies have described normobaric hyperoxia (100% $FiO_2$) as a method of delivering supernormal levels of $O_2$ to severe TBI patients (8, 27). Improvement in cerebral metabolism and reduced ICP has been described. The relative ease of administration and its inexpense require that normobaric hyperoxia be evaluated as an alternative treatment to HBO.

This is not a clinical outcome study. However, surrogate outcome variables which predict and correlate with clinical outcome will be studied. They are measured prior to initiation of therapy, during administration of therapy, and for 24 hours following therapy. Continuously monitored outcome variables include ICP, $PtO_2$, microdialysate lactate, glucose, pyruvate, and glycerol. CBF, $AVDO_2$, $CMRO_2$, CSF lactate, F2-isoprostanes, and bronchial lavage fluid (IL-8 and IL-6 assays) are being obtained once before treatment, during treatment, and at one and six hours post-treatment. The results of the trial will allow a direct comparison of HBO and normobaric hyperoxia in terms of their treatment efficacy on the surrogate outcome variables as well as their relative toxicity. In addition, post-treatment effects will be compared statistically to pre-treatment values. The duration of the effect will be determined. Traumatic brain injury is very heterogenous in terms of lesions and severity. The study will allow us to determine which severe TBI patients respond to therapy in terms of their GCS scores and lesion types.

The work described above by Daugherty and Zhou from the laboratory at the Medical College of Virginia has prompted a fourth treatment arm in this study (9, 10). That is a combination of HBO for 60 minutes at 1.5 ATA followed by three hours of 100% $FiO_2$ at 1.0 ATA. The hypothesis to be tested is that improvement in cerebral metabolism does not occur during the HBO treatment, but HBO treatment results in improved utilization of $O_2$ by restoring mitochondrial function in the hours following treatment.

Following completion and analysis of the above clinical trial, our goal is to use positron emission tomography (PET) scanning in testing the hypothesis that the optimum HBO treatment paradigm improves mitochondrial dysfunction and the energy depletion crisis which occurs following severe TBI in humans. Hovda and colleagues at UCLA have demonstrated a strong correlation between cerebral metabolism and neurologic outcome in TBI (104-106). Clinical improvement coupled to enhanced cerebral metabolism documented by PET scanning would provide strong evidence for the beneficial effect of HBO.

It remains to be seen whether the data accumulated will be compelling enough to institute HBO either alone or in combination with 100% $FiO_2$ as a standard treatment for severe TBI or whether a multicenter clinical outcome trial will be required. The authors are reasonably confident based on this review and their experience that in either case HBO will become a significant treatment for patients suffering a severe TBI.

# REFERENCES

1. Narayan RK, Michel ME, Ansell B, et al. Clinical trials in head injury. J Neurotrauma. 2002; 19(5):503-557.

2. Clifton GL, Miller ER, Choi SE, et al. Lack of effect of hypothermia in acute brain injury. N Engl J Med. 2001; 344:556-563.

3. Gaab MR, Trost HA, Akantara A, et al. Ultrahigh dexamethasone in acute brain injury. Results from a prospective randomized double-blind multicenter trial (GUDHIS). Zentralbl. Neurochir. 1994; 55:135-143.

4. Marshall LF, Maas AI, Marshall SB, et al. A multicenter trial on the efficacy of using Tirilazad mesylate in cases of head injury. J Neurosurg. 1998; 89:519-525.

5. Morris GF, Bullock R, Marshall SB, et al. Failure of the competitive N-methyl-D-aspartate antagonist Selfotel (CGS 19755) in the treatment of severe head injury: results of two phase III clinical trials. The Selfotel Investigators. J Neurosurg. 1999; 91:737-743.

6. Rockswold GL, Ford SE, Anderson DL, et al. Results of a prospective randomized trial for treatment of severely brain-injured patients with hyperbaric oxygen. J Neurosurg. 1992; 76:929-934.

7. Rockswold SB, Rockswold GL, Vargo JM, et al. The effects of hyperbaric oxygen on cerebral metabolism and intracranial pressure in severely brain-injured patients. J Neurosurg. 2001; 94:403-411.

8. Tolias CM, Reinert M, Seiler R, et al. Normobaric hyperoxia-induced improvement in cerebral metabolism and reduction in intracranial pressure in patients with severe head injury: a prospective historical cohort-matched study. J Neurosurg. 2004; 101:435-444.

9. Daugherty WP, Levasseur JE, Sun D, et al. Effects of hyperbaric oxygen therapy on cerebral oxygenation and mitochondrial function following moderate lateral fluid-percussion injury in rats. J Neurosurg. 2004; 101:499-504.

10. Zhou Z, Daugherty WP, Sun D, et al. Hyperbaric oxygen treatment protects mitochondrial function and improves cognitive recovery in rats following lateral fluid percussion injury. Accepted for publication, J Neurosurg.

11. Sukoff MH, Hollin SA, Espinosa OE, et al. The protective effect of hyperbaric oxygenation in experimental cerebral edema. J Neurosurg. 1968; 29:236-241.

12. Sukoff MH, Ragatz RE. Hyperbaric oxygenation for the treatment of acute cerebral edema. Neurosurgery. 1982; 10:29-38.

13. Miller JD and Ledingham IM. Reduction of increased intracranial pressure. Arch Neurol 1971; 24:210-216.

14. Holbach KH, Wassman H, Kolberg T. Verbesserte Reversibilität des traumatischen Mittelhirnsyndroms bei Anwendung der hyperbaren Oxygenierung. Acta Neurochir. 1974; 30:247-256.

15. Artru F, Chacornac R, Deleuze R. Hyperbaric oxygenation for severe head injuries: Preliminary results of a controlled study. Surgery. 1976; 14:310-318.

16. Graham DI, Adams JH, Doyle D. Ischaemic brain damage in fatal non-missile head injuries. J Neurol Sci. 1978; 39:213-34.

17. Bouma GJ, Muizelaar JP, Stringer WA, et al. Ultra-early evaluation of regional cerebral blood flow in severely head-injured patients using xenon-enhanced computerized tomography. J Neurosurg. 1992; 77:360-368.

18. Siesjo BK, Siesjo P. Mechanisms of secondary brain injury. Eur J Anaesthesiol. 1996; 13:247-268.

19. Krebs EG. Protein kinases. Curr Top Cell Regul. 1972; 5:99-133.

20. Muizelaar, JP. Cerebral blood flow, cerebral blood volume, and cerebral metabolism after severe head injury, in Becker and Gudeman (eds): Textbook of Head Injury. Philadelphia: W.B. Saunders, 1989, pp 221-240.

21. Waxman SG, Ransom BR, Stys PK. Non-synaptic mechanisms of Ca2+-mediated injury in CNS white matter. Trends Neurosci. 1991; 14:461-468.

22. Young W. Role of calcium in central nervous system injuries. J Neurotrauma. 1992; 9:S9-S25.

23. Siesjo BK. Basic mechanisms of traumatic brain damage. Ann Emerg Med. 1993; 22:959-969.

24. Krause GS, Kumar K, White BC, et al. Ischemia, resuscitation, and reperfusion: Mechanisms of tissue injury and prospects for protection. Am Heart J. 1986; 16:1200-1205.

25. Ikeda Y, Long DM. The molecular basis of brain injury and brain edema: The role of oxygen free radicals. Neurosurg. 1990; 27:1-11.

26. Siesjo BK, Agardh CD, Bengtsson F. Free radicals and brain damage. Cerebrovascular and Brain Metabolism Reviews. 1989; 1:165-211.

27. Menzel M, Doppenberg EM, Zauner A, et al. Increased inspired oxygen concentration as a factor in improved brain tissue oxygenation and tissue lactate levels after severe human head injury. J Neurosurg. 1999; 91:1-10.

28. Verweij BH, Muizelaar JP, Vinas FC, et al. Mitochondria dysfunction after experimental and human brain injury and its possible reversal with a selective N-type calcium channel antagonist (SNX-111). Neurol Res. 1997; 19:334-339.

29. Lifshitz J, Sullivan PG, Hovda DA, et al. Mitochondrial damage and dysfunction in traumatic brain injury. Mitochondrion xx. 2004; 1-9.

30. Signoretti S, Marmarou A, Tavazzi B, et al. N-Acetylaspartate reduction as a measure of injury severity and mitochondrial dysfunction following diffuse traumatic brain injury. J Neurotrauma. 2001; 18(10):977-991.

31. Verweij BH, Muizelaar P, Vinas FC, et al. Impaired cerebral mitochondrial function after traumatic brain injury in humans. J Neurosurg. 2000; 93(5):815-20.

32. Bergsneider M, Hovda DA, Shalmon E, et al. Cerebral hyperglycolysis following severe traumatic brain injury in humans: A positron emission tomography study. J Neurosurg. 1997; 86:241-251.

33. Valadka AB, Goodman JC, Gopinath SP, et al. Comparison of brain tissue oxygen tension to microdialysis-based measures of cerebral ischemia in fatally head-injured humans. J Neurotrauma. 1998A; 7:509-519.

34. Van den Brink WA, Van Santbrink H, Steyerberg EW, et al. Brain oxygen tension in severe head injury. Neurosurg. 2000; 46:868-876.

35. Zauner A, Doppenberg EMR, Woodward JJ, et al. Continuous monitoring of cerebral substrate delivery and clearance: Initial experience in 24 patients with severe acute brain injuries. Neurosurg. 1997; 41:1082-1091.

36. DeSalles AAF, Muizelaar JP, Young HF. Hyperglycemia, cerebrospinal fluid lactic acidosis, and cerebral blood flow in severely head-injured patients. Neurosurgery. 1987; 21:45-50.

37. Metzel E, Zimmermann WE. Changes of oxygen pressure, acid-base balance, metabolites and electrolytes in cerebrospinal fluid and blood after cerebral injury. Acta Neurochir. 1971; 25:177-188.

38. DeSalles AAF, Kontos HA, Becker DP, et al. Prognostic significance of ventricular CSF lactic acidosis in severe head injury. J Neurosurg. 1986; 65:615-624.

39. Murr R, Stummer W, Schürer L, et al. Cerebral lactate production in relation to intracranial pressure, cranial computed tomography findings, and outcome in patients with severe head injury. Acta Neurochir. 1996; 138:928-937.

40. Robertson CS, Narayan RK, Gokaslan ZL, et al. Cerebral arteriovenous oxygen difference as an estimate of cerebral blood flow in comatose patients. J Neurosurg. 1989; 70:222-230.

41. Lambertsen CJ, Kough RH, Cooper DY, et al. Oxygen toxicity. Effects in man of oxygen inhalation at 1 and 3.5 atmospheres upon blood gas transport, cerebral circulation and cerebral metabolism. J Appl Physiol. 1953; 5:471-486.

42. Kety SS, Schmidt CF: The nitrous oxide method for the quantitative determination of cerebral blood flow in man: theory, procedure and normal values. J Clin Invest. 1948; 27:476-483.

43. Illingworth C. Treatment of arterial occlusion under oxygen at two atmospheres pressure. Brit Med J. 1962; 2:1271

44. Smith G, Lawson S, Renfrew I, et al. Preservation of cerebral cortical activity by breathing oxygen at two atmospheres of pressure during cerebral ischemia. Surg Gynec Obstet. 1961; 113:13.

45. Jacobson I, Harper AM, McDowall DG. The effects of oxygen under pressure on cerebral blood flow and cerebral venous oxygen tension. Lancet 1963; 2:549.

46. Tindall GT, Wilkins RH, Odom GL. Effect of hyperbaric oxygenation on cerebral blood flow. Surg Forum. 1965; 16:414-416.

47. Saltzmann HA, Smith RL, Fuson HO, et al. Hyperbaric oxygenation. Monogr Surg Sci. 1965; 2:1.

48. Ingvar DH, Lassen, NA. Treatment of focal cerebral ischemia with hyperbaric oxygenation. Acta Neurol Scand. 1965; 41:92.

49. Whalen RE, Heyman A, Saltzman H. The protective effect of hyperbaric oxygenation in cerebral anoxia. Arch Neurol. 1966; 14:15.

50. Jacobson I and Lawson DD: The effect of hyperbaric oxygen on experimental cerebral infarction in the dog. J Neurosurg. 1963; 20:849.

51. Dunn JE and Connolly JM: Effects of Hypobaric and Hyperbaric Oxygen on Experimental Brain Injury. Natl Acad Sci Natl Res Council Publ. 1966; 1404:447-454.

52. Sukoff MH, Hollin SA, Jacobson JH. The protective effect of hyperbaric oxygenation in experimentally produced cerebral edema and compression. Surgery. 1967; 62:40-46.

53. Moody RA, Mead CO, Ruamsuke S, et al. Therapeutic value of oxygen at normal and hyperbaric pressure in experimental head injury. J Neurosurg. 1970; 32:51-54.

54. Wüllenweber R, Gött U, Holbach KH. rCBF during hyperbaric oxygenation, in Brock, Fieschi, Ingvar and Lassen (eds): Cerebral Blood Flow. Berlin: Springer, 1969, pp 270-272.

55. Mogami H, Hayakawa T, Kanai N, et al. Clinical application of hyperbaric oxygenation in the treatment of acute cerebral damage. J Neurosurg. 1969; 1:636-643.

56. Hayakawa T, Kanai N, Kuroda R, et al. Response of cerebrospinal fluid pressure to hyperbaric oxygenation. J Neurol Neurosurg Psychiatry. 1971; 34: 580-586.

57. Miller JD, Fitch W, Ledingham IM, et al. The effect of hyperbaric oxygen on experimentally increased intracranial pressure. J Neurosurg. 1970; 33:287-296.

58. Holbach KH, Schröder FK, Köster S. Alterations of cerebral metabolism in cases with acute brain injuries during spontaneous respiration of air, oxygen and hyperbaric oxygen. Surgery. 1972:158-160.

59. Holbach KH. Effect of hyperbaric oxygenation (HO) in severe injuries and in marked blood flow disturbances of the human brain, in Schürmann K (ed): Advances in Neurosurgery. Berlin-Heidelberg-New York: Springer, 1973, Vol 1, pp 158-163.

60. Holbach KH, Caroli A, Wassmann H. Cerebral energy metabolism in patients with brain lesions of normo- and hyperbaric oxygen pressures. J Neurol. 1977; 217:17-30.

61. Artru F, Philippon B, Gau F, et al. Cerebral blood flow, cerebral metabolism and cerebrospinal fluid biochemistry in brain-injured patients after exposure to hyperbaric oxygen. Surgery. 1976; 14:351-364.

62. Contreras FL, Kadekaro M, Eisenberg HM. The effect of hyperbaric oxygen on glucose utilization in a freeze traumatized rat brain. J Neurosurg. 1988; 68:137-141.

63. Mink RB, Dutka AJ. Hyperbaric oxygen after global cerebral ischemia in rabbits reduces brain vascular permeability and blood flow. Stroke. 1995; 26:2307-2312.

64. Siddiqui A, Davidson JD, Mustoe TA. Ischemic tissue oxygen capacitance after hyperbaric oxygen therapy: a new physiologic concept. Plast Reconstr Surg. 1997; 99:148-155.

65. Obrist WD, Langfitt TW, Jaggi JL, et al. Cerebral blood flow and metabolism in comatose patients with acute head injury. J Neurosurg. 1984; 61:241253.

66. Robertson CS, Contant CF, Gokaslan ZL, et al. Cerebral blood flow, arteriovenous oxygen difference, and outcome in head injured patients. J Neurol Neurosurg Psychiatry. 1992; 55:594-603.

67. Rogatsky GG, Kamenir Y, Mayevsky A. Effect of hyperbaric oxygenation on intracranial pressure elevation rate in rats during the early phase of severe traumatic brain injury. Brain Research. 2005; 1047:131-136.

68. Rogatsky GG, Sonn J, Kamenir Y, et al. Relationship between intracranial pressure and cortical spreading depression following fluid percussion brain injury in rats. J Neurotrauma. 2003; 20:1315-1325.

69. Niklas A, Brock D, Schober R, et al. Continuous measurements of cerebral tissue oxygen pressure during hyperbaric oxygenation – HBO effects on brain edema and necrosis after severe brain trauma in rabbits. J Neurological Sciences. 2004; 219:77-82.

70. Palzur E, Vlodavsky E, Mulla H, et al. Hyperbaric oxygen therapy for reduction of secondary brain damage in head injury: An animal model of brain contusion. J Neurotrauma. 2004; 21(1):41-48.

71. Shreiber DI, Bain AC, Ross DT, et al. Experimental investigation of cerebral contusion: histopathological and immunohistochemical evaluation of dynamic cortical deformation.
J Neuropathol Exp Neurol. 1999; 58:153-164.

72. Vlodavsky E, Palzur E, Soustiel JF. Hyperbaric oxygen therapy reduces neuro-inflammation and expression of matrix metalloproteinase-9 in the rat model of traumatic brain injury. Neuropath Appl Neurobio. 2006; 32:40-50.

73. Dixon CE, Lyeth BG, Povlishock JT, et al. A fluid percussion model of experimental brain injury in the rat. J Neurosurg. 1987; 67:110-119.

74. McIntosh TK, Vink R, Noble L, et al. Traumatic brain injury in the rat: characterization of a lateral fluid-percussion model. Neuroscience. 1989; 28:233-244.

75. Levasseur JE, Alessandri B, Reinert M, et al. Fluid percussion injury transiently increases then decreases brain oxygen consumption in the rat. J Neurotrauma. 2000; 17:101-112

76. Azbill RD, Mu X, Bruce-Keller AJ, et al. Impaired mitochondrial function, oxidative stress and altered antioxidant enzyme activities following traumatic spinal cord injury. Brain Res. 1997; 765:283-290.

77. Springer JE, Azbill RD, Carlson SL. A rapid and sensitive assay for measuring mitochondrial metabolic activity in isolated neural tissue. Brain Res Protoc. 1998; 2:259-263.

78. Neubauer RA. The effect of hyperbaric oxygen in prolonged coma. Possible identification of marginally functioning brain zones. Minerva Med Subaecquea ed Iperbarica. 1985a; 5:75.

79. Neubauer RA, Gottlieb SF. Hyperbaric oxygen for treatment of closed head injury. Southern Med J. 1994; 87(9):4.

80. Golden ZL, Neubauer R, Golden C, et al. Improvement in cerebral metabolism in chronic brain injury after hyperbaric oxygen therapy. Intern J Neuroscience. 2002; 112:119-131.

81. Barrett KF, Masel B, Patterson J, et al. Regional CBF in chronic stable TBI treated with hyperbaric oxygen. Undersea Hyperbaric Med Society. 2004; 31(4):395-406.

82. Barrett KF, Masel BE, Harch PG, et al. Cerebral blood flow changes in cognitive improvement in chronic stable traumatic brain injuries treated with hyperbaric oxygen therapy. Undersea Hyperbaric Med. 1998; 25:9.

83. Bullock RM, Mahon R. Hypoxia and traumatic brain injury. Neurosurgical forum.
J Neurosurg. 2006; 104:170-172.

84. Rockswold GL, Ford SE, Anderson BJR. Patient monitoring in the monoplace hyperbaric chamber. Hyperbaric Oxygen Rev. 1985; 6:161-168, 1985.

85. Weaver LK, Greenway L, Elliot CG. Performance of the Sechrist 500A hyperbaric ventilator in a monoplace hyperbaric chamber. J Hyperbaric Med 1988; 3(4):215-225.

86. Weaver LK: Management of critically ill patients in the monoplace hyperbaric chamber, in Kindwall EP, Whelan HT, eds. Hyperbaric medicine practice, 2nd edition. Flagstaff. Best Publishing Company 1999, 245-279

87. Weaver LK. Operational use and patient monitoring in the monoplace chamber, in Moon R, McIntrye N, eds. Respiratory Care Clinics of North America – Hyperbaric Medicine, Part I. Philadelphia: W.B . Saunders Company, 1999, 51-92

88. Klein J. Normobaric pulmonary oxygen toxicity. Anesth Analg. 1990; 70:195-207

89. Wispe JR, Roberts RJ. Molecular basis of pulmonary oxygen toxicity. Clin Perinatol. 1987; 14(3):651-656

90. Mantell LL, Horowitz S, Davis JM, et al. Hyperoxia-induced cell death in the lung – the correlation of apoptosis, necrosis, and inflammation. Ann NY Acad Sci. 1999; 887:171-180

91. DeForge LE, Preston AM, Takeuchi E, et al. Regulation of interleukin-8 gene expression by oxidant stress. J Biol Chem.1993; 5;268(34):25568-25576

92. Deaton PR, McKellar CT, Culbreth R, et al. Hyperoxia stimulates interleukin-8 release from alveolar macrophages and U937 cells: attenuation by dexamethasone. Am J Physiol. 1994; 267:L187-192

93. Muehlstedt SG, Richardson CJ, Lyte M, et al. Cytokines and the pathogenesis of nosocomial pneumonia. Surgery. 2001; 130(4):602-609; discussion 2001; 609-611

94. Bardin H, Lambertsen CJ. A quantitative method for calculating pulmonary toxicity. Use of the unit of pulmonary toxicity dose (UPTD). Institute for Environmental Medicine Report 1970. Philadelphia, University of Pennsylvania.

95. Wright WB. Use of the University of Pennsylvania Institute for Environmental Medicine procedure for calculation of cumulative pulmonary oxygen toxicity. US Navy Experimental Diving Unit, 1972; Report 2-72

96. Demopoulos HB, Flamm E, Seligman M, et al. Oxygen free radicals n central nervous system ischemia and trauma, in Autor AP (ed): Pathology of Oxygen. New York, Academic Press, 1982A, pp 127-155

97. Demopoulos HS, Flamm ES, Seligman ML, et al. Further studies on free-radical pathology in the major central nervous system disorders: Effect of very high doses of methylprednisolone on the functional outcome, morphology, and chemistry of experimental spinal cord impact injury. Can J Physiol Pharmacol. 1982B; 60:1415-1424

98. Ortega BD, Demopoulos HB, Ransohoff J. Effect of antioxidants on experimental cold-induced cerebral edema, in Reulen HJ, Schurmann K (eds): Steroids and Brain Edema. New York, Springer-Verlag, 1972, pp 167-175

99. Harabin AL, Braisted JC, Flynn ET. Response of antioxidant enzymes to intermittent and continuous hyperbaric oxygen. J Appl Physiol. 1990; 69:328-335

100. Noda X, McGeer PL, McGeer EML. Lipid peroxidase distribution in brain and effect of hyperbaric oxygen. J Neurochem. 1983; 40:1329-1332

101. Puglia CD, Loeb GA. Influence of rat brain superoxide dismutase inhibition by diethyldithiocarbamate upon the rate of development of central nervous system oxygen toxicity. Toxicol Appl Pharmacol. 1984; 75:258-264

102. Montine TJ, Beal MF, Cudkowicz ME et al. Increased CSF F2-isoprostane concentration in probable AD. Am Acad Neuro. 1999; 52;562-565

103. Pratico D, Barry OP, Lawson JA, et al. IPF2a-I: An index of lipid peroxidation in humans. Proc Natl Acad Sci USA. 1998; 95:3449-3454

104. Hattori N, Huang SC, Wu HM, et al. Correlation of regional metabolic rates of glucose with Glasgow Coma Scale after traumatic brain injury. J Nucl Med. 2003; 44(11):1709-1716

105. Glenn TC, Kelly DF, Boscardin WJ, et al. Energy dysfunction as a predictor of outcome after moderate or severe head injury: Indices of oxygen, glucose, and lactate metabolism.
J Cereb Blood Flow Metab. 2003; 23(10):1239-1250

106. Vespa PM, McArthur D, O'Phelan K, et al. Persistently low extracellular glucose correlates with poor outcome six months after human traumatic brain injury despite a lack of increased lactate: A microdialysis study. J Cereb Blood Flow Metab. 2003; 23(7):865-877.

# NOTES

CHAPTER 39

# NEUROLOGICAL ASPECTS OF HYPERBARIC MEDICINE

## CHAPTER THIRTY-NINE OVERVIEW

# NEUROLOGICAL ASPECTS OF HYPERBARIC MEDICINE

*Ann K. Helms, Valerie J. Bonne, Charles C. Falzon, Harry T. Whelan*

## INTRODUCTION

Since the early days of hyperbaric medicine, there has been interest in using HBO to treat neurologic disease. The exquisite sensitivity of neural tissue to hypoxia makes increased oxygenation attractive as a therapy for disease processes that induce ischemia, edema, and, more recently, apoptosis. This chapter addresses the evidence for using HBO to treat several neurologic diseases, which is an issue that has drawn significant interest and criticism from the press. It is important to note that none of the diseases mentioned in this chapter have received approval from the Food and Drug Administration (FDA) as indications for HBO.

## STROKE

The largest body of evidence involving the use of hyperbaric oxygen for neurologic illness is found in the field of cerebral ischemia, reviewed by Helms, et al. in 2005 (1). Ischemic stroke occurs when neural tissue receives inadequate vascular supply due to cerebral blood vessel occlusion. At the core, or center, of the infarct, blood flow is completely absent, causing neurons to die within a matter of minutes. The region of the brain that draws the most interest is the penumbra, where evidence has shown that blood flow is diminished, but not absent. The cells in this region remain viable for a prolonged period, and can be saved if adequate perfusion is restored. The only approved therapy for acute ischemic stroke presently available is Tissue Plasminogen Activator (tPA), which restores blood flow to the ischemic penumbra, but must be used within the first few hours of the onset of symptoms to be effective. There is also evidence that a percentage of the cells subjected to prolonged ischemia will inevitably undergo apoptosis, regardless of the efforts made to restore perfusion. As a result, there has been great interest in using HBO to treat ischemic stroke for its ability to improve the delivery of oxygen to deprived tissue and for the added benefit of its anti-inflammatory properties.

There is reasonable evidence from animal studies, involving mice, rats, gerbils, and cats, that focal cerebral ischemia may improve after treatment with HBO. Several studies have investigated the efficacy of using HBOT that is provided either immediately or delayed minutes to hours after temporary or permanent occlusion of cerebral vessels (2-13). Most studies administer a single, one hour-long treatment at doses ranging from 2 to 3 ATA, with a few giving similar treatments multiple times. The overwhelming majority of these studies showed a clinical benefit in the treatment group, such as decrease of infarct size, improved neurologic function, and increased survival. Only two studies failed to show any benefit from HBOT when it was given within the first several hours following the ischemic event (14, 15). Based on these studies, the therapeutic window is limited to the first six hours after restoring perfusion, as treatments given after this window provided no benefit. In addition, the window for observing any improvement from treatment may be even shorter in brains with a permanently occluded vessel (16, 17).

Analyses of brain tissue in HBO-treated animals suggest that treatment may provide an indirect benefit to ischemic tissue, in addition to increasing local oxygen levels. In animals treated with HBO, there was a significant decrease in neuronal shrinkage, edema and necrotic tissue, and, more importantly, fewer neurons showed evidence of undergoing apoptosis after ischemia (18-23). These findings indicate that HBO exposure initiates a lasting physiologic change by interrupting the apoptotic cascade that is triggered by the ischemia/reperfusion phenomenon. It also helps to explain studies that show a protective benefit to pre-treatment with HBO prior to ischemia (24-27).

Several human trials investigating the use of HBO for ischemic stroke have been performed. While most of these lacked controls, uniform standards for inclusion criteria and outcome measurement, or both, there are still three prominent randomized controlled studies that have evaluated HBO in ischemic stroke. Anderson, et al. enrolled patients up to 14 days after an ischemic stroke and gave multiple treatments of HBO at 1.5 ATA versus air at 1.5 ATA (28). After four months of treatments, examiners saw no difference in stroke size on either CT or graded neurologic exam. Nighoghossian, et al. also gave HBO at 1.5 ATA, although they limited enrollment to the first 24 hours after onset of symptoms and gave only one 60 minute treatment (29). Control patients were given a sham treatment of air at a minimal pressure increase. At one year, there was no difference in global function as measured by the modified Rankin scale, however, two other outcome measures, the Orgogozo and Trouillas scores, were significantly higher in the treatment group. The conflicting data from this study suggest that the effect of the regimen was minimal, if at all quantifiable. The most recent study in this field performed by Rusyniak, et al, also randomized patients in the first 24 hours after ischemia to receive one 60 minute treatment of either HBO at 2.5 ATA or 100% oxygen at 1.1 ATA (30). Patients in the "control" group showed a better outcome on two functional scales after three months of treatment, which suggests a potentially harmful effect of HBO, but an intention-to-treat analysis showed no statistical difference between the groups.

One might conclude from this that HBO is an ineffective treatment for ischemic stroke, however, it should be noted that these studies enrolled patients well after the therapeutic window of six hours that was suggested by previous animals studies had elapsed. Based on our present understanding of ischemia, one would not expect treatment after two weeks to be effective. Two of the three studies used a very low HBO dose of 1.5 ATA, which is well below the standard dose used for other therapeutic indications. In addition, the control groups in the studies performed by the Anderson and Rusyniak groups received higher doses of oxygen (air at 1.5 ATA and 100% oxygen at 1.1 ATA, respectively) than a patient breathing air, which might be considered intermediate therapy (28, 30).

Based on the studies just discussed, HBO cannot currently be recommended for the treatment of ischemic stroke outside of a research protocol. Considering the results that have been produced in animal models, it is imperative that follow-up studies be performed on human subjects to analyze the effects of HBO treatment within the first few hours following an ischemic event using higher doses of oxygen. Potential protocols should also include controls receiving oxygen treatments at percentages closely approximating room air to improve both the rigor of the study and the validity of their results. Until such time as these protocols are thoroughly investigated, there is no definitive answer regarding the role of HBO for the treatment of ischemic stroke.

## RADIATION INDUCED CEREBRAL NECROSIS

Radiation Induced Cerebral Necrosis (RIN) is a dreaded complication associated with the treatment of brain tumors. The neurologic signs and symptoms that result are often progressive and can be difficult to distinguish from tumor recurrence. The most common presentations involve cognitive changes such as short term memory loss, poor concentration, personality changes, and focal neurologic abnormalities such as hemi-paresis and aphasia.

Radiation injury can develop immediately after treatment, commonly resulting in transient worsening of neurologic symptoms and headaches. This is presumed to be due to both leaky capillaries and edema in the tumor bed, which is frequently reversible with steroid therapy. The symptoms that develop within a few weeks of radiation treatments are usually reversible, often without treatment. Radiation necrosis, however, develops months to years after radiation exposure, and is usually irreversible.

MRI scanning following radiation shows signal changes and enhancement that are difficult to distinguish from tumor recurrence. While imaging studies such as MR Spectroscopy, PET scanning, SPECT scanning, and MR perfusion studies can be used to distinguish between the two, a biopsy is required for definitive diagnosis. Pathologic examination shows necrosis of white matter and fibrinoid necrosis of blood vessels. This is theorized to be due to endothelial cell damage that induces a signaling cascade that causes ischemia and necrosis of white matter (31).

Treatment of radiation necrosis of the brain is difficult. Surgical resection can sometimes stop progression, and some benefit has been seen with anti-thrombotic medications, unfortunately, these therapies are performed with significant risks and therapeutic limitations (32). HBO has been very successful in treating soft tissue radiation injuries that are discussed in other sections of this text. Given that endothelial cell damage and microvascular ischemia are considered to be part of the injury cascade in RIN, hyperbaric oxygen therapy may be a viable treatment alternative.

There has been only one small, phase I-II randomized controlled study investigating the use of HBO in RIN. Hulshof, et al. randomized seven patients with cognitive deficits at least 1.5 years after brain irradiation to receive either 30 HBO treatments at 3.0 ATA for 115 minutes, or no treatment

(33). Using a battery of neuropsychological tests as outcome measures, they found a trend towards improved function at three months in the treatment group, but this result was not statistically significant. There have also been numerous anecdotal reports of efficacy and a few short series reporting positive results (34-39). In the largest series, reported only in abstract form, Warnick, et al. included 29 patients with RIN of the brain receiving HBO at 2.5 ATA over 90 minutes for 20-60 treatments (39). All of the patients in the study had focal, progressive neurological deficits with increasing steroid requirements and an MRI showing a ring-enhancing mass with surrounding edema. In this series, 27 of the 29 patients showed improvement or stabilization of symptoms, decreased steroid requirement, and improved MRI appearance. The two patients who worsened were shown to have tumor progression. Interestingly, the greatest benefit was noted in a subset of four patients with benign underlying pathology (meningioma and arteriovenous malformation [AVM]). Chuba, et al. also reported benefit in a group of 10 pediatric patients who underwent HBOT after a diagnosis of RIN and failure of traditional steroid therapy (40). All ten patients showed clinical improvement or stabilization both initially and at follow-up, while five of the six surviving patients showed continued improvement. The four deaths in this group were attributed to tumor progression.

The evidence suggests that in cases where either the patient is not improving on medical therapies, such as steroids and anti-thrombotics, or when surgical resection is not possible, HBO should be considered as a treatment option. Due to the lack of studies currently available in this field, there is a definite need for both more and larger randomized trials utilizing HBO for the treatment of RIN.

## TRAUMATIC BRAIN INJURY

Traumatic brain injury (TBI) is one of the leading causes of disability in the United States, effecting more than two million people yearly. Although the primary injury to the brain sustained at the time of the trauma is usually not reversible, it is the secondary injury occurring in the hours and days following the initial injury that provides more opportunities for treatment to preserve tissue and function. Unfortunately, the mechanisms by which these secondary injuries occur are not fully understood. In addition to the initial injury, the largest contributor to morbidity and mortality is cerebral ischemia resulting from post-traumatic hypoxia and hypotension. On a microscopic level, abnormalities of calcium and potassium homeostasis, mechanical membrane disruption, excitotoxicity, and altered glucose metabolism also contribute to cellular damage, which in turn cause edema and neuronal cell death. Cell death in the form of both necrosis and apoptosis occurs in the areas surrounding the primary injury, but can also occur at more distant areas. Increased intracranial pressure from edema, as well as from contusions and hemorrhages, contribute to secondary injury by increasing the level of ischemia, lead to herniation and death.

Treatment of TBI has traditionally focused on supportive care, but recent studies have changed their focus toward the prevention or reversal of secondary injury cascades. The largest advances in the field have been made regarding early intervention with a focus on minimizing the roles of hypotension and hypoxia, which play a limited role in the development of ischemia (41). Intracranial hypertension is treated with a combination of ventricular drainage, mannitol, intermittent hyperventilation, hypertonic saline, and barbiturates, although this is not always fully effective (42). Decompressive craniectomy can be useful, but there are several medical treatments that have been utilized to limit secondary injury including hypothermia, calcium channel blockers, anticonvulsants and other neuroprotectants with varying efficacy.

The interest in using HBO to treat TBI is based upon the premise that hypoxia, edema and apoptosis play significant role in the pathophysiology of the disease. HBO has been shown to decrease cerebral edema and to decrease cellular apoptosis after an ischemic event (8, 22, 23, 44-46). There have been several reports showing a benefit from HBO in TBI patients using surrogate markers that were expected to influence the outcome, including the effects of HBO on intracranial pressure that was studied by several teams (46-48). Although intracranial pressure (ICP) sometimes increased during the treatment, some persistent, albeit mild, decreases were seen in several patients. One study was able to correlate this decrease in ICP with clinical improvement, however, analysis of other surrogate markers, such as cerebral blood flow and metabolism, were less reliable as outcome measures (47-49).

Only a few studies have directly compared HBO to standard of care in TBI. In 1976, Artru et al. randomized 60 patients who were in coma after TBI for an average of 4.5 days after their injuries, and treated them at 2.5 ATA for 60 minutes daily over 10 days with a four day break repeated versus standard of care (50). At one year, the study showed non-significant trends towards shorter coma and higher rate of consciousness in the HBO group, and mortality was not affected. The only significant improvements were in a subgroup of young patients with brainstem injury who had higher rates of consciousness at one month, 67% versus control 11%. In 1974, Holbach alternated 99 patients in coma with acute midbrain syndrome to either standard care or HBO at 1.5 ATA and saw significant improvements in mortality (53% v. 74%) and good outcome on the Glasgow Outcome Scale (33% v. 6%) (51). More recently, Rockswold, et al. randomized 168 TBI patients between six and 24 hours after injury with GCS of nine or less to HBO at 1.5 ATA for 60 minutes every eight hours for two weeks versus standard care (52). At 12 months, blinded examiners saw no change in outcome among survivors, but there was a significant decrease in mortality (17% v. 32%) at one year. The smallest and most recent trial randomized patients at day three with a GCS of less than nine to HBO at 2.5 ATA for 400-600 minutes every four days for three or four treatments versus standard care (53). A markedly larger percentage of patients in the treatment group achieved a good outcome at six months (83% v. 30%).

At first glance this data might lead one to question why HBO is not now standard care for TBI. The problem with the above studies is that none were blinded, there were no sham controls, and there was extreme variability in criteria of inclusion, time of enrollment, and type of treatment given. In meta-analysis, there does appear to be a positive effect on mortality, but this too is limited by the quality and quantity of studies. More large, well-designed, rigorous studies are needed before HBO can be recommended as a treatment modality for traumatic brain injury.

## CEREBRAL PALSY

One of the more controversial uses of hyperbaric oxygen therapy involves the treatment of children with cerebral palsy. The first, and perhaps most difficult, part of any discussion of cerebral palsy (CP) is that it is a poorly defined entity. The term CP encompasses many causes and diagnoses that have a common presentation. Recently, an international symposium defined CP as "a group of disorders of the development of movement and posture, causing activity limitations that are attributed to non-progressive disturbances that occurred in the developing fetal or infant brain" (54).

CP presents as spasticity or motor impairment and can be characterized as hemiplegic, diplegic, or quadriplegic, each with a spectrum of symptoms ranging from mild to severe. Motor deficits are often accompanied by other neurologic deficits including visual and other sensory problems, mental retardation, learning disabilities and epilepsy. The deficits are non-progressive, but can fluctuate over time. There is no cure for CP and treatment has traditionally consisted of symptomatic therapy aimed at increasing function.

In the 1980s, Dr. Richard Neubauer suggested the theory of "idling neurons" in anoxic brain injury, based on SPECT scan evidence of hypofunctioning cortical neurons that were shown to have increased metabolism after HBO treatment (55). He also reported some improvements in patients with anoxic brain injury, closed head injuries, and stroke with HBO treatments (56-58). Despite being either uncontrolled series or case reports done in patients with injuries that would not be characterized as CP, these studies have been used to justify the administration of HBO to treat CP. The same group presented two cases of improvement after HBO in patients with CP, however, the study was not controlled and the cases were never reported in the literature (59).

There are only a few studies specifically looking at HBO treatment for CP. Montgomery, et al. evaluated 25 patients between the ages of three and eight years old with spastic diplegia (60). All patients received 20 treatments of 95% $O_2$ at 1.75 ATA and served as their own controls. They were evaluated by parental questionnaire as well as several evaluation scales. The patients showed significant improvement in gross and fine motor tasks and much greater improvement in spasticity. The study was the first evidence that HBO might be effective in CP, but was criticized for being uncontrolled and unblinded.

The only randomized, controlled study was by the same group reported in two papers evaluating HBO treatment of 111 children with CP (61, 62). In this study, all other therapies were withheld throughout the course of the trial and patients were randomized to 40 treatments lasting one-hour at either 1.75 ATA of HBO or sham treatment using air at 1.3 ATA. Investigator assessments of motor function, working memory, and attention, combined with parental evaluations, both immediately and at three months, showed significant improvement in both groups without a trend towards better function in the treatment arm. The benefits experienced by both groups were attributed to the placebo effect, but the study was criticized because the sham group received 1.3 ATA of air, or the equivalent of 28% $O_2$ by facemask, which some argue might provide a therapeutic benefit (63). A similar study was performed advocating the use of "low pressure hyperbaric oxygen therapy" for other "cerebral hypoperfusion" syndromes, including autism (64). In this small series, 40 one hour sessions of 1.3 ATA of air were given to 6 autistic children. Analysis of parental evaluations showed a therapeutic benefit in all six cases, but the utility of the results was limited since the study was uncontrolled and unblinded.

At this point, the only randomized study published shows no benefit to treating CP with HBO. While there are scattered reports of improvement in uncontrolled small series and case reports, the large placebo effect seen in the randomized study is concerning. Most reviewers agree that more research is needed before HBO therapy is offered to patients with CP and autism.

## MULTIPLE SCLEROSIS

Multiple sclerosis (MS) is a disease of the nervous system defined by inflammation and demyelination in the white matter of the brain and spinal cord. In its most common form, relapsing-remitting MS, presents with isolated attacks of neurologic symptoms such as visual loss, weakness, or numbness. For the first few years of the disease, patients are normal between attacks, but the cumulative effects of axonal damage in the brain results in permanent deficits. At some point during the disease course, patients experience a steady decline in function, which is termed secondary progressive MS. In another form of the disease, also known as primary progressive MS, patients experience permanent deficits from the onset of symptoms and decline progressively over several years. While the exact cause of MS is not clear, it is known that immune system dysfunction is involved, and that both environmental and genetic factors are presumed to contribute. There is no cure for the disease, however, acute attacks often respond well to treatment with intravenous steroids. Over the last ten years, patients with relapsing-remitting MS have benefited from several recently developed effective immunomodulatory therapies that decrease the attack rate and severity of the disease. Unfortunately, there are few known therapeutic options for primary or secondary progressive MS.

Interest in the use of HBO for MS was particularly high in the 1980s and 1990s when there were few therapies available. Several nonrandomized reports suggested a benefit from HBO for disability in MS (65-67). In response to that, a number of randomized controlled trials of various designs were performed to evaluate the efficacy of HBO in treating MS patients (68-77). All of the trials enrolled patients with "definite MS," but many used differing criteria while others defined a maximum level of disability for enrollment. Most of the studies also required patients to be stable symptomatically with no recent exacerbations. The doses given ranged from 1.75 to 2.5 ATA, but the most common was 2.0 ATA for 90 minutes, and in each trial 20 treatments were given, although a few gave "booster" treatments later on. Outcomes of the various studies included improvement on the expanded disability status scale (EDSS), bowel and bladder function, pyramidal function, number of exacerbations, changes in visual evoked potentials, and MRI appearance. Only one small study of 34 patients showed significant differences between the treatment and sham groups, with a decreased mean EDSS seen at the end of treatment and at six but not at 12 months after treatment (65). Two other studies showed small improvements in secondary outcomes of sphincter function and pyramidal function (69, 70, 73).

Other outcomes did not exhibit differences between treatment and sham groups in any study. A large registry of 312 MS patients treated at numerous sites did not show any significant improvement in the EDSS (78). A meta-analysis of these studies did not show any significant effect of HBO on the clinical presentation and progression of MS (79). Interestingly, it was noted that quite a few patients in the placebo groups in these studies claimed improvement which might explain the presumed benefit seen in uncontrolled studies.

Based on a more modern understanding of MS, the most important distinction to make regarding these studies is assessing both how the disease is defined and at what stage of the disease the patients were treated. In most cases, the patients enrolled at a chronic or advanced stage in the disease, and presented with significant disability. The average EDSS for these study groups was approximately five or six, which translates to the inability to work and requires some form of ambulatory assistance, such as a cane, for walking. Although the data available overwhelmingly denies any benefit to MS from HBO, it has not been proven that patients with early stages or milder forms of the disease would not benefit from such treatment.

## CONCLUSION

HBO has been suggested for use in a number of neurological disorders. There are many studies examining the effects of HBO treatment, but none have provided irrefutable evidence supporting any specific neurological disease as an indication for treatment. The case for the use of HBO in ischemic stroke is strong based on animal studies but has yet to be proven in clinical trials. There is data available supporting the use of HBO to treat Radiation Induced Cerebral Necrosis (RIN) on a case-by-case basis, however, larger studies are still warranted. Further study is also necessary to establish the efficacy of HBO in treatment of traumatic brain injury (TBI) because the evidence alleging any benefit is seen in only a small number of low quality studies. The evidence is also weak for the use of HBO in cerebral palsy (CP), where the only randomized study found no benefit, so its use cannot be supported. The most substantial evidence against HBO is found in studies to treat multiple sclerosis (MS), where it provides no clinical benefit.

# REFERENCES

1. Helms AK, Torbey MT, Whelan HT. Hyperbaric Oxygen Therapy of Cerebral Ischemia. Cerebrovasc Dis 2005;20:417-426.

2. Dong H, Xiong L, Zhu Z, Chen S, Hou L, Sakabe T. Preconditioning with hyperbaric oxygen and hyperoxia induces tolerance against spinal cord ischemia in rabbits. Anesthesiol 96:907-912. 2002.

3. Chang CF, Niu KC, Hoffer BJ, Wang Y, Borlongan CV. Hyperbaric oxygen therapy for treatment of postischemic stroke in adult rats. Exper Neurol 166:298-306.2000.

4. Veltkamp R, Siebing DA, Heiland S, Schoenffeldt-Varas P, Veltkamp C, Schwaninger M, Schwab S. Hyperbaric oxygen induces rapid protection against focal cerebral ischemia. Brain Res. 1037:134-138. 2005.

5. Kawamura S, Yausi N, Shirasawa M. Fukasawa H. Therapeutic effects of hyperbaric oxygenation on acute focal cerebral ischemia in rats. Surg Neurol 34:101-106.1990.

6. Veltkamp R, Warner DS, Domoki R, Brinkhous AD, Toole JF, Busija DW. Hyperbaric oxygen decreases infarct size and behavioral deficit after transient focal cerebral ischemia in rats. Brain Res 853:68-73.2000.

7. Badr AE, Yin W, Mychaskiw G, Zhang JH. Effect of hyperbaric oxygen on striatal metabolites: a microdialysis study in awake freely moving rats after MCA occlusion. Brain Research 916:85-90.2001.

8. Yin W, Badr AE, Myechaskiw G, Zhang JH. Down regulation of COX-2 is involved in hyperbaric oxygen treatment in a rat transient focal cerebral ischemia model. Brain Res. 926:165-171.2002.

9. Sunami K, Takeda Y, Hashimoto M, Hirakawa M. Hyperbaric oxygen reduces infarct volume in rats by increasing oxygen supply to the ischemic periphery. Crit Care Med 28:2831-2836.2000.

10. Mink RB, Dutka AJ. Hyperbaric oxygen after global cerebral ischemia in rabbits does not promote brain lipid peroxidation. Crit Care Med 23:1398-1404.1995.

11. Corkill G, Van Housen K, Hein L, Reitan J. Videodensitometric estimation of the protective effect of hyperbaric oxygen in the ischemic gerbil brain. Surg Neurol 24:206-210. 1985.

12. Burt JT, Kapp JP, Smith RR. Hyperbaric oxygen and cerebral infarction in the gerbil. Surg Neurol. 28:265-268.1987.

13. Reitan JA, Kien ND, Thorup S, Corkill G. Hyperbaric oxygen increases survival following carotid ligation in gerbils. Stroke 21:119-123. 1990.

14. Roos JA, Jackson-Friedman C, Lyden P. Effects of hyperbaric oxygen on neurologic outcome for cerebral ischemia in rats. Acad Emer Med 5:18-24.1998.

15. Hjelde A, Hjelstuen M, Haraldseth O, Martin JD, Thom SR, Brubakk AO. Hyperbaric oxygen and neutrophil accumulation/tissue damage during permanent focal cerebral ischaemia in rats. Eur J Appl Physiol 86:401-405.2002.

16. Weinstein PR, Anderson GG, Telles DA. Results of hyperbaric oxygen therapy during temporary middle cerebral artery occlusion in unanesthetized cats. Neurosurg 20:518-524. 1987.

17. Lou M, Eschenfelder CC, Herdegen T, Brecht S, Deuschl G. Therapuetic window for use of hyperbaric oxygenation in focal transient ischemia in rats. Stroke 35:578-583. 2004.

18. Rosenthal RE, Silbergleit R, Hof PR, Haywood Y, Fiskum G. Hyperbaric oxygen reduces neuronal death and improves neurological outcome after canine cardiac arrest. Stroke 34:1311-1316.2003.

19. Yang Z, Camporesi C, Yang X, Wang J, Bosco G, Lok J, Gorji R, Schelper RL, Camporesi EM. Hyperbaric oxygenation mitigates focal cerebral injury and reduces striatal dopamine release in a rat model of transient middle cerebral artery occlusion. Eur J App Physiol 87:101-107.2002.

20. Weinstein PR, Hameroff SR, Johnson PC, Anderson GG. Effect of hyperbaric oxygen therapy or dimethyl sulfoxide on cerebral ischemia in unanesthetized gerbils. Neruosurg 18:528-532. 1986.

21. Yin D, Zhou C, Kusaka I, Calvert JW, Parent AD, Nanda A, Zhang JH. Inhibition of apoptosis by hyperbaric oxygen in a rat focal cerebral ischemic model. J Cereb Blood Flow Metab 23:855-864. 2003.

22. Kondo A, Baba S, Iwaki T, Harai H, Koga H, Kimura T, Takmatsu J. Hyperbaric oxygenation prevents delayed neuronal death following transient ischaemia in the gerbil hippocampus. Neruopath Appl Neurobiol 22:350-360.1996.

23. Calvert JW, Yin W, Patel M, Badr A, Mychaskiw G, Parent AD, Zhang JH. Hyperbaric oxygenation prevented brain injury induced by hypoxia-ischemia in a neonatal rat model. Brain Res 951:1-8.2002.

24. Atochin DN, Fisher D, Demchenko IT, Thom SR. Neutrophil sequestration and the effect of hyperbaric oxygen in a rat model of temporary middle cerebral artery occlusion. Undersea & Hyperbar Med 27:185-190.2000.

25. Miljkovic-Lolic M, Silbergleit R, Fiskum G, Rosenthal RE. Neuroprotective effects of hyperbaric oxygen treatment in experimental focal cerebral ischemia are associated with reduced brain leukocyte myeloperoxidase activity. Brain Res 971:90-94.2003.

26. Wada K, Ito M, Miyazawa T, Katoh H, Nawashiro H, Shima K, Chigasaki H. Repeated hyperbaric oxygen induces ischemic tolerance in gerbil hippocampus. Brain Res 740:15-20.1996.

27. Wada K, Miyazawa T, Nomura N, Nawashiro H, Shima K. Preferential conditions for and possible mechanisms of induction of ischemic tolerance by repeated hyperbaric oxygenation in gerbil hippocampus. Neurosurg 49:160-167. 2001.

28. Anderson DC, Bottini AG, Jagiella WM, Westphal B, Ford S, Rockswold GL, Loewenson RB. A pilot study of hyperbaric oxygen in the treatment of human stroke. Stroke 22:1137-1142.1991.

29. Nighoghossian N, Trouillas P, Adeleine P, Salford F. Hyperbaric oxygen in the treatment of acute ischemic stroke: a double-blind pilot study. Stroke 26:1369-1372.1995.

30. Rusyniak DE, Kirk MA, May JD, Kao LW, Brizendine EJ, Welch JL, Cordell WH, Alonso RJ. Hyperbaric oxygen therapy in acute ischemic stroke results of the hyperbaric oxygen in acute ischemic stroke trial pilot study. Stroke 34:571-4.2003.

31. Giglio P, Gilbert MR, Cerebral Radiation Necrosis. Neurologist 9:180–188, 2003.

32. Glantz MJ, Burger PC, Friedman AH, Radtke RA, Massey EW, Schold SC. Treatment of radiation -induced nervous system injury with heparin and warfarin. Neurology 1994;44:2020–7.

33. Hulshof M, Stark N, Van der Kleij A, Sminia P, Smeding H, Gonzales D. Hyperbaric oxygen therapy for cognitive disorders after irradiation of the brain. Strahlentherapie und Onkologie 2002;178(4):192-8.

34. Kohshi K, Imada H, Nomoto S, Yamaguchi R, Abe H, Yamamoto H. Successful treatment of radiation-induced brain necrosis by hyperbaric oxygen therapy. Journal of the Neurological Sciences 209 (2003) 115– 117.

35. Tandon N, Vollmer DG, New PZ, Hevezi JM, Herman T, Kagan-Hallet K, et al. Fulminant radiation-induced necrosis after stereotactic radiation therapy to the posterior fossa. Case report and review of the literature. J Neurosurg 2001;95:507–12.

36. Takenaka N, Imanishi T, Sasaki H, Shimazaki K, Sugiura H, Kitagawa Y, Sekiyama S, Yamamoto M, Kazuno T. Delayed radiation necrosis with extensive brain edema after gamma knife radiosurgery for multiple cerebral cavernous malformations. Neurologia Medico-Chirurgica. 43(8):391-5, 2003.

37. Leber KA, Eder HG, Kovac H, Anegg U, Pendl G. Treatment of cerebral radionecrosis by hyperbaric oxygen therapy. Stereotact Funct Neurosurg 1998;70(suppl 1):229– 36.

38. McPherson CM. Warnick RE, Results of contemporary surgical management of radiation necrosis using frameless stereotaxis and intraoperative magnetic resonance imaging. Journal of Neuro-Oncology. 68(1):41-7, 2004.

39. Warnick RE, Gessell LB, Breneman JC, Albright RE, Racadio J, Mink S: Hyperbaric oxygen is an effective treatment for radiation necrosis of the brain. Neurosurgery 51: 560, 2002.

40. Chuba PJ, Aronin P, Bhambhani K, Eichenhorn M, Zamarano L, Cianci PM, et al. Hyperbaric oxygen therapy for radiation-induced brain injury in children. Cancer 1997;80:2005– 12.

41. Brain Trauma Foundation New York: Guideline for prehospital management of traumatic brain injury. Available at: http://www2.braintrauma.org/guidelines/index.php. Accessed 2001.

42. Aarabi B, Eisenberg HM, Murphy K, Morrison C, Weinmann M. Traumatic brain injury: management and complications. In: Textbook of Neurointensive Care Layton. AJ, Gabrielli A and Friedman WA eds. Saunders Publishing, Philadelphia, PA 2004.

43. Atochin DN, Fisher D, Demchenko IT, Thom SR. Neutrophil sequestration and the effect of hyperbaric oxygen in a rat model of temporary middle cerebral artery occlusion. Undersea & Hyperbar Med 27:185-190.2000.

44. Omae T, Ibayashi S, Kusuda K, Nakamura H, Yagi H, Fujishima M. Effects of high atmospheric pressure and oxygen on middle cerebral blood flow velocity in humans measured by transcranial doppler. Stroke 29:94-97.1998.

45. Zhilyaev SY, Moskvin AN, Platonova TF, Gutsaeva DR, Churilina IV, Demchenko IT. Hyperoxic vasoconstriction in the brain is mediated by inactivation of nitric oxide by superoxide anions. Neurosci Behav Phys 33:783-787.2003.

46. Sukoff MH, Ragatz RE. Hyperbaric oxygenation for the treatment of acute cerebral edema. Neurosurg 10:29-38. 1982.

47. Hayakawa T, Kanai N, Kuroda R. Response of cerebrospinal fluid pressure to hyperbaric oxygenation. Journal of Neurology, Neurosurgery and Psychiatry 1971;34(5):580-6.

48. Rockswold SB, Rockswold GL, Vargo JM, Erickson CA, Sutton RL, Bergman TA, Biros MH. Effects of hyperbaric oxygenation therapy on cerebral metabolism and intracranial pressure in severely brain injured patients. J Neurosurg 95:544-546.2001.

49. Neubauer RA, Gottlieb SF, Pevsner NH. Hyperbaric oxygen for treatment of closed head injury. Southern Medical Journal 1994;87(9):933-6.

50. Artru F, Chacornac R, Deleuze R. Hyperbaric oxygenation for severe head injuries. Preliminary results of a controlled study. European Neurology 1976;14(4):310-18.

51. Holbach KH, Wassmann H, Kolberg T. Improved reversibility of the traumatic midbrain syndrome using hyperbaric oxygen. Acta Neurochirurgica (Wien) 1974;30(3-4):247-56.

52. Rockswold GL, Ford SE, Anderson DC, Bergman TA, ShermanRE. Results of a prospective randomized trial for treatment of severely brain-injured patients with hyperbaric oxygen. Journal of Neurosurgery 1992;76(6):929-34.

53. Ren H, Wang W, Ge Z. Glasgow coma scale, brain electrical activity mapping and Glasgow outcome score after hyperbaric oxygen treatment of severe brain injury. Chinese Journal of Traumatology 2001;4(4):239-41.

54. Executive Committee for the Definition of Cerebral Palsy. Developmental Medicine & Child Neurology 2005, 47: 571–576.

55. Neubauer RA, Kagan RL, Gottlieb SF, James P. Delayed metabolism or reperfusion in brain imaging after exposure to hyperbaric oxygenation – a therapeutic indicator. Proceedings of the XV Annual Meeting of the European Undersea Biomedial Society, Eilat, Israel, Sept. 17-21, 1989.

56. Neubauer RA. The effect of hyperbaric oxygen in prolonged coma: possible identification of marginally functioning brain zones. Med Subacquea ed Iperbarica 1985; 5: 75-79.

57. Neubauer RA, Gottlieb SF, Pevsner NH. Hyperbaric oxygen for treatment of closed head injury. Southern Med J 1994; 87: 933-35.

58. Neubauer RA, James P. Cerebral oxygenation and the recoverable brain. Neurol Res 1998; 20 (supp 1): S33-36.

59. Neubauer RA, Uszler J, James P. Hyperbaric oxygen: the recoverable brain in certain pediatric patients: 8th International Child Neurology Congress, Ljubliana, Slovenia, Sept 13-18, 1998.

60. Montgomery D, Goldberg J, Amar M, et al. Effects of hyperbaric oxygen therapy on children with spastic diplegic cerebral palsy: a pilot project. Undersea Hyperb Med 1999;26(4):235-242.

61. Collet JP, Vanasse M, Marois P, et al. Hyperbaric oxygen for children with cerebral palsy: a randomised multicentre trial. Lancet 2001;357:582-586.

62. Hardy P, Collet JP, Goldberg J, et al. Neuropsychological effects of hyperbaric oxygen therapy in cerebral palsy. Dev Med Child Neurol 2002;44:436-446.

63. Neubauer RA. Hyperbaric oxygen therapy for cerebral palsy. Lancet 2001; 357: 2052.

64. Rossignol DA, Rossignol LW. Hyperbaric oxygen therapy may improve symptoms in autistic children. Medical Hypotheses (2006) 67, 216–228.

65. Meneghetti G, Sparta S, Rusca F, Facco E, Martini A, Comacchio F, Schiraldi C. Hyperbaric oxygen therapy in the treatment of multiple sclerosis. A clinical and electrophysiological study in a 2 year follow-up. Riv Neurol. 1990 Mar-Apr;60(2):67-71.

66. Webster CJ, MacIver C, Allen S, Murray S. The chief scientist reports ... hyperbaric oxygen for multiple sclerosis patients. Health Bull (Edinb). 1989 Nov; 47(6):320-31.

67. Zannini D, Formai C, Bogetti B, Sereni G. 40 cases of multiple sclerosis treated with hyperbaric oxygen therapy. Minerva Med. 1982 Nov 3;73(42):2939-45.

68. Fischer BH. Marks M. Reich T. Hyperbaric-oxygen treatment of multiple sclerosis. A randomized, placebo-controlled, double-blind study. New England Journal of Medicine. 308(4):181-6, 1983.

69. Barnes MP. Bates D. Cartlidge NE. French JM. Shaw DA. Hyperbaric oxygen and multiple sclerosis: short-term results of a placebo-controlled, double-blind trial. Lancet. 1(8424):297-300, 1985.

70. Barnes MP. Bates D. Cartlidge NE. French JM. Shaw DA. Hyperbaric oxygen and multiple sclerosis: final results of a placebo-controlled, double-blind trial. Journal of Neurology, Neurosurgery & Psychiatry. 50(11):1402-6, 1987.

71. Lhermitte F. Roullet E. Lyon-Caen O. Metrot J. Villey T. Bach MA. Tournier-Lasserve E. Chabassol E. Rascol A. Clanet M. et al. Double-blind treatment of 49 cases of chronic multiple sclerosis using hyperbaric oxygen. Revue Neurologique. 142(3):201-6, 1986.

72. Harpur GD. Suke R. Bass BH. Bass MJ. Bull SB. Reese L. Noseworthy JH. Rice GP. Ebers GC. Hyperbaric oxygen therapy in chronic stable multiple sclerosis: double-blind study. Neurology. 36(7):988-91, 1986 Jul.

73. Oriani G, Barbieri S, Cislaghi G, Albonico G, Scarlato G, Mariani C, et al. Long-term hyperbaric oxygen in multiple sclerosis: a placebo-controlled, double-blind trial with evoked potentials studies. Journal of Hyperbaric Medicine 1990;5:237-45.

74. Confavreux C, Mathieu C, Cacornac R, Aimard G, Devic M. Hyperbaric oxygen in multiple sclerosis. La Presse Medicale 1986;15(28):1319-22.

75. Wiles CM. Clarke CR. Irwin HP. Edgar EF. Swan AV. Hyperbaric oxygen in multiple sclerosis: a double blind trial. British Medical Journal Clinical Research Ed.. 292(6517):367-71, 1986.

76. Wood J. Stell R. Unsworth I. Lance JW. Skuse N. A double-blind trial of hyperbaric oxygen in the treatment of multiple sclerosis. Medical Journal of Australia. 143(6):238-40, 1985.

77. Neiman J. Nilsson BY. Barr PO. Perrins DJ. Hyperbaric oxygen in chronic progressive multiple sclerosis: visual evoked potentials and clinical effects. Journal of Neurology, Neurosurgery & Psychiatry. 48(6):497-500, 1985

78. Kindwall EP. McQuillen MP. Khatri BO. Gruchow HW. Kindwall ML. Treatment of multiple sclerosis with hyperbaric oxygen. Results of a national registry. Archives of Neurology. 48(2):195-9, 1991 Feb.

79. Bennett M, Heard R. Hyperbaric oxygen therapy for multiple sclerosis. Cochrane Database of Systematic Reviews. 3, 2006.

# NOTES

CHAPTER 40

# HYPERBARIC OXYGEN IN ACUTE MYOCARDIAL INFARCTION IN ANIMALS AND MAN

## CHAPTER FORTY OVERVIEW

# HYPERBARIC OXYGEN IN ACUTE MYOCARDIAL INFARCTION IN ANIMALS AND MAN

*Myrvin H. Ellestad, George B. Hart, Joseph Myslinski*

## INTRODUCTION

Boerema's classic paper "Life Without Blood," published in 1960, where pigs had their blood replaced with plasma expanders at three atmospheres atmospheric absolute (ATA) showed no adverse effect, despite the fact that the pigs' hemoglobin level was essentially zero (1). This encouraged the medical community to seriously examine HBO. In the last thirty years, randomized, controlled studies have moved HBO from a suspect medical treatment to the standard of care for certain medical conditions.

HBO is currently considered the standard of care for CO poisoning, cerebral arterial gas embolism, osteoradionecrosis, decompression sickness, and clostridial gas gangrene. It is also considered an adjunct to care for: acute exceptional blood loss anemia, acute thermal burns, compromised skin grafts or skin flaps, crush injury, compartment syndrome, necrotizing soft-tissue infections, non-clostridial gas gangrene, radiation tissue damage, refractory osteomyelitis, selected problem wounds, and selected refractory mycosis.

The success of HBO in acute ischemic conditions led to its consideration in the treatment of acute myocardial infarction. Significant advances have been made in the management of acute myocardial infarction (AMI) during the past 30 years. The widespread acceptance of coronary care units during the 1960s helped lower AMI mortality from 30% to 15%. Thrombolytic agents have further reduced the death rate to 6-7%. Yet, despite optimal and timely therapy, AMI often leads to irreversible myocardial damage. Arrhythmias, a significant cause of mortality and morbidity, are now less of a problem, but improvement in left ventricular function is still suboptimal. Can hyperbaric oxygen (HBO) offer an added benefit to current therapy? To help answer that question, a brief history of HBO in the management of AMI will be reviewed.

## STUDIES THROUGHOUT HISTORY

The 1950s saw many AMI patients dying of ventricular fibrillation. Feeling that these arrhythmias were the result of decreased oxygen tension at the margin of the ischemic myocardium, Smith and Lawson examined the effect of HBO on the acutely ischemic canine heart in their 1958 landmark article (2). Dogs underwent surgical ligation of the circumflex artery and were then randomized to receive one hour of 100% $O_2$ either at 2 ATA or 1 ATA. After a 2-hour observation period, 6 of 10 normobaric dogs had died of ventricular fibrillation (VF), whereas only 1 of 10 had died in the hyperbaric group. These results were reproduced in 1962 in an extended study (3).

The next important study also used a canine coronary artery ligation model (4). After ligating the mid-LAD (left anterior descending artery), dogs received 6 hours of oxygen at either 3 ATA or 1 ATA. The hearts were then removed and stained to identify areas of anoxia. Not surprisingly, the HBO group was noted to have 50-75% less ischemic myocardium than the control group (4). This reduction in anoxic myocardium is attributable not only to the increased $pO_2$ and tissue diffusion of oxygen, but also to the fact that collateral blood flow supplies 60-80% of the original blood flow to areas bordering ischemic myocardium and at least 15-20% of the original blood flow to the center of infarcted areas (5).

During the 1960s, other articles appeared showing benefit from HBO in the acute myocardial infarction (MI) setting. Meijne showed that HBO led to regression of EKG findings of AMI in rabbits that had undergone ligation of the anterior descending coronary artery (6). Pretreatment with HBO at 2 ATA (in conjunction with induced hypothermia) allowed dogs to withstand total circulatory arrest for longer periods (sometimes for as much as 30 minutes) without neurologic deficit (7).

In a diffuse myocardial injury model (induced by intracoronary injection of microspheres), HBO blunted the decreases in cardiac output and aortic pressure, and significantly improved the 24-hour survival, compared to dogs not undergoing HBO therapy (77% vs. 31%) (13). Peter et al., from Duke University, utilized a gradually constricting band of Ameroid around a swine coronary artery. This model, HBO (1.25 ATA for 32 hours), prolonged survival over controls (46 hours vs. 21 hours) (9). Two other projects described reduced injury with hyperbaric oxygen therapy in animals subjected to norepinephrine or isoproterenol-induced myocardial insult (10, 11).

However, the data was not always so compelling. Chardack et al. utilized a canine coronary artery ligation model and found that, although survival increased with increasing atmospheres, the improvment survival did not reach statistical significance, even at 4 atmospheres (12). Others failed to show any beneficial effects of HBO therapy, either with a coronary artery ligation model or a diffuse myocardial damage model (13, 14).

Whalen and Saltzman wrote an excellent review article in 1968 on hyperbaric oxygen and its use in AMI (15). They noted that animal studies were encouraging, but results could not be extrapolated to humans: dogs have a different coronary circulation than humans; animals usually have no underlying coronary artery disease; the HBO regimen used in these studies are inappropriate for people; and the time interval between coronary occlusion and HBO is unrealistically short.

The first case report of a human undergoing HBO therapy after AMI was described by Moon in 1964. This patient developed cardiogenic shock and, with HBO intermittently over 48 hours, ultimately had a successful outcome (16). However, it was not until 1966 that the first randomized trial with humans took place. Cameron reported on 50 patients that received either HBO at 2 ATA or normobaric 100% oxygen. Six patients died in each group, but the HBO group had five of the seven patients with cardiogenic shock. It is difficult to determine whether HBO had any benefit in this small study (17). Cameron also studied the hemodynamic effects of HBO in a subset of ten MI patients. As with normal subjects, HBO reduced cardiac output and increased systemic vascular resistance. Unlike HBO in normal patients, heart rate in the MI patients did not change significantly. Rather, the reduced cardiac output in MI patients undergoing HBO therapy was attributed to a decrease in stroke volume. Nonetheless, mean arterial pressure still rose in MI patients. Furthermore, MI patients with elevated lactate levels had reductions in these levels with HBO therapy. These results point out one of many paradoxes associated with HBO therapy: decreased cardiac output, but improved tissue oxygen delivery.

Another interesting study was published in 1969, which examined the use of HBO in 40 patients with severe acute MIs (18). It was not a controlled study and was not widely known. Fourteen of the forty patients were in pulmonary edema, 12 had blood pressures of 90 systolic or less, and 5 had recent ventricular fibrillation. All underwent HBO at 2 ATA for 2 hours, alternating with air at 1 ATA, for four days. Only 3 patients died during the four days of HBO therapy; all developed asystole during the air breaks. Three additional patients died prior to discharge (two with asystole and one with VF), giving a mortality rate of 15% for this subset of "severe" MI patients. There were no serious arrhythmias during HBO therapy; instead, HBO provided a significant antiarrhythmic effect.

The biochemical effects of HBO during AMI was examined by Kline et al. (19). HBO at 3 ATA was found to decrease myocardial oxygen consumption, reduce excess myocardial lactate production, and narrow the oxygen difference between coronary artery and coronary sinus blood.

In 1973, a larger randomized study involving 208 patients was reported (20). These patients received either traditional AMI care, or traditional AMI care plus a 48-hour HBO protocol of 2 hours of 100% oxygen at 2 ATA, alternating with 1 hour of air at 1 ATA. The last half-hour of the HBO cycle was spent decompressing to the surface. No significant difference in mortality between the two groups was found during hospitalization, but the HBO group was clinically sicker than the control group. Taking this into account, HBO reduced mortality by 50% in the most critical patients, and appeared beneficial to older patients, women, those with extensive cardiac history, or those presenting with cardiogenic shock. In those patients with a Peel index of severity of greater than 10 (on a 0-28 scale), the chances of leaving the hospital alive rose from 13% to 56%, when tandomized to the HBO group (p=0.03). An interesting phenomenon was the repeated resolution of high-grade AV block with HBO, only to have the block reappear during the hour of breathing air on the surface.

The advent of surgical revascularization prompted some researchers to apply HBO to temporary occlusion states. Kawamura et al. temporarily occluded the LAD for 2 hours in dogs, and then examined their hearts after 5 days. Histologic examination revealed that the HBO-treated dogs had a significant reduction in the percentage of infarcted tissue compared to control dogs. In addition, repair of necrotic myocardium had begun by 5 days in the HBO-group, whereas the control group had little evidence of repair (21).

Thrombolytic therapy, now generally accepted for AMI patients, can also lead to reperfusion injury. Animal studies reveal myocardial generation of oxygen-derived radicals is minimal during ischemia, but significant during reperfusion. Furthermore, the addition of superoxide dismutase and catalase prior to reperfusion improved cardiac function helps minimize post-reperfusion CPK levels (22). The major culprit responsible for myocardial reperfusion injury appears to be the neutrophil. Depletion of WBCs with antiserum limited myocardial injury, after temporary coronary artery occlusion in dogs (23). It now appears that areas of post-ischemic hypocontractility ("stunned myocardium") are the result of reperfusion injury (24).

The study on simultaneous HBO and t-PA, by Thomas and his group in Cleveland, has generated considerable interest (25). Briefly, an LAD thrombus was artificially induced with an intracoronary copper coil in dogs. After two hours of angiographically, confirmed occlusion, one of four therapies were instituted: no treatment; HBO at 2 ATA for 90 minutes; t-PA for 90 minutes; or HBO plus t-PA for 90 minutes. The animals were then sacrificed and the hearts stained to identify areas of maximal, moderate and no injury.

The control group had 36% of the myocardium with maximal injury and 24% with moderate injury; the HBO-only group had 9% of the heart with maximal injury and 44% with moderate injury. The t-PA only group had 6% of the heart with maximal injury and 47% with moderate injury. The combined HBO plus t-PA group had only 1% of the heart with maximal injury and 12% with moderate injury.

Compared to the control group, CPK levels after 4 hours were unchanged in the HBO-only group, 10 times higher in the t-PA-only group, and only 2 times higher in the combined group. Reperfusion arrhythmias in the combined group were only 1/5th as frequent as the t-PA-only group. Restored enzyme activity was 36% in the HBO-only group, 47% in the t-PA only group and 97% in the combined group. Thus, the effects of simultaneous t-PA and HBO appear to be synergistic. Needless to say, if these results hold up in human studies, HBO should become a necessity in most hospitals.

The report in 1997 by Shandling et al. on 64 patients randomized to t-PA and HBO, or t-PA alone, revealed a marked improvement in the time to pain relief over the t-PA-only group (264 min vs 775 min) and reduction in 12-hour CPK levels (224 vs 1,635). There is also a trend towards improved left ventricular (LV) ejection fraction that did not reach significance (26). The prominence of inferior MIs may be one reason why the beneficial affect was not reflected in a significant improvement in ejection fraction.

## CURRENT RESEARCH

Currently, it is difficult to determine which AMI patients will improve their ejection fraction following early surgical revascularization. A recent study claims that hyperbaric oxygen might be used in the subacute MI setting to help identify stunned and hibernating myocardium (27). SPECT-thallium exercise scintigraphy identified ventricular segments with normal, reversible, or fixed abnormalities. Echocardiography was then performed prior to and after a 30-minute course of HBO therapy, and LV segmental contraction was graded.

Ventricular segments that improved contraction following HBO potentially represent hibernating myocardium. These segments can then be analyzed for myocardial viability by SPECT-thallium. In this fashion, the researchers are able to identify 20% of the damaged ventricular segments as representing hibernating myocardium. Although this is the first direct evidence to preoperatively determine which patients might benefit from early surgical revascularization, it could be an extremely valuable test for cardiologists and cardiovascular surgeons.

HBO appears to offer significant benefit when given after reperfusion. But the critical question remains: How soon after reperfusion is established must HBO be given in order to have benefit? One group, from Alabama, helped answer this question in a roundabout way (28). Sterling and his colleagues believe HBO use during reperfusion would increase free-radical generation and lead to more injury. To test their hypothesis, they divided rabbits into six groups. All rabbits underwent coronary artery occlusion for 30 minutes and were then reperfused for 3 hours. The HBO protocol here used 100% oxygen at 2.5 ATA during: 1) none of the stages (control breathing 100% oxygen at 1 ATA); 2) the 30 minutes of occlusion only; 3) the 3 hours of reperfusion only; 4) the entire occlusion and reperfusion stages; 5) the final 150 minutes of reperfusion only (the late-HBO reperfusion group); and 6) none of the stages (pressure control group breathed 40% oxygen at 2.5 ATA). When not undergoing HBO, all rabbits breathed 100% oxygen at 1 ATA.

The results surprised the researchers. Rather than finding increased infarct sizes in the HBO groups, they found that HBO afforded considerable protection against ischemia. Myocardial infarct size from the control rabbits averaged 41%, but only 15% in the HBO groups. All groups appeared to have equal reductions in infarct size, except for the late-HBO reperfusion group. This group of rabbits underwent 30 minutes of occlusion and 30 minutes of reperfusion at 1 ATA, and then received HBO. This 30-minute delay in administering HBO was crucial, as these animals fared no better than the control groups. The authors concluded that there is a critical time period in reperfusion in which HBO must be administered to be protective. They also were converted to "believers" and conducted further studies in this area.

Other recent studies provide a clue to why HBO is protective in reperfusion injury. The bulk of the evidence points to oxygen-derived free radicals as the agents responsible for reperfusion injury. It is not surprising that many prominent researchers argue against the use of HBO in this setting, as they felt it would add "fuel to the fire" and lead to even more damage. Yet, studies continue to clearly indicate a benefit with HBO when used in this setting.

In the last few years, a clearer picture of HBO and reperfusion injury is beginning to emerge. Simpson showed that reperfusion injury could be prevented by the use of monoclonal antibodies to inhibit neutrophil adherence to the damaged endothelium (29). It is now believed that HBO prevents neutrophil adherence by preventing the activation or "up regulation" of CD-18 receptors (30). These special receptors make it possible for the leukocyte to adhere to the site of injury. Without leukocyte adherence, there is a marked decrease in the generation of free radicals. So, HBO appears to break a critical link in the chain of events that characterize reperfusion injury. Whether this will ultimately translate into widespread clinical use of HBO is yet unknown.

A multicenter study combined 112 cases from 5 centers (31). Sixty-six had inferior MIs and 46 had anterior infarcts. All patients received either tPA or streptokinase, and were randomized to thrombolysis alone, or 2 hours of HBO plus thrombolysis. The left ventricular ejection fraction (LVFE) on discharge was 51.7% in the HBO group, and 48.4% in the controls. These trends are encouraging but not statistically different. As in an earlier study, the time to pain relief and the peak CPK were reduced in those receiving HBO. The fact that there were only 3 deaths suggests the trial only included patients with smaller infarctions; thus, it may be that those who might benefit the most were often not treated. When comparing the ejection fraction benefits of HBO in anterior versus inferior infarcts, however, we are unable to demonstrate a significant difference. The centers contributing cases are:

Long Beach Memorial Medical Center, Long Beach, California
Zemum Clinical Hospital Center, U.y Belgrade, Yugoslavia
Northridge Heart Institute, Northridge, California
Indian River Memorial Hospital, Vero Beach, Florida
Richland Memorial Hospital, Columbia, South Carolina

The most impressive finding, in both this study and the earlier one, was the rapid resolution of ST elevation once the patients were under 2 atmospheres of pressure. See Figures 1a thru 1d. This suggests a beneficial effect from the hyberbaric oxygen not observed with the thrombolysis alone.

## TREATMENT PROTOCOL

Patients with classical acute myocardial infarction, identified by a typical pain pattern and ST elevation, were offered the opportunity to be included. The thrombolytic was either tPA or streptokinase.

The tPA dose was 100 mg IV with 12 mg given as a bolus, and 20 mg per hour given following this. Streptokinase is administered at a dose of 1.5 million units over a 60-minute period. All patients are given enteric coated aspirin (325 mg) immediately. Patients who were given tPA were given 5,000 units of heparin immediately at the end of the tPA infusion. Heparin was then titrated to maintain a partial thromboplastic time between 60 and 90 seconds for 3 days. Those receiving streptokinase were not given heparin.

Patients randomized to HBO are immediately transported to the hyperbaric unit after the thrombolytic is started, and pressurized to 2 ATA, equivalent to 33 feet of sea water pressure, breathing 100% $O_2$. Pressurization usually takes about 30 minutes. They remain at pressure for 60 minutes, and are decompressed to surface pressure over a 30-minute period.

Monitoring of the ECG, noninvasive blood pressure, and other vital signs must be the same as in the CCU. The ability to take 12-lead ECGs in the

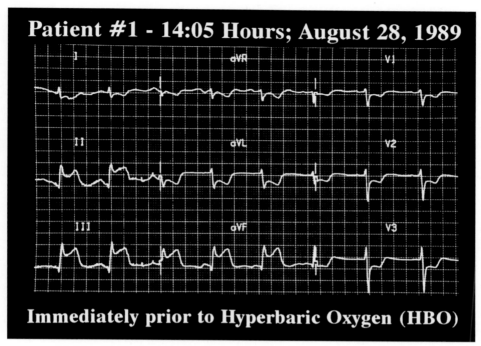

Figure 1A. ECG taken immediately prior to starting therapy.

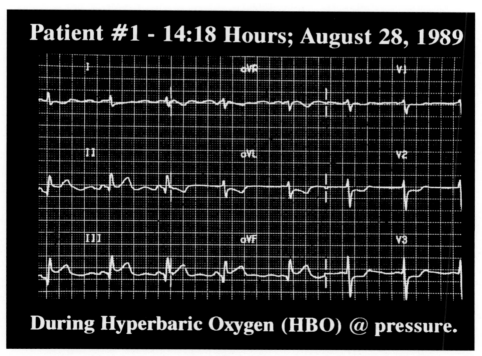

Figure 1B. ECG taken just as patient reached full pressure of 2 atmospheres. Chest pain also subsided at this time.

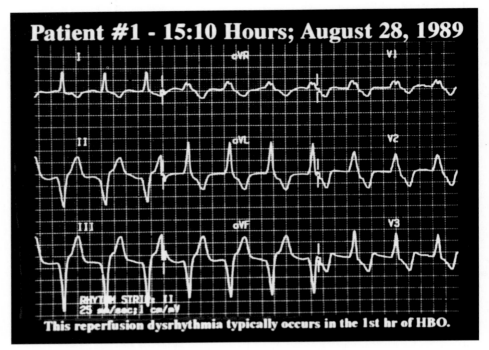

Figure 1C. 52 minutes after figure 1b patient developed an idioventricular tachycardia. We believe this was a reperfusion arrhythmia. It subsided about 2 minutes after its inception. Blood pressure was maintained during the arrhythmia.

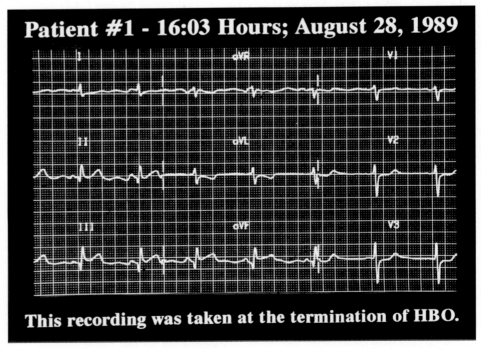

Figure 1D. Two hours after intiation of HBO the ST elevation has almost completely resolved.

chamber is very important. After removal from the chamber, they are transported to the CCU and monitored and treated, in the usual manner, depending on their clinical status.

## CONCLUSION

Hyperbaric oxygen in the setting of acute myocardial infarction has come of age, and has moved from the animal lab to the realm of human therapy. The study by Shandling, et al. (26) and the subsequent multicenter study (31), demonstrate that it is technically feasible, clinically safe and possibly beneficial. Some of the questions remaining to be answered are:

1. What is the optimum time window?
2. Will it be more beneficial for anterior vs. inferior MI?
3. Will it reduce mortality and improve ventricular function?
4. What is the optimum HBO protocol?
5. What are the most important mechanisms of its effect?

It is hoped that new studies will shed more light on this interesting approach to therapy.

## REFERENCES

1. Boerema I, Meijne NG, Brummelkamp WH, et al. Life without blood. J Cardiovasc Surg 1960;1:133-146.

2. Smith G, Lawson DA. Experimental coronary arterial occlusion: effects of the administration of oxygen under pressure. Scot Med J 1958;3:346-350.

3. Smith G, Lawson DA. The protective effect of inhalation of oxygen at two atmospheres absolute pressure in acute coronary arterial occlusion. Surg Gyn Obst 1962;114:320-322.

4. Trapp WG, Creighton R. Experimental studies of increased atmospheric pressure on myocardial ischemia after coronary ligation. J Thor Cardiovasc Surg 1964;47(5):687-692.

5. Jugdutt BI, Hutchins GM, Bulkley BH, Becker LC. Myocardial infarction in the conscious dog: three dimensional mapping of infarct, collateral flow and region at risk. Circulation 1979;60:1141-1150.

6. Meijne NG, Bulterijs A, Eloff SJ. An experimental investigation into the influence of administration of oxygen under increased atmospheric pressure upon coronary infarction. J Cardiov Surg 1963;4:521-525.

7. Illingsworth C. Treatment of arterial occlusion under oxygen at two atmospheres pressure. Brit Med J 1962;1271-1275.

8. Jacobson JH, Wang MC, Yamaki T, Kline HJ, Kark AE, Kuhn LA. Hyper6;23:169-172.

9. Peter RH, Rau RW, Whalen RE, Entman ML, McIntosh HD. Effect of hyperbaric oxygenation on coronary artery occlusion in pigs. Proceedings of the third international conference on hyperbaric medicine. 1965;395-401.

10. Violago F, Penn I. The effect of hyperbaric oxygen on I-noradrenal in induced myocardial necrosis. Canad J Surg 1966;9:419-422.

11. Kennedy JH, Alousi M, Homi J. The protective effect of hyperbaric oxygenation upon isoproterenol-induced myocardial necrosis in syrian hamsters. Med Thorac 1966;23:169-172.

12. Chardack WM, Gage AA, Federico AJ, Cusick JK, Matsumoto PJH, Lanphir EH. Reduction by hyperbaric oxygenation of the mortality from ventricular fibrillation following coronary artery ligation. Circ Res 1964;15:497-502.

13. Robertson HF. The effect of hyperbaric oxygen on myocardial infarction in dogs. Canad J Surg 1966;9:81-84.

14. Holloway DH, Whalen RE, Saltzman HA, McIntosh HD. Hyperbaric oxygenation in the treatment of acute coronary artery embolization in dogs. J Lab Clin Med 1965;66:596-603.

15. Whalen RE, Saltzman HA. Hyperbaric oxygen in the treatment of acute myocardial infarction. Prog Cardiovasc Dis 1968;10:575-583.

16. Moon AJ, Williams KG, Hopkinson WI. A patient with coronary thrombosis treated with hyperbaric oxygen. Lancet 1964;1:18-20.

17. Cameron AJ, Gibb BH, Ledingham IMcA, McGuinnes JB. A controlled clinical trial of hyperbaric oxygen in the treatment of acute myocardial infarction. In: Ledingham IMcA ed. Hyperbaric Oxygenation: Proceedings of the Second International Congress. London: ES Livingston; 1965:277.

18. Ashfield R, Drew CE, Gavey CJ. Severe acute myocardial infarction treated with hyperbaric oxygen: report on forty patients. Postgrad Med J 1969;45:648-653.

19. Kline HJ, Marano AJ, Johnson CD, Goodman P, Jacobson JH III, Kuhn LA. Hemodynamic and metabolic effects of hyperbaric oxygenation in myocardial infarction. J Appl Path 1970;28:256-263.

20. Thurston JG, Greenwood TW, Bending MR, Connor H, Curwen MP. A controlled investigation into the effects of hyperbaric oxygen on mortality following acute myocardial infarction. Quart J Med 1973;168:751-770.

21. Kawamura M, Sakakibara K, Sakakibara B, et al. Protective effect of hyperbaric oxygen for the temporary ischemic myocardium: macroscopic and histologic data. Cardiov Res 1976;10:599-604.

22. Otani H, Engelman RM, Rousou JA, Breyer RH, Lemeshow S, Das DK. Cardiac performance during reperfusion improved by pretreatment with oxygen free-radical scavengers. J Thorac Cardiov Surg 1986;91:290-295.

23. Romson JL, Hook BG, Kunkel SL, Abrams GD, Schork A, Lucchesi BR. Reduction of the extent of ischemic myocardial infarction by neutrophil depletion in the dog. Circulation 1983;67:1016-1023.

24. Marban E. Myocardial stunning and hibernation: the physiology behind the colloquialisms. Circulation 1991;83:681-688.

25. Thomas MP, Brown LA, Sponseller DR, Williamson Se, Diaz JA, Guyton DP. Myocardial infarct size reduction by the synergistic effect of hyperbaric oxygen and recombinant tissue plasminogen activator. Amer Heart J 1990;120(4):791-800.

26. Shandling AH, Ellestad MH, Hart GB, et al. Hyperbaric oxygen and thrombolysis in myocardial infarction. Amer Heart J 1997;134:544-50.

27. Swift PC, Turner JH, Oxer HF, O'Shea JP, Lane GK, Wollard KV. Myocardial hibernation identified by hyperbaric oxygen treatment and echocardiography in postinfarction patients: comparison with exercise thallium scintigraphy. Amer Heart J 11992;124:1151-1158.

28. Sterling DL, Thornton JD, Swafford A, et al. Hyperbaric oxygen limits infarct size in ischemic rabbit myocardium in vivo. Circulation 1993;88:1931-1936.

29. Simpson RJ, Todd RF, Fantone JG, Mickelson JK, Griffin JD, Lucchesi BR. Reduction of experimental canine myocardial reperfusion injury by a monclonal antibody (antiCDmo1, anti-CD11b) that inhibits leukocyte adhesion. J Clinical Invest 1988;81:624-629.

30. Thom SR. Functional inhibition of leukocyte b2 integrins by hyperbaric oxygen in carbon monoxide-mediated brain injury in rats. Toxic Appl Pharm 1993;123:248-256.

31. Stavitsky Y, Shandling AH, Ellestad MH, Hart GB, VanNatta B, Messenger, JC, Strauss M, Dekleva MN, Alexander JM, Mattice M, Clarke D. Hyperbaric oxygen and thrombolysis in myocaridal infarction: the "Hot MI" randomized multicenter study. Cardiology: 1998;90:131-136.

# NOTES

CHAPTER 41

# HYPERBARIC OXYGEN IN THE TREATMENT OF HANSEN'S DISEASE

## CHAPTER FORTY-ONE OVERVIEW

# Hyperbaric Oxygen in the Treatment of Hansen's Disease

*David A. Youngblood*

## INTRODUCTION

Hansen's disease is a chronic infection caused by mycobacterium leprae with a spectrum ranging from the paucibacillary forms (indeterminate, polar tuberculoid, and tuberculoid) to multibacillary forms (borderline, borderline lepromatous, and lepromatous). The latter group is characterized by greater infectivity, cellular immunodeficiency in the host, and a tendency to relapse despite prolonged drug therapy. The clinical attack rate among close family contacts exposed to the multibacillary form of the disease is less than 10%, and the paucibacillary form is essentially noninfective (7).

The prevalence of Hansen's disease in the world today as estimated by reports to the World Health Organization (WHO) is about eleven million (2), but this takes no account of the number of countries where Hansen's disease is endemic but reliable health statistics are lacking. The Leprosy Study Center of London estimates that the total number exceeds 15-16 million. Fewer than 20% of these cases are considered to be under treatment (2).

Effective drug therapy in Hansen's disease began in the 1950s with the introduction of dapsone (DDS: 4, 4-Diaminodiphenyl sulphone). This remains the primary drug for the control of Hansen's disease in most of the world since it is relatively inexpensive and side effects are minimal. Secondary resistance to dapsone was first reported in 1964 (7) and primary dapsone resistance in previously untreated patients appeared in the 1970s (13). Resistance rates of up to 40% have been reported.

Rifampin (Rifampicin), clofazimine, and ethionamide have been recommended in a combined regimen with dapsone to retard the development of resistance. These drugs, unfortunately, have some undesirable side effects, and they are expensive, requiring foreign exchange credits, which may be limited in developing countries where Hansen's disease is endemic. Despite the use of a combined regimen, the emergence of drug resistance so far seems inevitable, and the predicted development of a vaccine probably remains decades away. Hyperbaric oxygen therapy has yet to prove its potential as an effective adjunct in the treatment of Hansen's disease.

## BACKGROUND

The first formal report of the favorable effect of HBO on Hansen's disease was presented by A. Ozorio de Almeida and Eduardo Rabello before the Brazilian National Academy of Medicine on November 25, 1937. The same paper was read by invitation before the Brazilian Dermatological Society on December 6, 1937. The following year, a paper by E. Rabello and A. Ozorio de Almeida entitled *Essai de Traitement de Lepre Par L'Oxygène Sous Pression* (10) appeared in the journal **Société Francaise de Dermatologie and Syphiligraphie**. This is believed to be the first published report on the use of HBO in the treatment of Hansen's disease. It was followed in the same year by Ozorio de Almeida and Enrique Moura Costa's paper, *Treatment of Leprosy by Oxygen under High Pressure Associated with Methylene Blue* in the **Revista Brasileira de Leprologia** (7).

Ozorio de Almeida and his associates had noted clinical improvement in Hansen's disease patients participating in an experimental HBO anticancer therapy. During these studies the two investigators noted that methylene blue intensified the toxic effect of oxygen upon various organisms. Finding that Mycobacterium leprae fixes methylene blue, they predicted that the effect of HBO on the bacillus could be intensified without adversely affecting the human host.

The treatment of Hansen's disease patients with the combination of HBO and methylene blue commenced in August of 1937. By November, nine patients had been treated on a variety of oxygen regimens at pressures between 3.0 and 3.5 ATA for durations of 70-80 minutes per treatment and a cumulative average of 10 chamber hours per patient. Post-treatment clinical changes consisted of a marked decrease in skin infiltration, a disappearance of tubercles, a gain in weight, and general improvement. The bacteria decreased in number and their morphology was altered. In six cases the bacilli disappeared completely. A. Ozorio de Almeida and his colleague, Enrique Moura Costa, claimed that oxygen under pressure plus methylene blue was the most effective treatment regimen for Hansen's disease of their era (7).

More than thirty years elapsed before reports on the use of HBO in Hansen's disease reappeared. On August 15, 1969, at the Second National Reunion of the Argentine Society of Leprology in Formosa, Argentina, Doctor Felix F. Wilkinson (15) and his colleagues presented a report on their results using HBO in the leprotomous form of Hansen's disease. They were unaware of the previous Brazilian studies at the time of their presentation, but the published version, *Conclusiones Preliminares Sobre el Uso del Oxígeno Hiperbarico en Lepra Lepromatosa* from the Revista de Leprologia included a preface which acknowledged the pioneering work of Ozorio de Almeida and his colleagues in Brazil.

Interest in the application of HBO in the treatment of Hansen's disease apparently was confined to Argentina until the Fifth International Hyperbaric Conference in Vancouver, B.C., in 1973 where Dr. Sebastian A. Rosasco (11), representing his colleagues, reported on 200 patients with the leprotamous form of the disease who had been treated with 3 ATA of oxygen for one hour twice daily for three consecutive days. Drug therapy was stopped at the time of treatment and not resumed. Ten patients available for 5-year follow-up showed no signs of recurrence. Dr. Rosasco's presentation stirred international interest.

In the U.S.A., Dr. Sheldon Gottlieb recognized their findings as confirmation of his earlier predictions on the possible use of HBO in the treatment of Hansen's disease (3). With the advent of the mouse footpad as an animal model (12) to evaluate the efficacy of drug therapy in the disease, Drs. Hart and Levy conducted an unpublished trial on the effect of HBO on the growth of Mycobacterium leprae. Their experiment did not demonstrate any effect of HBO on the growth of the organism in the mouse footpad model (4).

Repeated attempts were made to communicate with the researchers in Argentina during the 1970s, but only Kindwall was successful. Dr. Kindwall received an impressive set of before-and-after-treatment photographs. Then all contact was lost during the long period of civil strife in Argentina during the late 1970s.

Fortunately, the author found Drs. Wilkinson and Rosasco in Buenos Aires, Argentina, in July of 1981. Frustrated by the continual skepticism and occasional ridicule from their leprologist colleagues, the Argentine investigators had all but abandoned efforts to find support for a formal clinical trial complete with long-term follow-up, although they continued to treat occasional charity patients. Armed with their published and unpublished data on the use of HBO in Hansen's disease, the author returned to Washington, D.C., where Dr. Charles Shilling and Ms. Nancy Riegle-Hussey obtained funding from the Max and Victoria Dreyfuss Foundation for a pilot study which would attempt to replicate and refine the work of the South American researchers.

The pilot study protocol required patients with a recent diagnosis of the leprotamous form of Hansen's disease and no previous or current drug therapy. After an appropriate medical evaluation, a pretreatment biopsy would be obtained, analyzed, and inoculated into the footpads of a control group of mice. The patient would be treated with HBO for one hour at 3 ATA twice daily for five days. Following the completion of this HBO regimen, a second biopsy from the same site would be implanted in the footpads of a post-treatment mouse group. After an incubation period of approximately ten months, tissue specimens from the footpads of both groups of mice would be harvested and analyzed to compare the viability, morphology, and relative number of bacteria between the control and treatment groups.

Due to administrative changes at the National Hansen's disease Center in Carrville, Louisiana, the study was never implemented as planned. The author (17) treated only one patient under the protocol, a 30-year-old native of South Texas who had never been out of the United States. He presented with moderate facial edema and reddish macular lesions over the trunk. By the third day of treatment there was a centripetal blanching of the truncal lesions and the facial edema had disappeared. The skin biopsies were shipped to the laboratory at the National Hansen's disease Center and inoculated into the footpads of ten mice for each group for studies of viability and bacterial propagation. Eight months later mice from each group were studied. There was no significant difference in the bacterial density in the footpads of mice from either the pretreatment or the post-treatment samples

(The patient had been placed on a conventional drug regimen following the completion of his experimental HBO therapy, and he made a rapid clinical recovery.)

Interest had also been stimulated in other parts of the world: during the Fifth International Conference on Hyperbaric Medicine in Aberdeen, Scotland, in 1977, Dr. Sheldon Gottlieb exchanged ideas with Dr. R.R. Pai of Bombay, India, on the possibility of conducting clinical trials in that country. These plans were interrupted, however, by Dr. Pai's unfortunate illness, but he did communicate in 1980 that preliminary studies in Bombay had included 33 patients treated with HBO supplemented with Rifamicin (Rifampin) and Dapsone, stating in a letter to Dr. Gottlieb that "...Just as the effect of HBO in certain leprosy cases is spectacular, there are others where the effect is debatable...unless an adequate number of patients is studied, I do not think it would be worthwhile presenting a paper on this subject..." (8).

Meanwhile, Mokashi from Bombay reported in a personal communication to Dr. K.K. Jain on the results of a controlled study in a group of twenty drug resistant Hansen's disease patients, half of which received HBO at 2.5 ATA twice daily for three days after drug therapy had been halted. On follow-up at 8 months, the biopsy specimens from the HBO-treated patients were all negative, whereas no changes were present in the non-HBO control group (6).

In Argentina Dr. Wilkinson (14, 16) and his colleagues continued to follow a few of their original patients as well as treat occasional new cases, including two patients with the paucibacillary tuberculoid form, one of which demonstrated a disappearance of the lesions within 15 days following the second HBO series, but no reports appeared in the literature until Wilkinson et al. (1987) presented their findings from a double-blind study in which 10 patients with the leprotamous form of Hansen's disease receiving DDS, clofazimine and Rifampicin were randomly allocated to a 3 ATA HBO group or an air control group. They reported a statistically significant reduction in the bacillary population in the HBO-treated group (15).

There are rumours of clinical studies elsewhere in the world: Brazil, India, and Latvia, but none have appeared in the literature except for the report by M. Bertholds et al. (1), from Riga, Latvia, regarding the failure of HBO to induce or enhance free radical activity in one patient with the leprotamous form of Hansen's disease (1).

## DISCUSSION

HBO is not a "magic bullet" that kills Mycobacterium leprae. In the few mouse footpad experiments it has shown no tendency to inhibit the growth of the bacteria. The beneficial effect of HBO on the multibacillary forms of Hansen's disease in the human host could be a combination of factors: a mild alteration in immune response, interference in some fashion with the oxygen metabolism of this obligate intracellular parasite, or perhaps some improvement in leukocyte function. Although the clinical effect may have been spectacular in some cases, much of the benefit could have been secondary. In looking at the larger series, the overall effect of HBO is less impressive.

But perhaps we have been side-tracked to some extent by our enthusiasm for the discoveries reported from Argentina. In attempting to continue in the direction of their investigations, we apparently overlooked the important details of Ozorio de Almeida's (7) work which preceded the independent discoveries in Argentina.

By 1937, Ozorio de Almeida had already observed the beneficial effects of HBO alone on Hansen's disease among subjects participating in an entirely separate study of the effects of HBO on cancer. The observation intrigued him, but he apparently did not feel that the beneficial effects of HBO were likely to be of clinical significance unless they could be amplified by some synergistic drug. He chose methylene blue because it was known to increase the toxic effect of oxygen on living organisms and it is firmly fixed by the Mycobactium leprae bacillus and held fast while the remainder of the drug is rapidly eliminated from the human host. At that point, he reasoned, high-dose HBO could be administered with devastating effect to the bacillus and little or no harm to the human host.

Methylene blue is a dye and so is clofazimine. Perhaps the elegant strategy employed by Ozorio de Almeida could be utilized in a similar fashion using clofazimine or a related chemical. Furthermore, we know now that the generation time for Mycobacterium leprae is very long – around 12 days in the mouse foot pad and perhaps even longer in the human. If the combined or synergistic effects of HBO and the experimental drug happen to be limited to a particular phase in the lifespan of the bacillus, it could be that all previous treatment protocols have halted the HBO prematurely. It would seem that we might need to apply our treatment protocol for at least two weeks in order to measure the effects of the HBO and experimental drug combination on all of the maturation phases of Mycobacterium leprae. These approaches merit further study.

## CONCLUSION

Despite the decades of frustration and false promises, the role of HBO in Hansen's disease remains to be determined.

## REFERENCES

1. Bertholds M, Andreyev G, Goldstein N. "Effect of hyperbaric oxygen on free radical activity in a patient with leprotamous leprosy." J of Hyperbaric Med. 1989;4 (3):131-134.

2. Browne SG. "The control of Hansen's disease - chimera and prospects." Bull et Memoires. Royal Acad Med of Belgium. 1970;3151:208-218.

3. Gottlieb SF. "The possible use of high pressure oxygen in the treatment of leprosy and tuberculosis." Dis Chest. 1963;44 (2):215-217.

4. Gottlieb SF "Oxygen under pressure and microorganisms." In: Hyperbaric Oxygen Therapy. JC Davis, TK Hunt (Eds.) Bethesda, MD: Undersea Medical Society, 1977;79-99.

5. Harboe M. Tropical and Geographical Medicine. New York: McGraw-Hill, 1984;799-808.

6. Jain KK. Textbook of Hyperbaric Medicine. Toronto: Hogrefe and Huber, 1990;184-186.

7. Ozorio de Almeida A and De Moura Costa H. "Treatment of leprosy by oxygen under high pressure associated with methylene blue." Revista Brasileira de Leprologia. 1938;6:237-265.

8. Pai RR. Personal Communication to SF Gottlieb, June 4, 1980.

9. Pettit JH, Rees RJ. "Sulphone resistance in leprosy: An experimental and clinical study." Lancet, 1964;2:673-674.

10. Rabello E and Ozorio de Almeida A. "Essai de traitement de la lepre par l'oxygène sous pression." Soc Francaise de Dermatologie et Syphiligraphie. 1938;5:810-823.

11. Rosasco SA, Wilkinson FW and Calori B. "Hyperbaric oxygen and Mycobacterium leprae: Preliminary report on 200 cases." Fifth International Conf Proc. Vancouver, B.C., Simon Fraser University, 1974.

12. Shepard CC. "The experimental disease that follows the injection of human leprosy bacilli into footpads of mice." J Exp Med. 1960;112:445-454.

13. Shepard CC. "Leprosy Today." New Eng. J. Med. 1982;307 (26):1640-1641.

14. Wilkinson FF. "Respuesta de la forma clinica tuberculoide al oxígeno hiperbarico." Leprologia. 1970;15 (2):69-70.

15. Wilkinson FF, Rosasco Palau SA, Besuschio S, Calori BA, Bertholds M. "Hyperbaric oxygen (HBO) as a complementary treatment of patients with multibacillary leprotamous leprosy." Japanese J Leprosy. 1987;56:159-165.

16. Wilkinson FF, Rosasco SA, Calori BA, Equia OF, Rubio RA. "Conclusiones preliminares sobre el uso del oxígeno hiperbarico en lepra lepromatosa." Revista de Leprologia. 1970;7 (5):459-471.

17. Youngblood DA. "Hyperbaric oxygen in the treatment of Hansen's disease." HBO Review. 1984;5 (4):244-250.

# INDEX

# A

# G

# H

# I

# J

# N

# O

# W

# Z